SECOND EDITION

PHARMACOLOGY
for PHARMACY TECHNICIANS

Kathy Moscou, RPh, MPH
Program Manager and Lecturer, International Pharmacy Graduate Program
University of Toronto, Leslie Dan Faculty of Pharmacy
Toronto, Ontario, Canada
Former Director, Pharmacy Technician Program (1989–2006)
North Seattle Community College
Seattle, Washington

Karen R. Snipe, CPhT, MEd
Pharmacy Technician Program Coordinator
Department Head, Diagnostic and Imaging Services
Trident Technical College
Charleston, South Carolina

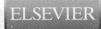

3251 Riverport Lane
St. Louis, Missouri 63043

PHARMACOLOGY FOR PHARMACY TECHNICIANS   ISBN: 9780323084970

Library of Congress Cataloging-in-Publication Data

Moscou, Kathy.
    Pharmacology for pharmacy technicians / Kathy Moscou, Karen R. Snipe.—2nd ed.
       p. ; cm.
    Includes bibliographical references and index.
    ISBN 978-0-323-08497-0 (pbk.)
    I. Snipe, Karen R.   II. Title.
    [DNLM: 1. Pharmaceutical Preparations.   2. Pharmacists' Aides. QV 55]
    615.1'9—dc23
                                                    2012033782

Vice President and Publisher: Andrew Allen
Executive Content Strategist: Jennifer Janson
Senior Content Development Specialist: Kelly Brinkman
Publishing Services Manager: Hemamalini Rajendrababu
Project Manager: Divya Krish
Designer: Brian Salisbury

Printed in China

Last digit is the print number: 9   8   7   6   5   4   3   2   1

Reviewers

Michelle Arkayus, CPhT
Pharmacy Technician Instructor
Everest Institute
Gahanna, Ohio

Angel Decatur, BS, CPhT
Pharmacy Technician Instructor
Everest College
Thornton, Colorado

Rachel Eskridge, CPhT, BA
Pharmacy Technician Program Director
St. Louis College of Health Careers
Fenton, MO

Marlene Fearon, BSN, OCN
Registered Nurse
Leisureworld
Brampton, Ontario

Muy Heak Lair, CPhT
Licensed Certified Pharmacy Technician, Lead Pharmacy
    Technician Instructor
Corinthian Colleges
West Valley City, Utah

Mary Lichtenberg, CPhT
Pharmacy Technician Instructor
Remington College
Cleveland, Ohio

Marcy May, MEd, CPhT, PhTR
Adjunct Associate Professor
Austin Community College
Austin, Texas

Joshua J. Neumiller, PharmD, CDE, CGP, FASCP
Assistant Professor
Washington State University
Spokane, Washington

Richard R. Nunez, RPhT, CPhT
Director of Pharmacy
Everest College, Kentfield Hospital Pharmacy Staff
San Francisco, California

Becky Schonscheck, BS, CPhT
Home Office Program Manager, Pharmacy Technician
Anthem Education Group
Phoenix, Arizona

Stephen M. Setter, PharmD, CGP, CDE
Geriatric Consultant Pharmacist
GeriMed Consulting
Spokane, Washington

Lisa Thompson, RPT, CPhT
Pharmacy Technician Instructor
Everest University
Pharmacy Technician Program
Pompano Beach, Florida

Preface

The pharmacy technician profession has been growing by leaps and bounds because of the increase in the number of prescriptions written, the aging of the population, and the increasing number of new pharmacies. The role of the pharmacy technician has expanded to address the growing need for pharmaceutical services, coupled with increasing requirements for pharmacists to provide cognitive services and direct patient care. It does not matter in which type of pharmacy setting one is employed, a basic understanding of pharmacology is needed to assist the pharmacist effectively in the dispensing of medications and education of the clients of the pharmacy. To this end, *Pharmacology for Pharmacy Technicians* seeks to provide a body of knowledge that will enable the pharmacy technician to understand the principles of pharmacology and apply them to the daily activities and challenges presented in all pharmacy practice settings.

Background

This book was conceived and developed by both a pharmacist and pharmacy technician involved in the training of pharmacy technicians who saw the need for a comprehensive pharmacology text that would provide knowledge and applications for students in the field of pharmacy practice.

Who Will Benefit from This Book?

Pharmacology for Pharmacy Technicians provides students with comprehensive coverage of pharmacology and also gives the instructor the tools necessary to present this information effectively. Today's pharmacy technicians are increasingly called on to perform highly technical tasks that were previously the responsibility of the pharmacist. In all practice settings, pharmacy technicians are required to perform their duties and maintain accuracy and professionalism. Given the volume of medication doses currently dispensed, pharmacy technicians need to understand the general principles of pharmacology to be able to assist the pharmacist in spotting medication errors, drug interactions, and therapeutic duplication. Knowledge of pharmacology will increase the pharmacy technician's brand and generic name recognition. Moreover, the study of pharmacology will help pharmacy technicians identify duplicate drugs and drug interactions and can speed the process of identifying the drug requested for refill when the patient can't remember the drug name.

Why Is This Book Important to the Profession?

Although there are many pharmacology texts on the market geared toward pharmacy technicians, this textbook seeks to go beyond the basic required knowledge to provide current drug information, tools to enhance learning, and Tech Alerts and Tech Notes that are key to preventing medication errors in a way that is easily understood and grasped by the reader.

Organization

Pharmacology for Pharmacy Technicians is organized to support teaching of a two-term (semester or quarter) pharmacology course. The text is organized to provide an integrated approach to the understanding of pharmacology and pharmacotherapy. Unit I provides the basic foundation for understanding pharmacology and includes content on pharmaceutics, pharmacokinetics, and pharmacodynamics. Unit II through Unit XI are organized according to body systems—the nervous system, musculoskeletal system, ophthalmic and otic systems, cardiovascular system, endocrine system, genitourinary system, respiratory system, and integumentary system. An overview of common disorders of each body system is described, including symptoms. This will help students understand why a given medication is useful for treatment of the condition. The mechanism of action for drugs is also presented. It builds on basic information presented in Unit I and aids in understanding pharmacotherapeutics. Duplicate entries of some drugs are found throughout the text for those that are prescribed for the treatment of more than one medical condition as the rationale for usage may differ according to the medical condition being treated. Each chapter contains a list of basic terminology, chapter summary, review questions, and critical thinking exercises. Common endings of drug classifications are provided to aid in memorizing drugs and their use.

Distinctive Features

Pharmacology for Pharmacy Technicians makes extensive use of tables and figures to enhance learning. U.S. and Canadian brand names are provided for each generic name product. Available strengths and dosage forms are placed in tables along with photographs of many of the top 200 selling drugs to aid in product identification.

Additional unique features include common endings of drug classifications, warning labels for every drug, Tech Alerts for drug look-alike and sound-alike issues, and Tech Notes for important need to know information. As compared with other pharmacology texts, *Pharmacology for Pharmacy Technicians* is comprehensive and contains descriptions of hundreds of pharmaceuticals.

Learning Aids

A variety of pedagogical features are included in the book to aid in learning:
- **Learning Objectives.** These are listed at the beginning of each chapter and clearly outline what students are expected to learn from the chapter materials.
- A list of **Key Terms** follows the Learning Objectives, identifies new terminology, and makes it easier for students to learn the new vocabulary. Learning this new terminology is vital to success on the job.
- **Tech Alerts** are found in the margins of the text and alert the student to drug look-alike and sound-alike issues.
- Helpful **Tech Notes** are presented throughout the chapters and provide critical, need to know information regarding dispensing concerns and interesting points about pharmacology.
- **Mini drug monographs** with pill photos are provided for every body system and in every drug classification chapter. These include generic and trade names, strength of medication, route of administration, dosage form, dosing schedule, and warning labels.
- A **Chapter Summary** is found at the end of each chapter that summarizes the key concepts of the chapter.
- **Review Questions** further enhance student review and retention of chapter content by testing them on the key content within the chapter.
- The **Technician's Corner** provides critical thinking exercises that help students prepare for on the job experiences by challenging them to pull together a collection of facts and information to reach a conclusion.
- The **Bibliography** provides a list of sources that students and instructors can use for additional information on the chapter's topic.

ANCILLARIES
For the Instructor
EVOLVE

We are offering several assets on Evolve (http://evolve.elsevier.com/Moscou/pharmacology) to aid instructors:
- Test Bank: An ExamView test bank of 700 multiple-choice questions that features rationales, cognitive levels, and page number references to the text. This can be used as a review in class or for test development.
- PowerPoint Presentations: One PowerPoint presentation per chapter. These can be used as is or as a template to prepare lectures.
- Image Collection: All the images from the book are available in JPEG format and can be downloaded into PowerPoint presentations. These can be used during lectures to illustrate important concepts.
- Text Answer Key: All the answers to the Review Questions and Technician's Corner questions from the text.

- Workbook Answer Key: All the answers to the Workbook exercises.
- **TEACH:** Including lesson plans and PowerPoint slides, all available via Evolve. TEACH provides instructors with customizable lesson plans and PowerPoints based on learning objectives. With these valuable resources, instructors will save valuable preparation time and can create a learning environment that fully engages students in classroom preparation. The lesson plans are keyed chapter by chapter and are divided into logical lessons to aid in classroom planning. In addition to lesson plans, instructors will have unique lecture outlines in PowerPoint with talking points, thought-provoking questions, and unique ideas for lectures.

FOR THE STUDENT
Student Workbook

The student workbook includes:
- Fill-in-the-blank exercises, multiple-choice questions, matching questions, and true-false questions reinforce the concepts presented in the textbook.
- Research activities teach students how to keep current with an ever-changing industry.
- Critical thinking exercises help students apply the knowledge that they learn in class to real-life scenarios, including testing their knowledge of pharmacy calculations.

Evolve

The student resources on Evolve include:
- Two comprehensive mock examinations, which includes more than 350 questions to check students' knowledge and comprehension.
- An English-Spanish audio glossary that helps students master key terms while also reinforcing word meanings.
- Several appendices, which feature additional information relevant to pharmacology, including the top 200 selling drugs, the top 30 selling herbals, abbreviations commonly used in the pharmacy, and abbreviations that shouldn't be used.
- *Mosby's Essential Drugs for Pharmacy Technicians:* Detailed drug monographs, including full-color pill photos, for the top 200 drugs dispensed in the United States.
- Interactive exercises, which include drag-and-drop exercises and fill-in-the-blank questions.
- An image bank of pill photos that shows the top 200 selling drugs.

Note to the Student

Pharmacology for Pharmacy Technicians was created to provide pharmacy technicians with a strong foundation in pharmacology. As you proceed through this text, you will notice that key concepts are repeated to reinforce learning. Review the key terms before you begin to read the chapter; this will help you understand the chapter better. The chapter summary provides a synopsis of key concepts in each chapter. You will want to refer often to the tables of brand and generic names as this knowledge of brand and generic names is critical for your profession. The drug photos of the top 200 selling drugs will help you learn to identify commonly prescribed medicines; familiarity with product appearance helps reduce medication errors. You may also find this text useful in other pharmacy technician courses.

Acknowledgments and Dedication

The education of pharmacy technicians to assume ever-expanding professional responsibilities has been the focus of most of my professional career. This book is dedicated to all my former students at North Seattle Community College, whom I have challenged and hopefully inspired to achieve their best, for themselves and the profession. I dedicate this book to my husband, Gervan Fearon, who has supported me throughout the arduous process of writing this textbook, and my children, Gyasi and Chi Moscou-Jackson, who have started their own professional careers. Finally, I would like to thank my co-author, Karen Snipe, for her enthusiasm and motivation throughout the writing of this book, and the Pharmacy Technician Educators Council and other organizations for encouraging the development of instructional materials for pharmacy technicians.

— *Kathy Moscou*

I would like to thank my family; without their continuous support, I would not have pursued this project. And I'd like to say thank you to my writing partner, Kathy, whose encouragement was priceless throughout this project. I dedicate this text to my pharmacy technician students for inspiring me to write teaching materials that are relevant and pertinent to their training.

— *Karen Snipe*

Acknowledgments and Dedication

Table of Contents

Introduction to Pharmacology

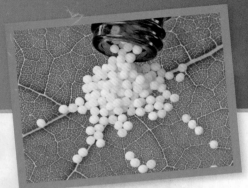

Fundamentals of Pharmacology

KEY TERMS

Bioavailability: The fraction of the administered drug dose that enters the systemic circulation and is available to produce drug effect.

Biopharmaceuticals: Pharmaceuticals derived from biological sources (e.g., proteins, gene sequences) and manufactured using biotechnology methods such as recombinant DNA technology.

Controlled substance: Drug whose possession and distribution are restricted because of its potential for abuse as determined by federal or state law. Controlled substances are placed in schedules according to their abuse potential and effects if abused.

Dosage form: Drug formulation (e.g., capsule, tablet, solution).

Dose: Amount of a drug required for one application or administration.

Dosing schedule: How frequently a drug dose is administered (e.g., "four times a day").

Drug: Substance used to diagnose, treat, cure, prevent, or mitigate disease in humans or other animals. (U.S. Food and Drug Administration, 2012).

Drug delivery system: Dosage form or device designed to release a specific amount of drug.

Enteral: Drug dosage form that is administered orally.

Homeopathic medicine: Drugs that are administered in minute quantities to stimulate natural body healing systems.

Legend drugs: Drugs that are required by state or federal law to be dispensed by a prescription only. Prescriptions must be written for a legitimate medical condition and issued by a practitioner authorized to prescribe.

Materia medica: Medicinal materials.

Over-the-counter (OTC) drugs: Drugs that may be obtained without a prescription.

Parenteral: Drug dosage form that is administered by injection or infusion.

Pharmacognosy: Science dealing with the biological, biochemical features of natural drugs and their constituents. It is the study of drugs of plant and animal origins.

Pharmacology: Study of drugs and their interactions with living systems, including chemical and physical properties, toxicology, and therapeutics.

Pharmacotherapy: Use of drugs in the treatment of disease.

Toxicology: Science dealing with the study of poisons.

Pharmacology

Pharmacology is the study of drugs and their interactions with living systems, including chemical and physical properties, *toxicology*, and therapeutics. Knowledge of *pharmacology* is essential to the accurate, effective, and efficient performance of the responsibilities of pharmacy technicians. Pharmacy technicians educated in pharmacology have the skills to properly identify the drug from a patient's profile when refills are requested and the patient does not remember the drug name. Less time is spent searching for drugs when pharmacy technicians have good brand and generic name recognition. Pharmacy technicians possessing substantial knowledge of pharmacology may be able to reduce dispensing errors associated with look-alike or sound-alike drugs, incorrect drug or strength, incorrect dosage form, and improper dosing schedule. Knowledge of pharmacology facilitates selection of warning labels for drugs dispensed. Pharmacy technicians who possess a good knowledge of pharmacology understand the importance of recognizing drug interactions, therapeutic duplication, and excessive dose alerts screened by the computer. Overall, pharmacy technicians who have a working knowledge of pharmacology can perform duties within their scope of practice with greater independence.

History of Medicines and Their Use

Plants have been collected, cultivated, and harvested for their healing properties and used in the treatment of illness for centuries. Contributors to the current knowledge about drugs span the globe. Records dating as early as 3000 BC document the pharmacological knowledge by the people of ancient Egypt, Mesopotamia, India, and China. Papyrus Ebers (1550 BC), which was found in Egypt and describes more than 700 medical compounds and lists more than 811 prescriptions, is thought to be a copy of an ancient manuscript that dates to 3000 BC. More than 800 clay tablets have been unearthed describing more than 500 remedies in Mesopotamia (Persian Gulf 2500 BC), and Emperor Shen Nung is credited with writing the *Pen T'sao Ching* (2750 BC) in which more than 1000 medicinal compounds are described and 11,000 prescription remedies are listed. The *Dravyaguna* (2500 BC) is an ancient Aryuvedic manuscript (India) of *materia medica* (medicinal materials) and includes sources, descriptions, criteria for identification, properties, methods for preparation, and therapeutic uses of hundreds of medicinal herbs. Some of the medicinal compounds described in these ancient manuscripts are still used today for essentially the same purposes. For example, castor oil and tincture opii were described in *Papyrus Ebers*.

Theophratus (300 BC), the "father of pharmacology," was a Greek physician known for his accurate observation of medicinal plants. By the first century, Dioscorides, another Greek physician, described approximately 600 medicinal plants in *De Materia Medica*. Aloe, belladonna, ergot, and opium are a few of the medicines described in the manuscript that are still in use today.

Since the 20th century, research into medicines and the introduction of new drugs and vaccines have grown exponentially. Antiinfective agents, the discovery of insulin and its use for the treatment of diabetes, and antiretroviral drugs for the treatment of HIV/AIDS have all been discovered since the 1930s. The Human Genome Project, a study of human genes, has provided data useful in understanding diseases that are caused by genetic defects or linked to heredity. The study of genes has also enabled scientists to develop new genetically modified drugs, such as human insulin. Bioengineering is the process used to produce *biopharmaceuticals*.

A pharmacology timeline is shown in Box 1-1.

BOX 1-1   **Pharmacology Timeline**

3000 BC: Imhotep, Egyptian god of medicine

2750 BC: Emperor Shen Nung (China) is credited with writing the *Pen T'sao Ching*. More than 1000 medicinal compounds are described, and 11,000 prescription remedies are listed.

2500 BC: The *Dravyaguna*, an ancient Aryuvedic manuscript of medicinal materials, sources, descriptions, criteria for identification, properties, methods for preparation, and therapeutic uses of hundreds of medicinal herbs, is written in India.

1550 BC: *Papyrus Ebers*, thought to be a copy of an ancient Egyptian manuscript that dates back to 3000 BC, describes more than 700 medical compounds and lists more than 811 prescriptions.

1000 BC: Charaka described more than 2000 medicinal substances (including mercury compounds, e.g., merthiolate), methods to improve palatability, and metrology (measurements and dosages).

400 BC: Hippocrates, the "father of medicine"

300 BC: Theophratus, the "father of botany," was a Greek physician known for his accurate observation of medicinal plants.

AD 100: Dioscorides, the "father of pharmacology," a botanist and pharmacologist, authored *Dioscorides Herbal*.

AD 120 to 200: Galen, the "father of pharmacotherapy," promoted Humoral theory, the dominant theory of disease and treatment for more than 1500 years. This theory states that illness is caused by an imbalance of "humors" and is treated with Simples, Composites, and Entities.

AD 1000: Avicenna Ibn Sina, known as the "Persian Galen," whose writings unified pharmaceutical and medicinal knowledge of his time and whose teachings were accepted in the West until the 17th century.

AD 1500s: Paracelsus, the "father of the pharmaceutical revolution," promoted the concept that disease is a chemical abnormality treated with chemicals. Introduced laudanum, a drug derived from opium that deadens pain.

Indians of the Americas had pharmacological knowledge of up to 1200 plants, including:
    West Indies: guaiacum (evergreen tree)
    South America: cocaine (cocoa leaves), curare
    Mexico: jalap (laxative)
    Peru: quinine (cinchona)
    Brazil: balsam Tolu (expectorant)

AD 1700s: William Withering (United Kingdom) isolated digitalis from foxglove.

Edward Jenner (United Kingdom) developed the vaccine against cowpox. His research led to the development of the smallpox vaccine.

Bernard Courtois (France) discovered iodine, used to treat goiter and to decrease mucus (mucolytic).

Joseph Caventou and Pierre Pelletier (France) discovered quinine, which is used to treat malaria.

Johannes Buchner (Germany) identified salicin from willow bark (ASA) and nicotine in tobacco (niacin).

Emil von Behring (Germany) worked with antitoxins, resulting in diphtheria and tetanus vaccine.

Gregor Mendel (Austria), a famous scientist and monk, discovered the basis of genetics and how genes are woven into heredity.

1800s: Frederich Serturner (Germany) extracted morphine from opium.

Louis Pasteur's experiments showing that microorganisms can cause disease and heat can kill them became the basis of "germ theory."

1900s: Frederick Banting and Charles Best (Canada) discovered that insulin lowers blood sugar levels and can be used to treat diabetes.

Gerhardt Domagk (Germany) introduced the sulfonamide Prontosil, the first antiinfective agent.

Alexander Fleming (United States) discovered penicillin, a chemical produced by a fungus.

Beyer (United States) was instrumental in the development of thiazide diuretics, derivatives of sulfonamides, and other drugs.

2000s: Pfizer (United States) was instrumental in developing linezolid, a synthetic antibiotic in the oxazolidinone class.

Sanofi-Aventis (Europe) developed telithromycin, a semisynthetic erythromycin derivative.

TABLE 1-1   **Drugs and Their Sources**

Classification	Source	Generic Name	Use
Plant	Foxglove Chinchona Opium poppy	Digitalis Quinine Morphine	Heart failure (CHF) Malaria Pain
Animal	Thyroid gland Pancreas	Thyroid, USP Pancreatin	Hypothyroidism Digestive aid
Mineral	Silver Gold	Silver sulfadiazine Auranofin	Burns (anti-infective) Arthritis
Synthetic	Synthetic opioid Red azo dye	Fentanyl Sulfonamides	Pain Infection
Bioengineering (recombinant DNA technology)	Isolated DNA + *Escherichia coli* bacteria	Hepatitis B vaccine* Human insulin†	Hepatitis B prevention Diabetes mellitus

*Source of hepatitis B vaccine is viral DNA copied into a yeast cell.
†Source of human insulin is isolated DNA + *Escherichia coli* bacteria.

ORIGIN OF DRUGS

Pharmacognosy, a term derived from the Greek words *pharmakon* ("drug") and *gnosis* ("knowledge"), is the branch of science dealing with the study of the natural origin of drugs. Pharmacognosy is the study of the constituents of natural drugs that are responsible for their effects. A ***drug*** is a substance that affects the normal function or structure of humans or animals and may be used to diagnose, treat, mitigate, cure, or prevent disease. Drugs may come from natural or synthetic origins. Natural drugs may be derived from plants (e.g., digitalis, quinine), animals (e.g., thyroid USP, pepsin), or minerals (e.g., silver nitrate). Some natural drugs are administered in their crude form; however, most frequently, the chief active ingredient(s) are extracted from the crude source.

Synthetic drugs may be a chemical modification of a natural drug or manufactured entirely from chemical ingredients unrelated to the natural drug. The synthetic drug may be equally potent or more potent. Fentanyl is a synthetically manufactured analgesic that is more potent than the natural drug, morphine (a naturally occurring analgesic derived from the opium poppy). Drugs may also be produced via the process of bioengineering. Erythropoietin and human insulin are examples of biopharmaceuticals. Table 1-1 details common origins of drugs.

What Is Pharmacology?

Pharmacognosy and pharmacology are both sciences that involve the study of medicinal substances. However, the science of pharmacology involves the action of drugs on humans and animals. The aim of drug therapy is to diagnose, treat, cure, or lessen the symptoms of disease. The study of pharmacology applies knowledge of properties of drugs, mechanism of drug action, anatomy and physiology, and pathology. Selection of the appropriate drug for a patient in the proper ***dose*** and ***dosage form***, administered at an appropriate dosing schedule, requires knowledge of pharmacology. The drug dose is the amount of drug units given for a single administration (e.g., two tablets, one teaspoonful). The ***dosing schedule*** is the number of times the drug dose is administered per day.

WHAT IS PHARMACOTHERAPY?

Pharmacotherapy is defined as the use of drugs in the treatment of disease. Contrasting philosophies about pharmacotherapy exist. Allopathic medicine, sometimes called Western medicine, is a system of medical practice in which the goal of pharmacotherapy is to fight disease by using drugs or surgery that produces effects different from or incompatible with those produced by the disease being treated. In ***homeopathic medicine*** drugs are administered in minute quantities to produce effects similar to the disease in healthy persons, yet stimulate the body's natural healing systems in individuals with disease.

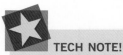

TECH NOTE!
Some common beverages and foods are natural drugs. Coffee and tea contain the drug caffeine. Ginger and peppermint contain ingredients that can reduce nausea.

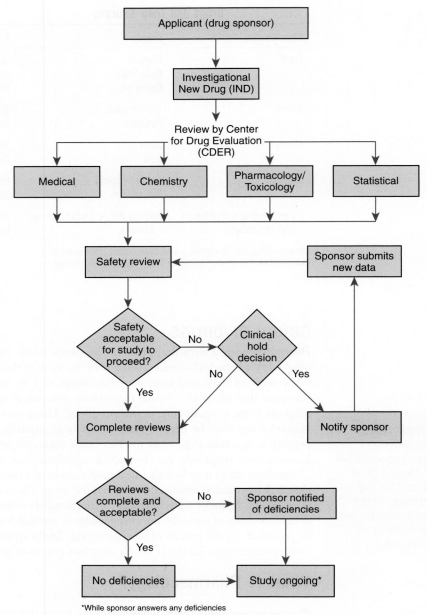

FIGURE 1-1 The Investigational New Drug process.

*While sponsor answers any deficiencies

RESEARCH AND DEVELOPMENT

In 1906 the Pure Food and Drug Act was passed to protect the public from ineffective and harmful drugs. This act was expanded in 1938, and standards for allowing new drugs onto the market were set. Today, it can take several years to move a new drug from the idea phase to making it available to the public. Thousands of chemical compounds may be tested before one is discovered that can produce the desired effects with an acceptable level of adverse effects.

There are many steps in the drug development process (Figure 1-1). The steps from the test tube to production and distribution of a new drug involve preclinical research, clinical studies, new drug application process, and review. Manufacturers of new drugs must submit data showing that their drug is reasonably safe before a preliminary small-scale clinical study is approved. Preclinical research is conducted to determine a pharmacological profile for the drug and acute toxicity of the drug in at least two species of animals. Upon completion of the preclinical phase, drug manufacturers file an Investigational New Drug (IND) application. Only approved INDs move to the clinical study phase.

There are three clinical study phases (Figure 1-2). In phase 1 clinical trials, the drug is administered to a small number of healthy volunteers who are enrolled in the clinical study. Preliminary information about the drug's pharmacology, mechanism of action, and efficacy (effectiveness in humans in a controlled clinical trial) is gathered in phase 1. If appropriate, the drug enters phase 2 clinical studies. Phase 2 studies are controlled trials with a limited number of patients with the condition to be treated. During this phase, data are collected to determine the drug's efficacy and the drug's side effects in patients with the disease. Phase 3 clinical studies involve hundreds to a few thousand patients. Drug safety is evaluated, and the benefit of taking the drug is compared with the risks associated with taking the drug. If safety and efficacy are shown, the drug begins the new drug application process and then moves on to review. An accelerated process exists to speed drug development and review when the drug provides significant benefit over existing therapies or a life-threatening illness is present. Additional safety information is collected in the postmarketing phase. Phase 4 trials are studies that are conducted after the drug is marketed to the public to determine safety and effectiveness when the drug is used in "real-world" conditions.

In 1992, the Prescription Drug User Fees Act was passed to allow companies to pay a fee to the U.S. Food and Drug Administration (FDA) in return for a faster review period. The Prescription Drug User Fees Act (PDUFA) was renewed in 1997, 2002, and 2007. The FDA Amendments Act, passed in 2007, permits PDUFA user fees to be used for risk management and communication, increased the FDA's responsibility to adopt a more proactive approach to pharmacovigilance, and set guidelines for postmarket clinical studies.

Drug approval and marketing of new drugs are also regulated in Canada. The Therapeutic Products Directorate approves prescription drugs in Canada, and the Marketed Health Products Directorate is responsible for postmarket drug safety. Preclinical and phase I to IV clinical studies are also required in Canada. A Notice of Compliance (NOC) or NOC/c (approval with conditions) must be issued before a new drug can be marketed in Canada. Prescription drugs are issued a Drug Identification Number (DIN).

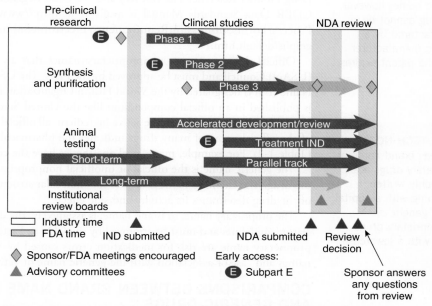

FIGURE 1-2 The pre-clinical and clinical phases of the new drug development process. (From The New Drug Development Process, Food and Drug Administration: The new drug development process. [http://www.fda.gov/Drugs/DevelopmentApprovalProcess/SmallBusinessAssistance/ucm053131.htm])

TABLE 1-2   Examples of Common Endings to Official Drug Names

Classification	Common Ending	Prototypical Drug
Benzodiazepine	-zepam -zolam	Diazepam Alprazolam
Corticosteroid	-sone -lone	Prednisone Prednisolone
Nonsteroidal anti-inflammatory drug (NSAID)	-profen -olac	Ibuprofen Ketorolac
β-Adrenergic blocking drug (β-blocker)	-olol	Propranolol
H₂ receptor antagonist	-tidine	Cimetidine
Proton pump inhibitor	-prazole	Omeprazole
Calcium channel blockers (dihydropyridines)	-dipine	Nifedipine
Macrolide antiinfective	-thromycin	Erythromycin

TABLE 1-3   Examples of Chemical, Generic, and Proprietary Names

Generic Name	Chemical Name	Brand Name
fluoxetine HCI	(±)-N-Methyl-3-phenyl-[(α,α,α-trifluoro-p-tolyl)oxy]propylamine	Prozac
acetaminophen	N-(4-Hydroxyphenyl)acetamide	Tylenol
ibuprofen	(±)-2-(p-isobutylphenyl)propionic acid	Motrin

TECH NOTE!

Every drug has a generic name; however, the drug cannot be manufactured by a generic manufacturer until the patent expires.

TECH NOTE!

Whereas brand name or proprietary drugs are commonly written beginning with a capital letter, generic or nonproprietary drugs begin with a lowercase letter.

DRUG NOMENCLATURE

All drugs are identified by a generic name, a chemical name, and a proprietary name. The name of a new drug is made according to standards set by the Center for Drug Evaluation and Research (CDER). The standards published in the CDER Data Standards Manual (DSM) are used by the Drug Product Reference File (DPRF) and the Drug Registration and Listing System (DRLS). (The CDER Data Standards Manual is available at http://www.fda.gov/Drugs/DevelopmentApproval Process/FormsSubmissionRequirements/ElectronicSubmissions/DataStandardsManualmono graphs/default.htm.)

Official drug names are nonproprietary names that are selected by the U.S. Adopted Name (USAN) Council and must be approved by the FDA. The USAN and International Non-proprietary Name (INN) designated by the World Health Organization is usually identical. The drug name that is published in an official compendium like the United States Pharmacopoeia is the official name. If a drug contains more than one active ingredient, all official drug names must be listed. The ending of the official name of many drugs indicates the pharmacological class to which the drug belongs (Table 1-2). For example, many local anesthetics have the common ending "-caine."

The generic name is the official or unofficial nonproprietary name commonly used to designate the drug. The chemical name describes the molecular structure of the drug. The chemical structure of the drug determines its activity and side effects.

The proprietary name, or brand name, is assigned by the drug manufacturer according to nomenclature guidelines and must be approved by the CDER. Factors considered when selecting a suitable proprietary name are risk for medication errors caused by existing "look-alike" and "sound-alike" names and ease of association with the generic name or active ingredient name (Table 1-3).

COMPARISONS BETWEEN BRAND NAME DRUGS AND GENERIC DRUGS

The innovator of a new drug may apply for patent protection. If awarded, the manufacturer is given up to 20 years' exclusive rights to manufacture and distribute the new drug. The manufacturer selects a brand name for the drug according to CDER recommendations. When the drug is off patent, other drug companies may manufacture a generic equivalent. Generic drugs contain the same active ingredient as the original manufacturer's drug in the same strength and in the same dosage form. Generic drugs may contain different inactive ingredients. Occasionally, these inactive ingredients result in slight differences between brand name and generic products that affect how much of the drug is available to produce drug action or how quickly drug effect is produced. Generic drugs that are not significantly different from the innovator's product receive an "A" rating from the FDA and may be substituted for the brand name product according to state and federal product substitution laws.

Generic drugs are always less expensive than brand name drugs. In many states and provinces, pharmacists routinely dispense generic drugs. Most prescription drug insurance plans require that generic drugs be dispensed; brand name drugs are only dispensed when the prescriber insists that a brand name drug is necessary.

Drug Legislation

The Pure Food and Drug Act (1906) was the first significant legislation passed to protect the public from harmful and ineffective drugs in the United States. Over the years, many more laws have been passed that regulate drug manufacture and distribution. The Durham-Humphrey Amendment (1951) established the distinction between *legend drugs* and drugs that could safely be used by the public without supervision by a health care provider. Legend drugs can only be obtained by prescription, whereas *over-the-counter (OTC) drugs* do not require a prescription. "Rx only" (U.S.) and "Pr" (Canada) must be printed on the manufacturer's product label for all prescription drugs. The Kefauver-Harris Amendment (1962) requires that all drugs be safe and effective before they are made available to the public. INDs are limited to drug study participants until clinical studies have shown them to be safe and effective. The Drug Price Competition Act and Patent Restoration Act (1984) encouraged the creation of generic drugs by streamlining the drug approval process for drugs no longer patented. A patent gives exclusive production rights to manufacturers of proprietary drugs for up to 20 years. When a patent has expired, manufacturers of generic drugs may produce and market the drug. Generic manufacturers are not required to conduct additional studies to prove safety and effectiveness but instead are permitted to rely on safety data submitted by the manufacturer of the proprietary drug. There is a transitional status between Rx only and OTC drugs known as behind-the-counter (BTC) drugs in the United States and Canada. BTC drugs are classified in National Association of Provincial Regulatory Authority (NAPRA) Schedule II in Canada. BTC drugs may be sold without prescription, but access is restricted and pharmacist intervention is required to ensure safe, appropriate use and to monitor misuse, abuse, chronic use, and the need for physician referral. Examples of BTC Schedule II drugs include iron supplements, insulin, lice treatments (e.g., pyrethrins), aspirin for pediatric use, nitroglycerin and exempt narcotics (e.g., Tylenol with codeine 8 mg). Examples of drugs that are sold BTC in both the United States and Canada are pseudoephedrine and Plan B. The FDA approved OTC access for Plan B for women 18 and older and a prescription requirement for women 17 years of age and younger. In Canada, Plan B is classified as Schedule II (BTC) and Schedule III (OTC). Where the product is stocked depends on directions for use found on the package labeling.

In the United States, the Combat Methamphetamine Epidemic Act of 2005 (CMEA) was passed to curb the illegal manufacture and use of "crystal meth." The CMEA was signed into law on March 6, 2006, to regulate, among other things, retail OTC sales of ephedrine, pseudoephedrine, and phenylpropanolamine products used to manufacture crystal meth. Purchase limits, placement of product out of direct customer access, sales logbooks, customer ID verification, employee training, and self-certification of regulated sellers are required provisions of the CMEA.

The Comprehensive Drug Abuse Prevention and Control Act, also known as the Controlled Substance Act (CSA), was passed by Congress in 1970. It regulates drugs that have a history for abuse in the United States. Access to *controlled substances* is more restrictive than access to legend drugs. Controlled substances are placed in Schedule C-I, C-II, C-III, C-IV, or C-V categories according to their abuse potential and effects if abused (Table 1-4). Controlled substance schedules are determined by federal and state laws.

Canada, similar to the United States, has passed legislation to limit the access to drugs with a potential for abuse. Narcotics, controlled drugs, and benzodiazepines and targeted substances

TABLE 1-4   **Controlled Substances (United States): Schedules, Classification, Dispensing Rules, and Examples**

Schedule	Classification	Dispensing Rules	Examples
C-I	The drug has a high potential for abuse. The drug has no currently accepted medical use in treatment in the United States.	Only with approved protocol or investigational use	Ecstasy, heroin, LSD, marijuana, PCP
C-II	The drug has a high potential for abuse. Abuse of the drug may lead to severe psychological or physical dependence The drug has an accepted medical use in treatment in the United States.	Written prescription (if called in or faxed in, a written prescription must follow within 72 hours) No refills allowed	Methylphenidate, codeine, meperidine, oxycodone, secobarbital
C-III	The drug has a potential for abuse less than that of C-II drugs. Abuse may lead to moderate or low physical dependence or high psychological dependence. The drug has an accepted medical use in treatment in the United States.	Written, oral, or faxed prescription Prescription expires within 6 months Refillable (no more than five refills within 6 months)	Codeine with acetaminophen, hydrocodone with acetaminophen, methyltestosterone, phendimetrazine
C-IV	The drug has a potential for abuse less than that of C-III drugs. Abuse may lead to limited physical dependence or psychological dependence relative to the C-III drugs. The drug has an accepted medical use in treatment in the United States.	Written, oral, or faxed prescription Prescription expires within 6 months Refillable (no more than five refills within 6 months)	Alprazolam, buprenorphine, butorphanol, diazepam, diethylpropion, pentazocine plus naloxone, phentermine, triazolam
C-V	The drug has a potential for abuse less than that of C-IV drugs. Abuse may lead to limited physical dependence or psychological dependence relative to C-IV drugs. The drug has an accepted medical use in treatment in the United States.	*Prescription:* Written, oral, or faxed prescription Prescription expires within 6 months Refillable (no more than five refills within 6 months) *OTC:* Rules vary for each state	Diphenoxylate plus atropine

LSD, Lysergic acid diethylamide; OTC, over the counter; PCP, phencyclidine.

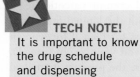

TECH NOTE!
It is important to know the drug schedule and dispensing requirements for prescription and BTC drugs.

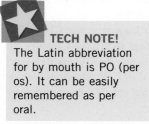

TECH NOTE!
The Latin abbreviation for by mouth is PO (per os). It can be easily remembered as per oral.

regulations are found in the Controlled Drug and Substances Act. Controlled drugs are identified by a Ⓒ symbol on the product label. Narcotics are identified by an Ⓝ symbol on the product label, and the symbol used to identify benzodiazepines and targeted substances is ℞C. Examples of narcotics, controlled substances, and benzodiazepines are found in Table 1-5.

Drug Dosage Forms and Delivery Systems

Drugs are formulated for delivery by mouth (oral), injection (parenteral), inhalation, or topical application to skin or a mucous membrane. Factors influencing the choice for drug formulation are chemical properties of the drug and human physiology. Chemical properties of the drug influence absorption, distribution, metabolism, and elimination of the drug in the body. Normal physiological processes can influence effectiveness of the drug. For example, drugs formulated for transdermal administration must have sufficient lipid solubility to enable the drug to pass through the cell membranes of skin and get to the site of action. Insulin is formulated for subcutaneous injection because it is composed of two amino acid strands and, if formulated for oral delivery, would be destroyed by the digestive enzymes that break down protein foods.

DOSAGE FORMS FOR ORAL (ENTERAL) ADMINISTRATION

Oral administration is safe, easy, and generally more economical than parenteral administration. Common oral formulations include tablets, capsules, solutions, emulsions, syrups, suspensions, and elixirs.

TABLE 1-5   Examples of Narcotics, Controlled Substances, and Benzodiazepines and Targeted Substances (Canada)

	Examples	Dispensing Rules
Narcotics	Codeine, meperidine, hydromorphone, morphine, oxycodone	Written or faxed prescription only No refills permitted Part fills allowed
Verbal narcotics	Narcotic preparations containing two or more non-narcotic ingredients (e.g., codeine + acetaminophen and caffeine)	Written, faxed, or verbal prescription No refills permitted Part fills allowed
Controlled substances	Amphetamines (e.g., Dexedrine), methylphenidate, (part I, schedule G), barbiturates (e.g., secobarbital) (part II), anabolic steroids (e.g., testosterone) (part III)	Written, faxed, or verbal prescription Refills permitted for part I controlled substances only when written on prescription Verbal refills permitted on part II and III controlled substances Part fills allowed
Benzodiazepines and targeted substances	Diazepam, clonazepam	Written, faxed, or verbal prescription Refills may be dispensed when authorized if less than 1 year has elapsed since the original prescription was issued

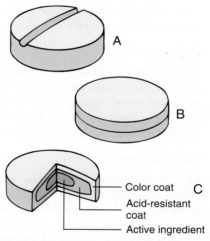

FIGURE 1-3 Enteric-coated tablets. **A,** Scored side. **B,** Unscored side. **C,** Interior of tablet. (From Clayton BD, Stock YN, Harroun RD: *Basic pharmacology for nurses*, ed 14, St Louis, 2007, Mosby.)

Tablets

Tablets are solid dosage forms containing one or more active ingredients plus binders and fillers. Binders are added to aid in compressing the drug into a tablet shape. Fillers make up the required bulk and help bind the tablet. Binders and fillers are inactive ingredients but may influence the rate of drug absorption. Tablets are formulated to deliver their contents immediately or over time. Types of tablets are listed below:

Repeat-action tablets are layered. The outer layer rapidly disintegrates in the stomach, and the inner layer dissolves in the small intestine.

Delayed-action tablets slow the release of drug to avoid stomach upset, improve absorption, or prevent drug destruction in the stomach.

Enteric-coated tablets are a type of delayed-action tablet (Figure 1-3). Enteric-coated tablets do not dissolve in the stomach. They release their contents in the small intestine.

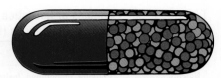

FIGURE 1-4 Capsules. (From Clayton BD, Stock YN, Harroun RD: *Basic pharmacology for nurses*, ed 14, St Louis, 2007, Mosby.)

Sustained-release and *time-release tablets* deliver their contents over time. Some drugs are formulated to deliver their contents over 24 hours and only need to be taken once a day. Sustained-release drugs should be swallowed whole; crushing may cause the contents to be released immediately. Sustained release and time release are patented processes.

Film coating and *sugar coating* tablets make them easier to swallow and improves taste.

Chewable tablets are formulated for people who have difficulty swallowing pills. Many children's medicines are available in a chewable dosage form.

Sublingual tablets and *buccal tablets* dissolve in the mouth. Sublingual tablets are dissolved under the tongue, and buccal tablets are dissolved in the cheek pouch. Many blood vessels are located in the mouth. Drugs that are destroyed by stomach acids or need to get into the bloodstream rapidly (e.g., nitroglycerin) may be formulated for sublingual or buccal administration.

Oral disintegrating tablets (ODTs) or *orodispersible tablets (ODTs)* are similar to sublingual tablets, but they disintegrate more rapidly (in <60 seconds) when placed on the tongue.

Troches and *lozenges* are dissolved in the mouth.

Thin film includes a thin layer of film that disintegrates or dissolves to release the drug and is applied to sublingual tablets (dissolves on the tongue), buccal tablets (absorption in the mouth), and extended-release tablets.

Capsules

Capsules are solid dosage forms containing one or more active ingredient plus binders and fillers (Figure 1-4). Capsules are formulated to deliver their contents immediately or over time. An osmotic controlled-release capsule (ORDS), delivers the drug through a rigid water-permeable membrane with one or more small holes. As the capsule passes through the body, the osmotic pressure of water entering the capsule pushes the active drug through the opening in the capsule.

Oral Liquids

Oral liquids include suspensions, solutions, syrups, elixirs, tinctures, and emulsions (explained below). Typically, they are water based. Drugs formulated in liquids are easy to swallow. Liquid medicines work more rapidly than tablets or capsules.

Suspensions contain small drug particles (solute) suspended in a solvent (Figure 1-5). Drug particles settle to the bottom of the bottle when suspensions are left standing. Solutions are dosage forms in which drug particles completely dissolve in the liquid. Solutions remain clear. Suspensions may be administered orally, topically, or rectally.

Syrups contain a high concentration of sucrose or other sugar.

Elixirs contain between 5% and 40% alcohol.

Tinctures may contain as little 17% alcohol or as much as 80% alcohol.

Emulsions are similar to suspensions. Drugs suspended in oil may be dispersed in water (O/W) or drugs suspended in water may be dispersed in oil (W/O).

DOSAGE FORMS FOR TOPICAL ADMINISTRATION

Solutions, suspensions, and emulsions are also formulated for topical application to the skin, eye, ear, and mucous membranes of the rectum and vagina. Topical dosage forms not previously described include ointments, creams, and suppositories.

Ointments are semisolid preparations containing petrolatum or another oily base (lanolin, wool fat). They soften dry, scaly skin and protect the skin by forming a barrier between the skin and harmful substances.

Creams are semisolid emulsions. Vanishing creams have high water content (O/W); cold cream is an oil-in-water emulsion (W/O).

TECH NOTE!
Pharmacy technicians must carefully read the labels of medications available for immediate release, sustained release, and delayed release to avoid errors. Many are available in the same strength.

TECH NOTE!
When suspensions are dispensed, a SHAKE WELL auxiliary label should be placed on the prescription bottle.

TECH NOTE!
Eye drops may be placed in the ear, but ear drops should not be used in the eye.

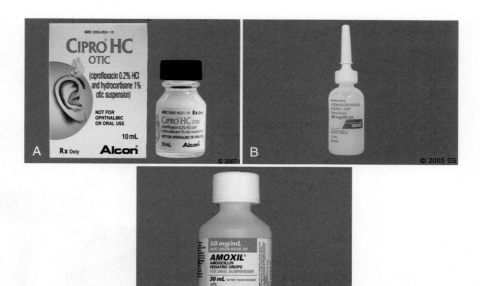

FIGURE 1-5 Suspensions. **A,** Otic suspensions. **B,** Rectal suspension. **C,** Oral suspension. (Copyright © Gold Standard, Inc., 2007.)

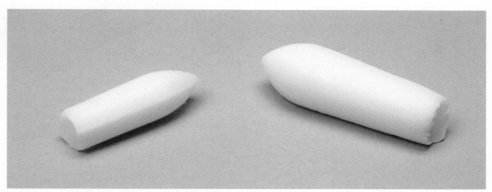

FIGURE 1-6 Typical shapes of suppositories. (Courtesy Rick Brady Riva, MD. From Lilley LL, Harrington S, Snyder JS: *Pharmacology and the nursing process*, ed 5, St Louis, 2007, Mosby.)

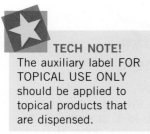

TECH NOTE!
The auxiliary label FOR TOPICAL USE ONLY should be applied to topical products that are dispensed.

TECH NOTE!
Patients should be advised to remove the foil or outer wrapper from the suppository before inserting it into the rectum or vagina.

Hydrogels contain up to 99% water and are a controlled-release ***drug delivery system***. They are used in transdermal implants (e.g., Histrelin) and wound dressings (e.g., Microsyn Skin and Wound Hydrogel).

Suppositories are solid or semisolid dosage forms intended to be inserted into a body orifice. They are shaped for vaginal, urethral, or rectal insertion. Suppositories melt at body temperature, dispersing the medicine (Figure 1-6).

Transdermal Drug Delivery Systems (Patches)

Transdermal patches are controlled-release devices that deliver medication across skin membranes into the general circulation (Figure 1-7). They produce systemic effects (throughout the body) in addition to local effects. Medicines formulated for transdermal application are used to treat angina (e.g., nitroglycerin), male hypogonadism (e.g., testosterone), menopause (e.g., estrogen), and pain (e.g., fentanyl).

DOSAGE FORMS FOR PARENTERAL ADMINISTRATION

Parenteral drugs are injected or infused (slowly injected) directly into a blood vessel, muscle, skin, or joint (Figure 1-8). Parenterally administered drugs enter the bloodstream, often producing

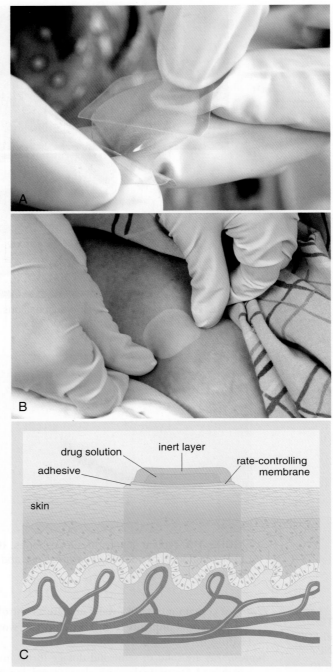

FIGURE 1-7 Transdermal patches. (**A** and **B**, Courtesy Rick Brady Riva, MD. From Lilley LL, Harrington S, Snyder JS: *Pharmacology and the nursing process*, ed 5, St Louis, 2007, Mosby. **C,** From Page C, et al: *Integrated pharmacology*, ed 3, Philadelphia, 2006, Mosby.)

TECH NOTE!
To avoid drug contamination, aseptic technique must always be followed when preparing drugs for parenteral administration.

rapid action. In the bloodstream, the side effects cannot be easily stopped. To avoid introducing contaminants that are harmful if injected into a patient, pharmacy technicians prepare parenterally administered using aseptic technique in a sterile environment. The following are examples of parenteral drugs:

Intravenous (IV) solutions are injected or infused directly into a vein and go immediately into the bloodstream.

Intramuscular (IM) solutions and suspensions are injected deep into a skeletal muscle.

Subcutaneous (subcut) solutions and suspensions are injected just beneath the skin.

Intraarticular solutions are injected directly into a joint.

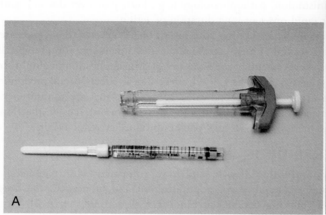
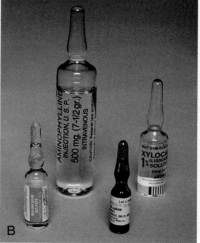

FIGURE 1-8 Typical containers for parenteral medications. A. Syringes, B. Vials (From Potter PA, Perry AG: *Basic nursing: theory and practice*, ed 3, St Louis, 1995, Mosby.)

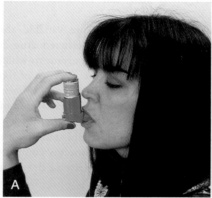
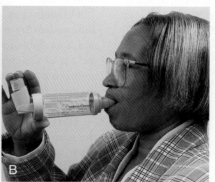

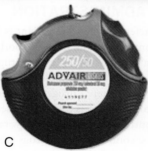

FIGURE 1-9 A, Proper use of an inhaler. **B,** Inhaler with spacer (also known as an aerochamber). (From Hopper T: *Mosby's pharmacy technician*, ed 2, St Louis, 2007, WB Saunders.) **C,** Accuhaler. (From Mason RJ, Broaddus C, et al: *Murray and Nadel's textbook of respiratory medicine*, ed 5, Philadelphia, 2010, Saunders.)

Intradermal solutions are injected into the dermal layer (allergy tests or tuberculosis vaccinations). *Intrathecal* solutions are injected directly into the cerebrospinal fluid.

DOSAGE FORMS FOR RESPIRATORY TRACT ADMINISTRATION

Solutions and suspensions are applied to mucous membranes of the nose as sprays or drops. Microfine powders, solutions, and gaseous drugs are inhaled into the lungs using a metered-dose aerosol inhaler (Figure 1-9) or a nebulizer. A nebulizer is a device that turns solutions into vapors that can be inhaled.

Routes of Administration

The formulation of a drug is largely controlled by the chemical properties of the drug and human physiology. The method of drug administration is determined by drug dosage form. When a drug is available for administration via more than one route, the selection of one route of administration over another is made according to the properties of the drug (e.g., lipid solubility, ionization), ease of administration, pathophysiology (e.g., kidney or liver disease), and therapeutic objectives (e.g., need for rapid onset or long duration of action).

The major routes of drug administration are ***enteral*** (oral), ***parenteral*** (IV, IM, subcut), inhalation, and topical. Enteral, parenteral, and inhalation routes typically produce systemic effects. Systemic effects extend beyond the area of drug application or administration. Drugs that are applied topically usually produce a local effect. Local effects occur predominantly at or near the site of application. These are general rules. Some drugs that are administered orally produce a local effect (e.g., antacids, neomycin), and some drugs administered by injection produce a local effect (e.g., local anesthetics). Transdermal patches produce systemic effects.

ENTERAL DRUG ADMINISTRATION

Oral administration is safe and easy compared with parenteral administration. No special techniques are required for administration and, if needed, the drug can be removed from the body via vomiting (emesis) or binding with activated charcoal. Drugs available for oral administration are generally less expensive than their parenteral dosage form. All orally administered drugs must disintegrate and dissolve into solution before they can be absorbed and distributed. This process is the pharmaceutical phase of drug disposition. Tablets and capsules contain binders and fillers that can influence the rate and extent of disintegration and dissolution.

Disadvantages of oral administration are variable absorption and decreased bioavailability. ***Bioavailability*** is the fraction of the administered drug dose that enters the systemic circulation and is available to produce drug effect. The extent to which a drug is absorbed and distributed to the site of action may be influenced by the presence of food in the stomach, which can delay the absorption of some drugs and aid the absorption of others. The first-pass effect, a process whereby the liver metabolizes a fraction of an administered dose of drug before it passes into the general circulation, also reduces bioavailability (see Chapter 2).

There are other disadvantages to oral administration. Drugs that are swallowed must pass through the gastrointestinal (GI) tract. Stomach contents contain powerful acids and digestive enzymes. These acids and enzymes can significantly decrease the amount of drug to be absorbed or inactivate some drugs (e.g., penicillin G, insulin).

PARENTERAL DRUG ADMINISTRATION

Parenteral administration is preferred when the patient is unable to swallow (e.g., unconscious) or is experiencing nausea and vomiting or the drug is poorly absorbed via an oral route. Medicines that are administered parenterally bypass the GI tract. Drugs administered parenterally directly enter the general circulation and therefore are not subject to degradation by GI and liver enzymes. The bioavailability of parenterally administered drugs is greater than that of orally administered drugs. An advantage of parenteral administration is the rapid onset of action. The amount of drug delivered parenterally can be carefully controlled by managing flow rates. The exact amount of drug circulating throughout the body cannot be controlled when drugs are administered orally. There are disadvantages to parenteral administration of drugs. Aseptic technique must be used when preparing drugs for parenteral administration to avoid introducing life-threatening contaminants into the patient's bloodstream. After a drug has been administered parentally, it cannot be recalled through vomiting. Table 1-6 compares the advantages and disadvantages of oral and parenteral administration.

Parenteral drugs must be administered using specialized techniques. Proper injection procedures must be followed to avoid harm to the patient (Figure 1-10). When a large volume of a drug is to be administered intravenously (injected into a vein) it must be injected slowly to avoid the destruction of red blood cells (hemolysis). Drugs formulated for intramuscular administration (injected into a muscle) may produce a rapid onset or a slow onset of action. Rapid-onset formulations are typically prepared in water-soluble solutions. Slow-onset, prolonged-duration-of-action formulations are suspended in oil or other nonaqueous vehicles (solvent). As the vehicle diffuses out of the muscle into which it has been injected, the drug is slowly deposited. The drug is slowly released from the muscle depot.

TECH NOTE!
It is important to apply warning labels to medications that inform the patient to TAKE WITH FOOD or TAKE ON AN EMPTY STOMACH.

TECH NOTE!
Pharmacy technicians must carefully read the labels of medications to avoid dispensing errors. Many drugs are available for immediate release and slow depot release. Many are available in the same strength.

TECH NOTE!
Please make sure to double-check your calculations for parenteral medications. After being administered, the drug cannot be recalled from the body.

TABLE 1-6   **Summary of Potential Advantages and Disadvantages of Oral versus Parenteral Administration**

Oral	Intravascular
Self-administration easy	Self-administration difficult
Safer; recall by emesis	No recall
Absorption slower	Absorption faster
Less expensive	Relatively expensive
Bioavailability lower	Bioavailability higher
Degraded by gastrointestinal enzymes	Not degraded by gastrointestinal enzymes
Subject to the "first-pass effect"	Not subject to the "first-pass effect"
Sterile preparation not critical	Aseptic product preparation critical

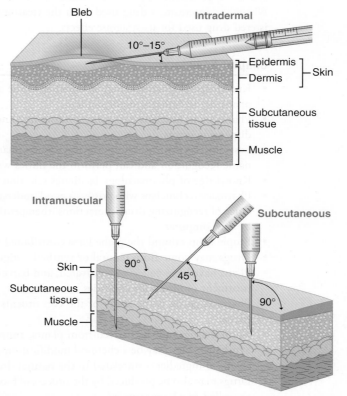

FIGURE 1-10 Forms of injection: intradermal injection, subcutaneous injection, and intramuscular injection. (From Kee JL, Hayes ER, McCuistion LE: *Pharmacology: a nursing process approach*, ed 5, St Louis, 2006, WB Saunders.)

Drugs intended for subcutaneous injection pose fewer risks than intravascular administration; however, aseptic technique must still be followed, and the site of injection must be rotated to avoid complications.

INHALATION

Inhalation is one of the most effective ways to rapidly deliver drug locally to cells of the respiratory tract and into the general circulation. Absorption problems that are encountered with oral administration are avoided. Some of the side effects associated with oral or parenteral administration are minimized. Inhalation is an effective method for the delivery of medications used to treat asthma and other respiratory disorders. Some medicines used to produce general anesthesia are administered by inhalation.

TRANSDERMAL DRUG ADMINISTRATION

Drugs that are formulated for transdermal administration are applied to the skin to produce systemic effects. Drugs such as nitroglycerin, estrogen, and testosterone are available for transdermal administration. Patients may experience systemic side effects and local side effects from drugs applied as transdermal patches. Local side effects such as skin irritation are often associated with the adhesives used to affix the patch to the skin and can be minimized by rotating the site where the patch is applied.

TOPICAL

Topically administered drugs typically produce a local effect. For example, hydrocortisone cream applied to the skin will reduce itchiness and redness associated with rashes without the systemic side effects associated with oral administration of the drug unless the drug is applied to a large percentage of body surface area. Side effects associated with topical administration are usually localized to the site of application. Topical administration is not exclusively used to produce a local effect. Nitroglycerin cream, a drug used to in the treatment of angina, is an example of topically administered drug used for its systemic effects.

Chapter Summary

- Knowledge of pharmacology is essential to the accurate, effective, and efficient performance of pharmacy technician responsibilities.
- Pharmacy technicians possessing a substantial knowledge of pharmacology may be able to reduce dispensing errors.
- Less time is spent searching for drugs when pharmacy technicians have good brand and generic name recognition and can perform the duties with greater independence.
- Knowledge of pharmacology facilitates selection of warning labels for drugs dispensed.
- Pharmacy technicians who possess a good understanding of pharmacology understand the importance of recognizing drug interactions, therapeutic duplication, and excessive dose alerts screened by the computer.
- People from around the globe have contributed to the knowledge of drugs.
- Drugs may come from natural or synthetic origins.
- Plants have been collected, cultivated, and harvested for their healing properties and used in the treatment of illness for centuries.
- Pharmacognosy is the study of the constituents of natural drugs that are responsible for their effects.
- Natural drugs may be derived from plants, animals, or minerals.
- Synthetic drugs may be a chemical modification of a natural drug or manufactured entirely from chemical ingredients unrelated to the natural drug.
- Drugs may also be produced by the process of bioengineering. Drugs produced by bioengineering are called *biopharmaceuticals*.
- Pharmacology is the study of the action of drugs on humans and animals.
- The new drug application process takes years to complete and includes preclinical research; clinical studies; phase 1, phase 2, and phase 3 drug trials; and phase 4 postmarket studies.
- The Food and Drug Administration regulates the new drug and IND process in the United States. The Health Products and Food Branch of Health Canada regulates the use of therapeutic drugs in Canada.
- The name of a new drug is made according to standards set by the Center for Drug Evaluation and Research.
- The generic name is the official or unofficial, nonproprietary drug name.
- The chemical name describes the molecular structure of the drug.
- The proprietary name, or brand name, is assigned by the drug manufacturer. Factors considered when selecting a suitable proprietary name are existing "look-alike" and "sound-alike" names and ease of association with the generic name or active ingredient name.

- Patent holders for new drugs are given up to 20 years of exclusive right to manufacture and distribute the new drug.
- Generic drugs contain the same active ingredient as the original manufacturer's drug in the same strength and in the same dosage form.
- Generic drugs may contain different inactive ingredients.
- Generic drugs are less expensive than brand name drugs.
- The Durham-Humphrey Amendment established the distinction between legend drugs and OTC drugs.
- The Kefauver-Harris Amendment requires all drugs be safe and effective before they are made available to the public.
- The Drug Price Competition Act and Patent Restoration Act encouraged the creation of generic drugs.
- Access to controlled substances is more restrictive than access to legend drugs because controlled substances may cause physical or psychological dependence.
- BTC drugs may be sold without a prescription, but access is restricted, and pharmacist intervention is required.
- Drugs are formulated for delivery by mouth, injection, inhalation, or topical application to skin or a mucous membrane. Factors influencing the choice for drug formulation are chemical properties of the drug and human physiology.
- The formulation of a drug is largely controlled by the chemical properties of the drug and human physiology.
- When a drug is available for administration by more than one route, the selection of one route of administration over another is made according to the properties of the drug, ease of administration, therapeutic objectives, and whether the patient has a preexisting disease.
- The major routes of drug administration are enteral (oral), parenteral (IV, IM, subcut), inhalation, and topical.
- The enteral, parenteral, and inhalation routes typically produce systemic effects.
- Topical administration is typically used to produce local effects but may be administered for systemic effects.
- Orally administered drugs must disintegrate and dissolve into solution before they can be absorbed and distributed. This process is called the pharmaceutical phase.
- Drugs that are swallowed must pass through the gastrointestinal tract. Acids in the stomach and digestive enzymes can inactivate some drugs (e.g., penicillin G).
- Medicines that are administered parenterally bypass the gastrointestinal tract. Drugs administered parenterally directly enter the general circulation and therefore are not subject to the degradation by gastrointestinal and liver enzymes.
- An advantage to parenteral administration is the rapid onset of action.
- Aseptic technique must be used when preparing drugs for parenteral administration to avoid introducing life-threatening contaminants into the patient's bloodstream.
- When a large volume of a drug is to be administered intravenously (injected into a vein) it must be injected slowly to avoid destruction of red blood cells (hemolysis).
- Drugs formulated for intramuscular administration (injected into a muscle) may produce a rapid onset or a slow-onset of action. Rapid-onset formulations are typically prepared in water-soluble solutions, and slow-onset, prolonged duration of action formulations are suspended in oil or other nonaqueous vehicles (solvent).
- Inhalation is one of the most effective ways to rapidly deliver drug locally to cells of the respiratory tract and into the general circulation. Inhalation is an effective method for delivery of medications used to treat asthma, other respiratory disorders, and general anesthetics.
- Drugs such as nitroglycerin, estrogen, and testosterone are formulated for transdermal administration (applied to the skin) but produce systemic effects.
- Transdermal patches may cause skin irritation, which is associated with the adhesive. Rotating the site of patch application can reduce risk of skin irritation.

1. Who was called the "father of pharmacology" and was a Greek physician known for his accurate observation of medicinal plants?
   a. Dioscorides
   b. Theophrastus
   c. Hippocrates
   d. Shen Nung

2. What is the study of the constituents of natural drugs that are responsible for their effects?
   a. Pharmacology
   b. Pharmacogenomics
   c. Pharmacognosy
   d. Pharmacokinetics

3. In 1906, what law was passed to protect the public from ineffective and harmful drugs?
   a. Pure Food and Drug Act
   b. Harrison Narcotic Act
   c. Pure Food Drug and Cosmetic Act
   d. none of the above

4. Which of the following drugs is *not* made from a plant?
   a. Morphine
   b. Fentanyl
   c. Quinine
   d. Digitalis

5. The study of pharmacology applies knowledge of
   a. Properties of drugs
   b. Mechanism of drug action
   c. Anatomy, physiology, and pathology
   d. All of the above

6. Which of the following is *not* a step in developing and receiving approval for a new drug?
   a. Preclinical research
   b. Clinical studies
   c. Marketing
   d. New drug application process and review

7. The official, non-proprietary name of the drug is the
   a. Generic name
   b. Trade name
   c. Brand name
   d. Chemical name

8. Which drugs can be obtained *only* by prescription?
   a. Herbal remedies
   b. Legend
   c. Compounded
   d. All of the above

9. Which of the following is *not* an oral formulation?
   a. Tablet
   b. Capsule
   c. Suspension
   d. Suppository

10. Parenterally administered drugs must be prepared using
    a. Aseptic technique in sterile environment
    b. Countertops cleaned with alcohol
    c. Patient carts in nursing units
    d. None of the above

TECHNICIAN'S
CORNER

1. The Kefauver-Harris Amendment (1962) requires all drugs to be safe and effective before they are made available to the public. Exactly what is involved in making a drug "safe and effective" for public use?
2. How would you explain to a client that a generic drug works just as well as a brand name drug?

Bibliography

Basch E, Ulbricht C: *Natural standard herb & supplement handbook: the clinical bottom line*, St Louis, 2005, Mosby.

Food and Drug Administration: *CDER data standards manual*. Retrieved from http://www.fda.gov/Drugs/DevelopmentApprovalProcess/FormsSubmissionRequirements/ElectronicSubmissions/DataStandardsManualmonographs/default.htm. Accessed Dec. 27, 2010.

Food and Drug Administration: *The new drug development process*. (http://www.fda.gov/cder/handbook)

Food and Drug Administration. (Feb. 2, 2012). Drugs@FDA Glossary of Terms. Retrieved April 6, 2012, from http://www.fda.gov/Drugs/InformationOnDrugs/ucm079436.htm?utm_campaign=Google2&utm_source=fdaSearch&utm_medium=website&utm_term=glossary&utm_content=1

Frederick H, Branding R Ph: Rahul Narula (ReedSmith) (http://www.nabp.net/events/assets/Branding12508NABP.pdf)

Goodman L, Gilman A: *The pharmacological basis of therapeutics*, ed 5, New York, 1975, Macmillan, pp 1-8.

Haas LF: Neurological stamp: Papyrus of Ebers and Smith, *J Neurol Neurosurg Psychiatry* 67:578, 1999.

Merck manual home edition: *Introduction: overview of drugs*. (http://www.merck.com/mmhe/sec02/ch010/ch010a.html)

National Library of Medicine, History of Medicine Division: *Classics of traditional Chinese medicine*. (http://www.nlm.nih.gov/hmd/chinese/emperors.html)

Shargel L, Mutnick A, Souney P, et al: *Comprehensive pharmacy review*, ed 4, Philadelphia, 2001, Lippincott Williams & Wilkins, pp 28-66.

Tyler V, Brady L, Robbers J: *Pharmacognosy*, ed 9, Philadelphia, 1988, Lea & Febiger, pp 1-6.

United States Drug Enforcement Administration: *Title 21: food and drugs, chapter 13: drug abuse prevention and control*. (http://www.dea.gov/pubs/csa.html)

Wiktorowicz ME, Lexchin J, Moscou K, et al: *Keeping an eye on prescription drugs, keeping Canadians safe. Active monitoring systems for drug safety and effectiveness in Canada and internationally*. Toronto, 2010, Health Council of Canada. (www.healthcouncilcanada.ca)

2

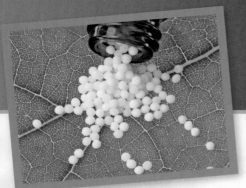

Principles of Pharmacology

LEARNING OBJECTIVES	1 Give a definition for each pharmacokinetic phase.
	2 Describe factors that influence each pharmacokinetic phase.
	3 Explain the importance of the first-pass effect.
	4 Describe the function of the blood-brain barrier.
	5 List major routes of drug elimination.
	6 Describe elimination half-life.
	7 Explain the importance of bioavailability to generic drug substitution.
	8 Learn the terminology associated with the principles of pharmacology.

KEY TERMS

Absorption: Process involving the movement of drug molecules from the site of administration into the circulatory system.

Bioavailability: The fraction of an administered dose that enters the systemic circulation in an unchanged form and is available to produce its effects.

Bioequivalent drug: Drug that shows no statistical differences in the rate and extent of absorption when it is administered in the same strength, dosage form, and route of administration as the brand name product.

Biotransformation: Process of drug metabolism in the body that transforms a drug to a more active, equally active, or inactive metabolite.

Diffusion: Passive movement of molecules across cell membranes from an area of high drug concentration to lower concentration.

Distribution: Process of movement of the drug from the circulatory system across barrier membranes to the site of drug action.

Duration of action: Time between the onset of action and discontinuation of drug action.

Elimination: Process that results in the removal of drug from the body.

Enzyme: Protein capable of causing a chemical reaction. Enzymes are involved in the metabolism of some drugs.

First-pass effect: Process whereby only a fraction of an orally administered drug reaches systemic circulation because much of the drug is metabolized in the liver to an inactive metabolite before entering the general circulation.

Half-life (t ½): Length of time it takes for the plasma concentration of an administered drug to be reduced by half.

Hydrophilic: Having a strong affinity for water; water loving. Able to dissolve in and absorb water.

Hydrophobic: Lacking an affinity for water; water hating. Resistant to wetting.

Ionization: Chemical process involving the gain or release of a proton (H^+). Ionized drug molecules may have a positive or negative charge.

Lipid: Fat like substance.

Lipophilic: Having an affinity for lipids; lipid loving.

Metabolism: Biochemical process involving transformation of active drugs to a compound that can be easily eliminated, or the conversion of prodrugs to active drugs.

Metabolite: Product of drug metabolism. Metabolites may be inactivated drugs or active drugs with equal or greater activity than the parent drug.

Microvilli: Brushlike border of each villus in the small intestine; increases the surface area for absorption.

Onset of action: Time it takes for drug action to begin.

Peak effect: Maximum drug effect produced by a given dose of drug after the drug has reached its maximum concentration in body.

Pharmaceutical alternative: Drug that contains the same active ingredient as the brand name drug; however, the strength and dosage form may be different.

Pharmaceutical equivalent: Drug that contains identical amount of active ingredient as brand name drug but may have different inactive ingredients, be manufactured in a different dosage form, and exhibit different rates of absorption.

Pharmacokinetics: Science dealing with what the body does to a drug, which includes the study of absorption, distribution, metabolism, and elimination.

Prodrug: Drug administered in an inactive form that is metabolized in the body to an active form.

Therapeutic alternative: Drug that contains different active ingredient(s) than the brand name drug yet produces the same desired therapeutic outcome.

Pharmacokinetics

The word ***pharmacokinetics*** is derived from the Greek words pharmaco ("drug") and kinesis ("movement"). Absorption, distribution, metabolism, and elimination are four pharmacokinetic phases. Drugs that are administered must be absorbed into the bloodstream and distributed to their site of action before they can begin to produce their effect. The body metabolizes the drug, and then it is eliminated. As a drug moves throughout the body, it undergoes changes that may increase or decrease its absorption, distribution, metabolism, or elimination. These pharmacokinetic phases control the intensity of the drug's effect and the duration of the drug action (Figure 2-1).

The length of time it takes for drug action to begin after a dose is administered is called the ***onset of action***. The onset of action is not achieved until the drug reaches the minimum concentration in the body needed to produce drug action. The maximum drug effect, or ***peak effect***, occurs after the maximum drug concentration after administration of a given dose of drug is reached in the body. The ***duration of action*** is the time between the onset of action and discontinuation of drug action. The duration of action is the amount of time the drug concentration remains within the therapeutic range (Figure 2-2).

Pharmacokinetic Phases

ABSORPTION

Absorption is the first pharmacokinetic phase. Absorption is the process that involves the movement of drug molecules from the site of administration, across cell membranes, and into the circulatory system of the body (blood or lymphatic system). Absorption may occur across the skin or cells that line blood vessels. How quickly or slowly a drug is absorbed is determined by the characteristics of the drug, the drug dosage form, the route of administration, human anatomy, and physiology. The amount of drug absorbed is also influenced by many factors. Absorption of drugs taken by mouth may be delayed when food is present in the stomach. Absorption of pills that have been swallowed does not begin until after the drug goes into solution, so factors effecting disintegration

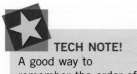
TECH NOTE!
A good way to remember the order of the pharmacokinetic phases is to use the acronym ADME.

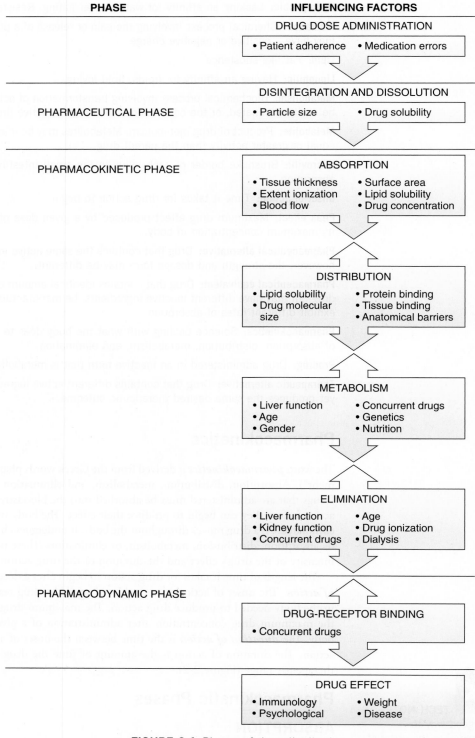

FIGURE 2-1 Phases of drug distribution.

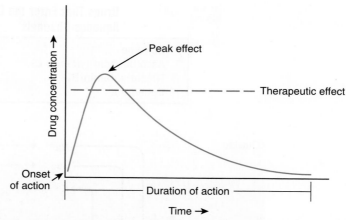

FIGURE 2-2 Onset of action, peak effect, duration of action, and therapeutic effect.

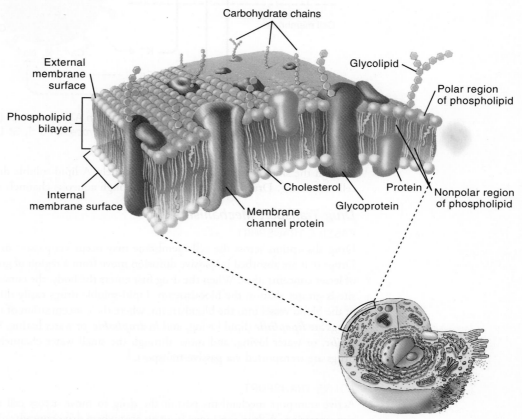

FIGURE 2-3 Plasma membrane. (From Thibodeau GA, Patton KT: *Anatomy and physiology*, ed 6, St Louis, 2007, Mosby.)

or dissolution of the drug (pharmaceutical phase) can decrease absorption (see Chapter 1). The ease in which the drug is able to cross cell membranes is a factor in how readily the drug is absorbed via oral, rectal, vaginal, and other routes of administration.

The Cell Membrane

Drug movement from the site of administration into the circulatory system depends on the ability of the drug to move across cell membranes. The cell membrane is a complex structure of *lipids*, protein, and water-filled channels (Figure 2-3). Movement across the cell membrane is restricted unless the drug can pass through the lipid layers of the cell membrane or is small enough to pass

BOX 2-1   **Drugs That Enter the Cell through Aqueous Channels**

- Caffeine
- Ascorbic acid (vitamin C)
- Niacin (vitamin B_3)
- Ephedrine

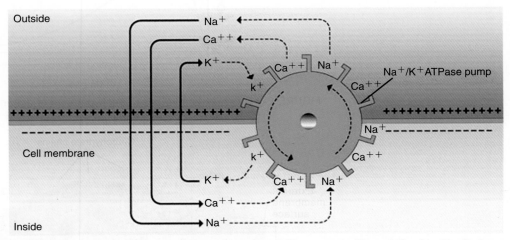

FIGURE 2-4 Active transport: sodium/potassium ATPase pump. (From Lilley LL, Harrington S, Snyder JS: *Pharmacology and the nursing process*, ed 5, St Louis, 2007, Mosby.)

through the small water-filled (aqueous) channels. A lipid-soluble drug can move easily across the cell membrane. Drugs that enter the cell through aqueous channels are listed in Box 2-1.

Drug Transport Mechanisms

PASSIVE TRANSPORT

Drug absorption across the cell membrane may occur via passive or active transport mechanisms. Drugs that are absorbed by passive diffusion move from a region of greater concentration to a region of lesser concentration. When the drug first enters the body, the concentration at the administration site is greater than in the bloodstream. Lipid-soluble drugs easily diffuse across the cell membrane of the blood vessel into the bloodstream, where the concentration of the drug is small. Lipid-soluble drugs are *lipophilic* (lipid loving) and *hydrophobic*, or water hating. Water-soluble drugs are *hydrophilic*, or water loving, and move through the small water channels in the cell membrane. Most drugs are transported via passive transport.

ACTIVE TRANSPORT

Active transport mechanisms permit the drug to move across cell membranes without regard to concentration. A drug can move from an area where drug concentration is low to an area where the concentration is high. Active transport takes energy and requires special carrier proteins or pumps to "carry the drug" across the cell membrane (Figure 2-4).

Factors Influencing Absorption

EFFECT OF PH ON DRUG ABSORPTION

Most drugs are either weak acids or weak bases. In solution, weak acids and weak bases exist between the ionized and the nonionized state. In solution, weak acids (HA) disassociate, releasing a proton (H^+) and negatively charged anion (A^-).

$$HA \rightleftarrows H^+ + A^-$$

Weak bases also release a proton when they are in solution. Release of a proton results in an uncharged drug molecule.

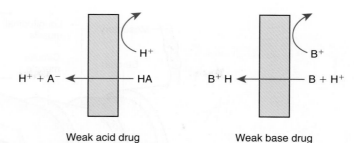

FIGURE 2-5 Weak acids and weak bases crossing cell membranes.

$$B^+H \rightleftarrows B + H^+$$

Weakly acidic drugs are more ionized when they are in basic solutions. When the drug is in an acidic solution, it is less ionized. Weakly basic drugs are more ionized when they are in acidic solution and less ionized in basic solution. This is important because as the drug travels throughout the body, it passes through acidic solutions (e.g., in the stomach) and basic solutions (e.g., in the small intestine). The ability of a drug to diffuse across the cell membrane depends on properties of the drug and the pH of the body fluid in which it is dissolved. The pH is a measure of how acidic or alkaline (basic) a solution is. A pH of 1 is very acidic (e.g., stomach acids [HCl]). A pH of 7 is neutral. Plasma has a pH between the range of 7.35 and 7.45. A pH of greater than 7 is alkaline.

Diffusion across the cell membrane is greatest when the drug is lipid soluble and nonionized (uncharged). When a weakly acidic drug such as phenobarbital is in the stomach, it is less ionized and can readily cross the cell membranes (Figure 2-5). Absorption is high. When the drug moves into the small intestine, ionization increases and absorption is reduced.

EFFECT OF BLOOD FLOW ON DRUG ABSORPTION

Absorption is greatest in areas of the body that have a good blood supply. Medications administered sublingually have good absorption because many blood vessels are located under the tongue. Absorption of orally administered drugs is greatest in the small intestine. The structure of the intestine is designed to perform the specialized job of absorption. Thousands of *microvilli* line the walls of the small intestine (Figure 2-6). The microvilli are filled with blood vessels. As the drug passes through the cell membrane of the microvilli, it is quickly absorbed into the bloodstream. Absorption of drugs that are injected intramuscularly or subcutaneously is increased when the patient applies heat to the muscle, exercises, or does some other activity to stimulate blood flow to the site of administration.

EFFECT OF SURFACE AREA ON DRUG ABSORPTION

Microvilli also increase the surface area of the small intestine, making it the largest absorbing surface in the body (Figure 2-7). The area for absorption in the small intestine is about 1000 times greater than that in the stomach.

EFFECT OF CONTACT TIME AT THE ABSORPTION SURFACE

Drug absorption increases the longer the drug is in contact with the absorbing surface. Drug absorption is decreased if the patient has diarrhea because of the rapid passage of contents through the gastrointestinal (GI) tract. Absorption of delayed release drugs can be increased when a drug is taken with food because of delayed gastric emptying.

EFFECT OF TISSUE THICKNESS ON ABSORPTION

Drug absorption is greater across single cell membranes than multiple cell layers because some drugs may become trapped in cell layers. As tissue thickness increases, the portion of the drug trapped in the cell layers increases.

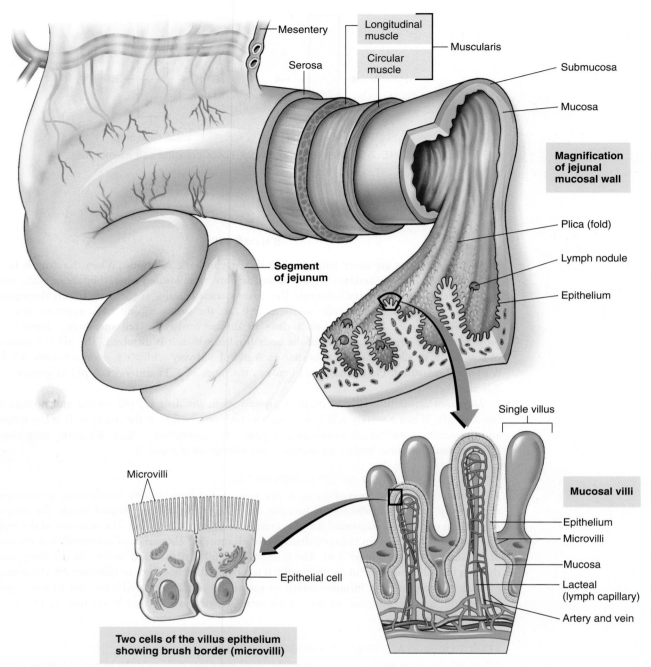

FIGURE 2-6 Wall of intestine with villi. (From Thibodeau GA, Patton KT: *Anatomy and physiology*, ed 6, St Louis, 2007, Mosby.)

DISTRIBUTION

Distribution is the process of movement of the drug from the circulatory system across barrier membranes to the site of drug action (Figure 2-8). It is the second pharmacokinetic phase. The volume of drug that is distributed is influenced by the properties of the drug, the extent of drug binding to blood proteins or tissue, the blood supply to the region, and the ability of the drug to cross natural body barriers. The drug may be distributed to water compartments of the body or to fat cells or proteins. Water compartments include plasma, extracellular fluid, and total body water.

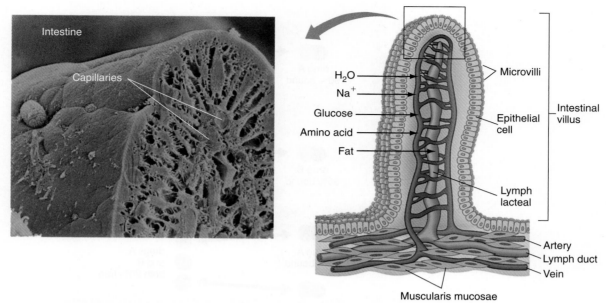

FIGURE 2-7 Intestinal villi showing absorbing surfaces. (From Thibodeau GA, Patton KT: *Anatomy and physiology*, ed 6, St Louis, 2007, Mosby.)

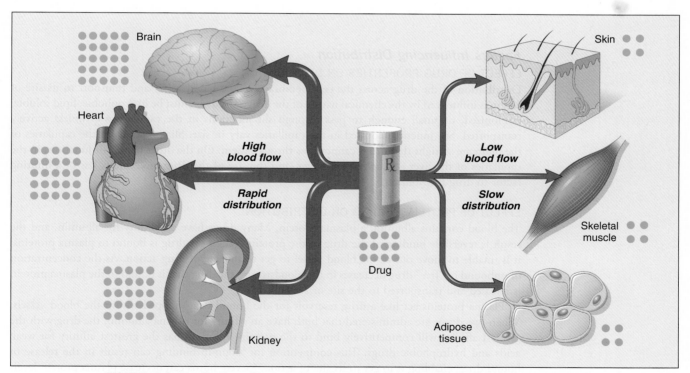

FIGURE 2-8 Distribution. (From Raffa RB, Rawls SM, Beyzarov EP: *Netter's illustrated pharmacology*, Philadelphia, 2005, WB Saunders.)

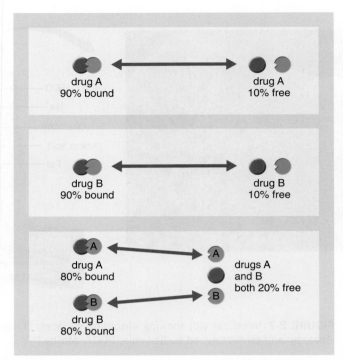

FIGURE 2-9 Protein binding and free fraction of drugs. (From Page C, et al: *Integrated pharmacology*, ed 3. Philadelphia, 2006, Mosby.)

Factors Influencing Distribution

EFFECT OF DRUG PROPERTIES ON DISTRIBUTION

Distribution of the drug across the cell membrane of the blood vessel and transport to its site of action is influenced by the chemical nature of the drug. The drug must be hydrophobic, lipid soluble, nonionized, or small enough to pass through slit junctions in the capillary wall unless actively transported. Slit junctions located in the capillaries vary in size. Slit junctions in the capillaries of the brain are so tight that drugs cannot pass through them. On the other hand, slit junctions in the capillaries of the liver and spleen are larger, and the size of the drug molecule is less of a limiting factor to drug distribution.

EFFECT OF PROTEIN BINDING ON DISTRIBUTION

The blood contains albumin, a plasma protein. Many drugs have an affinity for albumin, and the result is reversible binding of the drug to the protein. When the drug is bound to plasma proteins, it is unable to move out of the blood vessel to get to the site of drug action. As the concentration of unbound or "free" drug decreases in the bloodstream, the drug that is bound to the plasma protein is released and transported to the site of action.

Plasma proteins act like a drug reservoir for the bound drug trapped within the blood vessels. When two drugs are administered that both have an affinity for plasma albumin, the drug with the greatest affinity will competitively bind to the protein. Albumin has the greatest affinity for weak acids and hydrophobic drugs. This competition for albumin binding can result in the release of bound drug, enabling it to get to its site of action. (Severe burns can decrease plasma protein levels [hypoalbuminemia], which may alter the level of "free drug".) Competitive protein binding represents a mechanism for drug interactions (Figure 2-9).

ANATOMICAL BARRIERS TO DISTRIBUTION

Natural body barriers may limit access to the site of drug action. Anatomical structures that selectively limit drug access are the blood-brain barrier, blood-placenta barrier, and blood-testicular barrier.

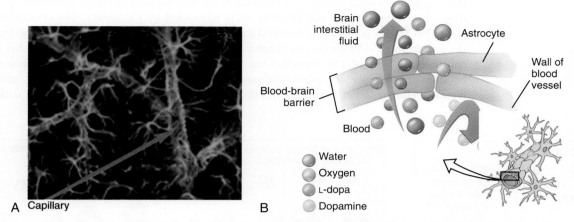

FIGURE 2-10 Barriers. (**A,** From Marie Simar Couldwell, MD, and Maiken Nedergaard. **B,** From Thibodeau GA, Patton KT: *Anatomy of physiology,* ed 6, St Louis, 2007, Mosby.)

TABLE 2-1   **Pregnancy Safety Categories**

Category	Description
Category A	Studies indicate no risk to human fetuses.
Category B	Animal reproductive studies indicate no risk; information in humans is reassuring.
Category C	Potential risk reported in animal reproduction studies or no studies conducted. Information in humans is not available. Potential benefits versus risk may warrant the use in pregnant women.
Category D	Possible fetal risk in humans reported; however, considering potential benefit versus risk, in selected cases, the use of these drugs in pregnant women may be warranted.
Category X	Fetal abnormalities reported, and positive evidence of fetal risk in humans is available from animal or human studies. These drugs should not be used in pregnant women.

Adapted From Lilley LL, Harrington S, Snyder JS: *Pharmacology and the nursing process,* ed 5, St Louis, 2007, Mosby and FDA (http://www.fda.gov/ohrms/dockets/ac/02/slides/3902s1-09-miller/sld009.htm).

The blood-brain barrier is composed of cells lining the capillaries of the brain that form tight junctions (Figure 2-10). The blood vessels in the brain are also surrounded by fatty structures called *glial feet* (also known as *astrocyte foot processes*). These structures limit the passage of ions between the capillaries and brain tissue. They permit passage of lipid-soluble, hydrophobic drugs into the brain and limit access of ionized hydrophilic drugs.

The blood-placenta barrier limits access of drugs taken by a pregnant woman to the fetus. Many drugs are able to cross the blood-placenta barrier, so it is important for pregnant women to ask their physicians or pharmacists about potential safety issues before taking a drug. There are five pregnancy safety categories (Table 2-1). Drugs classified in pregnancy safety category A have been shown to be safe when taken during pregnancy. Drugs listed in pregnancy safety category B have been shown to be safe when studied in animals, but no well-controlled studies in pregnant women have been conducted. Category C contains a list of drugs with reported adverse effects in animal fetuses. No information for humans is available. Adverse effects in humans may occur when drugs listed in pregnancy safety category D are taken, so the benefits of use must be balanced against the risks. Drugs listed in category X should be avoided because fetal abnormalities have been reported.

METABOLISM

Few drugs that are administered are eliminated unchanged. Most drugs are transformed by enzymes to a **metabolite**(s). An **enzyme** is a protein capable of causing a chemical reaction. A metabolite is a product of drug **metabolism**. **Biotransformation** is the process of drug metabolism in the body that transforms a drug to a more active, equally active, or inactive metabolite. The primary site of biotransformation is the liver; however, metabolism may occur in the intestines, lung, kidney, or other cells in the body. Microsomal enzymes in the liver are responsible for transforming lipophilic drugs to compounds that can be more easily eliminated by the kidney. The cytochrome P-450 (CYP450) system is frequently involved in this process. Drugs that interfere with the enzymes of the cytochrome P-450 system can enhance or inhibit the metabolism of other drugs that are taken concurrently (Figure 2-11). Phenobarbital, a drug used in the treatment of epilepsy, increases metabolic enzyme activity of other antiseizure medications (phenytoin, valproic acid), resulting in increased elimination of the drugs. This decreases their effectiveness. CYP450 activity is also found

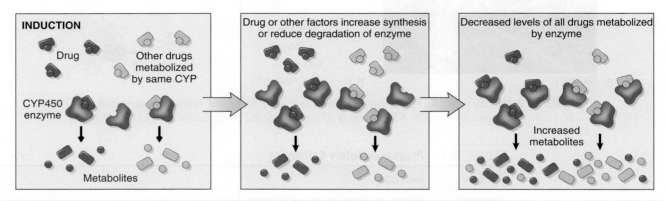

CYP	Inducers	Inhibitors
1A2	Smoking, charbroiled foods, cruciferous vegetables, insulin, modafinil, nafcillin, omeprazole, phenobarbital, primidone, rifampin	Amiodarone, anastrozole, cimetidine, ciprofloxacin, diltiazem, enoxacin, erythromycin, fluoroquinolones, fluvoxamine, grapefruit (juice), mexiletine, norfloxacin, ritonavir, tacrine, ticlopidine
2A6	Dexamethasone, phenobarbital	Methoxsalen, ritonavir, tranylcypromine
2B6	Cyclophosphamide, dexamethasone, phenobarbitol, phenytoin, primidone, rifampin	Efavirenz, nelfinavir, orphenadrine, ritonavir, thiotepa, ticlopidine
2C8/9	Dexamethasone, primidone, rifampin, secobarbital	Anastrozole, amiodarone, cimetidine, diclofenac, disulfiram, fluconazole, luvoxamine, flurbiprofen, fluvastatin, isoniazid, ketoprofen, lovastatin, metronidazole, omeprazole, paroxetine, phenylbutazone, ritonavir, sertraline, sulfinpyrazone, sulfonamides, sulfamethoxazole, trimethoprim, troglitazone, zafirlukast
2C19	Barbituates, rifampin	Cimetidine, ketoconazole, modafinil, omeprazole, oxcarbazepine, ticlopidine
2D6	Dexamethasone, quinidine, rifampin	Amiodarone, buproprion, celecoxib, chlorpromazine, chlorpheniramine, cimetidine, clomipramine, cocaine, doxorubicin, fluoxetine, fluphenazine, fluvoxamine, haloperidol, lomustine, metoclopramide, methadone, norfluoxetine, paroxetine, perphenazine, propafenone, quinidine, ranitidine, ritonavir, sertindole, sertraine, terbinafine, thioridazine, venlafaxine, vinblastine, vinorelbine
2E1	Acetone, ethanol, isoniazid	Disulfiram, ritonavir
3A4	Barbituates, carbamazepine, dexamethasone, efavirenz, macrolides, glucocorticoids, modafinil, nevirapine, oxcarbazepine, phenobarbital, phenylbutazone, pioglitazone, phenytoin, primidone, rifabutin, rifampin, St John's wort, sulfinpyrazone, troglitazone	Amiodarone, anastrozole, chloramphenicol, cimetidine, ciprofloxacin, clarithromycin, clotrimazole, danazol, delavirdine, diltiazem, erythromycin, fluconazole, fluoxetine, fluvoxamine, grapefruit juice, indinavir, itraconazole, ketoconazole, metronidazole, mibefradil, miconazole, nefazodone, nelfinavir, nevirapine, norfloxacin, norfluoxetine, omeprazole, paroxetine, propoxyphene, quinidine, ranitidine, ritonavir, saquinavir, sertindole, troglitazone, troleandomycin, verapamil, zafirlukast, zileuton

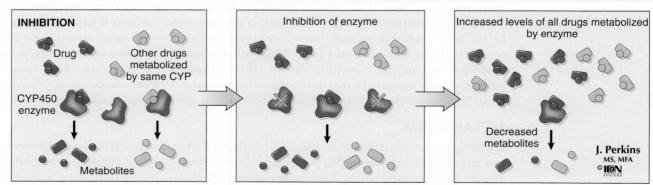

FIGURE 2-11 Metabolic enzyme induction and inhibition. (From Raffa RB, Rawls SM, Beyzarov EP: *Netter's illustrated pharmacology*, Philadelphia, 2005, WB Saunders.)

in the mucous membranes of the nose. Metabolic enzymes are found in saliva and are secreted by bacteria in the intestines.

Not all drugs are metabolized to inactive metabolites. Table 2-2 shows the potential products of metabolism.

Latanoprost is a drug that is used to treat glaucoma. It is an example of a drug that is metabolized in the eye rather than in the liver. It is also a good example of a prodrug. ***Prodrugs*** are drugs that are administered in an inactive form and must be metabolized to their active form. Drugs may be formulated as prodrugs to avoid side effects or to increase distribution to the site of action. Levodopa is a prodrug that is metabolized to dopamine in the brain. The drug is used to treat Parkinson's disease. Levodopa is able to cross the blood-brain barrier better than dopamine. Administration of the prodrug increases the volume of drug distributed into the brain. Adding the drug carbidopa to levodopa further increases the amount of drug that is converted to dopamine because carbidopa interrupts levodopa metabolism outside the brain.

"First-Pass Effect"

Orally administered drugs must pass into the hepatoportal circulation (liver) before entering the general circulation. The ***first-pass effect*** is a process whereby only a fraction of an orally administered drug reaches systemic circulation. Much of the drug is metabolized in the liver to an inactive metabolite before passing into the general circulation (Figure 2-12). Orally administered

TABLE 2-2   **Products of Metabolism**

Parent Drug	Example	Metabolite	Example
Active drug	6-Mercaptopurine	Inactive drug	6-Mercapturic acid
Active drug	Prednisolone Imipramine	Equally active drug	Prednisone Desipramine
Active drug	Diazepam Codeine	More active drug	Oxazepam Morphine
Inactive drug	Fosamprenavir Levodopa Fosinopril	Active drug	Amprenavir Dopamine Fosinoprilat

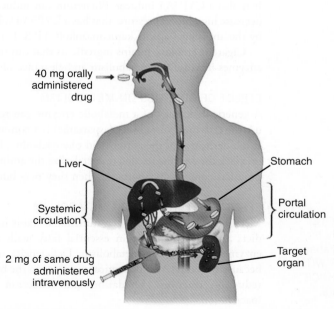

FIGURE 2-12 The first-pass effect. (From Lilley LL, Aucker RS: *Pharmacology and the nursing process*, ed 3, St Louis, 2001, Mosby.)

nitroglycerin is approximately 90% cleared during a single pass through the liver. Sublingual administration avoids the first-pass effect. Many blood vessels are located under the tongue, so drugs administered by this route can pass directly into the general circulation before passing through the liver. Morphine is also subject to the first-pass effect.

Factors Influencing Metabolism

When metabolism is increased, the duration of effect of many drugs is reduced. The onset of drug action begins with metabolism for prodrugs.

EFFECT OF LIVER FUNCTION ON METABOLISM

The liver is the primary site for metabolism. If the liver is functioning below capacity, metabolism is decreased. Drug doses should often be reduced in the presence of liver dysfunction.

EFFECT OF DISEASE ON METABOLISM

Diseases such as hepatitis decrease the metabolic capacity of the liver. The liver, however, is not the only site of metabolism. Lung disease and kidney disease can also reduce the ability of the body to metabolize drugs. Heart failure decreases blood flow to the liver, altering the extent of drug metabolism.

EFFECT OF AGE ON METABOLISM

Metabolism in the liver is decreased in elderly adults and in infants. Age-related changes in the liver decrease metabolic enzyme function in elderly adults. Metabolizing enzyme systems (cytochrome P-450 system [CYP450]) is not fully developed in infants; therefore, their ability to metabolize drugs is decreased. Infants and elderly adults generally require lower doses of drug to produce therapeutic effects.

EFFECT OF CONCURRENT ADMINISTRATION OF DRUGS (INTERACTIONS)

Administration of two or more drugs that both use the same metabolic pathways can alter the metabolism of each other. CYP450 isoform substrates are a large group of metabolic enzymes. The metabolism of many drugs is altered by the coadministration of CYP450 substrate inducers or inhibitors. Enzyme inducer–substrate binding increases metabolic enzyme activity, and enzyme inhibitor–substrate binding decreases metabolic enzyme activity. CYP 450 isoform substrates include CYP1A2, CYP2A6, CYP2B6, CYP2C8, CYP2C9, CYP2C19, CYP2D6, CYP2E1, and CYP3A4. Phenytoin is a drug used in the treatment of epilepsy. It contains CYP2C9 and CYP2C19 substrates. It is also a CYP3A4 inducer. Phenytoin can induce the metabolism of amlodipine, a drug used to decrease high blood pressure, that has a CYP3A4 substrate. The metabolism of phenytoin is inhibited by the antifungal agents ketoconazole (CYP2C19) and fluconazole (CYP2C9).

Cigarette smoke contains ingredients that can stimulate the activity of metabolic enzymes. These enzymes increase the metabolism and clearance of theophylline, a drug used to treat asthma.

EFFECT OF GENETICS ON METABOLISM

A genetic deficiency of a metabolic enzyme can reduce the body's ability to metabolize drugs that use the enzyme. NutraSweet (aspartame) is a common sweetener found in diet foods and beverages. It is a derivative of the amino acid phenylalanine. People diagnosed with the disorder phenylketonuria lack the enzyme needed to metabolize the amino acid phenylalanine to tyrosine. If they consume products containing aspartame, then they may build up toxic levels of phenylalanine.

EFFECT OF NUTRITION ON METABOLISM

Metabolism is decreased when nutritional status is severely depressed as in starvation. Low-protein diets and diets deficient in essential fatty acids can reduce the synthesis of drug-metabolizing enzymes and decrease metabolism. Deficiencies of vitamins and minerals can affect metabolism because they catalyze biochemical reactions in the body. For example, vitamin B_2 catalyzes oxidation-reduction reactions. Oxidation and reduction are metabolic processes that result in drug inactivation.

Foods can influence metabolism of drugs. Many drug interactions are linked to consumption of grapefruit juice. Grapefruit juice is an inhibitor of metabolic enzyme CYP3A4. When drugs that

TECH NOTE!
Be sure to apply the warning label stating: "DO NOT TAKE WITH GRAPEFRUIT JUICE" when appropriate.

have a CYP3A4 substrate, such as the anticholesterol drug lovastatin and the antiretroviral drug saquinavir, are taken with grapefruit juice, metabolism is reduced, and blood levels of the drugs can increase along with drug effects.

EFFECT OF GENDER ON METABOLISM

The rate of metabolism of some drugs varies between men and women, suggesting the sex hormones may influence metabolism. Men metabolize propranolol (a heart drug) faster than do women. Women metabolize acetaminophen (an analgesic) slightly faster than do men.

ELIMINATION

Elimination is the final pharmacokinetic phase. Elimination results in removal of the drug from the body and discontinuation of drug action. The three major routes of drug elimination are the kidney, lung, and bowel (Table 2-3).

The normal function of the kidney is to filter the blood and remove things that are foreign or harmful. This job is done by the nephrons of the kidney (Figure 2-13). Free drug (not bound to albumin) is transported to Bowman capsule, where it is filtered by the glomerulus. As the drug moves through the nephron to the distal convoluted tubule, its concentration increases. If the drug is nonionized, it may diffuse out of the nephron back into the systemic circulation and continue to produce drug action.

Factors Influencing Elimination

EFFECT OF KIDNEY FUNCTION ON ELIMINATION

Kidney dysfunction can have a profound effect on elimination of drugs from the body. Decreased kidney function decreases the extent of drug cleared and the rate of clearance. This can cause a buildup of drug in the body and produce toxic drug effects. Drugs that are highly eliminated via the kidneys require a reduction in dose to avoid toxicity when kidney function is reduced. When kidney function is critically reduced, dialysis is needed. Dialysis mechanically filters the blood and can increase drug elimination.

EFFECT OF DISEASE ON ELIMINATION

Lung disease decreases the body's capacity to eliminate drugs and their metabolites. Bowel disease may increase or decrease elimination. Crohn's disease causes excessive diarrhea, which speeds the elimination of drugs. When movement of contents of the bowel is slowed, drug elimination is delayed.

TABLE 2-3   **Routes of Drug Elimination**

	Eliminated in
Major Routes	
Kidney	Urine
Lung	Expired air
Bowel	Feces
Minor Routes	
Liver	Bile
Skin	Sweat
Eyes	Tears
Mouth	Saliva
Nose	Mucus
Penis	Semen
Breast	Breast milk

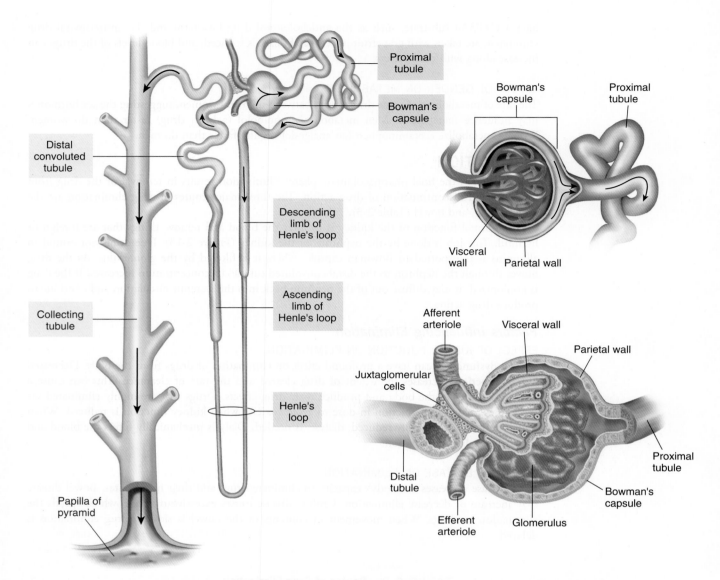

FIGURE 2-13 Nephron. (From Thibodeau GA, Patton KT: *Anatomy and physiology*, ed 6, St Louis, 2007, Mosby.)

EFFECT OF DRUG IONIZATION ON ELIMINATION

Changes in the acidity of the urine can influence the rate in which a drug is cleared from the body. Weakly acidic drugs are less ionized in acidic urine. As the pH of the urine becomes more basic, the ***ionization*** of acidic drugs increases. Weak bases are more ionized when the urine is acidic and less ionized when the urine is basic. Drugs that are ionized are eliminated in the urine. Nonionized drugs are reabsorbed back into the circulatory system to continue their drug action.

EFFECT OF CONCURRENT ADMINISTRATION OF DRUGS (INTERACTIONS)

Drug interactions can result in increased or decreased elimination of drugs. Pharmacists and health care providers may purposefully recommend coadministration of two drugs to delay elimination and prolong drug action or to speed elimination. Urinary acidifiers (e.g., vitamin C) decrease the elimination of acidic drugs. Urinary alkalinizers (e.g., sodium bicarbonate) decrease the elimination of basic drugs.

TABLE 2-4   **The Concept of Drug Half-Life**

Different Perspectives				Changing Values					
Drug concentration (mg/L)	100	50	25	12.5	6.25	3.125	1.563	0.782	0.391
Hours after peak concentration	0	8	16	24	32	40	48	56	64
Number of half-lives	0	1	2	3	4	5	6	7	8
Percentage of drug removed	0	50	75	88	94	97	98.437	99.128	99.609

Modified from Lilley LL, Harrington S, Snyder JS: *Pharmacology and the nursing process*, ed 5, St Louis, 2007, Mosby.

Elimination Half-Life (t ½)

Elimination **half-life (t ½)** refers to the time it takes for 50% of a drug to be cleared from the bloodstream (Table 2-4). It takes approximately eight half-lives to entirely eliminate a drug from the body. Every drug has a unique half-life that is dependent on characteristics of the drug (e.g., active metabolites). Knowledge of elimination half-life is important; it is an indicator of how long a drug will produce effects in the body. The half-life of a drug can be as short as a few minutes (e.g., drugs used to produce general anesthesia) or as long as several days (e.g., levothyroxine, a drug used to treat hypothyroidism). Drugs with long half-lives are dosed less frequently than are drugs with very short half-lives. Given the rate of elimination at any given time is proportional to the concentration at that time in first-order kinetics, the elimination half-life can be calculated by dividing the elimination rate constant (0.693) by proportionality constant (k):

$$t \frac{1}{2} = 0.693/k$$

BIOAVAILABILITY AND BIOEQUIVALENCE OF DRUGS

Bioavailability is defined as the rate and extent to which the active ingredient of an administered drug enters the systemic circulation, reaches the site of action, and is available to produce its effect. The bioavailability of a drug is influenced by drug absorption, the first-pass effect, and distribution to the site of action. The bioavailability of generic drugs is compared with the innovator's product to determine if the generic is bioequivalent. Tests are conducted to measure maximum concentration (C_{max}) of the drug in the bloodstream after a single dose is administered. The time it takes to reach maximum concentration (T_{max}) is also measured. A graph showing rise and fall of drug blood levels after the administration of a single dose of drug looks like a curve. The area under the curve (AUC) is a measure of the drug bioavailability. Bioavailability tests are conducted to determine if the generic drug achieves the same maximum blood concentration in the same time as the brand name drug. The generic is bioequivalent if no statistical differences are found in the rate and extent of absorption when the drug is administered in the same strength, dosage form, and route of administration as the brand name product (Figure 2-14).

PHARMACEUTICAL EQUIVALENTS AND PHARMACEUTICAL ALTERNATIVES

Pharmaceutical equivalents differ from bioequivalents. **Bioequivalent drugs** and pharmaceutical equivalent drugs both contain the same active ingredient in the same strength as the innovator's drug (brand name). Pharmaceutical equivalents may have different inactive ingredients, be manufactured in a different dosage form, and exhibit different rates of absorption than the brand name. **Pharmaceutical alternatives** contain the same active ingredient as the brand name product; however, the strength and dosage form may be different. A **therapeutic alternative** may contain different active ingredients yet produce the same desired therapeutic outcome.

TECH NOTE!
Product substitution laws regulate the dispensing of generic drugs. Only generics that are bioequivalent can be substituted and dispensed when brand name drugs are prescribed.

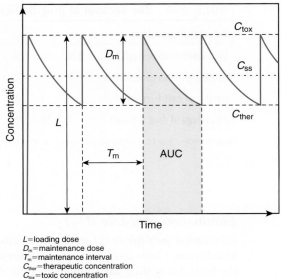

L = loading dose
D_m = maintenance dose
T_m = maintenance interval
C_{ther} = therapeutic concentration
C_{tox} = toxic concentration
C_{ss} = average steady state concentration
AUC = area under the curve

FIGURE 2-14 Plasma concentrations after repeated doses. (From Kalant H, Grant DM, Mitchell J: *Principles of medical pharmacology*, ed 7, Philadelphia, 2007, WB Saunders.)

Chapter Summary

- There are four pharmacokinetic phases: absorption, distribution, metabolism, and elimination.
- As a drug moves throughout the body, it undergoes changes that may increase or decrease its absorption, distribution, metabolism, or elimination.
- Pharmacokinetic phases control the intensity of the drug's effect and the duration of the drug action.
- The onset of drug action begins once the drug reaches the minimum concentration necessary to produce a therapeutic effect.
- The peak effect occurs when the maximum concentration of the drug is reached in the body.
- Duration of action is the time between the onset of action and discontinuation of drug action.
- The pharmaceutical phase of drug disposition involves drug disintegration and dissolution.
- Drugs administered parenterally enter directly into the general circulation; therefore, they are not subject to the first-pass effect and are not degraded by GI enzymes.
- The bioavailability of parenterally administered drugs is greater than orally administered drugs.
- Absorption is the process that involves the movement of drug molecules from the site of administration, across cell membranes, into the circulatory system of the body (blood or lymphatic system).
- Drugs are absorbed across cell membranes via active and passive transport mechanisms.
- Factors influencing absorption are chemical nature of the drug, pH, blood flow, surface area, and tissue thickness.
- Distribution is the process of movement of the drug from the circulatory system across barrier membranes to the site of drug action.
- Factors influencing distribution are the chemical nature of the drug, protein and tissue binding, and ability to move across anatomical barriers.
- Metabolism is a biochemical process involving enzymes that convert the administered drug to metabolites that are more active or less active than the original drug.
- Drugs that interfere with the enzymes of the cytochrome P-450 system can enhance or inhibit the metabolism of other drugs that are taken concurrently.
- First-pass metabolism describes a process whereby only a fraction of an orally administered drug reaches systemic circulation because the drug is metabolized in the liver to an inactive metabolite before passing into the general circulation.

- Factors influencing metabolism are liver function, diseases, age, drug interactions, genetics, nutrition, and gender.
- Elimination results in removal of the drug from the body and discontinuation of drug action.
- Factors influencing elimination are kidney function, diseases, drug ionization, and drug interactions.
- Elimination half-life (t ½) refers to the time it takes for 50% of a drug to be cleared from the bloodstream. It takes approximately eight half-lives to eliminate a drug from the body.
- Bioavailability is the rate and extent to which the active ingredient of an administered drug enters the systemic circulation, reaches the site of action, and is available to produce its effect.
- A generic drug is bioequivalent if no statistical differences are found in the rate and extent of absorption when the drug is administered in the same strength, dosage form, and route of administration as the brand name product.
- ***Pharmaceutical equivalents*** may have different inactive ingredients, be manufactured in a different dosage form, and exhibit different rates of absorption than the brand name.
- Pharmaceutical alternatives contain the same active ingredient as the brand name drug; however, the strength and dosage form may be different.
- A therapeutic alternative may contain different active ingredients yet produce the same desired therapeutic outcome.

REVIEW QUESTIONS

1. Name the four phases of pharmacokinetics.
   a. absorption, dissolution, catabolism, elimination
   b. absorption, distribution, metabolism, elimination
   c. assimilation, dissolution, metabolism, excretion
   d. assimilation, distribution, anabolism, excretion

2. Lipid-soluble drugs are _____.
   a. hydrophobic
   b. lipophobic
   c. lipophilic
   d. a and c

3. A process whereby the liver clears a portion of an administered dose of drug before it passes into the general circulation is known as the
   a. first-pass effect
   b. dissolution effect
   c. metabolite effect
   d. liver-pass effect

4. A drug that contains different active ingredient(s) than the brand name drug yet produces the same desired therapeutic outcome is called a therapeutic _____.
   a. equivalent
   b. alternative
   c. substitution
   d. replacement

5. The process that involves the movement of drug molecules from the site of administration, across cell membranes into the circulatory system of the body is known as
   a. distribution
   b. metabolism
   c. absorption
   d. elimination

6. Drugs are assigned to one of five categories according to their safety if taken during pregnancy. Which one of the following is the safest?
   a. category A
   b. category C
   c. category D
   d. category X

7. The metabolism of drugs via biochemical processes involving enzymes to metabolites is termed
   a. bioequivalence
   b. biotransformation
   c. bioavailability
   d. bioeffect

8. A drug that is administered in an inactive form and must be metabolized to its active form is called a(an)
   a. investigational drug
   b. metabolite
   c. prodrug
   d. none of the above

9. Which body organ serves as the primary site of the metabolism of drugs?
   a. kidney
   b. lungs
   c. stomach
   d. liver

10. The time it takes for 50% of the drug to be cleared from the bloodstream is termed the
    a. distribution half-life ($t\frac{1}{2}$)
    b. elimination half-life ($t\frac{1}{2}$)
    c. metabolism half-life ($t\frac{1}{2}$)
    d. absorption half-life ($t\frac{1}{2}$)

TECHNICIAN'S CORNER

What is the difference between bioavailability and bioequivalence?

Bibliography

Fulcher E, Soto C, Fulcher R: *Pharmacology: Principles and applications. A worktext for allied health professionals*, Philadelphia, 2003, WB Saunders, pp 21-22, 60-65, 83.

Indiana University School of Medicine: Cytochrome P450 Drug Interaction Table. Retrieved Dec 28, 2010, from http://medicine.iupui.edu/clinpharm/ddis/, 2009.

Lance L, Lacy C, Armstrong L, et al: *Drug information handbook for the allied health professional*, ed 12, Hudson, OH, 2005, APhA Lexi-Comp.

Page CP, Hoffman BB, Curtis MJ, et al: *Integrated pharmacology*, Philadelphia, 2005, Elsevier Mosby, pp 57-70.

Raffa RB, Rawls SM, Beyzarov EP: *Netter's illustrated pharmacology*, Philadelphia, 2005, WB Saunders, pp 10-11, 25-27.

Shargel L, Mutnick A, Souney P, et al: *Comprehensive pharmacy review*, ed 4, Baltimore, 2001, Lippincott Williams & Wilkins, pp 78-84, 42-65, 131-132.

3

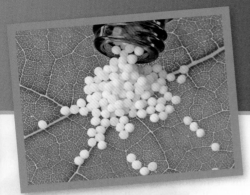

Pharmacodynamics

KEY TERMS

Affinity: Attraction that the receptor site has for the drug.

Agonist: Drug that binds to its receptor site and stimulates a cellular response.

Antagonist: Drug that binds to the receptor site and does not produce an action. An antagonist prevents another drug or natural body chemical from binding and activating the receptor site.

Drug-receptor theory: Theory that states that a drug must interact or bind with targeted cells in the body if drug action is to be produced.

Efficacy: Measure of a drug's effectiveness.

Hepatotoxicity: Serious adverse reaction that occurs in the liver.

Idiosyncratic reaction: Unexpected drug reaction.

Inverse agonist: Drug that has affinity and activity at the receptor site. The drug can turn "off" a receptor that is activated or turn "on" a receptor that is not currently active.

Mechanism of action: Manner in which a drug produces its effect.

Nephrotoxicity: Serious adverse effect that occurs in the kidney.

Noncompetitive antagonist: Drug that binds to an alternative receptor site that prevents the agonist from binding to and producing its desired action.

Partial agonist: Drug that behaves like an agonist under some conditions and acts like an antagonist under different conditions.

Pathophysiology: Study of structural and functional changes that are produced by disease.

Pharmacodynamics: Study of drugs and their action on the living organism.

Pharmacotherapeutics: Use of drugs in the treatment of disease. It is the study of factors that influence patient response to drugs.

Potency: Measure of the amount of drug required to produce a response. It is the effective dose concentration.

Receptor site: Location of drug-cell binding.

Therapeutic index (TI): Ratio of the effective dose to the lethal dose.

Pharmacodynamics

The previous chapter looked at how a drug is altered as it travels throughout the compartments of the body. ***Pharmacodynamics*** is the study of drugs and their action on a living organism. Pharmacodynamics looks at how the body responds to drugs that are administered. The ***mechanism of action*** (MOA) describes how the drug produces its effect. An understanding of ***pathophysiology*** and drug MOA will facilitate the selection of the best drug to treat each patient's medical condition. Pathophysiology is the study of disease in the body.

Drug-Receptor Interactions

According to ***drug-receptor theory***, drugs interact or bind with targeted cells in the body to produce pharmacological action. Most drugs bind with specific proteins in the body; however, they may also bind to carbohydrates, lipids, or enzymes. The location of drug-cell binding is called the ***receptor site***. Drug-receptor binding is similar to the action of a lock and key (Figure 3-1). The drug is the key, and the receptor site is the lock. The more similar the drug is to the shape of the receptor site, the greater is the ***affinity***, or attraction, that the receptor site has for the drug. When two or more drugs are administered, the receptor site will preferentially bind with the drug for which it has the greatest affinity (the drug that best fits the lock). Drug binding to the receptor is usually reversible. Most drugs spontaneously bind and disassociate with the receptor site.

Some drugs do not produce their actions by directly binding to a receptor site on the cell. They are able to produce a change in cell membrane stability or excitability through nonspecific mechanisms. Some general anesthetic gases produce their effects via nonspecific interactions.

SECOND MESSENGERS

Drug response does not always occur by stimulation of the primary drug receptor. In some cases, stimulation of the primary receptor causes a second receptor to be activated, and it is only after the release of the second messenger that the desired drug effect is produced.

TYPES OF DRUG-RECEPTOR INTERACTIONS

Drugs are described as agonist, partial agonist, antagonist, competitive antagonist, and noncompetitive antagonist based on their effect at the receptor site (Table 3-1).

Agonists

An ***agonist*** is a drug that binds to and activates the receptor site, eliciting a cellular response (Figure 3-2). Agonist binding may activate a receptor that was resting or turn off a receptor that was activated. ***Inverse agonists*** are drugs that have affinity at the receptor site but produce opposite actions (turn "off" a receptor that is activated or turn "on" a receptor that is not currently active). When two or more agonists are administered together, a competition for drug-receptor binding sites occurs. The drug with the greatest affinity will bind to the receptor site. The result of agonist binding may mimic the effects produced by binding of normal body chemicals to their target receptor. An example is the binding of barbiturates to their drug-receptor site. This mimics the effects produced by the

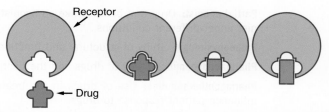

FIGURE 3-1 Drug-receptor interactions. (From Clayton BD, Stock YN, Harroun RD: *Basic pharmacology for nurses*, ed 14, St Louis, 2007, Mosby.)

TABLE 3-1 Summary of Effects of Drug-Receptor Binding

Interaction Term	Definition
Agonist	Drug binds to a receptor, and there is a response.
Partial agonist	Drug binds to a receptor, and there is a diminished response compared with that elicited by the agonist.
Antagonist	Drug binds to receptor, but there is no response. Drug prevents binding of agonists.
Competitive antagonist	Drug competes with the agonist for binding to receptor. If it binds, there is no response.
Noncompetitive antagonist	Drug combines with different parts of receptor and inactivates it, so agonist has no effect.

From Lilly LL, Harrington S, Snyder JS: *Pharmacology and the nursing process*, ed 5, St Louis, 2007, Mosby.

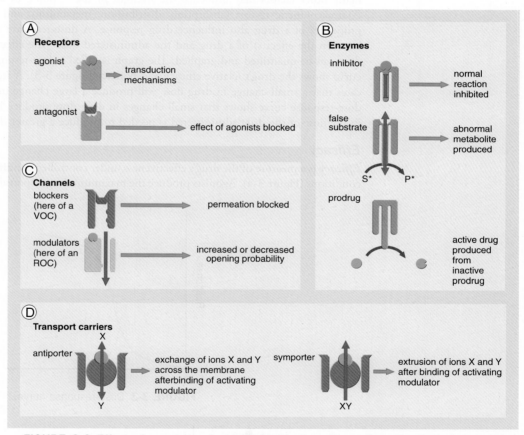

FIGURE 3-2 Effect of agonist and antagonist binding. (From Page C, et al: *Integrated pharmacology*, ed 3, Philadelphia, 2006, Mosby.)

neurotransmitter γ-aminobutyric acid (GABA), a chemical messenger of the nervous system, when it binds to its receptor site. Drug-receptor binding may also stimulate the release of a normal biological chemical. For example, when the drug amantadine is administered it stimulates the release of the neurotransmitter dopamine. An increase in dopamine levels reduces the symptoms associated with Parkinson disease.

Antagonists

Antagonists bind to the receptor site and do not activate the receptor. They prevent another drug or natural body chemical from binding by occupying or inactivating the receptor site. Antagonists block the actions of agonists, inverse agonists, and partial agonists.

Naloxone is an example of a pure antagonist. Administration reverses the effects of opiates (e.g., heroin) by occupying the receptor site and preventing the heroin from binding.

Noncompetitive antagonists bind to an alternative site than the agonist to prevent the agonist from binding the receptor. Noncompetitive antagonist binding results in inactivation of the receptor site.

Partial Agonists

A *partial agonist* behaves like an agonist under some conditions and acts like an antagonist under different conditions. The drug butorphanol (Stadol) is an example of a partial agonist. Partial agonists behave like antagonists in the presence of a high concentration of a full agonist or when administered after recent exposure to high concentrations of an agonist.

DOSE-RESPONSE RELATIONSHIP

Typically, increasing the drug dose will increase the cellular response and drug effect; however, many other factors may influence the strength of the response to a dose of administered drug. Pharmacokinetic factors (absorption, distribution, metabolism, and elimination) and individual properties of a drug also influence drug response. A dose-response curve shows the relationship between the effect(s) of a drug and the administered dose. The effects produced by a given drug dose can be quantified and graphed. The graph is called a dose-response curve. The dose-response curve shows the drug's relative efficacy and potency (Figure 3-3). A steep dose-response curve indicates that a small change in drug dose will produce a large change in the drug response. A flatter dose-response curve shows that small changes in drug dose produce little change. A large increase in the dose of the drug administered is needed to produce a greater drug response.

Efficacy

Efficacy is a measure of the drug's effectiveness under controlled conditions as opposed to real-world conditions (Figure 3-4). Agonists produce the maximum drug response. The drug response produced

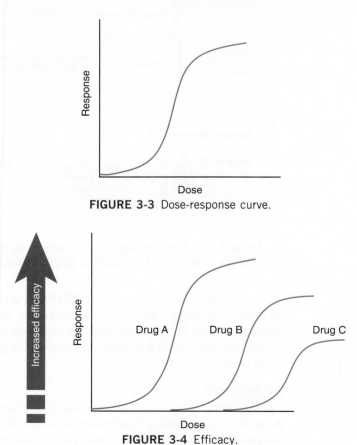

FIGURE 3-3 Dose-response curve.

FIGURE 3-4 Efficacy.

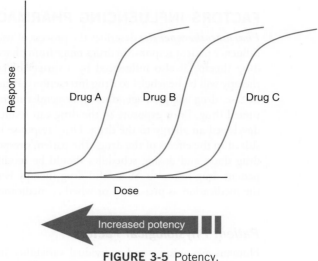

FIGURE 3-5 Potency.

by partial agonists is less than maximal. The efficacy of antagonists is measured by the extent to which they interfere with the effect of an agonist. Efficacy can be measured for each effect produced by a drug. It is not necessary for all drug-receptor sites to be occupied before the maximum drug effect is achieved.

Potency

Efficacy and *potency* are related. Drugs that have a high efficacy at a low dose are very potent. In other words, only a small dose is required to produce the maximum drug effect. Drugs that must be administered in very high doses to produce a minimal effect have low potency. In Figure 3-5, drug A is more potent than drug B and drug C because a lower dose produces an equal response.

Efficacy is more important than potency when determining usefulness of a drug unless the dose that is required to produce the therapeutic effect is so large that it is impractical to administer. When choosing between two equally effective drugs, pharmacokinetic factors, the disease, and the ability of the patient to tolerate the side effects of the drug become more important than the dose that is required to produce an effect.

Ceiling Effect

A graded dose-response curve shows that as the drug dose increases, the drug effect increases. Drug effects increase up to a ceiling. This ceiling effect may be reached when all drug receptors are saturated or when the maximum possible effect that could be produced is reached. For example, the ceiling effect for opioid analgesics is reached at the point when no more pain relief is achieved even if additional opioid is administered.

Therapeutic Index

All drugs produce toxic effects that can lead to death. When the lethal dose of a drug is close to the effective dose, the drug is not very safe. The safest drugs have a wide margin between the lethal dose and the effective dose. The *therapeutic index* (TI) is the ratio of the effective dose to the lethal dose; the formula is shown below. ED50 represents the effective dose for 50% of a population, and LD50 is the lethal dose for 50% of a population.

$$\text{Therapeutic Index (TI)} = \frac{\text{Lethal Dose (LD}_{50})}{\text{Effective Dose (ED}_{50})}$$

Digoxin, a drug used to treat heart disease, has a narrow TI. The drug dose needed to increase the force of heart contractions is similar to the drug dose that can cause the heart to stop beating. Another drug with a small TI is warfarin. The dose required to prolong blood clotting time is near the dose that causes hemorrhage and death. Patients respond differently to different doses of drug. Variation in patient response to a drug can become critical when the TI is narrow.

TECH NOTE!
Product substitution must be considered carefully when the therapeutic index is narrow or bioequivalency problems are present.

FACTORS INFLUENCING PHARMACOTHERAPEUTICS

Pharmacotherapeutics describes the process of using drugs in the treatment of disease. Factors that influence patient response to drugs range from pharmacokinetics to patient-specific factors. Successful drug therapy is also influenced by a variety of factors ranging from the patient's belief that the therapy will be beneficial to drug interactions. Patient-related factors such as the presence of chronic disease, drug allergies, age, obesity, or gender increase or decrease a person's response to an administered drug. Prior exposure to the drug can result in a heightened drug response if the patient has developed an allergy to the drug. Drug response is decreased when the patient has become desensitized to the effects of the drug. The patient's response to a drug is not always predictable; however, drug doses and dosing schedules should be modified to control for known factors that influence patient drug response. Successful drug therapy is strongly influenced by whether the patient takes the medication as prescribed or whether medication is taken at all.

Patient Physiological Factors

Humans are unique, and individual variability influences the outcome of drug therapy. Desired therapeutic effects are achieved when optimum drug doses are administered. Doses that are too low result in subtherapeutic effects. Doses that are too high result in toxic effects.

AGE

The human body undergoes physiological and hormonal changes between birth and death. Age-related changes influence how effectively the body is able to handle drugs. Neonates and infants have an underdeveloped capacity to absorb, distribute, metabolize, and eliminate drugs. The ability of the lungs, liver, and kidneys to process and eliminate drugs declines as humans age. Elderly adults and infants require lower drug doses.

WEIGHT

Drug doses for children are often calculated according to the child's weight; however, dose calculations based on body surface area are more accurate than those based on weight. Dose adjustments may need to be considered for obese or severely underweight adults. Drug doses must be increased in obese patients to produce therapeutic effects. Doses are decreased in severely underweight or emaciated adults and children to avoid toxic side effects.

GENDER

Gender may influence drug distribution and metabolism. The fat-to-muscle ratio varies between women and men and may influence the volume of drug distribution. Additionally, the rate of metabolism of some drugs varies between men and women, suggesting the sex hormones may influence metabolism.

GENETICS

Genetics influence enzyme and protein production in the body. Absence of certain enzymes can produce deadly side effects in people who take drugs that require the enzyme for metabolism and elimination.

DISEASE

The presence of disease can significantly influence pharmacotherapeutics. More severe drug reactions can occur in patients with kidney disease, liver disease, or lung disease because the ability to distribute, metabolize, and eliminate drugs may be compromised for certain drugs. The effects of a drug may diminish because the disease itself becomes more debilitating over time. Parkinson's disease is linked to destruction of dopamine-releasing nerve cells in the body. The ability of anti–Parkinson disease drugs to improve patient symptoms decreases as the disease progresses.

PREGNANCY

Drug response may be altered during pregnancy because of pregnancy-related physiological changes. Gastrointestinal (GI) motility slows, which can increase drug absorption and drug effects. The effects of pregnancy-related increases in blood volume, urination, and vomiting may alter drug absorption, distribution, and elimination that result in decreased drug response.

Immunological Factors

Excessive reactions can occur at any dose. Hypersensitivity reactions are extreme allergic reactions and can occur after a single dose of the drug or after multiple exposures to the drug. The reaction occurs because the patient develops antibodies to the drug. The presence of antibodies causes the release of histamine and other body chemicals that produce allergic symptoms. Symptoms may range from a mild rash to anaphylactic shock.

Desensitization

Repeated exposures to a drug may result in a decreased drug response. Desensitization is caused by changes to drug receptors (especially proteins) that decrease drug-receptor binding or reduce receptor site activation when binding occurs. When desensitization occurs, the effects can be limited to a single receptor or may influence multiple receptors. When drug-receptor binding involves a second messenger, the result may be desensitization to the effects that would have been produced by binding to multiple receptors (i.e., all of the receptors normally activated by binding of the drug to its primary receptor). Desensitization may be used therapeutically to minimize allergic reactions (e.g. allergy shots).

Idiosyncratic Reactions

Sometimes the response to a drug cannot be predicted. Unexpected drug reactions are known as *idiosyncratic reactions*.

Psychological Factors

Drug therapy is influenced by the patient's belief that the therapy will be beneficial. Studies have shown that sugar pills can produce the desired effect if the patient believes it will be effective. This is known as the placebo effect. Double-blind clinical studies are conducted to control for the placebo effect. In a double-blind study, some of the people in the study receive a drug containing active ingredient, and others receive a drug look-alike that does not contain active ingredients. Neither the people taking the drugs nor their care providers know who is receiving the real drug. This reduces the risk that drug effects reported are caused by placebo effect. This also decreases the likelihood that care providers will treat their patient differently because they know they are receiving the active drug. Increased attention can also improve patient outcomes.

Adverse Drug Reactions

Few drugs are so specific that they only produce their desired effect. Drugs produce desired effects (therapeutic effects) and undesired effects. Undesired effects are called adverse reactions. Approximately 10% of people who receive health care in industrialized countries will experience a preventable adverse drug reaction (ADR).

Adverse drug reactions have an impact on patients, family members, employers, pharmacies, health care facilities, and society. The cost of drug-related illness, hospitalization, and death in the United States is estimated to be more than $100 billion. In Canada, 2% of all hospitalized patients experience a preventable adverse drug event and 700 deaths per year are attributed to medication errors.

Some populations are more at risk for ADRs than others. The elderly have an increased risk for ADRs, because they are more likely to be on multiple-drug therapy and their capacity to metabolize and eliminate drugs is less than that of younger adults. Multiple-drug therapy (polypharmacy) is a risk factor for hospitalized patients, too. The average patient in the hospital is prescribed up to 10 drugs. The risk for drug side effects and drug interactions increases with the number of medications a person is administered.

ADRs may be localized and only occur at the site where the drug was administered. Other adverse reactions are widespread and occur throughout the body. Adverse effects may cause minor discomfort such as a rash, or they may be life threatening (e.g., coma and death).

Common adverse effects that occur in the central nervous system are drowsiness, dizziness, stimulation, or confusion. Life-threatening central nervous system effects include respiratory

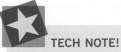

depression, coma, and death. ***Hepatotoxicity*** is a toxic adverse reaction that occurs in the liver. Some common drugs that can produce hepatotoxicity are acetaminophen and isoniazid (a drug used to treat tuberculosis). ***Nephrotoxicity*** is a serious adverse effect that occurs in the kidney. Nonsteroidal anti-inflammatory drugs such as ibuprofen and naproxen can produce nephrotoxicity.

ADRs also occur as a result of nonsterile drug preparation. Intravenous fluids and other parenterals must be prepared using aseptic technique. Failure to use aseptic technique can result in the introduction of contaminants, pathogens, and fever-causing agents into the solution. Prolonged illness or death may occur if the solution is injected into a patient.

TERATOGENICITY

ADRs that produce harm to a developing fetus are called teratogenic effects. To reduce possible harm to the fetus, pregnant women and their health care providers must weigh the risks versus the benefit of taking drugs. To assist in their decision-making, pregnancy safety categories have been created. Drugs with no known teratogenic effects in humans are listed in category A. Few drugs are found in category A. Drugs known to produce teratogenic effects are listed in category X (see Table 2-1). Similar risk may exist for drugs listed in categories C, D, and X, however when the risk is found in animal reproduction studies the drugs are classified in category C. There are no adequate, controlled tests in humans. Benefits do not outweigh the risk for drugs listed in category X.

CARCINOGENICITY

Drugs and natural products that stimulate the growth of cancers are classified as carcinogens. Carcinogenic drugs interact with DNA and produce permanent genetic mutations. Many of the drugs used to treat one type of cancer are capable of producing cancers in other areas. Drugs used to treat ovarian cancer increase the risk for acute nonlymphocytic leukemia (ANLL). Melphalan is a drug used to treat breast cancer that can increase the risk for ANLL. The synthetic estrogen diethylstilbestrol (DES) is no longer prescribed to women to prevent miscarriage because it increases the risks for breast and uterine cancer. The drug is still prescribed for the treatment of prostate cancer. Sassafras tea was widely used as a cleansing tea or tonic until it was discovered to be carcinogenic in the 1960s.

DEPENDENCE AND TOLERANCE

Patients taking controlled substances may develop dependence or tolerance to the drug's effects. Drugs are placed in controlled substance schedules according to their likelihood to produce physiological or psychological dependence. Patients who have developed dependence to a drug must continue to take the drug in order to prevent the onset of withdrawal symptoms. Once tolerance to a drug has developed, the patient must take increasing doses of the drug to produce the same effects as was previously produced by a lower dose. Tolerance may occur to the therapeutic effect or side effects. Tolerance develops to the sedation produced by some antiseizure drugs like clonazepam before tolerance develops to the desired antiseizure effects.

IMPROVING ADHERENCE TO DRUG THERAPY

Drug therapy is strongly influenced by whether the patient takes the medication as prescribed or whether medication is taken at all. Adherence to drug therapy is defined as taking the prescribed medication in the correct dose, at the right time, and without missed doses. Today, it is recognized that patients and their caregivers must be actively involved to making decisions about drug therapy. Patients who recognize the importance of the drug therapy and are involved in selecting the medication best suited for their individual needs are more likely to adhere to therapy.

Factors Influencing Adherence to Drug Therapy

Lack of adherence to drug therapy is associated with poor health outcomes. Understanding why medications are not taken as prescribed is important for the design of strategies to improve adherence. Strategies for improving adherence must be targeted at patients, caregivers, pharmacists, pharmacy technicians, clinicians, and other health care providers.

BELIEF THAT THERAPY IS BENEFICIAL

Adherence to the prescribed drug therapy is increased when patients believe therapy is beneficial. This is particularly important when the medication has substantial adverse effects. Hypertension is known as the silent killer because often no symptoms are present. Medications to treat hypertension may cause dizziness, upset stomach, impotence, or even depression, causing many patients to discontinue drug therapy. Adherence to drug therapy to avoid complications associated with untreated hypertension is essential.

ADVERSE DRUG REACTIONS

An adverse drug reaction (ADR) is an undesired side effect of a drug. An ADR may be mild (e.g., sedation and nausea) or severe (e.g., hepatotoxicity and seizures). ADRs are a principal cause of discontinuation of drug therapy. Even fear of potential adverse reactions is a sufficient disincentive for some patients to avoid taking their medications. Many drug formulations have been developed to minimize drug side effects. Enteric-coated formulations reduce the risk of stomach upset. GI side effects are avoided by use of drugs formulated for transdermal application.

Pharmacy technicians can assist pharmacists in reducing patients' anxiety about adverse reactions by alerting the pharmacists when patients have questions about pharmacotherapy and making certain patients receive pharmacist counseling for new medicines. Pharmacy technicians can also play a key role in helping patients limit adverse reactions by distributing patient drug information leaflets and affixing warning labels, also called auxiliary labels, to prescription vials, which are intended to ensure that the maximum benefits of drug therapy are achieved with minimum side effects. For example, taking medication with food or a glass of water can decrease the risk for upset stomach. Acting within their scope of practice, pharmacy technicians can assist pharmacists in providing drug information that may reduce the risk for drug side effects and increase adherence to prescribed drug therapy.

LACK OF ANY MEDICATION ADMINISTRATION ROUTINE

Adherence is improved when patients develop a regular routine for taking medicine. The pharmacist and pharmacy technician can work with patients to develop a routine for taking medications that fits the patient's lifestyle. Some pharmacies sell devices that prompt the patient to remember to take medicines.

UNDERSTANDING DOSING SCHEDULE

Dosing schedules must be convenient and understandable if patients are to avoid missed doses or taking double doses. Adherence to drug therapy increases in difficulty as the number of medications prescribed increases. Selection of drug formulations that are taken once a day may improve adherence. The pharmacy may also dispense the medicine compliance blister packs.

ABILITY TO AFFORD DRUG THERAPY

People with low socioeconomic status are at increased risk for low adherance. Poverty decreases the ability to afford medications and decreases access to health care when adverse events are experienced. When drug therapy is expensive, prescriptions may not be filled. When prescriptions are filled, patients may take less than the dose prescribed to make the prescription last longer. Pharmacy personnel can work with prescribers to ensure that effective and affordable drugs (e.g., generics) are prescribed and dispensed when appropriate. Pharmacy technicians can also contact insurance companies to obtain approval for nonformulary medicines.

REPORTING ADVERSE DRUG REACTIONS

Adverse drug reactions are reported to the U.S. Food and Drug Administration (FDA) by drug manufacturers, health care professionals, and consumers using the FDA Voluntary Reporting Form 3500 (Figure 3-6). The ADR reports are compiled into a computerized information database called the Adverse Event Reporting System (AERS). The reports are analyzed and used to update product labeling, send out a "Dear Health Care Professional" letter, or even reevaluate the drug approval decision. If reevaluation results in a decision to withdraw approval of the drug, then a recall will be issued. The AERS also issues safety alerts for drugs, biologics, devices, and dietary

TECH NOTE!
Many pharmacy computer systems now print auxiliary labels directly onto prescription labels using a different color for identification purposes.

TECH NOTE!
Extended-release (ER) medications promote patient adherence. Instead of taking medications three or four times a day, an ER, sustained-release (SR), or controlled-dose (CD) tablet may be taken once daily.

U.S. Department of Health and Human Services

MEDWATCH

The FDA Safety Information and
Adverse Event Reporting Program

For VOLUNTARY reporting of
adverse events, product problems and
product use errors

Page _____ of _____

Form Approved: OMB No. 0910-0291, Expires: 10/31/08
See OMB statement on reverse.

FDA USE ONLY

Triage unit
sequence #

PLEASE TYPE OR USE BLACK INK

A. PATIENT INFORMATION

1. Patient Identifier

   In confidence

2. Age at Time of Event, or
   Date of Birth:

3. Sex
   ☐ Female
   ☐ Male

4. Weight
   _____ lb
   or
   _____ kg

B. ADVERSE EVENT, PRODUCT PROBLEM OR ERROR

Check all that apply:

1. ☐ Adverse Event   ☐ Product Problem (e.g., defects/malfunctions)
   ☐ Product Use Error ☐ Problem with Different Manufacturer of Same Medicine

2. Outcomes Attributed to Adverse Event
   (Check all that apply)

   ☐ Death: _____ (mm/dd/yyyy)
   ☐ Life-threatening
   ☐ Hospitalization - initial or prolonged
   ☐ Required Intervention to Prevent Permanent Impairment/Damage (Devices)
   ☐ Disability or Permanent Damage
   ☐ Congenital Anomaly/Birth Defect
   ☐ Other Serious (Important Medical Events)

3. Date of Event (mm/dd/yyyy)

4. Date of this Report (mm/dd/yyyy)

5. Describe Event, Problem or Product Use Error

6. Relevant Tests/Laboratory Data, Including Dates

7. Other Relevant History, Including Preexisting Medical Conditions (e.g., allergies,
   race, pregnancy, smoking and alcohol use, liver/kidney problems, etc.)

C. PRODUCT AVAILABILITY

Product Available for Evaluation? (Do not send product to FDA)

☐ Yes   ☐ No   ☐ Returned to Manufacturer on: _____ (mm/dd/yyyy)

D. SUSPECT PRODUCT(S)

1. Name, Strength, Manufacturer (from product label)
   #1
   #2

2. Dose or Amount | Frequency | Route
   #1
   #2

3. Dates of Use (If unknown, give duration) from/to (or best estimate)
   #1
   #2

5. Event Abated After Use Stopped or Dose Reduced?
   #1 ☐ Yes ☐ No ☐ Doesn't Apply
   #2 ☐ Yes ☐ No ☐ Doesn't Apply

4. Diagnosis or Reason for Use (Indication)
   #1
   #2

8. Event Reappeared After Reintroduction?
   #1 ☐ Yes ☐ No ☐ Doesn't Apply
   #2 ☐ Yes ☐ No ☐ Doesn't Apply

6. Lot #
   #1
   #2

7. Expiration Date
   #1
   #2

9. NDC # or Unique ID

E. SUSPECT MEDICAL DEVICE

1. Brand Name

2. Common Device Name

3. Manufacturer Name, City and State

4. Model #
   Catalog #
   Serial #

   Lot #
   Expiration Date (mm/dd/yyyy)
   Other #

5. Operator of Device
   ☐ Health Professional
   ☐ Lay User/Patient
   ☐ Other:

6. If Implanted, Give Date (mm/dd/yyyy)

7. If Explanted, Give Date (mm/dd/yyyy)

8. Is this a Single-use Device that was Reprocessed and Reused on a Patient?
   ☐ Yes   ☐ No

9. If Yes to Item No. 8, Enter Name and Address of Reprocessor

F. OTHER (CONCOMITANT) MEDICAL PRODUCTS

Product names and therapy dates (exclude treatment of event)

G. REPORTER (See confidentiality section on back)

1. Name and Address

   Phone #
   E-mail

2. Health Professional? ☐ Yes ☐ No

3. Occupation

4. Also Reported to:
   ☐ Manufacturer
   ☐ User Facility
   ☐ Distributor/Importer

5. If you do NOT want your identity disclosed to the manufacturer, place an "X" in this box: ☐

FORM FDA 3500 (10/05)   Submission of a report does not constitute an admission that medical personnel or the product caused or contributed to the event.

FIGURE 3-6 Food and Drug Administration Voluntary Reporting Form 3500. (Courtesy U.S. Food and Drug Administration, Rockville, MD.)

supplements. Patient and consumer information sheets are also available from the FDA. In Canada, ADRs are also reported by drug manufacturers, consumers, and health professionals. ADRs are reported to the Canada Vigilance Program. ADR reporting forms can be obtained from the MedEffect Canada website (http://www.hc-sc.gc.ca/dhp-mps/medeff/report-declaration/index-eng.php).

Chapter Summary

- Pharmacodynamics looks at how the body responds to drugs that are administered.
- Drugs interact or bind with targeted cells in the body to produce pharmacological action.
- Drug-receptor binding is similar to a lock and key. The more similar the drug is to the shape of the receptor site, the greater is the affinity the receptor site has for the drug.
- Drug-receptor binding enhances or inhibits normal biological processes.
- An agonist is a drug that binds to its receptor site and stimulates a cellular response. Agonist binding may activate a receptor that was resting or turn off a receptor that was activated.
- Antagonists bind to the receptor site and prevent an agonist from activating the receptor. They prevent another drug or natural body chemical from binding by occupying or inactivating the receptor site. Binding may reverse the action of a currently administered drug.
- Partial agonists behave like antagonists in the presence of a high concentration of a full agonist or when administered after recent exposure to high concentrations of an agonist.
- Efficacy is a measure of the drug's effectiveness under controlled conditions rather than "real-world" conditions.
- Drugs that are administered in very low doses yet produce a maximum effect have high potency.
- The dose-response curve shows a drug's relative efficacy and potency. A steep dose-response curve indicates that a small change in drug dose will produce a big change in the drug response.
- The therapeutic index (TI) is ratio of the effective dose to the lethal dose. Safe drugs have a wide margin between the lethal dose and the effective dose.
- Successful drug therapy is influenced by a variety of factors. The patient's response to a drug is not always predictable.
- Age, gender, disease, pregnancy, weight, and genetics are patient-related factors that influence drug response.
- Drug allergies cause a heightened response to drugs and can occur after one or more exposures to a drug.
- Patients may become desensitized to the effects of drugs.
- Idiosyncratic reactions are unpredictable.
- Psychological factors can influence drug response. The placebo effect demonstrates that patients can experience drug effects even when no active drug has been administered.
- Drugs produce desired effects (therapeutic effects) and undesired effects. Undesired effects are called adverse reactions.
- Multiple-drug therapy increases risks for adverse drug reactions (ADRs). Elderly adults have increased risks for ADRs.
- ADRs can be mild or severe. Effects range from rash, upset stomach, and sedation to hepatotoxicity, teratogenicity, and anaphylactic shock.
- Dependence and tolerance are adverse reactions associated with controlled substances. When tolerance develops, the patient must take increasing doses of the drug to get the desired effect. When dependence has developed, patients must continue to take the drug to prevent withdrawal symptoms.
- Patients, caregivers, pharmacists, pharmacy technicians, clinicians, and other health care providers must work as a team to improve adherence to drug therapy.
- Adherence to drug therapy is influenced by patient belief that the therapy will be beneficial.
- Selection of effective, affordable medicines that have few side effects and that are dosed in convenient schedules improves adherence to drug therapy.

1. An _____ is a drug that binds to a receptor site and elicits cellular response.
   a. agonist
   b. antagonist
   c. alternative
   d. antimetabolite

2. All drugs produce toxic effects that can lead to death. The therapeutic _____ is the ratio of the effective dose to the lethal dose.
   a. equivalence
   b. derivative
   c. index
   d. window

3. The process of using drugs in the treatment of disease is called _____.
   a. pharmacodynamics
   b. pharmacotherapeutics
   c. pharmacokinetics
   d. pharmacognosy

4. What is the measure of a drug's effectiveness called?
   a. availability
   b. bioequivalence
   c. efficacy
   d. potency

5. Humans are unique, and individual variability influences the outcome of drug therapy. Name some physiological factors that influence drug therapy.
   a. age, weight, and gender
   b. genetics, disease, and pregnancy
   c. allergies, hypersensitivities, and desensitization
   d. both a and b

6. Toxic adverse reactions that cause hepatotoxicity occur in the _____, and toxic adverse reactions that cause nephrotoxicity occur in the _____.
   a. liver, lungs
   b. liver, kidneys
   c. kidneys, bladder
   d. kidneys, nephrons

7. _____ and _____ are associated with the use of controlled substances.
   a. Hypersensitivities and dependence
   b. Tolerance and toxicity
   c. Dependence and tolerance
   d. Toxicity and anaphylaxis

8. To which government agency are adverse reactions reported in the United States?
   a. DEA
   b. TJC
   c. CMS
   d. FDA

9. An adverse effect produced by drugs on fetuses is called _____.
   a. carcinogenic
   b. teratogenic
   c. pathogenic
   d. toxic

10. One drug that has a narrow therapeutic index is _____.
    a. acetaminophen
    b. penicillin
    c. digoxin
    d. melphalan

TECHNICIAN'S
CORNER

1. How can pharmacy technicians assist patients in reducing anxiety about adverse reactions?
2. Explain how people with low socioeconomic status are at an increased risk for adverse reactions.

Bibliography

Baker GR, Norton PG, Flintolf V, et al: The Canadian Adverse Events Study: The incidence of adverse events among hospital patients in Canada, *Can Med Assoc J* 170:1678-1686, 2004.

Edwards IR: The WHO World Alliance for Patient Safety: A new challenge or an old one neglected? *Drug Safety* 28:379-386, 2005.

FDA: *Summary of Proposed Rule on Pregnancy and Lactation Labeling*, 2009. Retrieved Aug 7, 2011, from http://www.fda.gov/Drugs/DevelopmentApprovalProcess/DevelopmentResources/Labeling/ucm093310.htm.

Gaber S: Principles of drug therapy in pregnancy and lactation. *Pharmacotherapeutics for advanced practice: a practical approach*, Lippincott, 2006, Williams & Wilkins, pp 49-54.

Lance L, Lacy C, Armstrong L, et al: *Drug information handbook for the allied health professional*, ed 12, Hudson, OH, 2005, APhA Lexi-Comp.

Page C, Curtis M, Sutter M, et al: *Integrated pharmacology*, Philadelphia, 2005, Elsevier Mosby, pp 57-70, 314.

Passarelli M, Jacob-Filho W, Figueras A: Adverse drug reactions in an elderly hospitalised population: Inappropriate prescription is a leading cause, *Drugs Aging* 22:767-777, 2005.

Raffa RB, Rawls SM, Beyzarov EP: *Netter's illustrated pharmacology*. Philadelphia, 2005, WB Saunders, pp 10-11, 21-23.

Ratajczak H: Drug-induced hypersensitivity: Role in drug development, *Toxicol Rev* 23:265-280, 2004.

Sorensen L, Stokes J, Purdie D, et al: Medication management at home: Medication-related risk factors associated with poor health outcomes, *Age Ageing* 34:626-632, 2005.

Tyler V, Brady L, Robbers J: *Pharmacognosy*, ed 9, Philadelphia, 1988, Lea & Febiger, p 486.

U.S. Food and Drug Administration: *Adverse Event Reporting System*. Retrieved from http://www.fda.gov/cder/aers/default.htm. Accessed June 2, 2006.

U.S. Food and Drug Administration: *Summary of Proposed Rule on Pregnancy and Lactation Labeling*, 2009. Retrieved Aug 7, 2011, from http://www.fda.gov/Drugs/DevelopmentApprovalProcess/DevelopmentResources/Labeling/ucm093310.htm.

Wu WK, Pantaleo N: Evaluation of outpatient adverse drug reactions leading to hospitalization, *Am J Health Syst Pharm* 60:253-259, 2003.

4

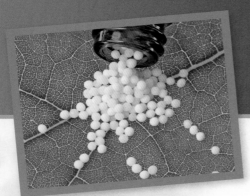

Drug Interactions and Medication Errors

KEY TERMS

Additive effect: Increased drug effect that is produced when a second similar drug is added to therapy that is greater than the effects produced by either drug alone.

Antagonism: Drug–drug interaction or drug–food interaction that causes decreased effects as when a pharmacological antagonist is administered to block the effect of another drug.

Drug–disease contraindication: No rationale for drug use; drug administration should be avoided because it may worsen the patient's medical condition.

Drug–drug interaction: Reaction that occurs when two or more drugs are administered at the same time.

Drug–food interaction: Altered drug response that occurs when a drug is administered with certain foods.

Medication error: Error made in the process of prescribing, preparing, dispensing, or administering drug therapy.

Potentiation: Process where one drug, acting at a separate site or via a different mechanism of action, increases the effect of another drug yet produces no effect when administered alone. Food can also potentiate the effects of a drug.

Synergistic effects: Drug–drug or drug–food interaction that produces an effect that is greater than would be produced if either drug were administered alone.

Therapeutic duplication: Administration of two drugs that produce similar effects and side effects. These drugs may belong to the same therapeutic class.

Drug Interactions

Drug effects are influenced by joint administration with foods and other drugs. The more drugs that are administered to a patient, the more likely it is that interactions will occur. Drug–drug interactions and drug–food interactions can increase or decrease the intended drug effects. They may also increase or decrease drug side effects. Drug interactions may produce life-threatening or minor undesired effects, or they may enhance the desired drug effect. Low doses of antidepressant drugs such as amitriptyline are administered along with pain medications such as hydrocodone to enhance pain relief. By administering these two drugs together, less hydrocodone is needed, and the patient's risk for development of tolerance and dependence from the hydrocodone is reduced. The study of pharmacology is important because it enables the prediction of the likelihood that a drug interaction may occur.

DRUG–DRUG INTERACTIONS

An interaction that occurs between two or more drugs administered at the same time is called a *drug–drug interaction*. Drug–drug interactions may increase or decrease the effect or side effects of the drug. Tetracycline and penicillin both treat infections. If the drugs are administered together, the infection-fighting ability of penicillin is reduced by the tetracycline. The antifungal action of ketoconazole is reduced if the drug is taken with antacids. Antiulcer drugs such as cimetidine increase the effects of alcohol. Amoxicillin reduces the effectiveness of oral contraceptives.

DRUG–FOOD INTERACTIONS

An interaction between an administered drug and food(s) consumed at the same time is called a *drug–food interaction*. The foods may contain enzymes, vitamins, or minerals that enhance or interfere with drug effects. The interaction may influence side effects, too. A classic example is the interaction between dairy products and the anti-infective tetracycline. Tetracycline binds with the calcium in milk or cheese, and its effect is diminished. Another example is levothyroxine, a synthetic thyroid hormone; its effect is decreased when iron supplements are taken. Grapefruit juice inhibits the metabolism of the cholesterol-lowering drug atorvastatin, thereby increasing the drug's effects.

ADDITIVE EFFECTS

Additive effects may occur when two drugs are administered concurrently. The increased effect is equal to the sum of the individual effects produced by each of the drugs alone. Many drug interactions produce additive effects. The sleeping pill lorazepam is administered to promote drowsiness. Alcoholic beverages also cause drowsiness. When alcoholic beverages are consumed together with lorazepam, additional drowsiness is caused. The sedation caused by lorazepam adds to the sedation caused by alcohol.

Additive effects can be described using the equation

$$1 + 1 = 2$$

SYNERGISTIC EFFECTS

Drug–drug interactions and drug–food interactions may produce synergistic effects. *Synergistic effects* result when two drugs administered together produce effects that are greater than would be produced if either drug were administered alone or would be seen with additive effects. Bleeding is a potential side effect of warfarin and aspirin. When warfarin and aspirin are administered together, excessive bleeding may occur.

Synergistic effects can be described using the equation

$$1 + 1 = 3$$

POTENTIATION

The process whereby one drug, or a food, increases the effects of another drug, yet does not produce any effect when administered alone, is called *potentiation*. Carbidopa exhibits no anti–Parkinson disease activity when administered alone. When added to levodopa, the anti–Parkinson disease effects of levodopa are increased. Carbidopa is able to decrease the destruction of levodopa in the

TECH NOTE!
The pharmacist should counsel a patient who has a prescription for amoxicillin and who is also taking oral contraceptives to use additional contraceptive measures while taking the antibiotic to prevent pregnancy.

gastrointestinal tract so more of the levodopa can get to its site of action in the brain. Grapefruit juice increases the effects of some antihypertensive drugs (e.g., diltiazem) because it inhibits metabolic enzymes. The action of the antifungal griseofulvin is increased when it is taken with fatty foods because food increases the absorption of the drug.

Potentiation can be described using the equation:

$$1 + 0 = 2$$

ANTAGONISM

Antagonism is a drug–drug interaction or drug–food interaction that causes decreased drug effects. Naloxone is administered to block the respiratory depression produced by morphine and heroin. Vitamin K is an antidote for the drug warfarin. It is administered in warfarin overdose to stop bleeding.

Antagonism can be described using the equation:

$$1 + 1 = 0$$

Mechanisms of Drug Interactions

Drug–drug interactions and drug–food interactions occur via many different mechanisms (Figure 4-1). Coadministration of drugs and foods can increase absorption, distribution, metabolism, or elimination and result in increased or decreased drug action or side effects. Epinephrine is added to local anesthetics to constrict blood vessels at the site of injection and thereby augment the local anesthetic effects at the injection site. Absorption of a drug can also be increased by administration of a second drug that speeds or slows movement within the gastrointestinal system. Prokinetic drugs such as metoclopramide stimulate movement through the stomach and increase the absorption of drugs that are primarily absorbed in the small intestine and decrease absorption of drugs that are absorbed in the stomach. Drugs that decrease the rate of gastric emptying or movement through the intestines, such as codeine and loperamide, can increase the absorption and effects of drugs (see Figure 4-1).

Drugs that are weak acids and weak bases are involved in many drug interactions. The absorption of cimetidine (H2 receptor antagonist) is decreased when taken with antacids because antacids make the pH more alkaline. Absorption of cimetidine is greatest in an acidic pH. Intravenous solutions of acids and bases are incompatible and, when combined, form solid particles (precipitate). For

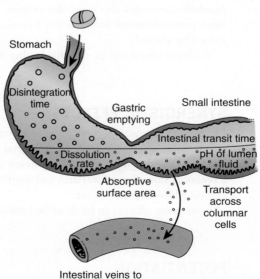

FIGURE 4-1 Factors involved in gastrointestinal drug interactions. (From Kalant H, Grant DM, Mitchell J: *Principles of medical pharmacology*, ed 7, Philadelphia, 2007, WB Saunders.)

example, if calcium gluconate is added to a solution of floxacillin sodium 2 g in normal saline, a thick white precipitation forms immediately. The resulting intravenous solution is not usable.

Displacement from protein binding sites is a mechanism for drug interactions that influences the distribution of a drug. Displacement increases the amount of drug that is free to get to its site of action and produce effects (see Figure 2-9). Warfarin is a drug that is highly protein bound. Even a small change in the percent of drug that is free to get to the binding site can increase drug effects and risk of hemorrhage. Sulfonamides are a class of anti-infectives that are also strongly protein bound. When a sulfonamide and warfarin are both administered, displacement occurs.

Interactions that alter the rate of drug metabolism are caused by induction or inhibition of metabolic enzymes. Barbiturates such as phenobarbital stimulate metabolic enzymes of other antiseizure medications (phenytoin, valproic acid). Grapefruit juice is a powerful inhibitor of metabolic enzyme CYP3A4 and potentiates the effect of anticholesterol drugs such as atorvastatin. H2 receptor antagonists alter the metabolism of alcohol. When drugs such as cimetidine and ranitidine are taken with alcohol, the effects of alcohol may be increased and may last longer (Table 4-1).

Some drug interactions influence elimination of drugs. Alteration of the pH of the urine can increase the elimination of a drug or enhance its reabsorption. Elimination of acidic drugs is increased when drugs that make the urine alkaline are administered. Elimination of alkaline drugs is increased when drugs that make the urine more acidic are administered.

Drug interactions that involve competition for a common transport system in the kidney can effect the elimination of some drugs. This describes the drug–drug interaction between penicillin and probenecid. When the drugs are administered together, elimination of penicillin is decreased.

Avoiding Undesired Drug Interactions

Studies indicate that between 7% and 22% of adverse drug reactions (ADRs) are caused by drug–drug interactions. Drug interactions that produce undesired effects should be avoided. Undesired drug interactions can result in cancellation of desired drug effect or reduced drug effect. At the opposite extreme, a drug interaction can produce toxic or harmful effects (Table 4-2). Failure to recognize drug interactions can harm the patient or prolong patient illness. It is the responsibility of pharmacists and pharmacy technicians to screen all prescriptions for potential drug interactions before dispensing the medication. Pharmacy technicians play a significant role in the screening process.

Pharmacy technicians play a key role in entering patient data into the pharmacy's prescription filling software. Data entered into the computer must be complete and accurate if the screening for drug interactions is to be effective. ***Drug–disease contraindications*** can be avoided by maintaining an up-to-date patient history of chronic and acute medical conditions. Computers prospectively screen for drug interactions so that adjustments can be made to the patient drug therapy before the drug is dispensed. When a drug–disease contradiction is identified by computer software, the pharmacy technician must alert the pharmacist so the significance of the computer-screened drug–disease contraindication can be evaluated. Drug–drug interactions can also be avoided by maintenance of an up-to-date patient profile. Pharmacy technicians and pharmacists should query patients about current nonprescription drug use as well as prescription drug usage. Information about prescriptions filled at other pharmacies should be obtained, if possible, and entered into the pharmacy's computer system.

Pharmacy technicians must also be knowledgeable of intravenous drug incompatibilities. Combining acidic intravenous solutions and alkaline solutions causes the precipitation of drug out of the solution. Intravenous solutions that contain precipitates cannot be used and must be destroyed.

Drug–food interactions can be avoided by counseling patients to avoid consuming foods that interact with their medications. Spacing the time between food consumption and medication administration is often sufficient to avoid an undesired interaction. Pharmacy technicians can play an active role in ensuring that appropriate warning labels are affixed to prescription containers.

Medication Errors

The National Coordinating Council for Medication Error Reporting and Prevention defines a ***medication error*** as "any preventable event that may cause or lead to inappropriate medication use

TECH NOTE!

When taking a patient's medication history, ask the following: "Are you taking any over-the-counter medications? Are you taking any herbal supplements or vitamins? What other prescription drugs are you taking?"

TABLE 4-1　Selected Substrates, Inhibitors, and Inducers of Specific Cytochromes P450 (CYPs)*

CYP Isoform	Substrate	Inhibitor	Inducer	CYP Isoform	Substrate	Inhibitor	Inducer
1A2	caffeine clozapine imipramine olanzapine theophylline zolmitriptan	amiodrone cimetidine ciprofloxacin fluvoxamine	broccoli Brussels sprouts insulin tobacco	2D6	amitriptyline amphetamine carvedilol codeine desipramine dextromethorphan duloxetine fluoxetine haloperidol imipramine ondansetron paroxetine propafenone risperidone thioridazine tamoxifen timolol tramadol venlafaxine	amiodarone bupropion celicoxib cimetidine clomipramine escitalopram fluoxetine methadone paroxetine ritonavir sertraline	dexamethasone rifampin
2B6	bupropion methadone	ticlopidine	phenobarbital rifampin				
2C8	torsemide repaglinide	gemfibrozil glitazones montelukast	rifampin				
2C19	amitriptyline carisoprodol clomipramine cyclophosphamide indomethacin omeprazole rabeprazole phenytoin progesterone propranolol	fluvoxamine ketoconazole lovastatin lansoprazole omeprazole probenecid sertraline sulfamethoxazole ticlopidine	carbamazepine norethindrone				
				2E1	acetaminophen chlorzoxazone ethanol	disulfiram	ethanol isoniazid
2C9	glyburide glipizide ibuprofen irbesartan losartan meloxicam phenytoin rosiglitazone tamoxifen tolbutamide warfarin	amiodarone fluconazole fluvastatin fluvoxamine isoniazid sulfamethoxazole zafirlukast	rifampin secobarbital	3A4/5	alprazolam amlodipine atorvastatin clarithromycin codeine cyclosporine diazepam diltiazem erythromycin estradiol indinavir lovastatin midazolam nifedipine nisoldipine progesterone ritonavir saquinavir sildenafil quinidine tamoxifen trazodone verapamil	amiodarone cimetidine clarithromycin diltiazem erythromycin fluvoxamine grapefruit juice indinavir itraconazole ketoconazole nefazodone nelfinavir ritonavir saquinavir verapamil	carbamazepine efavirenz nevirapine phenobarbital phenytoin pioglitazone rifampin St. John's wort

*This table can be used to anticipate some potential interactions between drugs that are substrates and those that are inhibitors or inducers.
(Adapted from Indiana University Department of Medicine [2009]. Cytochrome P 450 Drug Interaction Table: School of Medicine.)

or patient harm while the medication is in the control of the health care professional, patient, or consumer. Such events may be related to professional practice, health care products, procedures, and systems, including prescribing; order communication; product labeling, packaging, and nomenclature; compounding; dispensing; distribution; administration; education; monitoring; and use." Preventable medication errors are the cause of nearly 98,000 deaths in the United States annually and exceed deaths from motor vehicle crashes, breast cancer, and AIDS. Medication errors may also

TABLE 4-2   **Summary of Selected Drug Interactions**

Drug	Effects or Side Effects Increased by:	Effects or Side Effects Decreased by:
tetracycline		penicillin antacids dairy products
ketoconazole		antacids
alcoholic beverage	cimetidine	
oral contraceptives		amoxicillin
levothyroxine		iron supplements
triazolam	alcoholic beverages	
warfarin	aspirin	vitamin K
levodopa	carbidopa	
verapamil	grapefruit juice	
griseofulvin	fatty foods	
morphine		naloxone
lidocaine	epinephrine	
cimetidine		antacids
phenobarbital		phenytoin sodium bicarbonate
penicillin	probenicid	

result in hospitalization and account for increased medical costs, income loss, missed school days, and prolonged illness.

Medication errors are made by physicians, pharmacists, nurses, and pharmacy technicians in the health care setting. Medication errors typically occur in the process of ordering, transcribing, dispensing, and administering medications. Adverse drug events result from prescribing inappropriate medicines for patients, translating prescription orders, improper preparation and selection of drug to dispense, and improper drug administration. Medication errors may also be made by patients. Patient errors typically involve taking the wrong dose or forgetting to take a dose.

MEDICATION ERRORS MADE BY HEALTH CARE PROVIDERS WHO PRESCRIBE MEDICATION

Up to 57 out of 1000 medication orders have an error. Errors made in ordering medications are made by physicians, nurse practitioners, pharmacists, dentists, and other health professionals legally able to prescribe medicines. Medication errors associated with prescribers are often a result of miscommunication or misinformation.

Miscommunication

Miscommunication of the drug ordered may involve poor handwriting, confusion between drugs with similar names, misuse of zeros and decimal points, confusion of metric and other dosing units, or inappropriate abbreviations.

POOR HANDWRITING

Many jokes have been made about physicians' poor handwriting (often called "chicken scratch"); however, medication errors that are made because prescriptions were not decipherable are no laughing matter. When prescriptions are illegible, there may be confusion between drugs with similar names. Electronic prescribing has been shown to eliminate medications errors caused by illegible

TABLE 4-3   **Selected FDA, ISMP, and The Joint Commission List of Confused Drug Names**

Drug Name	Confused with Drug Name	Drug Name	Confused with Drug Name
acetaZOLAMIDE	acetoHEXAMIDE	FluPHENAzine	fluvoxaMINE
Adderall	Adderall XR, Inderal	HumaLOG	HumuLIN
Advair	Advicor	hydrALAZINE	hydrOXYzine
ALPRAZolam	LORazepam	HYDROcodone	oxyCODONE
Avandia	Coumadin	HYDROmorphone	morphine
buPROPion	busPIRone	Leucovorin calcium	Leukeran
carBAMazepine	OXcarbazepine	NovoLOG	NovoLIN, HumaLOG
Cardura	Coumadin	OxyCONTIN	oxyCODONE, MS Contin
CeleBREX	CeleXA, Cerebyx	PROzac	PriLOSEC
cloNIDine	KlonoPIN	predniSONE	prednisoLONE
DAUNOrubicin	DOXOrubicin, IDArubicin	Retrovir	ritonavir
Darvocet	Percocet	quiNIDine	quiNINE
Diabeta	Zebeta	Topamax	Toprol XL
Effexor	Effexor XR	traMADol	traZODone
cycloSERINE	cycloSPORINE	vinBLAStine	vinCRIStine
glyBURIDE	glipiZIDE	Wellbutrin SR	Wellbutrin XL
ePHEDrine	EPINEPHrine	Zantac	Xanax, ZyrTEC
fentaNYL	SUFentanil	ZyrTEC	ZyPREXA
FLUoxetine	DULoxetine/PARoxetine	NIFEdipine	niCARdipine

(Adapted from Institute for Safe Medication Practices. ISMP's list of confused drug names, 2010. [http://www.ismp.org/Tools/confuseddrugnames.pdf and Institute for Safe Medication Practices] and FDA and ISMP Lists of look-alike drug names with recommended tall man letters, 2011. [http://www.ismp.org/Tools/tallmanletters.pdf].)

handwriting and result in a sevenfold decrease in overall medication errors compared with handwritten prescriptions.

CONFUSION BETWEEN DRUGS WITH SIMILAR NAMES

Although the Center for Disease Evaluation and Research (CDER) tries to avoid assigning names to new drugs that are similar to existing drugs, sometimes this happens. Drugs with similar looking or sounding names are referred to as "look-alike/sound-alike drugs." According to the U.S. Food and Drug Administration (FDA) MedWatch, medication errors have been made involving Zyrtec and Zantac, Zantac and Xanax, Keppra and Kaletra, Flomax and Volmax, Zyprexa and Celexa, and Serzone and Seroquel. When prescribers fail to write legibly, confusion about the drug to dispense arises (Table 4-3).

MISUSE OF ZEROES AND DECIMAL POINTS

Orders for medication may be incorrect because the strength is written incorrectly or is illegible. Haloperidol is a drug used to treat schizophrenia. It is available as a 0.5-mg tablet and as a 5-mg tablet. If the decimal point to the left is illegible or the zero is omitted, there may be confusion about which strength to dispense. On the other hand, if the 5-mg tablet was ordered and the prescription was written as 5.0 mg, it could be confused with 50 mg. In both cases, if the error is not caught, the patient receives 10 times the desired dose (Figure 4-2).

CONFUSION OF METRIC AND OTHER DOSING UNITS OR INAPPROPRIATE ABBREVIATIONS

Prescriptions may be written using metric units or apothecary units. Medication errors have been caused by improper conversion between the two systems of measurement. For example, the apoth-

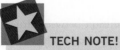

TECH NOTE!
To avoid medication errors, always place a zero in front of the decimal when calculating and recording doses that are less than 1 mL or 1 mg.

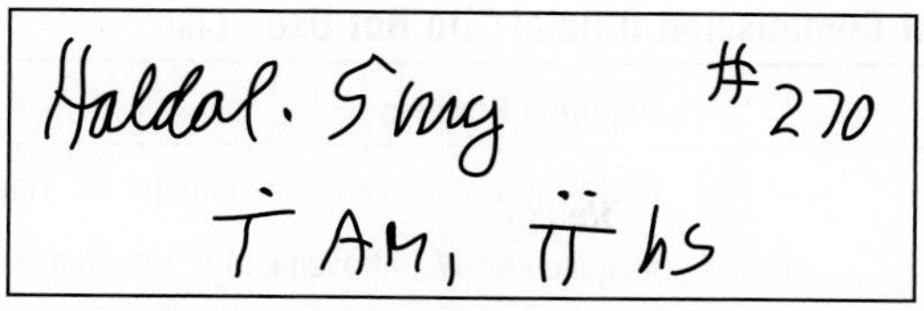

FIGURE 4-2 Decimal point error example.

ecary symbol for 1 dram (ʒi) has been interpreted as 3 mL, 4 mL, and 5 mL. Most pharmacists and pharmacy technicians interpret ʒi = 5 mL = 1 teaspoonful. Prescribers unfamiliar with apothecary symbols may confuse the symbol for ounce (ʒ) and dram (ʒ), causing toxic or subtherapeutic effects.

Misinformation

Medication errors made by prescribers occur because of lack of information or misinformation. Limited information about the patient occurs because no medical or drug history was taken or insufficient information was collected from the patient. Studies have shown that more than 25% of the prescribing errors made in hospitals are associated with incomplete medication histories being obtained at the time of admission. A complete history is needed of patients' allergies, other medicines they are taking, previous diagnoses, and laboratory results to prevent medication errors.

ERRORS OF OMISSION

An error of omission occurs when information is not collected or recorded in the patient's medical history. Studies have shown a 67% error rate in obtaining prescription medication histories. Medication histories taken by physicians were less accurate than histories taken by pharmacists. An incomplete drug history may be a cause for prescribing a drug similar to one currently being administered. This is called ***therapeutic duplication***. Therapeutic duplication may increase or decrease desired effects. If both drugs compete for the same drug receptor binding sites or the same transport systems, the drug with the greatest affinity will bind. If the drug bound to the receptor is less potent, a decreased desired effect results. Therapeutic duplication may cause an increase in adverse reactions. Omission of drug allergy information could result in a prescription written and filled for a medicine that may cause extreme harm to the patient. Errors of omission are a source of prescriptions written for drugs that are contraindicated because of the patient's disease state or allergies. An example of a drug–disease contraindication is the administration of the antidepressant bupropion to patients with a history of seizures. Patients can reduce their risk for drug interactions caused by errors of omission by filling all prescriptions at a single pharmacy. This pharmacy would have a record of the patient's complete medication history. Patients should also provide the pharmacy with a list of all regularly taken nonprescription drugs such as aspirin.

ERRORS OF COMMISSION

Commission errors result when a previously discontinued drug is accidentally restarted or a nonprescribed drug is accidentally added to the patient's medication history. This can occur when inaccurate drug histories are collected from caregivers (when the patient is too ill to provide his or her own drug history) or from patient confusion. When this occurs, unneeded drugs are taken, and the patient is at risk for adverse reactions.

Prescriptions written for the wrong strength or wrong dosing schedule are medication errors that are not specifically errors of omission or commission but do involve prescribers. This type of error occurs when the prescriber lacks familiarity with the drug that is being prescribed. The error may occur when drug dose and dosing frequency are determined according to patient weight and inaccurate weight information is given in the medical history.

MEDICATION ERRORS MADE BY HEALTH CARE PROVIDERS WHO DISPENSE MEDICATION

Pharmacists, pharmacy technicians, and pharmacy assistants make preventable medication errors, too! Medication errors made by pharmacy personnel usually involve transcribing errors, incorrect interpretation of prescription contents, improper product preparation, lack of prescription

TECH NOTE!
Pharmacy technicians should become familiar with the two following abbreviations: NKDA (no known drug allergies) and NDA (no drug allergies).

TABLE 4-4   The Joint Commission Official "Do Not Use" List*

Do Not Use	Potential Problem	Use Instead
U (unit)	Mistaken for "0" (zero), the number "4" (four), or "cc"	Write "unit"
IU (International Unit)	Mistaken for IV (intravenous) or the number 10 (ten)	Write "International Unit"
Q.D., QD, q.d., qd, QOD† (daily)	Mistaken for each other	Write "daily"
Q.O.D., QOD, q.o.d, qod (every other day)	Period after the Q mistaken for "I" and the "O" mistaken for "I"	Write "every other day"
Trailing zero (X.0 mg)‡	Decimal point is missed	Write X mg
Lack of leading zero (.X mg)	Decimal point is missed	Write 0.X mg
MS, MSO₄ and MgSO₄	Can mean morphine sulfate or magnesium sulfate; confused for one another	Write "morphine sulfate"
Additional Abbreviations, Acronyms, and Symbols for Possible Future Inclusion in the Official "Do Not Use" List		
< (greater than) and > (less than)	Misinterpreted as the number "7" (seven) or the letter "L"; confused for each other	Write "greater than" and "less than"
Abbreviations for drug names	Misinterpreted because of similar abbreviations for multiple drugs	Write drug names in full
Apothecary units	Unfamiliar to many practitioners; confused with metric units	Use metric units
@	Mistaken for the number "2" (two)	Write "at"
cc	Mistaken for U (units) when poorly written	Write "mL" or "milliliters"
μg	Mistaken for mg (milligrams) resulting in 1000-fold overdose	Write "mcg" or "micrograms"

*Applies to all orders and all medication-related documentation that is handwritten (including free-text computer entry) or on preprinted forms.
†QOD interpreted as "once daily" in Canada.
‡Exception: A "trailing zero" may be used only when required to demonstrate the level of precision of the value being reported, such as for laboratory results, imaging studies that report size of lesions, or catheter or tube sizes. It may not be used in medication orders or other medication-related documentation.
Courtesy of The Joint Commission, May 2010.

TECH NOTE!
Always check the original prescription against the prescription label and the NDC number or DIN on the stock medication chosen to ensure accuracy.

TECH NOTE!
When in doubt about what is written on a prescription, always get a second opinion. Never guess at what the medication might be. Ask for help to verify the drug in question.

monitoring, product labeling, and inaccurate dispensing. Some dispensing errors are caused by distractions in the pharmacy. The pharmacist or pharmacy technician filling a medication order may become distracted when his or her workflow is interrupted by the telephone ringing or by questions from a patient at the pharmacy counter.

Confusion of Metric and Other Dosing Units or Inappropriate Abbreviations

Serious medication errors have been caused by confusing abbreviations. This problem is so serious that The Joint Commission has recommended abolishment of the use of certain abbreviations and has published them in its official "do not use" list (Table 4-4).

Inaccurate Transcribing

Poor handwriting is responsible for many transcription errors. Medication orders received by the pharmacy must be translated and entered into the computer. If the order is illegible, the pharmacy must verify the order to prevent incorrect selection of the drug and strength ordered. Medication orders received by telephone or left on a computer messaging system are also subject to transcription errors. Verbal medication orders must be written down accurately or medication errors may result.

Insufficient Monitoring of Drug Therapy

Medication errors occur when a pharmacy fails to carefully monitor drug therapy. An important role of the pharmacist is to monitor the appropriateness of drug therapy. Pharmacy technicians assist the pharmacist with this task. Together they review each prescription to determine whether the medication ordered, dose, and dosing frequency are appropriate for the patient. Pharmacy technicians also help the pharmacist screen for drug interactions, drug–disease contraindications, and drug allergies. Monitoring drug therapy also reduces therapeutic duplication. Pharmacy technicians and

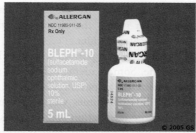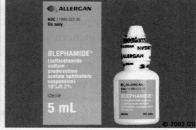

FIGURE 4-3 Example of similar packaging. (Copyright © Gold Standard, Inc., 2007.)

pharmacists work together to alert the prescriber when they see that two therapeutically equivalent drugs are ordered for the patient. Monitoring also prevents refills of discontinued medication

Improper Medication Preparation

Another medication error made by pharmacy staff is improper sterile and nonsterile compounding. Medications for parenteral administration must be prepared using aseptic technique. Medication errors associated with incorrect calculations occur, too. Combining incompatible drugs is also a source of medication errors.

Improper Labeling

Several medication errors involve improper labeling of drugs to be dispensed. A labeling error has occurred when the correct drug is selected but the container is labeled with the wrong drug name, dosage form, strength, or quantity. Putting the wrong patient's name on the label is also a labeling error. Incorrect or incomplete directions typed on the label are other preventable label errors.

Product Selection Errors

Selection of the wrong drug to dispense is a preventable error. This type of error most often occurs when drugs have similar names or similar packaging (Figure 4-3). Other product selection errors include dispensing the wrong strength or wrong dosage form.

Bagging Errors

Placing the correct prescription in the wrong patient's bag is a bagging error. Placing additional prescriptions into a patient's bag or omitting a prescription from the bag are bagging errors, too.

Miscellaneous Dispensing Errors

A properly filled prescription that is dispensed to the wrong patient is a medication error. This may occur when two customers have similar names. The pharmacy staff may incorrectly hear the name of the person who wants to pick up his or her prescription. The patient may incorrectly hear the name of the person the pharmacy staff has announced. This error is preventable. Always verify the name and identification of the person picking up a prescription.

MEDICATION ERRORS MADE BY HEALTH CARE PROVIDERS WHO ADMINISTER MEDICATION

Medication errors are made by health care providers and caregivers who administer medications. One error associated with drug administration can result in a drug being given to the wrong patient. Sometimes the correct drug is given to the right patient; however, the drug strength, dosing frequency, and dosage form are incorrect. This is a medication error, too.

MEDICATION ERRORS MADE BY PATIENTS

Medication errors are made by patients, too! Pharmacists, pharmacy technicians, and other health care providers can help patients prevent medication errors. Patients are often confused by generic and trade names. Their medicines may be labeled using the generic name in the hospital. The community pharmacy may label the same drug with the brand name. The patient may not realize the drugs are the same and take a double dose. A similar situation occurs when two similar medicines are prescribed by different physicians. The patient is unaware that taking both medicines is therapeutic duplication. Confusion is also the reason why patients refill medications that have been discontinued by their health care provider.

Two other medication errors are important to note. They are (1) taking too much medicine and (2) taking too little medicine. Some patients believe the saying, "If one pill is good, then two pills is better." Others do not realize the importance of taking medicines without missing doses. They do not realize that a chronic illness becomes worse or drug resistance can develop when doses are skipped. For some patients, the medication is too expensive, and they take less than the prescribed dose to try to "stretch" the prescription and make it last longer. Regardless of the reason, taking too little or too much medicine can negatively influence drug therapy outcomes.

Avoiding Medication Errors

Pharmacy technicians can play an important role in preventing medication errors. Some tips for preventing medication errors are:

- Always verify prescriptions with similar drug names. Verify spelling and strength.
- Always verify unfamiliar abbreviations or abbreviations published in The Joint Commission's "do not use" list or the National Coordinating Council for Medication Error Reporting and Prevention dangerous abbreviation list.
- Always confirm the drug, strength, and dosing schedule when prescriptions are written and the handwriting is illegible. Never guess.
- Avoid product selection errors by using the pull–dispense–review (PDR) system. Verify the drug name and NDC number. or DIN when selecting (pulling) the drug from the shelf. Check the drug name, strength, and dosage form against medication order. Confirm the drug a third time when returning the medicine to the shelf.
- Become familiar with the brand and generic names of commonly dispensed drugs.
- Become familiar with the strengths, dosage forms, and dosing frequencies of commonly dispensed drugs.
- Alert the pharmacist of all drug interactions and therapeutic duplications.
- Develop a routine to avoid errors associated with distractions.
- Check the identification of each person picking up prescriptions.
- Dispense patient information sheets as required.
- Affix warning labels to prescription vials as required.
- Verify all calculations.
- Check all labels for accuracy.

Chapter Summary

- Drug–drug interactions and drug–food interactions can increase or decrease intended drug effects.
- The more drugs that are administered to a patient, the more likely it is that interactions will occur.
- Drug–drug interactions may increase or decrease side effects of drugs.
- Foods may contain enzymes, vitamins, or minerals that enhance or interfere with drug effects.
- Additive effects are said to occur when the coadministration of two drugs results in increased side effects.
- Synergistic effects result when two drugs administered together produce effects that are greater than would be produced if either drug were administered alone.
- The process during which one drug or a food increases the effects of another drug yet does not produce any effect when administered alone is called potentiation.
- Antagonism is a drug–drug interaction or drug–food interaction that causes decreased drug effects.
- Coadministration of drugs and foods can increase absorption, distribution, metabolism, or elimination.
- Intravenous solutions of acids and bases are incompatible and, when combined, form solid particles (precipitate).

- Displacement from binding sites increases the amount of drug that is free to get to its site of action. Even a small change in the percent of drug that is free to get to the binding site can increase drug effects.
- Interactions that alter the rate of drug metabolism are caused by induction or inhibition of metabolic enzymes.
- Interactions that involve competition for a common transport system in the kidney can affect the elimination of some drugs.
- It is the responsibility of pharmacists and pharmacy technicians to screen all prescriptions for potential drug interactions before dispensing the medication.
- Drug–disease contradictions and drug–drug interactions can be avoided by maintaining an up-to-date history of each patients' chronic and acute medical conditions.
- Computers prospectively screen for drug interactions so adjustments can be made to the patient drug therapy before the drug is dispensed.
- Pharmacy technicians must also be knowledgeable of intravenous drug incompatibilities. Combining acidic intravenous solutions and alkaline solutions causes the precipitation of drug out of the solution.
- Medication errors in the health care setting typically occur in the process of ordering, transcribing, dispensing, and administering medications.
- Poor handwriting is responsible for many medication errors. When prescriptions are illegible, there may be confusion between drugs with similar names.
- Medication errors occur because of misplacement of zeros and decimal points.
- Medication errors have been caused by improper conversion between systems of measurement.
- Medication errors occur when pharmacists, pharmacy technicians, physicians, and other health care workers lack familiarity with the drug that is being prescribed.
- Medication errors made by pharmacy personnel usually involve transcribing errors, incorrect interpretation of prescription contents, improper product preparation, lack of prescription monitoring, product labeling, and inaccurate dispensing.
- Some dispensing errors are caused by distractions in the pharmacy.
- Medication errors made by patients can be minimized by proper education.
- Medication errors can be avoided by verifying prescriptions with similar drug names and unfamiliar abbreviations.
- Avoid product selection errors by using the pull–dispense–review (PDR) system and checking all labels for accuracy.
- Prevent medication errors by becoming familiar with brand and generic names and the strengths, dosage forms, and dosing frequencies of commonly dispensed drugs.
- Medication errors can be minimized by verifying all calculations.

REVIEW QUESTIONS

1. State whether the following statement is true or false: Drug–drug interactions may increase or decrease the effect or side effects of the drug.
   a. true
   b. false

2. _____ is the coadministration of two drugs results in increased side effects.
   a. Antagonistic
   b. Additive
   c. Adverse
   d. Absorption

3. When warfarin and aspirin are administered together, excessive bleeding occurs. This type of effect is _____.
   a. antagonistic
   b. idiosyncratic
   c. both a and b
   d. synergistic

4. Whose responsibility is it to screen all prescriptions for potential drug interactions before dispensing a medication?
   a. pharmacist
   b. technician
   c. pharmacist and technician
   d. pharmacy manager

5. Medication errors in the health care setting typically occur in the process of
   a. ordering medications
   b. transcribing medications
   c. dispensing and administering medications
   d. a, b, and c

6. Orders for medication may be incorrect because the strength is written incorrectly or is illegible. Which of the following is the correct way of writing the dose for digoxin?
   a. digoxin 0.25 mg
   b. digoxin 25 mg
   c. digoxin .25 mg
   d. digoxin 025 mg

7. All of the following are "checks" to ensure that the right medication is pulled from the pharmacy shelf when preparing a prescription EXCEPT_____
   a. Compare the NDC number or DIN with the computer-generated pharmacy label.
   b. Check with the pharmacy assistant every time a prescription is filled.
   c. Check the drug name against the medication order.
   d. Check the drug strength and dosage form against the medication order.

8. To which federal agency should medication errors be reported to using the program MedWatch?
   a. DEA
   b. FDA
   c. TJC
   d. CMS

9. Which agency developed a "do not use" abbreviation list to avoid medication errors?
   a. FDA
   b. DEA
   c. HIPAA
   d. TJC

10. Is the following statement true or false? "If one pill is good, than two pills is better."
    a. true
    b. false

TECHNICIAN'S CORNER

1. Look-alike/sound-alike drugs are responsible for dispensing errors. How might dispensing errors be avoided?
2. What should a pharmacy technician do if he or she is unsure about the name of a medication handwritten on a prescription?

Bibliography

Adubofour K, Keenan C, Daftary A, et al: Strategies to reduce medication errors in ambulatory practice, *J Natl Med Assoc* 96:1558, 2004.

Ashcroft D, Quinlan P, Blenkins A: Prospective study of the incidence, nature and causes of dispensing errors in community pharmacies, *Pharmacoepidemiol Drug Safety* 14:327-332, 2005.

Indiana University Department of Medicine: Cytochrome P 450 Drug Interaction Table: School of Medicine Division of Clinical Pharmacology. Retrieved Jan 3, 2011, from http://medicine.iupui.edu/clinpharm/ddis/table.asp, 2009.

Institute for Safe Medication Practices: ISMP's List of Confused Drug Names. Retrieved Jan 3, 2011, from http://www.ismp.org/Tools/confuseddrugnames.pdf, 2010.

Institute for Safe Medication Practices: FDA and ISMP Lists of Look-Alike Drug Names with Recommended Tall Man Letters. Retrieved Jan 3, 2011, from http://www.ismp.org/Tools/tallmanletters.pdf, 2011.

The Joint Commission: The official "Do Not Use" list. Retrieved from http://www.jointcommission.org/PatientSafety/DoNotUseList/. Accessed November 1, 2007.

Lance L, Lacy C, Armstrong L, et al: *Drug information handbook for the allied health professional*, ed 12, Hudson, OH, 2005, APhA Lexi-Comp.

National Coordinating Council for Medication Error Reporting and Prevention: Dangerous abbreviations. Retrieved from http://nccmerp.org. Accessed November 1, 2007.

Page C, Curtis M, Sutter M, et al: *Integrated pharmacology*, Philadelphia, 2005, Elsevier Mosby, pp 57-70.

Passarelli M, Jacob-Filho W, Figueras A: Adverse drug reactions in an elderly hospitalised population: Inappropriate prescription is a leading cause, *Drugs Aging* 22:767-777, 2005.

Rados C: Drug name confusion: Preventing medication errors, *FDA Consumer* 39:35, 2005, Health Module.

Shargel L, Mutnick A, Souney P, et al: *Comprehensive pharmacy review*, ed 4, Baltimore, 2001, Lippincott Williams & Wilkins, pp 78-84, 42-65, 131-132.

St Onge E, Dea M, Rose R: Medication errors and strategies to improve patient safety, *Drug Topics* 150:36, 2006.

Tam V, Knowles S, Cornish P, et al: Frequency, type and clinical importance of medication history errors at admission to hospital: A systematic review, *JAMC* 173(5), 2005.

U.S. Food and Drug Administration: Medication errors. Retrieved from http://www.fda.gov/cder/drug/MedErrors/default.htm. Accessed November 1, 2007.

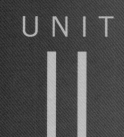

UNIT

II

Drugs Affecting the Autonomic Nervous System and Central Nervous System

LEARNING OBJECTIVES

1 List the divisions of the nervous system.

2 Describe the process of nerve impulse transmission.

3 Describe the function of neurotransmitters.

4 List neurotransmitters important to the autonomic nervous system.

5 Compare and contrast the fight-or-flight response with the rest and digest response.

KEY TERMS

Autonomic nervous system (ANS): Division of nervous system that controls the involuntary body functions; consists of sympathetic and parasympathetic divisions.

Central nervous system (CNS): Consists of the brain and spinal cord.

Glial cells: Form the blood-brain barrier and support the function of the neurons.

Neuron: Functional unit of the nervous system, which includes the cell body, dendrites, axon, and terminals.

Neurotransmitters: Proteins that transmits nerve signals from one neuron to another.

Parasympathetic nervous system: Division of ANS that functions during restful situations; rest and digest part of the ANS.

Peripheral nervous system (PNS): The division of the nervous system outside the brain and spinal cord.

Somatic nervous system: Division of the nervous system that carries information to the somatic effectors or skeletal muscles.

Sympathetic nervous system: Division of the ANS that functions during stressful situations; fight-or-flight part of the ANS.

Synapse: Gap between neurons where nerve information is transmitted from one neuron to another.

Overview

The nervous system is a complex communication system made up of the brain, spinal cord, and nerves that are organized to detect changes in the internal and external environment, evaluate that information, and possibly respond by initiating changes in muscles or glands. Messages are transmitted throughout the nervous system along nerve cells called neurons. Two main types of cells compose the nervous system, neurons and glia. *Neurons* conduct all the impulses that make the nervous system function. Glia, or glial cells, support the function of the neurons. All neurons consist of a cell body and its extensions, one axon, and many dendrites. At the end of every axon is a *synapse*, or space, that must be bridged for the impulse to continue on to its destination. Proteins called *neurotransmitters* are released as the impulses approach the synapse and provide the means for the impulse to cross the synapse. There are three types of neurons—afferent (sensory) neurons that transmit nerve impulses to the brain or spinal cord, efferent (motor) neurons that transmit nerve impulses away from the brain or spinal cords and toward the muscles and glands, and interneurons that conduct impulses from afferent neurons to efferent neurons. Interneurons are found only in the central nervous system (CNS).

Glial cells form the blood-brain barrier and support the function of the neurons by engulfing and destroying bacteria and cellular debris (phagocytosis), lining the fluid-filled ventricles of the brain, and producing fatty myelin sheaths that insulate nerve fibers.

Mechanism of Communication between Nerve Cells

NERVE IMPULSES

Neurons initiate and conduct signals called action potentials or nerve impulses. They exhibit both excitability and conductivity. A nerve impulse can be described as a wave of electrical fluctuation that travels along the neuron's plasma membrane. A synapse is the space between the *presynaptic neuron* and the *postsynaptic neuron* or effector site, such as a muscle, where a neurotransmitter is released to transmit the message from the presynaptic to the postsynaptic cell.

Neurotransmitters

Neurotransmitters are the means whereby neurons talk to each other and are commonly classified by their functions (excitatory or inhibitory) or by their chemical structure (small-molecule and large-molecule transmitters). Small-molecule transmitters are single amino acids and large-molecule transmitters are chains of 20 to 40 amino acids.

SMALL-MOLECULE TRANSMITTERS

Small-molecule transmitters are divided into four main chemical classes: *acetylcholine* (ACh), *amines* (e.g., serotonin, histamine), *catecholamines* (e.g., epinephrine, norepinephrine), and *hormones*. Norepinephrine and epinephrine are also classified as hormones because they are released directly into the bloodstream.

Divisions of the Nervous System

The nervous system is divided into two anatomical divisions, the central nervous system (CNS) and peripheral nervous system (PNS). The PNS is further subdivided into efferent and afferent divisions. The efferent division is subdivided again into the autonomic and somatic systems. The final subdivisions of the autonomic nervous system (ANS) are the parasympathetic and sympathetic systems.

CENTRAL NERVOUS SYSTEM

The CNS is composed of the brain and the spinal cord and is the principal integrator of sensory input and motor output.

Brain

There are six divisions of the brain—cerebellum, diencephalon, cerebrum, medulla oblongata (lowest part), pons (middle), and midbrain (upper)—collectively known as the brainstem.

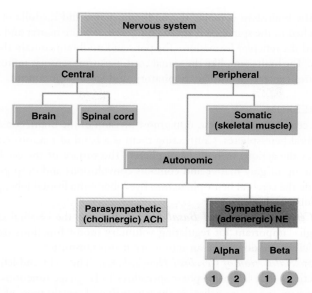

Divisions of the nervous system. (From Lilley LL, Harrington S, Snyder JS: *Pharmacology and the nursing process*, ed 5, St. Louis, 2007, Mosby.)

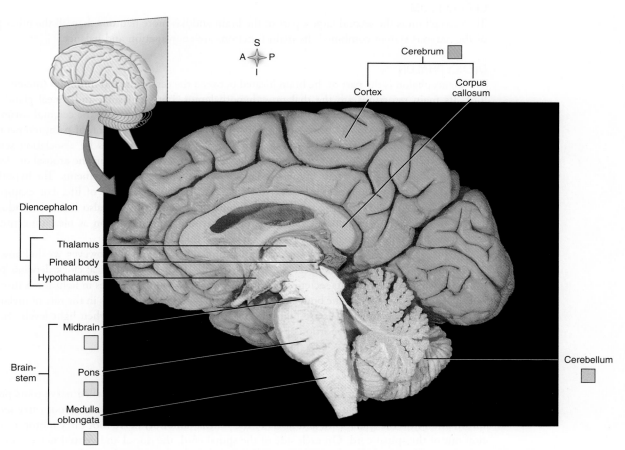

The brain. (From Vidic B, Suarez FR: *Photographic atlas of the human body*, St. Louis, 1984, Mosby.)

The brainstem contains the midbrain, pons, and medulla oblongata. The medulla oblongata is attached to the spinal cord and is composed of white matter and a network of gray and white matter called the reticular formation. The pons and midbrain contain the white matter and reticular formation. The brainstem, like the spinal cord, performs sensory, motor, and reflex functions and contains control centers for cardiac, respiratory, and vasomotor control.

CEREBRUM

The cerebrum, the largest, uppermost division of the brain, consists of two halves, the right and left cerebral hemispheres. Connecting them is a band of neurons called the corpus callosum that integrates the actions of both hemispheres. The surface of the cerebrum, called the cerebral cortex, is made up of gray matter and contains convolutions and deep grooves called fissures. These fissures divide the cerebral hemisphere into five lobes—the frontal lobe, parietal lobe, temporal lobe, occipital lobe, and insula.

Cerebral Tracts and Basal Nuclei. Beneath the cerebral cortex are the basal nuclei or basal ganglia, important for regulating voluntary motor functions (see Chapter 8). Normally, the basal nuclei secrete dopamine an inhibitory neurotransmitter.

Specialization of Cerebral Hemispheres. The right and left hemispheres specialize in different functions. The left hemisphere specializes in language functions and certain hand movements. The right hemisphere specializes in the perception of certain types of auditory stimuli, nonspeech sounds such as melodies, coughing, crying, and laughing. The left hemisphere functions better at tactile perception and perceiving visual and spatial relationships.

CEREBELLUM

The cerebellum is the second largest part of the brain and has more neurons than all the other parts of the nervous system combined. Its main functions are coordination and balance.

DIENCEPHALON

The diencephalon is the part of the brain located between the cerebrum and midbrain (mesencephalon). Its main structures are the thalamus, hypothalamus, optic chiasma, and pineal gland. The thalamus serves as a major relay station for sensory impulses on their way to the cerebral cortex and acts in the following way: (1) performs the function of conscious recognition of pain, temperature, and touch; (2) plays a part in the mechanisms responsible for emotions by associating sensory impulses with feelings of pleasantness and unpleasantness; (3) plays a part in the arousal or alerting mechanism; and (4) plays a part in mechanisms that produce complex movements. The hypothalamus performs many functions important for survival and the enjoyment of life. For example, it functions as a link between the psyche (mind) and the soma (body). It also links the endocrine system to the nervous system. Certain areas of the hypothalamus function as pleasure centers or reward centers for the primary drives such as eating, drinking, and sex.

The functions of the pineal gland are still not completely understood. However, we do know that is an important part of the biological clock mechanism. The body's biological clock depends partly on the pineal gland varying its secretion of the hormone melatonin. Changes in light levels throughout the day and night affect the body's circadian rhythm and trigger changes in the rate of melatonin secretion. When sunlight levels are high, melatonin secretion decreases; when light levels are low, melatonin levels increase proportionally.

Spinal Cord

The spinal cord lies within the spinal cavity. Two bundles of nerve fibers called nerve roots project from each side of the spinal cord. Fibers comprising the dorsal (posterior) nerve root carry sensory information into the spinal cord and fibers of the ventral (anterior) nerve root carry motor information out of the spinal cord. On each side of the spinal cord, the dorsal and ventral nerve roots join together to form a single mixed nerve called a spinal nerve. The spinal cord provides conduction routes to and from the brain and serves as a reflex center. Ascending tracts conduct sensory impulses up the cord to the brain and descending tracts conduct motor impulses down the cord from the brain to peripheral nerve pathways.

PERIPHERAL NERVOUS SYSTEM

The PNS consists of nerve tissue that lies in the periphery, or outer regions, of the nervous system. The PNS is made up of 31 pairs of spinal nerves that emerge from the spinal cord, the 12 pairs of cranial nerves that emerge from the brain, and all the smaller nerves that branch from the main nerves. The PNS includes all the nerve pathways outside the brain and spinal cord and all their individual branches. The PNS is composed of the ANS and somatic nervous system (SNS). The PNS has two functional divisions, the sensory (efferent) and motor (afferent) divisions. The SNS comprises of all the voluntary motor pathways outside the CNS, like the peripheral pathways to the skeletal muscles, which are somatic effectors.

Autonomic Nervous System

The ANS is a subdivision of the PNS and is also divided into two divisions, the sympathetic and parasympathetic systems. The ANS regulates involuntary actions such as the heartbeat, smooth muscle contraction, and glandular secretions that maintain homeostasis. The sympathetic and parasympathetic divisions produce opposite effects.

SYMPATHETIC SYSTEM

The major function of the **sympathetic system** is to serve as an emergency system. It is also called the fight-or-flight system. Whenever the body is undergoing physical or psychological stress, outgoing sympathetic signals increase greatly. Sympathetic impulses to the adrenal medulla stimulate the secretion of epinephrine and norepinephrine.

PARASYMPATHETIC SYSTEM

The **parasympathetic system** is the dominant controller of most autonomic effectors. Whereas the sympathetic system dominates during times of stress, the parasympathetic system dominates during time of rest and digest.

Somatic Nervous System

The somatic nervous system includes all the voluntary motor pathways outside the CNS. It contains the peripheral pathways to the skeletal muscles, termed the *somatic effectors*. All the somatic motor pathways involve a single motor neuron whose axon stretches from the cell body in the CNS all the way to the effectors (muscles) innervated by that neuron.

Transmitters and Receptors

NEUROTRANSMITTERS

Axon terminals of autonomic neurons release the neurotransmitters norepinephrine, epinephrine, and ACh. Neurons that release norepinephrine and epinephrine are known as adrenergic neurons and bind to adrenergic receptors. Cholinergic neurons release acetylcholine and bind to cholinergic receptors.

ADRENERGIC RECEPTORS

There are two types of adrenergic receptors, alpha (α) receptors and beta (β) receptors. Subtypes of these receptors are α_1, α_2, β_1, and β_2. The binding of norepinephrine to alpha receptors in the smooth muscle of blood vessels has a stimulating effect on the muscle that causes the muscle to constrict. The binding of norepinephrine to beta receptors in the smooth muscle of a different blood vessel produces opposite effects. The binding of norepinephrine to beta receptors in cardiac muscle has a stimulating effect that results in a faster and stronger heartbeat. The actions of norepinephrine and epinephrine are terminated in two ways. Most of the neurotransmitter molecules are taken back up by the synaptic knob of the postganglionic neurons, where they are broken down by the enzyme monoamine oxidase (MAO). The remaining neurotransmitter molecules are eventually broken down by another enzyme, catechol-*O*-methyltransferase (COMT).

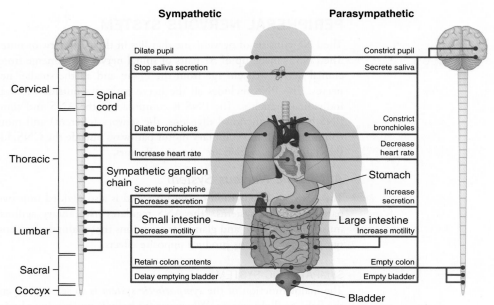

Peripheral nervous system: sympathetic and parasympathetic systems

CHOLINERGIC RECEPTORS

Acetylcholine binds to cholinergic receptors. The two main types of cholinergic receptors are nicotinic (N) receptors and muscarinic (M) receptors. Like the adrenergic receptors, cholinergic receptors have subtypes, such as nicotinic 1 (N_1), nicotinic 2 (N_2), muscarinic 1 (M_1), and muscarinic 2 (M_2). The action of ACh is quickly terminated through hydrolysis by the enzyme acetylcholinesterase.

Summary

The nervous system transmits information very rapidly by nerve impulses conducted from one area of the body to another. Injury or disease can destroy neurons. Diseases such as a cerebrovascular accident (CVA) or stroke may cause destruction of neurons in the motor area of the cerebrum caused by hemorrhage or lack of blood flow through cerebral blood vessels. Various degenerative diseases such as Alzheimer's disease may destroy neurons in the brain, resulting in dementia. Abnormal infectious proteins (prions) cause mad cow disease, which results in loss of nervous system function. Sudden bursts of abnormal neuron activity may produce seizures. A healthy nervous system is vitally important for normal physiological function.

Drugs Used to Affect the Autonomic and Somatic Nervous System

Drug	Primary Receptors	Primary Use
Examples of Cholinergics		
bethanechol	Cholinergic	Increase urination
pilocarpine	Cholinergic (eye)	Glaucoma
pyridostigmine	Cholinergic	Myasthenia gravis
galantamine	Cholinergic	Alzheimer's disease
Examples of Anticholinergics		
atropine	Cholinergic	Dilate pupils and increase heart rate
benztropine	Cholinergic	Parkinson's disease
ipratropium bromide	Cholinergic	Asthma
oxybutynin	Cholinergic	Incontinence
scopolamine	Cholinergic	Motion sickness
Examples of Sympathomimetics		
albuterol (salbutamol)	β_2	Asthma
clonidine	α_2	Hypertension
dobutamine	β_1	Cardiac stimulant
norepinephrine	α_1 and β_1	Shock
salmeterol	β_2	Asthma
Examples of Adrenergic Antagonists		
atenolol	β_1	Hypertension
carvedilol	α_1, β_1, and β_2	Hypertension
doxazosin	α_1	Hypertension
propranolol	β_1 and β_2	Angina and hypertension
terazosin	α_1	Benign prostatic hypertrophy and hypertension

Bibliography

Chabner E: *The language of medicine*, ed 9, 2010, Elsevier.
Patton K: *Survival guide for anatomy and physiology*, St. Louis, 2006, Mosby.
Thibodeau G, Patton K: *Anatomy and physiology*, ed 7, St. Louis, 2009, Mosby.

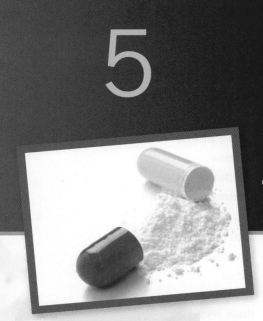

5

Treatment of Anxiety

LEARNING OBJECTIVES

1 Learn the terminology associated with anxiety and its treatment.
2 List and describe the function of neurotransmitters associated with symptoms of anxiety.
3 Classify medications used to treat anxiety.
4 Describe the mechanism of action for each class of drugs used to treat anxiety.
5 Identify significant drug look-alike/sound-alike issues.
6 Identify warning labels and precautionary messages associated with medications used to treat anxiety.

KEY TERMS

Anxiety: Condition associated with tension, apprehension, fear, or panic.

Anxiolytic: Drug used to treat anxiety.

Drug dependence: Person taking the drug must continue to take the drug in order to avoid the onset of physical or psychological withdrawal symptoms (or both).

Generalized anxiety disorder: Condition that is associated with excessive worrying and tension that is experienced daily for more than 6 months.

Obsessive-compulsive disorder: A condition associated with an inability to control or stop repeated unwanted thoughts or behaviors.

Panic disorder: Condition associated with repeated sudden onset of feelings of terror.

Phobia: Irrational fear of things or situations that produce symptoms of intense anxiety.

Posttraumatic stress disorder: Stress disorder that develops in persons who have participated in, witnessed, or been a victim of a terrifying event.

Tolerance: Increasing doses of a drug are required in order to achieve the same effects as were achieved previously at lower doses.

Overview

Anxiety disorder is the leading mental health illness and affects more than 40 million U.S. adults, according to Anxiety Disorders Association of America. The prevalence in Canada is 12% of the population. The cause of anxiety disorders may be environmental, biological, developmental, associated with socioeconomic conditions, or a combination of several of these individual factors.

There are four major types of anxiety disorders—generalized anxiety disorder, panic disorder, obsessive-compulsive disorder (OCD), and posttraumatic stress disorder (PTSD). Individuals diagnosed with anxiety disorders experience intense fear, apprehension, tension, or panic out of proportion to the actual threat or danger.

Certain physiological symptoms are diagnostic for individual anxiety disorders; however, some symptoms are common to all anxiety disorders. Common physiological symptoms include increased heart rate, palpitations, shortness of breath, rapid breathing, nausea, sweating, and dry mouth. All of these symptoms are associated with hyperactivity of the autonomic nervous system. More specifically, the physiological symptoms produced by anxiety are related to stimulation of the sympathetic nervous system and the parasympathetic nervous system.

GENERALIZED ANXIETY DISORDER

Although most adults will experience anxiety at one point in their lives, excessive worrying and tension that are experienced daily for longer than 6 months is an indication of *generalized anxiety disorder*. Generalized anxiety disorder affects up to 6.8 million Americans, according to Anxiety Disorders Association of America, and is the most common type of anxiety disorder. Approximately 1.1% of Canadians between the ages of 15 and 64 years are diagnosed with generalized anxiety disorder, and women are twice as likely as men to be diagnosed with generalized anxiety disorder.

PANIC DISORDER

Panic disorder affects approximately 6 million American adults and occurs twice as frequently in women than in men. It may be accompanied by major depression. Signs and symptoms of panic disorder include a sudden onset of terror, shortness of breath, increased heart rate, trembling, and nausea. The person may feel paralyzed by fear and unable to perform routine daily activities. If these symptoms occur at least four times in 4 weeks or if a single panic attack is followed by persistent fear of another attack, lasting for a minimum of 1 month, a diagnosis of panic disorder is made. Most symptoms of panic disorder last for only a few minutes.

Panic attacks may be triggered by a phobia. A *phobia* is an irrational fear of things or situations that produce symptoms of intense anxiety. Phobias cause the person to try to avoid the thing that is feared. Agoraphobia is a condition in which people become so fearful of situations that may produce "panicky feelings" that they isolate themselves or severely restrict their activities. Other more common phobias are claustrophobia (fear of being in confined spaces), aviophobia (fear of flying), and acrophobia (fear of heights). Nearly 15 million Americans are affected by social phobias. Social phobias cause affected individuals to shy away from social situations where they fear embarrassment or humiliation. Fear of public speaking or asking questions in a public forum setting is often associated with a social phobia. Approximately 8% of the populations of the United States and Canada have some type of phobia.

OBSESSIVE-COMPULSIVE DISORDER

Obsessive-compulsive disorder is a condition associated with an inability to control or stop repeated unwanted thoughts or behaviors. Individuals create rituals, which they perform repeatedly, to lessen anxieties about the things they fear. A person who fears germs may wash his or her hands excessively. The prevalence of OCD is 1.8% of the Canadian population between the ages of 15 and 64 years, according to the Public Health Agency of Canada Report on Mental Illness in Canada (2002). More than 2 million Americans are affected by OCD, and the lifetime incidence of OCD worldwide is 1.7% to 4%.

POSTTRAUMATIC STRESS DISORDER

Posttraumatic stress disorder may develop in persons who have participated in, witnessed, or been a victim of a terrifying event. According to Anxiety Disorders Association of America, nearly 8 million people in the United States have been diagnosed with PTSD. It may occur in soldiers who have committed atrocities or witnessed horrific events during wartime. Women, men, and children who have been sexually assaulted may develop PTSD. Up to 65% of men and 45.9% of women who have been sexually assaulted develop PTSD. PTSD is likely to develop at some point in the lifetimes of children who have been sexually abused. Some people have developed PTSD after natural disasters such as earthquakes and floods or human disasters such as airplane crashes. Depression, substance abuse, and anxiety disorders may accompany PTSD.

Neurochemistry of Anxiety

Pharmaceutical treatment of anxiety is achieved by administering drugs that affect the neurotransmitters γ-aminobutyric acid (GABA), serotonin (5-hydroxytryptamine [5-HT]), and norepinephrine (NE).

ROLE OF γ-AMINOBUTYRIC ACID

The mechanism of action for most *anxiolytics* is to potentiate the effects of GABA, a neurotransmitter, by enhancing the binding of GABA to GABA$_A$ and GABA$_B$ receptors. The anxiolytic agent binds to its specific receptor to produce this effect. Recall that GABA is the major inhibitory neurotransmitter in the nervous system. GABA$_A$ receptor binding causes chloride ion (Cl$^-$) channels to open, and GABA$_B$ receptor binding is coupled to G proteins. The influx of chloride ions results in hyperpolarization, which inhibits formation of action potentials. Ultimately, neuronal excitability is reduced, and nerve impulse transmission is decreased.

ROLE OF SEROTONIN

Serotonin, also known as 5-HT, also plays a role in the treatment of anxiety. Serotonin is a neurotransmitter, too. More than nine serotonin receptors have been identified. Most are located in the pons and midbrain. The receptor involved in the treatment of anxiety is 5-HT$_{1A}$. Activation of the 5-HT$_{1A}$ autoreceptors in the raphe region decreases firing of serotonergic neurons that are linked to anxiety-like behavior. Increasing 5-HT function decreases anxiety.

ROLE OF NOREPINEPHRINE

Norepinephrine is an important neurotransmitter for the sympathetic nervous system. It is responsible for mediating some of the adrenergic-related symptoms of anxiety.

Drugs Used to Treat Anxiety

Anxiety disorder is treated by the administration of anxiolytics and psychotherapy, including cognitive behavioral therapy. An anxiolytic is a drug that reduces symptoms of anxiety.

BENZODIAZEPINES

Benzodiazepines are the principal class of medications used in the treatment of anxiety (Table 5-1). They are indicated for short-term treatment of anxiety. Benzodiazepines are able to reduce anxiety even when taken in low doses. They reduce anxiety by depressing the limbic system and reticular formation. Other indications for benzodiazepines are panic attack, insomnia, seizure disorder, and muscle relaxation. These additional indications are listed under the description of individual benzodiazepines.

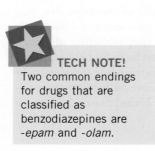

TECH NOTE!
Two common endings for drugs that are classified as benzodiazepines are *-epam* and *-olam*.

Mechanism of Action

Benzodiazepines bind to receptor sites on the GABA$_A$ complex. This increases the affinity of GABA to the GABA receptor. GABA receptor binding opens Cl$^-$ ion channels and lowers the neuronal membrane resting potential from −60 mV to −90 mV. This reduces neuronal excitability (Figure 5-1).

Pharmacokinetics

Benzodiazepines have a high degree of lipid solubility, which accounts for their rapid and complete absorption and enables the drugs to readily cross the blood-brain barrier. The duration of action varies from one benzodiazepine to another and may influence the selection of one benzodiazepine over another. A benzodiazepine that has a long duration of action may have long-lasting, unwanted side effects. The effects of some benzodiazepines may persist for up to 3 days (Table 5-2).

The benzodiazepines are fully metabolized, and some agents are metabolized to active metabolites (see Chapter 2). The half-life (t $\frac{1}{2}$) of the active metabolites can be several days and accounts for the long duration of action of some anxiolytics. The long duration of diazepam is associated with the formation of active metabolites.

TABLE 5-1   Benzodiazepines Used in the Treatment of Anxiety

Generic Name	U.S. Brand Name(s) Canadian Brand(s)	Dosage Forms and Strengths
alprazolam*	Alprazolam Intensol, Niravam, Xanax, Xanax XR Xanax, Xanax TS	**Solution (Alprazolam Intensol):** 1 mg/mL **Tablets (Xanax):** 0.25 mg, 0.5 mg, 1 mg, 2 mg **Tablets, triscored (Xanax TS):** 2 mg **Tablets, extended release (Xanax XR):** 0.5 mg, 1 mg, 2 mg, 3 mg **Tablets, disintegrating (Niravam):** 0.25 mg, 0.5 mg, 1 mg, 2 mg
clonazepam*	Klonopin Rivotril	**Tablets:** 0.5 mg, 1 mg, 2 mg **Tablets, disintegrating:** 0.125 mg, 0.25 mg, 0.5 mg, 1 mg, 2 mg
clorazepate*	Tranxene Generic	**Tablets:** 3.75 mg, 7.5 mg, 15 mg
diazepam*	Diastat, Diazepam Intensol, Valium Diastat, Diazemuls, Valium	**Rectal gel (Diastat):** 5 mg/mL as 2.5 mg†, 5 mg‡, 10 mg†, and 15 mg† prefilled syringe, 20 mg prefilled syringes‡ **Injection, IM emulsion (Diazemuls):** 5 mg/mL **Oral, solution:** 5 mg/5 mL **Oral concentrate (Diazepam Intensol):** 5 mg/mL **Tablets (Valium):** 2 mg, 5 mg, 10 mg
lorazepam*	Ativan Ativan	**Injection, solution (Ativan):** 2 mg/mL; 4 mg/mL **Solution, oral concentrate:** 2 mg/mL **Tablets (Ativan):** 0.5 mg, 1 mg, 2 mg
midazolam*	Generic Generic	**Injection, solution:** 1 mg/mL and 5 mg/mL **Syrup:** 2 mg/mL†
oxazepam*	Generic Generic	**Capsules:** 10 mg, 15 mg, 30 mg **Tablets:** 10 mg, 15 mg, 30 mg

IM, Intramuscular.
*Generic available.
†Strength available in the United States only.
‡Strength available in Canada only.

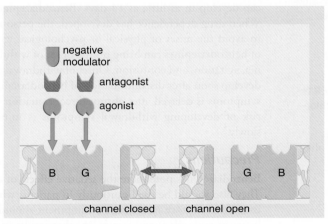

Mechanism of action of
G = GABA receptor site
B = benzodiazepine binding site

FIGURE 5-1 Anxiolytic agents. (From Page C, Curtis M, Sutter M, et al: *Integrated pharmacology*, ed 3, Philadelphia, 2006, Mosby.)

TABLE 5-2   **Half-lives of the Benzodiazepines**

Long Acting	
Chlorazepate	1-3 days
Diazepam	1-3 days
Chlordiazepoxide	1-3 days
Intermediate Acting	
Alprazolam	10-20 hours
Lorazepam	8-24 hours
Temazepam	Up to 25 hours
Short Acting	
Oxazepam	3-8 hours
Triazolam	3-8 hours

TECH NOTE!
Class IV drugs produce less risk for physical and psychological addiction than do Class I, II, and III drugs.

TECH ALERT!
Xanax, Zantac, and Zyrtec have look-alike/sound-alike issues. Immediate release and extended release have look-alike/sound-alike issues, too!

TECH ALERT!
Clorazepate immediate release and sustained release have look-alike/sound-alike issues.

TECH ALERT!
Clomipramine, chlorpromazine, and clomiphene have look-alike/sound-alike issues.

TECH ALERT!
Diazepam oral solution and oral concentrate have look-alike/sound-alike issues.

Adverse Reactions

Certain side effects are common to all benzodiazepines, but others are drug specific. All benzodiazepines produce some degree of sedation, ataxia, confusion, and reduced motor performance. Benzodiazepines can also interfere with cognitive functions and memory because they produce a type of amnesia. This side effect is sometimes used purposefully such as when benzodiazepines are used to reduce anxiety associated with dental or medical procedures. The person receiving the drug "forgets" the procedure, so anxiety associated with future procedures is reduced. Adverse reactions are dose dependent, and side effects increase as the dose increases. The therapeutic index for benzodiazepines is high. The lethal dose is approximately 1000 times greater than the typical therapeutic dose.

Tolerance and Dependence

All benzodiazepines are capable of producing tolerance and dependence, which is why they are classified as Class IV controlled substances in the United States. Benzodiazepines are categorized as a Targeted Substance in Canada and listed in Schedule IV of the Canadian Controlled Drugs and Substances Act.

Tolerance to a drug is said to have developed when the patient must take increasing doses to achieve the same effects as were achieved previously at lower doses. Tolerance to benzodiazepines can develop in as little as 14 days. Benzodiazepines are also known to produce *drug dependence*. When drug dependence has developed, the person taking the drug must continue to take the drug to avoid the onset of physical or psychological withdrawal symptoms (or both). Sudden cessation of benzodiazepines can bring on the onset of withdrawal symptoms such as tremors, anxiety, insomnia, agitation, and confusion. Onset of withdrawal symptoms is drug specific. Withdrawal symptoms develop soon after discontinuation of benzodiazepines with short half-lives. The onset of withdrawal symptoms is delayed after abrupt discontinuation of benzodiazepines that have long half-lives. The risk of developing withdrawal symptoms is minimized when benzodiazepines are discontinued slowly.

Precautions

Benzodiazepines potentiate the sedative effects of other central nervous system (CNS) depressants. They also should be used cautiously in patients who have liver disease. When midazolam is administered, respiratory resuscitation equipment should be readily available. There is a drug interaction between midazolam and cimetidine that results in increased midazolam levels.

AZAPIRONES

Buspirone is currently the only azapirone drug. Azapirones are effective in management of anxiety disorders (Table 5-3) and have a benefit over benzodiazepines because they do not produce tolerance or dependence.

TABLE 5-3 Azapirones Used in the Treatment of Anxiety

Generic Name	U.S. Brand Name(s)		Dosage Forms and Strengths
	Canadian Brand(s)		
buspirone*	BuSpar		**Tablets:** 5 mg, 7.5 mg[†], 10 mg, 15 mg[†], 30 mg[†]
	Generic		

*Generic available.
[†]Strength available in the United States only.

Mechanism of Action

The action produced by azapirones is believed to be caused by binding at dopamine (DA2) and serotonin (5-HT$_{1A}$) receptors. Azapirones are partial agonists at the 5-HT$_{1A}$ receptors. Drug-receptor binding at the presynapse is inhibitory and decreases neuronal firing. Azapirones have no effect on GABA receptors and lack CNS depressant activity.

Pharmacokinetics

Buspirone is the only drug in this class. The onset of action is slow, and maximum therapeutic effects are achieved 3 to 6 weeks after therapy has been initiated.

Buspirone is metabolized in the liver and eliminated in urine. The elimination half-life is between 2 and 3 hours. Food decreases first-pass metabolism in the liver and increases the drug's bioavailability.

Adverse Reactions

The most common adverse effects associated with buspirone therapy are dizziness, restlessness, headache, nausea, diarrhea, and insomnia. Buspirone produces only minimal sedation.

Precautions

Buspirone should be used with caution in patients with liver or kidney disease.

MISCELLANEOUS ANXIOLYTIC AGENTS

Hydroxyzine

Hydroxyzine is an antihistamine (see Chapter 29) that is also approved for the treatment of generalized anxiety disorders. It is a histamine-1 receptor antagonist. Hydroxyzine is also used in children and adults to reduce anxiety associated with dental and minor medical procedures. It produces a fair bit of sedation, but similar to buspirone, does not produce tolerance or dependence. Other side effects are dizziness, headache, dry mucous membranes, and urinary retention.

Hydroxyzine HCl and hydroxyzine pamoate are contraindicated in men with prostate disease and lactating women. Sedation is increased when the drug is taken with other CNS depressants or alcohol (Table 5-4).

ANTIDEPRESSANTS

Tricyclic antidepressants (TCAs), selective serotonin reuptake inhibitors (SSRIs), monoamine oxidase inhibitors (MAOIs), and serotonin noradrenaline reuptake inhibitors (SNRIs) are antidepressants prescribed for the treatment of anxiety disorders (see Chapter 6) (Table 5-5). Clomipramine, a TCA, is indicated for the treatment of OCD. Fluoxetine and sertraline are SSRIs and are indicated for OCD as well. Sertraline is also labeled for use in the treatment of panic disorder, social phobia, and PTSD. Venlafaxine is an SNRI and is used in the management of generalized anxiety disorders.

Treatment of OCD with antidepressants requires higher doses than the treatment of depression, and it takes a longer time for maximum benefits to be achieved. TCAs, similar to clomipramine, may take up to 6 weeks for full effects to be noticed. Maximum benefits of fluoxetine and sertraline are achieved in 1 to 3 weeks.

TABLE 5-4   Miscellaneous Drugs Used in the Treatment of Anxiety

Generic Name	U.S. Brand Name(s) / Canadian Brand(s)	Dosage Forms and Strengths
hydroxyzine HCl*	Generic only / Atarax	**Capsules:**[#] 10 mg, 25 mg, 50 mg **Injection, solution:** 25 mg/mL, 50 mg/mL **Syrup (Atarax):** 10 mg/5 mL **Tablets:**[##] 10 mg, 25 mg, 50 mg
hydroxyzine pamoate*	Vistaril / Not available	**Capsules:** 25 mg, 50 mg, 100 mg **Oral suspension:** 25 mg/5 mL

*Generic available.
[#]Available in Canada only.
[##]Available in the United States only.

TABLE 5-5   Antidepressants Used in the Treatment of Anxiety

Generic Name	U.S. Brand Name(s) / Canadian Brand(s)	Dosage Forms and Strengths
clomipramine*	Anafranil / Anafranil	**Capsules:**[†] 25 mg, 50 mg, 75 mg **Tablets:**[‡] 10 mg, 25 mg, 50 mg
escitalopram	Lexapro / Cipralex	**Oral:** 5 mg/5 mL **Tablets:** 5 mg,[@] 10 mg, 20 mg
fluoxetine*	Prozac, Prozac Weekly, Selfemra, Sarafem / Prozac	**Capsule (Prozac):** 10 mg, 20 mg, 40 mg **Capsulase (Prozac Weekly):** 90 mg **Oral solution:** 20 mg/5 mL **Tablets (Prozac):** 10 mg, 20 mg **Tablets, for PMS (Sarafem):** 10 mg, 20 mg
paroxetine*	Paxil, Paxil CR, Pexeva / Paxil, Paxil CR	**Oral suspension (Paxil):** 10 mg/5ml **Tablet, as HCl (Paxil):** 10 mg, 20 mg, 30 mg, 40 mg **Tablets, as mesylate (Pexeva):** 10 mg, 20 mg, 30 mg, 40 mg **Tablets, as controlled release (Paxil CR):** 12.5 mg, 25 mg, 37.5 mg
sertraline*	Zoloft / Zoloft	**Capsules:**[‡] 25 mg, 50 mg, 100 mg **Solution, oral concentrate:** 20 mg/mL[@] **Tablets:**[†] 25 mg, 50 mg, 100 mg
venlafaxine*	Effexor XR / Effexor XR	**Capsules, extended release (Effexor XR):** 37.5 mg, 75 mg, 150 mg **Tablets:**[@] 25 mg, 37.5 mg, 50 mg, 75 mg **Tablets, extended release:** 37.5 mg, 75 mg, 150 mg, 225 mg[†]

*Generic available.
[†]Strength available in the United States only.
[‡]Strength available in Canada only.
[@]Dosage form available only in the United States.

TECH ALERT!
Paxil and Taxol have look-alike/sound-alike issues. Paxil and Plavix have look-alike/sound-alike issues, too!

Mechanism of Action

SSRIs inhibit 5-HT reuptake into the presynaptic neuron increasing 5-HT availability at postsynaptic receptor sites. Sustained use of SSRIs desensitizes 5-HT$_{1A}$ autoreceptors in the raphe nuclei of the midbrain, allowing the receptors to recover sooner, increasing 5-HT released and inhibiting postsynaptic cell firing outside the raphe region. TCAs inhibit the reuptake of 5-HT and noradrenaline. MAOI binding increases synaptic availability of 5-HT, noradrenaline, and dopamine.

Adverse Reactions

Some adverse reactions are common to all the antidepressants used in the treatment of anxiety. Others are drug specific. Clomipramine may produce sedation or decreased alertness; fluoxetine, paroxetine, and sertraline may cause insomnia, decreased appetite, dry mouth, dizziness, and agitation or tremor; and paroxetine may also produce headache, nausea, diarrhea, and sexual dysfunction.

No tolerance or dependence is associated with any of the antidepressants. However, some serious side effects are possible. Clomipramine may produce seizures. Serotonin syndrome is a serious condition associated with the use of drugs such as sertraline and fluoxetine. Serotonin syndrome is potentially fatal and produces symptoms of confusion, agitation, diarrhea, tremors, increased blood pressure, and seizures. A detailed description of specific mechanisms of action and pharmacokinetics of these drugs will be discussed in Chapter 6.

BETA-ADRENERGIC ANTAGONISTS

Rapid heart rate is a common symptom of anxiety. Beta-adrenergic antagonists, also known as beta blockers, are administered to reduce palpitations. Beta-adrenergic antagonists are not approved by the U.S. Food and Drug Administration for the treatment of anxiety; however, the beta blockers (e.g., propranolol and nadolol) may be prescribed to control the symptoms that accompany anxiety and to prevent stage fright. Propranolol diminishes sympathetic activity in the brain. Recent studies suggest that propranolol may weaken the formation of stressful memories, making it useful in the treatment of PTSD however it is not yet FDA approved for this use.

Summary of Drugs Used in the Treatment of Anxiety Disorders

Generic Name	U.S. Brand Name	Usual Adult Oral Dose and Dosing Schedule	Warning Labels
Benzodiazepines			
alprazolam	Xanax	**Generalized anxiety disorder:** immediate release 0.5-4 mg daily (in 1-3 divided doses) **Panic disorder:** 1.5-10 mg/day (immediate release); 0.5-6 mg/day (extended release) **Anxiety associated with depression:** 2.5-3 mg/day in divided doses	MAY CAUSE DROWSINESS; MAY IMPAIR ABILITY TO DRIVE. AVOID ALCOHOL. MAY BE HABIT FORMING. DO NOT CRUSH, BREAK, OR CHEW (extended release).
clonazepam	Klonopin	**Panic disorder:** 0.25-1 mg twice a day (maximum, 4 mg/day)	
clorazepate	Tranxene	**Generalized anxiety disorder:** 7.5-15 mg 2-4 times/day (immediate release); 11.25-22.5 mg once daily (sustained release) **Ethanol withdrawal:** 30 mg dosed 2-4 times per day; increase up to maximum of 90 mg/day	
diazepam	Valium	**Anxiety disorder:** 2-10 mg 2-4 times/day (oral); 2-10 mg every 3-4 hours (IM, IV) **Ethanol withdrawal:** 5-10 mg IV every 3-4 hours as needed	
lorazepam	Ativan	**Anxiety and sedation:** Oral 1-10 mg daily in 2-3 divided doses **Preprocedure sedation:** 0.05 mg/kg IM (maximum, 4 mg/dose) or 0.044 mg/kg IV (maximum, 2 mg/dose)	

Continued

Summary of Drugs Used in the Treatment of Anxiety Disorders—cont'd

Generic Name	U.S. Brand Name	Usual Adult Oral Dose and Dosing Schedule	Warning Labels
midazolam	Generic	**Conscious sedation for preoperative procedures:** 0.5-2 mg slow IV every 2-3 minutes (maximum, 2.5-5 mg)	MAY CAUSE DIZZINESS AND DISORIENTATION. MAY CAUSE PAIN, SWELLING, OR REDNESS AT INJECTION SITE.
oxazepam	Generic	**Anxiety:** 10-30 mg 3-4 times a day **Ethanol withdrawal:** 15-30 mg 3-4 times a day	MAY CAUSE DROWSINESS; MAY IMPAIR ABILITY TO DRIVE. AVOID ALCOHOL. MAY BE HABIT FORMING. DO NOT CRUSH, BREAK, OR CHEW (extended release).
Azapirones			
buspirone	BuSpar	7.5-15 mg twice daily (maximum dose, 60 mg/day)	MAY CAUSE DROWSINESS; MAY IMPAIR ABILITY TO DRIVE. TAKE WITH FOOD.
Miscellaneous Anxiolytics			
hydroxyzine HCl	Atarax	**Anxiety:** 25-100 mg 4 times a day (maximum dose, 400 mg/day)	MAY CAUSE DROWSINESS; AVOID ALCOHOL MAY INTENSIFY THIS EFFECT.
hydroxyzine pamoate	Generic	**Ethanol withdrawal:** 50-100 mg IM 4 times a day **Preoperative sedation:** 50-100 mg as a single dose (oral); 25-100 mg (IM)	MAY IMPAIR ABILITY TO DRIVE.
Antidepressants Used in the Treatment of Anxiety Disorders			
clomipramine	Anafranil	**Obsessive-compulsive disorder:** 25-100 mg/day in divided doses (maximum, 250 mg/day)	MAY CAUSE DIZZINESS OR DROWSINESS; ALCOHOL MAY INTENSIFY THIS EFFECT. MAY IMPAIR ABILITY TO DRIVE. SWALLOW WHOLE; DO NOT CRUSH OR CHEW (delayed and extended release— Cymbalta, Prozac weekly, Paxil CR, Effexor XR). DO NOT DISCONTINUE WITHOUT MEDICAL SUPERVISION.
duloxetine	Cymbalta	**Generalized anxiety disorder:** 60 mg PO once daily	
escitalopram	Lexapro, Cipralex#	**Generalized anxiety disorder:** 10-20 mg once daily	
fluoxetine	Prozac	**Obsessive-compulsive disorder:** 20-80 mg/day **Panic disorder:** 20 mg/day (maximum, 60 mg/day)	
paroxetine	Paxil	**Generalized anxiety disorder:** 20-50 mg/day **Obsessive-compulsive disorder:** 20-60 mg/day **Panic disorder:** 10-60 mg/day (Paxil, Pexeva) or 12.75 mg/day (Paxil CR) **Posttraumatic stress disorder:** 12.5-25 mg daily (Paxil CR) **Social phobias:** 20 mg/day (Paxil) or 12.5-37.5 mg/day (Paxil CR)	
sertraline	Zoloft	**Obsessive-compulsive disorder:** 50 mg/day **Panic disorder, posttraumatic stress disorder, and social phobias:** 50 mg/day (up to 200 mg/day)	
venlafaxine	Effexor XR	**Generalized anxiety disorder, panic disorder, and social phobias:** 75-225 mg once daily; increase by 37.5 mg every 4-7 days	

#Available in Canada only.

Chapter Summary

- Anxiety disorders are the leading mental health illness.
- The cause of anxiety disorders may be environmental, biological, or developmental; associated with socioeconomic conditions; or a combination of several of these individual factors.
- The four major types of anxiety disorders are generalized anxiety disorder, panic disorder, obsessive-compulsive disorder (OCD), and posttraumatic stress disorder (PTSD).
- Common physiological symptoms include increased heart rate, palpitations, shortness of breath, rapid breathing, nausea, sweating, and dry mouth. All of these symptoms are associated with hyperactivity of the autonomic nervous system.
- Generalized anxiety disorder is associated with excessive worry and tension that are experienced daily for longer than 6 months.
- OCD is a condition associated with an inability to control or stop repeated unwanted thoughts or behaviors.
- Panic disorder is a condition associated with repeated sudden onset of feelings of terror.
- A phobia is an irrational fear of things or situations that produce symptoms of intense anxiety.
- Social phobias cause affected individuals to shy away from social situations where they fear embarrassment of humiliation. Fear of public speaking is an example of a social phobia.
- PTSD is a stress disorder that develops in persons who have participated in, witnessed, or been a victim of a terrifying event.
- Anxiety disorder is treated by the administration of anxiolytics and psychotherapy, including cognitive behavioral therapy.
- The mechanism of action for most anxiolytics is to enhance binding of γ-aminobutyric acid (GABA), a neurotransmitter, to $GABA_A$ and $GABA_B$ receptors.
- Benzodiazepines are the principal class of medications used in the treatment of anxiety and bind to receptor sites on the $GABA_B$ complex.
- GABA receptor binding opens Cl^- ion channels, which reduces neuronal excitability.
- The duration of action for benzodiazepines may be long acting, intermediate acting, or short acting.
- Benzodiazepines can produce a type of amnesia that causes the person receiving the drug to "forget," reducing anxiety associated with future dental or medical procedures.
- All benzodiazepines are capable of producing tolerance and dependence.
- When tolerance develops, increasing doses of a drug are required to achieve the same effects as were achieved a previously at lower doses. When drug dependence has developed, the person taking the drug must continue to take the drug to avoid the onset of or psychological withdrawal symptoms (or both).
- All benzodiazepines are scheduled Class IV controlled substances in the United States and are Targeted Substances in Canada.
- Withdrawal symptoms develop soon after discontinuation of benzodiazepines with short half-lives and are delayed after abrupt discontinuation of benzodiazepines that have long half-lives.
- Buspirone is an azapirone and is a partial agonist at 5-HT_{1A} receptor. These receptors are inhibitory at the presynapse, so stimulation causes decreased neuronal firing.
- Buspirone does not produce tolerance or dependence. Abrupt discontinuation does not produce withdrawal symptoms.
- Hydroxyzine is an antihistamine that is indicated for the treatment of anxiety. It is used in children and adults to reduce anxiety associated with dental and minor medical procedures.
- Tricyclic antidepressants, selective serotonin reuptake inhibitors, and monoamine oxidase inhibitors are antidepressants prescribed for the treatment of anxiety disorders.
- Serotonin syndrome is a potentially life-threatening adverse drug reaction caused by excessive serotonin that produces symptoms of confusion, agitation, diarrhea, tremors, increased blood pressure, and seizures.
- Beta-adrenergic antagonists are administered to reduce the palpitations associated with anxiety and are also useful for the management of stage fright.

REVIEW QUESTIONS

1. Is the following statement true or false? "Women are twice as likely as men to be diagnosed with generalized anxiety disorder."
   a. true
   b. false

2. The_____ treatment of anxiety is associated with increases in drug-receptor binding to the neurotransmitters γ-aminobutyric acid, serotonin, and norepinephrine.
   a. therapeutic
   b. psychological
   c. pharmacological
   d. physiological

3. Anxiety disorder is treated by the administration of _____ and psychotherapy.
   a. analgesics
   b. anxiolytics
   c. anti-inflammatories
   d. antipsychotics

4. Benzodiazepines are indicated for _____ treatment of anxiety.
   a. short-term
   b. long-term

5. _____ to a drug is said to have developed when the patient must take increasing doses to achieve the same effects as were achieved previously at lower doses.
   a. Dependence
   b. Addiction
   c. Tolerance
   d. none of the above

6. Which of the following benzodiazepines is indicated for the treatment of anxiety disorders, ethanol withdrawal, skeletal muscle relaxation, and seizure disorders?
   a. alprazolam
   b. clonazepam
   c. lorazepam
   d. diazepam

7. Buspirone is the only drug in this class.
   a. azapirone
   b. antihistamine
   c. amiodarone
   d. a and c

8. _____ is an antihistamine that is indicated for the treatment of anxiety.
   a. Promethazine
   b. Hydroxyzine
   c. Apresoline
   d. none of the above

9. Clomipramine, fluoxetine, and sertraline are antidepressants that are indicated for the treatment of
   a. panic disorders
   b. anxiety
   c. obsessive-compulsive disorder
   d. posttraumatic stress disorder

10. Rapid heart rate is a common symptom of anxiety. Beta-adrenergic antagonists are administered to reduce the palpitations. One example is
   a. propranolol
   b. Inderal
   c. nadolol
   d. all of the above

TECHNICIAN'S
CORNER

1. What happens if a patient stops using benzodiazepines abruptly?
2. What is the difference between tolerance and dependence on a drug?

Bibliography

Anxiety Disorders Association of America: Statistics and facts. Retrieved from http://www.adaa.org/AboutADAA/ PressRoom/StatsandFacts.asp. Accessed November 30, 2007.

Greenberg W, Aronson S: Obsessive-compulsive disorder. eMedicine 2007. Retrieved from http:// www.emedicine.com/med/topic1654.htm. Accessed February 15, 2008.

Lance L, Lacy C, Armstrong L, et al: *Drug information handbook for the allied health professional*, ed 12, Hudson, OH, 2005, APhA Lexi-Comp.

National Institute of Mental Health: *Anxiety disorders*. In U.S. Department of Health and Human Services (Ed.) (Vol. 09 3879), Bethesda, MD, 2009, Science Writing, Press & Dissemination Branch.

National Institute of Mental Health, Department of Health and Human Services, Public Health Service, National Institutes of Health: Facts about anxiety disorders. Retrieved from http://www.nlm.nih.gov/ medlineplus. Accessed June 15, 2006.

National Mental Health Information Center: Anxiety disorders. Retrieved from www.mentalhealth.samhsa.gov/ publications/allpubs/ken98-0045/default.asp.

Page C, Curtis M, Sutter M, et al: *Integrated pharmacology*, Philadelphia, 2005, Elsevier Mosby, pp 239-241.

Public Health Agency of Canada: A report on mental illness in Canada. Retrieved from http://www .phac-aspc.gc.ca/publicat/miic-mmac/chap_4_. Accessed June 15, 2006.

Raffa R, Rawls S, Beyzarov E: *Netter's illustrated pharmacology*, Philadelphia, 2005, WB Saunders, pp 65-66.

6

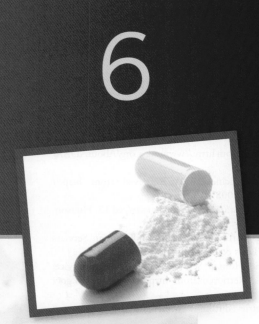

Treatment of Depression

LEARNING OBJECTIVES

1 Learn the terminology associated with depression and its treatment.

2 List and describe the function of neurotransmitters associated with symptoms of depression.

3 Classify medications used to treat depression.

4 Describe mechanism of action for each class of drugs used to treat depression.

5 Identify significant drug look-alike/sound-alike issues.

6 Identify warning labels and precautionary messages associated with medications used to treat depression.

KEY TERMS

Adjunct: Drug that is used to complement the effects of another drug.

Bipolar disorder: Mental health illness associated with sudden swings in mood between depression and periods of mania, racing thoughts, distractibility, and increased goal-directed behavior.

Enuresis: Bedwetting or uncontrollable urination during sleep.

Major depression: Mental health illness associated with persistent feelings of sadness, emptiness, or hopelessness that last for several weeks.

Monoamine oxidase: Enzyme found in the liver, intestine, and terminal neuron, responsible for degradation of monoamine neurotransmitters and dietary amines.

Serotonin syndrome: Potentially life-threatening adverse drug reaction that produces symptoms of confusion, agitation, diarrhea, tremors, increased blood pressure and is caused by excessive serotonin.

Overview

Depressive disorders affect nearly 23.8 million Americans in a given year, and at some time in their lives, one in 10 Canadians will be affected. Depression affects men, women, and children. Depressive disorder may be precipitated by hormonal changes (premenstrual syndrome, pregnancy, postpartum), substance abuse (alcohol and other drugs), or illnesses such as Parkinson's disease, heart attack, or thyroid dysfunction. Heredity plays a role as well, particularly in bipolar disorder because children born to a parent with bipolar disorder are at increased risk for the illness.

Depressive illness influences most aspects of a person's life and lifestyle. It affects self-esteem, mood, thoughts, eating, and sleeping. Depression reduces the ability to think and concentrate. Feelings of worthlessness or guilt often accompany depressive episodes. As many as 12% of depressed patients contemplate or attempt suicide. Without treatment, symptoms of depression can persist for a few weeks to years.

The three primary types of depressive disorders are major depression, bipolar disorder, and dysthymia. **Major depression** is also called *clinical depression* and is associated with persistent feelings of sadness, emptiness, or hopelessness. These feelings must persist for several weeks and are usually accompanied by a lack of interest in activities that were previously thought to be enjoyable, fatigue, irritability, and insomnia or hypersomnia. Sometimes the depression manifests itself in other physical ailments for which no treatments are able to cure or reduce symptoms. **Bipolar disorder**, formerly called *manic-depressive disorder*, is associated with sudden swings in mood between depression and periods of mania. Mania is associated with hyperactivity, racing thoughts, insomnia, distractibility, and increased goal-directed behavior. Manic periods can last for 1 or more weeks, during which time the person may sleep little and produce a prolific amount of work. Several well-known people such as Vincent Van Gogh are believed to have had bipolar disorder. Dysthymia produces symptoms that are similar to those of major depression; however, the symptoms are less severe. People diagnosed with dysthymia have symptoms that are chronic and, although not typically debilitating, keep the person from functioning well and feeling good.

The causes of depression are not completely known, but a deficiency of certain neurotransmitters is involved. This explains why people with depression cannot "pull themselves together" to get better. Drug treatment is aimed at restoring depleted neurotransmitters to normal levels.

Neurochemistry of Depression

BIOGENIC AMINE THEORY

According to the biogenic amine theory, clinical depression results from a decrease in monoamine neurotransmitters in the brain. This hypothesis was made upon the discovery that patients treated with drugs that deplete monoamine neurotransmitters stores in the neuron develop depression. Other evidence for the monoamine theory of depression is the laboratory finding that the concentration of monoamines and their metabolites is minimal in the cerebrospinal fluid of patients diagnosed with clinical depression. Evidence supports the fact that adrenergic receptors and serotonergic receptors are less sensitive in depressed persons so norepinephrine (NE) and serotonin (5-hydroxytryptamine [5-HT]) binding is decreased even when levels are normal. The γ-aminobutyric acid (GABA) receptor may also be involved in depression.

If depletion of monoamine neurotransmitters causes depression, what is the effect of excessive levels of these neurotransmitters? Bipolar affective disorder (BPAD), also known as mania, is believed to be associated with increased levels of monoamine neurotransmitters (Figure 6-1). The complete neurochemistry of BPAD is unclear.

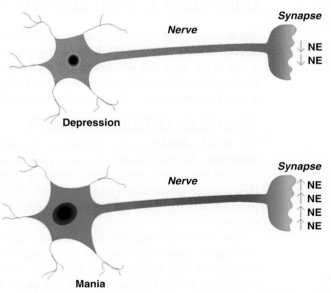

FIGURE 6-1 Biologic amine hypothesis. *NE,* Norepinephrine. (From Lilley LL, Harrington S, Snyder JS: *Pharmacology and the nursing process,* ed 5, St Louis, 2007, Mosby.)

The monoamine neurotransmitters that are thought to be depleted in clinical depression are NE, 5-HT, and dopamine (DA). All currently marketed antidepressants act to increase the levels of NE, 5-HT, or DA released into synapses within the brain or to increase neurotransmitter binding. Antidepressants are categorized according to the method that they use to potentiate the actions of NE, 5-HT, and DA. Some antidepressants are nonspecific, increasing the binding of more than one monoamine neurotransmitter, but other antidepressants are more specific and increase the binding of mainly one of the neurotransmitters.

ROLE OF NOREPINEPHRINE

The neurotransmitter NE plays an important role in the treatment of depression. It is widely distributed in the brain and in the periphery. Decreased levels in the brain are responsible for depression, and increased levels in the periphery can cause serious effects such as hypertension. Adrenergic neurons release NE. Most of the adrenergic neurons found in the central nervous system are found in the pons or midbrain. Because the effects of antidepressants are not immediate and increase over time, it is believed that their action may be linked to desensitization and down regulation in postsynaptic beta receptors.

ROLE OF SEROTONIN

Antidepressants that potentiate the activity of the neurotransmitter 5-HT play an important role in the treatment of depression. Serotonin is an excitatory neurotransmitter. More than nine 5-HT receptors have been identified. These 5-HT receptors influence G protein coupling and Na^+/K^+ channel operation. Serotonin receptors that have been well studied are $5-HT_{1A}$, $5-HT_{2A}$, $5-HT_{2C}$, and $5-HT_3$. Drugs that antagonize $5-HT_{2A}$ and $5-HT_{2C}$ receptors are used in the treatment of depression and negative-symptom schizophrenia. Drugs that antagonize $5-HT_3$ receptors are used to treat nausea. In addition to improved mood, 5-HT is involved in regulation of the sleep–wake cycle and pain perception.

ROLE OF DOPAMINE

There are five types of DA receptors. Binding to D2, D3, and D4 receptors is inhibitory, and binding to D1 and D5 is excitatory. Dopamine binding plays a lesser role in the treatment and management of depression compared with the neurotransmitters NE and 5-HT. Drugs that are used in the treatment of Parkinson's disease and schizophrenia potentiate the activity of DA (see Chapter 8).

Drugs Used to Treat Depression

The mechanism of action for drugs used to treat depression may differ, but all antidepressants are equally effective (Figure 6-2). Inhibition of the reuptake of specific monoamine neurotransmitters is one of the ways that antidepressants produce their effects. The other mechanism of action is to block the degradation of monoamine neurotransmitters. Selection of one antidepressant over another is based on the patient's ability to tolerate drug side effects.

TRICYCLIC ANTIDEPRESSANTS

The tricyclic antidepressants (TCAs) are the oldest class of medication used in the treatment of depression. The effectiveness of newer agents is compared with that of TCAs. As the name implies, all TCAs have a three-ring chemical structure (Figure 6-3). Because they all have a similar structure, they produce similar effects and similar side effects. The side chains attached to the rings affect the structure–activity relationship and account for differences in duration of action and adverse reactions.

The TCAs are used for the treatment and management of several medical conditions in addition to depression. They are also prescribed for *enuresis*, commonly known as bedwetting (imipramine and nortriptyline). Moreover, they are prescribed for the treatment of obsessive-compulsive disorder (clomipramine) and as an ***adjunct*** to other drug therapy for chronic pain (amitriptyline, nortriptyline).

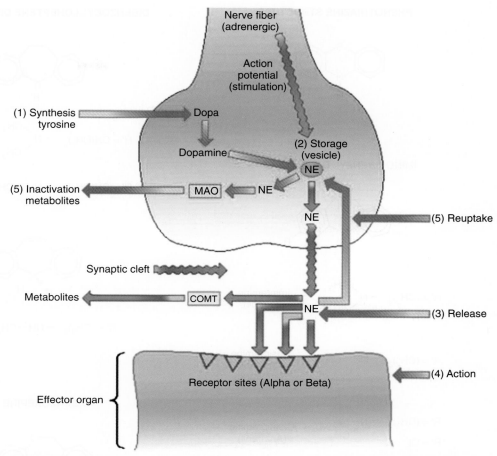

FIGURE 6-2 Site of neurotransmitter synthesis, storage, release, action, and inactivation. (From Lilley LL, Harrington S, Snyder JS: *Pharmacology and the nursing process*, ed 5, St Louis, 2007, Mosby.)

Mechanism of Action

In depression, sufficient neurotransmitters may be released into the synaptic cleft; however, the neurotransmitters may be returned to the neuron before binding occurs. The TCAs work by producing a nonspecific blockade of the reuptake of monoamine neurotransmitters. The TCAs block the reuptake of NE and 5-HT in the presynaptic neuron and in postsynaptic receptors. The TCAs also have some affinity for adrenergic, cholinergic (muscarinic), and histaminic postsynaptic receptors.

When the reuptake of NE and 5-HT back into the neuron is blocked, the neurotransmitters remain in the synaptic cleft longer. The longer the neurotransmitter remains in the synaptic cleft, the greater the opportunity for binding of the neurotransmitter to its receptor (Figure 6-4).

Pharmacokinetics

The TCAs are readily absorbed when administered orally. They are lipophilic so are widely distributed within the central nervous system. The onset of action, duration of action, and half-life ($t\frac{1}{2}$) vary among agents. The half-life of the TCAs can be as short as 4 hours (imipramine) and as long as 96 hours (nortriptyline). Their long half-lives are associated with their high degree of lipid solubility. The long duration of action of these agents permits once-daily dosing.

The TCAs are metabolized by microsomal enzymes in the liver. Several of the TCAs are metabolized to active metabolites. Amitriptyline is metabolized to nortriptyline, and desipramine is a metabolite of imipramine. They are ultimately eliminated in the urine.

Although the onset of action may be relatively short, maximum antidepressant benefit may take up to 6 weeks to be achieved.

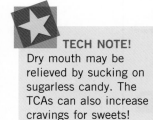

TECH NOTE!
Dry mouth may be relieved by sucking on sugarless candy. The TCAs can also increase cravings for sweets!

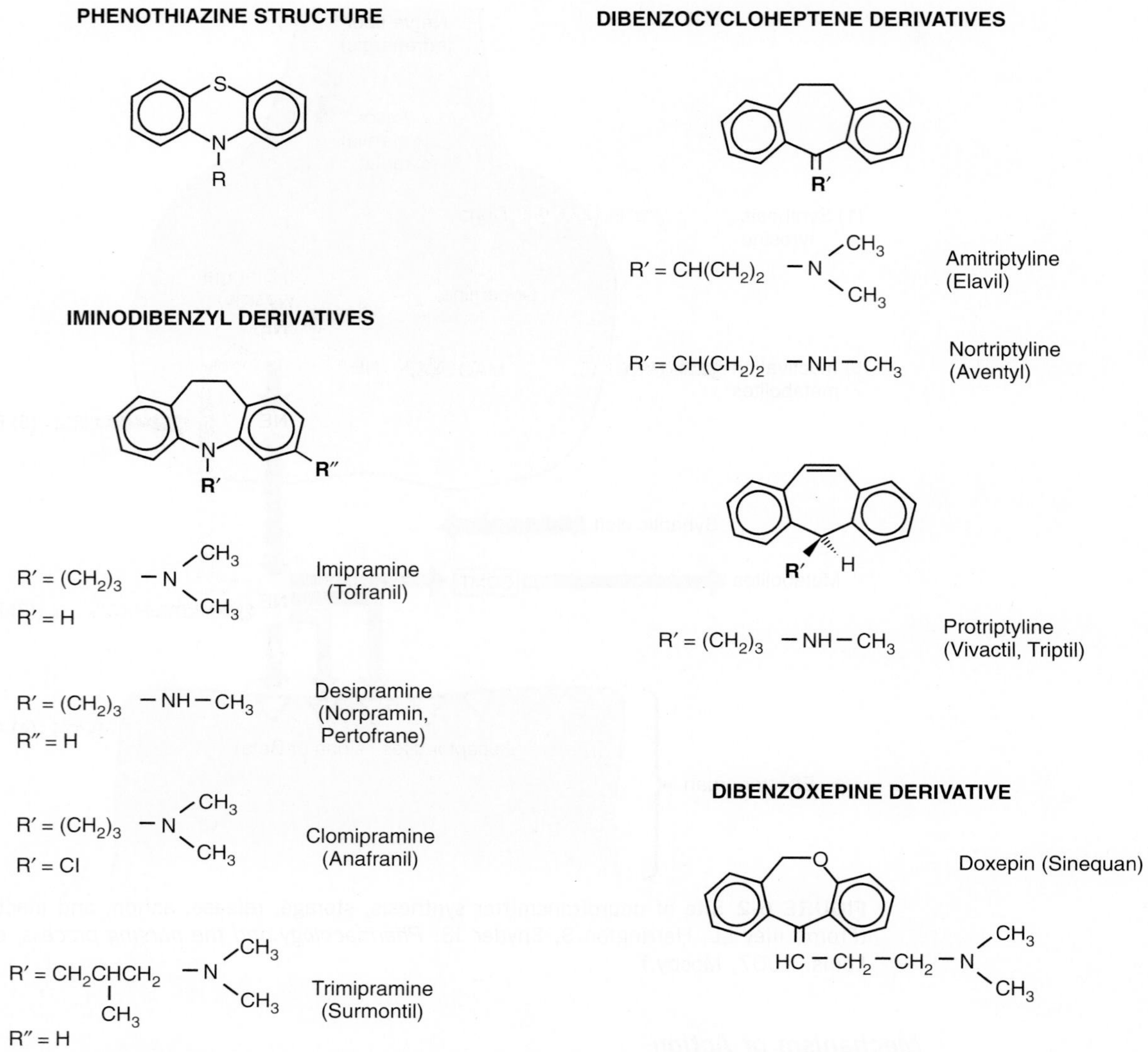

PHENOTHIAZINE STRUCTURE

DIBENZOCYCLOHEPTENE DERIVATIVES

$R' = CH(CH_2)_2$ —N$\begin{smallmatrix}CH_3\\CH_3\end{smallmatrix}$ Amitriptyline (Elavil)

$R' = CH(CH_2)_2$ —NH—CH$_3$ Nortriptyline (Aventyl)

IMINODIBENZYL DERIVATIVES

$R' = (CH_2)_3$ —N$\begin{smallmatrix}CH_3\\CH_3\end{smallmatrix}$ Imipramine (Tofranil)
$R' = H$

$R' = (CH_2)_3$ —NH—CH$_3$ Desipramine (Norpramin, Pertofrane)
$R'' = H$

$R' = (CH_2)_3$ —N$\begin{smallmatrix}CH_3\\CH_3\end{smallmatrix}$ Clomipramine (Anafranil)
$R' = Cl$

$R' = CH_2CHCH_2$ —N$\begin{smallmatrix}CH_3\\CH_3\end{smallmatrix}$ Trimipramine (Surmontil)
$|$
CH_3
$R'' = H$

$R' = (CH_2)_3$ —NH—CH$_3$ Protriptyline (Vivactil, Triptil)

DIBENZOXEPINE DERIVATIVE

Doxepin (Sinequan)

HC—CH$_2$—CH$_2$—N$\begin{smallmatrix}CH_3\\CH_3\end{smallmatrix}$

FIGURE 6-3 The three-ring structure of tricyclic antidepressants. (From Kalant H, Grant DM, Mitchell J: *Principles of medical pharmacology*, ed 7, Philadelphia, 2007, WB Saunders.)

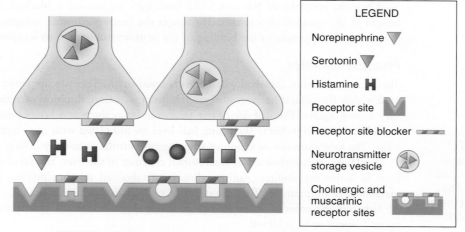

LEGEND

Norepinephrine ▽

Serotonin ▼

Histamine **H**

Receptor site ⋁

Receptor site blocker ▬

Neurotransmitter storage vesicle

Cholinergic and muscarinic receptor sites

FIGURE 6-4 Mechanism of action for tricyclic antidepressants.

Comparison of the Properties of the Tricyclic Antidepressants

Generic Name	Sedative Effects	Anticholinergic Activity	Hypotensive Effects	Cardiac Effects	Half-life (hr)	Reuptake Inhibition NE	5-HT
amitriptyline	High	High	Moderate-high	Moderate	8-24	++	++
clomipramine	Low	High	Moderate	Moderate	17-28	++	++++
desipramine	Low	Low-moderate	Moderate	Low	7-60	++++	+
doxepin	High	High	High	Moderate	6-28	++	+
imipramine	Moderate	Moderate	High	Moderate	4-18	++	+++
nortriptyline	Low-moderate	Low-moderate	Slight	Low	18-96	+++	+
protriptyline	Slight	Low-moderate	Low	Moderate	55-125	++++	+
trimipramine	High	Moderate-high	Moderate	Moderate	20-26	+	+

Key: + Low
++ Low-moderate
+++ Moderate
++++ High

Adapted from Kalant H, Grant D, Mitchell J: *Principles of medical pharmacology*, ed 7, Toronto, 2007, p 321, Saunders; Page CP, Curtis M, Sutter M, et al: Pharmacokinetic considerations with antidepressants. In *Integrated pharmacology*, Philadelphia, 2005, p 249, Saunders.

Tricyclic Antidepressants

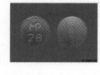

Generic Name	U.S. Brand Name(s) Canadian Brand(s)	Dosage Forms and Strengths
amitriptyline*	Generics / Elavil	**Tablets:** 10 mg, 20 mg, 50 mg, 75 mg, 100 mg[†], 150 mg[†]
desipramine*	Norpramin / Generic only	**Tablets:** 10 mg, 25 mg, 50 mg, 75 mg, 100 mg, 150 mg[†]
doxepin*	Generics, Prudoxin, Zonalon[§] / Sinequan, Zonalon[§]	**Capsules:** 10 mg, 25 mg, 50 mg, 75 mg, 100 mg, 150 mg **Solution, oral concentrate:** 10 mg/mL[†] **Cream:** 5% (Prudoxin, Zonalon)
imipramine*	Tofranil, Tofranil-PM / Tofranil	**Capsules, as pamoate (Tofranil-PM):** 75 mg, 100 mg, 125 mg, 150 mg **Tablets, as HCl (Tofranil):** 10 mg, 25 mg, 50 mg, 75 mg[‡]
nortriptyline*	Pamelor / Aventyl	**Capsules:** 10 mg, 25 mg, 50 mg, 75 mg[†] **Solution:** 10 mg/5 mL
protriptyline*	Vivactil / Not available	**Tablets:** 5 mg, 10 mg
trimipramine*	Surmontil / Generics only	**Capsules:** 12.5 mg[‡], 25 mg, 50 mg, 75 mg[‡], 100 mg

*Generic available
[†]Strength available in the United States only.
[‡]Strength available in Canada only.
[§]Prudoxin and Zonalon are topical dosage forms used for the treatment of itching.

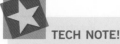

Adverse Reactions

The TCAs all have a similar structure, so the side effects of the drugs are similar. What varies is the degree to which a particular TCA will produce the side effect. For an example, all TCAs can produce sedation, but some TCAs, such as amitriptyline, have high sedative activity, but other TCAs, such as desipramine, have low sedative activity.

Adverse reactions of the TCAs are related to effects produced by increased binding to adrenergic, cholinergic, serotonergic, and histaminic receptors. A rise in NE levels is responsible for the increased cardiovascular activity caused by TCAs. On the other hand, postsynaptic adrenergic blockade is responsible for hypotension and reflex tachycardia caused by TCAs. Blockade of histaminic receptors can lead to sedation, weight gain, and hypotension. Blockade of cholinergic (muscarinic) receptors can lead to blurred vision, dry mouth, constipation, urinary retention, confusion, and delirium. The TCAs may also produce photosensitivity.

Precautions

Hypotension produced by the TCAs is a problem for elderly adults because they are at increased risk for fainting or falling. The TCAs have a narrow therapeutic index and can produce cardiotoxicity at doses that are six to eight times higher than the therapeutic dose.

SELECTIVE SEROTONIN REUPTAKE INHIBITORS

The SSRIs are the most widely prescribed antidepressants. They are categorized by their mechanisms of action rather than by their chemical structure. All are potent inhibitors of 5-HT and have little action on the reuptake of NE or DA. The SSRIs are also used in treating obsessive-compulsive disorder, premenstrual dysphoric disorder, and panic disorder and fluoxetine is also indicated for treatment of anorexia and bulimia.

Mechanism of Action

The SSRIs work by producing selective blockade of the reuptake of 5-HT at the synaptic cleft. Serotonin reuptake requires a specific transporter to move 5-HT across cell membranes, allowing for the specificity of the SSRIs. When reuptake is blocked, 5-HT remains in the synaptic cleft longer, thereby creating a greater opportunity for 5-HT binding to receptor sites.

The SSRIs are equally effective as TCAs yet they lack the cardiotoxic effects associated with the TCAs. This makes them the drugs of choice when heart disease is present.

Pharmacokinetics

The SSRIs are well absorbed from the gastrointestinal tract. They exhibit a high degree of protein binding. Fluoxetine, paroxetine, and sertraline are more than 94% protein bound. SSRIs are also extensively metabolized via the cytochrome P-450 (CYP450) isoenzyme system. Fluoxetine is metabolized to an active metabolite, which accounts for its long duration of action and relative increased length in time before reaching peak plasma levels. SSRIs interact with other drugs that are highly metabolized by CYP450 enzymes or exhibit extensive protein binding. These drug interactions may interfere with the rate of drug clearance of either the SSRI or drug that is administered with it.

Adverse Reactions

Insomnia is one of the more common side effects of SSRI administration. Fluoxetine and other SSRIs are dosed once daily in the morning to minimize nighttime sleeplessness. Other side effects include decreased appetite, nausea, agitation or anxiety, and diarrhea. Sexual dysfunction may occur as well. The most serious side effects are serotonin syndrome and suicidal ideation. Both conditions are potentially fatal. Suicidal ideation is persistent thoughts of suicide. Symptoms of **serotonin syndrome** are confusion, agitation, diarrhea, tremors, increased blood pressure, and seizures.

Precautions

The SSRIs are fairly well tolerated, but to avoid adverse reactions, the dose should be increased gradually to desired levels and the dose should be tapered to discontinue the drug. Serotonin

Comparison of Properties of Selective Serotonin Reuptake Inhibitors

Generic Name	Sedative Effects	Anticholinergic Activity	Cardiac Effects	Half-life (hr)	Receptor Blockade			Reuptake Inhibition	
					α_1	α_2	D_2	NE	5-HT
citalopram	Low	Low	Negligible	24-48	+	+/−	+/−	+	++++
fluoxetine	Low	Low	Negligible	48-72	+	+/−	+/−	+	+++
fluvoxamine	Low	Low	None	13-15	+	+/−	+	+/−	+++
paroxetine	Low	Low	Negligible	21	+	+/−	+	+	++++
sertraline	Low	Low	Negligible	24	++	+	+	+/−	++++

Selective Serotonin Reuptake Inhibitors

Generic Name	U.S. Brand Name(s) Canadian Brand(s)	Dosage Forms and Strengths
citalopram*	Celexa	Solution, oral: 10 mg/5 mL (240 mL)
	Celexa	Tablet: 10 mg, 20 mg, 40 mg
escitalopram	Lexapro	Solution, oral: 1 mg/mL (240 mL)
	Cipralex	Tablet: 5 mg†, 10 mg, 20 mg
fluoxetine*	Prozac, Prozac Weekly, Selfemra, Sarafem	Capsule (Prozac): 10 mg, 20 mg, 40 mg; (Selfemra): 10 mg, 20 mg
	Prozac	Capsule, delayed release (Prozac Weekly): 90 mg
		Oral solution (Prozac): 20 mg/5 mL
		Tablet, as HCl: 10 mg, 20 mg, 40 mg; (Sarafem): 10 mg, 15 mg, 20 mg
fluvoxamine*	Generics, Luvox CR	Capsule, extended release (Luvox CR): 100 mg, 150 mg
	Luvox	Tablet: 25 mg†, 50 mg, 100 mg
paroxetine*	Paxil, Paxil CR, Pexeva	Oral suspension (Paxil): 10 mg/5 mL
	Paxil, Paxil CR	Tablets, as HCl (Paxil): 10 mg, 20 mg, 30 mg, 40 mg†
		Tablets, as mesylate (Pexeva): 10 mg, 20 mg, 30 mg, 40 mg
		Tablets, as controlled release (Paxil CR): 12.5 mg, 25 mg, 37.5 mg†
		Oral suspension (Paxil): 10 mg/5 mL
		Tablets, as HCl (Paxil): 10 mg, 20 mg, 30 mg, 40 mg†
		Tablets, as mesylate (Pexeva): 10 mg, 20 mg, 30 mg, 40 mg
		Tablet, as controlled release (Paxil CR): 12.5 mg, 25 mg, 37.5 mg†
sertraline*	Zoloft	Solution, oral concentrate: 20 mg/mL†
	Zoloft	Tablets: 25 mg, 50 mg, 100 mg

*Generic available
†Strength available in the United States only.

syndrome can result from coadministration with the monoamine oxidase inhibitors (MAOIs). The SSRIs should be used cautiously in patients with liver disease.

MONOAMINE OXIDASE INHIBITORS

There are two forms of MAO, subtype A (MAO$_A$) and subtype B (MAO$_B$). Drugs that primarily interfere with the action of MAO$_A$ are used in the treatment of major depression and preferentially interfere with the metabolism of NE and 5-HT. MAO$_B$ is predominantly found in the brain. MAOIs that preferentially interfere with MAO$_B$ are used in the treatment of Parkinson's disease because they interfere with the metabolism of DA.

Mechanism of Action

The MAOIs interfere with the degradation of monoamine neurotransmitters and dietary amines (e.g., tyramine). Their mechanism of action is to block the action of the enzyme *monoamine oxidase* (MAO) (Figure 6-5). This enzyme is found in the terminal neuron, liver, and intestines. When no MAOI drugs are present, most of the NE, 5-HT, and DA released into the synaptic cleft is returned to the terminal neuron and inactivated by the MAO enzyme. When MAOIs are administered, neurotransmitter inactivation is inhibited, which results in more NE, 5-HT, and DA being available to bind at receptor sites.

Pharmacokinetics

The MAOIs are readily absorbed when taken orally, but elimination is slow. The drugs are categorized as reversible or irreversible inhibitors of MAO according to the time it takes for enzyme levels to return to normal when the drug is discontinued. It takes approximately 3 to 5 days for MAO levels to return to normal on discontinuation of reversible MAOIs. Recovery takes up to 2 weeks when irreversible MAOIs are administered.

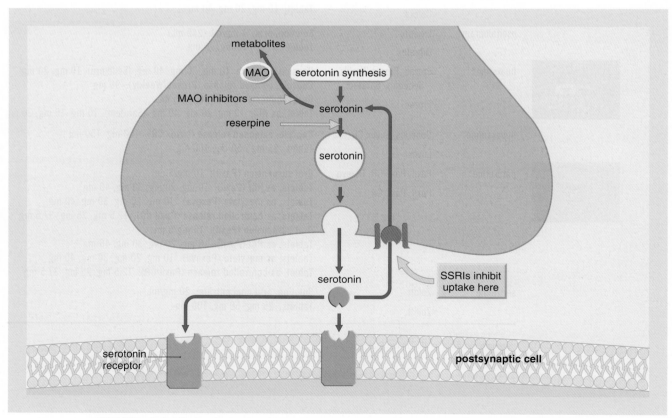

FIGURE 6-5 Mechanism of action of monoamine oxidase inhibitors. (From Page CP, Hoffman B, Curtis MJ, et al: *Integrated pharmacology*, ed 3, Philadelphia, 2006, Mosby.)

Monoamine Oxidase Inhibitors

Generic Name	U.S. Brand Name(s) Canadian Brand(s)	Dosage Forms and Strengths
moclobemide*,a	Not available	Tablets: 100 mg, 150 mg, 300 mg
	Manerix	
phenelzine^b	Nardil	Tablets: 15 mg
	Nardil	
tranylcypromine*,b	Parnate	Tablets: 10 mg
	Parnate	

*Generic available.
^aReversible MAOI.
^bIrreversible MAOI.

TABLE 6-1   **Foods and Beverages to Avoid while Taking Monoamine Oxidase Inhibitors**

Beverages	Chianti, and other red wines, alcohol-free beer, caffeine
Food	Cheeses (especially strong, aged, or processed varieties), sauerkraut, yogurt, raisins, bananas, sour cream, pickled herring, liver (especially chicken liver), dry sausage (including hard salami and pepperoni), canned figs, avocados, turkey, yeast extracts, fava beans, broad bean pods, chocolate
Seasonings	Soy sauce, papaya products (including certain meat tenderizers)

TECH NOTE!
Symptoms of hypertensive crisis are throbbing headache, neck stiffness, and palpitations.

Adverse Reactions

The MAOIs were first discovered in the 1950s, but the risk for serious side effects has limited their widespread use. Adverse reactions include sedation, dry mouth, urinary retention, constipation, orthostatic hypotension, impotence, and weight gain. The severity of these side effects is equal to or less than that of most TCAs. The most serious adverse reaction is hypertensive crisis.

Hypertensive crisis can be fatal and is caused by drug–drug and drug–food interactions with MAOIs. When MAOIs are not present, dietary amines (e.g., tyramine) are absorbed from the intestine and transported to the liver, where they are inactivated in the liver by the enzyme MAO. When MAOIs are administered, the effect of MAO in the liver is blocked, and tyramine is able to reach the general circulation. Tyramine travels to peripheral sympathetic nerve terminals, where it promotes the release of NE stores. Excess circulating NE causes blood pressure to rise to dangerously high levels and produces excessive stimulation of the heart.

Precautions

To avoid the risk of hypertensive crisis, patients taking MAOIs are advised to avoid eating certain foods and beverages (Table 6-1).

TECH NOTE!
Patients taking MAOIs should be given a list of tyramine-containing foods and a list of drugs to avoid.

SEROTONIN-NORADRENALINE REUPTAKE INHIBITORS

The TCAs and MAOIs are effective antidepressants; however, alternatives were desired that had fewer side effects and less potentially dangerous adverse reactions.

Duloxetine, desvenlafaxine and venlafaxine are serotonin-noradrenaline reuptake inhibitors (SNRIs). They inhibit the reuptake of 5-HT and NE. Dual inhibition of 5-HT and NE is more effective than inhibition of either serotonin or NE.

Adverse Reactions

Side effects are similar to those of SSRIs but, unlike the SSRIs, the SNRIs produce anticholinergic side effects and a modest increase in blood pressure and may cause hepatotoxicity. Common side effects of venlafaxine, desvenlafaxine, and duloxetine are nausea, headache, dry mouth, and dizziness. Sedation is common with venlafaxine and desvenlafaxine. Duloxetine may cause asthenia (weakness).

NORADRENALINE-DOPAMINE REUPTAKE INHIBITORS

Bupropion is classified as an aminoketone. Introduced in the 1970s as an alternative to TCAs, it does not cause drowsiness. Bupropion is rapidly absorbed and has weak effects on DA and NE reuptake.

Adverse Reactions

Although it is well tolerated, doses of bupropion that are greater than 450 mg/day or 150 mg/dose increase the risk for seizures in people with seizure disorders.

HETEROCYCLIC ANTIDEPRESSANTS

Mirtazapine is a heterocyclic antidepressant that increases NE and 5-HT release. The drug exhibits a high degree of protein binding (85%) and moderate bioavailability (50%). Mirtazapine is metabolized by hepatic microsomal enzymes and is subject to drug interactions involving activation and inhibition of CYP450 isozymes. Adverse reactions of mirtazapine are sedation, dry mouth, urinary retention, blurred vision, increased appetite, weight gain, and agranulocytosis. Trazodone is a heterocyclic antidepressant and is a weak inhibitor of 5-HT. Compared with TCAs, it produces moderate sedation and low anticholinergic activity. It may produce some cardiac stimulation. Side effects of trazodone are sedation, hypotension, nausea, and priapism (painful persistent erection).

Serotonin-Noradrenaline Reuptake Inhibitors, and Noradrenaline-Dopamine Inhibitors, and Other Antidepressants

| | U.S. Brand Name(s) | |
Generic Name	Canadian Brand(s)	Dosage Forms and Strengths
bupropion*	Wellbutrin, Wellbutrin SR, Wellbutrin XL, Zyban[1] Aplenzin	Tablets, as immediate release (Wellbutrin): 75 mg, 100 mg Tablets, as extended release 24-hour (Wellbutrin XL): 150 mg, 300 mg
	Wellbutrin SR, Wellbutrin XL, Zyban	Tablets, as hydrobromide, extended release (Aplenzin): 174 mg, 348 mg, 522 mg Tablets, as sustained release 12-hour (Wellbutrin SR): 100 mg, 150 mg, 200 mg
desvenlafaxine	Pristiq	Tablets, extended release: 50 mg, 100 mg
	Pristiq	
duloxetine	Cymbalta	Capsules, delayed release: 20 mg[†], 30 mg, 60 mg
	Cymbalta	
mirtazapine*	Remeron, Remeron SolTab	Tablets: 7.5 mg, 15 mg, 30 mg, 45 mg Tablets, orally disintegrating (Remeron SolTab, Remeron RD): 15 mg, 30 mg, 45 mg
	Remeron, Remeron RD	
trazodone*	Generics, Oleptro	Tablets: 50 mg, 68.25 mg[‡], 100 mg, 150 mg, 300 mg[†] Tablets, extended release 24-hour (Oleptro): 150 mg, 300 mg
	Generic only	
venlafaxine*	Effexor, Effexor-XR	Capsules, as extended release (Effexor-XR): 37.5 mg, 75 mg, 150 mg Tablets (Effexor): 25 mg, 37.5 mg, 50 mg, 75 mg, 100 mg Tablets, extended release: 37.5 mg, 75 mg, 150 mg, 225 mg
	Effexor, Effexor-XR	

*Generic available.
[1]Zyban is indicated for smoking cessation.
[†]Strength available in the United States only.
[‡]Strength available in Canada only.

Drugs Used to Treat Bipolar Disorder

Mood stabilizers are used in the treatment of bipolar disorder. All drugs currently indicated for the treatment of bipolar disorder have antimanic actions. Lithium is the oldest of these agents, introduced more than 50 years ago. Recently, selected medications used in the treatment of seizure have been discovered to exhibit antimanic properties. Most of the drugs currently indicated for the treatment of bipolar disorder are listed in U.S. Food and Drug Administration pregnancy category D.

Lithium is administered to reduce current symptoms of mania and depression as well as to prevent recurrence of future episodes. Lithium is thought to produce its effects by regulating cAMP (cyclic adenosine monophosphate), phosphoinositide, and calcium signal pathways. When signaling disturbances occur, lithium acts to restore order.

Lithium is rapidly absorbed from the gastrointestinal tract, which accounts for its rapid onset of action. The drug has a long half-life (24 hours), which increases the longer the patient is on lithium therapy. The half-life can double over the course of 1 year's continuous therapy. Lithium is not metabolized and is eliminated unchanged in the urine. Lithium has a narrow therapeutic index. A competitive interaction may occur between lithium and sodium in the kidneys that can result in

Drugs Used in the Treatment of Bipolar Disorder

Generic Name	U.S. Brand Name(s) Canadian Brand(s)	Dosage Forms and Strengths
lithium carbonate*	Lithobid Carbolith, Lithane	Capsules (Carbolith, Lithane): 150 mg, 300 mg, 600 mg Syrup, as citrate: 8 mEq/5 mL Tablets: 300 mg Tablets, extended release (Lithobid): 300 mg
divalproex sodium*	Depakote, Depakote ER, Depakote Sprinkle, Depacon Epival ECT	Capsules, sprinkles (Depakote Sprinkle): 125 mg Injection, solution (Depacon): 100 mg/mL Tablets, delayed release (Depakote, Epival ECT): 125 mg, 250 mg, 500 mg Tablets, extended release (Depakote ER): 250 mg, 500 mg
carbamazepine*	Carbatrol, Equetro, Epitol, Tegretol, Tegretol Chewable, Tegretol-XR Carbatrol, Equetro, Epitol, Tegretol, Tegretol Chewtabs	Capsules, extended release (Carbatrol, Equetro): 100 mg, 200 mg, 300 mg[†] Suspension: 100 mg/5 mL Tablets, chewable: 100 mg Tablets, extended release (Tegretol-XR): 100 mg, 200 mg, 400 mg
lamotrigine	Lamictal, Lamictal CD, Lamictal ODT, Lamictal XR Lamictal, Lamictal chewable	Tablets: 25 mg, 100 mg, 150 mg, 200 mg Tablets, as chewable (Lamictal CD): 2 mg[‡], 5 mg, 25 mg[†] Tablets, extended release (Lamictal XR): 25 mg, 50 mg, 100 mg, 200 mg Tablets, orally disintegrating (Lamictal ODT): 25 mg, 50 mg, 100 mg, 200 mg
fluoxetine + olanzapine	Symbyax Not available in Canada	Capsules: fluoxetine 25 mg + olanzapine 3 mg fluoxetine 25 mg + olanzapine 6 mg fluoxetine 25 mg + olanzapine 12 mg fluoxetine 50 mg + olanzapine 6 mg fluoxetine 50 mg + olanzapine 12 mg

*Generic available.
[†]Strength available in the United States only.
[‡]Strength available in Canada only.

lithium toxicity. Increased sodium intake can decrease lithium reabsorption. Dehydration can increase lithium reabsorption. Plasma lithium levels and renal function should be monitored regularly to avoid the development of lithium toxicity.

Early-onset side effects associated with lithium carbonate are sedation, nausea, increased urination, dry mouth, difficulty concentrating, and tremor. Adverse reactions associated with long-term use include weight gain, acne, impotence, hypothyroidism, rash, and hair loss.

Summary of Drugs Used in the Treatment of Depression

Generic Name	U.S. Brand Name	Usual Adult Oral Dose and Dosing Schedule	Warning Labels
Tricyclic Antidepressants			
amitriptyline	Generic	25-200 mg as a single daily dose (oral); 20-30 mg four times a day (IM)	MAY CAUSE DROWSINESS; ALCOHOL MAY INTENSIFY THIS EFFECT.
desipramine	Norpramin	150-200 mg/day (maximum dose, 300 mg/day in a single or divided doses)	MAY IMPAIR ABILITY TO DRIVE. DO NOT DISCONTINUE WITHOUT MEDICAL SUPERVISION.
doxepin	Sinequan	Initiate with 50-150 mg/day and gradually increase to 300 mg/day	AVOID PROLONGED EXPOSURE TO SUNLIGHT.
imipramine	Tofranil	Start with 25 mg 3-4 times a day (maximum dose, 300 mg/day)	MAY DISCOLOR URINE (BLUE-GREEN)—amitriptyline.
nortriptyline	Pamelor	25 mg 3-4 times per day up to 150 mg/day	
protriptyline	Vivactil	15-60 mg daily in 3-4 divided doses	
trimipramine	Surmontil	75-200 mg/day as a single bedtime dose	
Selective Serotonin Reuptake Inhibitors			
citalopram	Celexa	20-40 mg/day (maximum, 60 mg/day)	MAY IMPAIR ABILITY TO DRIVE. AVOID ALCOHOL.
escitalopram	Lexapro	20 mg/day	MAY CAUSE DIZZINESS.
fluoxetine	Prozac	20-40 mg/day or 90 mg/wk (Prozac Weekly)	SWALLOW WHOLE; DO NOT CRUSH OR CHEW (delayed release).
fluvoxamine	Generic	100 mg-300 mg daily (divide into 2 doses with larger dose at bedtime)	DO NOT DISCONTINUE WITHOUT MEDICAL SUPERVISION.
paroxetine	Paxil	20 mg/day (Paxil) Maximum dose: 50 mg/day 25 mg once daily (Paxil CR) Maximum dose: 62.5 mg/day	
sertraline	Zoloft	50-200 mg/day	
Monoamine Oxidase Inhibitors			
moclobemide	Manerix (Canada)	300-600 mg/day divided into two doses per day	TAKE WITH FOOD—moclobemide. AVOID ALCOHOL.
phenelzine	Nardil	15-90 mg 3 times a day	MAY CAUSE DIZZINESS OR DROWSINESS.
tranylcypromine	Parnate	30 mg/day in divided dose (maximum dose, 60 mg/day)	DO NOT DISCONTINUE WITHOUT MEDICAL SUPERVISION.

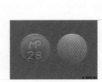

Summary of Drugs Used in the Treatment of Depression—cont'd

	Generic Name	U.S. Brand Name	Usual Adult Oral Dose and Dosing Schedule	Warning Labels
Serotonin-Noradrenaline Reuptake Inhibitors, Noradrenaline-Dopamine Reuptake Inhibitors, and Other Antidepressants				
	bupropion	Wellbutrin	For depression: 100 mg 2-3 times a day (immediate release); 150 mg twice a day (sustained release); 300 mg/day (extended release)	MAY CAUSE DIZZINESS OR DROWSINESS. MAY IMPAIR ABILITY TO DRIVE. AVOID ALCOHOL. TAKE WITH FOOD—trazodone, venlafaxine. SWALLOW WHOLE; DO NOT CRUSH OR CHEW (extended and sustained release). DO NOT DISCONTINUE WITHOUT MEDICAL SUPERVISION.
	duloxetine	Cymbalta	40-60 mg/day	
	mirtazapine	Remeron	15-45 mg/day (dosed at bedtime)	
	trazodone	Desyrel	150 mg 3 times a day (maximum dose, 600 mg/day)	
	venlafaxine	Effexor	75-375 mg/day in 2-3 divided doses (immediate release) or 75-225/day (extended release)	

Summary of Drugs Used in the Treatment of Bipolar Affective Disorder

	Generic Name	U.S. Brand Name	Usual Adult Oral Dose and Dosing Schedule	Warning labels
	lithium	Lithonate	900-1800 mg/day in 3-4 divided doses (immediate release) or 900-1200 mg/day in 2 divided doses (sustained release)	MAY CAUSE DIZZINESS OR DROWSINESS; MAY IMPAIR ABILITY TO DRIVE. AVOID ALCOHOL. TAKE WITH FOOD. DRINK PLENTY OF WATER—lithium, Symbyax. SWALLOW WHOLE; DO NOT CRUSH OR CHEW (controlled or slow release). AVOID PREGNANCY—divalproex, carbamazepine, lithium. DO NOT DISCONTINUE WITHOUT MEDICAL SUPERVISION. AVOID PROLONGED EXPOSURE TO SUN—Symbyax.
	divalproex sodium	Depakote	750-1500 mg/day in divided doses	
	carbamazepine	Tegretol	400 mg/day in 2 divided doses (maximum, 1600 mg per day)	
	lamotrigine	Lamictal	100 mg-200 mg/day	
	fluoxetine + olanzapine	Symbyax	25 mg fluoxetine/6 mg olanzapine every evening; may increase to 75 mg/18 mg	

Valproic acid, carbamazepine, and lamotrigine are antiseizure drugs with demonstrated efficacy in the treatment of bipolar disorder. They are indicated as an adjunct to lithium therapy or when lithium administration has not produced desired results. Side effects of valproic acid and its salts, divalproex sodium and sodium valproate, include sedation, nausea, ataxia, and liver dysfunction. The side effects of carbamazepine include sedation, dizziness, ataxia, and visual disturbances. Lamotrigine is used in the treatment of bipolar disorder and seizures, and side effects include sedation, nausea, ataxia, blurred vision, double vision, and rash. The use of valproic acid, carbamazepine, and lamotrigine in the treatment of seizure disorder is described in Chapter 9.

Aripiprazole (Abilify) is a dopamine system stabilizer that is used in the treatment of schizophrenia (see Chapter 7) and to manage agitation associated with bipolar disorder and is an adjunctive treatment for major depression. Drowsiness or insomnia, fatigue, and headache are the most common side effects. Tremor and extrapyramidal symptoms may also occur.

Chapter Summary

- Depressive disorders affect nearly 23.8 million Americans in a given year, and at some time in their lives, one in 10 Canadians will be affected.
- Depression affects self-esteem, moods, thoughts, eating, and sleeping; reduces the ability to think and concentrate; and produces feelings of worthlessness or guilt.
- Major depression is associated with persistent feelings of sadness, emptiness, or hopelessness.
- Bipolar disorder is associated with sudden swings in mood between depression and periods of mania.
- Dysthymia produces symptoms that are chronic and keep the person from functioning well.
- According to the biogenic amine theory, clinical depression results from a decrease in monoamine neurotransmitters in the brain.
- Bipolar affective disorder (mania) is believed to be associated with increased levels of monoamine neurotransmitters.
- Monoamine neurotransmitters associated with depression and bipolar disorder are norepinephrine (NE), serotonin (5-HT), and dopamine (DA).
- The mechanisms of action for drugs used to treat depression may differ; however, all antidepressants are equally effective.
- Inhibition of the reuptake of specific monoamine neurotransmitters is one of the ways antidepressants produce their effects. The other mechanism of action is to block the degradation of monoamine neurotransmitters.
- Selection of one antidepressant over another is based on the patient's ability to tolerate drug side effects.
- Tricyclic antidepressants (TCAs) are the oldest class of medication used in the treatment of depression.
- The TCAs are nonspecific reuptake inhibitors of monoamine neurotransmitters.
- The selective serotonin reuptake inhibitors (SSRIs) work by producing selective blockade of the reuptake of serotonin at the synaptic cleft.
- The SSRIs are equally effective as the TCAs yet lack the cardiotoxic effects associated with TCAs.
- The monoamine oxidase inhibitors (MAOI) interfere with the degradation of monoamine neurotransmitters and dietary amines (e.g., tyramine).
- Hypertensive crisis is a life-threatening adverse reaction caused by drug–drug and drug–food interactions with MAOIs.
- Lithium is administered to treat bipolar disorder. It reduces current symptoms of mania and depression and prevents recurrence of future episodes.
- Lithium has a narrow therapeutic index.

1. A mental health illness associated with persistent feelings of sadness, emptiness, or hopeless-ness that persists for several weeks is _____.
   a. bipolar disorder
   b. obsessive-compulsive disorder
   c. major depression
   d. schizophrenia

2. Antidepressants are categorized according to the method that they use to potentiate the actions of _____ neurotransmitters.
   a. norepinephrine
   b. serotonin
   c. dopamine
   d. a, b, and c

3. Antidepressants that are prescribed for enuresis, commonly known as bedwetting are
   a. SSRIs
   b. TCAs
   c. MAOIs
   d. GABAs

4. The most widely prescribed class of antidepressants is
   a. TCAs
   b. SSRIs
   c. MAOIs
   d. PPIs

5. The brand name for citalopram is
   a. Celexa
   b. Celebrex
   c. Cerebryx
   d. none of the above

6. Which SSRI is indicated for the treatment of major depression, anorexia and bulimia, obsessive-compulsive disorder, premenstrual dysphoric disorder, and panic disorder?
   a. Zoloft
   b. Lexapro
   c. Celexa
   d. Prozac

7. To avoid the risk of hypertensive crisis, patients taking _____ are advised to avoid eating certain foods containing tyramine.
   a. SSRIs
   b. TCAs
   c. MAOIs
   d. a and b

8. Two examples of MAOIs are
   a. Nardil
   b. Parnate
   c. Tofranil
   d. a and b

9. Bupropion is indicated for the treatment of depression and smoking cessation.
   a. true
   b. false

10. An example of a serotonin-noradrenaline reuptake inhibitor is
    a. fluoxetine
    b. sertraline
    c. venlafaxine
    d. nortriptyline

11. Valproic acid, carbamazepine, and lamotrigine are _____ drugs with demonstrated efficacy in the treatment of bipolar disorder.
    a. antiseizure
    b. antidepressant
    c. antimania
    d. antianxiety

12. The oldest drug used to treat bipolar disorder is _____.
    a. fluoxetine
    b. tranylcypromine
    c. lithium
    d. escitalopram

TECHNICIAN'S CORNER

1. For patients taking MAOI antidepressants, what kinds of foods can they eat?
2. What is the difference between "feeling blue" and major depression?

Bibliography

Kalant H, Grant D, Mitchell J: *Principles of medical pharmacology*, ed 7, Toronto, 2007, Elsevier Canada, A Division of Reed Elsevier Canada, pp 316-333.

Lance L, Lacy C, Armstrong L, et al: *Drug information handbook for the allied health professional*, ed 12, Hudson, OH, 2005, APhA Lexi-Comp.

National Institute of Mental Health: *Depression*, Bethesda, MD, 2002, National Institute of Mental Health, National Institutes of Health, U.S. Department of Health and Human Services. NIH Publication No. 02-3561.

National Institute of Mental Health: (January 21, 2011). The Numbers Count: Mental Disorders in America Retrieved January 22, 2011, from http://www.nimh.nih.gov/health/publications/the-numbers-count-mental-disorders-in-america/index.shtml.

Neurological protein may hold the key to new treatments for depression-*Press release*, Toronto, 2010, Centre for Addiction and Mental Health.

Page C, Curtis M, Sutter M, et al: *Integrated pharmacology*, Philadelphia, 2005, Elsevier Mosby, pp 239-241.

Statistics Canada: Mental health profiles. Retrieved from http://www.statcan.ca/english/freepub/82-617-XIE/tables.htm. Updated 2004. Accessed November 1, 2007.

7

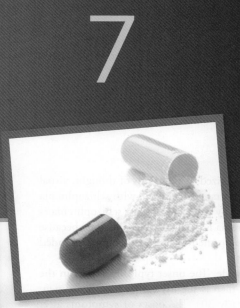

Treatment of Schizophrenia and Psychoses

LEARNING OBJECTIVES

1 Learn the terminology associated with schizophrenia.

2 Describe the symptoms of schizophrenia.

3 List and describe the function of neurotransmitters associated with the symptoms of schizophrenia and psychoses.

4 Classify medications used to treat schizophrenia and psychoses.

5 Describe the mechanism of action for each class of drugs used to treat schizophrenia and psychoses.

6 Identify warning labels and precautionary messages associated with medications used to treat schizophrenia and psychoses.

7 Identify significant drug look-alike/sound-alike issues.

KEY TERMS

Catatonia: Symptom of schizophrenia associated with unresponsiveness and immobility.

Delusion: Irrational thoughts or false beliefs that dominate a person's behavior and viewpoint and do not change even when evidence is provided that beliefs are not valid.

Extrapyramidal symptoms: Excessive muscle movement (motor activity) associated with use of neuroleptics that includes muscular rigidity, tremor, bradykinesia (slow movement), and difficulty in walking.

Hallucination: Visions or voices that exist only in the mind and cannot be seen or heard by others.

Negative symptoms: Sign of schizophrenia that is associated with decreased ability to think, plan, or express emotion.

Neuroleptic: Drug used to treat schizophrenia and psychoses.

Neuroleptic malignant syndrome: Potentially fatal reaction to administration of neuroleptics. Symptoms include stupor, muscle rigidity, and high temperature.

Positive symptoms: Hallucinations, delusions, or other unusual thoughts or perceptions that are symptoms of schizophrenia.

Postural hypotension: Drop in blood pressure caused by a change in posture.

Pseudoparkinsonism: Adverse reaction to the administration of neuroleptics characterized by symptoms mimicking Parkinson's disease.

Psychosis: Mental state characterized by disorganized behavior and thought, delusions, hallucinations, and a loss of touch with reality.

Schizophrenia: Type of psychosis characterized by delusions of thought, visual or auditory hallucinations (or both), and speech disturbances. Paranoid schizophrenia is characterized by delusions of persecution.

Tardive dyskinesia: Inappropriate postures of the neck, trunk, and limbs accompanied by involuntary thrusting of the tongue.

Overview

Schizophrenia is a chronic and major *psychosis* that is characterized by delusions of thought, visual or auditory hallucinations (or both), and speech disturbances. Persons diagnosed with schizophrenia often see visions or hear voices that cannot be seen or heard by others. Paranoid schizophrenia is characterized by delusions of persecution. Paranoid schizophrenia is particularly challenging because the patient may believe that the health care team is prescribing medicines and therapies intended to cause harm.

Schizophrenia affects about 1% of the population worldwide. The onset typically occurs in the late teens, after puberty begins, to the mid-20s; the onset in men is slightly earlier than in women, who may not develop symptoms until the mid-20s to the early 30s. The onset of symptoms after age 45 years is rare. Schizophrenia runs in families, and 10% of persons diagnosed with schizophrenia have a sibling or relative who has schizophrenia. If the sibling is an identical twin, the risk for schizophrenia increases to 40% to 65%. Environmental factors, exposure to viruses, fetal malnutrition, and substance abuse are also thought to influence the development of schizophrenia.

People diagnosed with schizophrenia often exhibit negative symptoms, positive symptoms, and cognitive symptoms. *Negative symptoms* are associated with a flat affect. This means that no visible sign of emotion is exhibited. Speech is monotonous, and no facial expressions are apparent. People exhibiting negative symptoms do not interact socially with others and communicate infrequently. *Positive symptoms* may appear as bizarre behavior. People diagnosed with untreated schizophrenia have often lost touch with reality. They may have delusions. *Delusions* are irrational thoughts or false beliefs that dominate a person's behavior. The person's viewpoint is unlikely to change even when evidence is provided that the beliefs are not valid. An example of a delusion is the belief that television characters are broadcasting personal messages to the person with schizophrenia. People with schizophrenia may also have visual or auditory *hallucinations*. They respond to visions and voices that only they can see. They may talk to themselves or, when speaking to others, may fail to complete sentences (their thoughts may be finished in their mind). Their thoughts are often disorganized. Cognitive symptoms associated with schizophrenia may interfere with the performance of routine activities of daily living. Memory loss may impede the person's ability to function on a job. Cognitive symptoms decrease the person's capacity to interpret information and make decisions.

Schizophrenia also produces physical symptoms. The person may be clumsy and appear catatonic or make repetitive movements. People who exhibit symptoms of *catatonia* are unresponsive and immobile.

Neurochemistry of Schizophrenia and Psychoses

Schizophrenia is thought to be associated with excess dopamine levels. Drugs capable of blocking transmission of signals in the dopaminergic system, located in the midbrain and hypothalamus, are used in the treatment of schizophrenia. Mesocortical dopamine tracts project to various emotional areas of the brain involved in cognition and regulation of motivation and emotion. The nigrostriatal pathway also originates in the midbrain and is involved in the control of excessive muscle movement. Treatments for schizophrenia that involve dopamine blockade can produce *pseudoparkinsonism*, Parkinson's disease–like symptoms (e.g., tremor and bradykinesia) as a side effect.

It is now known that other mechanisms of action may be involved in the treatment of schizophrenia. Other neurotransmitters that have been identified as playing a role in symptoms of schizophrenia include serotonin, cholecystokinin (CCK), neurotensin, γ-aminobutyric acid (GABA), and glutamate (Figure 7-1).

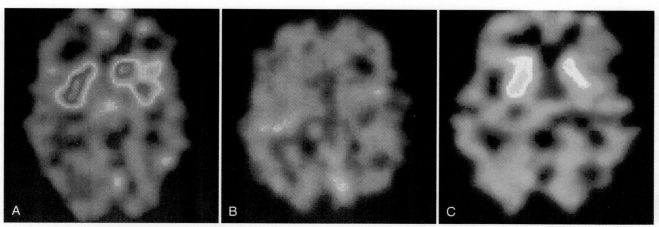

FIGURE 7-1 The cerebral distribution of dopamine receptors in treated and untreated schizophrenia. **A,** Striatal dopamine receptors in untreated schizophrenia. **B,** Complete blockade of receptors with typical neuroleptic. **C,** Partial blockade of receptors with equally effective dose of clozapine. (From Page CP, Hoffman BB, Curtis MJ, et al: *Integrated pharmacology,* ed 3, Philadelphia, 2006, Mosby.)

ROLE OF DOPAMINE

Of all the neurotransmitters involved in symptoms and treatment of schizophrenia, dopamine is considered most significant. All *neuroleptic* agents bind to dopamine receptors, and blockade of dopamine (D_2) receptors remains the primary therapeutic target for the treatment of schizophrenia. The greater the affinity the drug has for D_2 receptors, the more effective is the drug. Unfortunately, dopamine receptor blockade in the nigrostriatal tract produces Parkinson's disease–like symptoms (pseudoparkinsonism) that are associated with treatment using some classifications of neuroleptics. Some of the newer atypical neuroleptics have a lower affinity for D_2 receptors yet are clinically effective.

ROLE OF SEROTONIN

Serotonin (5-hydroxytryptamine [5-HT]) receptor blockade is a mechanism of action for some classifications of neuroleptics. Drugs that antagonize $5\text{-}HT_{2A}$ and $5\text{-}HT_{2C}$ receptors are useful in the treatment of negative symptoms of schizophrenia. Antagonism of $5\text{-}HT_{2A}$ receptors protects against long-term motor effects associated with some neuroleptic agents. Drugs that antagonize $5\text{-}HT_3$ receptors are also used to treat schizophrenia.

MISCELLANEOUS NEUROTRANSMITTERS AND SCHIZOPHRENIA

Cholecystokinin is a peptide neurotransmitter. It is believed to play a role in the release of dopamine and thought to be associated with the auditory hallucinations of schizophrenia. Neurotensin is a peptide neurotransmitter. Decreased level of neurotensin in the cerebrospinal fluid is thought to be associated with increased psychosis. Neuroleptic-induced increases in neurotensin is believed to improve negative symptoms of schizophrenia. The role of GABA is not fully understood; however, abnormalities of the GABA system are believed to be associated with working memory deficits in schizophrenia. GABAergic interneurons fail to synthesize and release enough GABA. Glutamate is an amino acid that acts as an excitatory neurotransmitter in the central nervous system. The role of glutamate in schizophrenia is not fully known; however, studies show that interference with glutamate signaling in the brain decreases psychosis.

Drugs Used to Treat Schizophrenia and Psychosis

Neuroleptics are classified by structure and function. Functionally, all neuroleptics fall into two classes based on their affinity for dopamine receptors. High-potency neuroleptics have a strong affinity for dopamine receptors. "Atypical" and low-potency neuroleptics have a weaker affinity for dopamine receptors and produce fewer side effects associated with blockade. Regardless of their potency, all of the neuroleptic agents are equally effective. Selection of agents is based on a balance between the achievement of the desired response and the patient's ability to tolerate drug side effects.

CONVENTIONAL "TYPICAL" NEUROLEPTICS AND "ATYPICAL" NEUROLEPTICS

Phenothiazines, butyrophenones, and thioxanthines are categorized as "conventional" neuroleptics. They are classified as low, medium, and high potency. The prototype for low-potency neuroleptics is chlorpromazine; medium potency, fluphenazine; and high potency, haloperidol. All other types of neuroleptics are categorized as "atypical." Clozapine (thienobenzodiazepines), risperidone (benzixasoles), and aripiprazole (quinolinones) are examples of atypical neuroleptics.

Mechanism of Action

Traditional neuroleptics block dopamine at postsynaptic receptor sites located in the basal ganglia, hypothalamus, limbic system, brainstem, and medulla. They have a strong alpha-adrenergic blocking action that accounts for the hypotension produced by traditional neuroleptics (Figure 7-2).

Atypical neuroleptics such as clozapine show strong affinity for serotonin receptors in addition to the dopaminergic receptor blockade. Aripiprazole, a quinolinone, is a dopamine system stabilizer. It is a partial dopamine (D_2) agonist with serotonin agonist (5-HT_{1A}) and antagonist (5-HT_{2A}) activity.

Pharmacokinetics

Traditional neuroleptics are well absorbed orally, rectally, and parenterally. They readily cross the blood-brain barrier because of their lipid solubility and are up to 90% bound to plasma proteins. They are rapidly metabolized in the liver and produce active metabolites that are stored in fatty tissue (tissue binding). Paliperidone is the active metabolite of risperidone. This reduces the bioavailability for oral routes of administration. Rectal and parenteral routes of administration have increased bioavailability. Neuroleptics are eliminated in the urine.

Several of the phenothiazines are available in slow release depot formulations for intramuscular injection. The therapeutic effects of fluphenazine deconoate and haloperidol persist for up to 4 weeks after injection.

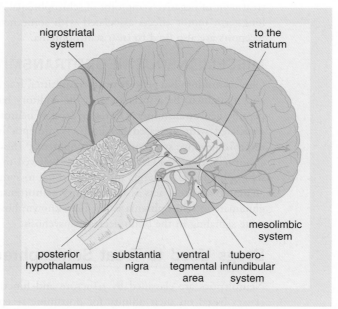

FIGURE 7-2 Dopamine pathways. (From Page CP, Hoffman BB, Curtis MJ, et al: *Integrated pharmacology*, ed 3, Philadelphia, 2006, Mosby.)

Many atypical neuroleptics are also actively metabolized in the liver. Coadministration of strong CYP3A4 inhibitors (e.g., ketoconazole) or inducers (rifampin) are contraindicated in patients taking lurasidone. Although not contraindicated, coadministration may require dosage adjustment in patients taking aripiprazole. Atypical neuroleptics are also available in dosage forms designed for rapid action (e.g., oral disintegrating tablets), extended-release tablets, and monthly intramuscular injection.

Adverse Reactions

Up to 80% of the people who are prescribed neuroleptics will experience adverse reactions (Table 7-1). Most adverse reactions are predictable and associated with dopaminergic, serotonergic, cholinergic, alpha-adrenergic, or histaminergic blockade (H1). Adverse effects are classified as central nervous system effects and peripheral nervous system effects. Sedation (histamine blockade), confusion, decreased ability to regulate body temperature, weight gain, increased appetite, and increased release of some endocrine hormones are central nervous system effects. Increased release of prolactin can produce pseudopregnancy-type symptoms. Extrapyramidal effects and tardive dyskinesia are associated with dopaminergic blockade and occur more frequently in elderly patients. **Extrapyramidal symptoms** are exhibited as excessive muscle movement. **Tardive dyskinesia** causes inappropriate postures of the neck, trunk, and limbs and is accompanied by involuntary thrusting of the tongue and lip smacking. There is no effective prevention or treatment for tardive dyskinesia.

Newer atypical neuroleptics such as ziprasidone and olanzapine have less risk for extrapyramidal symptoms, but they are associated with hyperglycemia and the onset of diabetes.

Peripheral nervous system adverse effects include blurred vision, dry mouth and urinary retention (cholinergic blockade), **postural hypotension**—a drop in blood pressure caused by a change in posture (alpha-adrenergic blockade), hepatotoxicity and jaundice, bone marrow depression, photosensitivity, and failure to ejaculate.

TABLE 7-1 **Comparison of Side Effects of Neuroleptics**

Generic Name	Sedative Effects	Anticholinergic Activity	Hypotensive Effects	Extrapyramidal Effects	Drug-Induced Diabetes	Drug-Induced Jaundice
High Potency						
Fluphenazine	+	+	+	+++	–	++
Thiothixene	+	+	+	+++	–	–
Trifluoperazine	+	+	+	+++	–	++
Medium Potency						
Loxapine	+		+	++	–	
Molindone	+		+	++	–	
Perphenazine	+		+	++	–	++
Low Potency						
Chlorpromazine	+++	+++	+++	+	–	++
Mesoridazine	+++	+++	+++	+	–	++
Thioridazine	+++	+++	+++	+	–	++
"Atypical"						
Quetiapine	+	+	+	++	++	–
Risperidone	+	+	+	++	+	–
Olanzapine	+++	+	+++	+/–	++	–

TECH ALERT!
The FDA requires a boxed warning be included in the labeling of all atypical neuroleptics stating the agents are associated with hyperglycemia and the onset of diabetes.

Precautions

Neuroleptic malignant syndrome is a life-threatening side effect of neuroleptic administration. It produces symptoms of muscle rigidity, increased body temperature (hyperthermia), fluctuating consciousness, and renal failure. Clozapine use is restricted because it can produce a fatal drop in white blood cells (agranulocytosis). Patients on clozapine therapy are required to have white blood cell levels monitored weekly when starting the medication.

Neuroleptic agents should be used cautiously in patients with seizure disorders. Low-potency agents and clozapine are most likely to induce seizures. The atypical neuroleptics are associated with an increased risk for diabetes and cardiovascular morbidity and mortality.

TYPICAL NEUROLEPTICS

Phenothiazines

Generic Name	U.S. Brand Name(s) / Canadian Brand(s)	Dosage Forms and Strengths
chlorpromazine*	Generic only	Injection, solution: 25 mg/mL
	Generic only	Tablets: 10 mg†, 25 mg, 50 mg, 100 mg, 200 mg†
fluphenazine*	Generic only	Elixir, as hydrochloride (U.S. only): 2.5 mg/5 mL
	Modecate	Injection, in oil as deconoate: 25 mg/mL, 100 mg/mL (Modecate) Injection, hydrochloride solution: 2.5 mg/mL Solution, oral concentrate (U.S. only): 5 mg/mL Tablets: 1 mg, 2 mg‡, 2.5 mg, 5 mg‡, 10 mg†
perphenazine*	Generic only	Liquid, oral concentrate (Canada only): 3.2 mg/mL
	Generic only	Tablets: 2 mg, 4 mg, 8 mg, 16 mg
thioridazine*	Generic only	Tablets: 10 mg, 25 mg, 50 mg, 100 mg
	Not available in Canada	
trifluoperazine*	Generic only	Syrup, oral (Canada only): 1 mg/mL, 10 mg/mL
	Generic only	Tablets: 1 mg, 2 mg, 5 mg, 10 mg

*Generic available.
†Strength available in the United States only.
‡Strength available in Canada only.

Butyrophenones

Generic Name	U.S. Brand Name(s) / Canadian Brand(s)	Dosage Forms and Strengths
haloperidol*	Generic only	Injection, oil, as deconoate: 50 mg/mL; 100 mg/mL
	Generic only	Injection, solution, as lactate: 5 mg/mL Solution, oral concentrate: 2 mg/mL Tablets: 0.5 mg, 1 mg, 2 mg, 5 mg, 10 mg, 20 mg

*Generic available.

Thioxanthenes

Generic Name	U.S. Brand Name(s) / Canadian Brand(s)	Dosage Forms and Strengths
thiothixene*	Navane	Capsules: 1 mg†, 2 mg, 5 mg, 10 mg, 20 mg†
	Navane	

*Generic available.
†Strength available in the United States only.

ATYPICAL NEUROLEPTICS

Adverse reactions for clozapine are sedation, headache, dizziness, nausea, weight gain, hypotension, and tachycardia. Agranulocytosis occurs in 1% to 2% of patients.

Dibenzodiazepines

Generic Name	U.S. Brand Name(s) Canadian Brand(s)	Dosage Forms and Strengths
clozapine*	Clozaril, Fazaclo Generics	Tablets (Clozaril): 25 mg, 50 mg, 100 mg, 200 mg Tablets, oral disintegrating (Fazaclo): 12.5 mg, 25 mg, 100 mg, 150 mg, 200 mg

*Generic available.

THIENOBENZODIAZEPINES

Olanzapine is used in the treatment and management of schizophrenia and bipolar disorder. Adverse reactions are sedation, headache, dizziness, nausea, weight gain, hyperglycemia and diabetes, hypotension, and tachycardia. Extrapyramidal symptoms occur rarely at high doses.

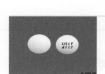

Thienobenzodiazepines

Generic Name	U.S. Brand Name(s) Canadian Brand(s)	Dosage Forms and Strengths
olanzapine*	Zyprexa, Zyprexa Relprevv, Zyprexa Zydis Zyprexa, Zyprexa Zydis	Injection, powder for reconstitution: 10 mg Injection, extended-release powder (Zyprexa Relprevv): 210 mg, 300 mg, 405 mg Tablets: 2.5 mg, 5 mg, 7.5 mg, 10 mg, 15 mg, 20 mg Tablets, oral disintegrating (Zyprexa Zydis): 5 mg, 10 mg, 15 mg, 20 mg

*Generic available.

BENZISOXAZOLES

Risperidone, paliperidone, and iloperidone are used in the treatment and management of schizophrenia, and risperidone is also indicated for the treatment of bipolar disorder. Side effects include sedation, dizziness, dry mouth, nausea, tremor, hyperglycemia and diabetes, postural hypotension, urinary retention, sexual dysfunction, restlessness, and extrapyramidal symptoms (occurs rarely at high doses). The drugs may cause QT interval prolongation, so they should be used cautiously in patients with heart disease.

DIBENZOTHIAZEPINES

Quetiapine is used in the treatment and management of patients with schizophrenia and bipolar disorder. Side effects include sedation, headache, dizziness, hypotension, and impaired thermoregulation. Similar to other atypical neuroleptics, quetiapine may cause hyperglycemia and diabetes.

BENZOISOTHIAZOL DERIVATIVES

Lurasidone and ziprasidone are used in the treatment of patients with schizophrenia, and ziprasidone is also approved for the treatment of bipolar disorder. Side effects include sedation, headache, weight gain, dizziness, hypotension, impaired thermoregulation, and hyperglycemia and diabetes. Blood glucose levels should be monitored in patients with diabetes.

OTHER ATYPICAL NEUROLEPTICS

Aripiprazole in a dopamine system stabilizer and is partial dopamine agonist. Asenapine action is produced by antagonism of dopamine (D_2) and serotonin ($5\text{-}HT_{2A}$). The side effects of aripiprazole and asenapine include confusion, weight gain, nausea, dizziness, increased urination, hunger, thirst, impaired thermoregulation, and hyperglycemia. Blood glucose levels should be monitored in patients

Benzisoxazoles

Generic Name	U.S. Brand Name(s) Canadian Brand(s)	Dosage Forms and Strengths
iloperidone	Fanapt, Fanapt Titration pack	Tablets: 1 mg, 2 mg, 4 mg, 6 mg, 8 mg, 10 mg, 12 mg
	Not available in Canada	
risperidone*	Risperdal, Risperdal Consta, Risperdal M-tabs	Injection (Risperdal Consta): 12.5 mg, 25 mg, 37.5 mg, 50 mg (vials and prefilled syringes) Solution, oral: 1 mg/mL Tablets: 0.25 mg, 0.5 mg, 1 mg, 2 mg, 3 mg, 4 mg Tablet, oral disintegrating (Risperdal M-tablets): 0.5 mg, 1 mg, 2 mg, 3 mg, 4 mg
	Risperdal	
paliperidone	Invega, Invega Sustenna	Suspension, for extended-release injection (Invega Sustenna): 39 mg/0.25 mL†, 50 mg 0.5 mL‡, 78 mg/0.5 mL†, 75 mg/0.75 mL‡, 117 mg/0.75 mL†, 100 mg/1 mL‡, 150 mg/1.5 mL‡, 156 mg/1 mL†, 234 mg/1.5 mL Tablet, extended release (Invega): 1.5 mg†, 3 mg, 6 mg, 9 mg
	Invega, Invega Sustenna	

*Generic available.
†Strength available in the United States only.
‡Strength available in Canada only.

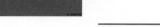

Dibenzothiazepines

Generic Name	U.S. Brand Name(s) Canadian Brand(s)	Dosage Forms and Strengths
quetiapine∞	Seroquel, Seroquel XR	Tablets: 25 mg, 50 mg, 100 mg, 200 mg, 300 mg, 400 mg† Tablets, extended release (Seroquel XR): 50 mg, 150 mg, 200 mg, 300 mg, 400 mg
	Seroquel, Seroquel XR	

∞Generic available in Canada.
†Strength available in the United States only.

Benzoisothiazol Derivatives

Generic Name	U.S. Brand Name(s) Canadian Brand(s)	Dosage Forms and Strengths
ziprasidone*	Geodon	Injection, powder for reconstitution:## 20 mg Tablets: 20 mg, 40 mg, 60 mg, 80 mg
	Zeldox	
lurasidone	Latuda	Tables: 40 mg, 80 mg
	Not available in Canada	

*Generic available.
##Available in the United States only.

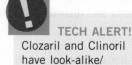

TECH ALERT!
Clozaril and Clinoril have look-alike/sound-alike issues.

TECH ALERT!
Zyprexa, Celexa, and Zyrtec have look-alike/sound-alike issues.

with diabetes. Aripiprazole may additionally cause insomnia, and asenapine may cause drowsiness. Aripiprazole and asenapine labeling have a boxed warning: Elderly patients with dementia-related psychosis treated with antipsychotic drugs are at an increased risk of death. Mortality is most commonly due to sudden heart failure, sudden death, or infection. Both drugs may produce suicidal thoughts and cause hyperglycemia and diabetes.

DIBENZOXAZEPINE

Loxapine is an atypical antipsychotic drug that is structurally similar to the antidepressant amoxapine. Adverse reactions include drowsiness, dizziness, photosensitivity, and hypotension.

TECH NOTE!
Risperidone oral solution should not be diluted with cola or tea.

TECH NOTE!
Dispense haloperidol, loxapine, risperidone, and aripiprazole oral solutions with the measuring device provided with packaging.

Other Atypical Neuroleptics

Generic Name	U.S. brand Name(s) Canadian Brand(s)	Dosage Forms and Strengths
aripiprazole	Abilify, Abilify Discmelt Abilify	Solution, for injection: 9.75 mg/1.3 mL## Solution, oral: 1 mg/mL## Tablets, disintegrating (Abilify Discmelt): 10 mg, 15 mg Tablets: 2 mg, 5 mg, 10 mg, 15 mg, 20 mg, 30 mg
asenapine	Saphris Not available in Canada	Tablets, sublingual: 5 mg, 10 mg

##Available in the United States only.

Dibenzoxazepines

Generic Name	U.S. Brand Name(S) Canadian Brand(s)	Dosage Forms and Strengths
loxapine*	Loxitane Loxapac IM	Capsules: 5 mg, 10 mg, 25 mg, 50 mg Injection (Loxapac IM): 50 mg/mL Solution, oral: 25 mg/mL

*Generic available.

Summary of Drugs Used in the Treatment of Psychosis

Generic Name	U.S. Brand Name	Usual Adult Oral Dose and Dosing Schedule	Warning Labels
Phenothiazines			
chlorpromazine	Generics	25-2000 mg/day in 1-4 divided doses (oral) or 300 mg-800 mg/day IM or IV (maintenance dose)	MAY CAUSE DROWSINESS; MAY IMPAIR ABILITY TO DRIVE; AVOID ALCOHOL. MAINTAIN ADEQUATE HYDRATION. AVOID PROLONGED EXPOSURE TO SUNLIGHT.
fluphenazine	Generics	Oral: 2.5-10 mg/day dosed every 6-8 hours (maximum, 10 mg/day) IM (as HCl): 2.5 mg-10 mg/day or IM (as deconoate) 12.5 mg every 3 weeks	DO NOT DISCONTINUE WITHOUT MEDICAL SUPERVISION. DILUTE ORAL CONCENTRATE BEFORE ADMINISTERING—chlorpromazine, fluphenazine.
perphenazine	Generics	4-16 mg 2-4 times a day (maximum, 64 mg/day)	MAY DISCOLOR URINE (PINK-REDDISH BROWN)—thioridazine. MAY CAUSE DRY MOUTH. CHEWING GUM OR SUCKING SUGARLESS CANDY MAY IMPROVE SYMPTOMS.
thioridazine	Generics	50-100 mg 3 times a day up to 800 mg/day divided in 2-4 doses	
trifluoperazine	Generics	Oral: 1-2 mg twice daily (maximum, 40 mg) IM: 1-2 mg every 4-6 hours (maximum, 6 mg/24 hours)	
Butyrophenones			
haloperidol	Generics	Oral: 0.5-5 mg 2-3 times/day (maximum, 30 mg/day) IM (lactate): 2-10 mg every 4-8 hours IM (deconoate): 15 mg-150 mg once every 4 weeks.	MAY CAUSE DROWSINESS; MAY IMPAIR ABILITY TO DRIVE; AVOID ALCOHOL. DO NOT DISCONTINUE WITHOUT MEDICAL SUPERVISION. DILUTE ORAL CONCENTRATE BEFORE ADMINISTRATION. MAINTAIN ADEQUATE HYDRATION. AVOID PROLONGED EXPOSURE TO SUNLIGHT.

Continued

Summary of Drugs Used in the Treatment of Psychosis—cont'd

Generic Name	U.S. Brand Name	Usual Adult Oral Dose and Dosing Schedule	Warning Labels
Thioxanthenes			
thiothixene	Navane	2 mg 3 times a day (maximum, 60 mg/day)	MAY CAUSE DROWSINESS; MAY IMPAIR ABILITY TO DRIVE; AVOID ALCOHOL. DO NOT DISCONTINUE WITHOUT MEDICAL SUPERVISION. MAINTAIN ADEQUATE HYDRATION. AVOID PROLONGED EXPOSURE TO SUNLIGHT.
Dibenzodiazepines			
clozapine	Clozaril	Begin 12.5 mg 1-2 times a day; increase to 300-400 mg/day (maximum, 600-900 mg/day)	MAY CAUSE DROWSINESS; MAY IMPAIR ABILITY TO DRIVE; AVOID ALCOHOL. MAINTAIN ADEQUATE HYDRATION. DO NOT DISCONTINUE WITHOUT MEDICAL SUPERVISION.
Thienobenzodiazepines			
olanzapine	Zyprexa	Start with 5-10 mg/day; increase to 10-30 mg/day (maximum, 30 mg/day)	MAY CAUSE DROWSINESS; MAY IMPAIR ABILITY TO DRIVE; AVOID ALCOHOL. MAINTAIN ADEQUATE HYDRATION. DO NOT DISCONTINUE WITHOUT MEDICAL SUPERVISION.
Benzisoxasoles			
iloperidone	Fanapt	Start 1 mg twice daily; increase to 2 mg twice daily on day 2; then increase by 2 mg twice daily up to 12 mg twice daily (day 7)	MAY CAUSE DROWSINESS; MAY IMPAIR ABILITY TO DRIVE; AVOID ALCOHOL. MAINTAIN ADEQUATE HYDRATION. DO NOT DISCONTINUE WITHOUT MEDICAL SUPERVISION. MAY CAUSE DRY MOUTH. CHEWING GUM OR SUCKING SUGARLESS CANDY MAY IMPROVE SYMPTOMS. ORAL SOLUTION MAY BE MIXED IN MILK, JUICE, WATER, OR COFFEE; AVOID CARBONATED BEVERAGES AND TEA—risperidone.
paliperidone	Invega	**Oral:** 6 mg once daily in the morning (maximum, 12 mg/day) **IM, extended release:** Initiate with 234 mg IM first dose followed by 156 mg IM 1 week later Maintenance dose, 117 mg IM per month (maximum, 234 mg/mo)	
risperidone	Risperdal	3 mg-6 mg/day (oral) or 25 mg every 2 weeks (IM)	
Dibenzothiazepines			
quetiapine	Seroquel, Seroquel XR	Start with 25 mg twice a day; increase to 300-800 mg/day dosed 2-3 times a day **Extended release:** 150-300 mg once daily; start with 50 mg once every evening and increase by 50 mg once daily	MAY CAUSE DROWSINESS: MAY IMPAIR ABILITY TO DRIVE; AVOID ALCOHOL. MAINTAIN ADEQUATE HYDRATION. DO NOT DISCONTINUE WITHOUT MEDICAL SUPERVISION.
Benzoisothiazol Derivatives			
lurasidone	Latuda	**Oral:** 40-160 mg once daily	MAY CAUSE DROWSINESS; MAY IMPAIR ABILITY TO DRIVE; AVOID ALCOHOL. DO NOT DISCONTINUE WITHOUT MEDICAL SUPERVISION. TAKE WITH FOOD. MAINTAIN ADEQUATE HYDRATION.
ziprasidone	Geodon	**Oral:** 20 mg twice daily (maximum, 80 mg twice daily) **IM:** 10 mg every 2 hours (maximum, 40 mg/day)	

Summary of Drugs Used in the Treatment of Psychosis—cont'd

Generic Name	U.S. Brand Name	Usual Adult Oral Dose and Dosing Schedule	Warning Labels
Dibenzoxazepines			
loxapine	Loxitane	20-100 mg/day divided into 2-4 doses per day	MAY CAUSE DROWSINESS; MAY IMPAIR ABILITY TO DRIVE; AVOID ALCOHOL. DO NOT DISCONTINUE WITHOUT MEDICAL SUPERVISION. AVOID PROLONGED EXPOSURE TO SUNLIGHT. MAINTAIN ADEQUATE HYDRATION.
Other Atypical Neuroleptics			
aripiprazole	Abilify	10-15 mg twice daily	KEEP MEDICATION IN BLISTER PACK UNTIL READY FOR USE—oral disintegrating tablets. MAY CAUSE DIZZINESS OR DROWSINESS; MAY IMPAIR ABILITY TO DRIVE; AVOID ALCOHOL. DO NOT DISCONTINUE WITHOUT MEDICAL SUPERVISION. MAINTAIN ADEQUATE HYDRATION. STORE IN REFRIGERATOR. DISCARD UNUSED MEDICINE 6 MONTHS AFTER OPENING.
asenapine	Saphris	Dissolve sublingually 5 mg twice daily	AVOID EATING OR DRINKING FOR 10 MINUTES AFTER DOSE. MAY CAUSE DROWSINESS; MAY IMPAIR ABILITY TO DRIVE; AVOID ALCOHOL. DILUTE SOLUTION BEFORE ADMINISTRATION. MAINTAIN ADEQUATE HYDRATION. DO NOT DISCONTINUE WITHOUT MEDICAL SUPERVISION. MAY CAUSE DRY MOUTH. CHEWING GUM OR SUCKING SUGARLESS CANDY MAY IMPROVE SYMPTOMS.

Chapter Summary

- Schizophrenia is a chronic and major psychosis characterized by delusions of thought, visual or auditory hallucinations (or both), and speech disturbances.
- Schizophrenia affects about 1% of the population worldwide.
- The onset typically occurs in the late teens after puberty begins to the mid-20s.
- Symptoms of schizophrenia in women may not develop until the mid-20s to early 30s.
- Schizophrenia is thought to be associated with excess dopamine levels.
- Drugs capable of blocking transmission of signals in the dopaminergic system, located in the midbrain and hypothalamus, are used in the treatment of schizophrenia.
- Other neurotransmitters that have been identified as playing a role in symptoms of schizophrenia include serotonin, cholecystokinin, neurotensin, GABA, and glutamate.
- The greater the affinity the drug has for D_2 receptors, the more effective is the drug.
- Dopamine receptor blockade in the nigrostriatal tract produces Parkinson's disease–like symptoms (pseudoparkinsonism) and is associated with treatment with some classifications of neuroleptics.

- Some of the newer atypical neuroleptics have a low affinity for D_2 receptors yet are clinically effective.
- Neuroleptics are classified by structure and function.
- Functional classifications for neuroleptics are based on their affinity for dopamine receptors. High-potency neuroleptics have a strong affinity for dopamine receptors. "Atypical" and low-potency neuroleptics have a weaker affinity for dopamine receptors and produce fewer side effects associated with blockade.
- Atypical neuroleptics such as clozapine show strong affinity for serotonin receptors in addition to dopaminergic receptor blockade.
- Atypical neuroleptics are associated with new-onset diabetes.
- Atypical neuroleptics are associated with increased mortality in elderly patients with dementia-related psychosis.
- Traditional neuroleptics are well absorbed orally, rectally, and parenterally; readily cross the blood-brain barrier; are up to 90% bound to plasma proteins; are rapidly metabolized in the liver to active metabolites; and are stored in fatty tissue.
- Typical and atypical neuroleptics are available in slow-release depot formulations for intramuscular injection, and the therapeutic effects persist for up to 4 weeks after injection.
- Up to 80% of the people who are prescribed neuroleptics will experience adverse reactions.
- Extrapyramidal effects and tardive dyskinesia are associated with dopaminergic blockade and occur more frequently in elderly patients.
- Neuroleptic malignant syndrome is a life-threatening side effect of neuroleptic administration.
- Clozapine use is restricted because it can produce a fatal drop in white blood cell levels (agranulocytosis).

REVIEW QUESTIONS

1. A symptom of schizophrenia that is associated with unresponsiveness and immobility is termed _____.
   a. dystonia
   b. ataxia
   c. catatonia
   d. neurolepnia

2. Schizophrenia runs in families.
   a. true
   b. false

3. Of all the neurotransmitters involved in symptoms and treatment of schizophrenia, _____ is most significant.
   a. norepinephrine
   b. dopamine
   c. serotonin
   d. epinephrine

4. Phenothiazines, butyrophenones, and thioxanthines are categorized as _____ neuroleptics.
   a. traditional (typical)
   b. nontraditional (atypical)

5. What causes inappropriate postures of the neck, trunk, and limbs and accompanied by involuntary thrusting of the tongue and lip smacking?
   a. extrapyramidal symptoms
   b. tardive dyskinesia
   c. hyperkinesia
   d. catatonia

6. The use of _____is restricted because it can produce a fatal drop in white blood cells (agranulocytosis).
   a. quetiapine
   b. clozapine
   c. olanzapine
   d. nifedipine

7. Which drug is used for the treatment of schizophrenia, tics, intractable hiccups, and Tourette's syndrome?
   a. haloperidol
   b. Mellaril
   c. Clozaril
   d. Seroquel

8. Hallucinations, delusions, or other unusual thoughts or perceptions are _____ symptoms of schizophrenia.
   a. positive
   b. negative

9. Selection of schizophrenia agents is based on a balance between achievement of desired response to the drug and the patient's ability to tolerate drug side effects.
   a. true
   b. false

10. Risperidone is available in which dosage forms?
    a. oral solution
    b. injection
    c. tablet
    d. a, b, and c

TECHNICIAN'S CORNER

1. The prevalence of schizophrenia in families in which a sibling or relative has schizophrenia is about 10 times higher than in the general population. What kind of genetic implications does this statement have?
2. Can one live a "normal" life when diagnosed with schizophrenia?

Bibliography

Elsevier: Gold standard clinical pharmacology, 2010. Retrieved April 21, 2012, from https://www.clinical pharmacology.com/.

FDA: FDA-Approved drug products, 2012. Retrieved April 21, 2012, from http://www.accessdata.fda.gov/scripts/cder/drugsatfda/index.cfm?fuseaction=Search.Search_Drug_Name.

Kalant H, Grant D, Mitchell J: *Principles of medical pharmacology*, ed 7, Toronto, 2007, Elsevier Canada, A Division of Reed Elsevier Canada, pp 303-315.

Lance L, Lacy C, Armstrong L, et al: *Drug information handbook for the allied health professional*, ed 12, Hudson, OH, 2005, APhA Lexi-Comp.

National Institute of Mental Health: Schizophrenia, Bethesda, MD, National Institute of Mental Health, National Institutes of Health, U.S. Department of Health and Human Services; Revised September 2009. Available at http://www.nimh.nih.gov/health/publications/schizophrenia/schizophrenia-booket-2009.pdf.

Page C, Curtis M, Sutter M, et al: *Integrated pharmacology*, Philadelphia, 2005, Elsevier Mosby, pp 242-247.

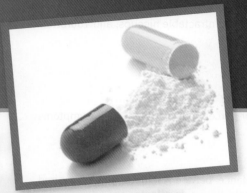

8

Treatment of Parkinson's Disease and Huntington's Disease

LEARNING OBJECTIVES

1 Learn the terminology associated with Parkinson's disease and Huntington's disease.

2 Compare and contrast the etiology of Parkinson's disease and Huntington's disease.

3 Compare and contrast the function of neurotransmitters associated with symptoms of Parkinson's disease and Huntington's disease.

4 Identify medications used to treat Parkinson's disease and Huntington's disease.

5 Describe mechanism of action for each class of drugs used to treat Parkinson's disease and Huntington's disease.

6 Identify warning labels and precautionary messages associated with medications used to treat Parkinson's disease and Huntington's disease.

7 Identify significant drug look-alike/sound-alike issues.

KEY TERMS

Acetylcholinesterase: Enzyme that degrades the neurotransmitter acetylcholine.

Basal ganglia: Subcortical nuclei located in the forebrain and brainstem that initiate, control, and modulate movement and posture.

Bradykinesia: Slowness in initiating and carrying out voluntary movements.

Cognitive functions: The ability to take in information via the senses, process the details, commit the information to memory, and recall it when necessary.

Huntington's disease: Progressive and degenerative disease of neurons that affects muscle movement, cognitive functions, and emotions.

Neurodegenerative disease: Disorder that results in progressive destruction of neurons.

Nigrostriatal pathways: Pathways located in the substantia nigra that stimulate and inhibit movement.

Parkinson's disease: Progressive disorder of the nervous system involving degeneration of dopaminergic neurons and causing impaired muscle movement.

Pseudoparkinsonism: Drug-induced condition that resembles Parkinson's disease.

Substantia nigra: Part of the basal ganglia containing clusters of dopamine-producing neurons.

Parkinson's Disease

Parkinson's disease is a progressive disorder of the nervous system involving degeneration of dopaminergic neurons in the basal ganglia and *nigrostriatal pathways* in the brain (Figure 8-1). The *basal ganglia* are composed of subcortical nuclei located in the forebrain (striatum and globus pallidus) and brainstem (substantia nigra and subthalamic nucleus). The basal ganglia are part of the extrapyramidal system that initiates, controls, and modulates movement and posture.

Loss of dopaminergic neurons results in reduction of available dopamine. Symptoms of Parkinson's disease are a result of an imbalance between dopamine and acetylcholine (ACh) (Figure 8-2). As the loss of dopaminergic neurons progresses, voluntary muscle movement diminishes.

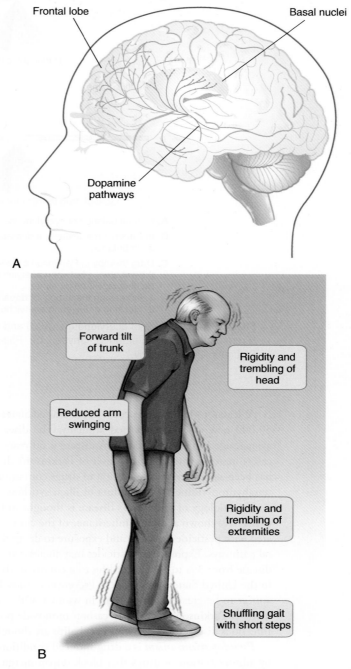

FIGURE 8-1 Dopaminergic pathways and signs of Parkinson's disease. (From Thibodeau GA, Patton KT: *Anatomy and physiology*, ed 6, St Louis, 2007, Mosby.)

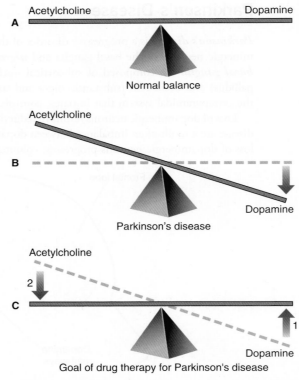

FIGURE 8-2 Balance of acetylcholine (ACh) and dopamine (DA) versus Parkinson's disease. (From Lilley LL, Harrington S, Snyder JS: *Pharmacology and the nursing process*, ed 5, St Louis, 2007, Mosby.)

At least 1 to 1.2 million people in the United States have Parkinson's disease (2007). Approximately 50,000 new cases are reported annually. The disease disproportionately affects elderly men. The average age at onset of Parkinson's disease is 60 years. The prevalence and incidence (number of new cases) increase with age. The onset of Parkinson's disease in persons under 40 years old is rare and has been associated with ingestion of drugs contaminated with MPTP (1-methyl-4-phenyl-1,2,3,6-tetrahydropyridine), a by-product of illicit synthesis of meperidine.

The etiology of Parkinson's disease is thought to be environmental; however, recent studies with twins have shown a familial inheritance of the chromosome 4 gene. Environmental causes are associated with pesticide exposure and exposure to drugs that destroy dopaminergic neurons in nigrostriatal pathways. Exposure to pesticides may increase the long-term risk for development of Parkinson's disease from 3% to 5%, according to a cohort study that reviewed surveys of 143,000 participants in the United States, the "Cancer Prevention Study II Nutrition Cohort" begun in 1982. The risks appear to be greater in men than in women. Other environmental toxins that may cause development of Parkinson's disease are carbon monoxide poisoning and heavy metal poisoning (mercury). Infectious diseases such as viral encephalitis are thought to be possible triggers for Parkinson's disease.

Pseudoparkinsonism is a drug-induced condition that resembles Parkinson's disease. It is caused by administration of drugs that block dopaminergic receptors in nigrostriatal pathways located in the basal ganglia. Examples of drugs that produce pseudoparkinsonism are neuroleptics (e.g., phenothiazines), administered to treat schizophrenia, and reserpine, a drug that is used to treat hypertension.

Characteristic signs of Parkinson's disease are ***bradykinesia*** and slowness in initiating and carrying out voluntary movements accompanied by muscle rigidity and tremors. When a person wishes to move her or his arm, the onset of movement is often delayed. When the forward motion begins, movements will be slow, rigid, and tremulous. Tremors are usually present at rest and may reduce the person's ability to perform skilled tasks. Postural and gait abnormalities are also typically present. The person walks with a characteristic shuffle. Other visible signs of Parkinson's disease are a blank facial expression, drooling, and speech impairment.

Cognitive functions may be impaired as well as motor functions. Parkinson's disease can cause memory loss, and affected persons may exhibit signs of dementia. Parkinson's disease can cause depression, too.

Parkinson's disease is treated by the administration of pharmaceuticals, exercise, and nutritional support.

NEUROCHEMISTRY OF PARKINSON'S DISEASE

Symptoms of Parkinson's disease are associated with an imbalance between dopamine and ACh (Figure 8-3). The amount of dopamine available for release diminishes as the disease progresses and degeneration of dopaminergic neurons increases. This results in unopposed cholinergic excitation and produces the tremors, muscle rigidity, and immobility associated with Parkinson's disease.

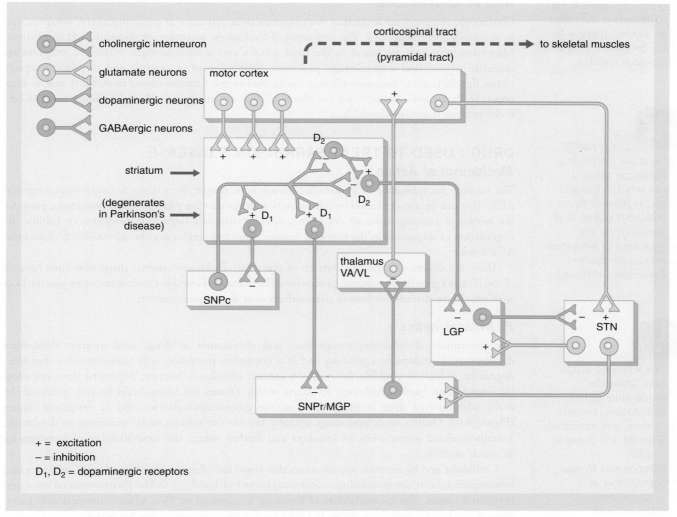

FIGURE 8-3 Summary of basal ganglia systems involved in Parkinson's disease. SNPc, substantia nigra pars compacta; VA/VL, ventroanterior/ventrolateral thalamic nuclei; SNPr/ MGP, substantia nigra pars reticula/medial globus pallidus; LGP, lateral globus pallidus; STN, subthalamic nucleus. (From Page C, Curtis M, Sutter M, et al: *Integrated pharmacology*, ed 6, Philadelphia, 2006, Mosby.)

Role of Dopamine

Dopaminergic neurons in the **substantia nigra** are involved in motor coordination. Dopamine regulates direct and indirect extrapyramidal pathways in the substantia nigra that modulate input to the motor cortex. As Parkinson's disease progresses, degeneration of dopaminergic neurons in nigrostriatal pathways increases, thereby reducing dopamine levels and dopamine action on GABAergic neurons. Compensatory systems in the basal ganglia involving GABAergic neurons are stimulated.

Role of γ-Aminobutyric Acid

Stimulation of GABAergic neurons by dopamine (D_1) sends signals that allow thalamic feedback to the motor cortex via the direct pathway that facilitate muscle movement. Stimulation of GABAergic neurons by dopamine (D_2) sends inhibitory feedback to the motor cortex via the indirect pathway. This results in impaired voluntary muscle movement.

Role of Glutamate

Large quantities of glutamate neurons are found in the cerebral cortex and exhibit excitatory control in the basal ganglia. Indirect and direct pathways are activated by glutamate neurons.

Role of Acetylcholine

Cholinergic receptors are located at the neuromuscular junction, at parasympathetic synapses, and in the brain and spinal cord. The two types of cholinergic receptors are nicotinic and muscarinic. Muscarinic receptors are found in the basal ganglia and substantia nigra. Nicotinic receptors are found in nigrostriatal dopaminergic pathways. Simulation of muscarinic and nicotinic receptors causes depolarization. Excessive stimulation of cholinergic neurons causes immobility and is what occurs in Parkinson's disease when the effects of ACh are unopposed. **Acetylcholinesterase** (AChE) is the enzyme that degrades ACh.

DRUGS USED TO TREAT PARKINSON'S DISEASE

Mechanism of Action

The strategy for treatment of Parkinson's disease is to restore the balance between dopamine and ACh. This can be accomplished by administering drugs that are synthesized to dopamine, promote the release of existing stores of dopamine, directly stimulate dopamine receptors, or inhibit the degradation of dopamine in the terminal neuron. Anticholinergics may be administered to decrease ACh levels.

There is a decrease in the effectiveness of most anti–Parkinson's disease drugs over time because of the disease's progressive neurodegeneration. The efficacy of levodopa and amantadine also declines with long-term therapy because of desensitization of dopamine receptors.

Pharmacokinetics

The absorption, distribution, metabolism, and elimination of drugs used to treat Parkinson's disease vary. Levodopa is a prodrug and is a dopamine precursor. It is administered rather than dopamine (which is available for use as a cardiac stimulant), because dopamine does not cross the blood-brain barrier. Although levodopa readily crosses the blood-brain barrier, much of the orally administered drug is metabolized in the gastrointestinal tract and in peripheral tissues (Figure 8-4). Only a small percentage actually reaches the neuron to be converted to dopamine. Sustained-release preparations of levodopa can further reduce the bioavailability of levodopa by as much as 30%.

Carbidopa and benserazide are adjuvants that boost the effectiveness of levodopa. Carbidopa and benserazide inhibit the metabolism (decarboxylation) of levodopa in the gastrointestinal tract and peripheral tissues. The bioavailability of levodopa is increased by 75% when combined with carbidopa. Catechol-*O*-methyltransferase (COMT) is the enzyme responsible for peripheral and central metabolism of catecholamines and metabolizes levodopa. Entacapone and tolcapone are COMT inhibitors and boost the bioavailability of levodopa by up to 50%.

A comparison of agents according to their mechanisms of action is given in Table 8-1.

TECH NOTE!
In addition to the treatment of Parkinson's disease, bromocriptine 0.8 mg (Cylcoset) is indicated as adjunct therapy for the treatment of type 2 diabetes mellitus.

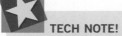

TECH NOTE!
Duodopa (carbidopa/ levodopa) gel is marketed in Canada and is infused by an intestinal pump. It is indicated for the treatment of advanced levodopa-responsive Parkinson's disease.

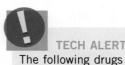

TECH ALERT!
The following drugs have look-alike/ sound-alike issues: amantadine, rimantadine, and ranitidine; Sinemet and Sinemet CR; Mirapex and Miralax; pramipexole and pramoxine; selegiline and sertraline; Eldepryl, Elavil, and enalapril

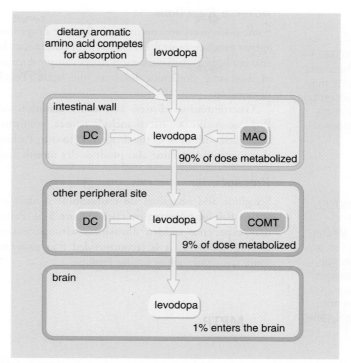

FIGURE 8-4 Disposition of orally administered levodopa. (From Page C, Curtis M, Sutter M, et al: *Integrated pharmacology*, ed 3, Philadelphia, 2006, Mosby.)

TABLE 8-1   **Comparison of Anti-Parkinson's Drugs**

Drug	Mechanism of Action	Time to Peak Concentration (hr)	Half-life (hr)
levodopa	Dopamine precursor	0.5-2	1-3
levodopa and carbidopa	Synthesis of dopamine inside the brain and blocking conversion outside the brain	1-2	
levodopa and benserazide	Synthesis of dopamine inside the brain and blocking conversion outside the brain	Unavailable	1.5
levodopa, carbidopa, and entacapone	Synthesis of dopamine inside the brain plus catechol-*O*-methyltransferase (COMT) inhibition	Unavailable	2.4
tolcapone	COMT inhibitor	2	2-3
amantadine	Stimulates release of dopamine from neuronal stores and decreases presynaptic reuptake; may have some anticholinergic activity	4-8	9.5-14.5
bromocriptine	Dopamine agonist	1-3	48
pramipexole	Dopamine agonist	1-2	8-12
ropinirole	Dopamine agonist	1-2	6
rasagiline	Blocks degradation of dopamine by inhibition of monoamine oxidase type B (MAOI$_B$)	1	3*
selegiline	Blocks degradation of dopamine by inhibition of monoamine oxidase type B (MAOI$_B$)	0.5-2	20
benztropine	Anticholinergic	Unknown	Unknown
trihexyphenidyl	Anticholinergic	1	5-10

*Does not correlate to duration of pharmacological effect.

TECH NOTE!
High-protein diets and iron supplements may decrease the absorption of Parkinson's drugs containing levodopa.

TECH NOTE!
Selegiline and rasagiline are MAOIs. Dispense with list of tyramine-containing foods and beverages to avoid. Dietary restrictions are not required for selegiline patches.

Adverse Reactions

Some side effects are common to all of the drugs used in the treatment of Parkinson's disease. Most agents produce central nervous system effects that include dizziness or lightheadedness, insomnia, and confusion. Anti-parkinson drugs can produce auditory and visual hallucinations as a function of increasing dopamine levels in the brain. People older than the age of 65 years are most susceptible.

Gastrointestinal distress is another common side effect of most of the drugs used to treat Parkinson's disease; effects include nausea, vomiting, and decreased appetite. Hypotension is also associated with most of the drugs used to treat Parkinson's disease. Many of the anti-parkinson drugs that increase dopamine also produce dry mouth and constipation.

Precautions

Selegiline and rasagiline are monoamine oxidase type B ($MAOI_B$) inhibitors and are associated with a risk for hypertensive crisis (Figure 8-5). Patients taking Prolopa (levodopa plus benserazide) may experience sudden drowsiness without warning and should be cautioned about risks for driving accidents. It is recommended that patients with diabetes test their blood glucose levels more frequently when taking Prolopa.

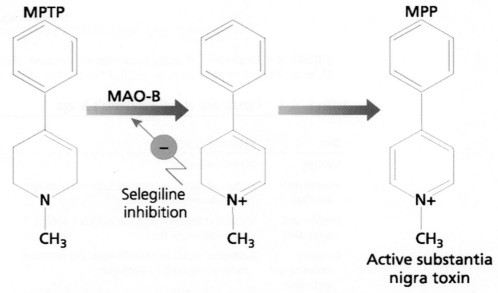

FIGURE 8-5 Selegiline inhibition. (From Lilley LL, Harrington S, Snyder JS: *Pharmacology and the nursing process*, ed 4, St Louis, 2005, Mosby.)

Drugs That Enhance Dopaminergic Activity

Generic Name	U.S. Brand Name(s)	Dosage Forms and Strengths
	Canadian Brand(s)	
amantadine*	Generics	Capsules: 100 mg
	Generics	Solution, oral: 50 mg/5 mL
		Tablets: 100 mg†
bromocriptine*	Parlodel	Capsules: 5 mg
	Generics	Tablets: 2.5 mg
carbidopa	Lodosyn	Tablets: 25 mg
	Not available	

Drugs That Enhance Dopaminergic Activity—cont'd

Generic Name	U.S. Brand Name(s) Canadian Brand(s)	Dosage Forms and Strengths
entacapone	Comtan	**Tablets:** 200 mg
	Comtan	
levodopa and carbidopa*	Parcopa, Sinemet, Sinemet CR	**Gel, intestinal (Duodopa):** 5 mg carbidopa + 20 mg levodopa per 1 mL **Tablets, extended release (Sinemet CR):** 25 mg carbidopa + 100 mg levodopa, 50 mg carbidopa + 200 mg levodopa **Tablets, immediate release (Sinemet):** 10 mg carbidopa + 100 mg levodopa, 25 mg carbidopa + 100 mg levodopa, 25 mg carbidopa + 250 mg levodopa **Tablets, immediate oral disintegrating (Parcopa):** 10 mg carbidopa + 100 mg levodopa, 25 mg carbidopa + 100 mg levodopa, 25 mg carbidopa + 250 mg levodopa
	Duodopa , Sinemet, Sinemet CR	
levodopa and benserazide	Not available	**Capsules:** 50 mg levodopa + 12.5 mg of benserazide 100 mg levodopa + 25 mg of benserazide 200 mg levodopa + 50 mg of benserazide
	Prolopa	
levodopa, carbidopa, and entacapone	Stalevo	**Tablets:** carbidopa 12.5 mg + levodopa 50 mg + entacapone 200 mg carbidopa 25 mg + levodopa 100 mg + entacapone 200 mg carbidopa 37.5 mg + levodopa 150 mg + entacapone 200 mg carbidopa 18.75 mg + levodopa 75 mg + entacapone 200 mg[‡] carbidopa 31.5 mg + levodopa 125 mg + entacapone 200 mg[‡]
	Stalevo	
pramipexole*	Mirapex, Mirapex ER	**Tablets:** 0.125 mg, 0.25 mg, 0.5 mg, 0.75 mg[†], 1 mg, 1.5 mg **Tablets, extended release (Mirapex ER):** 0.375 mg, 0.75 mg, 1.5 mg, 3 mg, 4.5 mg
	Mirapex	
rasagiline	Azilect	**Tablets:** 0.5 mg, 1 mg
	Azilect	
ropinirole*	ReQuip, ReQuip XL	**Tablets:** 0.25 mg, 0.5 mg[†], 1 mg, 2 mg, 3 mg[†], 4 mg[†], 5 mg **Tablets, extended release:** 2 mg, 4 mg, 6 mg, 8 mg, 12 mg
	ReQuip	
selegiline* (L-deprenyl)	Eldepryl, Zelapar	**Capsules (Eldepryl):** 5 mg **Tablets:** 5 mg **Tablets, oral disintegrating (Zelapar):** 1.25 mg
	Eldepryl	
tolcapone	Tasmar	**Tablets:** 100 mg, 200 mg
	Not available	

*Generic available.
[†]Strength available in the United States only.
[‡]Strength available in Canada only.

TECH ALERT!
Benztropine and
benzonatate have look-
alike/sound-alike issues.

DRUGS THAT REDUCE CHOLINERGIC ACTIVITY

Anticholinergics are administered as adjunctive treatment of Parkinson's disease and to lessen drug-induced extrapyramidal symptoms. Side effects are dizziness, sedation, confusion, dry mouth, blurred vision, constipation, urinary retention, heat intolerance, hypotension, and hallucinations.

Drugs That Reduce Cholinergic Activity

Generic Name	U.S. Brand Name(s) Canadian Brand(s)	Dosage Forms and Strengths
benztropine*	Cogentin	Injection: 1 mg/mL
	Cogentin	Tablets: 0.5 mg, 1 mg, 2 mg
trihexyphenidyl*	Generic only	Elixir: 2 mg/5 mL
	Generic only	Tablets: 2 mg, 5 mg

*Generic available.

Summary of Drugs Used in the Treatment of Parkinson's Disease

Generic Name	U.S. Brand Name	Usual Adult Oral Dose and Dosing Schedule	Warning Labels
Drugs That Increase Dopamine Levels			
amantadine	Generics	100 mg twice a day up to 300-400 mg/day	MAY CAUSE DIZZINESS; MAY IMPAIR ABILITY TO DRIVE.
bromocriptine	Parlodel	Start 1.25 mg twice/day; increase to 30-90 mg/day in 3 divided doses	AVOID ALCOHOL. DO NOT DISCONTINUE WITHOUT MEDICAL SUPERVISION.
entacapone	Comtan	200 mg up to 8 times a day	AVOID IRON SUPPLEMENTS WITHIN 2 HOURS OF DOSE—levodopa/
levodopa and carbidopa	Sinemet	**Immediate release:** carbidopa 25 mg/levodopa 100 mg 3-4 times a day (maximum, carbidopa 200 mg/levodopa 2000 mg) **Sustained release:** carbidopa 50 mg/levodopa 200 mg 2 times a day (maximum, carbidopa 400 mg/levodopa 1600 mg)	carbidopa, levodopa, carbidopa and entacapone, levodopa and benserazide. MAY CAUSE SUDDEN, EXCESSIVE DROWSINESS—Prolopa. SWALLOW WHOLE; DO NOT CRUSH OR CHEW (sustained release, Prolopa).
levodopa and benserazide	Prolopa	Initiate 1-2 capsules Prolopa (100-25 mg) 1-2 times a day; increase to 4-8 capsules daily in 4-6 divided doses	
levodopa, carbidopa and entacapone	Stalevo	Individualized (maximum, 1600 mg/day)	
pramipexole	Mirapex	Start 0.375 mg/day in 3 divided doses; increase to 1.5-4.5 mg/day	TAKE WITH FOOD—bromocriptine, Prolopa. AVOID FOODS HIGH IN TYRAMINE—
rasagiline	Azilect	0.5-1 mg once daily	rasagiline, selegiline. MAY DISCOLOR URINE—Stavelo,
ropinerole	ReQuip	Start 0.25 mg 3 times/day; increase weekly to a maximum 24 mg/day	tolcapone, entacapone, Sinemet. SWALLOW WHOLE; DO NOT CRUSH
selegiline	Eldepryl	5 mg twice a day or 10 mg once daily	OR CHEW—ReQuip XL, Mirapex ER.
tolcapone	Tasmar	100-200 mg 3 times a day	
Anticholinergics			
benztropine	Cogentin	0.5-6 mg/day in 1-2 divided doses	MAY CAUSE DROWSINESS; MAY IMPAIR ABILITY TO DRIVE.
trihexyphenidyl	Generics	5-15 mg/day in 3-4 divided doses	AVOID ALCOHOL. MAINTAIN ADEQUATE HYDRATION. DO NOT DISCONTINUE WITHOUT MEDICAL SUPERVISION.

Huntington's Disease

Huntington's disease is another progressive and degenerative disease of neurons that affects muscle movement, cognitive functions, and emotions. Huntington's disease is similar to Parkinson's disease in that it is associated with defects in the basal ganglia. Unlike Parkinson's disease, it produces excessive, abnormal muscle movement rather than immobility.

Huntington's disease is a hereditary disorder. It affects approximately one person in every 10,000. Children born to a parent who has Huntington's disease have a 50% chance of inheriting the gene for the disease. If the gene is inherited, the child will develop Huntington's disease at some point. Huntington's disease onset typically occurs in middle age; symptoms rarely occur after age 55. Juvenile onset is associated with rapid progression of symptoms and shorter life expectancy. Patients may live with the illness for 10 to 30 years.

Characteristic symptoms of Huntington's disease are tremors, rhythmic oscillations or circular movements around the ankles or wrists, and sudden abnormal movements. Movements are typically repetitive. The person may have speech impairment and difficulty swallowing and may exhibit facial grimaces. Choreiform movements are associated with Huntington's disease. Choreiform movements are unpredictable, irregular, and jerking.

Huntington's disease also causes emotional and intellectual changes. The person has difficulty concentrating, which worsens as the disease progresses. Irritability, mood swings, and depression are other symptoms of the disease. Cognitive impairment may appear as fixation on an idea, slowed thinking and responses, memory problems, and difficulty sequencing activities.

NEUROCHEMISTRY OF HUNTINGTON'S DISEASE

Huntington's disease causes defects in the basal ganglia that result in increased concentrations of dopamine coupled with a decrease in the activity of the enzymes glutamic acid decarboxylase and choline acetyltransferase. Glutamic acid decarboxylase is the enzyme that synthesizes GABA. Choline acetyltransferase is involved in the production of ACh. Deficient levels of ACh and GABA lead to hyperactivity of dopaminergic neurons in nigrostriatal pathways. The balance between GABA, ACh, and dopamine is upset, and this produces the excessive muscle movement associated with Huntington's disease.

DRUGS USED TO TREAT HUNTINGTON'S DISEASE
Mechanism of Action

Huntington's disease is primarily treated with drugs that decrease excessive dopaminergic activity. This is accomplished by depleting stores of dopamine in the neuron (e.g., tetrabenazine) and blockade of dopamine receptors (e.g., butyrophenones). Both mechanisms of action reduce dopamine levels.

DRUGS THAT DEPLETE STORES OF DOPAMINE IN THE NEURON
Drugs that deplete stores of dopamine are used for the treatment of Huntington's disease, Gilles de la Tourette syndrome, and tardive dyskinesia. Side effects of tetrabenazine are hypotension, sedation, constipation, dizziness, depression, and pseudoparkinsonism.

DRUGS THAT BLOCK DOPAMINE RECEPTORS
Haloperidol is indicated for the treatment of Huntington's disease, Tourette syndrome, and schizophrenia (see Chapter 7). Other neuroleptics, including pimozide and fluphenazine, have been

Drugs That Deplete Stores of Dopamine

Generic Name	U.S. Brand Name(s) Canadian Brand(s)	Dosage Forms and Strengths
tetrabenazine	Xenazine	Tablets: 12.5 mg[†], 25 mg
	Nitoman	

†Strength available in the United States only.

Drugs That Block Dopamine Receptors

Generic Name	U.S. Brand Name(s) / Canadian Brand(s)	Dosage Forms and Strengths
haloperidol*	Haldol, Haldol Deconoate / Generics	Injection, oil, as deconoate: 50 mg/mL; 100 mg/mL Injection, solution, as lactate: 5 mg/mL Solution, oral concentrate: 2 mg/mL Tablets: 0.5 mg, 1 mg, 2 mg, 5 mg, 10 mg, 20 mg

*Generic available.

Summary of Drugs Used in the Treatment of Huntington's Disease

Generic Name	U.S. Brand Name	Usual Adult Oral Dose and Dosing Schedule	Warning Labels
Drugs That Decrease Dopamine Levels			
tetrabenazine	Xenazine, Nitoman (Canada)	25-37.5 mg 2-3 times/day (maximum, 100 mg/day)	MAY CAUSE DROWSINESS; MAY IMPAIR ABILITY TO DRIVE; LIMIT ALCOHOL.
haloperidol	Haldol	Oral: 0.5-5 mg 2-3 times/day (maximum, 30 mg/day) IM, as lactate: 2-5 mg every 4-8 hours IM, as deconoate: 15-150 mg once every 4 weeks	DO NOT DISCONTINUE WITH MEDICAL SUPERVISION. DILUTE ORAL CONCENTRATE BEFORE ADMINISTRATION—haloperidol. MAINTAIN ADEQUATE HYDRATION—haloperidol. AVOID PROLONGED EXPOSURE TO SUNLIGHT—haloperidol.

administered to control choreiform movements but are not approved by the U.S. Food and Drug Administration for this purpose. Side effects include sedation, confusion, weight gain, increased appetite, blurred vision, dry mouth, urinary retention, constipation, postural hypotension, pseudoparkinsonism, extrapyramidal symptoms, tardive dyskinesia, photosensitivity, and sexual dysfunction.

Chapter Summary

- Parkinson's disease is a progressive disorder of the nervous system involving degeneration of dopaminergic neurons in the basal ganglia of the brain.
- The basal ganglia are part of the extrapyramidal system that initiates, controls, and modulates movement and posture.
- Symptoms of Parkinson's disease are a result of an imbalance between dopamine and acetylcholine.
- The average age at onset of Parkinson's disease is 60 years. Men are more often affected than women.
- Environmental exposures to pesticides, carbon monoxide poisoning, and heavy metal poisoning (mercury) can increase risk for Parkinson's disease.
- Infectious diseases, such as viral encephalitis and syphilis, and metabolic disorders, such as Wilson's disease, are also thought to cause Parkinson's disease.
- Neuroleptic drugs can cause pseudoparkinsonism, a drug-induced condition that resembles Parkinson's disease.
- Physical signs of Parkinson's disease are bradykinesia, muscle rigidity, tremors, postural and gait abnormalities, and walking with a characteristic shuffle. Other visible signs of Parkinson's disease are blank facial expression, drooling, and speech impairment.
- Parkinson's disease can be associated with memory loss, dementia, and depression.
- Symptoms of Parkinson's disease are associated with an imbalance between dopamine and acetylcholine.

- Levodopa is a prodrug and is a dopamine precursor.
- Carbidopa and benserazide are adjuvants that are combined with levodopa to inhibit the metabolism of levodopa in the gastrointestinal tract and peripheral tissues.
- The bioavailability of levodopa is increased up to 50%, and the elimination half-life is doubled when tolcapone is added to therapy.
- Tolcapone and entacapone inhibit catechol-O-methyltransferase (COMT), the enzyme responsible for metabolizing levodopa.
- Bioavailability is decreased by as much as 30% when sustained-release preparations are administered.
- People older than the age of 65 years are most susceptible to side effects of anti–Parkinson's disease drugs (e.g., dizziness, lightheadedness, insomnia, confusion, and hallucinations).
- Dizziness, hypotension, confusion, and gastrointestinal distress are common side effects of most of the drugs used to treat Parkinson's disease.
- Anticholinergic drug effects are dry mouth, blurred vision, constipation, and urinary retention.
- The effectiveness of anti-Parkinson's drugs decline over time due to the progressive nature of the disease. The efficacy of levodopa and amantadine also declines with long-term therapy because of desensitization of dopamine receptors.
- Selegiline and rasagiline are monoamine oxidase type B inhibitors (MAOI$_B$) and are associated with a risk for hypertensive crisis.
- Huntington's disease is a progressive and degenerative disease of neurons that affects muscle movement, cognitive functions, and emotions.
- Huntington's disease is similar to Parkinson's disease in that it is associated with defects in the basal ganglia.
- Huntington's disease is a hereditary disorder.
- Characteristic symptoms of Huntington's disease are tremors, rhythmic oscillations or circular movements around the ankles or wrists, and sudden abnormal movements.
- Choreiform movements are unpredictable, irregular, and jerking.
- Cognitive impairment may appear as fixation on an idea, slowed thinking and responses, and memory problems, along with difficulty sequencing activities.
- In Huntington's disease, the balance between GABA, acetylcholine, and dopamine is upset, which produces the excessive muscle movement associated with Huntington's disease.
- Huntington's disease is primarily treated with drugs that decrease excessive dopaminergic activity.

REVIEW QUESTIONS

1. Parkinson's disease is a progressive disorder of the nervous system involving degeneration of dopaminergic neurons in the basal ganglia and nigrostriatal pathways in the brain.
   a. true
   b. false

2. Approximately 5000 new cases of Parkinson's disease are reported annually.
   a. true
   b. false

3. Characteristic signs of Parkinson's disease are _____ and slowness in initiating and carrying out voluntary movements accompanied by muscle rigidity and tremors.
   a. hyperkinesia
   b. tardive dyskinesia
   c. bradykinesia
   d. neurokinesia

4. Symptoms of Parkinson's disease are associated with an imbalance between _____ and _____.
   a. epinephrine, dopamine
   b. dopamine, serotonin
   c. acetylcholine, norepinephrine
   d. dopamine, acetylcholine

5. _____ is a prodrug and is a dopamine precursor.
   a. Levodopa
   b. Carbidopa
   c. Cogentin
   d. ReQuip

6. The bioavailability of levodopa is increased by _____ % when combined with carbidopa.
   a. 25
   b. 50
   c. 75
   d. 95

7. _____ is a common side effect of most of the drugs used to treat Parkinson's disease.
   a. Headache
   b. Gastrointestinal distress
   c. Muscle spasms
   d. Flulike symptoms

8. Huntington's disease is similar to Parkinson's disease in that it is associated with defects in the brainstem.
   a. true
   b. false

9. Huntington's disease is treated with drugs that _____ excessive dopaminergic activity.
   a. increase
   b. decrease

10. This drug is indicated in the treatment of Huntington's disease, Gilles de la Tourette syndrome, and tardive dyskinesia.
    a. tetrabenazine
    b. benztropine
    c. fexofenadine
    d. a, b, and c

TECHNICIAN'S CORNER

1. Where is the location of the basal ganglia? How can one disease be caused by excessive dopamine and another disease be caused by a deficiency of dopamine?
2. The average age at onset of Parkinson's disease is 60 years. Have there been any cases of patients younger than 60 years contracting Parkinson's disease?

Bibliography

Ascherio A, Chen H, Weisskopf MG, et al: Pesticide exposure and risk for Parkinson's disease, *Annals of Neurology*, 60:197-203, 2006, Wiley-Liss, Inc., A Wiley Company.

Bourne C, Clayton C, Murch A, et al: Cognitive impairment and behavioural difficulties in patients with Huntinton's disease, *Nursing Standard* 20:41-44, 2006.

Elsevier: Gold Standard Clinical Pharmacology, 2010. Retrieved April 21, 2012, from https://www.clinical pharmacology.com/ accessed.

FDA: FDA Approved Drug Products, 2012. Retrieved April 21, 2012, from http://www.accessdata.fda.gov/scripts/cder/drugsatfda/index.cfm?fuseaction=Search.Search_Drug_Name.

Health Canada: Drug Product Database. Retrieved Feb 20, 2011, from http://www.hc-sc.gc.ca/dhp-mps/prodpharma/databasdon/index-eng.php, 2010.

Lance L, Lacy C, Armstrong L, et al: *Drug information handbook for the allied health professional*, ed 12, Hudson, OH, 2005, APhA Lexi-Comp.

National Institute of Neurological Disorders and Stroke: Huntington's disease, Bethesda, MD, NINDS, National Institutes of Health, U.S. Department of Health and Human Services. Updated January 2006. Retrieved at http://www.ninds.nih.gov/disorders/Huntington's/Huntington's.htm.

National Institute of Neurological Disorders and Stroke: Parkinson's's disease, Bethesda, MD, NINDS, National Institutes of Health, U.S. Department of Health and Human Services. Updated October 2004. Retrieved at http://www.ninds.nih.gov/disorders/Parkinson'ss_disease/detail_Parkinson's_disease.htm.

Page C, Curtis M, Sutter M, et al: *Integrated pharmacology*, Philadelphia, 2005, Elsevier Mosby, pp 242-247.

Raffa RB, Rawls SM, Beyzarov EP: *Netter's illustrated pharmacology*, Philadelphia, 2005, WB Saunders, pp 77-78.

U.S. Food and Drug Administration, U.S. Department of Health and Human Services, FDA News: FDA approves new treatment for Parkinson's's disease, Press releases P06-68, May 17, 2006. Retrieved at http://www.fda.gov/bbs/topics/NEWS/2006/NEW01373.html.

USP Center for Advancement of Patient Safety: Use caution: avoid confusion. USP Quality Review No. 79, Rockville, MD, April 2004, USP Center for Advancement of Patient Safety.

9

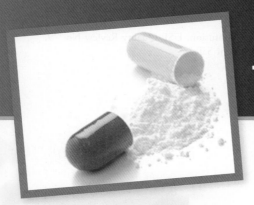

Treatment of Seizure Disorders

LEARNING OBJECTIVES

1 Learn the terminology associated with seizures.

2 Describe the etiology of seizure disorders.

3 Compare and contrast the function of neurotransmitters associated with symptoms of seizure disorders.

4 Classify medications used in the treatment of seizure disorders.

5 Identify significant drug look-alike/sound-alike issues.

6 Describe mechanism of action for each class of drugs used to treat seizure disorders.

7 Identify significant drug interactions.

8 Identify warning labels and precautionary messages associated with medications used to treat seizure disorders.

KEY TERMS

Anoxia: Lack of oxygen to the brain.

Aura: Unusual sensation, auditory, visual, or olfactory hallucination that is experienced just before the onset of a seizure.

Complex focal seizures: Seizure disorder that produces a blank stare, disorientation, repetitive actions, and memory loss.

Convulsions: Sudden contraction of muscles that is caused by seizures.

Eclampsia: A life-threatening condition that can develop in pregnant women that causes high blood pressure and seizures.

Epilepsy: A recurrent seizure disorder characterized by a sudden, excessive, disorderly discharge of cerebral neurons.

Febrile seizure: Seizure associated with a sudden spike in body temperature.

Generalized seizures: Seizures that spread across both cerebral hemispheres and include tonic-clonic, myoclonic, and petit mal seizures.

Gingival hyperplasia: Excess growth of gum tissue that may overgrow the teeth.

Hirsutism: Excessive growth of body hair (especially in women).

Myoclonic seizure: Seizure that is characterized by jerking muscle movements and is caused by contraction of major muscle groups.

Petit mal seizure: Absence seizure in which the person experiences a brief period of unconsciousness and stares vacantly into space.

Seizure threshold: A person's susceptibility to seizures.

Simple focal seizures: Seizure that affects only one part of the brain and causes the person to experience unusual sensations or feelings.

Status epilepticus: Medical emergency brought on by repeated generalized seizures that can deprive the brain of oxygen.

Tonic-clonic (grand mal) seizures: Generalized seizure that causes stiffening of the limbs, difficulty breathing, and jerking movements and is followed by disorientation and limbs that become limp.

Overview

Epilepsy is one of the oldest known brain disorders and was described as early as 3000 years ago in ancient Babylon. The word *epilepsy* is derived from the Greek word for "attack" because the ancient Greeks believed a person having a seizure was being attacked by demons. Approximately 1% of the population or 3 million people in the United States have epilepsy, and 200,000 new cases are diagnosed each year. The seizure risk increases with age. By 75 years, 3% of the population will have had a seizure caused by age-related cerebrovascular disease that deprives the brain of oxygen. Epilepsy is a type of seizure disorder that is associated with having experienced two or more seizures. Seizures are characterized by a sudden, excessive, disorderly discharge of cerebral neurons. Seizures may also be caused by conditions that range from injury to illness. Half of all seizures have no known cause. When the cause is known, the origin may be birth defects, infection (meningitis, AIDS), perinatal injury, malignant tumors, lead poisoning, head trauma or *eclampsia* (a life-threatening condition that can develop in pregnant women). Wearing seat belts, motorcycle helmets, and bike helmets can reduce the risk for seizures that are caused by head injury. The onset of a seizure may be preceded by an aura. An *aura* is an unusual sensation, auditory, visual, or olfactory hallucination that is experienced just before the onset of a seizure. In other words, the person may hear, see, or smell something distinctive immediately before the seizure activity begins. These signs of an upcoming seizure are important because it indicates the location of abnormal neuronal firing in the cerebrum.

Febrile seizures in children are associated with an infection causing a sudden spike in temperature; aggressive treatment with fever reducers is indicated to prevent more seizures. Most children who have febrile seizures will not develop epilepsy.

External causes of seizures include metabolic disturbance, hypoglycemia, electrolyte imbalance, drug and alcohol withdrawal, and use of drugs that lower the *seizure threshold*. Stroke and heart attack can cause seizures because the brain becomes deprived of oxygen (*anoxia*).

TECH NOTE!
Flashing or strobe lights such as those used in fire alarms systems can trigger seizures in individuals with epilepsy.

Seizure Classifications

There are two major seizure classifications (Figure 9-1), generalized seizures and focal or partial seizures. *Generalized seizures* spread across both of the cerebral hemispheres while partial seizures are confined to a single hemisphere. Tonic-clonic (grand mal) (Figure 9-2), myoclonic, and petit mal seizures are generalized seizures. *Tonic-clonic* and *myoclonic seizures* start with a stiffening of the limbs and difficulty breathing; are followed by jerking movements and loss of bladder and bowel control; and on conclusion (postictal phase), the limbs become limp and the person may be disoriented. The jerking muscle movement associated with grand mal seizures is sometimes referred to as a *convulsion*.

Petit mal seizures are also called absence seizures. This type of seizure is associated with a characteristic vacant or absent stare during the seizure. Absence seizures occur more commonly in children. They are barely noticeable to onlookers because no major muscle twitching is exhibited. *Status epilepticus* is a medical emergency and results from repeated, generalized seizures that deprive the brain of oxygen. Antiseizure medicines must be administered intravenously to persons with status epilepticus.

Approximately 60% of people with epilepsy have focal seizures. Focal (partial) seizures involve only one cerebral hemisphere. Focal seizures are classified as simple or complex. *Simple focal seizures* may cause the arms, face, or legs to twitch, and visual, olfactory, or auditory hallucinations may occur. *Complex focal seizures* often begin with a blank stare. The person becomes disoriented and engages in repetitive actions during the seizure. When the seizure is over, the person does not have any memory of the seizure. Psychomotor and temporal lobe seizures are complex partial seizures.

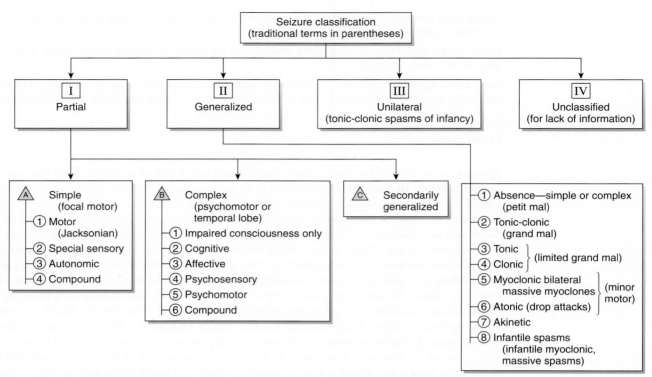

FIGURE 9-1 Classifications of seizures. (From Clayton BD, Stock YN: *Basic pharmacology for nurses*, ed 12, St Louis, 1997, Mosby.)

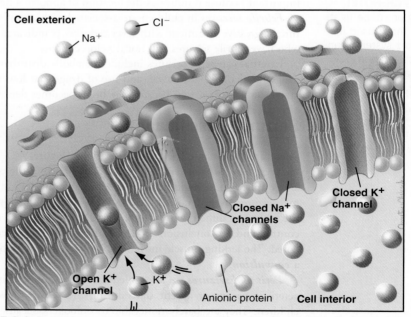

FIGURE 9-2 Role of ion channels. (From Thibodeau GA, Patton KT: *Anatomy and physiology*, ed 6, St Louis, 2007, Mosby.)

Neurochemistry of Seizures

When there is an abnormality in nerve signaling by neurotransmitters, seizures result. People with epilepsy have an abnormally high level of excitatory neurotransmitters coupled with a low level of inhibitory neurotransmitters. This accounts for the excess neuronal firing that occurs with seizure disorders. γ-Aminobutyric acid (GABA) is an inhibitory neurotransmitter that plays an important role in epilepsy. An excitatory neurotransmitter that plays a role in epilepsy is the amino acid glutamate. Some seizures are linked to a defect in the genes that control the ion channels that open and close to regulate the influx of chloride, sodium, and calcium into the neuron.

ION CHANNEL REGULATION

The aim of pharmaceutical treatment of seizure is to suppress seizure activity. This is accomplished by control of the voltage-dependent sodium channel. In the resting state, the neuron is more negative inside the cell and is surrounded by positive sodium, potassium, and calcium ions. Neuronal firing begins when the positive ions move from outside the neuron into the neuron. Neuronal firing is inhibited by drugs that delay the inflow of sodium ions. T-type voltage-dependent calcium channels are believed to be involved in initiation of seizure activity. Drugs that bind to T-type calcium channels inhibit absence (petit mal) seizures.

THE ROLE OF γ-AMINOBUTYRIC ACID

GABA is an inhibitory neurotransmitter. The GABA receptor regulates the movement of chloride ion into the neuron. Chloride ions are negatively charged. The influx of chloride ions inhibits formation of action potentials suppressing neuronal hyperactivity and seizures. GABAergic receptors are stimulated by dopamine (D_2), another inhibitory neurotransmitter.

Other neurotransmitters that play a role in the initiation of seizures are acetylcholine, norepinephrine, histamine, and glutamate.

Drugs Used to Treat Seizure Disorders

The goal of treatment of epilepsy and other seizure disorders is to reduce the incidence of seizures by suppressing seizure activity. Successful achievement of this therapeutic goal is dependent on correctly classifying the seizure type and selecting an appropriate drug for seizure type, with optimal drug administration and serum monitoring. Monodrug therapy is preferred to lower the incidence of adverse effects, reduce the incidence of drug interactions, improve adherence to drug therapy, and lower medication costs. Medications reduce seizure activity in approximately 80% of people diagnosed with epilepsy. The remaining 20% of people continue to experience seizures.

HYDANTOINS

Phenytoin (formerly diphenylhydantoin) was first introduced in 1938. It is used for the treatment of generalized (tonic-clonic) seizures, partial seizures, and status epilepticus. Fosphenytoin is used to treat status epilepticus and seizures occurring during neurosurgery.

Mechanism of Action

Phenytoin and fosphenytoin suppress seizure activity by binding to receptors on voltage-dependent sodium channels. They also reduce neuronal membrane permeability to calcium.

Pharmacokinetics

The absorption of phenytoin is variable and is influenced by particle size as well as by inactive ingredients in manufacturers' formulations. This influences bioavailability, which may result in an increase or a decrease in blood levels when switching between different manufacturers' formulations. Ninety percent of the drug is protein bound, so drug interactions involving protein binding are common. Phenytoin is primarily metabolized in the liver by cytochrome P450 enzymes. If enough phenytoin is administered to saturate metabolic enzymes, a secondary metabolic pathway is used. When this occurs, elimination is slowed, and excessive adverse reactions or toxicity can occur. Patients taking phenytoin must periodically have their blood levels monitored. Phenytoin acts as an inducer of metabolic enzymes in the liver; therefore, it can alter the rate of metabolism of other coadministered drugs that use the same metabolic system. For example, phenytoin can reduce the effectiveness of oral contraceptives as well as other antiseizure drugs. Drug interactions can also occur between phenytoin and erythromycin, isoniazid, and warfarin.

Fosphenytoin is converted to phenytoin by enzymes in the blood (phosphatases). It has a short half-life of approximately 8 minutes. Unlike phenytoin, which can be administered orally or parenterally, fosphentoin is only available for parenteral use and is administered intravenously or

TECH NOTE!
Therapeutic blood levels for phenytoin are best maintained by dispensing the same manufacturer's formulation every time a prescription is filled. Avoid switching if possible.

TECH NOTE!
Antiepileptic drugs may increase suicidal ideation and behavior. The U.S. Food and Drug Administration (FDA) issued an advisory to health care professionals and has required product labeling changes to warn of this adverse effect for Carbatrol, Celontin, Depakene, Depakote ER, Depakote sprinkles, Depakote tablets, Dilantin, Equetro, Felbatol, Gabitril, Keppra, Keppra XR, Klonopin, Lamictal, Lyrica, Mysoline, Neurontin, Peganone, Stavzor, Tegretol, Tegretol XR, Topamax, Tranxene, Tridione, Trileptal, Zarontin, and Zonegran and their generics.

TECH ALERT!
The following drugs have look-alike/sound-alike issues: Cerebyx, Celebrex, and Celexa; phenytoin and fosphenytoin; Dilantin and Diflucan

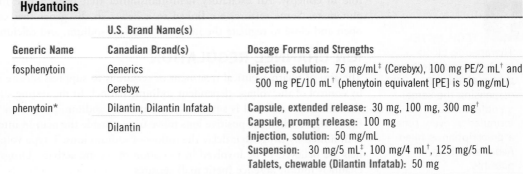

Hydantoins

Generic Name	U.S. Brand Name(s) / Canadian Brand(s)	Dosage Forms and Strengths
fosphenytoin	Generics	Injection, solution: 75 mg/mL‡ (Cerebyx), 100 mg PE/2 mL† and 500 mg PE/10 mL† (phenytoin equivalent [PE] is 50 mg/mL)
	Cerebyx	
phenytoin*	Dilantin, Dilantin Infatab	Capsule, extended release: 30 mg, 100 mg, 300 mg†
	Dilantin	Capsule, prompt release: 100 mg
		Injection, solution: 50 mg/mL
		Suspension: 30 mg/5 mL‡, 100 mg/4 mL†, 125 mg/5 mL
		Tablets, chewable (Dilantin Infatab): 50 mg

*Generic available.
†Strength available in the United States only.
‡Strength available in Canada only.

TECH NOTE!
Cerebyx is compatible in normal saline and dextrose.

TECH NOTE!
Dilantin is compatible in normal saline. Intravenous solution is stable for 14 hours at room temperature when diluted to 2 mg/mL. Dilantin chewable tablets should be followed by a glass of water.

TECH ALERT!
Depakote, Depakene, and Depakote ER have look-alike/sound-alike issues.

TECH NOTE!
Depakote sprinkles may be mixed into soft foods.

intramuscularly. Its advantage is that it produces more predictable serum concentrations when administered intramuscularly than phenytoin and is 100% bioavailable.

Adverse Reactions

Adverse reactions are dose dependent and are similar for phenytoin and fosphenytoin. Common side effects include nausea and vomiting, *hirsutism* (excessive growth of body hair, especially in women), *gingival hyperplasia* (excessive growth of gum tissue), ataxia, and sedation. The hydantoins can also produce slowed thinking. Infants born to women who took phenytoin during pregnancy may be born with cleft palate. Hydantoins may decrease folic acid, calcium, and vitamin D absorption; it may be necessary to supplement with vitamins.

Precautions

Phenytoin and fosphenytoin are known teratogens and are classified in FDA pregnancy risk category D.

VALPROATES

Valproates are described as "broad-spectrum" antiseizure drugs because they are effective in treating all types of seizures. They are one of the few antiseizure drugs indicated for the treatment of absence seizures. Valproates are also effective for treating general and focal (partial) seizures.

Mechanism of Action

One of the mechanisms of action for valproates and their derivatives is to enhance the inhibitory actions of GABA. Other mechanisms of action may be involved, including actions on potassium channels that result in membrane stabilization.

Pharmacokinetics

The effectiveness of all valproic acid derivatives is expressed as valproic acid activity. All are rapidly absorbed when administered orally and have 100% bioavailability. Valproates are up to 95% protein bound, so drug interactions involving protein binding must be considered when dispensing other drugs with them, including other antiseizure medicines such as phenobarbital and phenytoin.

Adverse Reactions

Common adverse reactions are gastrointestinal upset and sedation, although the valproates are less sedating than other drugs used to treat seizures. Other adverse effects are weight gain, hair loss, tremor, diplopia (double vision), bruising, irregular menstruation, and hepatotoxicity. Hepatotoxicity is rare, but when it occurs in children, it is potentially fatal.

Precautions

Valproates should be used cautiously in people with a history of liver disease. Up to 10% of the drug is passed in breast milk, limiting the use of valproates during lactation.

Valproates

Generic Name	U.S. Brand Name(s) / Canadian Brand(s)	Dosage Forms and Strengths
divalproex sodium* valproic acid*	Depacon, Depakene, Depakote Delayed Release, Depakote ER, Depakote Sprinkle, Stavzor Epival ECT	Capsules, as valproic acid (Depakene): 250 mg Capsules, as sprinkles (Depakote Sprinkle): 125 mg Capsules, delayed release (Stavzor): 125 mg, 250 mg, 500 mg Injection, solution (Depacon): 100 mg/mL Syrup, as valproic acid (Depakene): 250 mg/5 mL Tablets, as divalproex sodium delayed release (Depakote, Epival ECT): 125 mg, 250 mg, 500 mg Tablets, as divalproex sodium extended release (Depakote ER): 250 mg, 500 mg

*Generic available.

Iminostilbenes

Generic Name	U.S. Brand Name(s) / Canadian Brand(s)	Dosage Forms and Strengths
carbamazepine*	Carbatrol, Equetro, Epitol, Tegretol, Tegretol-XR Tegretol	Capsules, extended release (Carbatrol, Equetro): 100 mg, 200 mg, 300 mg Suspension (Tegretol): 100 mg/5 mL Tablets, chewable (Tegretol): 100 mg Tablets (Epitol, Tegretol): 200 mg Tablets, extended release (Tegretol-XR): 100 mg, 200 mg, 400 mg
oxcarbazepine	Trileptal Trileptal	Suspension: 300 mg/5 mL Tablets: 150 mg, 300 mg, 600 mg

*Generic available.

IMINOSTILBENES

There are only two antiseizure medications in this class, carbamazepine and oxcarbazepine. They are used to treat generalized and complex focal seizures. Neither drug is useful in the management of absence seizures. Carbamazepine is also used in the management of neuropathic pain caused by trigeminal neuralgia (see Chapter 10) and bipolar disorder (see Chapter 6).

Mechanism of Action

Carbamazepine is structurally similar to tricyclic antidepressants. The mechanism of action is not completely understood; however, it is believed to work by binding to voltage-dependent sodium channels.

Pharmacokinetics

Oral absorption and distribution of carbamazepine are moderately slow and are influenced by drug formulation. Differences in inactive ingredients and particle size can alter rates of absorption. Peak levels of the drug are not achieved until 6 to 8 hours after administration. Carbamazepine is metabolized in the liver. Over time, it begins to induce the same enzymes that metabolize it, causing serum levels to fluctuate. Erratic serum blood levels can result in poor seizure control. This may be minimized by administration of controlled release formulations.

Adverse Reactions

Side effects of carbamazepine and oxcarbazepine include nausea, vomiting, dizziness, sedation, unsteadiness (ataxia), bruising, jaundice, and double vision (diplopia).

Precautions

Carbamazepine should be protected from light and moisture. Moisture can decrease the potency by as much as 30%.

γ-AMINOBUTYRIC ACID ANALOGS

Gabapentin, pregabalin, tiagabine, and vigabatrin are administered for the treatment of general and partial (focal) seizures. All are ineffective in treating absence seizures. Gabapentin and pregabalin are also used to treat herpes-related nerve pain (see Chapter 10).

Mechanism of Action

Gabapentin was structurally designed to bind to $GABA_A$ receptors and act as an agonist; however, it turns out that this is not the mechanism of action for the drug. Gabapentin binds to voltage-dependent sodium channels and increases GABA turnover without binding to the GABA receptor. Pregabalin is structurally related to gabapentin, but its mechanism of action is different. Pregabalin reduces neuronal calcium currents by binding to calcium channels rather than to sodium channels. Tiagabine blocks the reuptake of GABA in the synapse, and vigabatrin enhances GABA activity by binding to GABA transaminase (GABA-T), the enzyme that inactivates GABA.

Pharmacokinetics

The oral absorption of gabapentin and tiagabine is rapid. Whereas gabapentin has lower bioavailability (60%) than tiagabine (90%) and has little protein binding, tiagabine is nearly 95% protein bound (i.e., making it susceptible to drug interactions involving protein binding). Gabapentin is primarily eliminated by the kidneys. Vigabatrin has a short half-life, but the effects of GABA-T binding persist even after blood levels of the drug declines.

Adverse Reactions

Drug-related side effects for gabapentin and tiagabine are dizziness, confusion, drowsiness, fatigue, ataxia, and nausea. Whereas tiagabine may cause anorexia, gabapentin may increase appetite. Double vision, blurred vision, dry mouth, and constipation are also associated with gabapentin. Vigabatrin can cause irreversible tunnel vision, limiting its use.

Precautions

Antacids decrease the absorption of gabapentin by 20%. The absorption of tiagabine is reduced by foods that have a high fat content.

GABA Analogs

Generic Name	U.S. Brand Name(s) / Canadian Brand(s)	Dosage Forms and Strengths
gabapentin*	Horizant, Neurontin / Neurontin	Capsules: 100 mg, 300 mg, 400 mg; Solution, oral: 250 mg/5 mL; Tablets: 600 mg, 800 mg; Tablets, extended release (Horizant): 600 mg
pregabalin	Lyrica / Lyrica	Capsules: 25 mg, 50 mg, 75 mg, 100 mg, 150 mg, 200 mg, 225 mg, 300 mg
tiagabine	Gabatril / Not available	Tablets: 2 mg, 4 mg, 12 mg, 16 mg, 20 mg
vigabatrin	Sabril / Sabril	Powder for oral suspension: 0.5-g packets; Tablets: 500 mg

*Generic available.

Succinimides

Generic Name	U.S. Brand Name(s)	Dosage Forms and Strengths
	Canadian Brand(s)	
ethosuximide*	Zarontin	Capsules (Zarontin): 250 mg
	Zarontin	Solution, oral: 250 mg/5 mL
		Syrup (Zarontin): 250 mg/5 mL
methsuximide	Celontin	Capsules: 300 mg
	Celontin	

*Generic available.

SUCCINIMIDES

Ethosuximide and methsuximide are indicated for the treatment of absence seizures. They are two of only a few drugs that target absence seizures.

Mechanism of Action and Pharmacokinetics

Ethosuximide inhibits T-type voltage-dependent calcium channels. The drug is well absorbed orally and reaches peak plasma concentrations within 3 to 7 hours after administration. Unlike many of the other antiseizure drugs, it is not protein bound and is completely metabolized by the liver. It has a long elimination half-life, approximately 40 hours. Drug interactions with phenytoin result in increased phenytoin levels, and interactions with valproic acid cause decreased ethosuximide clearance.

Adverse Reactions

Common side effects associated with ethosuximide are sedation, dizziness, unsteadiness, nausea, vomiting, and photophobia. Rarely, the drug causes liver and kidney damage.

BARBITURATES

Phenobarbital was the first drug used to treat seizures. It is indicated in the treatment of generalized tonic-clonic seizures and partial seizures and is administered to children to control febrile seizures. Amobarbital, mephobarbital, and primidone are also administered to treat tonic-clonic seizures. Pentobarbital is indicated for the treatment of status epilepticus and acute control of tonic-clonic seizures from meningitis, tetanus, ethanol withdrawal, eclampsia, and poisons.

Mechanism of Action

Barbiturates enhance GABA at GABA_A receptors by binding to a barbiturate receptor linked to chloride ion channels. This results in an influx of chloride ions into the neuron, which inhibits neuronal excitability.

Pharmacokinetics

Oral absorption of phenobarbital is moderately slow; however, the drug is readily distributed throughout the central nervous system because of its high degree of lipid solubility. It has 100% bioavailability. It is metabolized in the liver, as is primidone, another barbiturate that is administered to treat seizures. Primidone is metabolized to phenobarbital. Phenobarbital is capable of self-inducing the enzymes that metabolize it and many other drugs such as phenytoin and valproic acid. It is implicated in many drug interactions involving enzyme induction.

Adverse Reactions

Sedation, unsteadiness, confusion, nausea, hypotension, tolerance, and dependence are adverse effects associated with barbiturates. Serious side effects are megaloblastic anemia and respiratory depression. Phenobarbital may produce hyperactivity, rather than sedation, in children.

Barbiturates

Generic Name	U.S. Brand Name(s) / Canadian Brand(s)	Dosage Forms and Strengths
amobarbital*	Amytal / Not available	Powder for injection: 500 mg
mephobarbital	Mebaral / Not available	Tablets: 32 mg, 50 mg, 100 mg
pentobarbital	Nembutal / Veterinary use only	Injection, solution: 50 mg/mL
phenobarbital*	Luminal / Generics	Elixir: 20 mg/5 mL Injection, solution (Luminal): 60 mg/mL, 65 mg/mL, 130 mg/mL[†], 30 mg/mL, 120 mg/mL[‡] Solution, oral: 20 mg/5 mL Tablets: 15 mg, 30 mg, 60 mg, 100 mg
primidone*	Mysoline / Generics	Tablets: 50 mg[†], 125 mg[‡], 250 mg

*Generic available.
[†]Strength available in the United States only.
[‡]Strength available in Canada only.

Benzodiazepines Used in the Treatment of Seizures

	Generic Name	U.S. Brand Name(s) / Canadian Brand(s)	Dosage Forms and Strengths
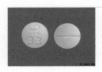	clonazepam*	Klonopin / Rivotril	Tablets (Klonopin, Rivotril): 1 mg[†], 0.5 mg, 2 mg Tablets, disintegrating: 0.125 mg, 0.25 mg, 0.5 mg, 1 mg, 2 mg
	clorazepate*	Tranxene / Generics	Tablets: 3.75 mg, 7.5 mg, 15 mg
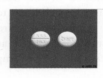	diazepam	Diastat, Diastat AcuDial, Valium / Diastat, Diazemuls, Valium	Injection, solution: 5 mg/mL Injection, emulsion (Diazemuls): 5 mg/mL Solution, oral: 5 mg/5 mg Rectal gel (Diastat): 2.5 mg, 5 mg[‡], 10 mg, 20 mg Tablets (Valium): 2 mg, 5 mg, 10 mg

*Generic available.
[†]Strength available in the United States only.
[‡]Strength available in Canada only.

BENZODIAZEPINES

Benzodiazepines are indicated for the treatment of status epilepticus (intravenous diazepam), absence seizures and myoclonic seizures (clonazepam), and partial seizures (clorazepate). Benzodiazepines bind to receptor sites on the GABA$_A$ complex. This increases the affinity of GABA to the GABA receptor. GABA receptor binding reduces neuronal excitability by opening chloride (Cl$^-$) ion channels and lowering the neuronal membrane resting potential. The mechanism of action and pharmacokinetics of benzodiazepines are discussed in detail in Chapter 5. Sedation, unsteadiness, confusion, impaired learning, tolerance, and dependence are adverse effects common to benzodiazepines. Intravenous diazepam can cause respiratory depression.

OTHER BROAD-SPECTRUM ANTISEIZURE DRUGS

Lamotrigine, levetiracetam, topiramate, and zonisamide are newer broad-spectrum antiseizure drugs. They are indicated for the treatment of generalized (tonic-clonic) and focal (partial) seizures.

TECH ALERT!
The following drugs have look-alike/sound-alike issues: Keppra and Kaletra; Lamictal, Lamisil, and Lomotil; lamotrigine and Lamivudine; Topamax and Toprol-XL

Mechanism of Action and Pharmacokinetics

Lamotrigine, zonisamide, and topiramate act by inhibiting voltage-dependent sodium channels. Additional mechanisms of action for zonisamide are inhibition of T-type calcium channels and GABA binding. Additional mechanisms of action for topiramate include antagonism of non-NMDA (N-methyl-D-aspartate) glutaminergic receptors and acting as a GABA agonist. The mechanism of action for levetiracetam is not fully known.

Lamotrigine, levetiracetam, and topiramate are rapidly absorbed orally. Oral absorption of zonisamide is slow to moderate. All of the drugs have greater than 95% bioavailability. Protein binding is less than 50% for all of these drugs, so there are fewer drug interactions than with some of the other antiseizure medications. Lower doses of lamotrigine are required when taken with valproic acid. Higher doses are required when taken with enzyme-inducing drugs.

Lacosamide was approved for the treatment of seizures in 2008. Its mechanism of action is not completely known, but it exhibits activity on voltage-gated sodium channels that decreases neuronal excitement. Lacosamide is indicated for the treatment of partial seizures.

Adverse Effects

Lamotrigine, levetiracetam, topiramate, and zonisamide may produce sedation and dizziness. Lamotrigine and topiramate also produce nausea and ataxia. Additional side effects of lamotrigine are blurred vision, double vision, and rash. Levetiracetam and topiramate may also produce weakness. Side effects of topiramate also include lack of concentration, headache, and heart palpitations. Zonisamide may produce nausea, rash, and kidney stones in addition to sedation. The most common side effects of lacosamide are drowsiness, headache, fatigue, and nausea.

TECH NOTE! Pregabalin is a C-V controlled substance.

TECH NOTE! Lacosamide (Vimpat) is a C-V controlled substance in the United States and may produce euphoria.

Miscellaneous

Generic Name	U.S. Brand Name(s) / Canadian Brand(s)	Dosage Forms and Strengths
lacosamide	Vimpat / Vimpat	Injection, solution: 10 mg/mL; Solution, oral: 10 mg/mL; Tablets, oral: 50 mg, 100 mg, 150 mg, 200 mg

Broad-Spectrum Antiseizure Drugs

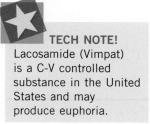

Generic Name	U.S. Brand Name(s) / Canadian Brand(s)	Dosage Forms and Strengths
lamotrigine*	Lamictal, Lamictal CD, Lamictal ODT kit, Lamictal XR / Lamictal	Tablets (Lamictal): 25 mg, 100 mg, 150 mg, 200 mg; Tablets, as chewable (Lamictal CD): 2 mg‡, 5 mg, 25 mg; Tablets, extended release (Lamictal XR): 25 mg, 50 mg, 100 mg, 200 mg; Tablets, oral disintegrating (Lamictal ODT): 25 mg, 50 mg, 100 mg, 200 mg
levetiracetam*	Keppra, Keppra XR / Keppra	Injection, solution: 100 mg/1 mL†; Solution, oral: 100 mg/mL†; Tablets: 250 mg, 500 mg, 750 mg, 1000 mg†; Tablets, extended release (Keppra XR): 500 mg, 750 mg
topiramate*	Topamax / Topamax	Capsules, sprinkle: 15 mg, 25 mg; Tablets: 25 mg, 50 mg, 100 mg, 200 mg
zonisamide	Zonegran / Not available	Capsules: 25 mg, 50 mg, 100 mg

*Generic available.
†Strength available in the United States only.
‡Strength available in Canada only.

Summary of Drugs Used for the Treatment of Seizures

Seizure Type	Drugs Used for the Treatment of Seizures		
Generalized (myoclonic and tonic-clonic)	amobarbital[§] carbamazepine[§] clonazepam[^] diazepam[§] fosphenytoin[§]	lamotrigine[§] levetiracetam mephobarbital[§] phenobarbital phenytoin[§]	primidone[§] topiramate valproic acid
Partial seizures	carbamazepine clorazepate diazepam fosphenytoin gabapentin lacosamide	lamotrigine levetiracetam oxcarbazepine phenobarbital phenytoin pregabalin	primidone tiagabine topiramate valproic acid vigabatrin zonisamide
Absence seizures	clonazepam ethosuximide mephobarbital	methsuximide valproic acid	
Status epilepticus	diazepam IV fosphenytoin IV lorazepam IV	pentobarbital IV phenobarbital IV phenytoin IV	

[^] myoclonic seizures only.
[§]tonic-clonic seizures only

Summary of Drugs Used in the Treatment of Seizures

Generic Name	U.S. Brand Name	Usual Adult Oral Dose and Dosing Schedule	Warning Labels
Hydantoins			
fosphenytoin	Cerebyx	**Status epilepticus:** IV loading dose: 15-20 mg/kg (PE) administered at rate of 100-150 mg/min **Nonemergent maintenance dose:** 4-6 mg/kg (PE)/day administered IM or IV	MAY CAUSE DROWSINESS; MAY IMPAIR ABILITY TO DRIVE. AVOID ALCOHOL. DO NOT DISCONTINUE WITHOUT MEDICAL SUPERVISION. SWALLOW WHOLE; DO NOT CRUSH OR CHEW—sustained release. TAKE WITH FOOD—Phenytoin. AVOID PREGNANCY. AVOID ANTACIDS AND CIMETIDINE— phenytoin. SHAKE WELL—suspension.
phenytoin	Dilantin	**Status epilepticus:** IV loading dose: 15-25 mg/kg; maintenance 300 mg/ day in 3 divided doses **Neurosurgery:** 100-200 mg administered every 4 hours during surgery **Generalized/partial seizures (oral):** Loading dose: 10-20 mg/kg in 3 divided doses **Maintenance:** 300 mg/day in 3 divided doses (immediate release) or 1-2 doses (extended release)	
Valproates			
valproic acid and derivatives	Depakene, Depakote	**Seizures (oral):** Start 10 mg-15 mg/ kg/day in 1-3 divided doses, increase up to 1000 mg-2500 mg/ day Note: regular and delayed-release formulations are dosed 2-4 times a day; extended-release formulations are dosed once daily	MAY CAUSE DIZZINESS OR DROWSIINESS; MAY IMPAIR ABILITY TO DRIVE. AVOID ALCOHOL. TAKE WITH FOOD. AVOID PREGNANCY. SWALLOW WHOLE; DO NOT CRUSH OR CHEW—extended release. DO NOT DISCONTINUE WITHOUT MEDICAL SUPERVISION.

Summary of Drugs Used in the Treatment of Seizures—cont'd

Generic Name	U.S. Brand Name	Usual Adult Oral Dose and Dosing Schedule	Warning Labels
Iminostilbenes			
carbamazepine	Tegretol	Start 200 mg twice a day; increase to 1200-1600 mg/day in 3-4 divided doses (maximum, 2400 mg/day)	MAY CAUSE DIZZINESS OR DROWSINESS; MAY IMPAIR ABILITY TO DRIVE. AVOID ALCOHOL.
oxcarbazepine	Trileptal	Start 600 mg twice a day; increase to 2400 mg/day	TAKE WITH FOOD. SWALLOW WHOLE; DO NOT CRUSH OR CHEW—extended release. TAKE WITH A FULL GLASS OF WATER— chewable tablets. SHAKE WELL—suspension. DO NOT DISCONTINUE WITHOUT MEDICAL SUPERVISION. MAY DECREASE THE EFFECTIVENESS OF ORAL CONTRACEPTIVES.
GABA Analogs			
gabapentin	Neurontin	Start 300 mg 3 times/day; increase to 900-1800 mg/day	MAY CAUSE DIZZINESS OR DROWSINESS; MAY IMPAIR ABILITY TO DRIVE. AVOID ALCOHOL. TAKE WITH FOOD.
pregabalin	Lyrica	150-600 mg dosed 2-3 times a day	AVOID ANTACIDS WITHIN 2 HOURS OF DOSE—gabapentin.
tiagabine	Gabatril	Start 4 mg once daily; increase up to 56 mg/day in 2-4 divided doses	DO NOT DISCONTINUE WITHOUT MEDICAL SUPERVISION.
vigabatrin	Sabril	Start 1 g once daily; increase up to 2-3 g/day	SHAKE WELL; DISCARD WITHIN 30 DAYS OF RECONSTITUTION—vigabatrin suspension
Succinimides			
ethosuximide	Zarontin	Start 250 mg twice a day; increase up to 1500 mg/day	MAY CAUSE DIZZINESS OR DROWSINESS; MAY IMPAIR ABILITY TO DRIVE. AVOID ALCOHOL.
methsuximide	Celontin	Start 300 mg/day; increase by 300 mg/wk up to a maximum of 1200 mg/day in 3-4 divided doses	TAKE WITH FOOD. DO NOT DISCONTINUE WITHOUT MEDICAL SUPERVISION.
Barbiturates			
amobarbital	Amytal	**Refractory tonic-clonic seizures:** 65-500 mg administered as a single IV dose	MAY CAUSE DROWSINESS; MAY IMPAIR ABILITY TO DRIVE. AVOID ALCOHOL.
pentobarbital	Nembutal	**Status epilepticus—for mechanically ventilated patients only:** 10-15 mg/kg IV over 1 hr (maximum total loading dose, 30 mg/kg) followed by 0.5-1 mg/kg/hr IV titrated by 0.5 mg/kg/hr as needed	MAY BE HABIT FORMING. DO NOT DISCONTINUE WITHOUT MEDICAL SUPERVISION.
mephobarbital	Mebaral	200 mg at bedtime up to 600 mg/day in 2-4 divided doses	
phenobarbital	Luminal	**Status epilepticus:** IV loading dose 15-30 mg/kg; start maintenance dose after 12-24 hours **Seizure maintenance:** Oral or IV 1-3 mg/kg/day dosed 2-3 times a day	
primidone	Mysoline	750-1500 mg/day in 3-4 divided doses	

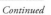

Continued

Summary of Drugs Used in the Treatment of Seizures—cont'd

Generic Name	U.S. Brand Name	Usual Adult Oral Dose and Dosing Schedule	Warning Labels
Benzodiazepines			
clonazepam	Klonopin	1.5 mg 3 times a day (maximum, 20 mg/day)	MAY CAUSE DROWSINESS; MAY IMPAIR ABILITY TO DRIVE. AVOID ALCOHOL. MAY BE HABIT FORMING. DO NOT CRUSH, BREAK, OR CHEW— extended-release clorazepate.
clorazepate	Tranxene	**Partial seizures:** 7.5 mg 2-3 times a day up to 90 mg/day	
diazepam	Valium	**Status epilepticus and drug-induced seizures:** 5-10 mg every 10-15 minutes IV up to 30 mg per 8-hour period	
Broad-Spectrum Antiseizure Drugs			
lamotrigine	Lamictal	300-500 mg/day in 2 divided doses (maximum, 700 mg/day)	MAY CAUSE DIZZINESS OR DROWSINESS; MAY IMPAIR ABILITY TO DRIVE. AVOID ALCOHOL. DO NOT DISCONTINUE WITHOUT MEDICAL SUPERVISION. MAINTAIN ADEQUATE HYDRATION— zonisamide.
levetiracetam	Keppra	Start 500 mg twice daily; increase to 3000 mg/day	
topiramate	Topamax	Start 25 mg-50 mg/day in 2 divided doses; increase to 400 mg/day (maximum, 1600 mg/day)	
zonisamide	Zonegran	Start 100 mg/day; increase to 400 mg/day (maximum, 600 mg/day)	
Miscellaneous			
lacosamide	Vimpat	Start 50 mg twice daily; increase in weekly intervals up to a maximum 400 mg/day	MAY CAUSE DIZZINESS OR DROWSINESS; MAY IMPAIR ABILITY TO DRIVE. AVOID ALCOHOL. STORE AT ROOM TEMPERATURE; DISCARD UNUSED PORTION 7 WEEKS AFTER OPENING—oral solution.

Chapter Summary

- Epilepsy was described as early as 3000 years ago in ancient Babylon.
- About 1% of the population has epilepsy.
- Epilepsy is a type of seizure disorder that is characterized by a sudden, excessive, disorderly discharge of cerebral neurons.
- People with epilepsy have an abnormally high level of excitatory neurotransmitters coupled with a low level of inhibitory neurotransmitters.
- Half of all seizures have no known cause.
- Causes of seizures include birth defects, infection (meningitis, AIDS), tumors, head trauma, high fevers, hypoglycemia, drug and alcohol withdrawal, and cerebrovascular disease.
- The incidence of seizures caused by head injury can be reduced by wearing seat belts, motorcycle helmets, and bike helmets.
- Whereas generalized seizures spread across both of the cerebral hemispheres, partial seizures are confined to a single hemisphere.

- Status epilepticus is a medical emergency that results from repeated generalized seizures that deprive the brain of oxygen.
- Status epilepticus is treated with intravenous medications.
- Some seizures are linked to a defect in the genes that control the ion channels that open and close to regulate the influx of chloride, sodium, and calcium into the neuron.
- Neuronal firing is inhibited by drugs that delay the inflow of sodium ions. Drugs that bind to T-type calcium channels inhibit absence (petit mal) seizures.
- The GABA receptor regulates the movement of chloride ion into the neuron, which inhibits the formation of action potentials, neuronal hyperactivity, and seizures.
- The goal of treatment of epilepsy and other seizure disorders is to reduce the incidence of seizures by suppressing seizure activity.
- Medications reduce seizure activity in approximately 80% of people diagnosed with epilepsy.
- Therapeutic blood levels for phenytoin are best maintained by dispensing the same manufacturer's formulation each time a prescription is filled.
- Carbamazepine should be protected from light and moisture. Moisture can decrease the potency by as much as 30%.
- Antacids decrease the absorption of gabapentin by 20%. The absorption of tiagabine is reduced by foods that have a high fat content.
- A few drugs are effective for treating absence seizures; they are ethosuximide, valproic acid, and clonazepam.
- Barbiturates and benzodiazepines used in the treatment of seizures are controlled substances.
- Lamotrigine, levetiracetam, topiramate, and zonisamide are broad-spectrum antiseizure drugs.
- Lacosamide is indicated for the treatment of partial seizures.
- Drug therapy with antiepileptic drugs increases the risk for suicide ideation and behavior.

REVIEW QUESTIONS

1. One of the oldest known brain disorders described as early as 3000 years ago in ancient Babylon is
   - a. schizophrenia
   - b. epilepsy
   - c. depression
   - d. fainting

2. Febrile seizures in children are associated with an _____, causing a sudden spike in temperature.
   - a. injury
   - b. injection
   - c. infection
   - d. a, b, and c

3. The only major seizure classification is generalized seizures.
   - a. true
   - b. false

4. A medical emergency that results from repeated generalized seizures and deprives the brain of oxygen is called
   - a. status epilepticus
   - b. myoclonic epilepticus
   - c. grand mal epilepticus
   - d. tonic-clonic status

5. The goal of treatment of epilepsy and other seizure disorders is to reduce the incidence of seizures by _____ seizure activity.
   - a. stopping
   - b. sedating
   - c. suppressing
   - d. shocking

6. This drug is used in the management of generalized and partial seizures, status epilepticus, and seizures after head trauma or neurosurgery.
   a. tiagabine
   b. carbamazepine
   c. valproic acid
   d. fosphenytoin

7. One of the few drugs indicated for the treatment of absence seizures is
   a. phenytoin
   b. gabapentin
   c. carbamazepine
   d. ethosuximide

8. What benzodiazepine is indicated for the treatment of status epilepticus, drug-induced seizures, and anxiety?
   a. diazepam
   b. clonazepam
   c. lorazepam
   d. alprazolam

9. Phenytoin was the first drug that was used to treat seizures.
   a. true
   b. false

10. An unusual sensation or, auditory, visual, or olfactory hallucination that is experienced just before the onset of a seizure is called a(n)
   a. halo
   b. aura
   c. vision
   d. hallucination

TECHNICIAN'S CORNER

1. If you see someone experiencing a seizure, what would you do?
2. What would be the best advice you can give a patient with epilepsy about his or her medication?

Bibliography

FDA: Suicidal Behavior and Ideation and Antiepileptic Drugs. Retrieved February 27, 2011, from http://www.fda.gov/Drugs/DrugSafety/PostmarketDrugSafetyInformationforPatientsandProviders/ucm100190.htm. 2009.

Elsevier: Gold Standard Clinical Pharmacology, 2010. Retrieved April 22, 2012, from https://www.clinicalpharmacology.com/ accessed.

FDA: FDA Approved Drug Products, 2012. Retrieved April 22, 2012, from http://www.accessdata.fda.gov/scripts/cder/drugsatfda/index.cfm?fuseaction=Search.Search_Drug_Name.

Health Canada: Drug Product Database. Retrieved Feb 27, 2011, from http://www.hc-sc.gc.ca/dhp-mps/prodpharma/databasdon/index-eng.php. 2010.

Kalant H, Grant D, Mitchell J: Principles of medical pharmacology, ed 7, Toronto, 2007, Elsevier Canada, A Division of Reed Elsevier Canada, pp 223-235.

Lance L, Lacy C, Armstrong L, et al: Drug information handbook for the allied health professional, ed 12, Hudson, OH, 2005, APhA Lexi-Comp.

National Institute of Neurological Disorders and Stroke: Seizures and epilepsy: Hope through research, Bethesda, MD, National Institute of Neurological Disorders and Stroke, National Institutes of Health, U.S. Department of Health and Human Services. Updated February 24, 2011. NIH Publication No. 04-156.

Page C, Curtis M, Sutter M, et al: Integrated pharmacology, Philadelphia, 2005, Elsevier Mosby, pp 257-259.

Raffa RB, Rawls SM, Beyzarov EP: Netter's illustrated pharmacology, Philadelphia, 2005, WB Saunders, pp 67-70.

USP Center for Advancement of Patient Safety: Use caution: avoid confusion. USP Quality Review No. 79, Rockville, MD, April 2004, USP Center for Advancement of Patient Safety.

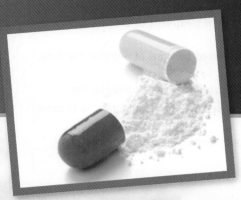

10

Treatment of Pain and Migraine Headache

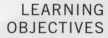

KEY TERMS

Acute pain: Sudden pain that results from injury or inflammation and is usually self-limiting.

Acupuncture: Nonpharmacological treatment for pain that involves the application of needles to precise points on the body.

Analgesic: Drug that reduces pain.

Arthritis: Condition that is associated with joint pain.

Biofeedback: Nonpharmacological treatment for pain that involves relaxation techniques and gaining self-control over muscle tension, heart rate, and skin temperature.

Breakthrough pain: Pain that occurs in between scheduled doses of analgesics.

Cephalgia: Head pain.

Chronic pain: Pain that persists for a long period of time that is worsened by psychological factors and is resistant to many medical treatments.

Cluster headache: Intensely painful vascular headache that occurs in groups and produces pain on one side of the head.

Cyclooxygenase-2 inhibitor: Analgesic, antiinflammatory drug that preferentially blocks cyclooxygenase-2, an enzyme that produces prostaglandin, which is a substance involved in mediating pain.

Diabetic neuropathy: Peripheral nerve disorder caused by diabetes and causing numbness, pain, or tingling in the feet or legs.

147

Dysphoria: Feeling of emotional or mental discomfort, restlessness, and depression; the opposite of euphoria.

Endorphins, enkephalins, and dynorphin: Substances released by the body in response to painful stimuli that act as natural painkillers.

Euphoria: State of intense happiness or well-being; the opposite of dysphoria.

Hyperalgesia: Heightened sensitivity to pain that can result from treatment of chronic pain with high-dose opioids.

Inflammation: A response to tissue irritation or injury that is marked by signs of redness, swelling, heat, and pain.

Migraine: Vascular headache that is often accompanied by nausea and visual disturbances.

Neuropathic pain: Type of pain associated with nerve injury caused by trauma, infection, or chronic diseases such as diabetes.

Nociceptors: Thin nerve fibers in skin, muscle, and other body tissues that carry pain signals.

NSAID: Nonsteroidal anti-inflammatory drug.

Opiate naïve: No current exposure to opioids.

Opioid: Naturally occurring or synthetically derived analgesic with properties similar to those of morphine.

PCA: Patient-controlled analgesia.

Plasticity: Ability of the brain to restructure itself and adapt to injury.

Shingles: Reoccurring and painful skin rash caused by the herpes zoster virus.

Substance P: Peptide that is involved in the production of pain sensations and controls pain perception.

Trigeminal neuralgia: Painful condition that produces intense, stabbing pain in areas of the face innervated by branches of the trigeminal nerve.

Overview

Most people will experience some type of physical pain in their lifetime. *Acute pain* is triggered by an injury, burn, infection, or some other stimuli and is self-limiting. *Chronic pain* may persist for years and is often inadequately controlled by pharmaceuticals or other pain management therapies. There is a strong psychological component to pain that is frequently underestimated. Psychological factors can influence a person's tolerance for pain and can determine whether the outcome of treatment is successful. To reduce anxieties associated with pain that result in higher doses of pain medications, patients may be permitted to control the frequency of administration of their doses of pain medications. Patient-controlled analgesia (*PCA*) is done using a device that is connected to the patient's intravenous line. The patient pushes a button to deliver a measured dose of pain medication.

Pain is often categorized by its origin. *Neuropathic pain* is associated with a nerve injury caused by trauma, infection, or chronic disease such as diabetes. Chronic pain is often of neuropathic origin. Nociceptive pain may be visceral or somatic in origin and is caused by stimulation of nociceptors in viscera (lungs, gastrointestinal [GI], heart) or skin, muscle, soft tissue, or bone (somatic). *Nociceptors* are thin nerve fibers located in the skin, muscle, and other body tissues that carry pain signals. The division of pain into distinct categories is somewhat simplistic because multiple pathophysiological mechanisms are probably involved. Because untreated pain can affect all body systems, increasing heart rate, anxiety, ischemia, muscle spasms, and decreasing immune response and intestinal motility, a multimodal approach to pain management is recommended. It is important to determine whether the pain has a neuropathic origin because the response to opioid analgesics is less with neuropathic pain than with nociceptive pain.

Pain may be referred. This means that the place where pain symptoms are most strongly felt may be different than the actual origin of the painful stimuli. Pain can also be triggered as part of an immune system response to fighting disease. Cytokines are a type of protein that is released as a response to injury. Cytokines cause inflammation that can result in pain at the inflammatory site.

Conditions That Produce Pain

NOCICEPTIVE ORIGIN

Inflammation

Inflammation is an important source of pain. ***Inflammation*** is a response to tissue irritation or injury that is marked by signs of redness, swelling, heat, and pain. When an injury occurs, phospholipase A_2 enzyme activity increases, stimulating the release of arachidonic acid from tissue membrane phospholipids. Arachidonic acid is activated by cyclooxygenase (COX), an enzyme involved in the biosynthesis of prostaglandins. Prostaglandins are important mediators of pain. Arthritis, muscle or nerve damage, and even infection can produce painful inflammation.

Arthritis

Arthritis is a condition that produces joint pain. Rheumatoid arthritis, osteoarthritis, and gout are all arthritic conditions. The cause and treatment of each of these arthritic conditions vary. Osteoarthritis is the most common of all arthritic conditions. It is the leading cause of musculoskeletal pain. Symptoms of osteoarthritis are joint pain, stiffness, swelling, and crepitus (creaking joints). Pain may occur after activity or at rest. Risk factors for osteoarthritis are previous joint injury or surgery, obesity, increasing age, muscle weakness, and occupations that involve excessive joint use. Inflammation of the fluid that surrounds the joint (synovial fluid) contributes to the pain associated with osteoarthritis.

Low Back Pain

Nearly one-third of adults will experience low back pain in any given year, making it one of the most common types of pain. Despite its high prevalence, only 20% of people experiencing low back pain seek medical attention.

Acute low back pain produces symptoms that last less than 6 weeks. Chronic low back pain can persist indefinitely and may produce leg pain or widespread body pain or restrict spinal movement.

Burns

Severe burns can produce excruciating pain. Third-degree burns are the most severe because the skin has been destroyed. First-degree burns are less severe than second- or third-degree burns.

Trauma

Musculoskeletal pain may be caused by trauma. Sport injuries, motor vehicle accidents, and workplace or home accidents can result in painful sprains, fractures, burns, cuts, and bruises.

NEUROPATHIC ORIGIN

Diabetic Neuropathy

Uncontrolled diabetes can lead to damage to peripheral nerves. Nerve damage results in numbness, pain, or tingling of the feet or legs. Symptoms of ***diabetic neuropathy*** become more severe as the disease progresses.

Phantom Limb

Patients who have had a limb amputated may describe pain in the area where the limb was removed. It is believed that although the limb is no longer present, the nerves that innervated the limb are remapped or rewired, permitting nerve messages to continue to be received. The ability of the brain to restructure itself and adapt to injury is called ***plasticity***.

Shingles

Shingles produces a reoccurring and painful skin rash and is caused by the herpes zoster virus. The herpes zoster virus, which causes chicken pox, lays dormant in nerve endings until activated. Shingles cannot be cured.

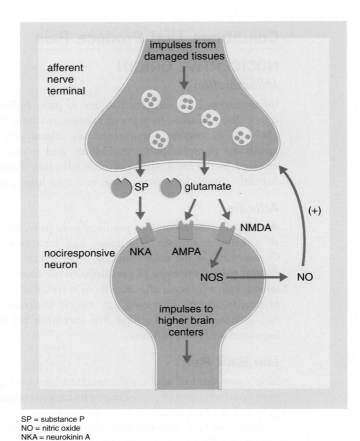

SP = substance P
NO = nitric oxide
NKA = neurokinin A

FIGURE 10-1 Mechanism of pain perception. (From Page C, Curtis M, Sutter M, et al: *Integrated pharmacology*, ed 3, Philadelphia, Mosby, 2006.)

Trigeminal Neuralgia

Trigeminal neuralgia produces headache and intense stabbing pain in areas of the face inner-vated by branches of the trigeminal nerve (lips, eyes, nose, scalp, forehead, upper jaw, and lower jaw). Approximately 1% to 2% of persons with multiple sclerosis develop trigeminal neuralgia.

Mechanism of Pain Signal Transmission

The pain message begins with stimulation of nociceptors in peripheral tissues. The signal is converted to an electrical impulse (transduction) that then travels to the dorsal horn of the spinal cord (trans-mission), where it is augmented or diminished by the release of neurotransmitters, amino acids, and neuropeptides (modulation) and then carried to the brain where the pain message is interpreted (perception) (Figure 10-1).

Neurochemistry of Pain

ROLES OF HISTAMINE, BRADYKININ, AND SEROTONIN

Histamine and bradykinin are released in response to tissue injury and are part of the immune system response. They produce inflammation, vasodilation, and pain. Bradykinin activates the enzyme (phospholipase A_2) that leads to the biosynthesis of prostaglandins. Prostaglandins are hormones that trigger pain response from peripheral nociceptors. Serotonin also stimulates nociceptors and causes pain when it is released by mast cells as part of the inflammatory response.

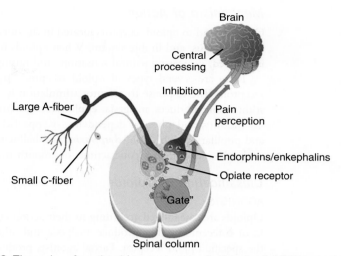

FIGURE 10-2 The role of endorphins and enkephalins in inhibiting pain perception. (Modified from Lilley LL, Harrington S, Snyder JS: *Pharmacology and the nursing process*, ed 5, St Louis, 2007, Mosby.)

ROLE OF GLUTAMATE

Glutamate is an amino acid neurotransmitter that binds to nociceptors carrying the pain message to higher brain centers. Glutamate enhances the response to painful stimuli.

ROLE OF SUBSTANCE P

Substance P is a peptide that is involved in the modulation of pain sensations and controls pain perception. It acts as a neurotransmitter at the junction between nociceptors in the dorsal route of the spinal cord and afferent nerve terminals that will transmit the pain message to the brain. Neurokinin A is another neuropeptide that is involved in pain perception and the transmission pain sensations.

ROLES OF ENDORPHINS, ENKEPHALIN, AND DYNORPHIN

Endorphins, enkephalin, and *dynorphin* are opioid peptides released by the body in response to painful stimuli. They bind to opioid receptors in the brain and spinal cord and block or dull the pain sensations by inhibiting the release of substance P and glutamate. They act like natural painkillers (Figure 10-2).

ROLE OF γ-AMINOBUTYRIC ACID

γ-Aminobutyric acid (GABA) also plays a role in controlling pain. When GABA binds to $GABA_B$ receptors located on presynaptic afferent nerve fibers, it reduces the release of glutamate and substance P. The effect of GABA is inhibitory on nociceptors, and pain sensations are reduced.

Drugs Used to Treat Pain

OPIOIDS

Opiates are naturally occurring substances that are derived from the opium poppy and have been used for more than 2000 years to induce sleep and *euphoria* and to relieve diarrhea. Morphine and heroin are examples of opiates. *Opioid* is a term used to describe a drug that acts like morphine, whether naturally occurring or synthetically derived. Opiates and opioid drugs produce analgesia. Drugs that produce *analgesia* reduce pain sensations and alter pain perception. Some opioid analgesics are also used to treat opioid dependence. When detoxification is achieved, a maintenance dose is continued. Methadone and buprenorphine are examples of opioid agonists that are administered for management of drug dependence. Opioid antagonists such as naltrexone are used to treat drug and alcohol dependence, too.

Mechanism of Action

Opioids bind to opioid receptors located in the dorsal route of the spinal cord, brainstem, thalamus, hypothalamus, and limbic system. When opioids bind to opioid receptors, nociceptive stimulation is reduced, decreasing painful sensations and raising the threshold for pain.

There are several types of opioid receptors: μ_1 and μ_2, κ_1, κ_2, and κ_3 as well as δ_1 and δ_2 receptors. The response to receptor stimulation is specific for each receptor type. Mu (μ) receptor stimulation produces analgesia, euphoria, respiratory depression, pupillary constriction, decreased GI motility, and physical dependence. Kappa (κ) receptor binding produces analgesia, sedation, and pupillary constriction, *dysphoria*, and hallucinations. Delta (δ) receptor stimulation produces analgesia and decreases contractions of smooth muscle.

Classification of Opioids

AGONISTS

Opioids are categorized according to their action at the opioid receptor. Opioid agonists activate μ, κ, or δ receptors. They produce analgesia and other adverse effects associated with stimulation of the specific opioid receptor. Partial agonists produce incomplete activation of the opioid receptor, producing less than maximum response.

ANTAGONISTS

Antagonists bind to the opioid receptor but do not activate it. They interfere with agonist binding. Antagonists are administered when reversal of the action of an opioid agonist is desired.

MIXED AGONIST/ANTAGONISTS

The response produced by some opioids is mixed. Sometimes the opioid behaves like an agonist and sometimes it behaves like an antagonist. Agonist activity is exhibited if the patient has had no recent exposure to an opioid agonist (*opiate naïve*). If the patient is currently taking an opioid agonist, the mixed agonist/antagonist exhibits antagonist activity.

Pharmacokinetics

The bioavailability of morphine is greater when administered parenterally than orally so lower doses are required to produce analgesia. If equianalgesic doses are administered, oral doses provide the same level of pain relief as parenterals. Oral absorption of opioid agonists, partial agonists, and mixed agonist/antagonist is varied. Many orally administered opioids exhibit significant first-pass metabolism. The average onset of action of orally administered opioids is approximately 30 minutes after administration. The onset of action of most parenterally administered opioids occurs within 10 to 15 minutes. A few opioids (meperidine, pentazocine, and butorphanol) begin working in less than 5 minutes. Peak effects are achieved between 30 minutes and 2 hours. The duration of action for immediate-acting opioids ranges between 2 and 6 hours (Table 10-1). The duration of action for controlled-release opioid analgesics may last for up to 72 hours (e.g., fentanyl patches). Patients who have been prescribed long-acting opioid dosage forms (e.g., Kadian, Exalgo) may also be prescribed short-acting opioids to control *breakthrough pain* that may occur between scheduled doses of the long-acting analgesic.

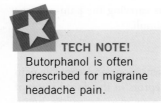

TECH NOTE!
Butorphanol is often prescribed for migraine headache pain.

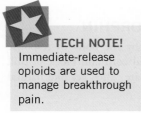

TECH NOTE!
Immediate-release opioids are used to manage breakthrough pain.

TABLE 10-1   **Comparison of Opioid Equivalent Doses, Onset, Peak, and Duration of Action**

Drug and Route	Equivalent Dose*	Onset (min)	Peak (min)	Duration (hr)
Buprenorphine				
IM	0.3 mg	15	60	Up to 6
IV	0.3 mg	<15	<60	Up to 6
SL	—	—	—	—

TABLE 10-1 **Comparison of Opioid Equivalent Doses, Onset, Peak, and Duration of Action—cont'd**

Drug and Route	Equivalent Dose*	Onset (min)	Peak (min)	Duration (hr)
Butorphanol				
IM	2 mg	10-30	30-60	3-4
IV	2 mg	2-3	30	2-4
Nasal spray	2 mg	—	—	—
Codeine				
PO	200 mg	30-45	60-120	4
IM	120 mg	10-30	30-60	4
Subcut	120 mg	10-30	30-60	4
Fentanyl				
IV	0.1 mg	—	—	1-1.5
Transdermal	—	—	—	72
Hydromorphone				
PO	7.5 mg	30	90-120	4
IM	1.5 mg	15	30-60	4-5
IV	1.5 mg	10-15	15-30	2-3
Subcut	1.5 mg	15	30-90	4
Levorphanol				
PO	4 mg	10-60	90-120	4-5
IM	2 mg	—	60	4-5
IV	2 mg	—	<20	4-5
Subcut	2 mg	—	60-90	4-5
Meperidine				
PO	300 mg	15	60-90	2-4
IM	75 mg	10-15	30-50	2-4
IV	75 mg	1	5-7	2-4
Subcut	75 mg	10-15	30-50	2-4
Methadone				
PO	20 mg	30-60	90-120	4-6
IM	10 mg	10-20	60-120	4-5
IV	10 mg	—	15-30	3-4
Morphine				
PO	60 mg	—	10-120	4-5
IM	10 mg	10-30	30-60	4-5
IV	10 mg	—	20	4-5
Subcut	10 mg	10-30	50-90	4-5
Oxycodone				
PO	30 mg	—	60	3-4

Continued

TECH ALERT!

The following drugs have look-alike/ sound-alike issues: codeine, Cardene, and Lodine; Lortab and Lorabid; Vicodin, Hycomine, and Hycodan; hydrocodone and hydromorphone; Demerol and Demadex; meperidine and morphine; Roxanol and Roxicet; Avinza, Evista, and Invanz

TECH NOTE!

Duragesic patches are worn for 72 hours and should be dispensed with instructions on proper storage and disposal to prevent accidental overdose or poisoning.

TECH ALERT!

Naloxone and naltrexone have look-alike/ sound-alike issues.

TECH NOTE!

Buprenorphine tablets may only be prescribed for the treatment of opioid dependency. Valid prescriptions are written by prescribers who have a DEA No. specifically for buprenorphine.

TABLE 10-1   **Comparison of Opioid Equivalent Doses, Onset, Peak, and Duration of Action—cont'd**

Drug and Route	Equivalent Dose*	Onset (min)	Peak (min)	Duration (hr)
Pentazocine				
PO	180 mg	15-30	60-90	3
IM	60 mg	15-20	30-60	2-3
IV	60 mg	2-3	15-30	2-3
SC	60 mg	15-20	30-60	2-3

*Dose in milligrams that produces an equivalent degree of analgesia as 10 mg of morphine.

TABLE 10-2   **Opioid-Induced Side Effects and Adverse Effects by Body System**

Body System	Side Effect or Adverse Effect
Central nervous system	Sedation, disorientation, euphoria, lightheadedness, dysphoria, lowered seizure threshold, and tremors
Cardiovascular system	Hypotension, palpitations, and flushing
Respiratory tract	Respiratory depression and aggravation of asthma
Gastrointestinal tract	Nausea, vomiting, constipation, and biliary tract spasm
Genitourinary tract	Urinary retention
Other	Itching, rash, and wheal information

From Lilley LL, Harrington S, Snyder JS: *Pharmacology and the nursing process*, ed 5, St Louis, Mosby, 2007.

Adverse Reactions

Adverse effects of opioid agonists, partial agonists, and mixed agonist/antagonists are determined by the extent to which they bind to specific opioid receptors. Morphine, codeine, and fentanyl are agonists primarily at μ receptors and produce euphoria, respiratory depression, pupillary constriction, constipation, and physical dependence. Pentazocine is a mixed agonist/antagonist that is a partial agonist at κ receptors and a weak antagonist at μ receptors. It produces sedation and pupillary constriction (Table 10-2). Side effects caused by acute use are sedation, constipation, and GI upset. Chronic use may additionally produce *hyperalgesia* (a heightened sensitivity to pain that can result from treatment of chronic pain with high-dose opioids), sexual dysfunction, and decreased immune response.

Precautions

Access to opioid agonists, partial agonists, and most mixed agonist/antagonists is restricted in the United States (Schedule C-I through C-V) and Canada (straight and verbal narcotics) because they produce tolerance and dependence.

OPIOID ANTAGONISTS

Opioid antagonists are indicated for reversal of respiratory depression caused by opioid use. Respiratory depression may be produced by drugs administered during surgery for general anesthesia or may occur in infants born to opioid-dependent women. The opioid antagonist naltrexone is also indicated for the treatment of opioid overdose and the management of drug and alcohol dependence. Naltrexone may produce drowsiness. The warning labels MAY CAUSE DROWSINESS, MAY IMPAIR ABILITY TO DRIVE, and AVOID ALCOHOL should be applied to prescription vials. Both naltrexone and naloxone can precipitate withdrawal symptoms in patients who are opioid dependent.

Opioid Agonists

Generic Name	U.S. Brand Name(s) / Canadian Brand Name(s)	Dosage Forms And Strengths	Controlled Substance Schedule
codeine*	Generics Codeine Contin	**Injection:** 15 mg/mL and 30 mg/mL **Syrup, oral:** 5 mg/mL‡ **Tablets, controlled release (Codeine Contin):** 50 mg, 100 mg, 150 mg, 200 mg **Tablets, as phosphate:**‡ 30 mg, 60 mg **Tablets, as sulfate:** 15 mg, 30 mg, 60 mg	C-II (US) Straight narcotic (Canada)
codeine and acetaminophen (APAP)*	Tylenol with Codeine No. 2, Tylenol with Codeine No. 3, Tylenol with Codeine No. 4, Tylenol with Codeine No. 1, Tylenol with Codeine No. 2, Tylenol with Codeine No. 3, Tylenol with Codeine No. 4	**Elixir:** APAP 120 mg and codeine 12 mg **Suspension:** APAP 120 mg and codeine 12 mg **Tablets (Tylenol with Codeine No. 1):** APAP 300 mg and codeine 8 mg† **Tablets (Tylenol with Codeine No. 2):** APAP 300 mg and codeine 15 mg† **Tablets (Tylenol with Codeine No. 3):** APAP 300 mg and codeine 30 mg† **Tablets (Tylenol with Codeine No. 4):** APAP 300 mg and codeine 60 mg †Also contains 15 mg caffeine in Canada	C-V (elixir only) C-III (US) Tylenol 1 (BTC schedule II in Canada) Tylenol 2, Tylenol 3 (verbal narcotic in Canada) Tylenol 4 (straight narcotic in Canada)
fentanyl*	ABSTRAL, Actiq, Duragesic, Fentora, Onsolis Duragesic	**Injection, solution (Sublimaze):** 50 mcg/mL **Lozenge (Actiq):** 200 mcg, 400 mcg, 600 mcg, 800 mcg, 1200 mcg, 1600 mcg **Oral dissolving film (Onsolis):** 200 mcg, 400 mcg, 600 mcg, 800 mcg, 1200 mcg **Tablets, buccal (Fentora):** 100 mcg, 200 mcg, 400 mcg, 600 mcg, 800 mcg **Tablets, sublingual (ABSTRAL):** 100 mcg, 200 mcg, 300 mcg, 400 mcg, 600 mcg, 800 mcg **Transdermal (Duragesic):*** 12 mcg, 25 mcg, 37 mcg†, 50 mcg, 75 mcg, 100 mcg	C-III (US) Straight narcotic (Canada)
hydrocodone and acetaminophen*	Anexsia, Lorcet, Lorcet Plus, Lortab, Norco, Stagesic, Vicodin, Vicodin ES, Vicodin HP, Zydone Not available	**Capsules (Stagesic):** 5 mg hydrocodone and 500 mg APAP **Elixir (Lortab):** 7.5 mg hydrocodone and 500 mg APAP/15 mL **Tablets (Anexsia):** 5 mg hydrocodone and 500 mg APAP; 7.5 mg/650 mg APAP **(Lorcet):** 10 mg/650 mg **(Lorcet Plus):** 7.5 mg/650 mg **(Lortab):** 5 mg/500 mg, 7.5 mg/500 mg, 10 mg/500 mg **(Norco):** 5 mg/325 mg, 7.5 mg/325 mg, 10 mg/325 mg **(Vicodin):** 5 mg/500 mg **(Vicodin ES):** 7.5 mg/750 mg **(Vicodin HP):** 10 mg/660 mg; **(Zydone):** 5 mg/400 mg, 7.5 mg/400 mg, 10 mg/400 mg	C-III (US)
hydrocodone and ibuprofen*	Reprexain, Vicoprofen Not available	**Tablets:** 2.5 mg/200 mg, 5 mg/200 mg, 7.5 mg/200 mg, 10 mg/200 mg	C-III

Continued

Opioid Agonists—cont'd

Generic Name	U.S. Brand Name(s) / Canadian Brand Name(s)	Dosage Forms And Strengths	Controlled Substance Schedule
hydromorphone*	Dilaudid, Dilaudid-HP, Exalgo	Capsules, controlled release (Hydromorph Contin): 3 mg, 6 mg, 12 mg, 18 mg, 24 mg, 30 mg	C-II (US) Straight narcotic (Canada)
	Dilaudid, Dilaudid-HP, Dilaudid-HP Plus, Dilaudin-XP, Hydromorph Contin, Hydromorph IR, Jurnista	Injection, powder for reconstitution (Dilaudid): 250 mg per vial Injection, solution: 1 mg/mL, 2 mg/mL, 4 mg/mL, 10 mg/mL (Dilaudid-HP), 20 mg/mL (Dilaudid-HP Plus), 50 mg/mL (Dilaudid-XP), 100 mg/mL Liquid, oral (Dilaudid): 1 mg/mL† Tablets, extended release (Exalgo, Jurnista): 4 mg‡, 8 mg, 12 mg†, 16 mg, 32 mg‡ Tablets, immediate release (Dilaudid, Hydromorph IR): 1 mg‡, 2 mg, 4 mg, 8 mg Suppository: 3 mg	
levorphanol*	Levo-Dromoran	Injection, solution: 2 mg/mL Tablets: 2 mg	C-II (US)
	Not available		
meperidine*	Demerol, Meperitab	Injection, solution (vials and prefilled syringe): 10 mg/mL, 25 mg/mL, 50 mg/mL, 75 mg/mL, 100 mg/mL Solution, oral: 50 mg/5 mL Tablets: 50 mg, 100 mg†	C-II (US) Straight narcotic (Canada)
	Demerol		
methadone*	Dolophine, Methadose	Injection, solution: 10 mg/mL Solution, oral: 5 mg/5 mL, 10 mg/5 mL Solution, oral concentrate (Methadose): 10 mg/mL Tablets (Dolophine): 1 mg‡, 5 mg, 10 mg, 25 mg‡ Tablets, dispersible (Methadose): 40 mg	C-II (US) Straight narcotic (Canada)
	Metadol		
morphine*	Astramorph/PF, Avinza, Duramorph, DepoDur, Kadian, MS Contin, Oramorph SR, Roxanol, Roxanol-T	Capsules, extended release (Avinza): 30 mg, 45 mg, 60 mg, 75 mg, 90 mg, 120 mg (M-Eslon): 10 mg, 15 mg, 130 mg, 60 mg, 100 mg, 200 mg Capsules, sustained release (Kadian): 10 mg, 20 mg, 30 mg†, 50 mg, 60 mg†, 80 mg†, 100 mg, 200 mg† Injection, extended release for epidural (DepoDur): 10 mg/mL Injection, epidural, intrathecal (Astramorph/PF, Duramorph): 0.5 mg/mL, 1 mg/mL Injection, solution: 1 mg/mL, 2 mg/mL, 4 mg/mL†, 5 mg/mL, 8 mg/mL†, 10 mg/mL, 15 mg/mL, 25 mg/mL Solution, oral: 20 mg/mL, 1 mg/mL‡, 5 mg/mL‡, 10 mg/mL‡, 10 mg/5 mL†, 20 mg/5 mL†, 100 mg/5 mL†	C-II (US) Straight narcotic (Canada)
	Kadian, M-Eslon, MS Contin, MS IR, Statex		

Opioid Agonists—cont'd

Generic Name	U.S. Brand Name(s) / Canadian Brand Name(s)	Dosage Forms And Strengths	Controlled Substance Schedule
		Solution, oral drops (Statex): 20 mg/mL, 50 mg/mL Suppositories: 5 mg, 10 mg, 20 mg, 30 mg Tablets, controlled release (MS Contin): 15 mg, 30 mg, 60 mg, 100 mg, 200 mg Tablets, immediate release (MS IR): 5 mg, 10 mg, 20 mg, 30 mg Tablets, sustained release (Oramorph SR): 15 mg, 30 mg, 60 mg, 100 mg	
morphine + naltrexone	Embeda Not available	Capsules, extended release: 20 mg morphine + 0.8 mg naltrexone 30 mg morphine + 1.2 mg naltrexone 50 mg morphine + 2 mg naltrexone 60 mg morphine + 2.4 mg naltrexone 80 mg morphine + 3.2 mg naltrexone 100 mg morphine + 4 mg naltrexone	C-II
oxycodone*	OxyContin, Oxydose, OxyFast, Roxicodone OxyNEO, Oxy IR, Supeudol	Capsules, immediate release: 5 mg Solution, oral: 5 mg/5 mL Solution, oral concentrate (Oxydose, OxyFast): 20 mg/mL Tablets, immediate release (Oxy IR, Supeudol): 5 mg, 10 mg, 15 mg[†], 20 mg, 30 mg[†] Tablets, extended release (OxyContin, OxyNEO): 10 mg, 15 mg, 20 mg, 30 mg, 40 mg, 60 mg, 80 mg	C-II Straight narcotic (Canada)
oxycodone and acetaminophen*	Endocet, Percocet, Roxicet, Tylox Endocet, Percocet, Percocet-Demi	Capsules (Tylox): 5 mg oxycodone/500 mg acetaminophen Solution, oral (Roxicet): 5 mg/325 mg/5 mL Tablets (Endocet, Percocet): 5 mg/325 mg, 7.5 mg/325 mg, 7.5 mg/500 mg, 10 mg/325 mg, 10 mg/650 mg (Percocet-Demi): 2.5 mg/325 mg	C-II (US) Straight narcotic (Canada)
oxycodone and aspirin	Endodan, Percodan Generics	Tablets: 5 mg oxycodone/325 mg aspirin	C-II
oxymorphone*	Opana, Opana ER Not available	Injection, solution (Opana): 1 mg/mL Tablets: 5 mg, 10 mg Tablets, extended release (Opana ER): 5 mg, 7.5 mg, 10 mg, 15 mg, 20 mg, 30 mg, 40 mg	C-II

*Generic available.
[†]Strength available in the United States only.
[‡]Strength available in Canada only.

Mixed Agonist/Antagonists

Generic name	U.S. Brand Name(s) / Canadian Brand(s)	Dosage Forms and Strengths	Controlled Substance Schedule
buprenorphine	Buprenex, Butrans, Subutex / Butrans	Injection, solution (Buprenex): 0.3 mg/mL Tablets, sublingual (Subutex): 2 mg, 8 mg Transdermal, weekly patch (Butrans): 5 mcg/hr, 10 mcg/hr, 20 mcg/hr	C-III
buprenorphine and naloxone	Suboxone / Suboxone	Tablets, sublingual: 2 mg buprenorphine and 0.5 mg naloxone, 8 mg buprenorphine and 2 mg naloxone	C-III
butorphanol*	Generics / Generics	Injection: 1 mg/mL, 2 mg/mL[†] Intranasal solution: 10 mg/mL	C-IV
nalbuphine*	Generics / Nubain	Injection, solution: 10 mg/mL, 20 mg/mL	Schedule G Controlled (Canada)
oxycodone and naloxone	Not available / Targin	Tablets: 5 mg, 10 mg, 20 mg	Straight narcotic (Canada)
pentazocine	Talwin / Talwin	Injection, solution: 30 mg/mL Tablets: 50 mg[‡]	Straight narcotic (Canada)
pentazocine and naloxone	Talwin NX / Not available	Tablets: 50 mg pentazocine + 0.5 mg naloxone	C-IV

*Generic available.
[†]Strength available in the United States only.
[‡]Strength available in Canada only.

Opioid Antagonists

Generic Name	U.S. Brand Name(s) / Canadian Brand(s)	Dosage Forms and Strengths	Usual adult dose
naloxone*	Generics / Generics	Injection, solution: 0.4 mg/mL, 1 mg/mL	0.4-2 mg IV every 2-3 minutes; repeat every 20-60 min
naltrexone*	ReVia, Vivitrol / ReVia	Powder, for injection (Vivitrol): 380 mg per vial Tablets (ReVia): 50 mg	Start 25 mg; 50 mg/day or 100-150 mg 3 times a week (up to 800 mg/day) 380 mg IM every 4 weeks (Vivitrol)

*Generic available.

Summary of Drugs Used to Manage Drug Dependence or Reverse Effects of Opioids

Generic Name	Dose	Onset[X] (min)	Duration[X] (min/hr)	Route
buprenorphine buprenorphine and naloxone	Opioid dependence Opioid dependence	30-60 PO	12 hours (2 mg) up to 72 hours (>16 mg)	IV, PO
methadone	Opioid dependence	30	24-36 hours	PO
naloxone	Reverse opioid-induced respiratory depression of overdose	2	30 minutes	IV
naltrexone	Alcohol dependence	15-30	50 mg (24 hours) 100 mg (48 hours) 150 mg (72 hours)	PO

[X]Varies according to dose and route of administration.

Summary of Opioid Analgesics

Generic Name	U.S. Brand Name	Usual Adult Oral Dose and Dosing Schedule	Warning Labels
Opioid Agonists			
codeine	Generics	Immediate release, IM and subcut injection: 15-120 mg every 4-6 hours Controlled release: 50-300 mg every 12 hours	MAY CAUSE DROWSINESS; MAY IMPAIR ABILITY TO DRIVE.
codeine and acetaminophen	Tylenol with Codeine #3	1-2 tablets every 4 hours (maximum, 4 g daily)	AVOID ALCOHOL. TAKE WITH FOOD.
fentanyl	Duragesic	For pain (opiate naïve): Apply one 25-100 mcg/hr transdermal system every 72 hours	MAY BE HABIT FORMING. TAKE EACH DOSE WITH A FULL GLASS OF
hydrocodone and acetaminophen	Vicodin	2.5-10 mg every 4-6 hours (maximum dose, hydrocodone 60 mg and APAP 4 g/day)	WATER. SWALLOW WHOLE; DO NOT CRUSH OR
hydrocodone and ibuprofen	Vicoprofen	1-2 tablets every 4-6 hours	CHEW—delayed release.
hydromorphone	Dilaudid	For pain (opiate naïve): IV: 0.2-0.6 mg every 2-3 hours PCA: 0.2 mg/mL Epidural: 1-1.5 mg (bolus); 0.05-0.075 mg/mL (infusion) Oral, controlled release: 3-30 mg every 12 hours Oral (immediate release): 2-8 mg every 3-4 hours	ROTATE SITE OF APPLICATION— transdermal.
levorphanol	Levo-Dromoran	For pain (opiate naïve): Oral: 2-4 mg every 6-8 hours IM and subcut: 1-2 mg every 6-8 hours	
meperidine	Demerol	For pain (opiate naïve): Oral, IM, and subcut: 50-150 mg every 2-4 hours IV: 5-10 mg every 5 minutes PCA: 5-25 mg on demand	
methadone	Dolophine	For pain (opiate naïve): Oral: 2.5-10 mg every 3-4 hours IV, IM, subcut: 2.5-10 mg every 8-12 hours Detoxification (oral): 15-40 mg/day	
morphine	MS Contin	For pain (opiate naïve): Oral (prompt release): 10-30 mg every 3-4 hours Oral (extended release and sustained release capsules): 1-2 times daily Controlled release (tablet): Every 8-12 hours IV: Start 2.5-5 mg every 3-4 hours; continuous infusion up to 80 mg/hr PCA: 0.5-2.5 mg, lock out interval: 5-10 minutes IM, subcut: 5-10 mg every 3-4 hours Epidural: 10 mg as a single dose	
oxycodone	OxyContin	For pain (opiate naïve): Immediate release: 5 mg every 6 hours Controlled release: 10-40 mg every 12 hours	
oxycodone and acetaminophen	Percocet, Tylox	1-2 tablets every 4-6 hours (maximum, 4 g APAP daily)	
oxymorphone	Numorphan	IM, IV, subcut: Start 0.5 mg; 1-1.5 mg every 4-6 hours Rectal: 5 mg every 4-6 hours	

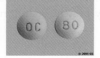

Continued

Summary of Opioid Analgesics—cont'd

Generic Name	U.S. Brand Name	Usual Adult Oral Dose and Dosing Schedule	Warning Labels
Mixed Agonist/Antagonists			
buprenorphine	Buprenex, Butrans	**Buprenex (opiate naïve): IM, IV:** 0.3 mg every 6-8 hours **Butrans:** Apply 1 patch every 7 days	MAY CAUSE DROWSINESS; MAY IMPAIR ABILITY TO DRIVE. AVOID ALCOHOL. MAY BE HABIT FORMING.
buprenorphine and naloxone	Suboxone	**Opioid dependence:** 4-24 mg/day titrated according to avoid withdrawal symptoms	
butorphanol	Stadol	**Acute pain (IM, IV):** 1-4 mg every 3-4 hours **Labor pain:** 1-2 mg within 4 hours of anticipated delivery	

TECH ALERT!
Product selection errors are common because of many strength combinations for hydrocodone and acetaminophen.

NONOPIOID ANALGESICS
Nonsteroidal Anti-inflammatory Drugs, Salicylates, and Acetaminophen

Nonsteroidal anti-inflammatory drugs (**NSAIDs**), salicylates (aspirin), and acetaminophen are widely used in the treatment of pain with or without inflammation. NSAIDs and aspirin have analgesic, anti-inflammatory, and antipyretic properties. An antipyretic is a drug that is capable of reducing fever. NSAIDs action and effectiveness are similar to those of aspirin (ASA).

MECHANISM OF ACTION
Similar to aspirin, NSAIDs decrease prostaglandin synthesis by inhibiting the action of COX. Most NSAIDs are not selective. They inhibit COX-1 and COX-2. COX-1 is expressed continuously, is found throughout the body, and is important for regulation of platelet aggregation and the biosynthesis of prostaglandins that protect the gastric mucosa. COX-2 is formed in selected cells as part of the immune response. COX-2 is involved in the biosynthesis of prostaglandins responsible for pain and inflammation. The analgesic effect of acetaminophen is thought to additionally be caused by inhibition of COX-3 in the brain.

TECH NOTE!
Ofirmev is a parenteral dosage form of acetaminophen approved by the U.S. Food and Drug Administration (FDA) in 2010.

PHARMACOKINETICS
Aspirin and NSAIDs are well absorbed orally. Aspirin is a weak acid (acetylsalicylic acid), and the rate of absorption varies according to the pH of stomach, small intestine, and urine. Enteric-coated aspirin is released in the pH of the intestine rather than in the stomach. Aspirin is eliminated in the urine. Acidification of the urine with vitamin C can increase rate of reabsorption, and sodium bicarbonate enhances elimination (see Chapter 2).

NSAIDs are structurally dissimilar; however, they are biologically similar. Oral absorption is good and bioavailability ranges between 80% and 99%. They are all highly protein bound, more than 97%, and they all are primarily eliminated in the urine.

ADVERSE REACTIONS
All of the NSAIDs and aspirin can produce nausea, GI bleeding, and ulceration. NSAIDs can cause fluid retention, leading to increased blood pressure. Some NSAIDs can produce dizziness. Serious side effects include salicylism (aspirin), hepatotoxicity (ketorolac), and agranulocytosis (indomethacin, flurbiprofen). Recently, selective COX-2 inhibitors rofecoxib (Vioxx) and valdecoxib (Bextra) were withdrawn from the market because of increased risk for heart attack and stroke. Celecoxib (Celebrex) remains the only selective COX-2 inhibitor currently in use. Acetaminophen can cause hepatotoxicity.

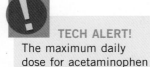

TECH ALERT!
The maximum daily dose for acetaminophen and aspirin is 4 G.

Commonly Used Nonopioid Analgesics

Generic Name	Brand Name	Usual Adult Dose	Side Effects	Warning Labels
Salicylates				
aspirin	Ecotrin, Bayer, Anacin	325-650 mg every 4-6 hours (maximum, 4 g/day)	GI upset, bleeding, tinnitus, salicylism	TAKE WITH FOOD.
diflunisal	Dolobid	250-500 mg twice a day	GI upset, rash, drowsiness, jaundice	TAKE WITH FOOD. MAY CAUSE DIZZINESS OR DROWSINESS. AVOID ASPIRIN AND RELATED DRUGS.
p-Aminophenol				
acetaminophen	Tylenol	325-650 mg every 4-6 hours (maximum, 4 g/day)	Skin, liver toxicity, kidney toxicity	
Indoles				
indomethacin	Indocin	25-50 mg 2-3 times a day	GI upset, headache, dizziness (drowsiness—sulindac), tinnitus, agranulocytosis (fatigue, apnea—indomethacin)	TAKE WITH FOOD. MAY CAUSE DIZZINESS OR DROWSINESS. AVOID ASPIRIN AND RELATED DRUGS.
sulindac	Clinoril	150-200 mg twice a day or 300-400 mg once a day		
etodolac	Lodine Lodine XL	200-400 mg every 6-8 hours 400-1000 mg once a day	GI upset, dizziness, drowsiness, palpitations	
Phenylpropionic Acid				
flurbiprofen	Ansaid	200-300 mg every 6-12 hours (maximum, 300 mg/day)	GI upset, headache, tinnitus, dizziness, kidney toxicity (ibuprofen)	TAKE WITH FOOD. MAY CAUSE DIZZINESS OR DROWSINESS. AVOID ASPIRIN AND RELATED DRUGS.
	Ocufen	1 drop in eye(s) every 30 minutes starting 2 hours before surgery		
ibuprofen	Motrin	200-800 mg every 4-8 hours (maximum, 3200 mg/day)		
ketoprofen	Orudis Oruvail (extended release)	50-75 mg 3-4 times a day 200 mg once a day		
oxaprozin	Daypro	600-1200 mg once a day		
Naphthylpropionic Acids				
naproxen	Naprosyn Naprosyn DS Napralen	**Immediate release:** Start 500 mg (Naproxen*)-550 mg (Anaprox); then 250-275 mg every 6-12 hours	GI upset, headache, tinnitus, rash, dizziness	TAKE WITH FOOD. MAY CAUSE DIZZINESS OR DROWSINESS. AVOID ASPIRIN AND RELATED DRUGS.
naproxen Na⁺	Anaprox Anaprox DS Napralen	**Delayed release** (EC Naprosyn): 375-500 mg twice daily **Controlled release** (Napralen): 750-1500 mg once daily (maximum 1500 mg/day)		

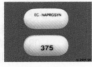

Continued

Commonly Used Nonopioid Analgesics—cont'd

Generic Name	Brand Name	Usual Adult Dose	Side Effects	Warning Labels
Naphthyalkanones				
nabumetone	Relafen	1000-1500 mg/day dosed 1-2 times/day	GI upset, dizziness, agranulocytosis	TAKE WITH FOOD. MAY CAUSE DIZZINESS OR DROWSINESS. AVOID ASPIRIN AND RELATED DRUGS.
Anthranilic acids				
meclofenamate	Meclomen (Canada)	50-100 mg every 4-6 hours (maximum, 400 mg/day)	GI upset, headache, dizziness, increased urination	TAKE WITH FOOD. MAY CAUSE DIZZINESS OR DROWSINESS. AVOID ASPIRIN AND RELATED DRUGS.
Pyrroleacetic Acid				
tolmetin	Tolectin	400-600 mg 3 times a day	GI upset, headache, dizziness, rash, liver toxicity (ketorolac), palpitations (tolmetin)	TAKE WITH FOOD. MAY CAUSE DIZZINESS OR DROWSINESS. AVOID ASPIRIN AND RELATED DRUGS.
ketorolac	Toradol Acular	**PO:** Start 20 mg; then 10 mg every 4-6 hours (maximum, 40 mg/day) **IM or IV:** 30 mg every 6 hours **Ophthalmic:** 1 drop 4 times a day		
Phenylacetic acid				
diclofenac	Voltaren Voltaren XR Voltaren Rapide (Canada)	**Immediate release:** 50 mg 2-4 times a day (oral) **Controlled release:** 100 mg once daily (maximum, 200 mg/day)	GI upset, pain, nausea and vomiting, ulceration	TAKE WITH FOOD. MAY CAUSE DIZZINESS OR DROWSINESS. AVOID ASPIRIN AND RELATED DRUGS.
Oxicams				
meloxicam	Mobic	7.5-15 mg once a day	GI upset, constipation or diarrhea, gas, dizziness, edema, GI bleeding, hypertension	TAKE WITH FOOD. MAY CAUSE DIZZINESS OR DROWSINESS. AVOID ASPIRIN AND RELATED DRUGS. SWALLOW WHOLE; DO NOT CRUSH OR CHEW. TAKE WITH A FULL GLASS OF WATER. SHAKE WELL— SUSPENSION.
piroxicam	Feldene	10-20 mg once a day		
COX-2 Inhibitors				
celecoxib	Celebrex	200 mg twice a day	GI upset, GI ulceration, heart attack, stroke	TAKE WITH FOOD. MAY CAUSE DIZZINESS OR DROWSINESS. AVOID ASPIRIN AND RELATED DRUGS.

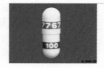

*550 mg naproxen Na = (500 mg naproxen base).

Drug Treatment for Neuropathic Pain

Neuropathic pain is associated with nerve injury caused by trauma, infection, or chronic diseases such as uncontrolled diabetes and is often treated with different drugs than are used to treat pain of nociceptive origin. Neuropathic pain is unique because pain sensations are felt even after the injury is healed. When nerves are damaged, the body may make adaptations to compensate for the nerve damage. These changes can lead to persistent nerve pain. Nerve injury can led to sensitization of nerve terminals. This lowers the threshold for neuron firing (action potential) and increases the response to stimuli. Nerve damage can result in a reorganization of nerves. The rewiring sometimes goes haywire, causing painful sensations even after limbs have been amputated. Another cause of neuropathic pain is changes in the sodium and calcium ion channels that result in increasing or decreasing levels of ions involved in neuronal firing. Nerve injuries can also cause a loss of inhibitory pathways such as the GABA pathways (described in Chapter 8).

Commonly Used to Treat Neuropathic Pain

Generic Name	Brand Name	Usual Adult Dose	Side Effects	Warning Labels
Antidepressants				
amitriptyline	Levate (Canada)	25-100 mg at bedtime	Sedation, dry mouth, urinary retention, nausea, blurred vision, photosensitivity	MAY CAUSE DROWSINESS; ALCOHOL MAY INTENSIFY THIS EFFECT. MAY IMPAIR ABILITY TO DRIVE. DO NOT DISCONTINUE WITHOUT MEDICAL SUPERVISION. MAY DISCOLOR URINE (BLUE-GREEN). AVOID PROLONGED EXPOSURE TO SUNLIGHT.
desipramine	Norpramin	150-200 mg/day in 1-2 doses		
imipramine	Tofranil	1-3 mg/kg/dose at bedtime		
Antiseizure Drugs				
gabapentin	Neurontin	300-1800 mg in 3 divided doses	Dizziness, confusion, fatigue, ataxia and nausea, double vision, blurred vision, dry mouth, and constipation	MAY CAUSE DROWSINESS; MAY IMPAIR ABILITY TO DRIVE. AVOID ALCOHOL. TAKE WITH FOOD. DO NOT DISCONTINUE WITHOUT MEDICAL SUPERVISION. SHAKE WELL.
pregabalin	Lyrica	50-100 mg 3 times a day		
carbamazepine	Tegretol	400-800 mg twice a day	Nausea, vomiting, sedation, dizziness, ataxia, bruising, jaundice, and visual disturbances	SWALLOW WHOLE; DO NOT CRUSH OR CHEW—controlled release. AVOID ANTACIDS WITHIN 2 HOURS OF DOSE—gabapentin, phenytoin. AVOID PREGNANCY—phenytoin.
Local anesthetics				
lidocaine	Generic only	Nerve block and postherpetic neuralgia** Maximum, 4.5 mg/kg/dose IV	Drowsiness, dizziness numbness, agitation, hypotension, heart block	MAY CAUSE DROWSINESS; MAY IMPAIR ABILITY TO DRIVE. AVOID ALCOHOL.
Topicals				
lidocaine	Lidoderm	1-3 patches up to 12 hours/day	Numbness, local irritation	ROTATE SITE OF APPLICATION— Lidoderm, Qutenza.
capsaicin	Zostrix, Qutenza	Apply 3-4 times a day	Burning, stinging	WASH HANDS AFTER USE— capsaicin.

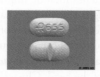

**Not FDA approved.

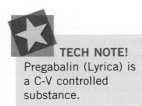

TECH NOTE!
Pregabalin (Lyrica) is a C-V controlled substance.

Drugs used in the treatment of neuropathic pain include antidepressants (amitriptyline, duloxetine), antiseizure drugs (gabapentin, lamotrigine), local anesthetics (lidocaine, mexiletine), and capsaicin. The tricyclic antidepressants are often used as first-line agents for the treatment of neuropathic pain. They inhibit the reuptake of neurotransmitters (e.g., norepinephrine and serotonin) at receptor sites in the spinal cord that are responsible for modulating pain sensation. Duloxetine is a serotonin-noradrenaline reuptake inhibitor that has been shown to be effective in reducing pain caused by fibromyalgia and diabetic neuropathy. There is little evidence to support the use of selective serotonin reuptake inhibitors for the management of neuropathic pain.

Gabapentin, pregabalin, and carbamazepine are antiseizure drugs that are used for the treatment of diabetic neuropathy, nerve pain caused by herpes virus infection, and trigeminal neuralgia. Topiramate enhances inhibitory effects of GABA in addition to its action on voltage-dependent sodium channels. These drugs are discussed in detail in Chapter 9.

Lidocaine is a local anesthetic used in the treatment of neuropathic pain. Lidocaine blocks sodium channels and may be administered intravenously or topically. Lidocaine patches are indicated for the treatment of nerve pain caused by herpes infection (shingles). Capsaicin is derived from chili peppers. It is applied topically and it depletes substance P from nerve terminals. It is indicated for the treatment of diabetic neuropathy and shingles.

Nondrug Treatment of Pain

The treatment of pain, especially chronic pain, requires a multimodal approach that includes drug therapy and nondrug therapy. Nondrug therapies that may be supportive are education, physical therapy, occupational therapy, *biofeedback*, cognitive behavioral therapy (counseling), *acupuncture*, chiropractic medicine, and transcutaneous electrical stimulation (TENS) (Figure 10-3). The TENS device delivers electrical impulses through the skin that causes contraction and numbness. This blocks the transmission of pain messages to the spinal cord by peripheral nerves. Cryotherapy (cold packs) and heat packs can reduce swelling, which can also decrease pain.

Headache

International Headache Society (IHS) classifications for primary headaches include migraine headache, tension-type headache, cluster headache, and trigeminal *cephalgia*. Tension headache is the most common of the primary headaches. It produces bilateral pain, affecting both sides of the head, is mild to moderate in intensity and is described as having a pressing or tightening quality. Left untreated, tension headaches may last for 30 minutes to up to 7 days. A *cluster headache* is a frequently reoccurring headache that produces severe pain on one side of the head. Cluster headaches may last 15 to 90 minutes and occur more frequently in men.

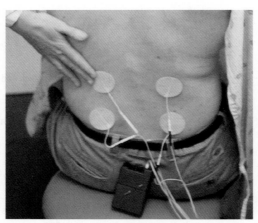

FIGURE 10-3 Transcutaneous nerve stimulation unit. (From Ignatavicius D, Workman L: *Medical-surgical nursing*, ed 5, Philadelphia, 2006, WB Saunders.)

Migraine Headache

In the United States, up to 18.2% of women and 6.5% of men experience migraine headaches annually. Up to 24% of Canadians will experience a migraine headache in their lifetime. Migraine headache occurs infrequently in children younger than 10 years of age; the onset is typically between 10 and 29 years old. The prevalence is greatest between 30 and 39 years old and tapers after 60 years old. The probability of developing migraines may be as high as 70% if both parents get migraine headaches.

Once thought to be a vascular headache, it is now believed that migraine pain occurs as a result of biochemical and hormonal changes involving serotonergic and adrenergic pain modulating systems. Serotonin is most commonly implicated; however, prostaglandins, catecholamines, histamine, substance P, and neuroexcitatory amino acids are also thought to play a role.

Migraine headaches are typically unilateral, affecting only one side of the head; however, the headache can spread to the opposite side. IHS classifications include migraine with aura, migraine without aura, menstrual migraine, and chronic migraine. Chronic migraine can occur from overuse of medicines used in the treatment of migraine. An aura is an unusual sensation that is experienced just before the onset of the migraine headache. An aura may present as a temporary flashing light, blind spots, double vision, a smell, paresthesia, weakness, or aphagia (loss of language).

Severe throbbing pain is characteristic of migraines, as are nausea, photophobia (eyes are sensitive to the light), and phonophobia (sensitivity to noise). Resting in a quiet area with the lights off can sometimes improve migraine symptoms. Physical activity worsens migraine symptoms. Acute migraine attacks can last between 4 and 72 hours; the average is 29 hours. Migraine headaches occur more frequently in women than in men.

PATHOPHYSIOLOGY OF MIGRAINE HEADACHES

Migraine headaches are triggered by numerous events, including stress, insufficient sleep, red wine, caffeine, strong odors, smoke, changes in the weather, and exposure to bright or flashing lights. The trigger sets off a series of events that starts with the release of vasoactive neuropeptides that cause blood vessels in the brain to first constrict and then dilate. The trigger produces vasospasms, which reduce blood flow to the brain. Platelets in the blood clump together and cause the release of serotonin, which further constricts blood vessels. This triggers afferent signals via the trigeminal nerve to release prostaglandins and other neurochemicals that dilate blood vessels, produce inflammation, and stimulate nociceptors. This causes the throbbing head pain characteristic of migraine headaches.

DRUG TREATMENT FOR MIGRAINE HEADACHE

Treatment of migraines is aimed at stopping the current migraine attack (abortive therapy) and preventing future migraines. Simple analgesics, combination analgesics, serotonin (5-hydroxytryptamine [5-HT]) agonists, ergot alkaloids, antidepressants (tricyclic antidepressants, selective serotonin reuptake inhibitors, and monoamine oxidase inhibitors), beta blockers, and antiseizure drugs are used in the treatment and prevention of migraine headaches. The overall goal of therapy is to treat attacks rapidly and consistently; decrease the frequency, intensity, and duration of headaches; restore the patient's ability to function; and minimize the use of rescue and backup medications with minimal adverse effects (Table 10-3).

TREATMENT OF ACUTE MIGRAINE HEADACHE

Simple Analgesics and Combination Analgesics

Simple analgesics (aspirin, acetaminophen, ibuprofen, and naproxen) are often effective in stopping mild to moderate migraine headaches if taken early and in high doses. The effective dose of aspirin or acetaminophen used to treat migraine headache (up to 1000 mg per dose) is higher than the usual dose recommended for the treatment of mild to moderate tension headache (325-650 mg per dose). Codeine, caffeine, and butalbital may be added to aspirin and acetaminophen to form combination analgesics. Simple analgesics and combined analgesics (aspirin and NSAIDs) reduce pain and decrease inflammation associated with migraine headache.

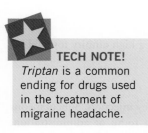

TECH NOTE!
Triptan is a common ending for drugs used in the treatment of migraine headache.

TABLE 10-3   **Quality of Evidence for Drugs Used in the Acute Treatment of Migraine Headache**

Drug Category	Drug	Quality of Evidence of Effectiveness*
Simple analgesics	acetaminophen	B
	aspirin	A
	ibuprofen	A
	naproxen Na$^+$	A
Combination analgesics	aspirin + acetaminophen + caffeine	A
	aspirin + butalbital + caffeine	C
Ergotamine and ergotamine combinations	ergotamine	B
	ergotamine + caffeine	B
	dihydroergotamine nasal spray	A
	dihydroergotamine subcut, IM, IV	B
Triptans	almotriptan, eletriptan, frovatriptan, naratriptan, rizatriptan, sumatriptan, zolmitriptan	A
Opioid analgesics	butorphanol nasal spray	A
	codeine + acetaminophen	A
	meperidine IM, IV	B

*Quality of the evidence (Grade A, B, or C [A = multiple well-designed randomized, clinical trials directly relevant to the recommendation; B = some evidence from randomized clinical trials, but the scientific support was not optimal; and C = the US Headache Consortium achieved consensus on the recommendation in the absence of relevant randomized, controlled trials.])

Triptans

The triptans are the most widely prescribed drugs for the treatment of migraine headaches. They are administered during an acute attack to lessen symptoms and to stop the headache from progressing to more severe migraine symptoms. They are administered at the first sign of an impending migraine (aura).

MECHANISM OF ACTION

The triptans are selective serotonin (5-HT) receptor agonists. They have a high affinity for 5-HT$_{1B}$ and 5-HT$_{1D}$ receptors, which stimulate vasoconstriction (Figure 10-4).

PHARMACOKINETICS

The triptans are available for administration via mouth, intranasally, and by injection. Subcutaneous injection produces the most rapid response and is the most effective route of administration; however, intranasal administration is also rapid and has fewer adverse reactions. Oral formulations have slower onsets of action. The half-lives of the triptans range between 2 hours and 25 hours. Triptans that have long half-lives, such as frovatriptan (24 hours) and naratriptan (8 hours), are more effective in reducing headache reoccurrence.

ADVERSE REACTIONS

The vasoconstriction caused by triptans is responsible for their therapeutic effects but can result in serious cardiac side effects, including arrhythmia, angina, coronary vasospasm, and myocardial infarction (heart attack). Vasoconstriction can also cause high blood pressure and stroke. Less serious and more common side effects are pain, tightness, and burning at the site of injection; dizziness; nausea; hot flashes; dry mouth; and fatigue.

TECH ALERT!
The following drugs have look-alike/sound-alike issues: Axert and Antivert; Amerge and Amaryl; sumatriptan and zolmitriptan; Maxalt and Maxair

Triptan Drugs: Mechanism of Action

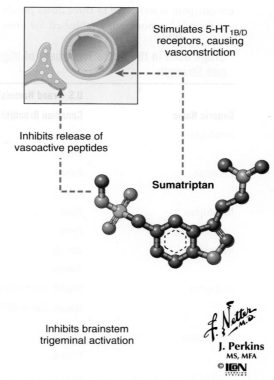

Stimulates 5-HT$_{1B/D}$ receptors, causing vasoconstriction

Inhibits release of vasoactive peptides

Sumatriptan

Inhibits brainstem trigeminal activation

J. Perkins
MS, MFA
© IGN

FIGURE 10-4 Mechanism of action for triptan drugs. (From Raffa RB, Rawls SM, Beyzarov EP: *Netter's illustrated pharmacology*, Philadelphia, 2005, WB Saunders.)

Comparison of Triptans

Generic Name (Brand Name)	Onset (min)	Repeat Time (hr)	Route	Headache* Effectiveness (%)	Dose (mg)§
almotriptan (Axert)	30	2	PO, tablet	57-68	25
eletriptan (Relpax)	30	2	PO, tablet	54-65	40
				68-77	80
frovatriptan (Frova)	30	2	PO, tablet	40	2.5
naratriptan (Amerge)	30	4	PO, tab	48	2.5
rizatriptan (Maxalt, Maxalt-MLT)	30	2	PO, tablet	73	10
		2	Wafer		
sumatriptan (Imitrex)	10-15	1	subcut	80-85	6
	15	2	Nasal	60-86	20
	30	2	PO, tablet	51-61	50
zolmitriptan (Zomig)	30	2	PO, tablet	59-69	2.5
		2	Wafer		
	10-15		Nasal	24-61	5

*Percentage patients reporting pain relief at 2 hours after dosing.
§Dose associated with headache effectiveness (%).

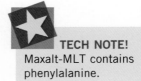

TECH NOTE!
Maxalt-MLT contains phenylalanine.

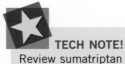

TECH NOTE!
Review sumatriptan nasal directions carefully—only one spray in one nostril is indicated.

PRECAUTIONS

The over use of triptans is limited. Nearly all triptans are restricted to two doses per 24 hours. Frovatriptan is restricted to three doses per 24 hours. The safety of treating more than four migraines per month has not been established for most of the triptans.

Drugs Used in the Acute Treatment of Migraine Headache: Triptans Dosage Forms and Strength

Generic Name	U.S. Brand Name(s) / Canadian Brand(s)	Dosage Forms and Strengths
almotriptan	Axert	Tablets: 6.25 mg, 12.5 mg
	Axert	
eletriptan	Relpax	Tablets: 20 mg, 40 mg
	Relpax	
frovatriptan	Frova	Tablets: 2.5 mg
	Frova	
naratriptan	Amerge	Tablets: 1 mg, 2.5 mg
	Amerge	
rizatriptan	Maxalt, Maxalt-MLT	Tablets (Maxalt): 5 mg, 10 mg
	Maxalt, Maxalt-RPD	Tablets, disintegrating (Maxalt-MLT): 5 mg, 10 mg
		Wafer (Maxalt-RPD): 5 mg, 10 mg
sumatriptan	Imitrex	Injection, as solution: 6 mg/mL (0.5 mL)
	Imitrex	Intranasal solution: 5 mg, 20 mg (100 µL unit dose spray device)
		Tablets: 25 mg[†], 50 mg, 100 mg
zolmitriptan	Zomig, Zomig-ZMT	Nasal solution: 5 mg/0.1 mL (0.1 mL)
	Zomig, Zomig-Rapimelt	Tablets: 2.5 mg, 5 mg[†]
		Tablets, disintegrating (Zomig-ZMT, Zomig-Rapimelt): 2.5 mg, 5 mg[†]
sumatriptan + naproxen Na[+]	Treximet	Tablets: 500 mg naproxen Na[+] + 85 mg sumatriptan
	Not available in Canada	

[†]Strength available in the United States only.

Summary of Triptans Used in the Treatment of Migraine Headaches

Generic Name	U.S. Brand Name	Usual Adult Oral Dose and Dosing Schedule	Warning Labels
almotriptan	Axert	**Oral:** 6.25-12.5 mg as a single dose; repeat dose in 2 hours if needed (maximum, 25 mg in 24 hours)	DO NOT EXCEED RECOMMENDED DOSAGE. IF NO IMPROVEMENT AFTER FIRST DOSE, DO NOT TAKE A SECOND DOSE.
eletriptan	Relpax	**Oral:** 20-40 mg as a single dose; repeat dose in 2 hours if needed (maximum, 80 mg in 24 hours)	
frovatriptan	Frova	**Oral:** 2.5 mg as a single dose; repeat dose in 2 hours if needed (maximum, 7.5 mg in 24 hours)	
naratriptan	Amerge	**Oral:** 1-2.5 mg as a single dose; repeat dose in 4 hours if needed (maximum, 5 mg in 24 hours)	
rizatriptan	Maxalt	**Oral:** 5-10 mg as a single dose; repeat dose in 2 hours if needed (maximum, is 30 mg [15 mg if also receiving propranolol] in 24 hours)	

Summary of Triptans Used in the Treatment of Migraine Headaches—cont'd

Generic Name	U.S. Brand Name	Usual Adult Oral Dose and Dosing Schedule	Warning Labels
sumatriptan	Imitrex	**Oral:** 25 mg, 50 mg, or 100 mg as a single dose; repeat dose in 2 hours if needed (maximum, 200 mg in 24 hours) **Nasal spray:** 1-2 sprays (5 mg, 10 mg), or 1 spray (20 mg) in one nostril; repeat dose in 2 hours if needed (maximum, 40 mg in 24 hours) **Subcut injection:** 6 mg as a single injection; repeat dose in 1 hour if needed	DO NOT INJECT MORE THAN 2 DOSES (6 MG) IN 24 HOURS. USE SPRAY IN ONE NOSTRIL ONLY. IF NO IMPROVEMENT AFTER FIRST DOSE, DO NOT TAKE A SECOND DOSE.
zolmitriptan	Zomig	**Oral:** 2.5-5 mg as a single dose; repeat dose in 2 hours if needed (maximum, 10 mg in 24 hours) **Nasal solution:** 1 spray as a single dose; repeat dose in 2 hours if needed	IF NO IMPROVEMENT AFTER FIRST DOSE, DO NOT TAKE A SECOND DOSE.
sumatriptan + naproxen Na+	Treximet	Take 1 tablet for migraine; may repeat dose in 2 hours if needed	DO NOT EXCEED 2 DOSES PER 24 HOURS. MAY CAUSE DIZZINESS OR DROWSINESS. SWALLOW WHOLE; DO NOT CUT, CRUSH, OR CHEW. TAKE WITH A FULL GLASS OF WATER.

Other Acute Treatments for Acute Migraine Headaches

Ergot alkaloids and 5-HT agonists are also prescribed as migraine abortive therapy. A summary of these agents is found in the following table.

Summary of Nontriptan Drugs Used to Treat Migraine Headaches

Generic Name	Brand Name	Usual Adult Dose	Side Effects	Warning Labels
Ergot alkaloids				
dihydroergotamine mesylate	D.H.E.	1 mg IM; repeat in 1 hour if needed (maximum, 6 mg/wk)	Numbness	DO NOT EXCEED RECOMMENDED DOSAGE.
	Migranal	1 spray in each nostril; repeat after 15 minutes if needed (maximum, 8 sprays/wk)		DO NOT ASSEMBLE SPRAYER UNTIL READY TO USE.
ergotamine tartrate	Ergomar	2 mg every 30 minutes until relief (maximum, 6 mg/day or 10 mg/week)	Nausea, vomiting, numbness, chest pain, abdominal pain	DO NOT EXCEED RECOMMENDED DOSAGE.
Opioid analgesics				
butorphanol	Stadol	1 spray in one nostril, may repeat in 60-90 minutes if needed (maximum, 4 doses/day)	Drowsiness, dizziness, nausea, constipation, dry mouth	MAY CAUSE DROWSINESS; MAY IMPAIR ABILITY TO DRIVE. AVOID ALCOHOL. TAKE WITH FOOD. MAY BE HABIT FORMING.
codeine 30 mg + acetaminophen	Tylenol #3	1-2 tablets every 4 hours (maximum, 4 g daily)	Drowsiness, dizziness, nausea, constipation	
meperidine	Demerol	75-100 mg IM at onset of headache	Drowsiness, dizziness, nausea, constipation, dry mouth	

Migraine Preventive Agents

Migraine preventive therapy is offered to persons that use abortive medication more than twice per week, or when acute-acting agents are contraindicated or have failed to relieve the headache. They are also offered to people who experience six or more migraine headaches per month. They may be offered to people experiencing only three to four migraines if the migraine produces moderate to severe impairment (requires bed rest). Beta blockers (see Chapter 22), tricyclic antidepressants (see Chapter 6), onabotulinumtoxinA (a neuromuscular blocker), neuromuscular blocking agents (see Chapter 13) and antiseizure drugs (see Chapter 9) are also prescribed for prophylaxis of migraine headaches.

Drugs Used for the Prevention of Migraine Headaches

Generic Name	U.S. Brand Name(s) Canadian Brand(s)	Dosage Forms and Strengths
β-blockers		
propranolol*	Inderal LA	Tablets: 10 mg, 20 mg, 40 mg, 60 mg, 80 mg
	Inderal LA	Tablets, extended release (Inderal LA): 60 mg, 80 mg, 120 mg, 160 mg
Valproates		
divalproex sodium	Depakote	Tablets: 250 mg, 500 mg
Tricyclic Antidepressants		
amitriptyline	Generics	Tablets: 10 mg, 20 mg, 50 mg, 75 mg, 100 mg†, 150 mg†
	Elavil	
Neuromuscular Blockers		
onabotulinumtoxinA	Botox	Powder for injection: 50 unit†, 100 units, 200 units†
	Botox	

*Generic available.
†Strength available in the United States only.

Summary of Drugs Used for the Prevention of Migraine Headaches

Generic Name	Brand Name	Usual Adult Dose	Side Effects	Warning Labels
β-Blockers				
propranolol	Inderal Inderal-LA	80-240 mg/day every 6 to 8 hours or 80-240 mg/day (long acting)	Hypotension, lethargy	MAY CAUSE DIZZINESS OR DROWSINESS AND IMPAIR ABILITY TO DRIVE.
Valproates				
divalproex Na+	Depakote	250 mg twice daily up to 1000 mg/day	Sedation, nausea, ataxia, and liver dysfunction	MAY CAUSE DROWSINESS AND IMPAIR ABILITY TO DRIVE. AVOID ALCOHOL. TAKE WITH FOOD.
Tricyclic Antidepressants				
amitriptyline	generics Elavil	30-150 mg/d (start at 25 mg/d, inc by 25 mg/wk)		MAY CAUSE DROWSINESS AND IMPAIR ABILITY TO DRIVE. AVOID ALCOHOL. TAKE WITH FOOD.
Neuromuscular Blockers				
onabotulinumtoxinA	Botox	155 Units administered IM as 5 Units/injection divided across 31 injection sites within 7 specific head and neck muscle areas	neck pain, stiffness, myestehenia, myalgia, muscle pain, pain at inj. site, botulism, blepharedema	

Chapter Summary

- Acute pain may be triggered by an injury, burn, infection, or some other stimuli and be self-limiting.
- Chronic pain may persist for years and is often inadequately controlled by pharmaceuticals.
- Psychological factors can influence a person's tolerance for pain and can determine whether the outcome of treatment is successful.
- Patient-controlled analgesia (PCA) permits patients to control the frequency of administration of their dose of pain medications.
- Neuropathic pain is associated with nerve injury caused by trauma, infection, or chronic diseases such as uncontrolled diabetes and is often treated with different drugs than other types of pain.
- Osteoarthritis, gout, burns, trauma, and low back pain are examples of pain with a nociceptor origin.
- Painful stimuli trigger the release of neurotransmitters, amino acids, and peptides that carry signals to increase sensitivity to the pain or to dull the painful sensations.
- Histamine, bradykinins, serotonin, prostaglandins, glutamate, and substance P are involved in the transmission of signals for pain sensation and pain perception.
- Endorphans, enkephalin, and dynorphin are the body's natural painkillers and bind to opioid receptors.
- Opioids are naturally occurring or synthetically derived drugs that act like morphine and are used to treat pain.
- Opioid receptors are mu (μ), kappa (κ), and delta (δ), and stimulation produces analgesia. The euphoria, dysphoria, respiratory depression, pupillary constriction, decreased gastrointestinal motility, and physical dependence associated with opioid use are linked to specific receptors.
- Opioid agonists activate μ, κ, or δ receptors.
- Antagonists bind to the opioid receptor but do not activate it.
- Mixed agonist/antagonists behave like an agonist when the patient has had no recent exposure to an opioid agonist (opiate naïve).
- Equianalgesic doses of opioids produce equivalent pain relief regardless of dosage form.
- Opioid agonists, partial agonists, and most mixed agonist/antagonists are restricted substances because they produce tolerance and dependence.
- Opioid antagonists and some mixed agonist/antagonists are used to treat drug dependence and opioid-induced respiratory depression.
- Nonsteroidal anti-inflammatory drugs (NSAIDs), acetaminophen, and aspirin are widely used in the treatment of pain with or without inflammation.
- NSAIDs and aspirin have analgesic, anti-inflammatory, and antipyretic properties.
- Acetaminophen does not reduce inflammation.
- Aspirin and NSAIDs decrease prostaglandin synthesis by inhibiting the action of cyclooxygenase (COX), an enzyme involved in the biosynthesis of prostaglandins. Prostaglandins are important mediators of pain.
- Most NSAIDs are not selective. They inhibit COX-1 and COX-2.
- Selective COX-2 inhibitors rofecoxib and valdecoxib were withdrawn from the market because of increased risk for heart attack and stroke.
- All of the NSAIDs and aspirin can produce nausea, gastrointestinal bleeding, and gastrointestinal ulceration.
- Enteric-coated aspirin is released in the pH of the intestine rather than in the stomach.
- Migraine headaches are triggered by numerous events, including stress, consumption of certain foods, red wine, caffeinated beverages, and exposure to bright or flashing lights.
- During a migraine, blood vessels in the brain dilate, produce inflammation, and stimulate nociceptors, causing the throbbing head pain characteristic of migraine headaches.
- Treatment of migraines is aimed at stopping the current migraine attack and preventing future migraines.
- Simple and combined analgesics, serotonin agonists, and ergot alkaloids are used in the treatment of acute migraine headache.
- Tricyclic antidepressants, selective serotonin reuptake inhibitors, monoamine oxidase inhibitors, beta blockers, and neuromuscular blocking agents antiseizure drugs can be used in the prevention of migraine headaches.

- Triptans are selective serotonin receptor agonists and are the most widely prescribed drugs for the treatment of acute migraine headaches.
- Triptans that have long half-lives, frovatriptan and naratriptan, are more effective in preventing headache reoccurrence.
- The use of triptans is restricted to a maximum of two or three doses per 24 hours. The safety of treating more than four migraines per month has not been established for most of the triptans.
- The vasoconstriction caused by triptans is partially responsible for their therapeutic effects but can result in serious effects, including arrhythmia, angina, myocardial infarction, and stroke.

REVIEW QUESTIONS

1. _____ pain may triggered by an injury, burn, infection, or some other stimuli and be self-limiting.
   a. Chronic
   b. Dull
   c. Acute
   d. Nerve

2. The most common of all arthritic conditions is _____.
   a. gout
   b. osteoarthritis
   c. rheumatoid arthritis
   d. ankylosis

3. _____ are hormones that trigger pain response from peripheral nociceptors.
   a. Histamines
   b. Serotonins
   c. Prostaglandins
   d. Norepinephrines

4. *Opiate* is a term used to describe _____ derived drugs that act like morphine.
   a. naturally
   b. synthetically
   c. both a and b
   d. none of the above

5. What U.S. controlled substance schedule does oxycodone fall into?
   a. C-II
   b. C-III
   c. C-IV
   d. C-V

6. Naloxone (Narcan), which is indicated for reversal of respiratory depression caused by opioid use and opioid overdose, is an example of an
   a. agonist
   b. antagonist

7. NSAIDs have analgesic, anti-inflammatory, and antipyretic properties.
   a. true
   b. false

8. The only COX-2 inhibitor that remains currently in use is
   a. rofecoxib, Vioxx
   b. valdecoxib, Bextra
   c. acetaminophen, Tylenol
   d. celecoxib, Celebrex

9. Migraine headaches are triggered by numerous events, including _____.
   a. stress or consumption of certain foods
   b. red wine or caffeinated beverages
   c. exposure to bright or flashing lights
   d. all of the above

10. _____ are the most widely prescribed drugs for the treatment of migraine headaches.
- a. Ergot alkaloids
- b. Antiseizure
- c. Antidepressants
- d. Triptans

TECHNICIAN'S CORNER

1. Describe the difference between neuropathic and muscular pain. Can they be intertwined?
2. A patient who has suffered for years with chronic pain asks, "Is there anything else I can do besides take pain medicines for my pain?" What can you tell the patient?

Bibliography

Adelman J, Lewit E: Comparative aspects of triptans in treating migraine, *Clin Cornerstone* 4:1-19, 2001.

Bennett M, Smith S, Torrance N, et al: Can pain be more or less neuropathic? *Comparison of symptom assessment tools with ratings of certainty by clinicians, International Association for the Study of Pain, Pain* 122:289-294, 2006.

DeMaagd G: The Pharmacological Management of Migraine, Part 1 Overview and Abortive Therapy, *P&T* 33(7), 2008.

Freeman-Wilson K: Methadone maintenance and other pharmacotherapeutic interventions in the treatment of opioid dependence, National Drug Institute, Drug Court Practitioner: Fact Sheet, April 2002, vol. III No. 1. Retrieved from http://www.ndci.org/publication/MethadoneFactSheet.pdf.

Gawel M, Aschoff J, May A, et al: Zolmitriptan 5 mg nasal spray: Efficacy and onset of action in the acute treatment of migraine—Results from Phase I of the REALIZE study, *Headache* 7-16, 2005.

Kalant H, Grant D, Mitchell J: *Principles of medical pharmacology*, ed 7, Toronto, 2007, Elsevier Canada, A Division of Reed Elsevier Canada, pp 236-251.

Kelmann L: *Pain characteristics of acute migraine attack, headache*, Ames, IA, 2006, Blackwell Publishing.

Kidd B: Osteoarthritis and joint pain: Topical review, International Association for the Study of Pain, *Pain* 123:6-9, 2006.

Lance L, Lacy C, Armstrong L, et al: *Drug information handbook for the allied health professional*, ed 12, Hudson, OH, 2005, APhA Lexi-Comp.

Lintzeris N, et al: National clinical guidelines and procedures for use of buprenorphine in the treatment of opioid dependency, 2006. Retrieved from http://www.nationaldrugstrategy.gov.au/internet/drugstrategy/publishing.nsf/Content/buprenorphine-abbrev.

Lipton RB, Bigal ME, Diamond M, et al: Migraine prevalence, disease burden, and the need for preventive therapy, *Neurology* 68:343-349, 2007.

Macfarlane G, Jones G, Hannaford P: Managing low back pain presenting in primary care: Where do we go from here? *International Association for the Study of Pain, Pain* 122:219-222, 2006.

Marcus D: Treatment of nonmalignant chronic pain, *Am Fam Phys* 61:1-8, 2000.

Matcher B, Young WB, Rosenberg JH, et al: Evidence-Based Guidelines for Migraine Headache in the Primary Care Setting: Pharmacological Management of Acute Attacks, US Headache Consortium, available online at: http://www.aan.com/professionals/practice/pdfs/gl0087.pdf.

National Institute of Neurological Disorders and Stroke: Pain: Hope through research, Bethesda, MD, NINDS, National Institutes of Health, U.S. Department of Health and Human Services. Updated June 2006. NIH Publication No. 01-2406.

Page C, Curtis M, Sutter M, et al: *Integrated pharmacology*, Philadelphia, 2005, Elsevier Mosby, pp 272-247.

Raffa RB, Rawls SM, Beyzarov EP: *Netter's Illustrated pharmacology*, Philadelphia, 2005, Saunders, p 85.

Teng J, Mekhail N: Neuropathic pain: Mechanisms and treatment options, World Institute of Pain, *Pain Pract* 3:8-21, 2003.

USP Center for Advancement of Patient Safety: Use caution: avoid confusion. USP Quality Review No. 79, Rockville, MD, April 2004, USP Center for Advancement of Patient Safety.

11

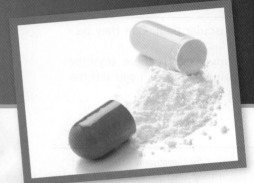

Treatment of Alzheimer's Disease

LEARNING OBJECTIVES

1 Learn the terminology associated with the treatment of Alzheimer's disease.

2 Describe the etiology of Alzheimer's disease.

3 Describe the function of neurotransmitters associated with symptoms of Alzheimer's disease.

4 Classify medications used in the treatment of Alzheimer's disease.

5 Describe mechanism of action for each class of drugs used to treat Alzheimer's disease.

6 Identify significant drug look-alike/sound-alike issues.

7 Identify warning labels and precautionary messages associated with medications used to treat Alzheimer's disease.

KEY TERMS

Acetylcholinesterase: Enzyme that degrades the neurotransmitter acetylcholine.

Alzheimer's disease: Neurodegenerative disease that causes memory loss and behavioral changes.

ApoE4 allele: Defective form of apolipoprotein E that is associated with Alzheimer's disease.

Dementia: Condition associated with a loss of memory and cognition.

Neurodegeneration: Destruction of nerve cells.

Neuroprotective: Protects nerve cells from damage.

Plaques: Substances composed of a protein called beta amyloid that fill the spaces between neurons and interfere with the transmission of signals between neurons.

Tangles: Twisted fibers made up of clumps of a protein called tau that interfere with nerve signal transmission.

Alzheimer's Disease

Alzheimer's disease is a neurodegenerative disease that causes memory loss and behavioral changes. According to the National Institutes of Health National Institute on Aging, up to 5.1 million Americans have Alzheimer's disease. Nearly 500,000 Canadians have Alzheimer's disease or a related dementia. The risk for Alzheimer's disease increases with advancing age. In fact, nearly 5% of the adult population 65 years of age will have Alzheimer's disease. That percentage doubles by age 70 years, and by age 85 years, nearly half of all men and women are estimated to have the disease. Although advancing age is an important risk factor for the development of Alzheimer's disease, *dementia* is not a normal part of the aging process.

Another risk factor for developing Alzheimer's disease is family history. Early-onset, familial Alzheimer's disease affects adults between 30 years and 60 years. Late-onset Alzheimer's is linked to

TABLE 11-1   **Comparisons Between Alzheimer's Disease and Normal Aging**

Alzheimer's Disease	Normal Aging
Making poor judgments and decisions a lot of the time	Making a bad decision once in a while
Problems taking care of monthly bills	Missing a monthly payment
Losing track of the date or time of year	Forgetting which day it is and remembering it later
Trouble having a conversation	Sometimes forgetting which word to use
Misplacing things often and being unable to find them	Losing things from time to time

Courtesy of the National Institute on Aging, Understanding Alzheimer's disease: what you need to know (http://www.nia.nih.gov/Alzheimer'ss/Publications/UnderstandingAD).

several nonhereditary genes. Apolipoprotein E (ApoE) helps carry cholesterol in the blood. Approximately 40% of people with Alzheimer's disease have a defective form of ApoE, although not everyone with a defective ***ApoE4 allele*** will develop the disease. Only 15% of people with the defective ApoE4 allele will develop Alzheimer's disease. In 2009, three new genes were discovered that are associated with the development of Alzheimer's disease: *CLU* (ApoJ/clusterin), *PICALM,* and *CRI* (complement receptor 1). *CLU* and *CRI* play a role in clearing beta amyloid out of the brain. Cell membrane proteins are recycled at the synapse by *PICALM.*

The most commonly reported symptom of Alzheimer's disease is forgetfulness. The person may not recall recent events or names of familiar people or things. This increases as the disease progresses and may interfere with the performance of activities of daily living such as personal hygiene. In the mid to late stages of Alzheimer's disease, the person may have difficulty reading, speaking, writing, and ambulating. The person may become anxious, angry, and aggressive. In addition, the person may be confused and wander, unable to find his or her way back to where he or she started. Many people confuse the differences between the normal aging process and Alzheimer's disease. Table 11-1 shows some comparisons between the disease and normal aging.

PATHOPHYSIOLOGY OF ALZHEIMER'S DISEASE

Alzheimer's disease causes damage to the hippocampus, the part of the brain that is involved in memory. The disease causes cholinergic nerve cells in the brain to die. The cerebral cortex shrinks in size, and the ability to think and function diminishes. Abnormal structures, called plaques and tangles, develop in the brain (Figure 11-1). ***Plaques*** are dense substances composed of a protein called beta amyloid. The plaques fill the spaces between neurons in the brain and interfere with the transmission of signals between the neurons. ***Tangles*** look like twisted fibers and are made up of clumps of a protein called tau. Tangles are also thought to block the transmission of messages between neurons. The accumulation of plaques and tangles also produces inflammation, which further damages neurons. Beta amyloid disrupts long-term potentiation (LTP), the mechanism the brain uses to store long-term memory.

Comorbid conditions such as cerebrovascular disease, high blood pressure, diabetes, sleep apnea, and Parkinson's disease are believed to speed the progression of Alzheimer's disease. Lewy bodies, abnormal clumps of protein, found in people with Alzheimer's disease, are also associated with Parkinson's disease. Sleep deprivation can increase beta amyloid deposits. Microvascular infarcts and inflammation, which block blood supply and nourishment to the brain, are common in patients with cerebrovascular disease, diabetes, and Alzheimer's disease.

ROLE OF NEUROTRANSMITTERS

Several neurotransmitters play a significant role in Alzheimer's disease. The most significant is acetylcholine (ACh). ACh levels gradually decline as the disease progresses producing the symptoms associated with Alzheimer's disease. Cholinergic pathways are involved in all aspects of cognition, or the ability to absorb, process, and use information. Recall that there are two types of cholinergic receptors, muscarinic and nicotinic (Figure 11-2). (See Unit II.) Stimulation of nicotinic receptors has been shown to play a role in Alzheimer's disease. Reduced nicotinic receptor function is correlated to impaired memory.

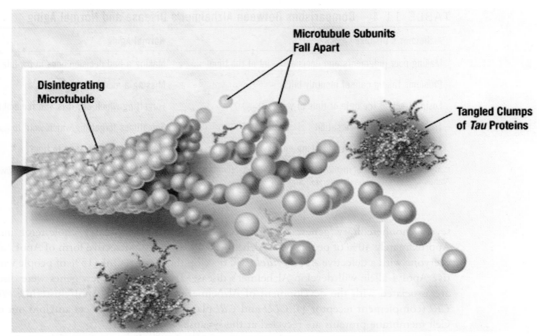

FIGURE 11-1 Disintegrating neurons and tangles. (Courtesy The Alzheimer's Disease Education and Referral Center, National Institute on Aging, Bethesda, MD.)

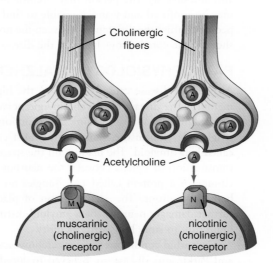

FIGURE 11-2 Muscarinic and nicotinic receptors. (From Thibodeau GA, Patton KT: *Anatomy and physiology,* ed 6, St. Louis, 2007, Mosby.)

Glutamate also plays a role in the development of Alzheimer's disease. Glutamate is an excitatory amino acid that is particularly active in the cerebral cortex and hippocampus (Figure 11-3) where binding to glutamatergic receptors is involved in memory formation and learning. There are three classes of glutamatergic receptors. The *N*-methyl-D-aspartate (NMDA) receptor is associated with memory and learning. Excess activity of this receptor is linked to Alzheimer's disease and is believed to contribute to the process of ***neurodegeneration***.

Other neurotransmitters that are believed to play a part in Alzheimer's disease are dopamine, norepinephrine, and serotonin.

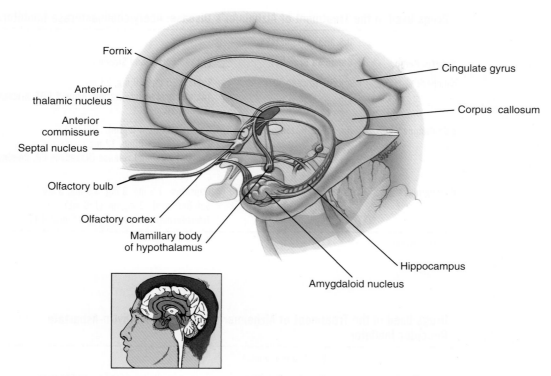

FIGURE 11-3 Parts of the brain controlling memory. (From Thibodeau GA, Patton KT: *Anatomy and physiology*, ed 6, St. Louis, 2007, Mosby.)

DRUG TREATMENT FOR ALZHEIMER'S DISEASE

Drugs that increase ACh levels at the synapse are used to treat Alzheimer's disease. Drugs that block glutamate activity are also used in the treatment of Alzheimer's disease. Three of the four drugs currently approved for the treatment of Alzheimer's disease are ***acetylcholinesterase*** (AChE) inhibitors; the other is an NMDA antagonist. AChE is an enzyme that degrades ACh. There are several types of AChEs. Two forms that are important to the treatment of Alzheimer's disease are AChE-S and AChE-R. AChE-R has been shown to be neuroprotective in human and animal studies. ***Neuroprotective*** agents protect nerve cells from damage. AChE-S appears to enhance the degeneration of cholinergic neurons. AChE inhibitors increase levels of ACh. They also increase the number and the activity of nicotinic receptors.

The AChE inhibitors are typically prescribed for the treatment of mild to moderate disease. The NMDA antagonist is prescribed for moderate to severe disease.

Mechanism of Action and Pharmacokinetics

Donepezil (Aricept), rivastigmine (Exelon), and galantamine (Razadyne, Reminyl) are AChE inhibitors. In addition to AChE inhibition, galantamine slightly increases glutamate activity.

Donepezil is highly protein bound and metabolized by CYP450 isoenzymes and thus subject to drug interactions with drugs that are similarly protein bound and metabolized by 2D6 and 3A4 hepatic enzymes. Donepezil is available as a swallowable tablet and an oral disintegrating tablet. Its bioavailability is not diminished by food, and donepezil may be taken without regard to meals. In contrast, the bioavailability of galantamine is delayed by food; however, the drug is nearly 90% bioavailable, and protein binding and CYP450 metabolism are minimal. Rivastigmine readily crosses the blood-brain barrier, where it is metabolized at central nervous system receptor sites; however, cholinesterase inhibition lasts up to 10 hours. Over a 24-hour period, 50% of the drug is released from rivastimine transdermal patches.

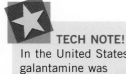

TECH NOTE!
In the United States, galantamine was formerly marketed under the brand name Reminyl but is now marketed as Razadyne.

TECH NOTE!
In 2010, the U.S. Food and Drug Administration agreed to review the new drug application for a transdermal dosage form of donepezil. The Aricept patch, if approved, will be dosed once weekly.

Drugs Used in the Treatment of Alzheimer's Disease: Acetylcholinesterase Inhibitors

Generic Name	U.S. Brand Name(s) Canadian Brand(s)	Dosage Forms and Strengths
donepezil*	Aricept, Aricept ODT Aricept, Aricept RDT	Tablets: 5 mg, 10 mg, 23 mg Tablets, oral disintegrating (Aricept ODT, Aricept RDT): 5 mg, 10 mg
galantamine*	Razadyne, Razadyne ER Reminyl ER	Solution, oral: 4 mg/mL (100 mL) Tablets: 4 mg, 8 mg, 12 mg Tablets, extended release (Razadyne ER, Reminyl ER): 8 mg, 16 mg, 24 mg
rivastigmine*	Exelon Exelon	Capsules: 1.5 mg, 3 mg, 4.5 mg, 6 mg Solution, oral: 2 mg/mL (120 mL) Transdermal patch: 4.6 mg, 9.5 mg/24 hr

*Generic available.

Drugs Used in the Treatment of Alzheimer's Disease: *N*-Methyl-D-Aspartate Receptor Inhibitor

Generic Name	U.S. Brand name(s) Canadian Brand(s)	Dosage Forms and Strengths
memantine*‡	Namenda, Namenda XR Ebixa	Solution, oral: 10 mg/5 mL† Tablets: 5 mg†, 10 mg Capsules (XR): 7 mg†, 14 mg†, 21 mg†, 28 mg†

*‡Generic in Canada only.
†Strength available in the United States only.

Summary of Drugs Used in the Treatment of Alzheimer's Disease

Generic Name	U.S. Brand Name	Usual Adult Oral Dose and Dosing Schedule	Warning Labels
donepezil	Aricept	Tablets/ODT: 5-23 mg once daily at bedtime	MAY CAUSE DIZZINESS OR DROWSINESS—donepezil, galantamine, rivastigmine, memantine.
galantamine	Reminyl	Tablets: 4-16 mg twice a day Extended release tablets: 8-24 mg once daily	TAKE WITH FOOD—galantamine, rivastigmine. DISSOLVE IN MOUTH—donepezil ODT.
rivastigmine	Exelon	Capsules/solution: 1.5-6 mg twice a day Transdermal patch: Apply one patch daily	DO NOT DISCONTINUE WITHOUT MEDICAL SUPERVISION. REMOVE OLD PATCH AND ROTATE SITE OF APPLICATION MAINTAIN ADEQUATE HYDRATION—galantamine.
memantine	Namenda	Tablets: 5-10 mg twice a day Capsules XR: 7-28 mg once daily	SWALLOW WHOLE; DO NOT CRUSH OR CHEW—donepezil (23 mg tab only), galantamine ER, memantine XR. MAY MIX SOLUTION WITH WATER, JUICE OR SODA ONLY—rivastigmine. CAPSULES MAY BE SPRINKLED ON APPLESAUCE—memantine XR.

TECH ALERT!

The following drugs have look-alike/sound-alike issues: Donepezil and Benazepril; Reminyl and Amaryl

TECH NOTE!

Dispense Razadyne solution with manufacturer's calibrated syringe.

Memantine (Namenda) blocks the actions of glutamate at NMDA receptor sites. This mechanism of action is theorized to protect the neuron from further damage. All dosage forms of memantine exhibit 100% bioavailability. The drug is minimally subject to drug interactions involving CYP450 isozymes; however, alkaline urine can decrease drug clearance by as much as 80%. Food has little effect on absorption, and memantine may be taken without regard to meals.

Adverse Reactions

Donepezil, galantamine, rivastigmine, and memantine can all produce abdominal pain and cramping, dizziness, diarrhea, nausea, and urinary incontinence. In some patients, donepezil and rivastigmine may increase urinary frequency. Tremor has been reported in all agents except donepezil. Pseudoparkinsonism has been reported with the use of rivastigmine and memantine. Myocardial infarction, erectile dysfunction, and suicide ideation have been reported with memantine.

NONPHARMACOLOGICAL MEASURES TO REDUCE RISKS FOR ALZHEIMER'S DISEASE

Head injury protection and adoption of a healthy lifestyle that includes reduction in cholesterol, adequate intellectual stimulation, and decreased obesity are modifiable factors the may reduce the risk for Alzheimer's disease. Social interaction keeps the brain stimulated. Some studies have shown that aerobic exercise can reduce risks for obesity, improve cognition, and reduce plaque formation. A diet that includes vegetables, legumes, fruits, cereals, olive oil, decreased saturated fats, dairy products, fish, lean meat, poultry, and antioxidants can reduce vascular disease, a comorbid condition linked to increasing the progression of Alzheimer's disease. Vitamin E, folate, selenium, and other antioxidants are being studied for their possible benefit in preventing Alzheimer's disease.

Summary

The effects of drugs used in the treatment of Alzheimer's disease diminish as the disease progresses and the brain produces less and less acetylcholine.

Chapter Summary

- Nearly 5 million Americans and 500,000 Canadians have Alzheimer's disease or disease-related dementia.
- Alzheimer's disease is a neurodegenerative disease that causes memory loss and behavioral changes.
- Risk factors for Alzheimer's disease are age and heredity.
- ApoE, *CRI*, *CLU*, and *PICALM* are genes linked to late-onset Alzheimer's disease.
- Alzheimer's disease causes damage to the part of the brain that is involved in memory.
- Abnormal structures called plaques and tangles form and interfere with the transmission of messages between neurons.
- Alzheimer's disease causes cholinergic nerve cells in the brain to die.
- The primary neurotransmitters involved in Alzheimer's disease are acetylcholine and glutamate.
- Alzheimer's disease is treated with drugs that increase acetylcholine levels that block glutamate activity.
- Acetylcholinesterase (AChE) is an enzyme that degrades acetylcholine (ACh).
- AChE inhibitors increase levels of ACh.
- Three of the drugs approved for the treatment of Alzheimer's disease are AChE inhibitors. They are donepezil (Aricept), rivastigmine (Exelon), and galantamine (Reminyl).
- Memantine (Namenda) blocks the actions of glutamate at the NMDA receptor.

TECH NOTE!

Rivastimine premixed solution must be consumed within 4 hours of mixing.

1. The most commonly reported symptom of Alzheimer's disease is _____.
   a. pain
   b. forgetfulness
   c. heart problems
   d. incontinence

2. Several neurotransmitters play a significant role in Alzheimer's disease. The most significant is _____.
   a. epinephrine
   b. serotonin
   c. norepinephrine
   d. acetylcholine

3. Drugs that increase _____ levels at the synapse are used to treat Alzheimer's disease.
   a. dopamine
   b. acetylcholine
   c. serotonin
   d. glutamate

4. Of the four drugs currently approved for the treatment of Alzheimer's disease, three of them are _____ inhibitors.
   a. acetylcholinesterase
   b. acetylcholine
   c. glutamate
   d. dopamine

5. Family history is not a factor for developing Alzheimer's disease.
   a. true
   b. false

6. Which Alzheimer's drug blocks the actions of glutamate?
   a. Aricept (donepezil)
   b. Namenda (memantine)
   c. Imitrex (sumatriptan)
   d. Exelon (rivastigmine)

7. All of the following are commonly reported side effects of drugs used to treat Alzheimer's disease EXCEPT
   a. abdominal cramping
   b. urinary retention
   c. diarrhea
   d. photosensitivity
   e. dizziness

8. A low-_____ diet may reduce the risk for Alzheimer's disease.
   a. sodium
   b. potassium
   c. cholesterol
   d. sugar

9. Comorbid conditions associated with increased progression of Alzheimer's disease include all of the following EXCEPT
   a. Parkinson's disease
   b. High blood pressure
   c. Diabetes
   d. Schizophrenia

10. The warning label MAY CAUSE DIZZINESS should be placed on prescriptions dispensed for Aricept and Namenda.
    a. true
    b. false

TECHNICIAN'S CORNER

1. According to the most current research, a brain-healthy diet is one that reduces the risk of heart disease and diabetes, encourages good blood flow to the brain, and is low in fat and cholesterol. What sort of physical, mental, and social activities can be added to daily living to delay the onset of Alzheimer's disease?

2. Family history is one of the contributing factors in Alzheimer's disease. Knowing that your uncle has Alzheimer's disease, what can you do to prevent this disease from affecting you?

Bibliography

Bren L: *Alzheimer's: searching for a cure, FDA Consumer magazine, US Food and Drug Administration, US Department of Health and Human Services.* March and May 2004, FDA publication No. 04-1318C rev.

Elsevier: Gold Standard Clinical Pharmacology, 2010. Retrieved March 7, 2011, from https://www.clinicalpharmacology.com/.

FDA: FDA Approved Drug Products, 2012. Retrieved April 28, 2012, from http://www.accessdata.fda.gov/scripts/cder/drugsatfda/index.cfm?fuseaction=Search.Search_Drug_Name.

Geerts H: Pharmacology of acetylcholinesterase inhibitors and *N*-methyl-D-aspartate receptors for the combination therapy in the treatment of Alzheimer's disease, *J Clin Pharmacol* 46:8S–16S, 2006.

Health Canada: Drug Product Database, 2010. Retrieved Feb 27, 2011, from http://www.hc-sc.gc.ca/dhp-mps/prodpharma/databasdon/index-eng.php.

Lance L, Lacy C, Armstrong L, et al: *Drug information handbook for the allied health professional,* ed 12, Hudson, OH, 2005, APhA Lexi-Comp.

National Institute on Aging: *Alzheimer's disease: fact sheet.* Bethesda, MD, 2005, ADEAR, National Institutes of Health, US Department of Health and Human Services, NIH publication No. 03-3431.

National Institute on Aging: *2009 Progress Report on Alzheimer's Disease: Translating New Knowledge,* 2010, US Department Health and Human Services, National Institutes of Health, NIH publication No. 10-7500.

National Institute on Aging: *Understanding Alzheimer's Disease: What You Need to Know,* June 2011, Department of Health and Human Services, National Institutes of Health NIH Publication No. 11-5441, Available at http://www.nia.nih.gov/Alzheimer's/Publications/UnderstandingAD/.

Nordberg A: Mechanisms behind the neuroprotective actions of cholinesterase inhibitors in Alzheimer's disease, *Alzheimer's Dis Assoc Disord* 20(suppl 1):S12-S18, 2006.

Page C, Curtis M, Sutter M, et al: *Integrated pharmacology.* Philadelphia, 2005, Mosby, pp 261-262.

Raffa R, Rawls S, Beyzarov E: *Netter's illustrated pharmacology.* Philadelphia, 2005, WB Saunders, pp 80-82.

Smetanin P, Kobak P, Briante C, et al: *Rising Tide: The Impact of Dementia on Canadian Society.* 2010, Alzheimer's Society of Canada.

USP Center for Advancement of Patient Safety: Use caution—avoid confusion, USP Quality Review No. 79, Rockville, MD, April 2004, USP Center for Advancement of Patient Safety.

12

Treatment of Sleep Disorders and Attention-Deficit Hyperactivity Disorder

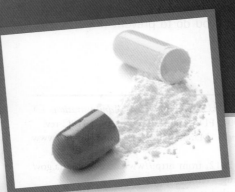

LEARNING OBJECTIVES

1 Learn the terminology associated with sleep disorders and attention-deficit hyperactivity disorder (ADHD).
2 Discuss the reasons why sleep is necessary.
3 Describe the phases of a normal sleep cycle.
4 Describe symptoms associated with sleep deprivation.
5 Describe the types of sleep disorders.
6 Describe the function of neurotransmitters associated with symptoms of sleep.
7 Classify medications used in the treatment of sleep disorders.
8 Describe mechanism of action for each class of drugs used to treat sleep disorders.
9 Identify warning labels and precautionary messages associated with medications used to treat sleep disorders.
10 Describe the etiology of ADHD.
11 Classify medications used in the treatment of ADHD.
12 Describe mechanism of action for each class of drugs used to treat ADHD.
13 Identify warning labels and precautionary messages associated with medications used to treat ADHD.
14 Identify significant drug look-alike/sound-alike issues.

KEY TERMS

Circadian rhythm: Biological change that occurs according to time cycles.

Disinhibition: Opposite of inhibited.

Hypnotic: Drug that induces sleep.

Insomnia: Condition characterized by difficulty falling asleep, staying asleep, or both.

Melatonin: Hormone that is released by the pineal gland that makes a person feel drowsy.

Non-REM sleep: Stages 1 through 4 of the sleep cycle.

Rebound hypersomnia: Condition associated with excessive sleep that follows long-term insomnia or the use of drugs that depress REM and non-REM sleep.

Rapid eye movement sleep: The stage of sleep when dreaming occurs.

Sedative: Drug that causes relaxation and promotes drowsiness.

Stimulant: Drug that increases activity in the brain and is used to treat ADHD and narcolepsy.

Sympathomimetic: Drug whose effects mimic the effects produced by stimulation of the sympathetic nervous system.

Overview

Sleep is a necessary biological function for the growth and maintenance of a healthy body. Sleep is needed for a healthy immune system and nervous system and for emotional and social functioning, as well as for physical and mental agility. Our memory is also improved when we get sufficient sleep.

The body's sleep cycle is influenced by circadian rhythms. **Circadian rhythms** are biological changes that occur according to time cycles. The human body operates on a 24-hour clock; however, this clock can be manipulated by external time cues. Sunlight is the primary external time cue. Changes in sunlight and darkness are picked up by the retina in the back of the eye. The retina sends signals to the pineal gland in the brain. The pineal gland controls the release of **melatonin**, a hormone that makes people feel drowsy in addition to regulating body temperature and hormone secretion. The fact that our normal sleep–wake cycle is linked to sunlight explains why people who work the night shift may feel uncontrollably drowsy in the middle of the night, and it explains why workplace accidents occur more frequently in the middle of the night than during the day.

The amount of time a person needs to sleep ranges between 5 and 16 hours per day. The amount of sleep needed can vary according to age. Infants may sleep up to 16 hours per day, teenagers require as much as 9 hours, and adults need as little as 5 to 8 hours. The patterns of sleep change as people age. Elderly adults often sleep for shorter time spans, sleep more lightly, and dream less than they did as young adults, although their overall sleep requirement may not change.

The normal sleep pattern involves five stages of sleep (Figure 12-1). *Stage 1* occurs first; during this stage, the person sleeps lightly and can be awakened easily. Sudden muscle contractions of the limbs may occur similar to when a person is startled while awake, and the eyes move slowly back and forth. In *stage 2,* sleep eye movements stop, and brain activity decreases. *Stage 3* and *stage 4* sleep are deep sleep. Brain activity slows (delta waves). It is difficult to wake someone from stage 3 or stage 4 sleep; if awakened, the person feels disoriented. The final stage of sleep is known as **rapid eye movement (REM) sleep** because of the characteristic eye movements that occur. This is the sleep cycle where dreaming occurs, and it lasts between 90 minutes and 110 minutes. REM sleep is crucial to normal emotional and physical functioning. Approximately 2 hours per night is spent in REM sleep. The thalamus and cerebral cortex actively communicate with each other during REM sleep. The cortex is the region of the brain involved in learning and interpretation of information.

Too little sleep causes symptoms of sleep deprivation. A drowsy feeling during the day with or without micro-sleeps and falling asleep within 5 minutes of lying down are signs of sleep deprivation. Studies show that sleep deprivation is dangerous and can cause motor vehicle accidents at a rate similar to driving under the influence of alcohol. As many as 100,000 motor vehicle accidents in the United States each year are attributed to sleep deprivation. Sleep deprivation can also trigger seizures, paranoia, and hallucinations.

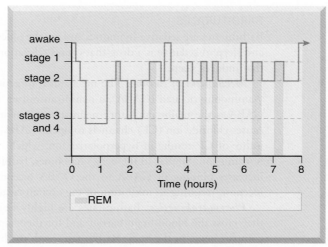

FIGURE 12-1 Normal sleep cycle. REM, rapid eye movement. (From Page C, et al: *Integrated pharmacology*, ed 3, Philadelphia, 2006, Mosby.)

Factors that contribute to the inability to get adequate sleep are numerous and include sleep apnea, restless legs syndrome, consumption of caffeinated beverages and foods near bedtime, use of prescription and nonprescription drugs, and chronic illness. Chronic illnesses that can interfere with sleep are gastroesophageal reflux disorder, angina, and chronic pain, among others.

Sleep Disorders

Millions of Americans have sleep disorders. The most common sleep disorders are insomnia, restless legs syndrome, sleep apnea, and narcolepsy. *Insomnia* affects nearly 60 million Americans each year and up to one-third of the world population. It is categorized according to the length of time the symptoms persist. Transient insomnia lasts less than 7 days, short-term insomnia lasts up to 3 weeks, and long-term insomnia lasts longer than 3 weeks and is often associated with a chronic condition such as pain.

As many as 12% of the people who say they have insomnia complain about periodic leg movements. Restless legs syndrome is reported in up to 12 million Americans and is more common in elderly adults. Diabetes, pregnancy, and anemia can also cause restless leg syndrome. Sleep apnea affects up to 18 million people in the United States. A Public Health Agency Canada survey (2009) revealed that 3% of Canadians older than 18 years have been diagnosed with sleep apnea and one in four reported having symptoms that are associated with high risk for sleep apnea. The condition is associated with an interruption in the supply of oxygen during sleep, which causes the person to awaken. Sleep apnea can increase the risk for cardiovascular disorders such as hypertension, myocardial infarction, and stroke. People with sleep apnea also have an increased risk for arrhythmias, heart failure, diabetes, and obesity. Rarely, sleep apnea is fatal. Sudden death occurs from respiratory arrest during sleep.

Narcolepsy is the least common of the sleep disorders. It is characterized by falling asleep suddenly and without warning. Attacks may last between a few seconds and 30 minutes. The disorder is usually hereditary but can be caused by brain trauma.

TREATMENT OF SLEEP DISORDERS
Insomnia

Pharmacological treatments for insomnia are recommended only for short-term use. Prescription drugs, nonprescription drugs, and natural remedies are commercially available, and all produce drowsiness that enables the person to drift off to sleep (improve sleep latency) and stay asleep (improve sleep maintenance). Prescription drugs that are used to treat insomnia are barbiturates, benzodiazepines, and other sedative-hypnotics. It is important to note that drugs that promote sleep do not result in a normal pattern of sleep. They alter *non-REM* and REM sleep. This can result in *rebound hypersomnia* and increased dreaming once the drugs are discontinued.

BARBITURATES

Barbiturates are sedative-hypnotics and are the oldest class of drugs prescribed to promote relaxation and sleep. A sedative is a drug that causes relaxation and promotes drowsiness. A hypnotic is a drug that induces sleep.

Mechanism of Action. The mechanism of action for barbiturates is to enhance binding of the γ-aminobutyric acid (GABA), a neurotransmitter, to $GABA_A$ and $GABA_B$ receptors (Figure 12-2). GABA is the major inhibitory neurotransmitter in the nervous system. $GABA_A$ receptor binding causes chloride ion (Cl^-) channels to open. $GABA_B$ receptor binding is coupled to G proteins. The influx of Cl^- results in hyperpolarization, which reduces neuronal excitability and nerve impulse transmission. Similar to the benzodiazepines, barbiturates bind to a specific receptor, which in turn increases binding of GABA to the GABA receptors. In addition, barbiturates block the AMPA receptor, resulting in inhibition of the excitatory action of glutamate.

Pharmacokinetics. Barbiturates are highly lipid soluble. This accounts for the ease in which they cross the blood-brain barrier and for their rapid redistribution out of the brain to other lipid compartments in the body. Barbiturates with the highest lipid solubility have the greatest degree of redistribution and the shortest duration of effect. An example is the general anesthetic thiopental. It is categorized as an ultra-rapid-acting barbiturate, and its effects last about 20 minutes.

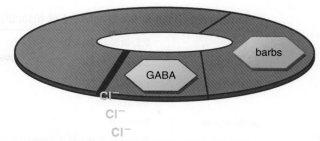

FIGURE 12-2 Barbiturate mechanism of action.

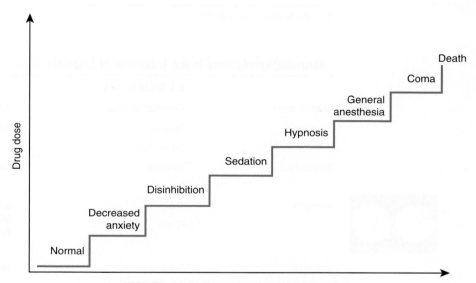

FIGURE 12-3 Dose effects of barbiturates.

Barbiturates are metabolized in the liver and are able to induce the hepatic enzymes of drugs that use the same metabolic enzyme pathway. They can also induce their own metabolic enzymes. Barbiturates are weak acids. Their elimination in urine is influenced by the pH of the urine. Increasing the pH of the urine will increase the elimination of barbiturates and is useful in managing barbiturate poisoning (see Chapter 2).

Adverse Reactions. The effects of barbiturates are dose dependent (Figure 12-3). Low doses produce decreased anxiety. As the dose increases, ***disinhibition*** occurs. This is followed by sedation. Higher doses produce somnolence or hypnosis. Increasing the dose produces general anesthesia. Toxic doses produce coma and death. Other adverse effects of barbiturates include ataxia, confusion, reduced motor performance, and hypotension.

Barbiturates can produce tolerance and dependence. When tolerance develops, the patient must take increasing doses to achieve the same effects as were achieved previously at lower doses. Barbiturates also produce drug dependence, causing the person taking the drug to continue to take the drug to avoid the onset of physical or psychological withdrawal symptoms (or both). For this reason, barbiturates are controlled substances. The controlled substance schedule is related to their abuse potential and their potential to produce physical or psychological dependence (see Chapter 1, Table 1-3). Amobarbital, pentobarbital, and secobarbital are C-II controlled substances. Phenobarbital and mephobarbital are C-IV controlled substances in the United States. Phenobarbital is no longer used for the short-term treatment of insomnia. Both phenobarbital and mephobarbital are used in the treatment of epilepsy (see Chapter 9). Barbiturates are also classified as controlled substances in Canada.

Barbiturates Used in the Treatment of Insomnia

| Generic Name | U.S. Brand Name(s) | Dosage Forms and Strengths |
	Canadian Brand(s)	
butabarbital	Butisol	Tablets: 30 mg, 50 mg
	Not available	Solution, oral: 30 mg/5 mL
pentobarbital	Nembutal	Injection, solution: 50 mg/mL, 65 mg/mL‡,
	Dorminal, Euthanyl (Veterinary use only)	200 mg/mL‡, 240 mg/mL‡, 340 mg/mL‡, 540 mg/mL‡
secobarbital	Seconal	Capsules: 50 mg, 100 mg
	Not available	

‡Strength available in Canada only.

Benzodiazepines Used in the Treatment of Insomnia

| Generic Name | U.S. Brand Name(s) | Dosage Forms and Strengths |
	Canadian Brand(s)	
estazolam*	Generics	Tablets: 1 mg, 2 mg
	Not available	
flurazepam*	Dalmane	Capsules: 15 mg, 30 mg
	Dalmane	
lorazepam*	Ativan	Solution, for injection: 2 mg/mL†, 4 mg/mL
	Ativan	Solution, oral: 2 mg/mL
		Tablets: 0.5 mg, 1 mg, 2 mg
quazepam	Doral	Tablets: 15 mg
	Not available	
temazepam*	Restoril	Capsules: 7.5 mg†, 15 mg, 22.5 mg†, 30 mg
	Restoril	
triazolam*	Halcion	Tablet: 0.125 mg, 0.25 mg
	Halcion	

*Generic available.
†Strength available in the United States only.

BENZODIAZEPINES

Benzodiazepines and other miscellaneous agents have largely replaced barbiturates for the treatment of insomnia. The benzodiazepines have a more desirable safety profile. Similar to barbiturates, the benzodiazepines decrease neuronal excitability by opening Cl⁻ channels. The mechanism of action, pharmacokinetics, and adverse reactions of benzodiazepines are discussed in detail in Chapter 5. Drugs with long half-lives may cause the user to feel groggy the morning after taking them.

MISCELLANEOUS DRUGS USED FOR THE TREATMENT OF INSOMNIA

Several newer agents are available for the treatment of insomnia that have a mechanism of action similar to that of benzodiazepines but are not classified as benzodiazepines. Zaleplon and zolpidem are classified as imidazopyridines (also called enzodiazepines). Eszopiclone and zopiclone are classified as cyclopyrrolone derivatives.

   Mechanism of Action and Pharmacokinetics. Zaleplon, zolpidem, eszopiclone, and zopiclone act on benzodiazepine receptors subtype v-1. They modulate the GABA-A receptor chloride channel

Miscellaneous Drugs Used for the Treatment of Insomnia

Generic Name	U.S. Brand Name(s) / Canadian Brand(s)	Dosage Forms and Strengths
doxepin	Silenor	Tablets: 3 mg, 6 mg
	Not labeled for insomnia in Canada	
eszopiclone	Lunesta	Tablets: 1 mg, 2 mg, 3 mg
	Not available	
ramelteon	Rozerem	Tablets: 8 mg
	Not available	
zaleplon*	Sonata	Capsules: 5 mg, 10 mg
	Not available	
zolpidem	Ambien, Ambien CR, Edluar, Zolpimist	Oromucosal spray (Zolpimist): 5 mg Tablets (Ambien): 5 mg, 10 mg Tablets, controlled release (Ambien CR): 6.25 mg, 12.5 mg Tablets, sublingual (Edluar): 5 mg, 10 mg Tablet, ODT (Sublinox): 10 mg
	Sublinox	
zopiclone*	Not available	Tablets: 5 mg, 7.5 mg
	Imovane	

*Generic available.

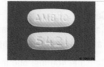

Half-life and Time to Peak Effect of Benzodiazepines and Miscellaneous Drugs Used in the Treatment of Insomnia

Generic Name	Time to Peak Effect (hr)	Half-life
Benzodiazepines		
flurazepam	1-2	1.5
nitrazepam (Canada)	2	15-40
temazepam	0.8-1.4	10-20
triazolam	1-2	1.5-5
Miscellaneous		
eszopiclone	1	6
zaleplon	1	1
zolpidem	1.6	2.5
zopiclone	<2	3.5-6

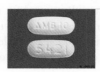

TECH ALERT! Ambien and Ambi 10 have look-alike/sound-alike issues.

to reduce neuronal excitability. Zaleplon's onset of action begins approximately 30 minutes after dosing, peaks within 1 hour, and lasts about 4 hours. Similarly, eszopiclone plasma concentration peaks within 1 hour. Zolpidem is available as an immediate-release tablet, controlled-release tablet, lingual spray, and sublingual tablet. Peak effects vary according to dosage form administered (≈50 minutes for the oral spray to 90 minutes for the oral tablet). Zolpidem is a biphasic controlled release formulation. Food reduces absorption, so zolpidem should be taken on an empty stomach.

Over-the-Counter Medications and Herbals Used in the Treatment of Insomnia

Generic Name	U.S. Brand Name(s) Canadian Brand(s)	Dosage Forms and Strengths
diphenhydramine*	Nytol Quickcaps, Simply Sleep, Sleep-Eze 3, Unisom SleepMelts, Unisom SleepGels, Sleepinal, Sominex	Capsules: 25 mg, 50 mg Solution, oral: 6.25 mg/5 mL‡, 12.5 mg/5 mL, 25 mg/5 mL Tablets: 25 mg, 50 mg Tablets, ODT (Unisom SleepMelts): 25 mg
	Extra Strength Nytol Quickgels, Extra Strength Nytol tabs, Jack & Jill Bedtime, Simply Sleep, Sleep-Eze	
doxylamine	Aldex AN, Doxytex, Unisom SleepTabs	Solution, oral: 2.5 mg/2.5 mL Suspension, oral: 2.5 mg/2.5 mL Tablets: 25 mg Tablets, chewable: 5 mg
	Unisom	
melatonin*	Generics	Capsules: 2.5 mg Capsules, extended release: 10 mg Tablet: 1 mg, 3 mg, 5 mg
	Generics	
valerian*	Generics	Capsule: 400 mg, 500 mg, 530 mg Extract: 50 mg, 250 mg
	Generics	

*Generic available.
‡Strength available in Canada only.

TECH NOTE!
Ramelteon is a selective melatonin receptor agonist that is used to treat insomnia. It is not a controlled substance.

It is claimed that zaleplon and zolpidem have less disruption of the normal stages of REM and non-REM sleep than do traditional benzodiazepines and barbiturates. Ramelteon is a selective melatonin receptor agonist. Melatonin is a hormone that regulates the circadian rhythm sleep–wake cycle. Ramelteon is indicated for insomnia caused by difficulty falling asleep. Diphenhydramine and doxylamine are over-the-counter drugs (OTC) that are used for short-term relief of insomnia. Both drugs have been used in pregnant women. Diphenhydramine is listed in U.S. Food and Drug Administration pregnancy category B. Antihistamines should be avoided in men who have benign prostatic hypertrophy and antihistamines may reduce the milk supply of breastfeeding women.

Adverse Effects of Miscellaneous Agents. Nearly all of the miscellaneous agents used in the treatment of insomnia are controlled substances and can produce tolerance and dependence. Sedation and dizziness are other side effects common to all. Zaleplon may also produce photosensitivity, and eszopiclone and zopiclone can produce a bitter or metallic taste. Ramelteon may cause sedation, headache, dizziness and gastrointestinal (GI) upset.

NATURAL REMEDIES FOR INSOMNIA
Several natural remedies have proven effectiveness for promoting sleep; they are melatonin and valerian root. Melatonin is a hormone that is produced by the pineal gland; it is sensitive to light changes and tells the body it is time to sleep. Doses of 3 mg to 5 mg have been used for treatment of short-term insomnia, and enhancement of sleep. The greatest evidence for efficacy of melatonin is in prevention of jet lag. The use of valerian root dates back more than 2000 years. Galen recommended it for the treatment of insomnia. A dose of 600 mg aqueous extract, taken 1 hour before bedtime, has been shown to be effective.

NONPHARMACOLOGICAL TREATMENTS
It is best to avoid the things that can cause sleeplessness when possible. Insomnia prevention tips include the following:
- Avoid stimulants close to bedtime.
  Caffeinated beverage such as colas, tea, chocolate, fortified water, OTC decongestants, and ephedra containing herbals are *stimulants* and can cause insomnia if consumed near bedtime.
- Adopt a regular sleeping schedule.
  A routine sleep schedule provides a cue that sleep time is approaching.

Summary of Drugs Used in the Treatment of Insomnia

Generic Name	U.S. Brand Name	Usual Adult Oral Dose and Dosing Schedule	Controlled Substance Schedule in United States	NAPRA Schedule in Canada	Warning Labels
Barbiturates					
butabarbital	Butisol	50-100 mg at bedtime	C-III		MAY CAUSE DROWSINESS; MAY IMPAIR THE ABILITY TO DRIVE. AVOID ALCOHOL. MAY BE HABIT FORMING.
pentobarbital	Nembutal	150-200 mg (IM)	C-II	C1	
secobarbital	Seconal	100-200 mg at bedtime	C-II		
Benzodiazepines					
estazolam	Generics	1 mg at bedtime	C-IV		MAY CAUSE DROWSINESS; MAY IMPAIR THE ABILITY TO DRIVE. AVOID ALCOHOL. MAY BE HABIT FORMING. TAKE 30 MINUTES BEFORE BEDTIME.
flurazepam	Dalmane	15-30 mg at bedtime	C-IV	TS	
lorazepam	Ativan	**For insomnia caused by anxiety:** 1-4 mg at bedtime as needed	C-IV	TS	
quazepam	Doral	15 mg at bedtime	C-IV		
temazepam	Restoril	15-30 mg at bedtime	C-IV	TS	
triazolam	Halcion	0.125-0.25 mg at bedtime	C-IV	TS	
Miscellaneous					
doxepin	Silenor	3-6 mg 30 minutes before bedtime			MAY CAUSE DROWSINESS; MAY IMPAIR THE ABILITY TO DRIVE—all. MAY CAUSE TEMPORARY MEMORY LOSS or SLEEP WALKING—ramelteon. TAKE ON AN EMPTY STOMACH—ramelteon. AVOID ALCOHOL—all. SWALLOW WHOLE; DO NOT CRUSH OR CHEW—extended release. DISSOLVE SUBLINGUALLY—Edluar, Sublinox. MAY BE HABIT FORMING—all targeted and controlled substances. AVOID PROLONGED EXPOSURE TO SUNLIGHT—zaleplon.
ramelteon	Rozerem	8 mg at bedtime			
zaleplon	Sonata	5-20 mg at bedtime	C-IV		
zolpidem	Ambien	5-10 mg at bedtime	C-IV		
eszopiclone	Lunesta	1-3 mg at bedtime	C-IV		
zopiclone‡	Imovane	5-7.5 mg at bedtime			

NAPRA, National Association of Pharmacy Regulatory Authorities.
‡Zopiclone (Imovane) is available in Canada.

Modafinil Use for the Treatment of Narcolepsy

Generic Name	U.S. Brand Name(s) Canadian Brand(s)	Dosage Forms and Strengths	Usual Adult Dose	U.S. Controlled Substance Schedule
armodafinil	Nuvigil Not available	Tablets: 50 mg, 150 mg, 250 mg	150-250 mg every morning	C-IV
modafinil*‡	Provigil Alertec	Tablets: 100 mg, 200 mg†	200-400 mg daily in divided doses in the morning and at noon.	C-IV

*‡Generic available in Canada only.
†Strength available in the United States only.

- Avoid daytime naps.
  Naps disrupt the normal sleep cycle.
- Create a safe comfortable sleeping environment, if possible.
  Fears about safety and extremes in temperature can prevent sleep.
- Do not go to bed hungry, if possible.
  Hunger can prevent sleep.
- Exercise 20 to 30 minutes each day (not at bedtime).
- Maximum benefits are achieved if exercise is performed 5 to 6 hours before bedtime. Exercise before bedtime can interfere with sleep.
- Do not lie in bed awake.
  If you do not fall asleep, get up and engage in a nonstimulating activity such as reading. Try to go to sleep again in about 10 minutes.

Narcolepsy

Narcolepsy is a relatively rare condition in which a person suddenly falls asleep, often in response to an emotional stimulus such as laughter or fear. The primary treatment for narcolepsy is the administration of stimulants. Stimulants used in the treatment of narcolepsy include amphetamine, methylphenidate, modafinil, and armodafinil. Modafinil and armodafinil are nonamphetamine stimulants. The drugs' mechanism of action is not fully known, but it is believed they stimulate alpha$_1$-adrenergic receptor sites. Modafinil and armodafinil are also prescribed for the treatment of sleep apnea. Amphetamine and methylphenidate are stimulants that are classified as **sympathomimetics**. A sympathomimetic is a drug that mimics the effects produced by stimulation of the sympathetic nervous system. A detailed discussion of amphetamine and methylphenidate is described in the section on treatment for attention-deficit hyperactivity disorder (ADHD).

SIDE EFFECTS AND PRECAUTIONS
The most common adverse effects produced by armodafinil and modafinil are headache, nausea, insomnia, and dizziness. The drugs may produce tolerance and dependence and are C-IV controlled substances in the United States. Stevens-Johnson syndrome, a fatal drug rash, has been linked to modafinil use. Armodafinil and modafinil may also decrease the effect of oral contraceptives. Warning labels listed below should be affixed to prescription vials for modafinil:
AVOID ALCOHOL.
MAY DECREASE THE EFFECT OF ORAL CONTRACEPTIVES.
MAY BE HABIT FORMING.

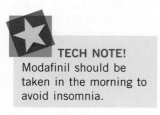

TECH NOTE!
Modafinil should be taken in the morning to avoid insomnia.

Attention-Deficit Hyperactivity Disorder

Attention-deficit hyperactivity disorder is the most commonly diagnosed childhood behavioral disorder. The percentage of school-age children reported to have ADHD in U.S. communities varies between 3% and 8%; in Canada, the percentage ranges between 5% and 10%. Although most statistics are gathered about children, ADHD affects adolescents and adults, too.

Look for signs of ADHD.

Put a check mark next to each one that sounds like your child. ☑

My child often…
- ☐ is moving something—fingers, hands, arms, feet, or legs.
- ☐ walks, runs, or climbs around when others are seated.
- ☐ has trouble waiting in line or taking turns.
- ☐ doesn't finish things.
- ☐ gets bored after just a short while.
- ☐ daydreams or seems to be in another world.
- ☐ talks when other people are talking.
- ☐ gets frustrated with schoolwork or homework.
- ☐ acts quickly without thinking first.
- ☐ is sidetracked by what is going on around him or her.

FIGURE 12-4 Checklist for signs of attention-deficit hyperactivity disorder. (Courtesy National Institute of Mental Health, Bethesda, MD.)

Symptoms of ADHD are also commonly observed in children without ADHD, making diagnosis challenging (Figure 12-4). These symptoms are hyperactivity, restlessness, an inability to sit still when required, impulsiveness, inattention, distractibility, forgetfulness, and an inability to complete tasks. All children sometimes exhibit these behaviors. A diagnosis of ADHD should only be made when these behaviors occur more frequently than would be expected for the child's age and if the behavior interferes with two or more areas of the child's life. These areas are defined as school, playground, home, community, and social relationships.

There are three subtypes of ADHD: they are predominantly hyperactive-impulsive, predominantly inattentive, and combined type. It is important to note that children who are diagnosed with predominantly inattentive type (attention-deficit disorder [ADD]) rarely exhibit hyperactivity and impulsiveness. Learning disorders such as dyslexia occur in approximately 20% to 30% of children with ADHD.

There is no single cause for ADHD. Genetics is most strongly linked to ADHD. Up to 25% of children who have a parent, sibling, or other close family relative with ADHD also have ADHD. The rate is only 5% in the general population.

Exposure to environmental agents such as cigarette smoke and alcohol during pregnancy has shown to increase the risk for ADHD. Exposure to high levels of lead-based paint also increases the risk. This is an important risk factor for children who live in older urban cities and attend school in old buildings that were painted with lead-based paint before it was banned. There is also an increased risk of ADHD in children who live in developing countries that still use leaded gasoline.

Some people believe that consumption of food additives and sugar can make ADHD worse. When placed on a diet that restricted these food additives, approximately 5% of children with ADHD showed improvement in symptoms.

PATHOPHYSIOLOGY OF ATTENTION-DEFICIT HYPERACTIVITY DISORDER

The part of the brain that is affected by ADHD is the frontal lobes of the cerebrum and the basal ganglia (see Unit II, p.72). The frontal lobe is the area of the brain involved in problem solving and planning. The basal ganglia are structures that transmit messages between the cerebrum and the

TECH ALERT!
The following drugs have look-alike/sound-alike issues: Adderall and Inderal; Ritalin, Ritalin SR, and Ritalin LA

TECH NOTE!
Adderall should be taken in the morning to avoid insomnia.

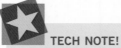

cerebellum and are involved in motor movement. Brain scans of children with ADHD show that these areas of the brain are smaller than those in children without ADHD.

TREATMENTS FOR ATTENTION-DEFICIT HYPERACTIVITY DISORDER

A variety of drug treatments are available for treating patients with ADHD; however, medications cannot cure ADHD. They only control symptoms. The most effective therapy for ADHD involves drug treatment in addition to behavioral therapy. The goal of behavioral therapy is to decrease anxiety and improve relationships and social skills.

Drugs Used for the Treatment of Attention-Deficit Hyperactivity Disorder

Generic Name	U.S. Brand Name(s) / Canadian Brand(s)	Dosage Forms and Strengths
amphetamine + dextroamphetamine*	Adderall, Adderall XR / Adderall XR	Capsules, extended release (Adderall XR): 5 mg, 10 mg, 15 mg, 20 mg, 25 mg, 30 mg Tablets: immediate release (Adderall): 5 mg, 7.5 mg, 10 mg, 12.5 mg, 15 mg, 20 mg, 30 mg
dextroamphetamine*	Dexedrine, ProCentra / Dexedrine, Dexedrine Spansule	Capsules, extended release (Dexedrine spansule): 5 mg, 10 mg, 15 mg Solution, oral (ProCentra): 1 mg/mL Tablets: immediate release (Dexedrine): 5 mg, 10 mg
dexmethylphenidate	Focalin, Focalin XR / Not available	Tablets: 2.5 mg, 5 mg, 10 mg
lisdexamfetamine	Vyvanse / Vyvanse	Capsules: 20 mg, 30 mg, 40 mg, 50 mg, 60 mg, 70 mg
methylphenidate*	Concerta, Daytrana, Metadate CD, Metadate ER, Methylin, Ritalin, Ritalin LA, Ritalin SR / Biphentin, Concerta, Ritalin, Ritalin SR	Capsules, biphasic extended release (Biphentin, Metadate CD, Ritalin LA): 10 mg, 20 mg, 30 mg, 40 mg, 50 mg, 60 mg (Biphentin, Metadate CD), 15 mg and 80 mg (Biphentin only) Solution, oral (Methylin): 2 mg/mL, 1 mg/mL Tablets, chewable (Methylin): 2.5 mg, 5 mg, 10 mg Tablets, extended release (Concerta): 18 mg, 27 mg, 36 mg, 54 mg Tablets, extended release (Metadate ER): 10 mg, 20 mg Tablets, immediate release (Ritalin): 5 mg†, 10 mg, 20 mg Tablets, sustained release (Ritalin SR): 20 mg Transdermal patch (Daytrana): 10 mg/9 hr, 15 mg/9 hr, 20 mg/9 hr, 30 mg/9 hr
atomoxetine	Strattera / Strattera	Capsules: 10 mg, 18 mg, 25 mg, 40 mg, 60 mg, 80 mg, 100 mg

*Generic available.
†Strength available in the United States only.

Pharmaceutical treatment of ADHD is achieved with the administration of amphetamines and nonamphetamine stimulants. Amphetamines behave differently in people who have ADHD than they do in people without ADHD. They decrease hyperactivity and improve focus rather than producing hyperactivity and a lack of focused behavior.

Mechanism of Action and Pharmacokinetics

Amphetamines are sympathomimetics structurally similar to norepinephrine. They work via three primary mechanisms: they stimulate the release of norepinephrine, block monoamine oxidase (further increasing catecholamine levels), and stimulate the release of dopamine. Increased stimulation of adrenergic receptors by norepinephrine is responsible for the increased alertness, responsiveness, wakefulness, and reduced awareness of fatigue associated with amphetamines.

Amphetamines are well absorbed from the GI tract, and their lipid solubility enables them to cross the blood-brain barrier. They are metabolized in the liver and eliminated in the urine. Lisdexamfetamine is a prodrug that is metabolized to dextroamphetamine. Amphetamines are manufactured in immediate-release, sustained-release, and extended-release dosage forms. The duration of action varies according to the dosage form administered. Atomoxetine is a nonamphetamine stimulant. It inhibits the reuptake of norepinephrine.

Summary of Drugs Used in the Treatment of Attention-Deficit Hyperactivity Disorder

Generic Name	Brand Name	Duration of Action (hr)	Usual Child Dosage	Approved Age
Amphetamines				
amphetamine + dextroamphetamine (Immediate release)	Adderall	6	5-20 mg/day (1-3 doses/day)	3+ years
amphetamine + dextroamphetamine (Extended release)	Adderall XR	12	5-20 mg every morning	
dextroamphetamine (Immediate release)	Dexedrine, Dextrostat	4	2.5-20 mg 1-2 times per day	3+ years
dexmethylphenidate	Focalin	6	2.5-20 mg/day given as 2 doses/day	6+ years
lisdexamfetamine	Vyvanse	12	30-70 mg once daily	6+
methylphenidate (Immediate release)	Ritalin	3-6	10-20 mg twice a day up to 60 mg/day	6+ years
methylphenidate (Extended release)	Concerta	12	18-54 mg once daily	6-12 years
			18-72 mg/day	13-17 years
	Ritalin LA	12	20 mg once a day up to 60 mg/day	6+
	Metadate CD	8	20 mg once a day up to 60 mg/day	6+
	Metadate ER	8	10-20 mg every 8 hours	6+
methylphenidate (Sustained release)	Ritalin SR	6-8	10-20 mg every 8 hours	6+
methylphenidate (Transdermal patch)	Daytrana	12	1 patch worn for 9 hours per day	6+
Nonamphetamine				
atomoxetine	Strattera	24	40-80 mg/day in 1-2 divided doses	6+

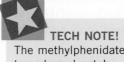

TECH NOTE!
The methylphenidate transdermal patch (Daytrana) should be worn for only 9 hours each day then removed.

Adverse Reactions

The most common side effects produced by amphetamines are decreased appetite, nausea, stomachache, anxiety, and irritability. They can also cause insomnia. Insomnia can be minimized if the last dose is taken before 6 PM. Sympathetic nervous system stimulation produced by amphetamines is responsible for these drugs' cardiovascular effects. Amphetamines can cause increased heart rate, palpitations, and arrhythmia. Other side effects produced by amphetamines are dizziness and tremor. Doses greater than therapeutic doses can produce amphetamine syndrome, a type of drug-induced psychosis.

Precautions

Amphetamines have a high abuse potential. They are all Schedule C-II controlled substances in the United States. They are also controlled in Canada (National Association of Pharmacy Regulatory Authorities schedule C1). Atomoxetine is not a controlled substance.

Chapter Summary

- Sleep is needed for a healthy immune system and nervous system and emotional and social functioning, as well as physical and mental agility.
- The body's sleep cycle is influenced by circadian rhythms.
- Our normal sleep–wake cycle is linked to changes in sunlight.
- The pineal gland controls the release of melatonin, a hormone that makes people feel drowsy.
- Infants may sleep up to 16 hours per day, teenagers require as much as 9 hours, and adults need as little as 5 to 8 hours. Patterns of sleep change as people age.
- There are five stages of sleep (four non–rapid eye movement [REM] stages and REM).
- Dreaming occurs during REM sleep and is crucial to normal emotional and physical functioning.
- Sleep deprivation contributes to workplace and motor vehicle accidents.
- Sleep apnea can increase the risk for hypertension, myocardial infarction, and stroke and is linked to arrhythmias, heart failure, diabetes, and obesity.
- Sleep apnea, restless legs syndrome, consumption of caffeinated beverages and foods, use of prescription and nonprescription drugs, and chronic illness can cause insomnia.
- Pharmacological treatment for insomnia is recommended for short-term use.
- Prescription drugs, nonprescription drugs, and herbal remedies are commercially available, and all produce drowsiness that enables the person to drift off to sleep and stay asleep.
- Prescription drugs used to treat insomnia are barbiturates, benzodiazepines, and other sedative-hypnotics.
- Drugs that promote sleep do not result in a normal pattern of sleep. They alter non-REM and REM sleep.
- Rebound hypersomnia and increased dreaming occur after the drugs are discontinued.
- Barbiturates decrease neuronal excitability by increasing GABA binding and blocking AMPA receptor binding.
- Barbiturates can produce tolerance and dependence.
- Several newer agents (e.g., zaleplon, zolpidem, eszopiclone, and zopiclone) are available for the treatment of insomnia that have a mechanism of action similar to that of benzodiazepines.
- Melatonin and valerian root are herbal remedies that have proven effectiveness for promoting sleep.
- Insomnia prevention tips include (1) avoid stimulants close to bedtime; (2) adopt a regular sleeping schedule; (3) avoid daytime naps; (4) create a safe comfortable sleeping environment, if possible; (5) do not go to bed hungry, if possible; (6) exercise; and (7) do not lie in bed awake.
- Stimulants are administered for the treatment of narcolepsy.
- Attention-deficit hyperactivity disorder (ADHD) is the most commonly diagnosed childhood behavioral disorder.
- Symptoms of ADHD are hyperactivity, restlessness, an inability to sit still when required, impulsiveness, inattention, distractibility, forgetfulness, and an inability to complete tasks.
- Genetics and environmental factors may increase the risk for ADHD.

- The most effective therapy for ADHD involves a combination of drug treatments and behavioral therapy.
- Pharmaceutical treatment of ADHD is achieved with the administration of amphetamines and nonamphetamine stimulants.
- Amphetamines behave differently in people who have ADHD than they do in people without ADHD.
- Amphetamines stimulate the release of norepinephrine, block monoamine oxidase, and stimulate the release of dopamine.
- The most common side effects produced by amphetamines are decreased appetite, nausea, stomachache, anxiety, insomnia, and irritability.
- Amphetamines have a high abuse potential and are controlled substances in the United States and Canada.
- The methylphenidate patch (Daytrana) should be applied to the hip area. It should not be worn for more than 9 hours per day.

REVIEW QUESTIONS

1. Not getting enough sleep does not affect the immune system, nervous system, or emotional and social functioning of the body.
   a. true
   b. false

2. Circadian rhythms are biological changes that occur according to _____ cycles.
   a. growth
   b. age
   c. time
   d. health

3. The pineal gland controls the release of _____, a hormone that makes people feel drowsy in addition to regulating body temperature and hormone secretion.
   a. serotonin
   b. melatonin
   c. dopamine
   d. acetylcholine

4. Narcolepsy is the most common of the sleep disorders.
   a. true
   b. false

5. Pharmacological treatment for insomnia is recommended for long-term use.
   a. true
   b. false

6. What dose of barbiturates produces sedation?
   a. low
   b. medium
   c. high
   d. it does not matter

7. Zaleplon and zolpidem are classified as _____.
   a. barbiturates
   b. benzodiazepines
   c. enzodiazepines
   d. amphetamines

8. The primary treatment for ADHD is administration of stimulants.
   a. true
   b. false

9. Pharmaceutical treatment of ADHD is achieved with the administration of _____.
   a. amphetamines
   b. nonamphetamine stimulants
   c. anxiolytics
   d. both a and b

10. Amphetamines have a high abuse potential and are classified as Schedule _____ controlled substances in the United States.
   a. C-I
   b. C-II
   c. C-IV
   d. C-III

TECHNICIAN'S CORNER

1. Does diet and lack of exercise or lack of attention have anything to do with the number of children diagnosed with ADHD?
2. What would you recommend to someone with a sleep disorder who does not want to take any sleep aids?

Bibliography

Elsevier: Gold Standard Clinical Pharmacology, 2010. Retrieved March 7, 2011, from https://www.clinical pharmacology.com/.

FDA: Drugs@FDA Approved Drug Products, 2012. Retrieved April 28, 2012, from http://www.accessdata.fda.gov/scripts/cder/drugsatfda/index.cfm?fuseaction=Search.Search_Drug_Name.

Health Canada: Drug Product Database, 2010. Retrieved March 7, 2011, from http://www.hc-sc.gc.ca/dhp-mps/prodpharma/databasdon/index-eng.php.

Kalant H, Grant D, Mitchell J: *Principles of medical pharmacology*, ed 7, Toronto, 2007, Elsevier Canada, A Division of Reed Elsevier Canada, pp 339-342.

Lance L, Lacy C, Armstrong L, et al: *Drug information handbook for the allied health professional*, ed 12, Hudson, OH, 2005, APhA Lexi-Comp.

National Institute of Mental Health: Attention deficit hyperactivity disorder, Bethesda (MD): February 2006, National Institute of Mental Health, National Institutes of Health, US Department of Health and Human Services. NIH publication No. 03-3572.

National Institute of Neurological Disorders and Stroke, National Institute of Health, U.S. Department of Health and Humans Services: Brain basics: understanding sleep, Bethesda, 2007, National Institute of Neurological disorders and stroke. NIH publication No. 06-3440-c.

Public Health Agency of Canada: Fast Facts from the 2009 Canadian Community Health Survey—Sleep Apnea Rapid Response, 2010. Retrieved March 5, 2011, from http://www.phac-aspc.gc.ca/cd-mc/sleepapnea-apneesommeil/pdf/sleep-apnea.pdf.

Raffa R, Rawls S, Beyzarov E: *Netter's illustrated pharmacology*, Philadelphia, 2005, WB Saunders, pp 80-82.

Romano E, Baillargeon R, Tremblay R: Prevalence of hyperactivity-impulsivity and inattention among Canadian children: findings from the first data collection cycle (1994-1995) of the National Longitudinal Survey of Children and Youth–Applied Research Branch, Strategic Policy, Human Resources Development–Canada, June 2002. Retrieved from http://www.sdc.gc.ca/en/cs/sp/sdc/pkrf/publications/research/2002-000170/page02.shtml.

USP Center for Advancement of Patient Safety: Use caution–avoid confusion, USP Quality Review No. 79. Rockville, MD, April 2004, USP Center for Advancement of Patient Safety.

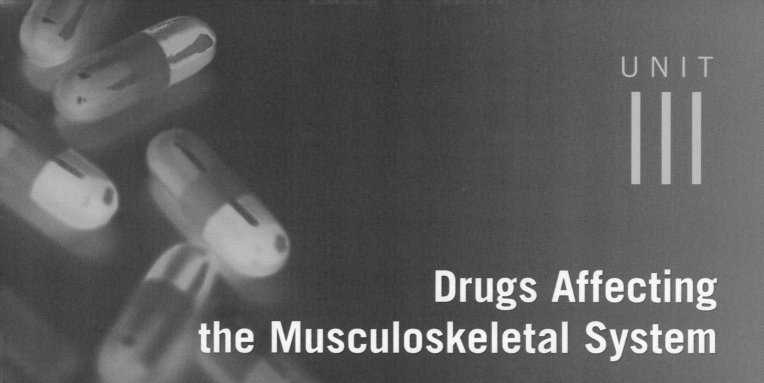

Drugs Affecting the Musculoskeletal System

LEARNING OBJECTIVES

1 Learn the terminology associated with the musculoskeletal system.
2 List the divisions and basic structure of the human skeleton.
3 Explain the differences in the types of joints of the skeleton.
4 Demonstrate knowledge of how muscles move the skeleton.
5 Describe the different arrangements of muscles.
6 Explain how the heart muscle works.
7 Describe the contraction and relaxation of muscles.

KEY TERMS

Acetylcholine: Neurotransmitter involved in muscle contraction.

Adenosine triphosphate: Nucleotide that supplies the energy required for muscle contraction.

Amphiarthroses: Slightly moveable joint (e.g., symphysis pubis in pelvic area).

Axial skeleton: Cranium, bones of face, ear, vertebral column, ribs, sternum, and hyoid.

Appendicular skeleton: Bone of upper extremities (arms, hands) and lower extremities (hip, legs, feet).

Diarthroses: Freely moveable joints (e.g., knee, hip, elbow, shoulder).

Fontanels: Soft spots found in a baby's skull.

Motor neuron: Connects to the sarcolemma to form a neuromuscular junction.

Neuromuscular junction: Space between motor neuron end plate and muscle sole plate that neurotransmitters must cross.

Peristalsis: Waves of contraction that move food along the digestive tract.

Sarcolemma: Plasma membrane of a muscle fiber.

Sarcomere: Basic contractile unit of the muscle cell.

Sarcoplasmic reticulum (SR): Networks of tubules and sacs contained in muscle cells.

Sinus cavity: Mucous-lined, air-filled spaces found in the frontal bone (frontal sinuses), sphenoid, ethmoid, maxillae (paranasal sinuses), and middle and inner ears (mastoid sinuses).

Synarthroses: Immovable joint (skull).

T tubules: Transverse tubules that extend across the sarcoplasm.

Anatomy and Physiology of the Skeleton

The human skeleton consists of two main divisions, the axial skeleton and appendicular skeleton. The *axial skeleton* consists of the cranium or brain case, bones of the face and ear, vertebral column, ribs, sternum, and hyoid. The *appendicular skeleton* contains the bones of the upper extremities (e.g., wrist, hand) and lower extremities (e.g., hip, kneecap, ankles).

SINUS CAVITY

The cranial and facial bones contain the frontal and paranasal sinuses. Another sinus cavity, the mastoid sinuses, is found in the middle and inner ear structures.

FETAL SKULL

The skull of the fetus and newborn infant has unique anatomical features not seen in the adult. The *fontanels*, or soft spots, provide additional space, which allows for molding of the head shape as the baby passes through the birth canal and for rapid brain growth that occurs in infancy without causing damaging increases in intracranial pressure. The fontanels close and the cranial bones fuse together as the skull reaches adult size.

VERTEBRAL COLUMN

The vertebral, or spinal, column forms the longitudinal axis of the skeleton. Joints between the vertebrae permit forward, backward, and sideways movement of the column. The vertebral column is divided into the cervical vertebrae, thoracic vertebrae, lumbar vertebrae, and sacrum.

RIBS

Twelve pairs of ribs together with the vertebral column and sternum form the thorax, which protects the heart and lungs. The ribs are named according to their articulation with the sternum (e.g., true ribs, false ribs, floating ribs). The first seven ribs attach to the sternum and are known as true ribs. The lower five ribs do not directly connect to the sternum and are known as false ribs. The last two false ribs have no ventral attachment and are called floating, fluctuating, or vertebral ribs.

APPENDICULAR SKELETON

The appendicular skeleton is divided into the upper and lower extremities. The upper extremities consist of the following bones: clavicle, scapula, humerus, radius and ulna, carpus (wrist), metacarpals (hand), and phalanges (fingers). The lower extremities consist of the following bones: hip, femur, tibia, fibula, patella (kneecap), tarsals (ankle), metatarsals, and phalanges (toes). The structure of the foot is similar to that of the hand. Strong ligaments and leg muscle tendons hold together the foot bones.

ARTICULATIONS

Articulations are joints or points of contact between two bones. Joints are classified on the basis of the amount of movement allowed. There are three major categories of joints: *synarthroses*—immovable (skull); *amphiarthroses*—slightly moveable (symphysis pubis in pelvic area); and *diarthroses*—freely moveable (knee, hip, elbow, shoulder). Ligaments, bands of fibrous tissue that connect bones to bones, are also present.

Muscular System

There are more than 600 muscles in the human body, which make up 40% to 50% of the body weight. This large mass of muscles is responsible for movement of the skeleton, heat production, and posture. Contraction or shortening of individual muscle cells is ultimately responsible for purposeful movement. There are three types of muscles—skeletal, smooth, and cardiac. Their movements power vital homeostatic mechanisms such as breathing, blood flow, digestion, and urine flow. A number of body systems support the function of muscle tissues.

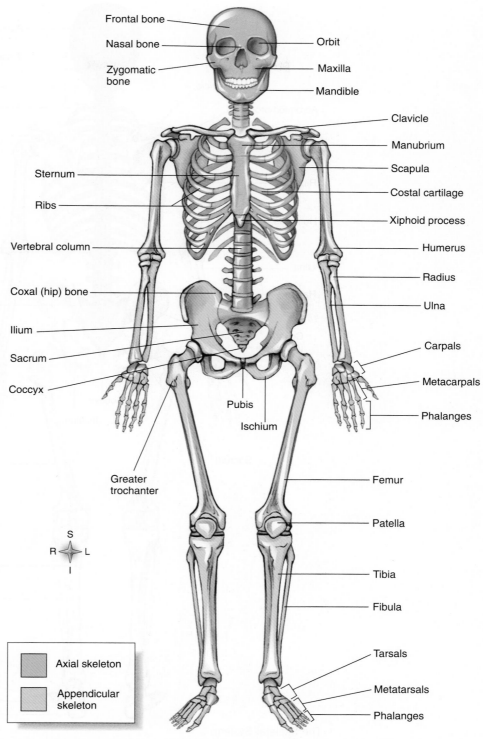

Frontal bone

Nasal bone

Zygomatic
bone

Orbit

Maxilla

Mandible

Clavicle

Manubrium

Scapula

Sternum

Costal cartilage

Ribs

Xiphoid process

Vertebral column

Humerus

Radius

Coxal (hip) bone

Ulna

Ilium

Sacrum

Carpals

Coccyx

Metacarpals

Pubis

Phalanges

Ischium

Greater
trochanter

Femur

Patella

S
R   L
I

Tibia

Fibula

Tarsals

Axial skeleton

Metatarsals

Appendicular
skeleton

Phalanges

The Skeletal System. (From Thibodeau G, Patton K: *Anatomy and physiology*, ed 6,
St. Louis, 2007, Mosby.)

Continued

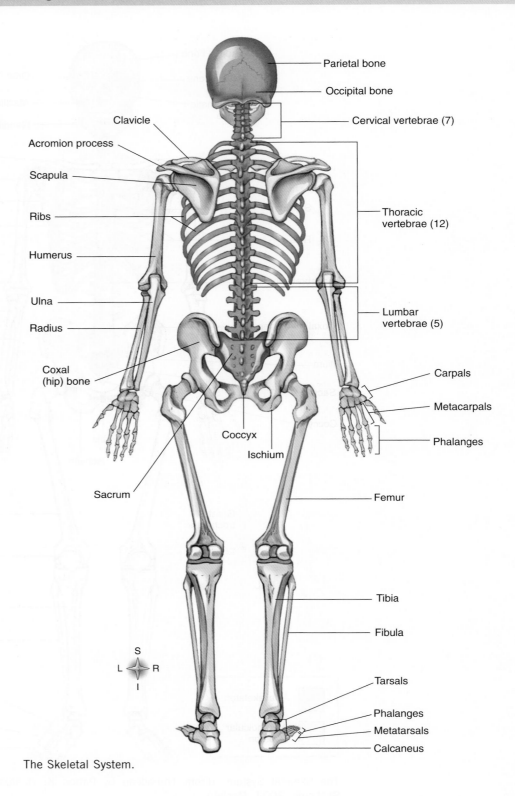

Parietal bone

Occipital bone

Cervical vertebrae (7)

Clavicle

Acromion process

Scapula

Ribs

Thoracic vertebrae (12)

Humerus

Ulna

Lumbar vertebrae (5)

Radius

Coxal (hip) bone

Carpals

Metacarpals

Coccyx

Phalanges

Ischium

Sacrum

Femur

Tibia

Fibula

S
L R
I

Tarsals

Phalanges

Metatarsals

Calcaneus

The Skeletal System.

GENERAL FUNCTIONS OF MUSCLES

Muscles are named as a result of location, points of attachment, and size. Energy for contractions comes from the nucleotide adenosine triphosphate (ATP). Glucose and oxygen are required for the efficient nutrient catabolism of muscle fibers. Without the presence of glucose and oxygen in the muscle cells, lactic acid is produced, which causes pain and stiffness in the joints.

FUNCTION OF SKELETAL MUSCLE TISSUE

Skeletal muscle tissue has three primary functions—excitability, contractility, and extensibility.
- Excitability: Ability of the muscle to be stimulated by a nervous impulse. Under normal circumstances, a skeletal muscle fiber remains at rest until is it stimulated by a signal from a special type of cell called a motor neuron.
- Contractility: The ability to contract or shorten allows muscle tissue to pull on bones and thus produce body movement.
- Extensibility: The ability to extend or stretch allows muscles to return to their resting length after having contracted.
  Skeletal muscle fibers usually contract to approximately 80% of their starting length.

CARDIAC MUSCLE

Cardiac muscle is found only in one organ of the body—the heart. It is also known as striated involuntary muscle. It is branched and forms junctions called intercalated discs with adjacent muscle fibers. Forming the bulk of the wall of each heart chamber, cardiac muscle contracts rhythmically and continuously to provide the pumping action necessary to maintain a relative constancy of blood flow through the internal environment.

SMOOTH MUSCLE

Smooth muscle cells form the muscular layer in the walls of many hollow structures such as the digestive, urinary, and reproductive tracts and the walls of large blood vessels. They cause *peristalsis* (waves of contraction) to move food along the digestive tract, assist the flow of urine to the bladder, and push a baby out of the womb during labor.

Steps of Muscle Contraction and Relaxation (Sliding Filament Model)

EXCITATION AND CONTRACTION

1. A nerve impulse reaches the end of a motor neuron and triggers the release of the neurotransmitter acetylcholine.
2. ACh diffuses across the neuromuscular junction and binds to ACh receptors on the motor endplate of the muscle fiber.
3. Stimulation of ACh receptors initiates an impulse along the sarcolemma through the T tubules to the sarcoplasmic reticulum (SR).
4. Calcium is released from the SR into the sarcoplasm, where it binds to troponin molecules in the thin myofilaments.
5. Tropomyosin molecules in the thin myofilaments shift and expose actin's active sites.
6. Energized myosin cross-bridges of the thick myofilaments bind to actin and use their energy to pull the thin myofilaments toward the center of the sarcomere. This cycle repeats itself many times per second, as long as ATP is available. Creatinine phosphate (CP) acts as a backup energy molecule when ATP needs to be resupplied.
7. As the filaments slide past the thick myofilaments, the entire muscle shortens.

RELAXATION

1. After the impulse is over, the SR begins actively pumping calcium into its sacs.
2. As calcium is stripped from troponin molecules in the thick myofilaments, tropomyosin returns to its position and blocks actin's active sites.
3. Myosin cross-bridges are prevented from binding to actin and thus can no longer sustain the contraction.
4. Because the thick and thin myofilaments are no longer connected, the muscle fiber may return to its longer resting length.

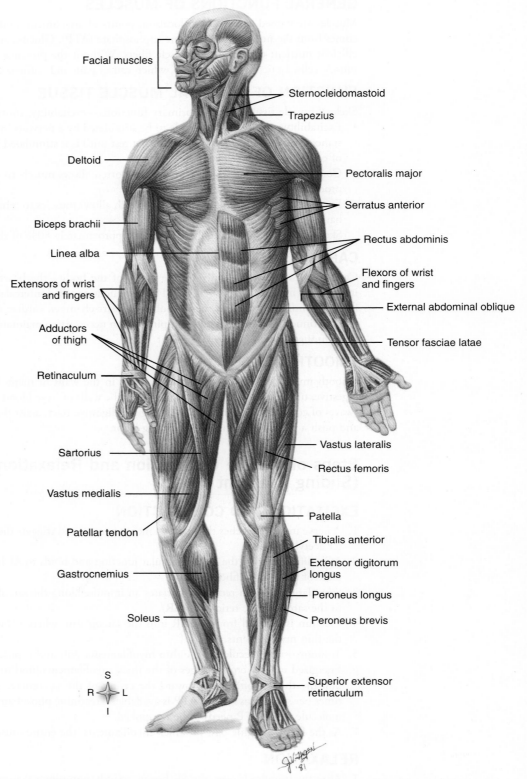

Facial muscles

Sternocleidomastoid

Trapezius

Deltoid

Pectoralis major

Serratus anterior

Biceps brachii

Rectus abdominis

Linea alba

Flexors of wrist
and fingers

Extensors of wrist
and fingers

External abdominal oblique

Adductors
of thigh

Tensor fasciae latae

Retinaculum

Sartorius

Vastus lateralis

Rectus femoris

Vastus medialis

Patella

Patellar tendon

Tibialis anterior

Extensor digitorum
longus

Gastrocnemius

Peroneus longus

Peroneus brevis

Soleus

Superior extensor
retinaculum

S
R L
I

The Muscular System. (From Thibodeau G, Patton K: *Anatomy and physiology*, ed 6,
St. Louis, 2007, Mosby.)

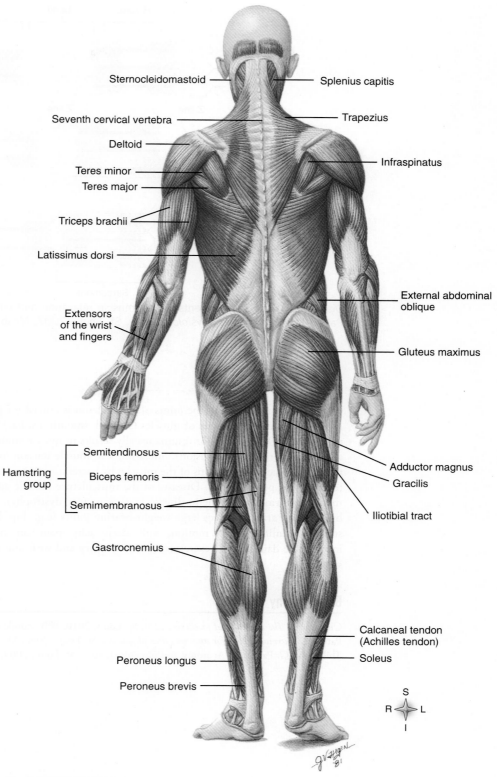

The Muscular System.

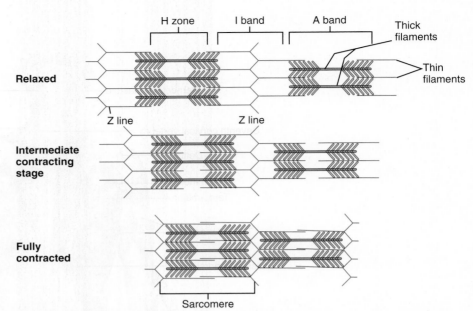

Diagram showing the filaments during muscle relaxation and contraction. (From Thibodeau G, Patton K: *Anatomy and physiology*, ed 6, St. Louis, 2007, Mosby.)

Summary

The proper functioning of the joints of the skeleton is crucial for purposeful movement. The function of all three major types of muscles (skeletal, smooth, cardiac) is integral to the function of the entire body. Overexertion or trauma usually results in muscle strain, sprain, muscle pain (myalgia), and muscle bruising (contusion). Stress-induced muscle tension in the head and neck can result in tension headaches. Infections of the muscles by bacteria, viruses, and parasites can produce myositis, tetanus, and poliomyelitis. Diseases of the musculature include autoimmune disorders (e.g., rheumatoid arthritis) and genetic disease (e.g., muscular dystrophy). Inflammatory disorders such as bursitis and arthritis affect large weight-bearing joints (e.g., hip, knees) characterized by morning stiffness, limited joint motion, and deep achy pain on movement. It is important to incorporate daily aerobic exercise to prevent injury and wear and tear of the skeletal and muscular systems.

Bibliography

Chabner E: *The language of medicine*, ed 9, St. Louis, 2010, WB Saunders.
Patton K: *Survival guide for anatomy and physiology*, St. Louis, 2006, Mosby.
Thibodeau G, Patton K: Anatomy and physiology, ed 7, St. Louis, 2009, Mosby.

13

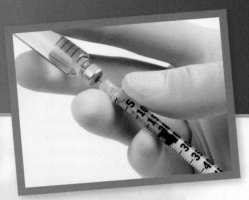

Neuromuscular Blockade

KEY TERMS

Acetylcholinesterase: Enzyme that degrades acetylcholine and reverses acetylcholine-induced depolarization.

Anaphylactic shock: Acute, life-threatening allergic reaction that produces peripheral vasodilation, bronchospasm, laryngeal edema, and airway obstruction.

Blepharoptosis: Condition that causes eyelid muscles to droop.

Botulinum toxin: Toxin produced by the bacterium *Clostridium botulinum* that causes muscle paralysis.

Central-acting muscle relaxants: Drugs that produce relaxation of muscles through central nervous system depression blocking nerve transmission between the spinal cord and muscles.

Depolarizing neuromuscular blockers: Drugs that act as agonists at acetylcholine receptor sites and produce sustained depolarization, causing the receptors to convert to an inactive state.

Diaphoresis (hyperhidrosis): Excessive sweating.

Endotracheal intubation: Process of inserting a tube into the trachea or windpipe to facilitate mechanical ventilation.

Endplate: Projection extending off the end of a motor neuron where the neurotransmitter acetylcholine is released.

Neuromuscular junction: Space between motor neuron endplate and the muscle soleplate that neurotransmitters must cross.

Nondepolarizing competitive blockers: Drugs that compete with acetylcholine for binding sites. When acetylcholine binding is inhibited, muscle contraction is blocked.

Peripheral-acting muscle relaxants: Drugs that block nerve transmission between the motor endplate and skeletal muscle receptors.

Soleplate: Portion of the membrane of muscle cells that receives messages transmitted by motor neurons.

Tetanus: Potentially fatal condition characterized by continuous muscle spasm that is caused by exposure to the nerve toxin produced by the bacterium *Clostridium tetani.* It is also known as "lockjaw."

Overview

Skeletal muscle contraction occurs as a response to communication between peripheral nerves and muscles. The neurotransmitter that is primarily responsible for transmitting messages between nerve cells and muscle cells is acetylcholine (ACh). The process of neuromuscular transmission begins with the release of ACh from vesicles located in the motor neuron endplate. The *endplate* is a projection extending off the end of one of the branches of the motor neuron. The end of the motor neuron may be divided into as many as 200 branches. ACh that is released from the neuron endplate binds to nicotinic receptor sites located in the muscle soleplate. The *soleplate* is the portion of the membrane of muscle cells that receives messages transmitted by motor neurons. The neuronal endplate does not physically touch the soleplate, so messages must travel across a 60-nm-wide space called the *neuromuscular junction* (Figure 13-1). The neuromuscular junction function is similar to the synaptic cleft in the central nervous system (CNS). Approximately 90% of the soleplate is composed of nicotinic receptors.

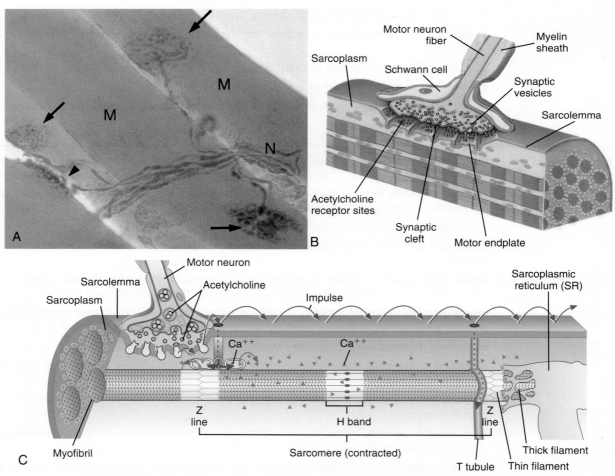

FIGURE 13-1 Excitation at the neuromuscular junction. (**A** from Leeson TS: *Text/atlas of histology*, Philadelphia, 1988, Saunders. **B** and **C** from Thibodeau GA, Patton KT: *Anatomy and physiology*, ed 6, St Louis, 2007, Mosby.)

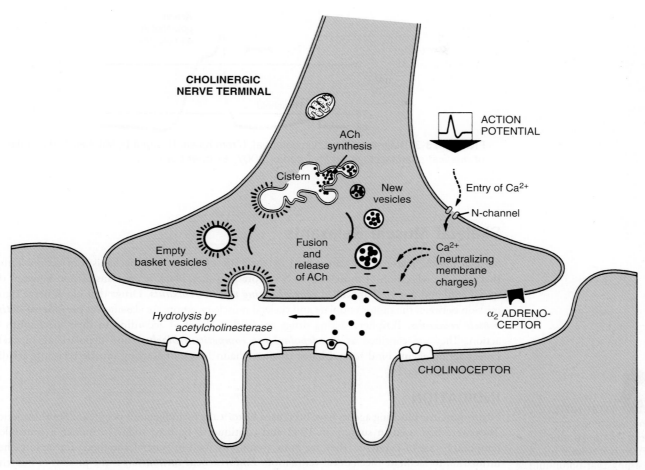

FIGURE 13-2 Acetylcholine synthesis and release. (From Kalant H, Grant D, Mitchell J: *Principles of medical pharmacology*, ed 7, Toronto, 2007, Elsevier Canada.)

Acetylcholine synthesis and release is a cyclical process (Figure 13-2). The process is stimulated by an influx of calcium into the neuronal endplate. Calcium entry occurs through voltage-regulated Na^+ channels. The influx of calcium raises the positive ions inside the cell, causing changes in the presynaptic membrane that result in the release of ACh from its storage vesicle. After ACh is released into the neuromuscular junction, a new vesicle begins to form in the presynaptic neuron. New ACh is synthesized in this vesicle. When the process is complete, the new vesicle filled with ACh buds off, awaiting a signal to release its contents.

Acetylcholine binding to nicotinic receptors opens sodium (Na^+), calcium (Ca^{2+}), and potassium (K^+) channels, increasing the endplate potential. When the endplate potential exceeds 15 mV, an action potential is produced (Figure 13-3).

Disassociation, or unbinding, of ACh from receptor sites inactivates and desensitizes the receptor site. The receptors are desensitized to more nerve contraction messages during the time it takes for the receptors to return to their preactivated state. Normally, between 10% and 20% of the nicotinic receptors are in an inactive state. Administration of neuromuscular blocking drugs leads to an increase in the percent of ACh receptor sites that are inactivated and results in relaxation of skeletal muscles. Drugs that decrease ACh release or deplete the neuron of ACh also cause relaxation of muscles. Examples of drugs or substances that decrease ACh release are ***botulinum toxin*** and magnesium. Black widow spider venom depletes neurons of ACh. Whereas high doses of ethanol decrease ACh release, low levels stimulate the release of ACh. Increased release of ACh produces skeletal muscle contraction. Calcium increases ACh release.

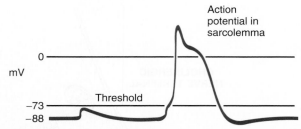

FIGURE 13-3 Diagram of an action potential. (From Kalant H, Grant D, Mitchell J: *Principles of medical pharmacology*, ed 7, Toronto, 2007, Elsevier Canada.)

Skeletal Muscle Relaxants

Skeletal muscle relaxants are categorized by their site of action and mechanism of action. Drugs that produce relaxation of muscles by CNS depression (i.e., block nerve transmission between the spinal cord and muscles) are called *central-acting muscle relaxants*. Drugs that block nerve transmission between the motor endplate and skeletal muscle receptors are classified as *peripheral-acting muscle relaxants*. Peripheral-acting drugs are further classified according to their mechanism of action. They are classified as *nondepolarizing competitive blockers* and depolarizing blockers. Direct-acting agents bind to and block calcium channels. Central-acting muscle relaxants are discussed in Chapter 14.

INDICATION

Neuromuscular blocking agents have been used historically by indigenous peoples of South America. They were first used in surgery in 1942 and continue to be used today to induce a controlled, temporary state of paralysis. They are most commonly used in general anesthesia for endotracheal intubation to facilitate mechanical ventilation. *Endotracheal intubation* is the process of inserting a tube down into the trachea or windpipe. Endotracheal tubes are inserted whenever complete blockade of muscle movement is required as in ocular surgery. Other uses for neuromuscular blocking are: management of status epilepticus, status asthmaticus, strychnine poisoning, *tetanus*, prevention of shivering in patients with severe burns and reduction of intracranial pressure "spikes" in patients with increased cranial pressure. OnabotulinumtoxinA, commonly known as Botox, is a neuromuscular blocking drug. Its use is becoming widespread, and it has been FDA approved for a variety of conditions, including temporary removal of wrinkles, treatment of excessive sweating (*diaphoresis*), spasticity, and chronic migraine (headache more than 15 days per month). Both onabotuliniumtoxinA and incobotulinumtoxinA are indicated for uncontrollable blinking (blepharospasms), cervical dystonia (abnormal head and neck position), and spasticity.

When neuromuscular blocking drugs are used during surgery, they should always be administered with analgesics to prevent pain. Their use should be closely monitored because these drugs can cause severe injury or death if misused. The degree of effectiveness of neuromuscular blockade should be measured using peripheral nerve stimulation and using devices that are made for monitoring of muscle twitching.

MECHANISM OF ACTION

The site of action of peripheral-acting muscle relaxants is the neuromuscular junction (Figure 13-4). Nerve transmission between the motor endplate and skeletal muscle receptors located at the soleplate is blocked and results in the inhibition of depolarization and repolarization activity in muscles.

Depolarizing Blockers

Depolarizing neuromuscular blockers are agonists at nicotinic receptors. They bind to ACh receptors, where they produce sustained depolarization, causing receptors to convert to their inactive state. The receptors become desensitized, and additional action potentials are prevented until the receptors return to their preactivated state. This prevents additional muscle contractions.

Succinylcholine is the only drug in this class. Similar to ACh, it is rapidly inactivated by cholinesterase enzymes. Cholinesterase enzymes are synthesized in the liver and are responsible for the breakdown of succinylcholine.

Pharmacology of Neuromuscular Transmission

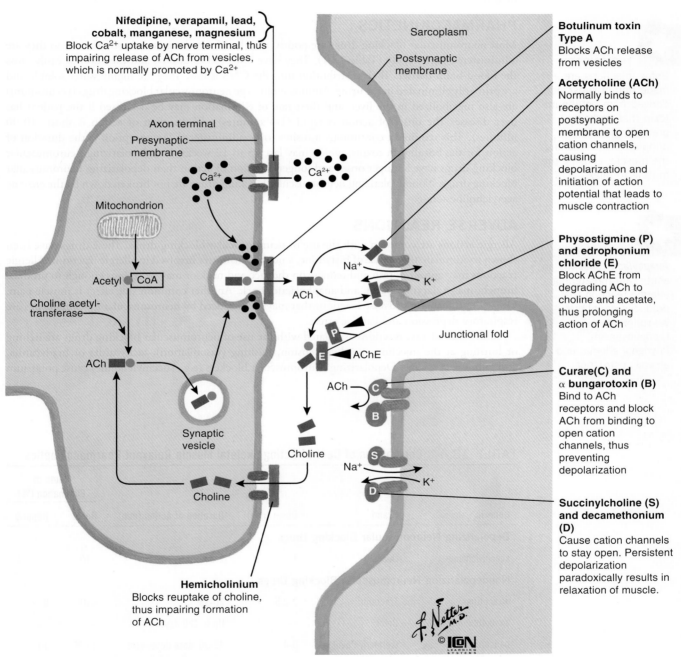

FIGURE 13-4 Mechanism of action of neuromuscular blocking drugs. (From Raffa R, Rawls S, Beyzarov E: *Netter's illustrated pharmacology*, Philadelphia, 2005, WB Saunders, pp 80-82.)

Nondepolarizing Neuromuscular Blockers

Most nondepolarizing neuromuscular blockers are competitive antagonists at prejunctional and postjunctional receptors. At low doses, they produce no effects of their own when they bind to receptor sites; instead, they compete with ACh for binding sites. When ACh binding is inhibited, muscle contraction is blocked. At high doses, nondepolarizing drugs interfere with Na⁺, Ca²⁺, and K⁺ channels that increase endplate potential. This further weakens neuromuscular transmission and reduces the actions of *acetylcholinesterase*, the enzyme that reverses ACh-induced depolarization. OnabotulinumtoxinA (Botox) blocks the release of ACh from storage vesicles in the presynaptic neuron.

PHARMACOKINETICS

Most neuromuscular blocking drugs are poorly absorbed from the gastrointestinal tract, so they are administered parenterally (Table 13-1). They have low lipid solubility, and they do not easily cross the blood-brain barrier. Their distribution into the CNS is low. They are highly water soluble and are primarily eliminated in the urine. Aminosteroid-type neuromuscular blocking drugs (vecuronium) are also metabolized in the liver, and their rate of elimination may be decreased if the patient has liver disease. The onset of action is rapid (1-4 minutes) and duration of action is short (10-90 minutes). This requires a continuous infusion to be administered. An exception is the duration of action for the botulinum toxins, which may last up to 12 weeks. Nondepolarizing neuromuscular blocking drugs have a longer onset and longer duration of action than depolarizing neuromuscular blocking drugs. Nondepolarizing neuromuscular blocking drugs are not broken down by the enzyme acetylcholinesterase.

ADVERSE REACTIONS

Allergic actions are common with the use of neuromuscular blocking drugs. These drugs have been shown to stimulate the release of histamine, a neurotransmitter involved in allergic reactions. Allergic reactions may appear as rash and redness on the face and neck or may be serious enough to produce bronchospasm, laryngospasm, and anaphylactic shock. Another common side effect is muscle pain. Other life-threatening adverse reactions that may be produced by neuromuscular blocking drugs are respiratory depression and cardiac arrest.

Additional adverse reactions associated with the use of neuromuscular blocking drugs are itching or burning at the injection site, hypotension, flushing (vasodilation), tachycardia or bradycardia, and pulmonary edema. Depolarizing neuromuscular blockers (e.g., succinylcholine) cause potassium

TABLE 13-1   Comparison of Central-Acting Skeletal Muscle Relaxant Pharmacokinetics

Generic	Brand	Onset (min)	Duration of Action (min)	Route of Elimination (%) Renal	Hepatic
Depolarizing Neuromuscular Blocking Drugs					
succinylcholine	Quelicin	1	2-3	<10	—
Nondepolarizing Neuromuscular Blocking Drugs					
atracurium	Tracrium	2-2.5	20-35	<10	0
onabotulinumtoxinA[π]	Botox	—	Up to 120 days	—	—
pancuronium	(Formerly Pavulon)	3-4	45-90, dose dependent	30-80	10
rocuronium	Zemuron	1-1.5	30-45	10-20	80-90
vecuronium	Norcuron	2.5-3	25-40	<25	20

[π]No available data.

Neuromuscular Blockers

Generic Name	U.S. Brand Name(s) / Canadian Brand(s)	Dosage Forms and Strengths
Depolarizing Neuromuscular Blocking Drugs		
succinylcholine*‡	Anectine, Quelicin	Injection, solution: 20 mg/mL, 100 mg/mL
	Quelicin	
Nondepolarizing Neuromuscular Blocking Drugs		
atracurium*	Generic	Injection, solution: 10 mg/mL
	Generic	
abobotulinumtoxinA	Dysport	Powder for injection: 300 units, 500 units
	Not available	
onabotulinumtoxinA	Botox, Botox Cosmetic	Powder for injection: 50 unit†, 100 units, 200 units†
	Botox, Botox Cosmetic	
rimabotulinumtoxinB	Myobloc	Injection, solution: 2500 units/0.5 mL
	Not available	5000 units/1 mL 10,000 units/2 mL
incobotulinumtoxinA	Xeomin	Powder for injection: 50 units†, 100-mg units
	Xeomin	
cisatracurium	Nimbex	Injection, solution: 2 mg/mL, 10 mg/mL†
	Nimbex	
pancuronium*	Generics	Injection, solution: 1 mg/mL, 2 mg/mL
	Generics	
rocuronium*	Zemuron	Injection, solution: 10 mg/mL
	Zemuron	
vecuronium*	Generics	Powder for injection: 10 mg, 20 mg
	Generics	

*Generic available.
*‡Generic available in Canada only.
†Strength available in the United States only.

channels to remain open, producing hyperkalemia and cardiac arrest. OnabotulinumtoxinA injections may produce muscle weakness in the injected muscles. This may cause droopy eyelid muscles (*blepharoptosis*), headache, nausea, flulike syndrome, redness, and muscle weakness.

Reversal of Neuromuscular Blockade

Drugs that reverse the effects of neuromuscular blockade must always be readily available any time neuromuscular blocking drugs are administered. Anticholinesterase drugs inhibit the action of ACh esterase at the neuromuscular junction. This causes ACh to accumulate and compete with the administered neuromuscular blocking drug for available receptor sites. Anticholinesterase drugs are most effective after the process of spontaneous recovery from neuromuscular blocking drugs has begun.

ADVERSE REACTIONS

Edrophonium and neostigmine may produce salivation, muscle twitching, muscle weakness, abdominal cramping, nausea, increased bronchial secretions, and difficulty breathing.

TECH NOTE!
Tubocurarine, formerly used in anesthesia, is the synthetic version of curare, a natural paralytic drug used by South American Indian hunters to immobilize prey.

Drugs That Reverse the Effects of Neuromuscular Blockade

Generic Name	U.S. Brand Name(s) / Canadian Brand(s)	Dosage Forms and Strengths
edrophonium	Enlon, Tensilon	Injection, solution: 10 mg/mL
	Tensilon	
neostigmine	Generics	Injection, solution: 0.5 mg/mL, 1 mg/mL, 2 mg/mL[‡]
	Prostigmin	Tablets (Prostigmin): 15 mg[‡]
pyridostigmine*	Mestinon, Mestinon Timespan, Regonol	Injection, solution: 5 mg/mL Syrup: 60 mg/5 mL[†]
	Mestinon, Mestinon SR	Tablets: 60 mg Tablets, sustained release (Mestinon SR, Mestinon Timespan): 180 mg
atropine + edrophonium	Enlon Plus	Solution, injection: 0.14 mg atropine + 10 mg edrophonium per 1 mL
	Not available	

*Generic available.
[†]Strength available in the United States only.
[‡]Strength available in Canada only

Summary of Neuromuscular Blocking Drugs

Generic Name	U.S. Brand Name	Usual Adult Oral Dose and Dosing Schedule	Warning Labels
succinylcholine	Quelicin	**Short surgeries IM:** 3-4 mg/kg **Rapid IV:** 0.3-1.1 mg/kg over 10-30 seconds **Continuous infusion:** 0.5-10 mg/min	KEEP REFRIGERATED. Before dilution: May store at room temperature for 14 days. After dilution to a concentration of 0.1% to 0.2%, the solution is stable 4 weeks in the refrigerator and 1 week at room temperature.
atracurium	Generics	**IV:** 0.4-0.5 mg/kg; then 0.08-0.1 mg/kg 20-45 minutes after initial dose and repeated every 15-25 minutes as needed **Continuous infusion:** 9-10 mcg/kg/min **Continuous infusion:** 11-13 mcg/kg/min	KEEP REFRIGERATED (2°–8° C); protect from freezing. Before dilution: May store at room temperature for 14 days. After dilution: Infusion solutions should be used within 24 hours of preparation.
abobotulinumtoxinA	Dysport	**Cervical dystonia:** 500 units IM in affected muscle every 12 weeks **Wrinkles:** 50 units IM in five divided injections	KEEP REFRIGERATED (2°–8° C); PROTECT FROM FREEZING. Before dilution: May store at room temperature for 14 days. After dilution: Refrigerated solutions should be used within 4 hours of preparation.
onabotulinumtoxinA	Botox	**Blepharospasm:** 1.25-2.5 units IM every 1-3 months **Cervical dystonia:** varies **Strabismus:** 1.25-5 units IM **Diaphoresis:** 50 units intradermal into armpit **Wrinkles:** 0.1 mL in five designated injection sites (maximum, 0.5 mL)	KEEP REFRIGERATED (2°–8° C); PROTECT FROM FREEZING. After dilution: Refrigerated solutions should be used within 4 hours of preparation.

Summary of Neuromuscular Blocking Drugs—cont'd

Generic Name	U.S. Brand Name	Usual Adult Oral Dose and Dosing Schedule	Warning Labels
incobotulinumtoxinA	Xeomin	**Blepharospasm:** 1.25-2.5 units IM every 1-3 months **Cervical dystonia:** 120 units IM in affected muscles	KEEP REFRIGERATED (2°-8° C). Before dilution: Powder may store at room temperature, refrigerator, or freezer. After dilution: Refrigerate and use within 24 hours; discard unused portion.
rimabotulinumtoxinB	Myobloc	**Cervical dystonia:** 2500-5000 units IM divided among affected muscles	KEEP REFRIGERATED; DO NOT FREEZE. After dilution: Use within 4 hours and discard unused portion. PROTECT FROM LIGHT.
cisatracurium	Nimbex	0.15-0.2 mg/kg IV	KEEP REFRIGERATED; DO NOT FREEZE (2°-8° C); protect from freezing. PROTECT FROM LIGHT. Once warmed to room temperature: Use within 21 days.
pancuronium	Generics	**IV:** Initiate 0.04-0.1 mg/kg or 0.05 mg/kg after succinylcholine **Maintenance:** 0.01 mg/kg 60-100 minutes after initial dose; then every 25-60 minutes	KEEP REFRIGERATED (5° C); PROTECT FROM FREEZING. DO NOT STORE IN PLASTIC SYRINGE. Before dilution: Refrigeration recommended; stable for 6 months if stored at room temperature.
rocuronium	Zemuron	**Intubation:** 0.6-1.2 mg/kg IV **Continuous infusion:** Initial 0.01-0.012 mg/kg/min up to 0.04-0.016 mg/kg/min	KEEP REFRIGERATED; PROTECT FROM FREEZING. Before dilution: If unopened, use within 60 days after removal from refrigerator. After dilution: Use within 24 hours and discard unused portion.
vecuronium	Norcuron	**Intubation:** 0.08-0.1 mg/kg (IV); prolonged surgery 0.01-0.015 mg 25-40 minutes after initial dose **Continuous infusion:** 0.0008-0.0012 mg/kg/min or 1 mcg/kg/min	KEEP REFRIGERATED; PROTECT FROM FREEZING. PROTECT FROM LIGHT. Before dilution: May store at room temperature. After dilution: Refrigerate and use within 24 hours if reconstituted with sterile water; use within 5 days if reconstituted with bacteriostatic water.

Strategies for Safe Use of Neuromuscular Blocking Agents

Neuromuscular blocking drugs are classified "high alert" by the Interdisciplinary Safe Medication Use Expert Committee of the United States Pharmacopoeia (USP) because improper use can result in permanent injury, respiratory arrest, and death. Problems associated with neuromuscular blocking drugs have been attributed to improper product selection, improper storage conditions, inappropriate dosing, improper labeling, and inadequate patient monitoring. Improper product selection is caused by similar product packaging and sound-alike drug names. Drug names that sound alike pose problems in dispensing regardless of the type of drug. Look-alike packaging is a problem that

Summary of Drugs Used to Reverse the Effects of Neuromuscular Blocking Drugs

Generic Name	U.S. Brand Name	Usual Adult Oral Dose and Dosing Schedule	Warning Labels
edrophonium	Enlon	10 mg over 30-35 seconds (IV); repeat in 5-10 minutes if needed up to 40 mg	STABLE AT ROOM TEMPERATURE.
neostigmine	Prostigmin	Reversal of nondepolarizing neuromuscular blockade: 0.5-2.5 mg (IV) to maximum 5 mg Bladder atony: 0.25-1 mg SC or IM every 3 hours for 5 doses	STABLE AT ROOM TEMPERATURE. PROTECT FROM LIGHT (injection solution). TAKE WITH FOOD or a FULL GLASS OF WATER (oral).
pyridostigmine	Mestinon	Myasthenia gravis: 60-1500 mg daily in divided doses (average, 600 mg)	

BOX 13-1 Safe Management of Neuromuscular Blocking Agents: Recommendations for Pharmacy Practice

PRODUCT SELECTION
- Procurement managers should select products that have distinctive names and packaging to avoid sound-alike/look-alike issues.

PRODUCT STORAGE
- Neuromuscular blocking drugs should be stored apart from other drugs.
- Storage of neuromuscular blocking drugs should be confined to primary care areas and pharmacy areas that care for mechanically ventilated patients.
- Storage conditions for undiluted and diluted solutions should be clearly marked.

LIMIT ACCESS
- Neuromuscular blocking drugs should be kept in sealed "intubation kits" or "anesthesia kits" until use is needed.
- Opened vials should be immediately discarded or returned to the seal kit after use.
- Neuromuscular blocking drugs should NOT be dispensed in unit dose carts or delivered to general nursing units unless in a sealed kit.
- Neuromuscular blocking drugs should be stored in a single access drawer when stored in drug storage devices such as Pyxis and AccuDose-Rx.
- Neuromuscular blocking drugs requiring refrigeration should be stored in a separate area away from other refrigerated drugs.

AUXILIARY LABELS OR WARNING LABELS
- Neuromuscular blocking drugs should always be dispensed with the auxiliary label "WARNING: Paralyzing agent. (Use requires mechanical ventilatory assistance.)"
- Overwraps should be considered for individual vials of neuromuscular blocking drugs stored outside of pharmacy and anesthesiology areas, especially drugs stored in the refrigerator.
- Affix preprinted syringe labels to syringes filled with neuromuscular blocking drugs at the time the drug is drawn up to avoid risks associated with unlabeled syringes.

ORDERING PRACTICES AND DISPENSING
- Contact prescriber for complete directions when medication orders for neuromuscular blocking agents are written with PRN directions.
- Verify patient identity and drug identity with bar-code readers when available.

Adapted from United States Pharmacopoeia Interdisciplinary Safe Medication Use Expert Committee recommendations.

can be attributed to drug manufacturers as well as pharmacies dispensing drugs (see Chapter 4). Neuromuscular blocking drugs may be repackaged for unit of use in institutional care settings. Infusion bags and syringes that have been prepared by the pharmacy look alike. Neuromuscular blocking drugs have been administered in the place of vaccines, intravenous flush solutions, and antibiotics by mistake. A pharmacy that fails to securely affix the label onto the infusion bag or syringe of a neuromuscular blocking drug has created a potentially life-threatening situation for a patient. Inaccurate sterile compounding has resulted in the dispensing of incorrect drug concentrations and incorrect doses placed in automated dispensing machines.

To prevent possible injury or death, the USP Interdisciplinary Safe Medication Use Expert Committee has compiled a list of recommendations for the safe use of neuromuscular blocking agents. The recommendations listed in Box 13-1 are modified for pharmacy-specific application.

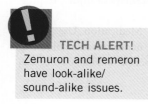

TECH ALERT!
Zemuron and remeron have look-alike/sound-alike issues.

Chapter Summary

- Skeletal muscle contraction occurs as a response to communication between peripheral nerves and muscles.
- The process of neuromuscular transmission begins with the release of acetylcholine (ACh) from vesicles located in the motor neuron endplate.
- ACh that is released from the nerve endplate binds to nicotinic receptor sites located in the muscle soleplate.
- The neuromuscular junction is the space between the neuron endplate and receptor sites in the muscle cell.
- Approximately 90% of the soleplate is composed of nicotinic receptors.
- ACh binding to nicotinic receptors opens sodium, calcium, and potassium channels, increasing the endplate potential.
- Unbinding of ACh from receptor sites desensitizes them to further nerve conduction messages during the time it takes for the receptors to return to their preactivated state.
- Neuromuscular blocking drugs cause skeletal muscle relaxation by increasing the percent of ACh receptor sites that are inactivated.
- Drugs that decrease ACh release or deplete the neuron of ACh also cause relaxation of muscles.
- Examples of drugs or substances that decrease ACh release are the botulinum toxins, magnesium, and high doses of ethanol.
- Peripheral-acting drugs are classified as nondepolarizing competitive blockers and depolarizing blockers.
- Depolarizing neuromuscular drugs are agonists at nicotinic receptors.
- Most nondepolarizing neuromuscular blockers are competitive antagonists at prejunctional and postjunctional receptors.
- Neuromuscular blocking drugs are most commonly used in general anesthesia for endotracheal intubation to facilitate mechanical ventilation.
- OnabotulinumtoxinA has been FDA approved to temporarily remove wrinkles, treat chronic migraine and treat excessive sweating. Both onabotulinumtoxinA and incobotulinumtoxinA are indicated for blepharospasms (uncontrollable blinking), cervical dystonia (abnormal head and neck position), and spasticity.
- The onset of action of neuromuscular blocking drugs is rapid (1-4 minutes), and the duration of action is short (10-90 minutes).
- Adverse reactions associated with the use of neuromuscular blocking drugs are hypotension, tachycardia, pulmonary edema, hyperkalemia, cardiac arrest, bronchospasm, and anaphylactic shock.
- Botulinum toxins type A injections can cause droopy eyelid muscles, headache, nausea, flulike syndrome, redness, muscle weakness, and pain at the injection site.
- Drugs that reverse the effects of neuromuscular blockade must always be readily available any time neuromuscular blocking drugs are administered.
- Anticholinesterase drugs cause ACh to accumulate and compete with the administered neuromuscular blocking drug for available receptor sites.

TECH NOTE!
Discard solutions of
doxacuronium that are
discolored or have
particles.

- Neuromuscular blocking drugs are classified "high alert" by the Interdisciplinary Safe Medication Use Expert Committee of the USP because improper use can result in permanent injury, respiratory arrest, and death.
- To prevent possible injury or death, the USP Interdisciplinary Safe Medication Use Expert Committee has compiled a list of recommendations for the safe use of neuromuscular blocking agents that includes suggestions for product selection, storage, limited access, auxiliary label use, ordering, and dispensing practices.

REVIEW QUESTIONS

1. The neurotransmitter that is primarily responsible for transmitting messages between nerve cells and muscle cells is _____.
   a. dopamine
   b. epinephrine
   c. acetylcholine
   d. GABA

2. Administration of neuromuscular _____ drugs leads to an increase in the percent of acetylcholine receptor sites that are inactivated and results in relaxation of skeletal muscles.
   a. blocking
   b. stimulating
   c. enhancing
   d. stabilizing

3. Botox has not been FDA approved for cosmetic use.
   a. true
   b. false

4. Most neuromuscular blocking drugs are poorly absorbed from the gastrointestinal tract so they are administered _____.
   a. topically
   b. enterally
   c. parenterally
   d. transdermally

5. Allergic actions may occur with the use of neuromuscular blocking drugs.
   a. true
   b. false

6. Neuromuscular blocking drugs are classified "_____" by the Interdisciplinary Safe Medication Use Expert Committee of the USP.
   a. dangerous
   b. high alert
   c. low alert
   d. use with caution

7. How should neuromuscular blocking drugs be stored?
   a. in alphabetical order on the shelf
   b. in the IV room
   c. with the fast movers
   d. apart from other drugs

8. Neuromuscular blocking drugs should always be dispensed with what auxiliary label?
   a. WARNING: Paralyzing agent. (Use requires mechanical ventilatory assistance.)
   b. WARNING: Allergic reactions possible.
   c. KEEP IN REFRIGERATOR UNTIL READY TO USE.
   d. FOR ONE TIME USE ONLY.

9. Which botulinum toxin is approved for cosmetic wrinkle removal?
   a. onabotulinumtoxinB
   b. incobotulinumtoxinA
   c. rimabotulinumtoxinB
   d. onabotulinumtoxinA

10. Medication errors can easily happen with nondepolarizing neuromuscular blocking drugs because _____.
    a. all packages look the same
    b. some drugs have look-alike/sound-alike names
    c. doses are all the same.
    d. all are made by same manufacturer

TECHNICIAN'S CORNER

1. Everyone wants to keep looking young. What solutions can you give a client other than using Botox for wrinkles?
2. You are in charge of inventory in the pharmacy and need to alert everyone about the potential of medication errors that can occur with neuromuscular blocking drugs. What would be the best way to alert everyone?

Bibliography

FDA: FDA Approved Drug Products, 2012. Retrieved April 29, 2012, from http://www.accessdata.fda.gov/scripts/cder/drugsatfda/index.cfm?fuseaction=Search.Search_Drug_Name.

Harboe T, Guttormsen A, Irgens A: Anaphylaxis during anesthesia in Norway—A 6-year single center follow-up study, *Anesthesiology* 102:897-903, 2005.

Health Canada: Drug Product Database. Retrieved April 29, 2012, from http://www.hc-sc.gc.ca/dhp-mps/prodpharma/databasdon/index-eng.php, 2010.

Kalant H, Grant D, Mitchell J: *Principles of medical pharmacology*, ed 7, Toronto, 2007, Elsevier Canada, A Division of Reed Elsevier Canada, pp 176-180.

Lance L, Lacy C, Armstrong L, et al: *Drug information handbook for the allied health professional*, ed 12, Hudson, OH, 2005, APhA Lexi-Comp.

Lewis C: Botox cosmetic: a look at looking good, U.S. Food and Drug Administration, FDA Consumer Magazine. Retrieved from http://www.fda.gov/fdac/features/2002/402_botox.htmL.

Matthey P, Wang P, Finegan B, et al: Rocuronium anaphylaxis and multiple neuromuscular blocking drug sensitivities, *CJA* 47(9):890-893, 2000.

Mehta S, Burry L, Fischer S, et al: Canadian survey of the use of sedatives, analgesics, and neuromuscular blocking agents in critically ill patients, *Crit Care Med* 34:374-380, 2006.

Parenteral drug therapy manual, Pharmaceutical Sciences, Vancouver General Hospital, Vancouver, BC. Retrieved from http://www.vhpharmsci.com/PDTM/.

Phillips M, Williams R: Improving the safety of neuromuscular blocking agents: a statement from the USP Safe Medication Use Expert Committee, *Am J Health Syst Pharm* 63:139-142, 2006.

Shapiro B, Warren J, Egol AB, et al: Practice parameters for sustained neuromuscular blockade in the adult critically ill patient, *Crit Care Med* 23:1601-1605, 1995.

Wood A: New neuromuscular blocking drugs, *N Engl J Med* 332, 1995.

14

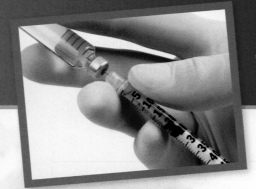

Treatment of Muscle Spasms

LEARNING OBJECTIVES

1 Learn the terminology associated with spasticity and its treatment.

2 Describe the signs and symptoms of spasticity.

3 List medical conditions that cause spasticity.

4 Describe the function of neurotransmitters associated with antispasticity drugs.

5 Classify medications used in the treatment of spasticity.

6 Describe the mechanism of action for each class of drugs used in the treatment of spasticity.

7 Identify significant drug look-alike/sound-alike issues.

8 Identify warning labels and precautionary messages associated with medications used to treat spasticity.

KEY TERMS

Amyotrophic lateral sclerosis: Degenerative disease that causes muscle wasting and muscle weakness. ALS is also known as Lou Gehrig's disease.

Cerebral palsy: Neurological disorder that affects muscle movement and coordination.

Clonus: Involuntary rhythmic muscle contraction that causes the feet and wrists to involuntarily flex and relax.

Lower motor neurons: Neurons that branch out from the spinal cord to the muscles and tissues of the body.

Multiple sclerosis: Autoimmune disease that causes progressive damage to nerves resulting in spasticity, pain, mood changes, and other physical symptoms.

Negative symptoms: Spasticity symptoms that can produce muscle weakness, decreased endurance, and reduction in the ability to make voluntary muscle movements.

Phenylketonuria: A disease marked by failure to metabolize the amino acid phenylalanine to tyrosine. It results in severe neurological deficits in infancy if untreated.

Positive symptoms: Spasticity symptoms that cause muscle spasms and hyperexcitable reflexes.

Sarcomere: Contracting unit of muscle fibers.

Spasticity: Motor disorder that causes increased muscle tone, exaggerated tendon jerks, and hyperexcitable muscles.

Upper motor neurons: Neurons that carry messages from the brain down to the spinal cord.

Overview

Spasticity is a debilitating motor disorder that affects up to 12 million people worldwide. Symptoms of spasticity are increased muscle tone, exaggerated tendon jerks, and hyperexcitability of the stretch reflex. These symptoms are collectively known as muscle spasms and are *positive symptoms* of spasticity. *Negative symptoms* associated with spasticity include muscle weakness, decreased endurance, and reduction in the capacity to make voluntary muscle movements. Spasticity interferes with the normal performance of activities of daily living. The ability for self-care is significantly impaired, and it can inhibit effective walking, cause fatigue and stiffness, disturb sleep, and increase risk for pressure ulcers and infections.

Stroke, spinal cord injury, cerebral palsy, muscle trauma (e.g., whiplash), multiple sclerosis, head injury, and metabolic diseases such as *amyotrophic lateral sclerosis* (ALS; Lou Gehrig's disease), and *phenylketonuria* can all cause spasticity. In fact, 65% to 78% of people with spinal cord injuries and 65% of people who have had a stroke will develop spasticity.

Spasticity can be aggravated by a variety of factors. Fatigue, pain, stress, fever, cold, constipation, immobility, and hormonal changes can all worsen symptoms of spasticity.

Pathophysiology of Spasticity

Any condition that can damage the brain or spinal cord can cause spasticity. Regardless of the cause, the progression to spasticity follows a specific pattern, and the degree of spasticity is related to the duration since the original injury. The four phases are (1) decreased muscle contractility; (2) excessive muscle tone and increased reflex activity lasting from days to years; (3) decreased reflex excitability; and (4) stiff, contracted muscles.

Conditions That Produce Spasticity

SPINAL CORD INJURY

Spinal cord injury may produce muscle paralysis and loss of tendon reflexes in the region below the level of spinal cord injury immediately after the injury. Within a few weeks, this period of spinal shock ends and is followed by a period of increased muscle tone, exaggerated tendon jerks, and involuntary muscle spasms. It is believed that spasticity develops because the neurons that branch out from the spinal cord to the muscles and tissues of the body (*lower motor neurons*) grow new synapses. The increase in the number of synapses causes a stronger reflex connection and a greater response to stretching of the muscle. Moreover, normal inhibitory control of sustained neuron firing is lost during the recovery period after spinal cord injury. What follows are unopposed motor neuron excitability and changes in endplate potential (see Chapter 13). Receptors become more sensitive to neurotransmitters and muscle changes cause altered contractility. Muscle fibers atrophy, the number of sarcomeres decreases, and connective tissue increases. *Sarcomeres* are units within muscle fibers responsible for muscle contraction (Figure 14-1).

Spinal cord injury also results in *clonus*, involuntary rhythmic muscle contraction that produces involuntarily flexing and relaxation of the feet and wrists.

STROKE

Stroke can cause a lesion to form in the brain or spinal cord that results in unopposed motor neuron excitability by normal inhibitory mechanisms.

CEREBRAL PALSY

Spasticity caused by *cerebral palsy* follows the same pathophysiological pathway as stroke and spinal cord injury. Treatment is complicated because spasticity impairs effective muscle movement in some people with cerebral palsy and helps maintain posture, making walking easier in other people.

AMYOTROPHIC LATERAL SCLEROSIS

People who have ALS exhibit predominantly negative symptoms of spasticity. *Upper motor neurons* (which carry messages from the brain down to the spinal cord) are damaged by decreased reuptake of the excitatory amino acid glutamate. This causes glutamate levels to accumulate and calcium to

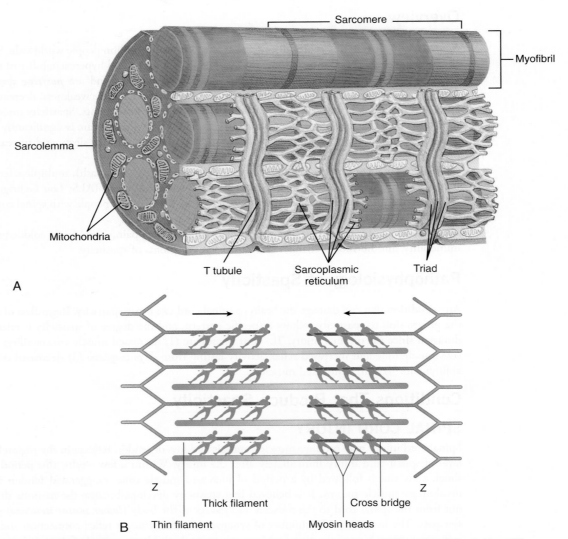

FIGURE 14-1 A, Sarcomere. **B,** Simplified sarcomere. (From Thibodeau GA, Patton KT: *Anatomy and physiology*, ed 6, St Louis, 2007, Mosby.)

TECH NOTE!
The myelin sheath around neurons acts as an electrical insulator and increases the velocity of impulse transmission.

flood into motor neurons (Figure 14-2). The influx of calcium raises the positive ions inside the cell, causing changes in the presynaptic membrane that result in the release of acetylcholine (ACh) from its storage vesicle (see Chapter 13). This ultimately causes desensitization of motor nerves, muscle weakness, and cell death.

MULTIPLE SCLEROSIS

Multiple sclerosis is an autoimmune disease that causes damage to myelinated nerves (see Figure 15-2). Lesions damage nerves in the central nervous system (CNS) and cause spasticity, pain, fatigue, dysfunction of the bladder and bowel, impotence, cognitive dysfunction, and changes in mood or depression. Nerve damage and symptoms get progressively worse over time.

MUSCLE STRAIN

Muscle strain, sprains, fibromyalgia, tension headache, low back pain, and neck pain can cause muscle spasm, stiffness, and pain. When spasms are present, it is typically related to local injury or irritation of a specific muscle group.

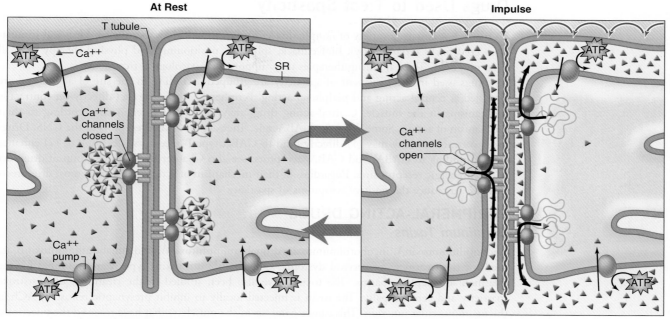

FIGURE 14-2 Storage and release of calcium ions in muscle cells. (From Thibodeau GA, Patton KT: *Anatomy and physiology*, ed 6, St Louis, 2007, Mosby.)

Neurotransmitters Involved in Spasticity

Spasticity is a symptom of upper motor neuron syndrome. The cause may be excess activity of neurotransmitters that carry excitatory messages, such as glutamate, or decreased activity or a deficiency of inhibitory transmitters, such as γ-aminobutyric acid (GABA) and glycine. Spasticity also may be accompanied by pain.

ROLE OF ACETYLCHOLINE

Acetylcholine is the neurotransmitter that is primarily responsible for transmitting messages between nerve cells and muscle cells. ACh binding to nicotinic receptors opens sodium (Na^+), calcium (Ca^{2+}), and potassium (K^+) channels, increasing the endplate potential and producing muscle contraction (see Figure 13-2).

ROLE OF γ-AMINOBUTYRIC ACID

GABA is the major inhibitory neurotransmitter in the nervous system. $GABA_A$ receptor binding causes chloride ion (Cl^-) channels to open. The influx of chloride ions results in hyperpolarization and inhibits formation of action potentials. $GABA_B$ receptor binding inhibits the release of excitatory neurotransmitters and substance P. Ultimately, neuronal excitability is reduced, and nerve impulse transmission is decreased. GABAergic receptors are stimulated by dopamine (D_2), another inhibitory neurotransmitter.

ROLE OF GLYCINE

Glycine is an inhibitory neurotransmitter. Defective glycine receptors are associated with a rare disease that causes an exaggerated startle reflex called hyperekplexia. This produces intense muscle contractions known as hypertonia.

ROLE OF GLUTAMATE

Voltage-dependent calcium channels are believed to be involved in spasticity. Glutamate is an excitatory amino acid responsible for the flow of calcium into motor neurons. Drugs that decrease glutamate availability are used to treat patients with ALS.

Drugs Used to Treat Spasticity

To manage spasticity, a variety of nonpharmaceutical treatments have been tried. Electrical stimulation, cold packs (cryotherapy), biofeedback, splinting, positioning, and physical therapy have all been proposed. These nondrug therapies may support pharmacological treatments.

Drugs used in the treatment of spasticity are grouped according to the site of action and are classified as central acting and peripheral acting. Peripheral-acting drugs act directly on contractile mechanisms in the muscle. Central-acting drugs may be further categorized according to their mechanism of action. Some drugs are GABAergic. They act on GABA receptors in the CNS. Drugs used to treat spasticity may (1) directly bind to GABA type B receptors ($GABA_B$), or (2) enhance GABA binding to $GABA_A$ and $GABA_B$ receptors (see also Chapter 8). Another group of drugs act at α_2-adrenergic receptor sites. Regardless of their mechanism of action, the goal of most drug treatments is to reduce the positive symptoms of spasticity.

PERIPHERAL-ACTING DRUGS
Botulinum Toxins

AbobotulinumtoxinA, incobotulinumtoxinA, onabotulinumtoxinA, and rimabotulinumtoxinB are used for the treatment of cervical dystonia. Only botulinum toxins type A are indicated for the treatment of blepharospasms. The toxins have also been studied in the treatment of poststroke spasticity and cerebral palsy. The toxin is injected locally to inhibit presynaptic release of ACh at the neuromuscular junction. This causes paralysis in the muscle(s) that have received the injections. The paralysis is reversed when the motor neuron sprouts new terminals that begin to release ACh. The onset of effect begins 3 to 7 days after injections are administered and lasts 3 to 6 months. Resistance develops with repeated use and injections, and the frequency of injection should be limited to no sooner than every 3 months. Botulinum toxins are discussed in detail in Chapter 13.

Dantrolene

Dantrolene is indicated for the treatment of spasticity associated with spinal cord injury, stroke, cerebral palsy, multiple sclerosis, and malignant hyperthermia. It reduces spasticity by weakening hyperexcited muscles. It acts directly on contractile mechanisms in skeletal muscle. Dantrolene inhibits the release of calcium from structures found in the muscle called the sarcoplasmic reticulum (see Figure 14-1), inhibiting calcium-dependent excitation–contraction (see Figure 14-2). The use of dantrolene in the treatment of some spastic conditions is limited because the drug produces muscle weakness. Muscle weakness is undesirable when treating spasticity associated with spinal cord injury or ALS. Other adverse effects produced by dantrolene include sedation, fatigue, diarrhea, and hepatotoxicity.

Peripheral-Acting Drugs Used for the Treatment of Spasticity

Generic Name	U.S. Brand Name(s)	Dosage Forms and Strengths
	Canadian Brand(s)	
dantrolene*	Dantrium, Revonto	**Capsules:** 25 mg, 50 mg[†], 100 mg
	Dantrium	**Injection, powder for reconstitution:** 20 mg

*Generic available.
[†]Strength available in the United States only.

CENTRAL ACTING DRUGS

Central-acting skeletal muscle relaxants reduce spasticity by binding to receptor sites that control motor movement in the brain and spinal cord. The mechanism of action of these drugs is to enhance the actions of GABA, an inhibitory neurotransmitter, or to stimulate α_2-adrenergic receptors.

GABAergic Drugs
DRUGS THAT BIND DIRECTLY TO GABA RECEPTORS

Baclofen is indicated for the treatment of spasticity associated with spinal cord injury and multiple sclerosis. Baclofen is structurally similar to the neurotransmitter GABA and is particularly useful

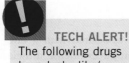

TECH ALERT!
The following drugs have look-alike/sound-alike issues: baclofen and bactroban; Lioresal, Lotensin, and lisinopril

in treatment of spasticity associated with spinal cord injury. By mimicking a naturally occurring inhibitory neurotransmitter, baclofen screens out unnecessary sensory messages coming from the environment.

Mechanism of Action and Pharmacokinetics. Baclofen acts as an agonist at $GABA_B$ receptor sites. It also decreases the release of excitatory neurotransmitters that cause muscle contractions and reduces pain linked to spasticity by inhibiting the release of substance P. The site of action for baclofen is the spinal cord, where it binds to presynaptic and postsynaptic receptors. GABA binding interrupts the flow of calcium and potassium ions into the nerve terminal, causing hyperpolarization of the nerve membrane and reduction of spinal reflexes. The ability of baclofen to cross the blood-brain barrier is limited, so its effectiveness is augmented by administering the drug intrathecally. Intrathecal solutions are injected directly into the cerebrospinal fluid (CSF), so the level of the drug in the CSF is increased. Surgery is required to implant the intrathecal delivery system. The pump needs to be refilled every 2 to 3 months and must be replaced every 4 to 5 years.

Adverse Reactions. Adverse reactions include dizziness, drowsiness, headache, nausea, orthostatic hypotension, confusion, and weakness. Sudden discontinuation can cause withdrawal symptoms. Rebound spasticity, hallucinations, itching, hyperthermia, and seizures are signs and symptoms of withdrawal syndrome.

DRUGS THAT ENHANCE GABA BINDING

Diazepam is classified as a central-acting agent because its site of action is the reticular formation of the brainstem and polysynaptic pathways in the spinal cord. Diazepam increases the binding of GABA to GABA receptors, decreasing the excitability of nerve terminals and hyperpolarizing the nerve. Diazepam is the most commonly used benzodiazepine for the treatment of spasticity, and it is effective in treating hyperactive reflexes and painful muscle spasms. It improves range of motion and decreases anxiety and sleeplessness—both conditions that can aggravate spasticity. Diazepam is a C-IV controlled substance in the United States and a targeted substance in Canada. A detailed discussion of the pharmacokinetics and adverse reactions of the benzodiazepines is found in Chapters 5 and 9.

TECH ALERT!
Diazepam and Ditropan have look-alike/sound-alike issues.

Central-Acting Drugs Used for the Treatment of Spasticity (Bind to GABA Receptors)

Generic Name	U.S. Brand Name(s) / Canadian Brand(s)	Dosage Forms and Strengths
baclofen*	Gablofen, Lioresal / Lioresal	**Solution, intrathecal injection (Lioresal):** 0.05 mg/mL, 0.5 mg/mL, 2 mg/mL **Tablets:** 10 mg, 20 mg

*Generic available.

Central-Acting Drugs Used for the Treatment of Spasticity (Enhance GABA Binding)

Generic Name	U.S. Brand Name(s) / Canadian Brand(s)	Dosage Forms and Strengths
diazepam*	Diastat, Diazepam Intensol, Valium / Diastat, Diazemuls, Valium	**Rectal gel (Diastat):** 5 mg/mL as 2.5 mg, 5 mg‡, 10 mg, 15 mg‡, and 20 mg prefilled syringes **Injection, IM emulsion (Diazemuls):** 5 mg/mL **Oral, solution:** 5 mg/5 mL **Oral concentrate (Diazepam Intensol):** 5 mg/mL **Tablets (Valium):** 2 mg, 5 mg, 10 mg

*Generic available.
‡Strength available in Canada only.

Centrally-Acting Drugs Used for the Treatment of Spasticity (α₂-Adrenergic Drugs)

Generic Name	U.S. Brand Name(s)	Dosage Forms and Strengths
	Canadian Brand(s)	
tizanidine*	Zanaflex	Capsules (US only): 2 mg, 4 mg, 6 mg
	Zanaflex	Tablets: 2 mg†, 4 mg

*Generic available.
†Strength available in the United States only.

TECH ALERT!
Tizanidine and nizatidine have look-alike/sound-alike issues.

TECH ALERT!
Cyproheptadine and cyclobenzaprine have look-alike/sound-alike issues.

TECH NOTE!
Skeletal muscle relaxants should not be combined with alcohol. Alcohol increases the CNS depression produced by the skeletal muscle relaxants, causing excessive drowsiness and decreased alertness.

TECH ALERT!
When carisoprodol is combined with codeine, it is a Schedule C-III controlled substance in the United States.

TECH ALERT!
The following drugs have look-alike/sound-alike issues: cyclobenzaprine, cyproheptadine, and cycloserine; metaxalone and metalazone

α₂-ADRENERGIC DRUGS

α₂-Adrenergic agonists (e.g., tizanidine) act like naturally occurring neurotransmitters. When α₂-adrenergic drugs are administered, they screen out unnecessary sensory messages that cause spasticity. They reduce muscle tone and the frequency of muscle spasms in people who have had spinal cord injuries, cerebral palsy, and stroke.

Mechanism of Action and Pharmacokinetics. Spasticity is reduced when α₂-adrenergic drugs are administered because the drugs prevent the release of excitatory neurotransmitters in the spinal cord and increase the actions of the inhibitory neurotransmitter glycine. α₂-Adrenergic agonists also cause hyperpolarization of motor neurons. Painful muscle spasms are diminished because α₂-adrenergic drugs interfere with the release of substance P, the neurotransmitter involved in the production of pain sensations and controlling pain perception (see Chapter 10).

Tizanidine is an α₂-adrenergic agonist. Tizanidine is structurally similar to the antihypertensive drug clonidine, but it produces fewer effects on the cardiovascular system.

Adverse Reactions. Tizanidine produces sedation, hypotension, and dizziness. The incidence of sedation is less with tizanidine than with clonidine. The drug reportedly can cause hepatotoxicity but is not associated with decreased muscle strength.

MISCELLANEOUS

Cyproheptadine is an antihistamine that is used in the treatment of spasticity associated with spinal cord injury as well as to treat baclofen withdrawal symptoms; however, this use is not approved by the U.S. Food and Drug Administration. Its mechanism of action appears to be linked to its effects on the neurotransmitters serotonin, histamine, and ACh.

Drugs Used to Treat Muscle Strain

Skeletal muscle relaxants are used to treat muscle stiffness, pain, and spasms associated with muscle tension, strain, sprains, or injury. Some, such as methocarbamol and orphenadrine, are additionally indicated for supportive therapy in tetanus. Drugs in this category include carisoprodol, chlorzoxazone, cyclobenzaprine, metaxalone, methocarbamol, and orphenadrine. These skeletal muscle relaxants are central acting; however, the mechanism of action is unknown. It is believed their actions may be related to their sedative effects on the CNS.

Common adverse effects associated with drugs used to treat muscle strain are dizziness, drowsiness, and blurred vision. Additional adverse effects are discoloration of urine—chlorzoxazone (orange to reddish purple) and methocarbamol (black, brown, or green).

Skeletal muscle relaxants should be used along with nonpharmaceutical therapies such as rest, exercise, cryotherapy, heat, and physical therapy.

Central-Acting Drugs Used for the Treatment of Muscle Strain

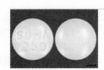
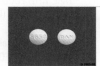

Generic Name	U.S. Brand Name(s) / Canadian Brand(s)	Dosage Forms and Strengths
carisoprodol*	Soma	Tablets: 250 mg, 350 mg
	Not available	
chlorzoxazone*	Parafon Forte DSC	Tablets: 500 mg (Parafon Forte DSC)
	Not available	
cyclobenzaprine*	Flexeril, Amrix	Capsules, extended release (Amrix): 15 mg, 30 mg
	Generics	Tablets: 5 mg[†], 7.5 mg[†], 10 mg
metaxalone	Skelaxin	Tablets: 800 mg
	Not available	
methocarbamol*	Robaxin	Tablets: 500 mg, 750 mg
	Robaxin	Solution, for injection: 100 mg/mL
orphenadrine*	Norflex	Solution, for injection: 30 mg/mL (2 mL)
	Norflex[§], Orphenace[§]	Tablets, extended release: 100 mg
Combination Products		
carisoprodol + aspirin*	Generics	Tablets: 200 mg carisoprodol + 325 mg aspirin
	Not available	
carisoprodol + aspirin + codeine*	Generics	Tablets: 200 mg carisoprodol + 325 mg aspirin + 16 mg codeine
	Not available	
chlorzoxazone + acetaminophen	Not available	Tablets: 250 mg chlorzoxazone + 300 mg acetaminophen
	Acetazone Forte, Back Aid Forte[§]	
chlorzoxazone + acetaminophen + codeine	Not available	Tablets: 250 mg chlorzoxazone + 300 mg acetaminophen + 8 mg codeine
	Acetazone Forte C8[§]	
methocarbamol + aspirin	Generic	Tablets: 400 mg methocarbamol + 325 mg aspirin; 400 mg methocarbamol + 500 mg aspirin
	Extra Strength Muscle and Backache Relief[§], Robaxisal[§], Robaxisal Extra Strength[§]	
methocarbamol + aspirin + codeine	Not available	Tablets: 400 mg methocarbamol + 500 mg aspirin + 8 mg codeine; 400 mg methocarbamol + 500 mg aspirin + 16.2 mg codeine; 400 mg methocarbamol + 500 mg aspirin + 32.4 mg codeine
	Robaxisal C 1/8[§], Robaxisal C ¼, Robaxisal C ½	
methocarbamol + acetaminophen	Not available	Tablets: 400 mg methocarbamol + 325 mg acetaminophen; 400 mg methocarbamol + 500 mg acetaminophen
	Extra Strength Tylenol Back Pain[§], Robaxacet[§], Robaxacet Extra Strength[§]	
methocarbamol + acetaminophen + codeine	Not available	400 mg methocarbamol + 325 mg acetaminophen + 8 mg codeine
	Robaxacet-8[§]	
methocarbamol + ibuprofen	Not available	Tablets: 500 mg methocarbamol + 200 mg ibuprofen
	Axum[§], Robax Platinum[§]	
orphenadrine + caffeine + aspirin	Generic	Tablets: 25 mg orphenadrine + 30 mg caffeine + 385 mg aspirin; 50 mg orphenadrine + 60 mg caffeine + 770 mg aspirin
	Not available	

*Generic available.
[†]Strength available in the United States only.
[§]Over the counter in Canada.

Summary of Drugs Used in the Treatment of Spasticity

Generic Name	U.S. Brand Name	Usual Adult Oral Dose and Dosing Schedule	Warning Labels
Central-Acting Skeletal Muscle Relaxants			
baclofen	Lioresal	**Oral:** 5 mg 3 times a day (maximum, 80 mg/day) **Intrathecal:** 25-100 mcg test dose, then 50-200 mcg infused via intrathecal pump over 24 hours	MAY CAUSE DIZZINESS OR DROWSINESS. MAY IMPAIR ABILITY TO DRIVE. AVOID ALCOHOL. TAKE WITH FOOD—baclofen. MAY DISCOLOR URINE—chlorzoxazone, methocarbamol. MAY BE HABIT FORMING—diazepam. SWALLOW WHOLE; DO NOT CRUSH OR CHEW—orphenadrine extended release.
carisoprodol	Soma	250-350 mg 4 times a day	
chlorzoxazone	Parafon Forte	250-500 mg 3-4 times a day	
cyclobenzaprine	Flexeril	5-10 mg 3 times a day	
diazepam	Valium	**Oral:** 2-10 mg 2-4 times a day **IM, IV:** 2-10 mg every 3 to 4 hours	
metaxolone	Skelaxin	800 mg 3-4 times a day	
methocarbamol	Robaxin	**Oral:** 1.5 g 4 times a day (up to 8 g/day) **IM, IV:** 1 g every 8 hours	
orphenadrine	Norflex	**Oral:** 100 mg twice a day **IM, IV:** 60 mg every 12 hours	
tizanidine	Zanaflex	2-4 mg 3 times a day (maximum, 36 mg/day)	
Direct-Acting Skeletal Muscle Relaxants			
dantrolene	Dantrium	25-100 mg 2-4 times a day	MAY CAUSE DIZZINESS OR DROWSINESS. MAY IMPAIR ABILITY TO DRIVE. AVOID ALCOHOL. PROTECT FROM LIGHT AND MOISTURE.

Chapter Summary

- Spasticity is a debilitating motor disorder that affects up to 12 million people worldwide.
- Symptoms of spasticity are increased muscle tone, exaggerated tendon jerks, and hyperexcitable reflexes.
- Spasticity interferes with the normal performance of activities of daily living.
- Stroke, spinal cord injury, cerebral palsy, muscle trauma, multiple sclerosis, head injury, and amyotrophic lateral sclerosis can all cause spasticity.
- Between 65% and 78% of people with spinal cord injuries and 65% of people who have had a stroke will develop spasticity.
- The progression to spasticity follows a specific pattern, and the degree of spasticity is related to the duration since the original injury.
- There are four phases to the development of spasticity: (1) decreased muscle contractility; (2) excessive muscle tone and increased reflex activity lasting from days to years; (3) decreased reflex excitability; and (4) stiff, contracted muscles.

- After a spinal cord injury, spasticity develops because neurons grow new synapses, and the increase in the number of synapses causes a stronger reflex response to stretching of the muscle.
- Spasticity impairs effective muscle movement in some people and helps maintain posture, making walking easier in other people.
- Spasticity may be caused by an excess of neurotransmitters that carry excitatory messages, such as glutamate, or decreased activity or a deficiency of inhibitory transmitters, such as GABA and glycine.
- Nonpharmaceutical treatments of spasticity are electrical stimulation, cold packs (cryotherapy), biofeedback, splinting, positioning, and physical therapy.
- Drugs used in the treatment of spasticity are grouped according to the site of action and are classified as central acting and peripheral acting.
- Peripheral-acting drugs act at the neuromuscular junction or directly on contractile mechanisms in the muscle.
- Botulinum toxins injected locally inhibit presynaptic release of ACh at the neuromuscular junction. This causes paralysis in the muscle(s) that received the injections. The paralysis is reversed when the motor neuron sprouts new terminals that begin to release ACh.
- Dantrolene is a peripheral-acting drug that acts directly on contractile mechanisms in skeletal muscle.
- Central-acting drugs primarily act on GABA receptors in the CNS or act at α_2-adrenergic receptor sites.
- Baclofen is a central-acting drug that looks and acts like GABA, a naturally occurring neurotransmitter.
- The ability of baclofen to cross the blood-brain barrier is limited. Its effectiveness is augmented by direct administration into CSF via a surgically implanted pump.
- Skeletal muscle relaxants are used to treat muscle stiffness, pain, and spasms associated with muscle tension, strain, sprains, or injury.

REVIEW QUESTIONS

1. Negative symptoms of spasticity are increased muscle tone, exaggerated tendon jerks, and hyperexcitability of the stretch reflex.
   - a. true
   - b. false

2. Any condition that can damage the _____ can cause spasticity.
   - a. brain
   - b. spinal cord
   - c. motor neurons
   - d. a, b, and c

3. People who have amyotrophic lateral sclerosis exhibit predominantly _____ symptoms of spasticity.
   - a. positive
   - b. negative
   - c. no
   - d. both b and c

4. The mechanism of action for drugs used to treat spasticity is to directly bind to or enhance the binding of _____.
   - a. GABA$_A$ receptors
   - b. GABA$_B$ receptors
   - c. GABA$_A$ and GABA$_B$ receptors
   - d. GABA$_D$ receptors

5. The effect of botulinum toxins in reducing spasticity lasts up to _____.
   - a. 2 weeks
   - b. 12 weeks
   - c. 8 weeks
   - d. 4 weeks

6. The ability of baclofen to cross the blood-brain barrier is limited so its effectiveness is augmented by administering the drug _____.
   a. intravenously
   b. intrapleurally
   c. intrathecally
   d. intraocularly

7. _____is the most commonly used benzodiazepine for the treatment of spasticity and it is effective in treating hyperactive reflexes and painful muscle spasms.
   a. Alprazolam
   b. Diazepam
   c. Clonazepam
   d. Lorazepam

8. Spasticity is reduced when α_2-adrenergic drugs are administered because the drugs prevent the release of inhibitory neurotransmitters in the spinal cord by increasing the actions of the excitatory neurotransmitter glycine.
   a. true
   b. false

9. Chlorzoxazone (Paraforon forte) discolors urine to what color?
   a. orange
   b. red
   c. reddish purple
   d. a and c

10. The brand name for cyclobenzaprine is _____.
    a. Benezil
    b. Flexeril
    c. Cyclodril
    d. Skelaxin

TECHNICIAN'S CORNER

1. Why does the blood-brain barrier prevent some drugs from entering the brain?
2. When should nonpharmaceutical treatments of spasticity be discontinued in favor of pharmaceutical treatments?

Bibliography

Adams MM, Hicks AL: Spasticity after spinal cord injury, *Spinal Cord* 43:577-586, 2005.

FDA: FDA Approved Drug Products, 2012. Retrieved April 29, 2012, from http://www.accessdata.fda.gov/scripts/cder/drugsatfda/index.cfm?fuseaction=Search.Search_Drug_Name.

Gallichio J: Pharmacologic management of spasticity following stroke, *Phys Ther* 84:973-981, 2004.

Health Canada: Drug Product Database, 2010. Retrieved March 25, 2011, from http://www.hc-sc.gc.ca/dhp-mps/prodpharma/databasdon/index-eng.php.

Honda M, Sekiguchi Y, Sato N, et al: Involvement of imidazoline receptors in the centrally acting muscle-relaxant effects of tizanidine, *Eur J Pharmacol* 445:187-193, 2002.

Lance L, Lacy C, Armstrong L, et al: *Drug information handbook for the allied health professional*, ed 12, Hudson, OH, 2005, APhA Lexi-Comp.

Ozcakir S, Sivrioglu K: Botulinum toxin in poststroke spasticity, *Clin Med Res* 5(2):132-138, 2007.

Patel D, Soyode O: Pharmacologic interventions for reducing spasticity in cerebral palsy, *Indian J Pediatr* 72:869-872, 2005.

USP Center for Advancement of Patient Safety: Use caution–avoid confusion, USP Quality Review No. 79, Rockville, MD, April 2004, USP Center for Advancement of Patient Safety.

Zafonte R, Lombard L, Elovic E: Antispasticity medications: uses and limitations of enteral therapy, *Am J Phys Med Rehabil* 83(suppl):S50-S58, 2004.

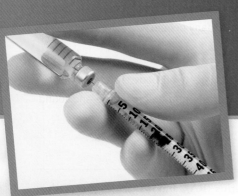

15

Treatment of Autoimmune Diseases That Affect the Musculoskeletal System

KEY TERMS

Antinuclear antibody: Autoantibody or abnormal antibody that attacks the nucleus of normal cells in the body.

Ataxia: Condition where the muscles fail to function in a coordinated manner.

Autoantibody: Abnormal antibody that attacks healthy cells and tissue.

Autoimmune disease: Disease that occurs when the immune system turns against the parts of the body it is designed to protect.

Dermatomyositis: Form of myositis that affects muscles and the skin.

Demyelination: Damage caused by recurrent inflammation of myelin that results in nervous system scars that interrupt communication between the nerves and the rest of the body.

Interferons: Antiviral proteins that enhance T-cell recognition of antigens (γ-interferon) and produce immune system suppression (α-interferon, β-interferon).

Multiple sclerosis: Autoimmune disease that causes progressive damage to nerves, resulting in spasticity, pain, mood changes, and other physical symptoms.

Myasthenia gravis: Autoimmune disease in which the immune system attacks the muscle cells at the neuromuscular junction and is characterized by muscle weakness.

Myelin: Fatty covering that insulates nerve cells in the brain and spinal cord.

Myositis: Autoimmune disease that causes chronic inflammation of the muscles.

Plaques: Patchy areas of inflammation and demyelination that disrupt nerve signals between the brain and the rest of the body.

Polymyositis: Form of myositis that affects multiple muscles, particularly the muscles closest to the trunk.

Rheumatoid arthritis: Chronic disease characterized by inflammation and remodeling of the joints.

Rheumatoid factor: Immunoglobulin (antibody) that is present in many people who have rheumatoid arthritis.

Synovium: Thin layer of tissue that lines the joint space.

Systemic lupus erythematosus: Autoimmune disease that affects nearly all body systems.

Tumor necrosis factor: Inflammatory cytokine released as part of the immune response and found in synovial fluid of people with rheumatoid arthritis.

Overview

Myasthenia gravis, multiple sclerosis (MS), rheumatoid arthritis (RA), and systemic lupus erythematosus (SLE) are examples of ***autoimmune diseases*** that affect the musculoskeletal system. An autoimmune disease occurs when the immune system turns against the parts of the body it is designed to protect. The body attacks its own cells, thinking they are germs or a harmful foreign substance.

No one knows exactly why autoimmunity develops. It is believed that several factors may be involved. The trigger may be exposure to a virus, environmental toxins, the sun, genetics, hormonal changes, drugs, pregnancy, or some combination of any of these things. What is known is that autoimmunity can affect any organ of the body. Autoimmune diseases that involve the muscles are dermatomyositis, myasthenia gravis, and polymyositis. Multiple sclerosis is an autoimmune disease that affects the nerves and causes muscle weakness and spasticity in addition to central nervous system (CNS) effects. Ankylosing spondylitis, RA, and SLE are autoimmune diseases involving the joints. SLE also commonly attacks the blood vessels, heart, lungs, nerves, brain, and skin in addition to the joints.

Description of Autoimmune Diseases Affecting the Musculoskeletal System

MYASTHENIA GRAVIS

Myasthenia gravis is an autoimmune disease that causes muscle weakness. The muscles are easily fatigued after even brief activity. Muscle weakness improves after periods of rest. Myasthenia gravis typically affects skeletal muscles of the face, neck, and limbs. Sometimes the muscles involved in breathing are affected.

Approximately 20 people per 100,000 worldwide have been diagnosed with myasthenia gravis. The onset of the disease typically occurs in women younger than 40 years and men older than 60 years; however, the onset can be triggered at any age, including infancy.

In myasthenia gravis, the body attacks and destroys receptor sites that bind acetylcholine (ACh) in the neuromuscular junction (Figure 15-1) (see Chapter 13). Fewer nicotinic receptor sites mean that there will be fewer muscle contractions, and when contractions occur, they will not be as strong. This is because the action potentials needed to generate contractions, as well as the strength of contractions generated, are dependent on the number of interactions between ACh and nicotinic receptors (see Chapter 13).

MYOSITIS

Myositis is an autoimmune disease that causes chronic inflammation of the muscles. It often begins with pain in the shoulders and hips; interferes with walking; and can progress to involve the muscles that affect breathing, swallowing, and speech. Dermatomyositis and polymyositis are specific forms of myositis. ***Polymyositis***, as its name describes, affects muscles in multiple parts of the body. Inflammation of muscles closest to the trunk is most common. The disease causes weakness, fatigue,

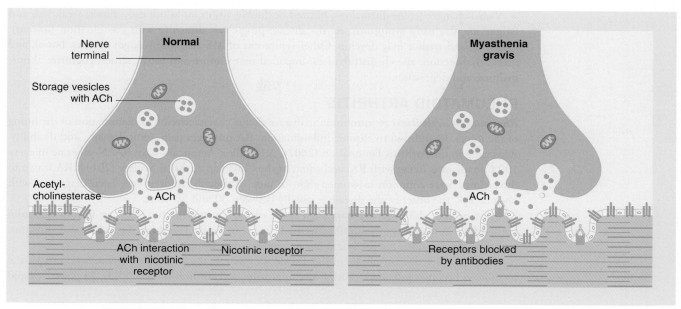

FIGURE 15-1 The effects of antibodies on the neuromuscular junction in myasthenia gravis. (From Page C, et al: *Integrated pharmacology*, ed 3, Philadelphia, 2006, Mosby.)

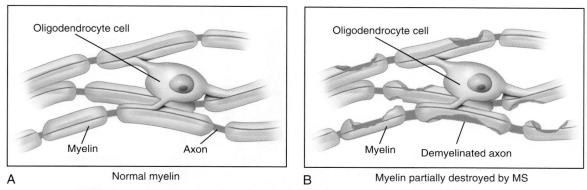

FIGURE 15-2 Effects of multiple sclerosis. (From Thibodeau GA, Patton KT: *Anatomy and physiology*, ed 6, St Louis, 2007, Mosby.)

and pain in the joints and muscles. ***Dermatomyositis*** causes inflammation and damage to muscles and skin. People with dermatomyositis develop a distinctive patchy, reddish rash on the eyelids, cheeks, bridge of the nose, back or upper chest, elbows, knees, and knuckles. It also causes fatigue and painful muscles and joints.

MULTIPLE SCLEROSIS

According to the World Health Organization (2008), Canada and the United States rank within the top five countries with the highest prevalence of ***multiple sclerosis*** (MS) in the world with nearly 135 of every 100,000 people with the disease. Higher income countries have more persons with MS than lower income countries. MS affects women more commonly than men (2 : 1), and the average age of onset is 30 years. As with many autoimmune diseases, MS is caused by a trigger that causes the body to start attacking its own cells. Some of the risk factors and triggers that are associated with MS are exposure to a virus, environmental factors, genetics, and malfunction of the blood-brain barrier that permits entry of antimyelin T cells produced by the immune system.

In MS, the insulating coating of nerves (***myelin***) is attacked (Figure 15-2). Reoccurring attacks of inflammation cause ***demyelination*** of nerves and result in lesions and scarring of the white matter of the brain. The scarring, known as ***plaques***, is responsible for the signs and symptoms of MS.

Visual changes (color distortions, blurred or double vision, or blindness), muscle weakness, and fatigue are also early symptoms. As the disease progresses, difficulty with coordination (*ataxia*), spasticity, and tremor may develop. Other symptoms of MS are pain; vertigo; bladder, bowel, and sexual dysfunction; speech disturbances; impaired temperature and touch senses; cognitive abnormalities; and depression.

RHEUMATOID ARTHRITIS

Rheumatoid arthritis is an autoimmune disease that is characterized by inflammation of the lining of the joints. In addition to chronic inflammation, RA produces pain, joint damage, and disability. According to the Arthritis Foundation (2007), 2.1 million Americans have RA. Nearly one in every 100 Canadians is living with RA, according to the Canadian Arthritis Society (2011). RA is two to three times more common in women than in men. Although children have been diagnosed with juvenile RA, the onset of the disease is usually between 30 and 50 years.

Most people who have RA have high levels of *rheumatoid factor* (RF), an immunoglobulin (antibody) that regulates other antibodies made by the body. RF is not specific to RA, so its presence is part of the diagnosis for RA but is not a definitive diagnostic tool.

There are three distinct phases of the disease. In phase 1, the joint lining (*synovium*) or synovial membrane becomes inflamed, causing swelling, pain, and stiffness (Figure 15-3). In phase 2, rapid

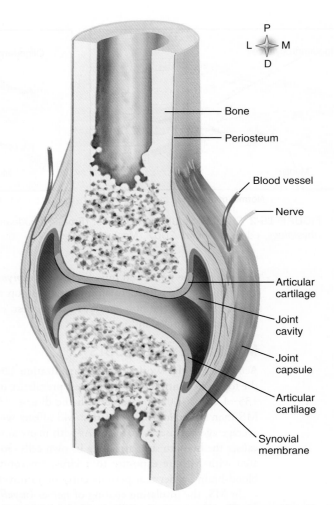

FIGURE 15-3 Synovial joint. (From Vidic B, Suarez FR: *Photographic atlas of the human body*, St Louis, 1984, Mosby.)

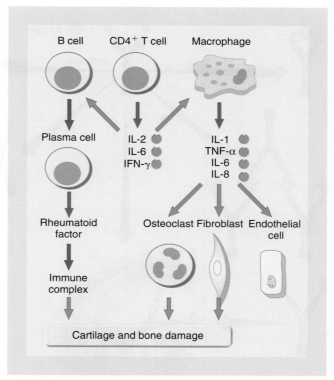

FIGURE 15-4 Cytokine network in the pathogenesis of rheumatoid arthritis. (From Page C, et al: *Integrated pharmacology*, ed 6, Philadelphia, 2006, Mosby.)

cell growth causes the synovium to thicken. In phase 3, inflamed cells in the synovium release enzymes that digest bone and cartilage. This results in more pain and disability. The damaging, chronic cycle of inflammation is stimulated by proinflammatory cytokines (Figure 15-4) such as interleukins (ILs) and ***tumor necrosis factor*** (TNF-α).

Rheumatoid arthritis causes more than joint problems. Other symptoms of RA are fatigue, weakness, flulike symptoms, nodules that form under the skin, muscle pain, decreased appetite, depression, and dry mouth.

SYSTEMIC LUPUS ERYTHEMATOSUS

Systemic lupus erythematosus is an autoimmune disease that affects nearly all parts of the body. The prevalence of SLE worldwide is approximately 20 to 150 per 100,000 people. Women between the ages of 15 and 25 years are more likely to get SLE than are men, and African American women are three times more likely to get SLE than are women of European descent.

It is not known what triggers the onset of SLE. As with other autoimmune diseases, it is likely that a combination of factors is responsible. Potential triggers include stress, viral infection, certain drugs, and sunlight. Heredity also appears to play a role. When SLE is triggered, the body produces antibodies that cause inflammation and damage healthy cells and organs. ***Antinuclear antibody*** (ANA) levels are elevated in people who have SLE. ANA attaches to the cell nucleus, causing the body's immune system to attack it as if it were a harmful bacteria or virus (Figure 15-5).

Systemic lupus erythematosus causes swollen and painful joints similar to RA. Unlike RA, it affects most other regions of the body, too, including the kidneys, heart, lungs, blood vessels, and skin. Inflammation of the kidney interferes with waste removal and causes swelling of the legs and feet. Inflammation of the lungs causes pain when breathing. Other signs and symptoms of SLE are muscle pain, fever, red rashes, hair loss, sun sensitivity, swollen glands, extreme fatigue, seizures, mouth ulcers, and poor circulation in fingers and toes.

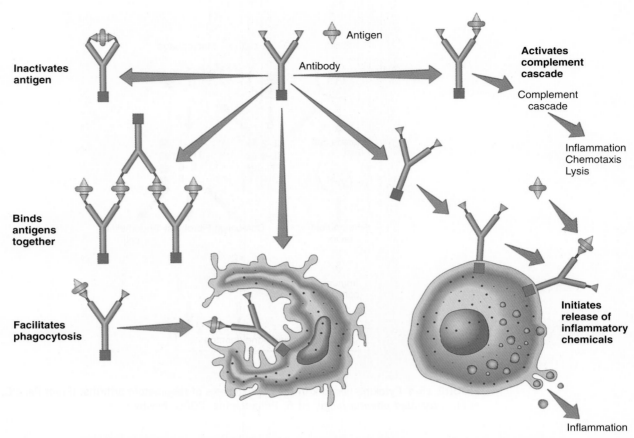

FIGURE 15-5 Actions of antibodies. (From Thibodeau GA, Patton KT: *Anatomy and physiology*, ed 3, St Louis, 2007, Mosby.)

Treatment of Autoimmune Diseases That Affect the Musculoskeletal System

Multiple sclerosis, myasthenia gravis, SLE, myositis, RA, and other autoimmune diseases that affect the musculoskeletal system are treated using pharmacological and nonpharmacological therapies. Drug therapy is aimed at suppressing inflammation, pain, and immune system response. Drugs used to suppress inflammation and reduce joint swelling and pain include glucocorticosteroids (e.g., dexamethasone and prednisone), nonsteroidal anti-inflammatory drugs (NSAIDs; e.g., celecoxib and naproxen), and salicylates (aspirin). Disease-modifying antirheumatic drugs (DMARDs) are an important group of drugs that slow the progression of RA and SLE by modifying biological response. Immunosuppressive drugs (e.g., azathioprine and methotrexate), TNF inhibitors (e.g., etanercept and infliximab), IL antagonists (e.g., anakinra), the antimalarial hydroxychloroquine, and even gold salts are classified as DMARDs. ***Interferons*** (IFNs) and monoclonal antibodies (*mabs*) are biological response modifiers used in the treatment of MS (IFNs) and RA (*mabs*).

Treatment goals are also aimed at minimizing further nerve or joint destruction, preservation of body functions, and prevention of disability. Additional medications are administered to control disease-specific symptoms such as spasticity, muscle weakness, fatigue, nerve pain, or rashes.

ANTI-INFLAMMATORIES AND ANALGESICS
Glucocorticosteroids

Glucocorticosteroids are prescribed to suppress inflammation, reduce flare-ups, and treat pain associated with MS, myasthenia gravis, SLE, myositis, and RA (Figure 15-6). Glucocorticosteroids have

TECH ALERT!
The following drugs have look-alike/ sound-alike issues: hydrocortisone, cortisone, and hydrocodone; Medrol and Mebaral; methylprednisolone and medroxyprogesterone; prednisone, prednisolone, Pramosone, and primodone

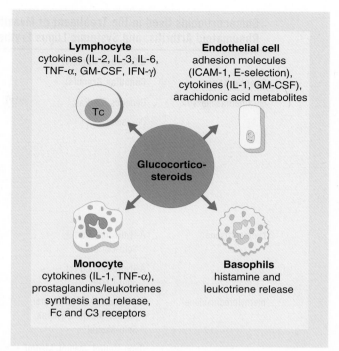

FIGURE 15-6 Suppressive effects of glucocorticosteroids on immune and inflammatory response. (From Page C, et al: *Integrated pharmacology*, ed 3, Philadelphia, 2006, Mosby.)

immunosuppressive actions, and they inhibit the synthesis of antibodies that are responsible for attacking the body's healthy cells. They decrease the accumulation of cells that mobilize to fight when the body believes it is under attack, such as leukocytes and T cells. They interfere with the binding of antibodies to receptor sites on the cell surface. Glucocorticosteroids are also used to restore the effectiveness of the blood-brain barrier to screen out antibodies harmful to brain cells and nerves. Glucocorticosteroids are potent anti-inflammatory drugs, too. They decrease the synthesis of proinflammatory substances—prostaglandins (see Chapter 10), leukotrienes, cytokines, arachidonic acid, and macrophages—that are released as part of the inflammatory response and cause swelling, pain, irritation, and other effects. Glucocorticosteroids may also be prescribed for the treatment of ulcerative colitis, allergic reactions, cerebral edema, or septic shock or used as a diagnostic agent for endocrine disorders (see Unit IX, Introduction to the Endocrine System).

PHARMACOKINETICS
The absorption, distribution, metabolism, and elimination of glucocorticosteroids used in the treatment of MS, myasthenia gravis, SLE, myositis, and RA vary according to the dosage form administered. In general, oral dosage forms are well absorbed in the gastrointestinal (GI) tract and are readily distributed. Metabolism occurs in the liver. Glucocorticosteroids are eliminated in urine.

ADVERSE REACTIONS
The adverse effects produced by glucocorticosteroids are numerous and affect all body systems. In the CNS, they cause insomnia and euphoria. In the cardiovascular system, they produce edema and hypertension. In the endocrine system, they may produce hyperglycemia, leading to diabetes. Short-term use of glucocorticosteroids can also cause nausea and weight gain. Other adverse drug effects are osteoporosis, acne, cataracts, poor wound healing, increased risk of infection, and ulceration in the GI tract.

Glucocorticoids Used in the Treatment of Myasthenia Gravis, Multiple Sclerosis, Rheumatoid Arthritis, and Systemic Lupus Erythematosus

Generic Name	U.S. Brand Name(s) Canadian Brand(s)	Dosage Forms and Strengths
dexamethasone*	Generics, DexPak Dexasone	Elixir: 0.5 mg/5 mL Solution for injection: 4 mg/mL and 10 mg/mL, 24 mg/mL[†] Solution, oral: 0.5 mg/5 mL Solution, oral concentrate: 1 mg/mL Tablets: 0.25 mg[†], 0.5 mg, 0.75 mg, 1 mg[†], 1.5 mg[†], 2 mg, 4 mg, 6 mg[†] Tablets (DexPak, TaperPak): 1.5 mg (51 tablets on taper dose card)
hydrocortisone*	A-Hydrocort, Cortef, Solu-Cortef A-Hydrocort, Cortef, Solu-Cortef	Injection, powder for reconstitution (A-Hydrocort, Solu-Cortef): 100 mg, 250 mg, 500 mg, 1000 mg Injection, solution: 50 mg/mL Tablets: 5 mg[†], 10 mg, 20 mg
methylprednisolone*	A-Methapred, Depo-Medrol, Medrol, Medrol Dosepak, Solu-Medrol Depo-Medrol, Medrol, Medrol Dosepak, Solu-Medrol	Injection, powder for reconstitution (A-Methapred, Solu-Medrol): 40 mg, 125 mg, 500 mg, 1000 mg Injection, suspension (Depo-Medrol): 20 mg/mL, 40 mg/mL, 80 mg/mL Tablets: 2 mg[†], 4 mg, 8 mg[†], 16 mg, 32 mg[†] Tablets (Medrol Dosepak): 4 mg (21 tablet taper dose)
prednisone*	Generics, Prednisone Intensol Winpred	Solution, oral: 1 mg/mL Solution, oral concentrate (Prednisone Intensol): 5 mg/mL Tablets: 1 mg, 2.5 mg[†], 5 mg, 10 mg[†], 20 mg[†], 50 mg

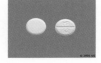

*Generic available.
[†]Strength available in the United States only.

PRECAUTIONS

Glucocorticosteroids may initially produce muscle weakness. This is a serious problem for people with myasthenia gravis given that muscle weakness is a symptom of the disease. Alternate-day therapy can minimize some adverse effects caused by glucocorticosteroids. Long-term use of glucocorticosteroids may increase the need for potassium; vitamins A, B6, C, and D; folate; calcium; zinc; and phosphorous supplementation.

NONSTEROIDAL ANTI-INFLAMMATORY DRUGS

Nonsteroidal anti-inflammatory drugs and aspirin (ASA) are widely used in the treatment of pain and inflammation associated with RA, myasthenia gravis, SLE, myositis, and MS. Aspirin and NSAIDs inhibit the release of prostaglandins, important mediators of pain (see Chapter 10). Prostaglandins are substances that stimulate a cascade of events that result in inflammation. Aspirin and NSAIDs block the activity of the enzyme cyclooxygenase (COX-1 and COX-2), interfering with the synthesis of prostaglandin.

Celecoxib remains the only COX-2 inhibitor available for sale in the United States and Canada. As per U.S. Food and Drug Administration (FDA) requirements, manufacturers of all NSAIDs must print a boxed warning in the package insert describing the risk for cardiovascular toxicity and GI ulceration. The pharmacokinetics, adverse reactions, and precautions for NSAIDs are discussed in detail in Chapter 10.

TECH ALERT!
The following drugs have look-alike/sound-alike issues:
Celebrex, Celexa, and Cerebyx;
naprosyn, Naprelan, and Niaspan;
Anaprox and Avapro

Selected Nonsteroidal Anti-inflammatory Drugs Used in the Treatment of Myasthenia Gravis, Multiple Sclerosis, Rheumatoid Arthritis, and Systemic Lupus Erythematosus

Generic Name	U.S. Brand Name(s) / Canadian Brand(s)	Dosage Forms and Strengths
celecoxib*	Celebrex	Capsules: 50 mg†, 100 mg, 200 mg, 400 mg†
	Celebrex	
ibuprofen*	Advil, Motrin, Motrin IB	Caplets, capsules, gelcap, tablets (Advil, Motrin IB): 100 mg†¶, 200 mg†¶
	Advil, Advil Junior Strength, Axum, Motrin IB	Suspension, oral: 100 mg/5 mL†¶§
		Suspension, oral drops: 40 mg/mL§
		Tablets, chewable: 50 mg, 100 mg
		Tablets: 300 mg§, 400 mg§, 600 mg, 800 mg†
naproxen*	Aleve, Anaprox, Anaprox DS, EC-Naprosyn, Naprelan	Suspension, oral (Naprosyn): 125 mg/5 mL
		Tablets (Naprosyn): 250 mg, 375 mg, 500 mg
	Anaprox, Anaprox DS, Naprosyn, Naprelan	Tablets, enteric coated (EC-Naprosyn): 375 mg, 500 mg
		Tablet, extended release (Naprelan): 375 mg, 500 mg, 750 mg†
		Tablets (as sodium): 220 mg¶§ (Aleve), 275 mg (Anaprox), 550 mg (Anaprox DS)

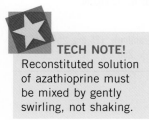

*Generic available.
†Strength available in the United States only.
¶Over the counter in the United States.
§Over the counter in Canada.

DISEASE-MODIFYING ANTIRHEUMATIC DRUGS

Disease-modifying antirheumatic drugs are used in the treatment of MS, myasthenia gravis, SLE, myositis, and RA to slow disease progression rather than provide symptomatic relief. Selected immunosuppressives, TNF inhibitors, IL antagonists, the antimalarials, lefluonomide, gold salts, penicillamine, and sulfasalazine are all DMARDs and are described in this chapter.

IMMUNOSUPPRESSIVES

TECH NOTE! Reconstituted solution of azathioprine must be mixed by gently swirling, not shaking.

Immunosuppressive drugs interfere with the formation of immune cells by damaging RNA and DNA needed for cell replication. They may also block immune system response to autoantibodies. An *autoantibody* is an abnormal antibody that attacks healthy cells and tissue.

Azathioprine, cyclophosphamide, cyclosporine, methotrexate, and mitoxantrone are treatments for MS, RA, myasthenia gravis, and SLE.

Azathioprine is used in the treatment of RA, myasthenia gravis, and SLE. The mechanism of action is to block purine synthesis and cause DNA damage. Azathioprine also suppresses T cell–mediated immune system responses.

Cyclophosphamide is used in the treatment of patients with RA and SLE. It interferes with DNA synthesis and cell replication. It inhibits B-cell antibody production and T-cell activity, suppresses cytokine and immunoglobulin production, and suppresses the antigen-induced response to T cells. Because of toxicity, cyclophosphamide is reserved for severe, active disease. Cyclophosphamide is also prescribed for the treatment of leukemia, lymphomas, and multiple cancers (breast, ovarian, endometrial, and testicular) and to prevent rejection of bone marrow transplants.

Cyclosporine is used with azathioprine or glucocorticosteroids to treat severe RA and severe corticosteroid-resistant SLE, myasthenia gravis, and other autoimmune diseases affecting the musculoskeletal system. Cyclosporine selectively interferes with T-cell proliferation and IL production. The result is a decreased immune system response to autoantibodies. Cyclosporine is also prescribed for the prevention of organ transplant rejection, for psoriasis, and to increase tear production in patients with keratoconjunctivitis sicca.

Disease-Modifying Antirheumatic Drugs

Generic Name	U.S. Brand Name(s) / Canadian Brand(s)	Dosage Forms and Strengths
Tumor Necrosis Factor-α Inhibitors		
adalimumab	Humira	Injection, solution: 40 mg/0.8 mL,
	Humira	20 mg/0.4 mL (1 mL prefilled syringe)
certolizumab pegol	Cimzia	Powder, for injections: 400 mg per vial
	Cimzia	Solution, for injection: 200 mg/mL
etanercept	Enbrel	Injection, powder for reconstitution: 25 mg
	Enbrel	Injection, solution: 50 mg/mL (0.98 mL prefilled syringe)
golimumab	Simponi	Solution for injection: 50 mg/0.5 mL prefilled syringe
	Simponi	
infliximab	Remicade	Injection, powder for reconstitution: 100 mg
	Remicade	
Interleukin Antagonists		
anakinra	Kineret	Injection, solution: 100 mg/0.67 mL (1 mL prefilled syringe)
	Kineret	
Miscellaneous		
leflunomide	Arava	Tablets: 10 mg, 20 mg
	Arava	
sulfasalazine*	Azulfidine, Azulfidine EN-tabs	Tablets (Azulfidine): 500 mg
	Salazopyrin, Salazopyrin EN-tabs	Tablets, enteric coated (Azulfidine EN-tab): 500 mg
auranofin	Ridaura	Capsules: 3 mg
	Ridaura	
gold sodium thiomalate	Aurolate	Injection, solution: 50 mg/mL
	Myochrysine	
penicillamine	Cupramine, Depen Titratable	Capsules (Cupramine): 125 mg, 250 mg
	Cupramine, Depen	Tablets (Depen): 250 mg

*Generic available.

Methotrexate was one of the first drugs used for the treatment of RA, and it continues to be used as monotherapy or along with other DMARDs. Methotrexate is also used to treat SLE. It works by inhibiting the formation of folates that are needed for purine synthesis; thus, folic acid supplementation is prescribed with methotrexate. Methotrexate also decreases cytokine and immunoglobulin production and COX-2 activity, reducing both inflammation and immune system activity. In addition to RA, methotrexate is prescribed for the treatment of leukemias; neoplasms; psoriasis; breast, lung, and head and neck cancer; GI tract and testes cancers; and osteosarcoma.

Mitoxantrone in used in the treatment of MS and interferes with DNA repair and RNA synthesis, effectively reducing the growth and spread of immune cells and decreasing the progression of the disease. Mitoxantrone is listed as an FDA pregnancy category D drug. Mitoxantrone is also prescribed for the treatment of leukemia, breast and prostate cancer, and pediatric sarcoma.

Precautions and Adverse Reactions

Adverse reactions to azathioprine include nausea, vomiting, infections, hepatotoxicity, cytopenias, and myelosuppression. Cyclophosphamide may produce alopecia, nausea, infertility, infections,

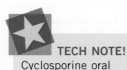

TECH NOTE!
Cyclosporine oral solution must be dispensed in a glass container. Dispense the same manufacturer's product each time (bioavailability issues).

Immunosuppressives Used in the Treatment of Myasthenia Gravis, Multiple Sclerosis, Rheumatoid Arthritis, and Systemic Lupus Erythematosus

Generic Name	U.S. Brand Name(s) Canadian Brand(s)	Dosage Forms and Strengths
azathioprine*	Azasan, Imuran	Injection, powder for reconstitution: 50 mg‡, 100 mg†
	Imuran	Tablets: 25mg†, 50 mg, 75 mg† and 100 mg†
cyclophosphamide*	Generics	Injection, powder for reconstitution: 200 mg‡, 500 mg†, 1 g, 2 g
	Procytox	Tablets: 25 mg, 50 mg
cyclosporine* (ciclosporin)	Gengraf, Neoral, Restasis, Sandimmune	Capsules, modified (Gengraf, Neoral): 10 mg‡, 25 mg, 50 mg, 100 mg
	Neoral, Sandimmune	Capsules, nonmodified (Sandimmune): 25 mg, 100 mg
		Emulsion, ophthalmic (Restasis): 0.05%
		Solution, for injection, (Sandimmune): 50 mg/mL
		Solution, oral, modified (Gengraf, Neoral): 100 mg/mL
		Solution, nonmodified: 100 mg/mL
methotrexate*	Rheumatrex, Trexall	Injection, powder for reconstitution: 1000 mg†
	Methotrexate	Injection, solution: 10 mg/mL, 25 mg/mL
		Tablets: 2.5 mg (Rheumatrex), 5 mg, 7.5 mg, 10 mg, 15 mg (Trexall)
		Tablets (Rheumatrex Dose Pack): 2.5 mg (4 cards with 2, 3, 4, 5, or 6 tablets each)
mitoxantrone	Novantrone	Injection, solution: 2 mg/mL
	Generics	

*Generic available.
†Strength available in the United States only.
‡Strength available in Canada only.

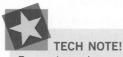

TECH NOTE!
For cyclosporine solution for injection: Do not refrigerate. Protect from light. DILUTE SOLUTION AND USE IMMEDIATELY. Stable for 6 hours in plastic IV bags or 24 hours in glass.

TECH ALERT!
The following drugs have look-alike/sound-alike issues: cyclosporine, cyclo-serine, and cyclophosphamide; Gengraf and Prograf; Neoral and Nizoral

hemorrhagic cystitis, bladder cancer, hypoglycemia, and bone marrow depression. Adverse reactions to cyclosporine include kidney toxicity, infections, nausea, abdominal pain, mouth sores, gingival hyperplasia, headache, hirsutism, weight gain, hepatotoxicity, and hypertension. Methotrexate's side effects include nausea, vomiting, diarrhea, GI ulceration, rash, photosensitivity, hair loss, bone marrow depression, hepatotoxicity, renal toxicity, and stomach pain. Adverse reactions to mixantrone include nausea and vomiting, hair loss, palpitations, leukopenia, blue urine or sclera (white part of the eye), menstrual irregularities, skin rash, mouth sores, dizziness, and drowsiness.

TUMOR NECROSIS FACTOR-α INHIBITORS

Tumor necrosis factor-α inhibitors are used in the treatment of RA. TNF is a cytokine that is released by cells that mobilize to fight what the body believes is a harmful invasion. High levels of TNF are found in the synovial fluid of people with RA, and the factor is responsible for joint-damaging inflammation. TNF-α inhibitors are genetically engineered drugs that block the inflammatory process triggered by high concentrations of TNF. They prevent cell lysis (destruction) and release of the substances that cause inflammation. Monoclonal antibodies used in the treatment of RA are adalimumab, certolizumab, golimumab, and infliximab. They bind to TNF-α and interfere with the inflammatory process by reducing mediators of the inflammatory response. Etanercept is a fusion protein that inhibits TNF-α.

Precautions

In some cases, the body recognizes the nonhuman proteins and produces antibodies to the drug, resulting in allergic and immune system reactions such as anaphylactic shock. All TNF-α inhibitors increase the risk for opportunistic infections. The most commonly reported opportunistic infections associated with TNF-α inhibitors are tuberculosis and fungal infections. TNF-α inhibitors are known to cause the onset of MS in susceptible people and should be avoided if preexisting MS is suspected. TNF-α inhibitors are associated with the development of secondary cancers.

Adverse Reactions

In addition to opportunistic infections, adverse reactions common to all "-mabs" are rash, pruritus, nausea, headache, and injection site redness and itchiness. Redness, itching, and swelling at the injection site are the most common side effects of etanercept. Similar to monoclonal antibodies, etanercept may increase risk for infection and produce anaphylactic shock.

INTERLEUKIN ANTAGONISTS

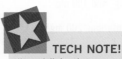

TECH NOTE!
"-mab" is the common ending for monoclonal antibody drugs (e.g., TNF-α inhibitors and IL inhibitors).

Multiple sclerosis, RA, SLE, and other autoimmune diseases have been associated with increased serum levels of ILs. Anakinra is a genetically engineered IL-1 receptor antagonist. It is approved for the treatment of RA. Anakinra interferes with the binding of ILs that promote inflammatory responses. Drug-receptor binding results in fewer lymphocytes and macrophages in synovial fluid. Adverse reactions to anakinra include redness or irritation at the injection site, infections, and bone or muscle weakness.

ANTIMALARIALS

Antimalarials have anti-inflammatory and analgesic properties that are useful in the management of RA and SLE. They are used to treat joint pain, skin rashes, and inflammation of the lungs associated with SLE. Hydroxychloroquine has been shown to reduce SLE flare-ups.

Although the exact mechanism of action is unknown, antimalarials are known to accumulate inside cell structures, where they raise the pH and interfere with processes that are normally stimulated when the body thinks its own cells are harmful antigens. An antigen is a substance that stimulates an immune response (see Figure 15-5).

The most common adverse reaction is GI irritation; however, chloroquine and hydroxychloroquine can cause permanent damage to the retina, resulting in blindness. This adverse reaction is associated with long-term chronic use (greater than 10 years) at doses greater than 400 mg/day. Additional adverse reactions include nausea, stomach pain, visual disturbances, and tinnitus.

ADDITIONAL DISEASE-MODIFYING ANTIRHEUMATIC DRUGS

Leflunomide is approved for the treatment of RA and selectively blocks the replication of lymphocytes by interfering with pyrimidine synthesis. Leflunomide's effectiveness is enhanced when used along with methotrexate, but the FDA issued a box warning advising that the combination may increase the risk for liver toxicity. Additive effects are achieved because together they block both pathways in the cell division process for lymphocytes (purine and pyrimidine synthesis). Adverse reactions include nausea, diarrhea, rash, hair loss, liver dysfunction, and fetal toxicity.

Sulfasalazine is used in the treatment of RA. It is classified as a DMARD and was developed by combining an anti-infective agent (sulfapyridine) with an aspirin-like anti-inflammatory agent (5-aminosalicylic acid). It was once believed that RA was caused by a bacterial infection. Sulfasalazine slows the progression of RA. Sulfasalazine takes about 2 to 3 months to produce maximum effects.

Antimalarials Used in the Treatment of Systemic Lupus Erythematosus and/or Rheumatoid Arthritis

Generic Name	U.S. Brand Name(s) Canadian Brand(s)	Dosage Forms and Strengths
chloroquine*	Aralen	**Tablets:** 250 mg, 500 mg (Aralen 500 mg)[†]
	Generics	
hydroxychloroquine*	Plaquenil	**Tablets:** 200 mg (155 mg base)
	Plaquenil	

*Generic available.
[†]Strength available in the United States only.

Common side effects are GI upset, increased sensitivity to sunlight, allergy, crystalluria, impaired folic acid absorption, and damage to white blood cells (cytopenias).

Gold compounds are used in the treatment of RA; however, their use is limited because of side effects, cost, and lack of sustained effectiveness. Gold compounds are believed to affect the function of B cells and macrophages, part of the immune system response. They decrease the release of antibodies and cytokines and inhibit the action of collagenase. Gold compounds may be delivered by mouth or intramuscular injection. The onset of action is slow, and it can take 4 to 6 months before maximum effectiveness is achieved. Gold compounds can produce temporary remission in about 50% of the people who respond favorably to the drug. The drug is most effective when administered along with other DMARDs such as methotrexate. Adverse reactions to auranofin and gold sodium thiomalate include itching rash, metallic taste, sore mouth, photosensitivity, cytopenias, interstitial pneumonia, and proteinuria.

Penicillamine has anti-inflammatory actions and alters immune system response. This makes it useful in the treatment of RA. It inhibits T-cell function and blocks collagen cross-linking. Adverse reactions include rash, GI upset, and nephrotoxicity.

BIOLOGICAL RESPONSE MODIFIERS

Autoimmune diseases are caused by a defective immune system response that causes the body to attack its own normal healthy cells. Biological response modifiers act to inhibit or modify immune system response. They inhibit the release of cells that mobilize to fight what the body believes is a harmful invasion and inhibit the release of substances that produce inflammation. Chronic inflammation can cause degeneration of nerves, bones, and muscles. Biological response modifiers interfere with the activity of immune system mediators such as cytokines, leukocytes, B cells, and T cells. Many DMARDs are biological response modifiers, including immunosuppressives, TNF inhibitors, and IL antagonists. Biological response modifiers not previously described include IFNs and the fusion protein abatacept.

MONOCLONAL ANTIBODIES

Not all monoclonal antibodies used in the treatment of RA are TNF-α inhibitors. The monoclonal antibody rituximab depletes circulating B cells and tocilizumab inhibits IL-6. They interfere with the inflammatory process by reducing mediators of the inflammatory response. Rituximab is indicated for the treatment of RA when TNF-α inhibitor therapy has been unsuccessful. Tocilizumab may be administered with methotrexate or given as monotherapy. It is approved for the treatment of RA and juvenile RA. Infusion reactions can occur with rituximab and tocilizumab and may be fatal. The drugs may increase the risk for infection, and live vaccines should be avoided.

INTERFERONS

There are approximately 2000 IFN receptors on each normal and malignant cell. These receptors recognize and bind IFNs, proteins with antigenic properties. IFN-β1a and IFN-β1b are first-line therapies for the treatment of MS. They alter the actions of T cells and B cells and other cytokines that produce immune response and inflammation. They reduce the development of the brain lesions

TECH ALERT!
The following drugs have look-alike/sound-alike issues: methotrexate and mitoxantrone; sulfasalazine, sulfadizine, and sulfisoxazole; Ridura and Cardura; penicillamine and penicillin

TECH NOTE!
Drug vials and cytotoxic waste (e.g., cyclophosphamide, mitoxantrone, methotrexate, and azathioprine), including bags, sets, tubing, and gloves, must be properly disposed of in the cytotoxic waste containers.

Biological Response Modifiers Used in the Treatment of Rheumatoid Arthritis

Generic Name	U.S. Brand Name(s) / Canadian Brand(s)	Dosage Forms and Strengths
abatacept	Orencia	Powder, for injection: 250 mg per vial
	Orencia	
rituximab	Rituxan	Solution, for injection: 100 mg/10 mL, 500 mg/50 mL
	Rituxan	
tocilizumab	Actemra	Solution, for injection: 80 mg/4 mL, 200 mg/10 mL, 400 mg/20 mL
	Actemra	

Interferons Used in the Treatment of Multiple Sclerosis

Generic Name	U.S. Brand Name(s) Canadian Brand(s)	Dosage Forms and Strengths
interferon β1a	Avonex, Rebif	Injection, powder for reconstitution (Avonex): 33 mcg
	Avonex, Rebif	Injection, solution (Avonex): 30 mcg/0.5 mL (0.5 mL prefilled syringe)
		Injection, solution (Rebif): 22 mcg/0.5 mL and 44 mcg/0.5 mL (0.5 mL prefilled syringe)
interferon β1b	Betaseron, Extavia	Injection, powder for reconstitution: 0.3 mg
	Betaseron, Extavia	

Miscellaneous Drugs Used in the Treatment of Multiple Sclerosis

Generic Name	U.S. Brand Name(s) Canadian Brand(s)	Dosage Forms and Strengths
dalfampridine	Ampyra	Tablets, extended release: 10 mg
	Not available	
fingolimod^	Gilenya	Capsules: 0.5 mg
	Gilenya	
glatiramer^	Copaxone	Solution, for injection: 20 mg/mL prefilled syringe
	Copaxone	
natalizumab	Tysabri	Solution, for injection: 300 mg/15 mL
	Tysabri	

^Biological response modifiers.

that cause disability in people who have MS. Adverse reactions of IFN-β1a and IFN-β1b include flulike symptoms, headache, fatigue, weight loss, anorexia, and neutropenia.

FUSION PROTEINS

Abatacept, similar to etanercept, is a fusion protein that is used to treat RA. Unlike the TNF-α inhibitor etanercept, abatacept blocks T-cell activation. Abatacept is only recommended in patients who have not improved on combined methotrexate therapy or nonbiologic DMARD therapy. The most common side effects of abatacept are headache, dizziness, nausea, and hypertension. Abatacept may increase risk for infection and produce anaphylactic shock, and its use is associated with the development of cancers.

MISCELLANEOUS DRUGS USED FOR THE TREATMENT OF MULTIPLE SCLEROSIS

Glatiramer is also administered for the treatment of relapsing-remitting MS. The exact mechanism is unknown. Injection site irritation and chest pain are the most common side effects. Other adverse effects are flulike syndrome, sweating, back pain, headache, and nausea. Fingolimod is used in the treatment of relapsing-remitting MS. It blocks the movement of lymphocytes into the peripheral bloodstream. Fingolimod may cause bradycardia and heart block after the initial dose, so patients are observed for up to 6 hours after the first dose. More commonly, it causes cough, diarrhea, back pain, and weight loss. It may also elevate triglycerides and liver enzymes.

DRUGS USED TO IMPROVE MUSCLE STRENGTH
Cholinesterase Inhibitors

Cholinesterase inhibitors block the destruction of acetylcholine at the neuromuscular junction, increasing the amount available to bind at receptors and improving muscle strength. Cholinesterase inhibitors are used to treat muscle weakness in patients with myasthenia gravis. Side effects of neostigmine and pyridostigmine include nausea, vomiting, abdominal cramps, diarrhea, hypersalivation, increased bronchial secretions, and hypotension.

Potassium Channel Blockers

Dalfampridine is used to improve walking in patients with multiple sclerosis. It is a potassium channel blocker. The drug increases action potential in demyelinated nerves. Side effects include insomnia, headache dizziness, seizures, and balance disorders. Dalfampridine may also increase the risk for urinary tract infections.

CONTROL OF DISEASE-RELATED SYMPTOMS IN AUTOIMMUNE DISEASES AFFECTING THE MUSCULOSKELETAL SYSTEM

Multiple sclerosis, myasthenia gravis, RA, SLE, and myositis produce symptoms secondary to inflammation, brain lesions, and nerve degeneration. MS can cause spasticity, fatigue, optic neuritis, trigeminal neuralgia, and bladder and sexual dysfunction. Drug therapy for spasticity is covered in detail in Chapter 14, fatigue in Chapter 12, and trigeminal neuralgia in Chapter 10. A summary of the drugs used to treat secondary symptoms of autoimmune diseases affecting the musculoskeletal system is given in Table 15-1.

Cholinesterase Inhibitors Used in the Treatment of Myasthenia Gravis

Generic Name	U.S. Brand Name(s) / Canadian Brand(s)	Dosage Forms and Strengths
neostigmine	Generics	Solution, for injection: 0.5 mg/mL, 1 mg/mL, 2mg/mL
	Prostigmin	Tablets: 15 mg‡
pyridostigmine	Mestinon, Mestinon Timespan, Regonol	Solution, for injection: 5 mg/mL
	Mestinon, Mestinon SR	Syrup, oral: 60 mg/5 mL / Tablets: 60 mg / Tablet, extended release: 180 mg

TABLE 15-1 **Drugs Used to Treat Specific Symptoms of Myasthenia Gravis, Multiple Sclerosis, Rheumatoid Arthritis, and Systemic Lupus Erythematosus**

Acute Symptom	Drug	Disease
Inflammation, joint swelling	**Glucocorticosteroids** dexamethasone hydrocortisone methylprednisolone prednisone	Myasthenia gravis (MG) Multiple sclerosis (MS) Rheumatoid arthritis (RA) Systemic lupus erythematosus (SLE) Myositis—all glucocorticosteroids listed
	NSAIDs celecoxib ibuprofen naproxen	MG, MS, RA, SLE—all NSAIDs listed
	Antimalarials hydroxychloroquine chloroquine	RA RA
Pain	aspirin acetaminophen NSAIDs opioids antidepressants	MS, RA, SLE, myositis, MG—all agents listed

TABLE 15-1   **Drugs Used to Treat Specific Symptoms of Myasthenia Gravis, Multiple Sclerosis, Rheumatoid Arthritis, and Systemic Lupus Erythematosus—cont'd**

Acute Symptom	Drug	Disease
Spasticity	**Peripheral-acting skeletal muscle relaxants**	
	dantrolene	MS
	Central-acting skeletal muscle relaxants	
	baclofen	MS
	diazepam	MS
	tizanidine	MS
Fatigue	amantadine*	MS
	pemoline*	MS
	antidepressants*	MS
Trigeminal neuralgia	carbamazepine	MS
Muscle weakness	neostigmine	MG
	pyridostigmine	MG
	dalfampridine	MS
Slow disease progression	**Disease-modifying antirheumatic drugs**	
	Immunosuppressives	
	azathioprine	RA (SLE, MG)*
	cyclophosphamide	(RA, SLE, myositis)*
	cyclosporine	RA
	methotrexate	RA, SLE
	mitoxantrone	MS
	Tumor necrosis factor inhibitors	
	adalimumab	RA
	certolizumab	RA
	etanercept	RA
	golimumab	RA
	infliximab	RA
	tocilizumab	RA
	Interleukin antagonists	
	anakinra	RA
	Other	
	gold salts	RA
	hydroxychloroquine	RA
	lefluonomide	RA
	penicillamine	RA
	sulfasalazine	RA
	Biological response modifiers (non DMARD)	
	Interferons	
	interferon β1a	MS
	interferon β1b	MS
	Other	
	abatacept	RA
	fingolimod	MS
	glatiramer	MS
	rituximab	RA
	tocilizumab	RA

*Unlabeled use.

Usual Dosage and Warnings for Drugs Used in the Treatment of Myasthenia Gravis, Multiple Sclerosis, Rheumatoid Arthritis, and Systemic Lupus Erythematosus

Generic Name	U.S. Brand Name	Usual Adult Oral Dose and Dosing Schedule	Warning Labels
dexamethasone	Generics	**MS:** **Oral:** 16 mg/day given in 4 divided doses for 5 days **Myasthenia gravis, RA, SLE:** **Oral:** 0.75-9 mg/day given in 2-4 divided doses	TAKE WITH FOOD. DO NOT DISCONTINUE ABRUPTLY. TAKE AT THE SAME TIME EACH DAY. TAKE WITH A FULL GLASS OF WATER.
hydrocortisone	Cortef	**Myasthenia gravis, MS, SLE:** **Oral:** 20-240 mg once daily or on alternate days **IM:** 15-240 mg once daily or on alternate days	
methylprednisolone	Medrol	**MS:** 200 mg once daily PO for 7 days followed by 80 mg every other day for 1 month or 160 mg IM or IV daily for 1 week followed by 64 mg PO, IV, or IM every other day for 1 month **Myasthenia gravis:** 12-20 mg PO daily for 1-3 months; may increase dose 4 mg every 2-3 days up to maximum 40 mg/day **RA, SLE:** 4-48 mg PO daily in 4 divided doses or 10-120 mg IM or 10-40 mg IV infused over several minutes	
prednisone	Generics	**Myasthenia gravis:** Initially, 15-20 mg/day PO; increase by 5 mg every 2-3 days as needed (maximum, 60 mg/day) **RA:** 5-30 mg PO once daily **SLE:** 20-300 mg/day PO in 2-3-divided doses (acute) **Maintenance:** 10-20 mg once daily or 20-40 mg every other day	
NSAIDs			
celecoxib	Celebrex	**Osteoarthritis:** 200 mg/day in 1-2 divided doses **RA:** 100-200 mg twice a day	TAKE WITH FOOD. AVOID ASPIRIN AND RELATED PRODUCTS. MAY CAUSE DIZZINESS OR DROWSINESS. SWALLOW WHOLE; DO NOT CRUSH OR CHEW—EC-Naprosyn.
ibuprofen	Motrin	**Inflammatory disease, RA:** 400-800 mg 3-4 times a day (maximum, 3200 mg/day)	
naproxen	Anaprox, Naprosyn	**RA, osteoarthritis:** 500-1000 mg/day in 2 divided doses up to 1500 mg	

Continued

Usual Dosage and Warnings for Drugs Used in the Treatment of Myasthenia Gravis, Multiple Sclerosis, Rheumatoid Arthritis, and Systemic Lupus Erythematosus—cont'd

Generic Name	U.S. Brand Name	Usual Adult Oral Dose and Dosing Schedule	Warning Labels
Antimalarials			
chloroquine	Aralen	RA: 250 mg (150 mg base) daily until maximal response; then taper to discontinue (usually 3-6 weeks)	AVOID ANTACIDS (and kaolin products) WITHIN 2 HOURS OF DOSE. TAKE WITH FOOD. AVOID PROLONGED EXPOSURE TO SUNLIGHT.
hydroxychloroquine	Plaquenil	RA: 400-600 mg/day; when optimal response is reached (4-12 weeks), reduce dose to 200-400 mg/day SLE: Begin 400 mg (310 mg base) 1-2 times daily; maintenance, 200-400 mg/day	
Immunosuppressives			
azathioprine	Imuran	RA: 1 mg/kg/day for 6-8 weeks; increase every 4 weeks up to 2.5 mg/kg/day	TAKE WITH FOOD. AVOID PREGNANCY.
cyclophosphamide	Cytoxan	SLE: 1-3 mg/kg PO once daily or 0.5-1 mg/m² IV monthly for 6 months; then every 2-3 months RA: 1.5-2.5 mg/kg PO once daily or 0.5-1 mg/m² IV monthly for 6 months; then every 2-3 months	TAKE WITH A FULL GLASS OF WATER. TAKE AT THE SAME TIME EACH DAY. SWALLOW WHOLE; DO NOT CRUSH OR CHEW—cyclosporine, cyclophosphamide. AVOID PREGNANCY.
cyclosporine (ciclosporin)	Neoral, Sandimmune	RA: Begin 2.5 mg/kg/day in 2 divided doses; increase 0.5 mg to 0.75 mg/kg/day after 8 weeks if inadequate response; maximum dose, 4 mg/kg/day	AVOID ASPIRIN and NSAIDs—cyclophosphamide. AVOID ALCOHOL—cyclosporine. AVOID GRAPEFRUIT JUICE—cyclosporine. AVOID PREGNANCY.
fingolimod	Gilenya	MS: 0.5 mg PO once daily	AVOID PREGNANCY.
methotrexate	Rheumatrex	RA: 7.5 mg PO once a week or 2.5 mg every 12 hours for 3 doses/week (maximum, 20 mg/wk) SLE: 5-10 mg IV or IM once weekly up to 50 mg per week	TAKE WITH A FULL GLASS OF WATER. AVOID ALCOHOL. AVOID ASPIRIN and NSAIDs. AVOID PROLONGED EXPOSURE TO SUNLIGHT. AVOID PREGNANCY.
mitoxantrone	Novantrone	MS: 12 mg/m² IV infused once every 3 months	AVOID ASPIRIN and NSAIDs. MAY DISCOLOR URINE, NAILS, OR THE WHITES OF THE EYES (blue-green). AVOID PREGNANCY.

Usual Dosage and Warnings for Drugs Used in the Treatment of Myasthenia Gravis, Multiple Sclerosis, Rheumatoid Arthritis, and Systemic Lupus Erythematosus—cont'd

Generic Name	U.S. Brand Name	Usual Adult Oral Dose and Dosing Schedule	Warning Labels
Interferons			
interferon β1a	Avonex, Rebif	**MS:** 30 mcg IM (Avonex) once weekly **MS:** 44 mcg subcut (Rebif) 3 times a week	REFRIGERATE; DO NOT FREEZE. WARM PREFILLED SYRINGES TO ROOM TEMP BEFORE USING.
interferon β1b	Betaseron	**MS:** 0.25 mg subcut every other day	AVOID PREGNANCY.
Monoclonal Antibodies			
adalimumab	Humira	**RA:** 40 mg subcut every other week (if not taking methotrexate 40 mg/wk)	PROTECT FROM LIGHT. REFRIGERATE; DO NOT FREEZE.
certolizumab	Cimzia	**RA:** 400 mg subcut, given as two 200-mg subcut injections at weeks 0, 2, and 4; then 200 mg subcut every other week	REFRIGERATE POWDER AND RECONSTITUTED PRODUCT. ROTATE SITE OF INJECTION.
golimumab	Simponi	**RA:** 50 mg subcut once monthly	ROTATE SITE OF INJECTION. DO NOT SHAKE PREFILLED SYRINGE.
infliximab	Remicade	**RA:** 3 mg/kg at 2 and 6 weeks after first dose; repeat in 8 weeks; if IV infusion, 3-10 mg/kg; repeat at 4- or 8-week intervals	REFRIGERATE; DO NOT FREEZE. GENTLY SWIRL RECONSTITUTED PRODUCT; DO NOT SHAKE AFTER MIXING, DISCARD ANY UNUSED PORTION.
rituximab	Rituxan	**RA:** 1000 mg IV on days 1 and 15; repeat every 16-24 weeks based on clinical evaluation	REFRIGERATE VIALS. GENTLY INVERT IV BAG TO MIX TO AVOID FOAMING. AFTER MIXING, DISCARD ANY UNUSED PORTION.
tocilizumab	Actemra	**RA:** 4 mg/kg IV every 4 weeks; maximum, 8 mg/kg	REFRIGERATE VIALS. GENTLY INVERT IV BAG TO MIX TO AVOID FOAMING. AFTER MIXING, DISCARD ANY UNUSED PORTION.
Other Biological Response Modifiers			
abatacept	Orencia	**RA:** 1000 mg IV every 2 weeks; beginning week 8, administer 1000 mg every 4 weeks	USE WITHIN 24 HOURS OF MIXING; DISCARD UNUSED PORTION.
anakinra	Kineret	**RA:** 100 mg subcut once daily	ROTATE SITE OF INJECTION. GENTLY SWIRL TO DISSOLVE. REFRIGERATE. PROTECT FROM LIGHT.

Continued

Usual Dosage and Warnings for Drugs Used in the Treatment of Myasthenia Gravis, Multiple Sclerosis, Rheumatoid Arthritis, and Systemic Lupus Erythematosus—cont'd

Generic Name	U.S. Brand Name	Usual Adult Oral Dose and Dosing Schedule	Warning Labels
etanercept	Enbrel	**RA:** 25 mg subcut twice weekly or 50 mg once weekly	ROTATE SITE OF INJECTION. GENTLY SWIRL TO DISSOLVE. REFRIGERATE. PROTECT FROM LIGHT.
glatiramer	Copaxone	**MS:** 20 mg subcut once daily	REFRIGERATE; DO NOT FREEZE. PROTECT FROM LIGHT.
DMARDs			
leflunomide	Arava	**RA:** Start 100 mg/day for 3 days; decrease to 20 mg/day	AVOID PROLONGED EXPOSURE TO SUNLIGHT—auranofin, sulfasalazine.
sulfasalazine	Azulfidine	**RA:** Start 500-1000 mg/day; increase to 2000-3000 mg/day in 2 divided doses (enteric-coated tablets)	MAINTAIN ADEQUATE HYDRATION—sulfasalazine.
auranofin	Ridura	**RA:** 6 mg/day in 1-2 divided doses (maximum, 9 mg/day)	MAY DISCOLOR URINE (or skin)—orange-yellow, sulfasalazine.
gold sodium thiomalate	Aurolate	**RA:** Start 10 mg/week (IM); increase to 25-50 mg/wk until 1000-mg cumulative dose has been reached; if effective, continue 25-50 mg every 2-3 weeks for 2-20 weeks; then once every 3-4 weeks indefinitely	DISCARD IF DARKENED (solution should be clear or pale yellow).
penicillamine	Cupramine	**RA:** 125-250 mg/day (maximum, 1500 mg/day)	TAKE ON AN EMPTY STOMACH.

Chapter Summary

- An autoimmune disease occurs when the immune system attacks its own cells, thinking they are germs or a harmful substance.
- Triggers for autoimmunity may be exposure to a virus, environmental toxins, the sun, genetics, hormonal changes, drugs, pregnancy, or some combination of any of these things.
- Myasthenia gravis, multiple sclerosis (MS), rheumatoid arthritis (RA), and systemic lupus erythematosus (SLE) are examples of autoimmune diseases that affect the musculoskeletal system.
- In myasthenia gravis, the body attacks and destroys receptor sites in the neuromuscular junction that bind acetycholine (ACh), resulting in muscle weakness.
- Myositis causes chronic inflammation of the muscles.
- Myelin, the insulating coating of nerves, is attacked in MS.
- MS causes muscle weakness; fatigue; spasticity; pain; bladder, bowel, and sexual dysfunction; speech disturbances; and depression.
- RA is characterized by inflammation of the lining of the joints.
- RA is more common in women than in men.
- SLE affects nearly all parts of the body and produces swollen, painful joints similar to RA.
- Other signs and symptoms of SLE are muscle pain, fever, red rashes, hair loss, sun sensitivity, swollen glands, extreme fatigue, seizures, mouth ulcers, and poor circulation in the fingers and toes.

- Drug therapy for autoimmune diseases affecting the musculoskeletal system is aimed at suppressing inflammation, pain, and immune system response. Treatment goals are also aimed at minimizing further nerve or joint destruction, preservation of body functions, and prevention of disability.
- Glucocorticosteroids are prescribed to suppress inflammation, reduce flare-ups, and treat pain.
- Glucocorticosteroids have immunosuppressive actions and they inhibit the synthesis of antibodies that are responsible for attacking the body's healthy cells.
- Nonsteroidal anti-inflammatory drugs (NSAIDs) and aspirin (ASA) are widely used in the treatment of pain and inflammation.
- Celecoxib is the only selective cyclooxygenase-2 (COX-2) inhibitor still available for use in the United States and Canada. Its use is restricted in Canada.
- Selective COX-2 inhibitors increase the risk for cardiovascular toxicity and gastrointestinal ulceration.
- Antimalarials have anti-inflammatory and analgesic properties that are useful in the management of RA and SLE.
- Biological response modifiers act to inhibit the release of cells that mobilize to fight what the body believes is a harmful invasion and inhibit the release of substances that produce inflammation.
- Biological response modifiers interfere with the activity of cytokines, leukocytes, B cells, and T cells.
- Immunosuppressive drugs interfere with the formation of immune cells by damaging RNA and DNA needed for cell replication.
- Interferon- β1a (IFN-β1a) and interferon β1b are first-line therapies for the treatment of MS, and they alter the actions of T cells and B cells and other cytokines that produce immune response and inflammation.
- Tumor necrosis factor-α (TNF-α) inhibitors are genetically engineered drugs that block the inflammatory process triggered by high concentrations of TNF.
- MS, RA, SLE, and other autoimmune diseases have been associated with increased serum levels of interleukins (ILs).
- IL-1 receptor antagonists interfere with the binding of ILs that promote inflammatory responses.
- Methotrexate blocks purine synthesis needed for lymphocyte cell proliferation, reducing inflammation and immune system activity.
- Leflunomide interferes with pyrimidine synthesis, and when used along with methotrexate, both pathways in the cell division process for lymphocytes are blocked.
- Sulfasalazine is a combination of an anti-infective agent and an aspirin-like anti-inflammatory agent, and it is used to treat RA.
- Gold compounds are used in the treatment of RA and work by decreasing the release of antibodies and cytokines and inhibiting the action of collagenase, actions that are part of the immune response.
- Penicillamine is used in the treatment of RA because it has anti-inflammatory actions and alters immune-system response.
- Cholinesterase inhibitors improve muscle strength in patients with myasthenia gravis. They block the destruction of ACh at the neuromuscular junction.

1. A disease that occurs when the immune system turns against the parts of the body it is designed to protect is called a(an) _____.
   a. autoimmune disease
   b. viral disease
   c. immune disease
   d. bacterial disease

2. Which of the following is *not* an example of an autoimmune disease?
   a. myasthenia gravis
   b. rheumatoid arthritis
   c. osteoarthritis
   d. systemic lupus erythematosus

3. In myasthenia gravis, the body attacks and destroys receptor sites in the neuromuscular junction that bind _____.
   a. dopamine
   b. epinephrine
   c. GABA
   d. acetylcholine

4. Systemic lupus erythematosus is an autoimmune disease that affects nearly _____ parts of the body.
   a. one-fourth of the
   b. all
   c. the trunk
   d. one-half of the

5. _____ are prescribed commonly to suppress inflammation, reduce flare-ups, and treat pain associated with multiple sclerosis, myasthenia gravis, systemic erythematosus, myositis, and rheumatoid arthritis.
   a. Mineralocorticoids
   b. Glucocorticosteroids
   c. Anabolic steroids
   d. All of the above

6. Aspirin and NSAIDs inhibit the release and block the activity of _____.
   a. prostaglandins
   b. COX-1
   c. COX-2
   d. all of the above

7. _____ response modifiers interfere with the activity of cytokines, leukocytes, B cells, and T cells.
   a. Biological
   b. Microbiological
   c. Neurological
   d. Protein

8. Tumor necrosis factor-α inhibitors are _____ engineered drugs that block the inflammatory process triggered by high concentrations of tumor necrosis factor.
   a. chemically
   b. biologically
   c. genetically
   d. neurologically

9. Which of the following drugs is indicated for the treatment of active rheumatoid arthritis, ankylosing spondylitis, and chronic plaque psoriasis?
   a. Enbrel
   b. Remicade
   c. Humira
   d. Kineret

10. Gold compounds can produce permanent remission in about 50% of the people who respond favorably to the drug.
    a. true
    b. false

TECHNICIAN'S CORNER

1. Celebrex is the only prescriptive COX-2 inhibitor left on the market. Discuss the FDA's or Health Canada's role in identifying postmarket drug safety issues.
2. What are some nonpharmacological therapies for autoimmune diseases?

Bibliography

Arthritis Foundation Disease Center: Rheumatoid arthritis: overview. Retrieved from http://www.arthritis.org/conditions/DiseaseCenter/RA/ra_overview.asp.

Crayton H, Rossman H: Managing the symptoms of multiple sclerosis: a multimodal approach, *Clin Ther* 28, 2006.

Doan T, Massarotti E: Rheumatoid arthritis: an overview of new emerging therapies, *J Clin Pharmacol* 45:751-762, 2005.

Elsevier: Gold Standard Clinical Pharmacology. Retrieved April 2, 2011, from https://www.clinical pharmacology.com/, 2010.

FDA: Drugs@FDA. Retrieved May 4, 2012, from http://www.accessdata.fda.gov/scripts/cder/drugsatfda/index.cfm?fuseaction=Search.Search_Drug_Name, 2012.

Fox R, Bethoux F, Goldman M, et al: Multiple sclerosis: advances in understanding, diagnosing, and treating the underlying disease, *Cleve Clin J Med* 73:91-102, 2006.

Health Canada: Drug Product Database. Retrieved March 29, 2011, from http://www.hc-sc.gc.ca/dhp-mps/prodpharma/databasdon/index-eng.php, 2010.

Kalant H, Grant D, Mitchell J: *Principles of medical pharmacology*, ed 7, Toronto, 2007, Elsevier Canada, A Division of Reed Elsevier Canada, pp 548-549, 553-554, 595-596.

Lance L, Lacy C, Armstrong L, et al: *Drug information handbook for the allied health professional*, ed 12, Hudson, OH, 2005, APhA Lexi-Comp.

Myasthenia Gravis Foundation of America Inc.: Clinical Overview of MG. Retrieved March 28, 2011, from http://www.myasthenia.org/HealthProfessionals/ClinicalOverviewofMG.aspx, 2006, June 2010.

National Institute of Arthritis and Musculoskeletal and Skin Diseases: *Autoimmunity*, Bethesda, MD, 2002, NIAMS, National Institutes of Health, U.S. Department of Health and Human Services. NIH Publication No. 02-4858. Retrieved from http://www.niams.nih.gov/hi/topics/autoimmune/autoimmunity.htm.

National Institute of Arthritis and Musculoskeletal and Skin Diseases: *Systemic lupus erythematosus*, Bethesda, MD, 2003, NIAMS, National Institutes of Health, U.S. Department of Health and Human Services. NIH publication No. 03-4178. Retrieved from http://www.niams.nih.gov/hi/topics/lupus/slehand-out/index.htm.

National Institute of Neurological Disorders and Stroke: *Multiple sclerosis: hope through research*, Bethesda, MD, 2006, NINDS, National Institutes of Health, U.S. Department of Health and Human Services. NIH publication No. 96-75. Retrieved from http://www.ninds.nih.gov/disorders/multiple_sclerosis/multiple_sclerosis_pr.htm.

National Institute of Neurological Disorders and Stroke: *Myasthenia gravis fact sheet*, Bethesda, MD, 2011, NINDS, National Institutes of Health, U.S. Department of Health and Human Services. NIH publication No. 10-768. Retrieved from http://www.ninds.nih.gov/disorders/myasthenia_gravis/detail_myasthenia_gravis.htm.

Page C, Curtis M, Sutter M, et al: *Integrated pharmacology*, Philadelphia, 2005, Mosby, pp 228-233, 336-341, 445-452.

Pharmaceutical Sciences, Vancouver General Hospital, Vancouver, British Columbia, Canada: Parenteral drug therapy manual, Retrieved from http://www.vhpharmsci.com/PDTM/.

Raffa R, Rawls S, Beyzarov E: *Netter's illustrated pharmacology*, Philadelphia, 2005, WB Saunders, p 79.

Torpy J: Myasthenia gravis, *JAMA* 293:1940, 2005.

USP Center for Advancement of Patient Safety: *Use caution–avoid confusion, USP Quality Review No. 79*, Rockville, MD, April 2004, USP Center for Advancement of Patient Safety.

World Health Organization: *Atlas multiple sclerosis resources in the world 2008*, Geneva, 2008, WHO Press.

Wright B, Bharadwaj S, Abelson A: Systemic Lupus Erythematosus. Retrieved April 2, 2011, from http://www.clevelandclinicmeded.com/medicalpubs/diseasemanagement/rheumatology/systemic-lupus-erythematosus/, 2010.

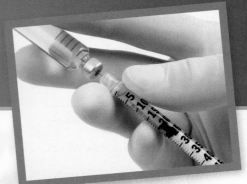

16

Treatment of Osteoporosis and Paget's Disease of the Bone

KEY TERMS

Bone mineral density: Test measurement that is taken to determine the degree of bone loss.

Bone resorption: Process during which bone is broken down into mineral ions (e.g., calcium).

Osteoblasts: Cells responsible for bone formation, deposition, and mineralization of the collagen matrix of bone.

Osteoclasts: Cells responsible for bone resorption.

Osteolysis: Dissolution or degradation of bone.

Osteopenia: Decrease in bone mineral density that places people at increased risk of developing osteoporosis.

Osteoporosis: Chronic, progressive disease of bone characterized by loss of bone density and bone strength and resulting in increased risk for fractures.

Remodeling: Process of continual turnover of bone.

Osteoporosis

Osteoporosis is the most common disease of bone. It affects 10 million men and women in the United States and up to 1.4 million people in Canada. It affects women more often than men, and eight in 10 people with the disease are women. *Osteoporosis* is a chronic, progressive disease of bone characterized by loss of bone density and bone strength, resulting in an increased fracture risk. The risk for osteoporosis increases with age, increasing from 4% of women ages 50 to 59 years up to 52% by age 80 years. *Osteopenia* is a condition whereby *bone mineral density* (BMD) is decreased. Osteopenia affects up to 34 million people in the United States. People with osteopenia are at increased risk of developing osteoporosis.

Osteoporosis is responsible for more than 1.5 million fractures annually in the United States. The most common are fractures of the vertebrae of the spine (700,000) and hips (300,000 in hips), although fractures of the wrists, feet, toes, and forearm also occur. The lifetime risk for fractures in people older than 50 years is one in two women and one in four men regardless of ethnic background. Fractures caused by osteoporosis are classified according to health outcomes as low-impact or fragility fractures. Low-impact osteoporosis fractures are often caused by falls or other trauma. Fragility fractures may occur in the absence of trauma and can occur from simply coughing or sneezing.

PATHOPHYSIOLOGY OF OSTEOPOROSIS

Primary osteoporosis is associated with the aging process. Up until the age of 30 or 40 years, the percentage of bone formed is greater than the percentage of bone lost. After menopause, women have a dramatic shift in the ratio between bone formation and bone loss, with bone loss exceeding bone formation. In men, this process is more gradual until the age 65 or 70 years; then the rates of bone loss for men and women are about equal.

Bone formation and loss is a carefully controlled process and is regulated from birth to death. The process is called *remodeling* (Figure 16-1). Osteoclasts and osteoblasts are cells that are involved in the bone turnover process. *Osteoblasts* are responsible for bone formation, deposition, and mineralization of the collagen matrix of bone. *Osteoclasts* are responsible for bone resorption. *Bone resorption* is the process whereby bone is broken down (*osteolysis*) into mineral ions (e.g., calcium).

Bone turnover is linked to levels of calcium in the blood (Figure 16-2). Ninety-nine percent of total body calcium is located in the skeleton; therefore, bones are a reservoir for calcium when serum levels are too low.

If serum calcium levels are too low, hormones are released to transfer calcium stored in bones back into serum. When blood levels are too high, hormones are released to reduce serum calcium and deposit excess in bones. The hormones principally responsible for regulation of serum calcium levels are parathyroid hormone (PTH), calcitonin, and vitamin D. PTH is secreted by the parathyroid gland when intestinal absorption of calcium and renal reabsorption of calcium are insufficient to maintain the required calcium balance. PTH mobilizes calcium from bone, increasing serum calcium levels by transferring calcium from bone to blood. Calcitonin reduces serum calcium levels by storing excess in the bone. Vitamin D enhances calcium absorption and is one of the hormones involved in the formation of osteoclasts. PTH and sex hormones are also associated with osteoclast formation. Other hormones linked to the regulation of bone formation and bone loss are estrogen, progesterone, luteinizing hormone, and androgens. Estrogen and progesterone levels are lowered in postmenopausal women, and testosterone levels are reduced in men as part of the normal aging process, which in part explains why calcium absorption decreases as men and women age.

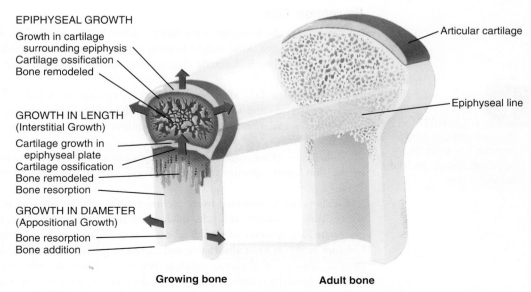

EPIPHYSEAL GROWTH
Growth in cartilage
  surrounding epiphysis
Cartilage ossification
Bone remodeled

Articular cartilage

Epiphyseal line

GROWTH IN LENGTH
(Interstitial Growth)

Cartilage growth in
  epiphyseal plate
Cartilage ossification
Bone remodeled
Bone resorption

GROWTH IN DIAMETER
(Appositional Growth)

Bone resorption
Bone addition

Growing bone   **Adult bone**

FIGURE 16-1 Bone remodeling. (From Thibodeau GA, Patton KT: *Anatomy and physiology*, ed 6, St Louis, 2007, Mosby.)

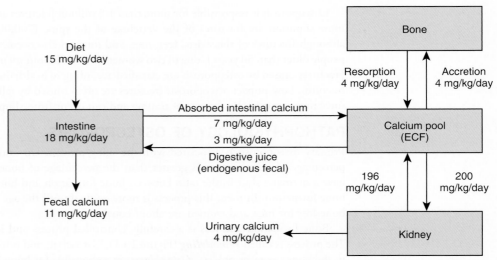

FIGURE 16-2 Calcium level fluctuations between bone, kidneys, intestines, and calcium reservoirs. (From Kalant H, Grant D, Mitchell J: *Principles of medical pharmacology*, ed 7, Toronto, 2007, Elsevier Canada.)

CONDITIONS THAT PRODUCE OSTEOPOROSIS

Osteoporosis can be classified as primary or secondary. Secondary osteoporosis may be related to another disease process or can be drug induced. Some of the diseases that can produce secondary osteoporosis include hyperthyroidism, hyperparathyroidism, rheumatoid arthritis, systemic lupus erythematosus, multiple myeloma, inflammatory bowel disease, renal insufficiency, Parkinson's disease, multiple sclerosis, chronic obstructive pulmonary disease, and AIDS. Some of the conditions associated with bone loss are shown in Box 16-1.

Drugs that can induce osteoporosis are administered for a wide variety of diseases. They are used in the treatment of autoimmune diseases of the musculoskeletal system, seizures, prostate cancer, bipolar disorder, hypothyroidism, kidney disease, and other conditions. Alcohol abuse can also produce osteoporosis. Examples of some of the drugs that can produce bone loss leading to osteoporosis are shown in Box 16-2.

Prevention Tips

It is best to lay the foundation for healthy dense bones early in life, although bone health can be improved at any age. Mild weight-bearing exercise along with a diet rich in vitamin D and calcium is key to strong bones. Lifestyle changes that reduce alcohol consumption and smoking are also important.

Recommended daily allowances (RDAs) for calcium are listed in Table 16-1. The Osteoporosis Society of Canada and the (U.S.) National Osteoporosis Foundation recommend that postmenopausal women and men at risk for fractures ingest 1200 mg of calcium and 800-1000 IU of vitamin D each day.

Milk, leafy green vegetables, and soybeans contain calcium, and vitamin D is produced by the skin upon exposure to sunlight. Foods rich in calcium and vitamin D are given in Table 16-2.

Calcium can be obtained from calcium supplements in addition to food. Calcium supplements are available as calcium chloride, calcium citrate, calcium carbonate, calcium lactate, and calcium gluconate. The amount of elemental calcium contained in these calcium salts varies (Table 16-3). Calcium citrate is most absorbable and easiest to tolerate; however, calcium carbonate provides the greatest amount of elemental calcium per tablet. Calcium carbonate should be taken on a full stomach. Food increases absorption and decreases upset stomach. Calcium citrate may be taken without regard to food.

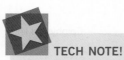

TECH NOTE!
Physical activity can improve bone health, but most people are not active enough.

BOX 16-1   **Diseases and Conditions That May Cause Bone Loss**

- HIV/AIDS
- Ankylosing spondylitis
- Blood and bone marrow disorders
- Chronic obstructive pulmonary disease
- Cushing's syndrome
- Cystic fibrosis
- Diabetes
- Eating disorders, especially anorexia nervosa and malnutrition
- Female athlete triad: loss of menstrual periods, an eating disorder, and excessive exercise
- Gastrectomy, including gastrointestinal bypass procedures
- Hyperparathyroidism
- Hyperthyroidism
- Hypocalcemia and hypophosphatemia
- Inflammatory bowel disease, including Crohn's disease and ulcerative colitis
- Kidney disease that is chronic and long lasting
- Liver disease, including biliary cirrhosis
- Malignancies, including lymphoma, leukemia, and multiple myeloma
- Malabsorption syndromes, including celiac disease
- Organ transplants
- Ovarian failure
- Polio and postpolio syndrome
- Premature menopause (before 45 years old)
- Reduced mobility diseases, including multiple sclerosis, muscular dystrophy, Parkinson's disease, spinal cord injuries, stroke
- Rheumatoid arthritis
- Sickle cell anemia and thalassemia
- Testosterone deficiency
- Thyrotoxicosis

Adapted from National Osteoporosis Foundation. (2011). Diseases and Conditions That May Cause Bone Loss.   Retrieved July 8, 2012, from http://www.nof.org/node/233.
U.S. Department of Health and Human Services. (2004). The 2004 Surgeon General's Report on Bone Health and Osteoporosis: What it Means to You. In U.S. Department of Health and Human Services (Ed.): Office of the Surgeon General.

BOX 16-2   **Drugs That Can Produce Bone Loss**

- Antiandrogens (flutamide and nilutamide)
- Aromatase inhibitors
- Cyclosporine
- Depo-medroxyprogesterone acetate
- Gonadotropin-releasing hormone agonists (leuprolide)
- Glucocorticosteroids
- Lithium
- Methotrexate
- Anticonvulsants (e.g., phenytoin)
- Thiazolidinediones

TABLE 16-1   **Your Body Needs Calcium**

If This Is Your Age	Then You Need This Much Calcium Each Day (mg)*
0-6 months	210
6-12 months	270
1-3 years	500
4-8 years	800
9-18 years	1300
18-50 years	1000
Older than 50 years	1200

*One cup of milk or fortified orange juice has about 300 mg of calcium.
Courtesy of NIH: The 2004 Surgeon General's Report on Bone Health and Osteoporosis.
http://www.ncbi.nlm.nih.gov/books/NBK44687

TABLE 16-2   **Calcium Calculator**

Food	Calcium (mg)	Points
Fortified oatmeal, 1 packet	350	3
Sardines, canned in oil, with edible bones, 3 oz	324	3
Cheddar cheese, 1½ oz shredded	306	3
Milk, nonfat, 1 cup	302	3
Milkshake, 1 cup	300	3
Yogurt, plain, low-fat, 1 cup	300	3
Soybeans, cooked, 1 cup	261	3
Tofu, firm, with calcium, 6 oz	204	2
Orange juice, fortified with calcium, 6 oz	200-260 (varies)	2-3
Salmon, canned, with edible bones, 3 oz	181	2
Pudding, instant (e.g., chocolate, banana) made with 2% milk, ½ cup	153	2
Baked beans, 1 cup	142	1
Cottage cheese, 1% milk fat, 1 cup	138	1
Spaghetti, lasagna, 1 cup	125	1
Frozen yogurt, vanilla, soft serve, ½ cup	103	1
Ready-to-eat cereal, fortified with calcium, 1 cup	100-1000 (varies)	1-10
Cheese pizza, 1 slice	100	1
Fortified waffles, 2	100	1
Turnip greens, boiled, ½ cup	99	1
Broccoli, raw, 1 cup	90	1
Ice cream, vanilla, ½ cup	85	1
Soy or rice milk, fortified with calcium, 1 cup	80-500 (varies)	1-5

Points Needed	Your Total Today
Babies and toddlers (ages 0-3)········2-5	
Children (ages 4-12)·················8	
Teens····························13	
Adults younger than age 50 years······10	
Adults older than age 50 years········12	

Courtesy of NIH: U.S. Department of Health and Human Services. (2004). The 2004 Surgeon General's Report on Bone Health and Osteoporosis: What it Means to You. In U.S. Department of Health and Human Services (Ed.): Office of the Surgeon General..

TABLE 16-3   Percent Elemental Calcium per Calcium Salt

Calcium Salt	Percent Elemental Calcium per Tablet	Strength Commercially Available (mg)	No. of Tablets Needed to Obtain Recommended Dose of 1200 to 1500 mg/day
Calcium carbonate	40	500-600	2-3
Calcium chloride	27	—	—
Calcium citrate	21	—	8
Calcium lactate	13	42.25-84.5	16
Calcium gluconate	9	45-90	16
Calcium phosphate	—	600	2-3
Oyster shell (calcium carbonate)	—	250-1250	1-6

TECH NOTE!
Calcium can inhibit absorption of some medicines, such as iron and levothyroxine. Warning labels should instruct patients to avoid calcium within 2 hours of any other medication taken by mouth.

TECH ALERT!
The following drugs have look-alike and sound-alike issues: Fosamax and Flomax; Aredia and Adriamycin; Actonel and Actos

Paget's Disease of Bone

Paget's disease is most common in men older than 55 years. The disease is most common in the United Kingdom, Australia, New Zealand, and North America and is uncommon in Africa, Asia, and Scandinavia. Approximately 2-3% of Americans and 3% of Canadians have Paget's disease. The cause is unknown, yet it is believed that genetics, viral infection (paramyxoviruses), and environmental factors are involved.

PATHOPHYSIOLOGY OF PAGET'S DISEASE OF THE BONE

Paget's disease is a progressive disease of bone. The disease produces irregular activity of osteoclasts and osteoblasts. Excessive bone resorption in focal areas is followed by increased bone formation, resulting in enlarged bones that are structurally weak. Effects of the disease tend to be localized and most commonly affect the pelvis, lumbar sacral spine, skull, femur, or tibia; however, Paget's disease may be widespread throughout the body, and the entire skeleton may be affected.

Paget's disease causes deformities such as bowed legs, pain, arthritis, deafness, and (rarely) cranial nerve palsies. Pain may be constant or intermittent. Intermittent pain is typically associated with weight bearing or localized microfractures. When pain is constant, it may even occur at rest.

Drugs Used for the Treatment of Osteoporosis and Paget's Disease of Bone

The goals of pharmacological treatment for osteoporosis are to increase bone density and to reduce risks for future fractures. Pharmacological agents are categorized as antiresorptive (inhibit bone resorption) or anabolic (promote bone formation).

Paget's disease is also treatable; however, treatment is recommended for patients who have symptoms of bone pain and localized neurological involvement. Treatment is also recommended when the vertebrae, femur, and base of the skull are involved because of risks for fractures and deafness.

ANTIRESORPTIVE AGENTS

The majority of the drugs used to treat osteoporosis and Paget's disease are antiresorptive agents. They suppress bone turnover and loss. Antiresorptive agents are further classified by their structure and mechanism of action. Classifications of antiresorptive agents are bisphosphonates, calcitonin, and estrogens.

Bisphosphonates

Most of the bisphosphonates are used for the treatment of Paget's disease and osteoporosis. Alendronate, risedronate, and ibandronate have been shown to reduce vertebral fractures by up to

40% to 50% and hip fractures by 20% to 50%. Intravenous zoledronic acid has been shown to reduce the relative risk of vertebral fractures by up to 70% and also reduces relative risk for hip fractures. Ibandronate is approved by the U.S. Food and Drug Administration (FDA) for Paget's disease, and etidronate, pamidronate, and tiludronate are not FDA approved for treatment of osteoporosis.

MECHANISM OF ACTION AND PHARMACOKINETICS

Bisphosphonates inhibit osteoclast activity, the cells responsible for bone resorption. Bisphosphonates interfere with recruitment, differentiation, and action of osteoclasts. There are two groups of bisphosphonates. The nitrogen-containing bisphosphonates (alendronate, pamidronate, risedronate) are more potent than the non–nitrogen-containing agents (etidronate, tiludronate). Pamidronate and zoledronic acid are bisphosphonates that are administered via intravenous infusion.

The bisphosphonates are poorly absorbed in the gastrointestinal tract, and food further reduces absorption. All but ibandronate must be taken on an empty stomach at least 30 minutes before the first meal or beverage of the day. Ibandronate must be taken 60 minutes before the first meal. Between 50% and 80% of the drug is eliminated unchanged in the urine within 24 hours of dosing. The remainder permanently binds to bone. Bisphosphonates are available in dosage forms for daily (alendronate, risedronate, ibandronate), weekly (alendronate, risedronate), monthly (risedronate, ibandronate), and yearly (zoledronic acid) dosing. Patient adherence is improved when the medication is dosed once weekly. Zoledronic acid is administered as a single dose annually for osteoporosis treatment or every 2 years when administered for prevention. In one study, it was shown to be as effective as a daily risedronate therapy at 6 months after the drug was infused. It is administered as a single dose to induce remission in Paget's disease.

ADVERSE REACTIONS

Common adverse effects associated with bisphosphonates are painful swallowing, heartburn, diarrhea, nausea, and vomiting. Less common adverse reactions are musculoskeletal pain, atypical fractures, osteonecrosis or erosion of the jaw bone, and eye inflammation. Studies are ongoing to evaluate whether bisphosphonates increase the risk for cancer of the esophagus.

PRECAUTIONS

To prevent injury to the esophagus by bisphosphonates, the patient should sit or stand upright for 30 to 60 minutes (depending on the agent) after taking the medication. Each tablet should be taken with 6 to 8 oz of water. Calcium and vitamin D supplementation is recommended in conjunction with bisphosphonates but should not be administered at the same time. Multivitamins with iron, calcium supplements, and antacids should be avoided within 2 hours of administration of the prescribed bisphosphonate dose.

Selective Estrogen Receptor Modulators

Selective estrogen receptor modulators (SERMs) treat and prevent further destruction of bone architecture. They are indicated for treatment in postmenopausal women.

MECHANISM OF ACTION AND PHARMACOKINETICS

Raloxifene is indicated for the treatment and prevention of osteoporosis. It is a SERM that produces an agonist effect in bone and lipid metabolism and an antagonist effect in the breast and uterus. It has been shown to reduce new fractures of the vertebrae by 30% to 50% over 3 years but has no effect on hip fractures.

Only 2% of the amount of raloxifene administered is bioavailable. First-pass metabolism and protein binding limit the amount of drug absorbed to produce a therapeutic effect.

ADVERSE REACTIONS

Side effects common to raloxifene are hot flashes, leg cramps, peripheral edema, stroke, and venous thromboembolism (VTE). To reduce the risk for VTE, raloxifene should be discontinued at least 72 hours before and during prolonged immobilization (e.g., bed rest, after surgery) until the patient is fully ambulatory.

TECH NOTE!
The FDA issued a safety announcement regarding labeling changes for Reclast (zolendronic acid) in September 2011. Reclast should not be used in patients with evidence of renal impairment as it may increase the risk for developing renal failure. A second label change has been approved to warn patients: "The safety and effectiveness of Reclast for the treatment of osteoporosis is based on clinical data of three years' duration. The optimal duration of use has not been determined. Patients should have the need for continued therapy re-evaluated on a periodic basis."

TECH NOTE!
The FDA issued a safety announcement regarding labeling changes for bisphosphonates in October 2010. They recommend that bisphosphonates be discontinued in patients experiencing a femoral shaft fracture; otherwise, patients should continue with therapy and report any hip or thigh pain.

Bisphosphonates

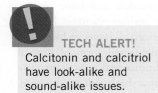

Generic Name	U.S. Brand Name(s) Canadian Brand(s)	Dosage Forms and Strengths
alendronate	Fosamax Fosamax	Solution, oral: 70 mg/75 mL Tablets: 5 mg, 10 mg, 40 mg Tablets, weekly: 35 mg, 70 mg
etidronate	Didronel Didronel	Tablets: 200 mg, 400 mg[†]
ibandronate	Boniva Not available	Solution, for injection: 1 mg/mL Tablets, monthly: 150 mg
pamidronate	Aredia Aredia	Powder, for injection: 30 mg, 90 mg Solution, for injection: 3 mg/mL, 6 mg/mL, 9 mg/mL
risedronate	Actonel, Atelvia Actonel	Tablets: 5 mg, 30 mg, 150 mg Tablets weekly: 35 mg Tablets, delayed release, weekly: 35 mg
tiludronate	Skelid Not available	Tablets: 200 mg
zoledronic acid	Reclast, Zometa Zometa	Solution, for injection: 4 mg/5 mL (Zometa), 5 mg/100 mg (Reclast)
Combinations		
alendronate + cholecalciferol	Fosamax Plus D Fosavance	70 mg alendronate + 2800 international units vitamin D 70 mg alendronate + 5600 international units vitamin D
etidronate + calcium carbonate	Not available Generics	Tablets: 400 mg etidronate + 500 mg calcium carbonate

[†]Strength available in the United States only.

Selective Estrogen Receptor Modulators

Generic Name	U.S. Brand Name(s) Canadian Brand(s)	Dosage Forms and Strengths
raloxifene[∞]	Evista Evista	Tablets: 60 mg

[∞]Generic available in Canada.

TECH ALERT!
Calcitonin and calcitriol have look-alike and sound-alike issues.

Calcitonin

Calcitonin is a hormone that is secreted by the thyroid gland and inhibits the rate of bone turnover stimulated by release of PTH. It lowers serum calcium levels by decreasing intestinal absorption of calcium and increasing renal elimination of calcium. These actions make calcitonin useful for the treatment of Paget's disease. The effectiveness of calcitonin in the treatment of osteoporosis is related to its ability to increase BMD. It has been shown to reduce vertebral fracture risk by 33% to 36% over 3 years but has not proven effective in decreasing hip fractures.

Miscellaneous

Generic Name	U.S. Brand Name(s)	Dosage Forms and Strengths
	Canadian Brand(s)	
calcitonin*	Fortical, Miacalcin	Nasal solution (Miacalcin): 200 units per actuation (spray)
	Calcimar, Caltine, Miacalcin NS	Solution, for injection: 100 units/mL (Caltine), 200 units/mL

*Generic available.

Absorption of calcitonin from intramuscular and subcutaneous injection sites is rapid, and the half-life of calcitonin is short (20 minutes). The bioavailability of calcitonin when administered intranasally is 3% to 50%. Local adverse reactions are mainly irritation of the nose or injection site.

HORMONE REPLACEMENT THERAPY

Estrogens with or without progestins decrease bone turnover, bone loss, and fractures and are indicated for prevention of osteoporosis rather than treatment. Hormone replacement therapy (HRT) is not a first-line therapy for the prevention of osteoporosis because of the increased risk for coronary heart disease, stroke, thromboembolism, and breast and uterine cancers.

Estrogen deficiency occurs with the onset of menopause and increases osteoclast activity. Osteoclasts are responsible for bone resorption. Hormone replacement restores estrogen levels and inhibits the effects of estrogen deficiency on cytokines that regulate the formation of osteoclasts. Cytokines involved in osteoclast regulation are interleukins (IL-1, IL-6) and tumor necrosis factor (TNF). HRT also has beneficial effects on BMD and reduces the relative risk for vertebral and hip fractures up to 34%. Increases in BMD are dose dependent; higher doses produce increased BMD. Increases in BMD occur with oral and transdermal dosage forms.

Estrogens and progestins that are prescribed for HRT in the treatment of osteoporosis are estradiol and estradiol combined with levonorgestrel, norethindrone, or norgestimate; conjugated estrogens and conjugated estrogens combined with medroxyprogesterone; esterified estrogens; and estropipate. HRT is also indicated for the treatment of menopausal symptoms (hot flashes, vaginal dryness and atrophy), postmenopausal urogenital symptoms (urgency, dysuria), abnormal uterine bleeding, hypoestrogenism, and breast and prostate cancer (palliation). These drugs are discussed in detail in Chapter 34. Adverse reactions include headache, nausea, rash at the site of patch application, coronary heart disease, depression, stroke, thromboembolism, and breast and uterine cancer.

Anabolic Agents

Parathyroid hormone analogues increase the rate of bone remodeling, thicken structural units of bone (ostens), and produce bone architecture that closely resembles normal bone. They decrease osteoblast cell death, allowing the balance between bone formation and bone resorption to shift toward bone formation. This is an improvement over bisphosphonates because alendronate, risedronate, and etidronate only prevent further destruction of bone architecture. They do not restore normal structure. Teriparatide is a genetically engineered form of human PTH and the only drug currently available in this category. It is administered subcutaneously and injected daily. It is indicated for postmenopausal women and men at high risk for fracture. Despite its benefits, use is limited because of risks for osteosarcoma. Other adverse reactions associated with teriparatide use are orthostatic hypotension, dizziness, headache, hypercalcemia, leg cramps, nausea, arthralgias, hyperuricemia, and gout. Safety when used beyond 2 years has not been determined.

TECH ALERT!
Raloxifene has a boxed warning stating that it can increase the risk for VTE and death from stroke.

TECH ALERT!
The following drugs have look-alike and sound-alike issues: Alora and Aldara; Estraderm and Testoderm; Estratab and Estratest

TECH ALERT!
Because of the potential risk for osteosarcoma, the FDA requires a boxed warning for teriparatide stating that its use is limited to patients for whom the benefit outweighs the risk.

Hormone Replacement Therapy[&]

Generic Name	U.S. Brand Name(s) Canadian Brand(s)	Dosage Forms and Strengths
estradiol*	Alora, Climara, Estrace, Estraderm, Femtrace, Gynodiol, Menostar, Vivelle-Dot Climara, Estrace, Estraderm, Estradot, Oesclim	Tablets, oral (Estrace, Gynodiol): 0.5 mg, 1 mg, 2 mg (1.5 mg Gynodiol only), 0.45 mg, 0.9 mg, 1.8 mg (Femtrace) Transdermal patch, biweekly (Alora, Estraderm, Estradot, Oesclim, Vivelle Dot): 0.025 mg/24 hr, 0.0375 mg/24 hr, 0.05 mg/24 hr, 0.075 mg/24 hr, 0.1 mg/24 hr Transdermal patch, weekly (Climara): 0.025 mg/24 hr, 0.0375 mg/24 hr, 0.05 mg/24 hr, 0.06 mg/24 hr, 0.075 mg/24 hr, 0.1 mg/24 hr and 0.014 mg/24 hr (Menostar)
estradiol + levonorgestrol	Climara Pro Climara Pro	Transdermal patch: estradiol, 0.045 mg + levonorgestrel, 0.015 mg per 24 hr
estradiol + norethindrone	Activella, Combipatch, Mimvey Activelle, Estalis	Tablets: estradiol 0.5 mg + norethindrone 0.1 mg (Activella, Activelle LD); estradiol 1 mg + 0.5 mg norethindrone 0.5 mg (Activella, Activelle, Mimvey) Transdermal Patch, bi-weekly (Combipatch, Estalis): 50 mcg estradiol + norethindrone acetate 140 mcg; estradiol 50 mcg/day + norethindrone acetate 250 mcg
estradiol + norgestimate	Prefest Not available	Tablets: estradiol 1 mg (15 pink tablets) + estradiol 1 mg + norgestimate 0.09 mg (15 white tablets)
Conjugated estrogens*	Cenestin, Enjuvia, Premarin C.E.S., Premarin	Tablets (Premarin): 0.3 mg, 0.45 mg[†], 0.625 mg, 0.9 mg[†], 1.25 mg Tablets, synthetic A (Cenestin): 0.3 mg, 0.45 mg, 0.625 mg, 0.9 mg, 1.25 mg Tablets, synthetic B (Enjuvia): 0.3 mg, 0.45 mg, 0.625 mg, 0.9 mg, 1.25 mg
estrogens + medroxyprogesterone	Premphase, Prempro Premplus	Tablets (Premphase): conjugated estrogens 0.625 mg (14 maroon tablets) and 0.625 mg conjugated estrogen + 5 mg medroxyprogesterone (14 blue tablets) Tablets (Prempro): 0.3 mg conjugated estrogen + 1.5 mg medroxyprogesterone; 0.45 mg conjugated estrogen + 1.5 mg medroxyprogesterone; 0.625 mg conjugated estrogen + 2.5 mg medroxyprogesterone; 0.625 mg conjugated estrogen + 5 mg medroxyprogesterone
estrogens esterified	Menest Estragyn	Tablets: 0.3 mg, 0.625 mg, 1.25 mg, 2.5 mg
estropipate	Generics Ogen	Tablets: 0.625 mg (0.75 mg estropipate), 1.25 mg (1.5 mg estropipate), 2.5 mg (3 mg estropipate)

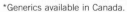

*Generics available in Canada.
[†]Strength available in the United States only.
[&]See Chapter 34 for other dosage form strengths.

Anabolic Agents

Generic Name	U.S. Brand Name(s) Canadian Brand(s)	Dosage Forms and Strengths
teriparatide	Forteo Not available	Solution, for injection: 20 mcg/dose (prefilled syringe)

RECEPTOR ACTIVATOR OF NUCLEAR FACTOR KAPPA-BETA LIGAND INHIBITORS

Denosumab is a monoclonal antibody that inhibits receptor activator of nuclear factor κ-beta ligand (RANKL) binding. Denosumab binding to RANKL results in inhibition of osteoclast activation, decreases bone resorption, and reverses bone remodeling from destruction to bone formation. Denosumab is indicated for postmenopausal women at risk for osteoporosis. Bone mass and strength in trabecular bone are observed. Denosumab is administered subcutaneously twice a year. Adverse reactions include increased risk for infection, hypocalcemia, skin rashes, osteonecrosis of the jaw, and fracture healing complications.

Monoclonal Antibody

Generic Name	U.S. Brand Name(s) Canadian Brand(s)	Dosage Forms and Strengths
denosumab	Prolia, Xgeva Prolia	Solution, for injection: 60 mg/mL (Prolia), 120 mg/1.7 mL (Xgeva)

Usual Dosage and Warnings for Drugs Used in the Treatment of Osteoporosis and Paget's Disease

Generic Name	U.S. Brand Name	Usual Adult Oral Dose and Dosing Schedule	Warning Labels
Bisphosphonates			
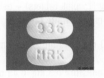 alendronate	Fosamax	**Osteoporosis, prevention:** 5 mg once a day or 35 mg once weekly **Osteoporosis, treatment:** 10 mg once a day or 70 mg once weekly **Paget's disease:** 40 mg once daily for 6 months	STAND OR SIT UPRIGHT FOR AT LEAST 30 MINUTES AFTER TAKING DOSE; DO NOT LIE DOWN— alendronate, etidronate, risedronate, tiludronate.
ibandronate	Boniva	**Osteoporosis:** 2.5 mg once a day or 150 mg once monthly or administer 3 mg IV bolus every 3 months	STAND OR SIT UPRIGHT FOR A LEAST 1 HOUR AFTER TAKING DOSE; DO NOT LIE DOWN— ibandronate.
etidronate	Didronel	**Paget's disease:** 5 mg to 10 mg/kg/ day for up to 6 months or 11 mg to 20 mg/kg/day up to 3 months; re-treat if needed after a drug-free period of 90 days	TAKE 30 MINUTES BEFORE THE FIRST MEAL OF THE DAY WITH 6 TO 8 OZ OF WATER.
pamidronate	Aredia	**Paget's disease:** 30 mg infused in 500 mL ½ NS or NS over 4 hours for 3 days in a row	TAKE 1 HOUR BEFORE FIRST MEAL OF THE DAY—ibandronate.
 risedronate	Actonel	**Osteoporosis:** 5 mg once a day, 35 mg once weekly, 75 mg once daily for 2 days a month, or 150 mg once a month **Paget's disease:** 30 mg once a day for 2 months; re-treat if needed after a 2-month drug-free period	AVOID DAIRY PRODUCTS AND ANTACIDS CONTAINING CALCIUM, MAGNESIUM, OR IRON WITHIN 2 HOURS OF DOSE.
tiludronate	Skelid	**Paget's disease:** 400 mg daily for 3 months	TAKE 1 HOUR BEFORE FIRST MEAL OF THE DAY—ibandronate.
zoledronic acid	Zometa	**Paget's disease:** 5 mg as a single dose infused over at least 15 minutes **Osteoporosis:** ** 5 mg IV once yearly	TAKE ON AN EMPTY STOMACH— etidronate, tiludronate.

Usual Dosage and Warnings for Drugs Used in the Treatment of Osteoporosis and Paget's Disease—cont'd

Generic Name	U.S. Brand Name	Usual Adult Oral Dose and Dosing Schedule	Warning Labels
Bisphosphonate Combinations			
alendronate + cholecalciferol	Fosamax Plus D	1 tablet once weekly	
Selective Estrogen Receptor Modulators			
raloxifene	Evista	60 mg/day	TAKE WITH OR WITHOUT FOOD.
Hormone Replacement Therapy			
estradiol	Estrace	Prevention of osteoporosis: Oral: 0.5 mg/day (3 weeks on and 1 week off) Transdermal patch, as Climara, Menostar: 1 patch once weekly Transdermal patch, as Alora, Estraderm, Estradot, Vivelle-Dot: 1 patch twice weekly	TAKE WITH FOOD. ROTATE SITE OF APPLICATION—patch. STORE IN SEALED FOIL POUCH AT ROOM TEMPERATURE—CombiPatch.
estradiol + levonorgestrol	Climara Pro	Prevention of osteoporosis: Apply 1 patch weekly	
estradiol + norethindrone	Activella, Combipatch	Prevention of osteoporosis: Tablets (Activella): 1 tablet daily Transdermal patch (Combipatch, Estalis): 1 patch twice a week	
conjugated estrogens	Premarin	Prevention of osteoporosis: 0.3 mg cyclically or daily	
estrogens esterified	Menest	Prevention of osteoporosis: 0.3 mg cyclically or daily (maximum, 1.25 mg/day)	
estropipate	Ogen	Prevention of osteoporosis: 0.75 mg daily for 25 days of a 31-day cycle	
estradiol + norgestimate	Prefest	Prevention of osteoporosis: 1 mg estradiol daily for 3 days (pink tablet) followed by 1 mg estradiol + norgestimate 0.09 mg once daily for 3 days (white tablet); repeat continuously	
estrogens + medroxyprogesterone	Premphase, Prempro	Prevention of osteoporosis: Premphase: 0.625 mg conjugated estrogen days 1 through 14 (maroon tablet), 0.625 mg conjugated estrogen + 5 mg medroxyprogesterone days 15 through 28 (blue tablet) Prempro: 0.3 mg conjugated estrogen + 1.5 mg medroxyprogesterone daily up to 0.625 mg conjugated estrogen + 5 mg medroxyprogesterone daily	

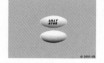

Continued

Usual Dosage and Warnings for Drugs Used in the Treatment of Osteoporosis and Paget's Disease—cont'd

Generic Name	U.S. Brand Name	Usual Adult Oral Dose and Dosing Schedule	Warning Labels
Calcitonin Hormone			
calcitonin	Miacalcin	**Osteoporosis:** 100 units/day (IM, SC) or 1 spray in 1 nostril (200 units/day) (intranasal) **Paget's disease:** Start 100 units/day (IM, SC); maintenance 50 to 100 units every 1 to 3 days	1 spray intranasally daily, alternating nostrils each day
Monoclonal Antibody			
denosumab	Prolia, Xgeva	**Osteoporosis:** 60 mg SC every 6 months	REFRIGERATE. DO NOT SHAKE. PROTECT FROM LIGHT.
Parathyroid Hormone Analogue			
teriparatide	Forteo	**Osteoporosis:** 20 mcg SC once a day	REFRIGERATE; DO NOT FREEZE. DISCARD AFTER 28 DAYS OF OPENING.

**Not FDA approved.

Chapter Summary

- Osteoporosis is a chronic, progressive disease of bone characterized by loss of bone density and bone strength and resulting in increased fracture risk.
- The lifetime risk for fractures in people older than age 50 years is one in two women and one in four men.
- Low-impact osteoporosis fractures can occur from falls or trauma; fragility fractures may occur from simply coughing or sneezing.
- Primary osteoporosis is associated with the aging process.
- Secondary osteoporosis may be caused by diseases or drugs.
- Glucocorticoids use can cause osteoporosis.
- After menopause, women's rate of bone loss exceeds the rate of bone formed. The rate of bone loss for men and women is equal after age 65 to 70 years.
- Bone formation and loss is a carefully controlled process and is regulated from birth to death.
- Osteoblasts are responsible for bone formation, and osteoclasts are responsible for bone resorption.
- Ninety-nine percent of total body calcium is located in the skeleton; therefore, bones are a reservoir for calcium when serum levels are too low.
- The hormones principally responsible for regulation of serum calcium levels are parathyroid hormone, calcitonin, and vitamin D.
- Other hormones linked to the regulation of bone formation and bone loss are estrogen, progestins, luteinizing hormone, and androgens.
- Paget's disease is also a progressive disease of bone.
- Paget's disease is characterized by excessive bone resorption in focal areas followed by increased bone formation that results in enlarged bones that are structurally weak.
- Paget's disease can cause bone deformities, pain, fractures, and deafness.
- Paget's disease is most common in men older than 55 years.
- A three-point program is recommended to prevent and treat osteoporosis; it includes lifelong nutritional calcium and vitamin D intake, exercise (weight bearing and strength training), and pharmacotherapy.
- Pharmacological agents used in the treatment of osteoporosis or Paget's disease are categorized as antiresorptive (inhibit bone resorption) or anabolic (promote bone formation).

- Bisphosphonates, calcitonin, SERMs, and estrogen are antiresorptive agents.
- Parathyroid hormone is an anabolic agent.
- Bisphosphonates must be taken on an empty stomach at least 30 to 60 minutes (depending on the agent) before the first meal or beverage of the day.
- Patients taking oral bisphosphonates must sit upright or stand for at least 30 to 60 minutes after dosing to avoid possible esophageal ulceration.
- Calcium and vitamin D supplementation is recommended in conjunction with bisphosphonate and RANKL therapy.
- Mild weight-bearing exercise along with a diet rich in vitamin D and calcium is key to strong bones.
- Lifestyle changes that reduce alcohol consumption and smoking are also important for bone health.

REVIEW QUESTIONS

1. A chronic, progressive disease of bone characterized by loss of bone density and bone strength and resulting in increased fracture risk is called _____.
   a. rheumatoid arthritis
   b. osteoporosis
   c. brittle bone disease
   d. osteosarcoma

2. Alcohol abuse can also produce osteoporosis.
   a. true
   b. false

3. Paget's disease is most common in women older than 55 years.
   a. true
   b. false

4. The goals of osteoporosis treatment are to _____ bone density and to _____ risks for future fractures.
   a. decrease, reduce
   b. increase, reduce
   c. reduce, remove
   d. decrease, reduce

5. The majority of the drugs used to treat osteoporosis and Paget's disease are _____ agents.
   a. absorption
   b. antifracture
   c. antiresorptive
   d. anticalcium

6. Only some of the bisphosphonates are indicated for the treatment of Paget's disease.
   a. true
   b. false

7. _____is a selective estrogen receptor modulator (SERM) indicated for the treatment and prevention of osteoporosis in postmenopausal women and prevents further destruction of bone architecture.
   a. Fosamax
   b. Evista
   c. Boniva
   d. Osteo-cal

8. Hormone replacement therapy is the first-line therapy for the prevention of osteoporosis because of the increased risk for coronary heart disease, stroke, thromboembolism, and breast and uterine cancer.
   a. true
   b. false

9. A diet rich in vitamin _____ and _____ is key to strong bones.
   a. C, calcium
   b. D, sodium
   c. D, calcium
   d. B, iron

10. The use of teriparatide, a genetically engineered form of human parathyroid hormone and the only drug currently available in this category, is limited because of risks for _____.
    a. fractures
    b. osteosarcoma
    c. pituitary tumors
    d. all of the above

TECHNICIAN'S CORNER

1. Mild weight-bearing exercise along with a diet rich in vitamin D and calcium is key to strong bones that resist fractures. Come up with a 10-day plan of meals and exercises for a client who is menopausal and overweight.
2. Why are lifestyle changes that reduce alcohol consumption and smoking so important to prevent osteoporosis or Paget's disease?

Bibliography

Alibhai S, Rahman S, Warde P, et al: Prevention and management of osteoporosis in men receiving androgen deprivation therapy: a survey of urologists and radiation oncologists, *Urology* 68:126-131, 2006.

American Pharmacists Association: new approaches to the management of osteoporosis, *Pharmacy Today* 13(1):1-12, 2010.

Cranney A, Papaioannou A, Zytaruk N, et al; for the Clinical Guidelines Committee of Osteoporosis Canada: Parathyroid hormone for the treatment of osteoporosis: a systematic review, *CMAJ* 175:52-59, 2006.

Elsevier: Gold Standard Clinical Pharmacology. Retrieved April 8, 2011, from https://www.clinicalpharmacology.com, 2010.

FDA: FDA Joint Reproductive Health Drugs Advisory Committee and Drug Safety and Risk Management Advisory Committee Meeting on the long term use of bisphosphonates for the treatment and prevention of osteoporosis. Retrieved May 6, 2012, from http://www.fda.gov/downloads/AdvisoryCommittees/CommitteesMeetingMaterials/Drugs/DrugSafetyandRiskManagementAdvisoryCommittee/UCM270963.pdf, 2011.

http://www.fda.gov/Safety/MedWatch/SafetyInformation/SafetyAlertsforHumanMedicalProducts/ucm229244.htm—Bisphosphonates (Osteoporosis Drugs): Label Change—Atypical Fractures Update.

FDA: FDA Drug Safety Communication: Ongoing safety review of oral osteoporosis drugs (bisphosphonates) and potential increased risk of esophageal cancer. Retrieved May 5, 2011, from http://www.fda.gov/Drugs/DrugSafety/ucm263320.htm, 2011.

Gold D, Alexander I, Ettinger M: How can osteoporosis patients benefit more from their therapy? Adherence issues with bisphosphonate therapy, *Ann Pharmacother* 40:1143-1150, 2006.

Health Canada: Drug Product Database. Retrieved April 8, 2011, from http://www.hc-sc.gc.ca/dhp-mps/prodpharma/databasdon/index-eng.php, 2010.

International Osteoporosis Foundation: Facts and statistics about osteoporosis and its impact. Retrieved April 9, 2011, from http://www.iofbonehealth.org/facts-and-statistics.html#factsheet-category-23, 2010.

Kalant H, Grant D, Mitchell J: *Principles of medical pharmacology*, ed 7, Toronto, 2007, Elsevier Canada, A Division of Reed Elsevier Canada, pp 860-861, 878-889.

Lance L, Lacy C, Armstrong L, et al: *Drug information handbook for the allied health professional*, ed 12, Hudson, OH, 2005, APhA Lexi-Comp.

Langston A, Ralston S: Management of Paget's disease of bone, *Rheumatology* 43:955-959, 2004.

Mauck K, Clarke B: Diagnosis, screening, prevention, and treatment of osteoporosis, *Mayo Clin Proc* 81:662-672, 2006.

Newman E, Matzko C, Olenginski T, et al: Glucocorticoid-Induced Osteoporosis Program (GIOP): a novel, comprehensive, and highly successful care program with improved outcomes at 1 year, *Osteoporos Int* 17:1428-1434, 2006.

Reid I, Miller P, Lyles K, et al: Comparison of a single infusion of zoledronic acid with risedronate for Paget's disease, *N Engl J Med* 353:898-908, 2005.

U.S. Department of Health and Human Services: *The 2004 Surgeon General's Report on bone health and osteoporosis: what it means to you*, Washington, DC, 2004, U.S. Department of Health and Human Services, Office of the Surgeon General.

Walsh J: Paget's disease of bone: clinical update, *MJA* 181:262-265, 2004.

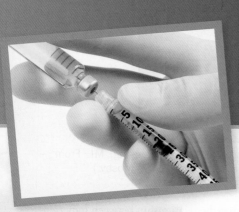

17

Treatment of Hyperuricemia and Gout

Overview

Hyperuricemia is a condition in which urate levels build up in the blood serum. *Urates* are the product of the metabolism of *purines*. Between 5% and 8% of men in the United States have asymptomatic hyperuricemia (serum urate in excess of 6.8 mg/dL). Population studies show that the rate of hyperuricemia in men is greater than in women until menopause, when the rates equalize. Before puberty, boys and girls both have low serum urate levels.

Medical Conditions Associated with Hyperuricemia

Hyperuricemia is associated with several medical conditions. *Gout* is the primary disease associated with hyperuricemia, but increased serum urates are also associated with cardiovascular disease, chronic kidney disease, hyperlipidemia, insulin resistance, and obesity. Up to 12% of persons with hypertension have gout, and 20% to 40% of people with untreated hypertension also have hyperuricemia. Resistance to the flow of blood through vessels, peripheral resistance, and renal vascular

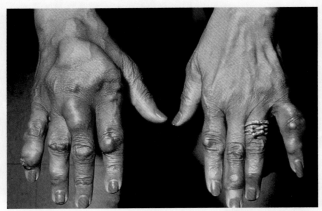

FIGURE 17-1 Gouty arthritis. (Courtesy Lanny L. Johnson, MD, East Lansing, MI. From Thibodeau GA, Patton KT: *Anatomy and physiology*, ed 6, St Louis, 2007, Mosby.)

resistance are increased in hypertension and gout. It is likely that the relationship between hypertension and hyperuricemia is attributable to decreased renal clearance resulting in accumulation of urate. Hyperuricemia can cause kidney disease and make preexisting kidney disease worse.

Hyperuricemia has been shown to increase the risk of coronary heart disease and stroke partly because of its role in producing hyperlipidemia. Hyperlipidemia causes atherosclerosis, a buildup of lipids in arteries that results in arterial occlusion. Patients with congestive heart failure do worse if they have hyperuricemia.

The relationship between hyperuricemia, obesity, and insulin resistance is interesting. Serum urate levels tend to be elevated in obesity because of increased production of urates accompanied by decreased renal clearance, leading to increased risk for gout. Hyperuricemia is a risk factor for diabetes, and obesity is associated with increased insulin resistance. Weight loss reduces hyperuricemia and insulin resistance. Exposure to lead in the environment can also increase the risk for development of gout.

PATHOPHYSIOLOGY OF GOUT

Gout affects about 1% of the U.S. population and 3% of the Canadian population. It is up to 4 times more common in men than in women. In fact, gout is rare in premenopausal women. Gout or gouty arthritis accounts for 5% of all arthritis and is the disease most commonly associated with hyperuricemia. The disease is caused when urate crystals are deposited in joints, where they produce inflammation and pain. Deposits of uric acid are called *tophi* (singular, tophus) and look like lumps under the skin around the joints and at the rim of the ear (Figure 17-1).

The joints most commonly affected are the big toe, foot, ankle, knee, wrist, finger, and elbow. Consumption of foods or beverages high in dietary purines can produce a flare-up of gout symptoms. For example, beer consumption increases the risk of an acute attack, perhaps because beer contains high levels of purine.

Some people with gout will experience sharp needle-like painful symptoms, but some people will have no symptoms at all. Acute gout attacks will resolve spontaneously in 7 to 10 days without treatment; however, people with symptoms may benefit from treatment. Chronic gout develops over a period of years and may cause permanent joint or kidney damage. Treatment is recommended when patients have symptoms, are being treated for malignancy, or are at risk for development of kidney stones.

DRUGS USED TO TREAT GOUT

Drugs prescribed for the treatment of gout include analgesics, anti-inflammatories, uricosurics, and inhibitors of uric acid synthesis. A **uricosuric** is a drug the increases the renal clearance of urates.

Analgesics and Anti-inflammatory Drugs

The principal anti-inflammatories and analgesics used for the treatment of acute gout are nonsteroidal anti-inflammatory drugs (NSAIDs), corticosteroids, and colchicine. Colchicine is one of the oldest agents use to treat gout, but it is most commonly used today when NSAIDs and corticosteroids do not control symptoms. Colchicine may be used in chronic gout to prevent symptoms. It penetrates inflammatory cells and inhibits their ability to respond normally to the site of irritation. It inhibits histamine release and blocks cell division. Common adverse reactions associated with the use of colchicine include nausea, vomiting, and diarrhea. Other adverse reactions are alopecia, bone marrow suppression, renal failure, intravascular coagulation, and death.

Nonsteroidal anti-inflammatory drugs and glucocorticosteroids are used in the treatment of gout. The most commonly prescribed NSAID is indomethacin; however, diclofenac, ketoprofen, tolmetin, meclofenamate, and naproxen are also administered. The cyclooxygenase-2 (COX-2) inhibitor cele-

Anti-inflammatories Used in the Treatment of Gout

Generic Name	U.S. Brand Name(s) / Canadian Brand(s)	Dosage Forms and Strengths
colchicine*‡	Colcrys	Tablets: 0.6 mg, 1 mg‡
	Generics	
NSAIDs, COX-2 Inhibitors		
indomethacin	Indocin	(See Chapters 10 and 15)
	Generics	
sulindac	Clinoril	
	Generics	
ibuprofen**	Motrin	
	Generics only (600 mg)	
ketoprofen**	Orudis, Oruvail (extended release)	
	Generics	
naproxen	Naprosyn, EC-Naprosyn	
	Naprosyn, Naprosyn E, Naprosyn SR	
naproxen Na+	Anaprox, Anaprox DS	
	Anaprox, Anaprox DS	
Glucocorticosteroids		
dexamethasone*	Dexamethasone Intensol,	(See Chapter 15)
	Dexasone	
hydrocortisone*	A-Hydrocort, Cortef, Solu-Cortef	
	A-Hydrocort, Cortef, Solu-Cortef	
methylprednisolone*	A-Methapred, Depo-Medrol, Medrol, Solu-Medrol	
	Depo-Medrol, Medrol, Solu-Medrol	
prednisone*	Prednisone Intensol,	
	Winpred (Canada)	
triamcinolone	Aristospan, Kenalog-10, Kenalog-40, Trivaris	
	Kenalog-10, Kenalog-40	

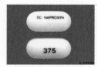

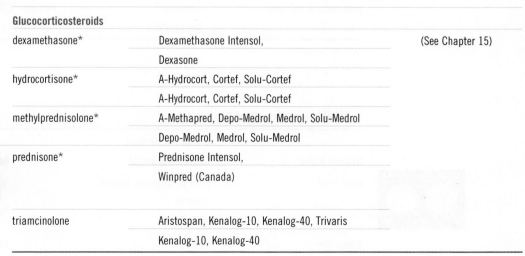

*Generic available.
‡Strength available in Canada only.
**Not FDA approved.
*‡Generic available in Canada only

coxib may also be prescribed for the treatment of acute gout. Oral prednisone and intraarticular injections of corticosteroids may sometimes be given when only one or two joints are involved. NSAIDs and glucocorticosteroids are discussed in depth in Chapters 10 and 15.

Uricosurics

Uricosurics are drugs that increase the clearance of uric acid. Probenecid is a uricosuric used in the treatment of gout. It inhibits the reabsorption of uric acid in the renal tubules and thereby promotes the elimination of urates. Nausea, vomiting, and worsening of preexisting kidney stones are adverse reactions to probenecid.

Inhibitors of Uric Acid Synthesis

XANTHINE OXIDASE INHIBITORS

Xanthine oxidase inhibitors block the final enzymatic step in the synthesis of uric acid. Urate-lowering drugs are indicated for patients who experience frequent attacks of gout. Allopurinol is a xanthine oxidase inhibitor and is effective in reducing hyperuricemia produced by gout secondary to malignancy or when drug induced. Thiazide diuretics (e.g., hydrochlorothiazide) and aspirin are known to increase urate levels. Allopurinol is readily absorbed when administered orally and is easily eliminated in the urine. Nausea, drowsiness, headache, diarrhea, and an itchy skin rash are adverse reactions linked to allopurinol use. Febuxostat (Uloric) is a selective xanthine oxidase inhibitor approved by the U.S. Food and Drug Administration (FDA) in 2009 for the treatment of patients with chronic hyperuricemia and gout. It is more selective than allopurinol. Gout flare-ups have been reported when drug therapy is initiated. Other adverse reactions are nausea, vomiting, and changes in appetite. Cardiovascular events have been reported with febuxostat including angina, myocardial infarction, stroke, and atrial fibrillation. Rhabdomyolysis, the breakdown of muscle tissue that can lead to acute renal failure, has also been reported and patients are advised to report muscle pain.

Uricosurics Used in the Treatment of Gout

Generic Name	U.S. Brand Name(s) Canadian Brand(s)	Dosage Forms and Strengths
probenecid*	Generics	Tablets: 500 mg
	Benuryl	
Combination		
probenecid + colchine*	Generics	Tablets: 500 mg probenecid + 0.5 mg colchine
	Not available	

*Generic available.

Inhibitors of Uric Acid Synthesis

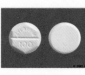

Generic Name	U.S. Brand Name(s) Canadian Brand(s)	Dosage Forms and Strengths
allopurinol*	Aloprim, Zyloprim, Lopurin	Injection, powder for reconstitution (Aloprim): 500 mg
	Zyloprim,	Tablet (Zyloprim): 100 mg, 300 mg
febuxostat	Uloric	Tablets: 40 mg†, 80 mg
	Uloric	

*Generic available.
†Strength available in the United States only.

Metabolism of Uric Acid
RECOMBINANT URATE OXIDASE ENZYMES

A new class of drugs is available for the treatment of chronic gout. Recombinant urate oxidase enzymes lower uric acid levels by metabolizing uric acid to the water-soluble benign purine metabolite allantoin, which is excreted in the urine. Pegloticase (Krystexxa) was FDA approved in 2010 for patients with chronic gout. Rasburicase (Elitek) is indicated for the treatment of hyperuricemia in patients receiving chemotherapy resulting in elevated uric acid. Pegloticase and rasburicase are administered intravenously. Patients experience infusion reactions such as rash, itching, redness, and anaphylaxis. Additional adverse reactions of pegloticase include nausea and vomiting, constipation or diarrhea, fatigue, arthralgia, upper respiratory infection, fever, heart failure, and hypotension.

Recombinant Urate Oxidase Inhibitors

Generic Name	U.S. Brand Name(s) Canadian Brand(s)	Dosage Forms and Strengths
pegloticase	Krystexxa	Solution, for injection: 8 mg/mL
	Not available	
rasburicase	Elitek	Powder, for injection: 1.5 mg/vial
	Fasturtek	

Nonpharmacological Therapy

A diet low in purines has been recommended to prevent gout attacks (Box 17-1). Foods high in purines are meat (especially liver), fish (anchovies), dried beans and peas, and gravies. Beer and spirits are also known to increase purine levels. Low-fat dairy products have low purine levels. Prevention tips include weight loss, decrease meat consumption, drink skim milk daily, and reduce alcohol consumption (especially beer).

Usual Dosage and Warnings for Drugs Used in the Treatment of Gout

Generic Name	U.S. Brand Name	Usual Adult Oral Dose and Dosing Schedule	Warning Labels
Anti-inflammatories			
colchine	Generics	Oral, prevention: Begin 0.6 mg twice a day; decrease to 0.6 mg every other day or 3 times a week Oral, acute attack: 0.6-1.2 mg every 1-2 hours until relief or 3 doses; wait 3 days before re-treatment IV, acute attack: Begin 1-2 mg, decrease to 0.5 mg every 6 hours until relief (maximum, 4 mg); wait 7 days before another treatment with any dosage form of colchicine	AVOID ALCOHOL. TAKE WITH LOTS OF WATER.
Uricosuric			
probenecid	Generics	250 mg twice a day for 1 week; increase as frequently as 250 mg to 500 mg/day up to maximum of 2 to 3 g/day if needed	TAKE WITH FOOD. TAKE WITH LOTS OF WATER. AVOID ASPIRIN.

Continued

Usual Dosage and Warnings for Drugs Used in the Treatment of Gout—cont'd

Generic Name	U.S. Brand Name	Usual Adult Oral Dose and Dosing Schedule	Warning Labels
Inhibitors of Uric Acid Synthesis			
allopurinol	Zyloprim	**Gout:** 200-600 mg/day orally; start with 100 mg/day and increase weekly **Hyperuricemia:** 600-800 mg/day orally in 2-3 divided doses for 2-3 days before starting chemotherapy **IV:** 200-400 mg/m²/day as single IV infusion or divided at 6-, 8-, or 12-hour intervals	TAKE WITH FOOD. AVOID ALCOHOL. MAY CAUSE DIZZINESS OR DROWSINESS. TAKE WITH LOTS OF WATER (10-12 GLASSES/DAY).
febuxostat	Uloric	**Chronic hyperuricemia with gout:** 40-80 mg/day	TAKE WITH A GLASS OF WATER.
Recombinant Urate Oxidase Enzyme			
pegloticase	Krystexxa	**Chronic gout:** 8 mg IV over 2 hours every 2 weeks	MIX BY GENTLY INVERTING IV BAG; DO NOT SHAKE. REFRIGERATE DILUTED SOLUTION. USE WITHIN 4 HOURS OF RECONSTITUTION—pegloticase.
rasuricase	Elitek, Fasturtek	**Management of uric acid levels in patients receiving anticancer therapy:** 0.2 mg/kg as a 30-minute infusion once daily for up to 5 days	

BOX 17-1   Purine Content of Foods

Foods considered high in purine content include:
- Alcoholic beverages
- Fish, seafood, and shellfish, including anchovies, sardines, herring, mussels, codfish, scallops, trout, and haddock
- Meats, such as bacon, turkey, veal, and venison, and organ meats such as liver and sweetbreads

Foods considered moderate in purine content include:
- Meats such as beef, chicken, duck, pork, and ham
- Crab, lobster, oysters, and shrimp
- Vegetables and beans such as asparagus, cauliflower, kidney beans, lentils, lima beans, peas, mushrooms, and spinach
- Grains: oatmeal, whole wheat bread, and cereal

Foods considered low in purine content include:
- Dairy products: Skim milk and cheese
- Eggs
- Fruit and most vegetables (except those listed above)
- Grains: enriched bread and cereal

Chapter Summary

- Hyperuricemia is a condition in which urate levels build up in the blood serum.
- Gout affects about 1% of the population and is the primary disease associated with hyperuricemia.
- Gout and hyperuricemia are more common in men than in women.
- Gout is rare in children before puberty and in women before menopause.
- Hyperuricemia is also associated with cardiovascular disease, chronic kidney disease, hyperlipidemia, insulin resistance, and obesity.
- Acute gout attacks will resolve spontaneously in 7 to 10 days without treatment.

- The joints most commonly affected by gout are the big toe, foot, ankle, knee, wrist, finger, and elbow. Urate crystals are deposited in joints causing inflammation and pain.
- Drugs prescribed for the treatment of gout include analgesics, anti-inflammatories, uricosurics, and inhibitors of uric acid synthesis.
- A uricosuric is a drug the increases the renal clearance of urate crystals.
- NSAIDS and glucocorticosteroids are used to reduce pain and inflammation in gout.
- Colchicine is the oldest drug used for the treatment of acute gouty arthritis pain.
- Probenecid is a uricosuric used in the treatment of gout.
- Allopurinol, a xanthine oxidase inhibitor, blocks the final enzymatic step in the synthesis of uric acid.
- Diets low in purines have been recommended to prevent gout attacks. Meat, fish, beer, and spirits are known to increase purine levels.
- Beer consumption increases risks of an acute attack, perhaps because beer contains high levels of purines.
- Pegloticase and rasburicase are recombinant urate oxidase enzymes that convert uric acid to a water-soluble purine that is excreted in the urine.

REVIEW QUESTIONS

1. _____is the most common symptom associated with increased serum urate levels.
   a. Pain
   b. Bladder infection
   c. Nausea
   d. Vomiting

2. _____is the primary disease associated with hyperuricemia.
   a. Arthritis
   b. Gout
   c. Osteoporosis
   d. Kidney stones

3. There is a relationship between hypertension and hyperuricemia.
   a. true
   b. false

4. Weight loss has no effect on hyperuricemia and insulin resistance.
   a. true
   b. false

5. Drugs prescribed for the treatment of gout include _____.
   a. analgesics
   b. anti-inflammatories
   c. uricosurics and inhibitors of uric acid synthesis
   d. all of the above

6. The most commonly prescribed NSAID for gout is _____.
   a. indomethacin
   b. diclofenac
   c. ketoprofen
   d. tolmetin

7. The oldest drug used in the treatment of gout is _____.
   a. naproxen
   b. allopurinol
   c. colchicine
   d. ketoprofen

8. Diets _____ in purine have been recommended to prevent gout attacks.
   a. high
   b. low

9. The brand name for allopurinol is _____.
   a. Zyban
   b. Zomig
   c. Zyloprim
   d. Zyrtec

10. A uricosuric is a drug that decreases the renal clearance of urates.
    a. true
    b. false

TECHNICIAN'S
CORNER

1. Beer consumption increases risks of an acute gout attack, perhaps because beer contains high levels of purine. Will nonalcoholic beer have the same effect?
2. Diets that are low in purine have been recommended to prevent gout attacks. What foods would you recommend that patients with gout include as part of their diet?

Bibliography

Becker M, Jolly M: Hyperuricemia and associated diseases, *Rheum Dis Clin North Am* 32:275-293, 2006.

Elsevier: Gold Standard Clinical Pharmacology. Retrieved April 16, 2011, from https://www.clinical pharmacology.com/, 2010.

FDA: FDA Approved Drug Products. Retrieved June 25, 2012, from http://www.accessdata.fda.gov/scripts/cder/drugsatfda/index.cfmfuseaction=Search.Search_Drug_Name, 2012.

Health Canada: Drug Product Database. Retrieved April 16, 2011, from http://www.hc-sc.gc.ca/dhp-mps/prodpharma/databasdon/index-eng.php, 2010.

Kalant H, Grant D, Mitchell J: *Principles of medical pharmacology*, ed 7, Toronto, 2007, Elsevier Canada, A Division of Reed Elsevier Canada, p 381.

Lance L, Lacy C, Armstrong L, et al: *Drug information handbook for the allied health professional*, ed 12. Hudson, OH, 2005, APhA Lexi-Comp.

National Institute of Arthritis and Musculoskeletal and Skin Diseases: *Questions and answers about gout*, Bethesda, MD, 2002, NIAMS, National Institutes of Health, US Department of Health and Human Services. NIH publication No. 02-5027. Retrieved at www.niams.nih.gov/hi/topics/gout/gout.htm.

Page C, Curtis M, Sutter M, et al: *Integrated pharmacology*, Philadelphia, 2005, Mosby, pp 450-451.

Pohar S, Murphy G, *Febuxostat for prevention of gout attacks [Issues in emerging health technologies issue 87]*, Ottawa, 2006, Canadian Agency for Drugs and Technologies in Health.

Underwood M: Diagnosis and management of gout, *BMJ* 332:1315-1319, 2006.

USP Center for Advancement of Patient Safety: *Use caution–avoid confusion*, USP Quality Review No. 79, Rockville, MD, April 2004, USP Center for Advancement of Patient Safety.

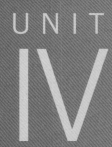

IV

Treatment of Diseases of the Ophthalmic and Otic Systems

LEARNING
OBJECTIVES

1 Learn the terminology associated with the eye and ear.

2 Learn the basic anatomy and physiology of the eye and ear.

3 Differentiate between the different parts of the eye and the ear.

4 Understand the function of the accessory structures of the eye.

5 Describe the processes of seeing and hearing.

6 Differentiate between the process of hearing and the sense of balance.

Accommodation: Ability of the lens to contract and relax to adjust for vision to see things from close up.

Aqueous humor: Portion of anterior cavity that lies in front of the lens and is filled with a clear watery liquid.

Astigmatism: Irregular curvature of the cornea or lens that results in the inability to form a well-focused image in the eye.

Cerumen: Ear wax.

Conduction impairment: Blocking of air waves as they are conducted through the external and middle ears to the sensory receptors of the inner ear.

Hyperopia: Farsightedness.

Myopia: Nearsightedness.

Presbycusis: Common in older adults; causes degeneration of nerve tissue in the ear and vestibular nerve.

Presbyopia: Farsightedness caused by the aging process

Refraction: Deflection or bending of light rays through the cornea, aqueous humor, lens, and vitreous humor.

Tear deficiency: Also known as dry eyes.

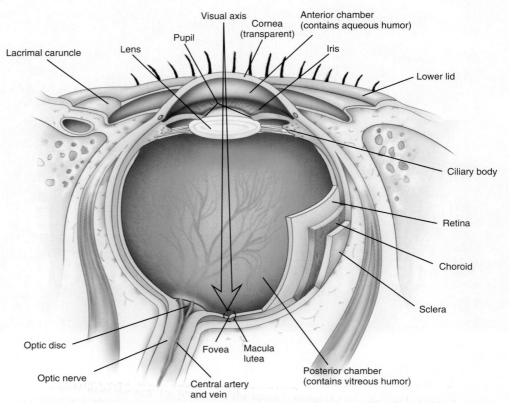

The eye. (From Thibodeau G, Patton K: *Anatomy and physiology*, ed 9, St. Louis, 2010, Mosby.)

Overview of Anatomy and Physiology of the Eye

One of the most important sensations involved in maintaining homeostasis is vision. Vision allows us to activate and respond to a multitude of warning systems and provides us with almost constant feedback in an ever-changing environment.

STRUCTURE OF THE EYE

The eye is divided into different parts and layers. Three layers of tissue compose the eyeball: the *fibrous layer*—sclera and cornea; the *vascular layer*—the choroids, ciliary body, and iris; and the *inner layer*—retina, optic nerve, and retinal blood vessels.

The fibrous layer or the anterior portion of the sclera is called the *cornea* and lies over the colored portion of the eye, the iris. The cornea is transparent, but the rest of the *sclera* is white and opaque and is known as the white of the eye. No blood vessels are found in the cornea or in the lens.

The vascular layer of the eye is characterized by many blood vessels and a large amount of pigment and contains the ciliary body, pupil, and retina. The *ciliary body* is composed of ciliary muscles and ciliary processes; it functions to hold and suspend the lens in place; the *iris*, or colored portion of the eye, has an opening in the middle called the *pupil* that controls the amount of light entering the eye by adjusting its size. The inner layer contains the *retina*, the innermost coat of the eyeball, which is made up of three layers of neurons that constitute our visual receptors. One type of receptor contains rods and cones. *Rods* function best for night vision and *cones* help us see color. The *optic disc*, or blind spot, contains no rods or cones and is located at the posterior end of the eyeball.

CAVITIES AND HUMORS

The eyeball is also divided into two cavities, the anterior and posterior cavities. The anterior cavity lies at the front of the lens and is filled with a clear watery liquid called the *aqueous humor*. The posterior cavity lies at the back of the lens and contains a soft gelatin-like material called the ***vitreous humor***. Both the aqueous and vitreous humors help maintain the intraocular pressure of the eye to keep it from collapsing.

MUSCLES

There are two types of eye muscles, extrinsic and intrinsic. The ***extrinsic eye muscles*** are skeletal and voluntary muscles that move the eyeball in any desired direction. Four of them are straight (superior, inferior, medial, and lateral rectus), and two of them are oblique (superior and inferior). ***Intrinsic eye muscles*** (iris and ciliary muscles) are smooth muscles located in the eye that control involuntary movement. The iris regulates the size of the pupil and the ciliary muscle controls the shape of the lens.

ACCESSORY STRUCTURES

Accessory structures of the eye include the eyebrows, eyelashes, eyelids, and lacrimal apparatus. The eyebrows and eyelashes give some protection against the entrance of foreign objects into the eye and help shade the eye and provide at least minimal protection from direct light. The eyelids consist mainly of voluntary muscles and skin, with a border of thick connective tissue. A mucous membrane called the ***conjunctiva*** lines each lid and continues over the surface of the eyeball, where it is transparent. The ***lacrimal apparatus*** secretes tears and drains them from the surface of the eyeball; it consists of the lacrimal glands, lacrimal ducts, lacrimal sacs, and nasolacrimal ducts. ***Tear deficiency***, also known as dry eyes, is a common disorder associated with aging, environmental conditions, and disease (e.g., rheumatoid arthritis). It causes eye irritation, blurred vision, redness, excessive tearing, and a gritty feeling in the eye. Dry eyes can be treated with nonprescription drugs.

PROCESS OF SEEING

For vision to occur, an image must be formed on the retina and nerve impulses must be conducted to the visual areas of the cerebral cortex for interpretation. Formation of the retinal image involves four processes that focus light rays so that they form a clear image on the retina:

- Refraction: Deflection or bending of light rays through the cornea, aqueous humor, lens, and vitreous humor. Nearsightedness (***myopia***), farsightedness (***hyperopia***), and ***astigmatism*** are errors of refraction.
- Accommodation of the lens: The ability of the lens to contract and relax to adjust for vision to see things from close-up to afar. For near vision, the ciliary muscle is contracted and the lens is bulging; for far vision, the ciliary muscle is relaxed and the lens is comparatively flat. As people grow older, they tend to become farsighted (***presbyopia***) because lenses lose their elasticity and therefore their ability to bulge and accommodate for near vision.
- Constriction of the pupil: Muscles of the iris play an important part in the formation of clear retinal images. Constriction of the pupil occurs simultaneously with accommodation of the lens for near vision. The pupil also constricts in bright light to protect the retina from stimulation that is too intense or too sudden.
- Convergence: The movement of the two eyeballs inward so that the visual axes come together at the object viewed. Convergence of the eye, single binocular vision, occurs when light rays from an object fall on the corresponding points of the two retinas.

Overview of the Anatomy and Physiology of the Ear

The ear is divided into three anatomical parts—the external ear, middle ear, and inner ear. The ear has dual sensory functions, hearing and balance, or equilibrium. The stimulation or trigger for hearing and balance is the activation of hair cells, receptors that transmit nerve impulses and are perceived in the brain as sound or balance.

EXTERNAL EAR

The external ear or outer ear has two divisions, the auricle or pinna and the ***external auditory meatus*** (ear canal). The auricle is the visible appendage on the side of the head surrounding the opening of the external auditory meatus. The external auditory meatus travels into the temporal bone, ending at the ***tympanic membrane*** or eardrum, which stretches across the inner end of the

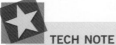

TECH NOTE
Pharmacy technicians are susceptible to dry eyes while performing sterile preparation of IV products in the laminar flow hood. Application of eye products such as Refresh Tears, Lacrilube, or other isotonic solutions can help prevent discomfort caused by the constant flow of air from the hood.

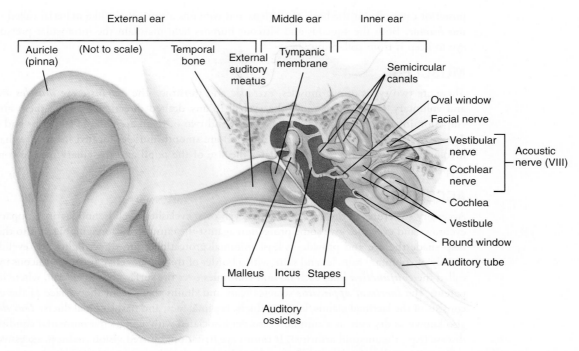

The ear. (From Thibodeau G, Patton K: *Anatomy and physiology*, ed 6, St. Louis, 2007, Mosby.)

canal, separating it from the middle ear. **Cerumen**, a waxlike substance, is secreted by modified sweat glands in the auditory canal.

MIDDLE EAR

The middle ear (tympanic cavity) is a tiny epithelium-lined cavity hollowed out of the temporal bone. It contains the three auditory ossicles—the **malleus** (hammer), **incus** (anvil), and **stapes** (stirrup). The handle of the malleus is attached to the surface of the tympanic membrane and the head is attached to the incus, which in turn attaches to the stapes. There are two openings into the inner ear, the oval window into which the stapes fit and the round window, which is covered by a membrane, the middle ear (tympanic cavity) opens into the auditory (eustachian) tube. The **eustachian tube** is composed partly of bone, cartilage, and fibrous tissue and is lined with mucus. It extends from the middle ear into the **nasopharynx** and functions to equalize pressure between the inner and outer surfaces of the tympanic membrane.

INNER EAR

The inner ear, or **labyrinth,** consists of two main parts, the bony labyrinth and a membranous labyrinth. The bony labyrinth consists of the vestibule and the semicircular canals (balance) and cochlea (hearing). The membranous labyrinth consists of the utricle and saccule inside the vestibule, the cochlear duct inside the cochlea, and the membranous semicircular canals inside the bony ones. The membranous labyrinth is filled with a clear fluid called endolymph and is surrounded by another fluid called the perilymph.

COCHLEA AND COCHLEAR DUCT

The word *cochlea* means snail; inside the cochlea is the membranous cochlear duct, the only part of the inner ear concerned with hearing. The hearing sense organ named the **organ of Corti** contains sensory neurons that extend to form the cochlear nerve that conduct impulses to the brain and produce the sensation of hearing. Hearing results from the stimulation of the auditory area of the cerebral cortex.

HEARING IMPAIRMENT

Hearing problems can be divided into two basic categories, conduction impairment and nerve impairment. **Conduction impairment** refers to the blocking of airwaves as they are conducted through the external and middle ear to the sensory receptors of the inner ear. Causes of conduction impairment are waxy buildup of cerumen, foreign objects in the external auditory meatus, tumors, and other matter. **Nerve impairment** may be inherited or acquired and results in insensitivity to sound. **Presbycusis**, common in older adults, causes degeneration of nerve tissue in the ear and vestibular nerve. Chronic exposure to loud noise damages receptors in the organ of Corti.

Summary

Healthy vision requires the formation of an image on the retina—refraction, stimulation of rods and cones, and conduction of nerve impulses to the brain. Malfunction of any of these processes can disrupt normal vision. Conditions such as myopia, hyperopia, presbyopia, and astigmatism can be corrected by using corrective lenses or refraction surgery. Cataracts (cloudy spots on the eye's lens) may also interfere with focusing and can be removed by surgery. Infections of the eye such as conjunctivitis or pink eye may be caused by bacterial infection, viral infection, or allergies. Disorders of the retina such as retinal detachment may be caused by aging, an eye tumor, or blows to the head; degeneration of the retina may cause nyctalopia or night blindness, which results from a deficiency of vitamin A. Diabetes mellitus may cause diabetic retinopathy and damage to the optic nerve. Glaucoma (excessive intraocular pressure) is caused by an abnormal accumulation of aqueous humor. A stroke can also cause visual impairment when resulting tissue damage occurs in the region of the brain that processes visual information. The leading cause of permanent blindness in older adults is macular degeneration; its exact cause is unknown. Some risk factors include cigarette smoking and a family history of the disorder.

Hearing impairment may be caused by conduction impairment (the blocking of sound waves travelling from the outer ear to inner ear) or nerve impairment resulting in insensitivity to sound because of inherited or acquired nerve damage. An accumulation of cerumen (earwax) may impede the conduction of sound waves, which results in conduction impairment. Infections of the ear such as external otitis or swimmer's ear is common in athletes. It can be bacterial or fungal in origin and is usually associated with prolonged exposure to water. Otitis media, common in children, may be caused by an infection of the throat that travels up through the eustachian tube, which connects to the middle ear. Because the inner ear contains nerve receptors for hearing and equilibrium, nerve damage may cause Ménière's disease, characterized by vertigo (sensation of spinning), tinnitus (ringing of the ear), and progressive nerve deafness.

The eye and ear are special sense organs that rely on optimal nerve conduction to function properly. Impairment of the eye and ear can be somewhat preventable, but aging plays a part in their degeneration of function.

Bibliography

Chabner E: *The language of medicine*, ed 7, St. Louis, 2009, Saunders.
Patton K: *Survival guide for anatomy and physiology*, St. Louis, 2010, Mosby.
Thibodeau G, Patton K: Anatomy and physiology, ed 9, St. Louis, 2010, Mosby.

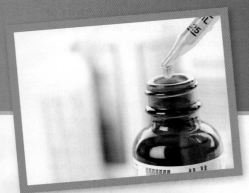

18

Treatment of Glaucoma

KEY TERMS

Angle-closure glaucoma: Sudden increase in intraocular pressure caused by obstruction of the drainage portal between the cornea and iris (angle); that can rapidly progress to blindness.

Aqueous humor: Fluid made in the front part of the eye.

Central vision: What is seen when you look straight ahead or when you read.

Cornea: Clear part of the eye located in front of the iris.

Intraocular pressure: Inner pressure of the eye. Normal intraocular pressure ranges from 12 to 22 mm Hg.

Iris: Colored part of the eye that can expand or contract to allow the right amount of light to enter the eye.

Open-angle glaucoma: Disorder characterized by elevated pressure in the eye that can lead to permanent blindness.

Optic nerve: Bundle of nerve fibers located in the back of the eye that connects the retina to the brain.

Peripheral vision: Sometimes called "side vision," this is usually the first area of vision to be lost with glaucoma.

Tonometry: Use of a device to measure the pressure in the eye.

Trabecular meshwork: Small openings around the outer edge of the iris that form meshlike drainage canals surrounding the iris and sometimes referred to as the Schlemm canal.

Glaucoma

More than 4 million Americans are estimated to have glaucoma, and half are unaware that they have the disease. According to the 2002 to 2003 National Population Health and Community Health Survey in Canada, approximately 409,000 Canadians older than the age of 20 years had glaucoma. The global prevalence of glaucoma is estimated to be greater than 70 million people, according to World Health Organization. This number is expected to increase to 80 million by 2020, making glaucoma the second leading cause of blindness worldwide. The prevalence of glaucoma increases with age, growing steadily after age 60 years. Having a family history for glaucoma also increases the risk. Neurovascular glaucoma is associated with diabetes, which is discussed in Chapter 33. African Americans are also six to eight times more likely to have glaucoma than whites. Persons of Asian and Hispanic ancestry are also at higher risk for the disease.

PATHOPHYSIOLOGY

There are actually several types of glaucoma; all are associated with progressive damage to the structures in the eye responsible for vision. *Peripheral vision* is first to be lost. The person gradually loses the ability to see images from the sides, top, or bottom of the eye(s). Eventually, only *central vision* remains (Figure 18-1).

Open-angle glaucoma is the most common and results from abnormal accumulation of *aqueous humor* (Figure 18-2). This in turn causes excessive *intraocular pressure* (IOP) and causes degeneration of the *optic nerve*. Sometimes damage to the optic nerve can occur in the absence of increased IOP. When this happens, low-tension or normal-tension glaucoma is said to be the cause. The unit of measure for IOP is millimeters of mercury (mm Hg).

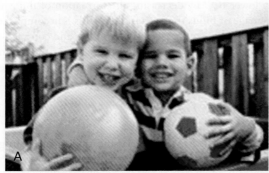 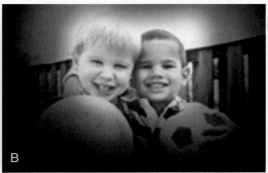

FIGURE 18-1 Glaucoma. **A,** Normal vision. **B,** Glaucoma. (Courtesy of U.S. National Institutes of Health National Eye Institute.)

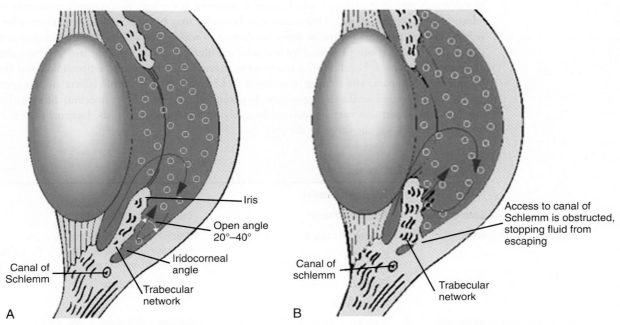

FIGURE 18-2 A, Aqueous humor: flow. **B,** Aqueous humor: obstruction. (From Clayton BD, Stock YN, Harroun RD: *Basic pharmacology for nurses*, ed 14, St Louis, 2007, Mosby.)

Intraocular pressure rises rapidly to dangerously high levels when a person has narrow-angle or *angle-closure glaucoma*. Normally, aqueous fluids drain from the eye through an opening in the eye where the *cornea* and *iris* meet. This region is called the angle (see Figure 18-2). When the angle becomes obstructed as occurs with inflammation or partial blockage of the *trabecular meshwork*, aqueous humor drainage is impaired, and there is a sudden increase in eye pressure. Pain and nausea may occur. If untreated, blindness can result in as little as a few days. Children born with defects in the structure of the angle of the eye may develop congenital glaucoma. Children with congenital glaucoma often have cloudy eyes, light sensitivity, and excessive tearing. If treated promptly, impaired vision may be avoided.

DIAGNOSIS

Tonometry is a diagnostic test that is performed to measure IOP. There are two types of devices used to perform tonometry. A tonometer is placed on the cornea, and gentle pressure is applied after first applying numbing drops to the eye, modern tonometers releases a puff of air into the eye to measure IOP. Eye drops that dilate the pupil may be adminstered to enable viewing of the retina to see if damage is evident.

TREATMENT

Drugs used in the treatment of glaucoma can be divided into two main classifications according to their method of action. Drugs may lower IOP by decreasing the formation of fluids that build up in the eye, or they may promote drainage of fluids that accumulate. This is accomplished by actions on parasympathetic or sympathetic nerves that control secretion of fluids and contraction of muscles that block fluid drainage. More than a single agent may be administered for the treatment of glaucoma. When two drops are administered, the second drop should be placed in the eye at least 5 to 10 minutes after the first agent.

Drugs That Decrease Aqueous Humor Formation

β-ADRENERGIC ANTAGONISTS

β-Adrenergic antagonists, also called beta blockers, are the classification of most drugs commonly used for the treatment of open-angle glaucoma. They are also administered for the treatment of intraocular hypertension. Stimulation of β-adrenergic receptors on ciliary cells increases secretion of aqueous humor. β-Adrenergic antagonists decrease aqueous humor formation by inhibiting the action of epinephrine and norepinephrine on β-adrenergic receptors located on the muscle and on blood vessels within the ciliary body. Betaxolol, however, is the only β-adrenergic antagonist that is selective for β_1-receptor sites. This means that betaxolol may be safer for use in patients who have asthma, congestive heart failure, or other conditions in which blockade of β_2-receptor sites is undesirable. Adverse reactions produced by betaxolol are blurred vision, light sensitivity (photophobia), dizziness, and nausea. Local adverse reactions to carteolol, levobunolol, metipranolol, and timolol include burning, pain, and itching in addition to blurred vision. Systemic effects are less common and include dizziness, weakness, depression, hypotension, decreased heart rate, and difficulty breathing. Systemic absorption may be reduced by applying finger pressure to the lacrimal sac for 1 to 2 minutes after placing the drops in the eyes.

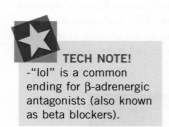
TECH NOTE!
-"lol" is a common ending for β-adrenergic antagonists (also known as beta blockers).

β-Adrenergic Antagonists

Generic Name	U.S. Brand Name(s) Canadian Brand(s)	Dosage Forms and Strengths
betaxolol*	Betoptic, Betoptic S	Solution, ophthalmic (Betoptic): 0.5%
	Betoptic S	Suspension, ophthalmic (Betoptic S): 0.25% Tablets: 10 mg[†], 20 mg[†]
carteolol*	Ocupress	Solution, ophthalmic: 1%
	Not available	
levobunolol*	Betagan	Solution, ophthalmic: 0.25%, 0.5%
	Betagan	

β-Adrenergic Antagonists—cont'd

Generic Name	U.S. Brand Name(s) Canadian Brand(s)	Dosage Forms and Strengths
metipranolol*	Optipranolol	Solution, ophthalmic: 0.3%
	Not available	
timolol hemihydrate*	Betimol	Solution, ophthalmic: 0.25%, 0.5%
	Not available	
timolol maleate*	Istalol, Timoptic, Timoptic in OcuDose, Timoptic Ocumeter, Timoptic XE	Solution, gel forming (Timoptic XE): 0.25%, 0.5% Solution, ophthalmic (Timoptic): 0.25%, 0.5%
	Timoptic, Timoptic XE	Solution, preservative free (Timoptic in OcuDose): 0.25%, 0.5% Tablets: 5 mg, 10 mg, 20 mg

Combinations		
timolol + brimonidine*	Combigan	Solution, ophthalmic: 0.2% brimonidine + 0.5% timolol
	Combigan	

*Generic available.
†Strength Available in the United States only.

α-ADRENERGIC AGONISTS

α-Adrenergic receptor agonists are used for the prevention and treatment of increased IOP. There are two α-adrenergic receptors in the eye (α_1 and α_2). Administration of α_1-adrenergic receptor agonists reduces blood flow in the ciliary body, and administration of α_2-adrenergic receptor agonists reduces the formation of aqueous humor. Administration of α_2-adrenergic agonists produces effects similar to administration of α-adrenergic antagonists. Adverse reactions produced by apraclonidine and brimonidine may be systemic as well as local. Local reactions include blurred vision, decreased night and distance vision, dry eyes, and irritated eyelids. Systemic effects are drowsiness and headache.

α-Adrenergic Agonists

Generic Name	U.S. Brand Name(s) Canadian Brand(s)	Dosage Forms and Strengths
apraclonidine*	Iopidine	Solution, ophthalmic: 0.5%, 1%
	Iopidine	
brimonidine*	Alphagan P	Solution, ophthalmic: 0.1%†, 0.15% (Alphagan P), 0.2% (Alphagan)
	Alphagan, Alphagan P	

*Generic available.
†Strength available in the United States only.

CARBONIC ANHYDRASE INHIBITORS

Carbonic anhydrase inhibitors are indicated for the treatment of open-angle glaucoma. Acetazolamide and methazolamide are also indicated for prevention of secondary acute angle-closure glaucoma and short-term treatment of angle-closure glaucoma when surgery must be delayed. Oral and parenteral dosage forms are used for the treatment of edema and centrencephalic epilepsy and prevention of altitude sickness. Their use in the treatment of glaucoma is based on the fact that they inhibit carbonic anhydrase, an enzyme responsible for speeding up the first step in the process of the conversion of carbon dioxide and water to bicarbonate. It is found in many parts of the body, including the ciliary structures of the eye. The production of aqueous humor depends on the transport of bicarbonate and sodium ions. Administration of carbonic anhydrase inhibitors decreases the rate of production of aqueous humor, thereby decreasing IOP. Adverse effects of acetazolamide and methazolamide include dizziness, drowsiness, potassium loss, frequent urination, kidney stones, a tingling

TECH NOTE!
To minimize systemic side effects, patients are advised to apply gentle pressure to the lacrimal sac for 1 to 2 minutes after the administration of eye drops.

TECH ALERT!
The following drugs have look-alike and sound-alike issues: Iopidine and Lodine; brominidine and bromocriptine

TECH NOTE!
Generic brimonidine 0.2% is *not* substitutable for Alphagan P, which is currently only available in 0.1% and 0.15% strengths.

TECH NOTE!
"-zolamide" is a common ending for carbonic anhydrase inhibitors.

Carbonic Anhydrase Inhibitors

Generic Name	U.S. Brand Name(s) Canadian Brand(s)	Dosage Forms and Strengths
acetazolamide*	Diamox Sequels	Capsule, sustained release (Diamox Sequels): 500 mg[†]
	Generics	Injection, powder for reconstitution: 500 mg
		Tablets: 125 mg[†], 250 mg
brinzolamide	Azopt	Suspension, ophthalmic: 1%
	Azopt	
dorzolamide*	Trusopt Ocumeter	Solution, ophthalmic: 2%
	Trusopt, Trusopt PF	
methazolamide*	Generics	Tablets: 25 mg[†], 50 mg
	Generics	
Carbonic Anhydrase Inhibitor Combination		
brinzolamide + timolol	Not available	Suspension, ophthalmic: 1% brinzolamide + 0.05% timolol
	Azarga	
dorzolamide and timolol*	Cosopt	Solution, ophthalmic: 2% dorzolamide and 0.5% timolol
	Cosopt, Cosopt PF	

*Generic available.
[†]Strength available in the United States only.

BOX 18-1   Directions for Preparing Echothiopate Iodide Eye Drops

- Use aseptic technique.
- Tear off aluminum seals and remove and discard rubber plugs from both the drug and diluent containers.
- Pour the diluent into the drug container.
- Remove the dropper assembly from its sterile wrapping. Holding the dropper assembly by the screw cap and WITHOUT COMPRESSING RUBBER BULB, insert it into drug container and screw down tightly.
- Shake for several seconds to ensure mixing.

TECH NOTE!
Carbonic anhydrase inhibitors may cause allergic reactions in people who have allergies to sulfonamide anti-infective agents.

TECH ALERT!
Acetazolamide and acetohexamide have look-alike and sound-alike issues.

TECH ALERT!
Isopto Carbachol and Isopto Carpine have look-alike and sound-alike issues.

sensation in the fingers and toes, bitter or metallic taste, nausea, impotence, and depression. Brimzolamide and dorzolamide produce primarily local adverse effects that include blurred vision; a bitter taste in the mouth; and burning or stinging, dry eyes. Less common reactions are irritation, discharge from the eyes, soreness, headache, and dizziness.

Drugs That Increase Aqueous Humor Drainage

Miotics are drugs that promote drainage of the aqueous humor. They produce this effect via a variety of mechanisms of action. Cholinergic agonists, acetylcholinesterase inhibitors, and prostaglandin analogues all promote drainage of accumulated levels of aqueous humor and reduce IOP.

CHOLINERGIC AGONISTS AND CHOLINESTERASE INHIBITORS

Cholinergic agonists are used to treat glaucoma and intraocular hypertension and to contract the pupil (miosis) during surgery. Cholinergic agonists bind to receptor sites and produce effects that mimic the neurotransmitter acetylcholine. Binding produces parasympathetic nervous system effects in the eye such as contraction of ciliary muscles and results in miosis. Pilocarpine is a cholinergic agonist that is used in the treatment of open- and closed-angle glaucoma. Cholinergic agonists also produce dilation of the trabecular meshwork to decrease IOP (see Figure 18-2, *B*). Pilocarpine (Salagen) is also used to treat xerostomia (dry mouth).

Echothiophate iodide is a cholinesterase inhibitor. Cholinesterase inhibitors block the enzyme that deactivates acetylcholine (see Chapter 13). This prolongs the effects of acetylcholine and administered cholinergic agonists. Adverse reactions include blurred vision, change in near or distance vision, difficulty in seeing at night or in dim light, headache, twitching of the eyelids, and watering of the eyes. For preparation instructions, see Box 18-1.

Cholinergic Agonists

Generic Name	U.S. Brand Name(s) Canadian Brand(s)	Dosage Forms and Strengths
carbachol*‡	Miostat	Solution, ophthalmic (Isopto Carbachol): 1.5%, 3%
	Isopto Carbachol, Miostat	Solution, for injection (Miostat): 0.01% Tablets: 2 mg*‡
pilocarpine*	Isopto Carpine, Pilopine HS, Salagen	Gel, ophthalmic (Pilopine HS): 4% Solution, ophthalmic (Isopto Carpine): 1%, 2%, 4%, 6%‡
	Akarpine, Diocarpine, Isopto Carpine, Pilopine HS, Salagen	Tablets (Salagen): 5 mg, 7.5 mg

Cholinesterase Inhibitor

echothiophate iodide	Phospholine iodide	Powder for reconstitution: 0.125% (6.25 mg)
	Not available	

*Generic available.
*‡Generic available in Canada only.
‡Strength Available in Canada only.

Prostaglandin Analogues

Generic Name	U.S. Brand Name(s) Canadian Brand(s)	Dosage Forms and Strengths
bimatoprost	Latisse, Lumigan	Solution, ophthalmic: 0.01%, 0.03%
	Latisse, Lumigan, Lumigan RC	
latanoprost*	Xalatan	Solution, ophthalmic: 0.005%
	Xalatan	
travoprost	Travatan Z	Solution, ophthalmic: 0.004%
	Travatan Z	
Combination		
latanoprost + timolol	Not available	Solution, ophthalmic: 0.5% timolol + 0.005% latanoprost
	Xalcom	
travoprost + timolol	Not available	Solution, ophthalmic: 0.5% timolol + 0.004% travoprost
	DuoTrav	

*Generic available.

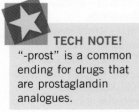

TECH NOTE!
"-prost" is a common ending for drugs that are prostaglandin analogues.

PROSTAGLANDIN ANALOGUES

Bimatoprost, latanoprost, and travoprost are prostaglandin analogues and are prodrugs. They mimic the action of prostaglandin F2α and therefore relax the ciliary muscles to permit drainage of aqueous humors. Prostaglandin analogues directly dilate the trabecular meshwork to promote drainage. The use of prostaglandin analogues can cause changes in the color or pigmentation of the eyes and may thicken eyelashes. Bimatoprost, latanoprost and travoprost may produce decreased vision, eye irritation, eye pain, itchy eyes, redness of eye, dry eyes, sun sensitivity, watery eyes, and permanent changes in eye pigmentation.

Miscellaneous

The use of marijuana is controversial. Some studies have shown it can reduce IOP. Marijuana is a Schedule I (C-I) controlled substance, and possession is a federal crime despite passage of regulation authorizing medical use in some states.

Summary of Drugs Used to Treat Glaucoma

Generic	Brand Name	Usual Dose	Warning Labels
Decrease Aqueous Humor Formation			
β-Adrenergic Antagonists			
betaxolol	Betoptic	**Open-angle glaucoma:** Instill 1 drop twice a day in affected eye(s)	SHAKE WELL—betaxolol suspension. WASH HANDS BEFORE USE; AVOID CONTAMINATION OF TIP—all. REMOVE CONTACT LENSES BEFORE USE; WAIT AT LEAST 15 MINUTES BEFORE REINSERTING—all. STORE AT ROOM TEMPERATURE—all. PROTECT FROM LIGHT—all. DO NOT DISCONTINUE WITHOUT MEDICAL SUPERVISION—all.
carteolol	Ocupress	**Open-angle glaucoma:** Instill 1 drop twice a day in affected eye(s)	
levobunolol	Betagan	**Open-angle glaucoma:** Instill 1-2 drops in affected eye(s) 1-2 times a day 0.25% or once daily 0.5%.	
metipranolol	Optipranolol	**Open-angle glaucoma:** Instill 1 drop in affected eye(s) twice daily	
timolol maleate	Timoptic, Timoptic XE	**Open-angle glaucoma:** Timoptic: Instill 1 drop twice daily in affected eye(s) Timoptic XE, Istalol: Instill 1 drop daily in the morning	
timolol hemihydrate	Betimol	**Open-angle glaucoma:** Instill 1 drop twice daily in affected eye(s)	
α-Adrenergic Agonists			
apraclonidine	Iopidine	Instill 1-2 drops in affected eye(s) 3 times a day	STORE AT ROOM TEMPERATURE—all. PROTECT FROM LIGHT—all. WASH HANDS BEFORE USE; AVOID CONTAMINATION OF TIP—all. REMOVE CONTACT LENSES BEFORE USE; WAIT AT LEAST 15 MINUTES BEFORE REINSERTING—all. DO NOT DISCONTINUE WITHOUT MEDICAL SUPERVISION—all.
brimonidine	Alphagan	Instill 1 drop in affected eye(s) 3 times a day	
brimonidine + timolol	Combigan	Instill 1 drop in affected eye(s) 2 times a day	
Carbonic Anhydrase Inhibitors			
acetazolamide	Diamox Sequels	**Oral (sustained release):** 500 mg twice daily **Oral (immediate release):** 250 mg 1-4 times a day **IV:** 250-500 mg; may repeat in 2-4 hours up to a maximum of 1 g/day (acute angle-closure glaucoma)	TAKE WITH FOOD—acetazolamide, methazolamide. SWALLOW WHOLE; DO NOT CRUSH OR CHEW—sustained-release capsule. MAY CAUSE DIZZINESS OR DROWSINESS—acetazolamide, methazolamide. SHAKE WELL—brinzolamide, brinzolamide + timolol. REMOVE CONTACT LENSES BEFORE USE; WAIT AT LEAST 15 MINUTES BEFORE REINSERTING—brinzolamide, dorzolamide, dorzolamide + timolol.
brinzolamide	Azopt	Instill 1 drop 3 times a day	
dorzolamide	Trusopt	Instill 1 drop 3 times a day	
brinzolamide + timolol	Azarga	Instill 1 drop 2 times a day	
dorzolamide + timolol	Cosopt	Instill 1 drop twice a day	

Summary of Drugs Used to Treat Glaucoma—cont'd

Generic	Brand Name	Usual Dose	Warning Labels
methazolamide	Neptazane	**Oral:** 50-100 mg 2-3 times a day	WASH HANDS BEFORE USE; AVOID CONTAMINATION OF TIP—brinzolamide, dorzolamide, dorzolamide + timolol. STORE AT ROOM TEMPERATURE—brinzolamide, dorzolamide, dorzolamide + timolol. PROTECT FROM LIGHT—brinzolamide, dorzolamide, dorzolamide + timolol. DO NOT DISCONTINUE WITHOUT MEDICAL SUPERVISION—brinzolamide, dorzolamide, dorzolamide + timolol.

Increase Drainage of Aqueous Humor

Cholinergic Agonists

Generic	Brand Name	Usual Dose	Warning Labels
carbachol	Isopto Carbachol	Instill 1-2 drops up to 3 times a day	WASH HANDS BEFORE USE; AVOID CONTAMINATION OF TIP—all. DO NOT DISCONTINUE WITHOUT MEDICAL SUPERVISION—all. STORE AT ROOM TEMPERATURE—carbachol. DO NOT WEAR CONTACT LENSES—carbachol. REFRIGERATE; DO NOT FREEZE—pilocarpine gel.
pilocarpine	Pilocar, Pilopine HS	**Solution:** Instill 1-2 drops up to 6 times a day **Gel:** Apply 0.5 inch in lower conjunctival sac at bedtime	

Cholinesterase Inhibitor

Generic	Brand Name	Usual Dose	Warning Labels
echothiophate	Phospholine Iodide	**Open-angle glaucoma:** Instill 1 drop twice a day	REFRIGERATE OR STORE RECONSTITUTED SOLUTION FOR UP TO 4 WEEKS AT ROOM TEMPERATURE.

Prostaglandin Analogs

Generic	Brand Name	Usual Dose	Warning Labels
bimatoprost	Lumigan	Instill 1 drop once daily in the evening	WASH HANDS BEFORE USE; AVOID CONTAMINATION OF TIP—all. REMOVE CONTACT LENSES BEFORE USE; WAIT AT LEAST 15 MINUTES BEFORE REINSERTING—all. DO NOT DISCONTINUE WITHOUT MEDICAL SUPERVISION—all. REFRIGERATE; DO NOT FREEZE—latanoprost, latanoprost + timolol. STORE AT ROOM TEMPERATURE—bimatoprost, travoprost, travoprost + timolol.
latanoprost	Xalatan	Instill 1 drop once daily in the evening	
travoprost	Travatan	Instill 1 drop in affected eye(s) once daily in the evening	
latanoprost + timolol	Xalcom	**Open-angle glaucoma:** Instill 1 drop in affected eye(s) once daily	
travoprost + timolol	DuoTrav	**Open-angle glaucoma:** Instill 1 drop in affected eye(s) once daily	

Nondrug Treatment

LASER SURGERY

Laser surgery may be performed to reduce IOP. There are three forms of laser surgery for glaucoma. Laser peripheral iridotomy creates a new drainage hole in the iris, permitting fluids to drain out of the eye. Laser trabeculoplasty unblocks existing channels, and laser cyclophotocoagulation, a type of laser surgery that is performed to reduce the amount of fluid entering the eye, is indicated for people who have severe glaucoma and have not responded to standard glaucoma surgery. Laser cyclophotocoagulation partially destroys the tissues that make the fluid in the eye.

Chapter Summary

- Glaucoma is the second leading cause of blindness worldwide.
- The percentage of the population that will develop glaucoma increases with advancing age.
- The prevalence of glaucoma in persons with diabetes is greater than that in persons without diabetes.
- There are actually several types of glaucoma: open-angle, angle-closure, low-tension, and secondary glaucoma.
- The most common form of glaucoma is open-angle glaucoma.
- Glaucoma can cause degeneration of the optic nerve.
- Increased IOP is caused by a buildup of aqueous humor and is a symptom of glaucoma.
- The aqueous humor accumulates when the angle formed by the iris and the cornea is reduced and drainage of fluid is blocked.
- Drugs used in the treatment of glaucoma can be divided into two main classifications according to their method of action: drugs that decrease formation of aqueous humor and drugs that promote drainage of aqueous humor.
- Drug classifications that decrease formation of the aqueous humor are beta blockers, α-adrenergic agonists, and carbonic anhydrase inhibitors.
- Drug classifications that promote drainage of the aqueous humor are cholinergics, cholinesterase inhibitors, and prostaglandin analogues.
- Miotics are drugs that cause contraction of the pupil. Drugs that promote drainage of the aqueous humor produce miosis.

REVIEW QUESTIONS

1. Glaucoma is the leading cause of blindness worldwide.
   a. true
   b. false

2. The most common form of glaucoma is _____.
   a. open angle
   b. closed angle
   c. narrow angle
   d. wide angle

3. The mechanism of action of drugs used in the treatment of glaucoma is_____.
   a. lower intraocular pressure by decreasing the formation of fluids
   b. promote drainage of fluids that accumulate
   c. lower intraocular pressure by increasing the formation of fluids
   d. a and b

4. The classification of the drug(s) most commonly used for the treatment of glaucoma is _____.
   a. α-adrenergic antagonists
   b. β-adrenergic antagonists
   c. carbonic anhydrase inhibitors
   d. prostaglandins

5. "-zolamide" is a common ending for which class of drugs?
   a. α-adrenergic antagonists
   b. β-adrenergic antagonists
   c. carbonic anhydrase inhibitors
   d. prostaglandins

6. Miotics are drugs that are used to decrease the drainage of the aqueous humor.
   a. true
   b. false

7. This drug is a β-adrenergic antagonist indicated for the treatment of open-angle glaucoma.
   a. latanoprost
   b. acetazolamide
   c. epinephrine
   d. timolol

8. Cholinergic agonists produce constriction of the trabecular meshwork and decrease intraocular pressure.
   a. true
   b. false

9. Select the FALSE statement about latanoprost.
   a. It must be stored in the refrigerator.
   b. It may increase pigmentation in the eye.
   c. It must be metabolized to its biologically active form.
   d. It must be premixed before use.

10. Laser surgery is not recommended to reduce intraocular pressure.
    a. true
    b. false

TECHNICIAN'S CORNER

1. The medical use of marijuana is controversial. What are your views on this subject? Give three pros and three cons for the medical use of marijuana.
2. The prevalence of glaucoma in a person with diabetes is greater than in persons without diabetes. What can be done to help diabetic patients to decrease the chance of developing glaucoma?

Bibliography

Bourne R: Worldwide glaucoma through the looking glass, *Br J Ophthalmol* 90:253-254, 2006.

Centers for Disease Control and Prevention: Prevalence of visual impairment and selected eye diseases among persons aged ≥50 years with and without diabetes–United States 2002, *MMWR Morb Mortal Wkly Rep* 53:1069-1071, 2004.

Chabner D: *The language of medicine*, ed 8, Philadelphia, 2007, WB Saunders.

Glaucoma Research Foundation: Glaucoma Facts & Stats. Retrieved May 1, 2011, from http://www.glaucoma.org/glaucoma/glaucoma-facts-and-stats.php, 2011.

Elsevier: Gold Standard Clinical Pharmacology. Retrieved April 30, 2011, from https://www.clinicalpharmacology.com/, 2010.

FDA: FDA Approved Drug Products. Retrieved May 13, 2012, from http://www.accessdata.fda.gov/scripts/cder/drugsatfda/index.cfm?fuseaction=Search.Search_Drug_Name, 2012.

The Glaucoma Foundation: About glaucoma. Retrieved from http://www.glaucomafoundation.org/education_content.php?i=7, 2006.

Health Canada: Drug Product Database. Retrieved May 1, 2011, from http://www.hc-sc.gc.ca/dhp-mps/prodpharma/databasdon/index-eng.php, 2010.

Lance L, Lacy C, Armstrong L, et al: *Drug information handbook for the allied health professional*, ed 12, Hudson, OH, 2005, APhA Lexi-Comp.

Mayo Clinic: Glaucoma. Retrieved May 1, 2011, from http://www.mayoclinic.com/health/glaucoma/DS00283, 2010.

National Eye Institute: *Glaucoma: what you should know*, Bethesda, MD, 2006, NEI, National Institutes of Health, U.S. Department of Health and Human Services. NIH publication No. 03-651. Retrieved from http://www.nei.nih.gov/health/glaucoma/glaucoma_facts.asp.

Page C, Curtis M, Sutter M, et al: *Integrated pharmacology*, Philadelphia, 2005, Mosby, pp 523-534.

Patton K: *Survival guide for anatomy and physiology*, St Louis, 2006, Mosby.

Quigley H, Broman A: The number of people with glaucoma worldwide in 2010 and 2010, *Br J Ophthalmol* 90:262-267, 2006.

Raffa R, Rawls S, Beyzarov E: *Netter's illustrated pharmacology*, Philadelphia, 2005, WB Saunders, p 48.

Thibodeau GA, Patton KT: *Anatomy and physiology*, ed 6, St Louis, 2007, Mosby.

USP Center for Advancement of Patient Safety: Use caution–avoid confusion, USP Quality Review No. 79, Rockville, MD, April 2004, USP Center for Advancement of Patient Safety.

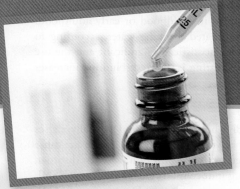

19

Treatment of Disorders of the Ear

KEY TERMS

Cerumen: Waxlike substance that is secreted by modified sweat glands in the ear.

Equilibrium: Steadiness or balance accompanied by a sense of knowing where the body is in relationship to surroundings.

Labyrinth: Bony structure in the inner ear consisting of three parts (vestibule, cochlea, and semicircular canals) and involved in balance.

Ménière's disease: Chronic inner ear disease associated with intermittent buildup of fluid in the inner ear that causes hearing loss and vertigo.

Otitis: Inflammation of the ear.

Otitis media: Infection of the middle ear.

Otoliths: Calcium carbonate crystals found in the utricle and saccule of the inner ear.

Otosclerosis: Hardening of the bones of the middle ear.

Ototoxicity: Damage or toxicity to the ear or eighth cranial nerve (associated with hearing).

Presbycusis: Bilateral hearing loss linked to aging and often accompanied by tinnitus.

Saccule: Saclike inner ear structure that senses vertical motion of the head.

Tinnitus: Intermittent or continuous whistling, crackling, squeaking, or ringing noise in the ears.

Tympanic membrane: Eardrum.

Utricle: Saclike inner ear structure that senses forward and backward motion and side-to-side motion of the head.

Vertigo: Feeling of spinning in space (dizziness and loss of balance).

Disorders Affecting Hearing

DISORDERS RESULTING IN HEARING LOSS
Otosclerosis

Otosclerosis is a disorder that causes destruction of bones in the ear (see Figure 19-1 for the anatomy of the ear). Bones that are typically affected are the stapes. Immobilization of the stapes footplate causes conduction hearing loss. Otosclerosis appears as tinnitus in childhood or early adulthood. The incidence of otosclerosis is lower in areas that have fluoridated drinking water, according to some epidemiologic studies. However, the differences are not statistically significant and the use of sodium fluoride to prevent bone destruction and preserve hearing is debated. Fluoride increases bone density by increasing bone mineralization.

Sudden Sensorineural Hearing Loss

Sudden sensorineural hearing loss (SSHL) progresses rapidly (hours to days) and typically causes hearing loss in only one ear. Other symptoms of SSHL may be vertigo and tinnitus. The exact cause of SSHL is unknown; however, it is believed it may be caused by a viral infection, vascular disorder, tumor, or rupture of the inner ear membrane or may be drug induced. Drugs that can cause SSHL are loop diuretics, aminoglycosides, anti-infectives, and antineoplastic agents. Drug-induced SSHL may disappear when the drug is stopped.

Treatment of SSHL involves the use of glucocorticosteroids (see Chapter 15). The best response occurs when hearing loss is moderate. Mild hearing loss resolves spontaneously without treatment, and no benefit is observed when hearing loss is severe. Vasodilating drugs and plasma expanders (e.g., normal saline, 5% glucose) may also be prescribed.

Autoimmune Hearing Loss

Autoimmune diseases such as multiple sclerosis can cause SSHL, but sometimes autoimmune hearing loss occurs in the absence of any other disease. Progression occurs over several months, and hearing loss may occur in both ears. Glucocorticosteroids such as prednisone are used in treatment (see Chapter 15).

DISORDERS RESULTING IN IMPAIRED PERCEPTION OF SOUND
Tinnitus

Tinnitus is a condition that can cause intermittent or continuous whistling, crackling, squeaking, or ringing noise in the ears. Sometimes it is described as ringing in the ear. It may be caused by

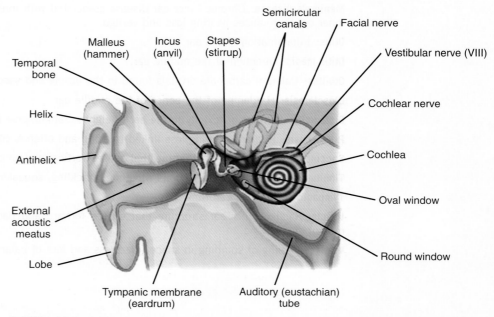

FIGURE 19-1 Anatomy of the ear. (From Lilley LL, Harrington S, Snyder JS: *Pharmacology and the nursing process*, ed 5, St Louis, 2007, Mosby.)

disease or *presbycusis* (bilateral hearing loss caused by aging), or it may be induced by drugs or noise. Tinnitus may be the first sign of *ototoxicity*. Alcohol and salicylates (aspirin) are the most common causes of drug-induced tinnitus.

Tinnitus is treated by masking the noise using a noise generator or stress management and avoiding alcohol or things that make tinnitus worse. Medications may produce some symptom relief if tinnitus is severe. Drugs that have been used are benzodiazepines (see Chapter 5) and tricyclic antidepressants (see Chapter 6).

Sense of Balance

The sense organs involved in balance or *equilibrium* are found in the vestibule and the three semicircular canals of the *labyrinth* (see Figure 19-1). The sense organs located in the *utricle* and *saccule* function in static equilibrium. They sense the position of the head relative to gravity, acceleration, or deceleration of the body. The sense organs associated with the semicircular canals function in dynamic equilibrium to maintain balance when the head or body itself is rotated or suddenly moved. Fluids in the semicircular canals shift when the body is in motion to inform the direction and speed of rotation. The superior, posterior, and horizontal semicircular canals inform whether movement is up or down and side to side.

Disorders of Sense of Balance and Motion

DISORDERS RESULTING IN IMPAIRED PERCEPTION OF MOTION
Vertigo

Our perception of balance and movement is a function of input from our eye, inner ear, and sense receptors on the skin and skeleton. The body integrates the input it gets from these sources and compares it with previous experience. *Vertigo* is a balance disorder that is caused by a neural mismatch or sensory conflict. When our eyes tell us our body should be moving yet our body remains still, such as when we watch a movie of a roller coaster, a sensory conflict occurs. Similarly, when we read a book in a car that is moving, our inner ear and skin receptors tell us we are in motion, yet our eyes are fixed on the book that is not moving. Again, a sensory conflict occurs. Sensory conflicts may also occur from an inner ear infection, especially if only one ear is involved and one ear receives motion signals and the other ear receives none or a different signal. Head trauma, degeneration of otolith organs (benign positional vertigo), inflammation of the vestibular nerve, bacterial infection of the labyrinths, brainstem or cerebral pathology, Ménière's disease, or motion sickness may also produce vertigo.

Vertigo and other balance disorders produce symptoms of dizziness or spinning, nausea and vomiting, blurred vision, disorientation, and a feeling of falling.

Benign Paroxysmal Positional Vertigo

Benign paroxysmal positional vertigo (BPPV) is the number 1 cause of vertigo, accounting for approximately 20% of all cases. It occurs after trauma to the inner ear, infection, or degeneration of otolith organs. *Otoliths* are calcium carbonate crystals found in the utricle and saccule of the inner ear. When otoliths dislodge, the debris moves to the lowest part of the posterior semicircular canal each time the head shifts position. The shifting of the otoliths produces vertigo, nausea, and nystagmus.

Ménière's Disease

Ménière's disease is the second most common cause of vertigo. It is a chronic inner ear disease associated with intermittent buildup of fluid in the inner ear. It is characterized by tinnitus, progressive nerve deafness, and vertigo. The cause is unknown.

Ménière's disease is treated by administering medicines and with diet and lifestyle changes. Reducing sodium, caffeine, nicotine, and alcohol consumption may be helpful. Aminoglycoside anti-infectives such as gentamicin and streptomycin are sometimes used, but their use is controversial because they can cause ototoxicity. Diuretics may also be prescribed to reduce endolymph fluid accumulation in the ear and other body fluids. Diuretics are discussed in Chapter 22.

TECH ALERT!
Dimenhydrinate and diphenhydramine have look-alike/sound-alike issues.

TREATMENT OF DISORDERS OF THE EAR
Vertigo and Ménière's Disease

Many of the treatments for vertigo, Ménière's disease, and other balance disorders do not involve drug therapy. Physical therapy is the treatment of choice for BPPV. Physical therapy is used to manipulate the head and shift otoliths that have dislodged. A low-sodium diet and lifestyle changes that restrict alcohol consumption are useful for the treatment of Ménière's disease.

When drug therapy is indicated, antihistamines are most widely used and may be prescribed in tablet, transdermal patches, and rectal suppository dosage forms. This is most likely because centrally acting antihistamines have anticholinergic actions that can moderate symptoms of motion sickness. Acetylcholine and histamine are excitatory neurotransmitters involved in the control of vomiting (emesis). Nausea and vomiting are common symptoms of vertigo. Moreover, antihistamines and anticholinergics are vestibular suppressants. Vestibular suppression is useful because it reduces the eye activity responsible for symptoms of vertigo. Administration of vestibular suppressants is not recommended when treatment for vertigo involves physical manipulation of the head and "retraining" of vestibular pathways.

Agents used to manage vertigo and Ménière's disease are betahistine, dimenhydrinate, diphenhydramine, and meclizine. Side effects common to all of these drugs are sedation, dry mouth, urinary retention, and blurred vision. Transdermal patches may produce local irritation, burning, or pain at the site where the patch is applied. Dry mouth, thickened bronchial secretions, and urinary retention may be produced, limiting their use in patients with prostate disease, asthma, and other conditions. Use should be limited in lactating women because the drugs may reduce the supply of breast milk.

Auralgia

Ear pain, also called auralgia or otalgia, is a symptom of **otitis** externa, **otitis media**, swimmer's ear, and many other disorders, including viral myringitis (inflammation of the **tympanic membrane**), temporomandibular joint disorders, referred pain from abscessed teeth, and others. It is treated by administration of topical analgesics, local anesthetics, or oral analgesics. Corticosteroids such as hydrocortisone, are combined with otic agents to reduce inflammation and pain. Local anesthetics numb or anesthetize the ear canal and tympanic membrane, further reducing pain and irritation.

Agents Used to Manage Vertigo and Ménière's Disease

Generic Name	U.S. Brand Name(s) Canadian Brand(s)	Dosage Forms and Strengths
betahistine*	Not available	Tablets: 8 mg, 16 mg, 24 mg
	Serc	
cyclizine	Marezine	Tablets: 50 mg
	Not available	
dimenhydrinate*	Dramamine (OTC), Trip Tone (OTC)	Solution: 3 mg/mL, 15 mg/5 mL (Gravol)
	Gravol (OTC), Nauseatol (OTC), Travel tabs (OTC)	Solution, for injection (Gravol): 10 mg/mL, 50 mg/mL Suppositories (Gravol): 25 mg, 100 mg Tablets: 15 mg‡, 50 mg Tablets, chewable: 15 mg‡, 50 mg
meclizine*	Antivert, Bonine Medivert, Dramamine Less Drowsy Formula (OTC)	Tablets: 12.5 mg, 25 mg, 50 mg and 30 mg (Medivert) Tablets, chewable: 25 mg
	Bonamine	
scopolamine*	Transderm Scōp	Transdermal patch: 1.5 mg/72 hr
	Not available	

*Generic available.
‡Strength available in Canada only.

Usual Dosage and Warning Labels for Agents Used to Treat Vertigo and Ménière's Disease

Generic	Brand	Usual Dose	Warning Labels
betahistine	Serc (Canada only)	**Vertigo:** 8-16 mg 3 times a day	MAY CAUSE DROWSINESS; MAY IMPAIR ABILITY TO DRIVE. AVOID ALCOHOL. MAINTAIN ADEQUATE FLUID INTAKE. OBSERVE GOOD ORAL HYGEINE. ROTATE SITE OF PATCH APPLICATION— scopolamine. TAKE WITH FOOD—betahistine.
dimenhydrinate	Dramamine	**Vertigo, motion sickness, nausea, and vomiting:** 50-100 mg every 4-6 hours (maximum, 400 mg/day)	
meclizine	Antivert	**Motion sickness:** 25-50 mg 1 hour before travel; repeat in 12-24 hours as needed **Vertigo:** 25-100 mg/day in divided doses	
scopolamine	Transderm Scōp	**Motion sickness:** Place patch behind ear every 72 hours as needed	

Pharmacological Treatments for Miscellaneous Ear Conditions

Generic Name	U.S. Brand Name(s) Canadian Brand(s)	Dosage Forms and Strengths
Analgesics		
antipyrine and benzocaine*	Aurodex, Auroguard, Dolotic, Oto Care Otic, Otoalgan Auralgan	**Solution, otic:** antipyrine 5.4% and benzocaine 1.4%

*Generic available.

When the ear is inflamed, otic drops can produce stinging. This can be minimized by administering suspensions rather than solutions containing alcohol if this option is available. Otic drops should also be warmed to room temperature before administering into the ear. Sweet olive oil is a home remedy for ear pain. The oil has no analgesic properties, but the warmed oil may be soothing and dislodge cerumen, which may be the cause of the pain.

Water-Clogged Ears and Swimmer's Ear
Water-clogged ears and swimmer's ear are different conditions that are sometimes confused. Water-clogged ears are caused by fluids that accumulate in the ear after swimming or showering. Swimmer's ear produces inflammation and infection of the external ear after prolonged exposure to water along with damage to the lining of the ear canal. Damage to the lining typically occurs when the person uses a rigid object to remove water from the ears. Swimmer's ear produces acute pain, itching, and a foul-smelling discharge from the ear.

Both conditions cause earache. Nonprescription drying agents are safe and effective for treatment of water-clogged ears. Alcohol (Auro Dri) and mild acidic solutions of vinegar (acetic acid) dry excess water and soothe the eardrum. Alcohol-containing eardrops may produce stinging if the ears are inflamed.

Cerumen Impaction
Cerumen (earwax) is a normal and necessary substance produced by the ear. It functions to reduce the risk for bacterial infections in the ear because earwax has a pH of 6.5 and is bactericidal. Cerumen repels water and helps to keep the ear dry during swimming and bathing. It lubricates the skin of the external ear canal and provides a barrier to entry of airborne substances (dust, insects) into the ear canal.

The healthy ear continuously replaces old cerumen. If cerumen becomes impacted, it can produce hearing loss, pressure, and ear pain. This condition is more common in people who wear hearing aids or regularly place earplugs and earphones in the ear. A cotton-tipped applicator or other small sharp object should never be used to remove earwax. These objects can cause accidental perforation of the eardrum (tympanic membrane).

TECH ALERT!
The U.S. Food and Drug Administration issued a public warning in 2011, that the use of benzocaine in the mouth (mucus membranes and gums) is associated with methemoglobinemia; a rare, but potentially fatal serious condition.

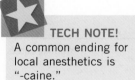

TECH NOTE!
A common ending for local anesthetics is "-caine."

TECH NOTE!
The pH is a measure of how acidic or alkaline (or basic) a solution is. A pH of 1 indicates that the solution is very acidic (e.g., stomach acids [HCl]). A pH of 7 is neutral. Plasma pH ranges between 7.35 and 7.45. A pH of greater than 7 is considered alkaline.

Treatments for Water-Clogged Ears and Swimmer's Ear

Generic Name	U.S. Brand Name(s) Canadian Brand Name(s)	Dosage Forms and Strengths
acetic acid solution*	Vosol	Solution, otic: 2%
	Burrow's Otic (OTC)	
Combination Otic Drops		
acetic acid + hydrocortisone solution*	Acetasol HC, Otomycet, Vosol HC	Solution, otic: 2% acetic acid + 1% hydrocortisone
	Not available	
isopropyl alcohol + glycerin*	Auro-Dri Ear-Water Drying Aid (OTC), Swim-Ear Ear-Water Drying Aid (OTC)	Solution, otic: 95% isopropyl alcohol and glycerin 5%
	Auro-Dri Ear-Water Drying Aid (OTC)	

*Generic available.

Cerumenolytics Used to Aid in Earwax Removal

Generic Name	U.S. Brand Name(s) Canadian Brand Name(s)	Dosage Forms and Strengths
carbamide peroxide (also known as urea hydrogen peroxide)*	Auro Earache Relief (OTC), Auro Ear drops (OTC), Debrox (OTC)	Solution, otic: 6.5%
	Murine Earwax Removal System (OTC)	
triethanolamine polypeptide oleate-condensate	Generics only	Solution, otic: 10%
	Cerumenex (OTC)	

*Generic available.

Summary of Drugs Used to Treat Miscellaneous Conditions of the Ear

Generic	Brand	Usual Dose	Warning Labels
Analgesics			
antipyrine and benzocaine	Aurodex	Instill 1-2 drops in ear canal and place a cotton pledgette in external ear 3-4 times a day or up to every 1-2 hours until pain relieved	FOR THE EAR.
Drying Agents			
acetic acid solution	Generics	Instill 4-6 drops in ear canal. Repeat every 2-3 hours as needed	FOR THE EAR.
isopropyl alcohol and glycerin	Auro-Dri Ear-Water Drying Aid	**Water-clogged ears:** Instill 4-5 drops in affected ear(s)	
Cerumenolytics			
carbamide peroxide	Debrox (OTC)	**Earwax removal:** Instill 5-10 drops twice daily for up to 4 days	FOR THE EAR.
triethylanolamine polypeptide oleate-condensate	Generics	**Earwax removal:** Fill ear canal; insert cotton pledgette; leave in for 15-30 minutes; then flush with warm water	FOR THE EAR.

Agents used to remove excess cerumen are called cerumenolytics. Emollients and carbamide peroxide are the principal ingredients found in cerumenolytics. Emollients are used to soften the wax, enabling it to slide out of the ear. Olive oil, mineral oil, and glycerin are emollients found in otics for earwax removal.

Peroxide-based products are used to break up the earwax and bubble away the debris. Carbamide peroxide 6.5% (over the counter [OTC]) and triethanolamine polypeptide oleate-condensate (OTC in Canada) are agents available to remove earwax.

After administration of emollients or peroxide-based agents, the affected ear is gently cleansed (irrigated) with warm water to remove cerumen that has become dislodged. Ear irrigation is performed using a bulb syringe.

Chapter Summary

- Perception of balance and movement is a function of input from the eyes, inner ear, and sense receptors on the skin and skeleton.
- The semicircular canals located in the inner ear control the sense of equilibrium or balance.
- Otosclerosis and autoimmune diseases such as multiple sclerosis and SSHL are conditions that can cause hearing loss.
- SSHL is treated with glucocorticosteroids.
- Otosclerosis also causes ringing in the ears (tinnitus).
- Tinnitus is a condition that produces ringing in the ear.
- Tinnitus may be drug induced. Aspirin and alcohol are common drugs that can cause tinnitus.
- Aminoglycoside anti-infectives (gentamicin) and loop diuretics can cause ototoxicity.
- BPPV is the number 1 cause of vertigo.
- Ménière's disease is the second most common cause of vertigo.
- Vertigo is a balance disorder that is caused by a neural mismatch or sensory conflict.
- Vertigo can occur from head trauma or degeneration of otolith organs, inflammation of the vestibular nerve, bacterial infection of the labyrinths, brainstem or cerebral pathology, or Ménière's disease.
- Vertigo and other balance disorders produce symptoms of dizziness or spinning, nausea and vomiting, blurred vision, disorientation, and a feeling of falling.
- Treatment of balance disorders may involve physical therapy, diet, and lifestyle changes.
- When drug therapy is indicated, antihistamines are most widely used.
- Antihistamines have anticholinergic actions that can moderate symptoms of motion sickness but produce urinary retention and other side effects that limit their use in patients with prostate disease or asthma or in women who are lactating.
- Other side effects that are common to all antihistamine drugs are sedation, dry mouth, and blurred vision.
- One scopolamine transdermal patch placed behind the ear prevents motion sickness for up to 3 days.
- Ear pain, also called auralgia or otalgia, is a symptom of otitis externa, otitis media, and many disorders of the ear such as viral myringitis, temporomandibular joint disorders, referred pain from abscessed teeth, and others.
- Ear pain is treated by administration of topical analgesics, local anesthetics, or oral analgesics.
- When the ear is inflamed, otic suspensions are more soothing than solutions that contain alcohol.
- Water-clogged ears and swimmer's ear are different conditions that are sometimes confused.
- Swimmer's ear produces inflammation and infection of the external ear.
- Nonprescription drying agents are safe and effective for treatment of water-clogged ears.
- Cerumen (earwax) is a normal and necessary substance produced by the ear.
- Cerumen is bactericidal and water repellant, and it provides a barrier to entry of airborne substances and lubricates the skin of the external ear canal.
- A cotton-tipped applicator or other small sharp object should never be used to remove earwax.
- Emollients and carbamide peroxide are the principal ingredients found in cerumenolytics.
- After administration of emollients or peroxide-based agents, the affected ear is gently cleansed (irrigated) with warm water to remove cerumen that has become dislodged.

1. The number 1 cause of vertigo accounting for approximately 20% of all cases is _____.
   a. overdose of aspirin and alcohol
   b. water in the ear
   c. benign paroxysmal positional vertigo
   d. constant diving

2. Presbycusis, common in _____, causes degeneration of nerve tissue in the ear and vestibular nerve.
   a. people with diabetes
   b. elderly adults
   c. middle-aged adults
   d. children with birth defects

3. Treatment of sudden sensorineural hearing loss involves the use of what type of medications?
   a. anti-inflammatories
   b. mineralocorticoids
   c. glucocorticosteroids
   d. stimulants

4. The most common cause for drug-induced tinnitus is _____.
   a. noise
   b. aspirin
   c. alcohol
   d. b and c

5. Which drug treatment for vertigo is available in a "patch" form?
   a. diphenhydramine
   b. scopolamine
   c. dimenhydrinate
   d. betahistine

6. Corticosteroids such as hydrocortisone are combined with _____ agents to reduce inflammation and pain in the ear.
   a. optic
   b. otic
   c. glaucoma
   d. ocular

7. Swimmer's ear produces inflammation and infection of the _____ ear after prolonged exposure to water along with damage to the lining of the ear canal.
   a. internal
   b. inner
   c. external
   d. semicircular canals

8. A cotton-tipped applicator or other small sharp object should be used to remove earwax.
   a. true
   b. false

9. Olive oil, mineral oil, and glycerin are emollients found in otics for removal of _____.
   a. ear wax
   b. fluid
   c. bacteria
   d. foreign material

10. Carbamide peroxide 6.5% is an approved agent for _____ removal.
    a. earwax
    b. fluid
    c. bacteria
    d. foreign material

TECHNICIAN'S
CORNER

1. How does ear candling work to remove unwanted cerumen or debris from the ear? What risks are associated with this practice?
2. What other home remedies have you heard of for helping with ear pain?

Bibliography

Chabner D: *The language of medicine*, ed 8, Philadelphia, 2007, WB Saunders.

Cruise AS, Singh A, Quiney RE: Sodium fluoride in otosclerosis treatment: review. *J Laryngol Otol* 2010;124(6):583-586. Epub 2010 Feb 18.

FDA: http://www.fda.gov/Drugs/DrugSafety/ucm250040.htm.

Hain T, Uddin M: Pharmacological treatment of vertigo, *CNS Drugs* 17:85-100, 2003.

National Institute on Deafness and Other Communication Disorders: *Balance disorders*, Bethesda, MD, 2006, NIDCD, National Institutes of Health, US Department of Health and Human Services. Retrieved from http://www.nidcd.nih.gov/health/balance/pages/balance_disorders.aspx.

Mayo Clinic: Tinnitus. Retrieved May 11, 2011, from http://www.nlm.nih.gov/medlineplus/tinnitus.html, 2010.

Mayo Clinic: Ménière's Disease: Treatment and Drugs. Retrieved May 15, 2011, from http://www.mayoclinic.com/health/menieres-disease/DS00535/DSECTION=treatments-and-drugs, 2010.

Page C, Curtis M, Sutter M, et al: *Integrated pharmacology*, Philadelphia, 2005, Mosby, pp 539-544.

Patton K: *Survival guide for anatomy and physiology*, St Louis, 2006, Mosby.

Thibodeau GA, Patton KT: *Anatomy and physiology*, ed 6, St Louis, 2007, Mosby.

Uppal S, Bajaj Y, Coatesworth AP: Otosclerosis 2: the medical management of otosclerosis. *Int J Clin Pract* 2010;64(2):256-265.

USP Center for Advancement of Patient Safety: Use caution–avoid confusion, USP Quality Review No. 79, Rockville, MD, April 2004, USP Center for Advancement of Patient Safety.

Vartiainen E, Karjalainen S, Nuutinen J, et al: Effect of drinking water fluoridation on hearing of patients with otosclerosis in a low fluoride area: a follow-up study. *Otol* 1994;15(4):545-548.

20

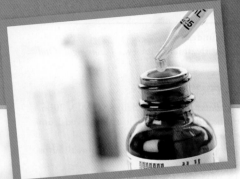

Treatment of Ophthalmic and Otic Infections

LEARNING
OBJECTIVES

1 Learn the terminology associated with eye and ear infections.
2 List and describe infections of the eye.
3 List and categorize medications used in the treatment of eye infections.
4 List and describe infections of the ear.
5 List and categorize medications used in the treatment of ear infections.
6 Identify significant drug look-alike and sound-alike issues.

KEY TERMS

Blepharitis: Chronic disease of the eye that produces distinctive flaky scales that form on the eyelids and eyelashes.

Conjunctivitis (pink eye): Common, self-limiting ailment that causes itching, burning, and teary outflow.

Cytomegalovirus retinitis: Viral opportunistic infection of the eye that can cause pain and blindness.

Fusarium keratitis: Rare fungal infection that occurs in soft contact lens wearers and can result in blindness.

Helminthes: Parasitic worms that can cause eye infection and blindness.

Herpes simplex keratitis: Painful eye infection caused by herpes virus that can lead to blindness.

Herpes zoster ophthalmicus: Painful eye infection caused by herpes virus that can lead to blindness.

Iritis: Condition associated with inflammation of the iris.

Keratitis: Severe infection of the cornea that may be caused by bacteria or fungi.

Otitis externa: Inflammation of the ear canal or external ear.

Otitis media: Inflammation of the middle ear typically caused by viral or bacterial infection.

Otorrhea: Discharge coming from the external auditory canal or inside of the canal.

Photopsia: Condition similar to floaters and associated with flashes of light.

Stye: Painful lump located on the eyelid margin caused by an acute self-limiting infection of the oil glands of the eyelid.

Uveitis: Serious eye condition that produces inflammation of the uvea and can cause scarring of the eye and blindness if untreated.

Vitreous floaters: Particles that float in the vitreous and cast shadows on the retina and appear as spots, cobwebs, or spiders.

300

Bacterial Infections of the Eye

BLEPHARITIS

Blepharitis is a chronic disease of the eye. It is also known as granulated eyelids because of the distinctive flaky scales on the eyelids and eyelashes produced by the condition. There are two forms of blepharitis, anterior blepharitis and posterior blepharitis. Anterior blepharitis affects the outside of the eyelid where the eyelashes are attached and is caused by bacteria (*Staphylococcus*) and scalp dandruff. Posterior blepharitis affects the inside of the eyelid and is caused by dysfunction of the oil glands in the eyelid, seborrhea, psoriasis (Figure 20-1), and acne rosacea.

Symptoms of blepharitis are eye pain or burning, excessive tearing, feeling of "something in the eye," light sensitivity, blurred vision, dry eye, and flaky scales on the eyelids and eyelashes. Complications of blepharitis are stye and tear film abnormalities.

Blepharitis is self-treated by applying clean warm compresses to the eyelids to loosen the scales followed by cleansing the eyelids with a mild eyelid scrub. Anti-infective ointments, corticosteroid eye drops, and artificial tears may also be used to manage the symptoms of blepharitis. Aminoglycoside anti-infectives are used in the treatment of blepharitis and include gentamicin, neomycin, and tobramycin.

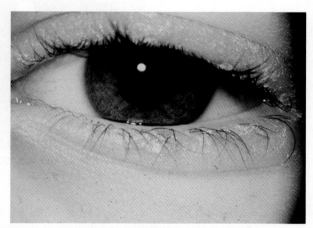

FIGURE 20-1 Psoriatic blepharitis. (Courtesy of the Cogan Collection, National Eye Institute/ National Institutes of Health.)

CONJUNCTIVITIS

Conjunctivitis (pink eye) is a common ailment that causes itching, burning, and teary outflow and is caused by allergies, bacteria, or a virus. Viral and allergic conjunctivitis is typically self-limiting and resolves without treatment with anti-infective agents. Conjunctivitis in newborns may be caused by exposure to a sexually transmitted infection and is treated preventatively by administering antibiotic drops at birth. Conjunctivitis of bacterial origin is contagious and is treated with antibiotic eye drops or orally administered anti-infectives. Various pathogens such as *Chlamydia trachomatis*, *Staphylococcus aureus*, *Streptococcus pneumoniae*, and *Haemophilus influenzae* bacteria may be the causative agents for bacterial infections. Antibacterial agents that are used in treatment include aminoglycosides, sulfonamides, quinolones, and macrolides. The antiviral trifluridine is used to treat keratoconjunctivitis attributable to herpes simplex type 1 virus (Figure 20-2).

IRITIS

Iritis is a condition associated with inflammation of the iris (Figure 20-3). Most causes of iritis are unknown; known causes are herpes virus, autoimmune disease, eye trauma, infectious disease (histoplasmosis, toxoplasmosis, syphilis, tuberculosis), and juvenile rheumatoid arthritis.

Symptoms of iritis include redness, blurred vision, inflammation, pain, and light sensitivity. Iritis is treated with the administration of corticosteroids (to reduce inflammation) and mydriatics (to

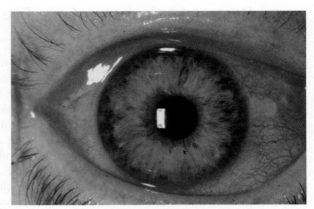

FIGURE 20-2 Viral conjunctivitis. (Courtesy of the Cogan Collection, National Eye Institute/National Institutes of Health.)

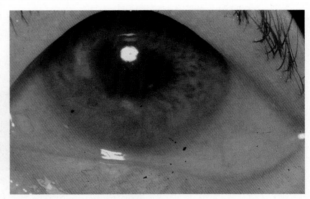

FIGURE 20-3 Iritis with rosacea keratitis. (Courtesy of the Cogan Collection, National Eye Institute/National Institutes of Health.)

reduce painful swelling). Mydriatics act on the dilator muscle and arterioles of the conjunctiva to produce vasoconstriction and dilation of the pupil. Antivirals also may be administered if the iritis is caused by a viral infection.

KERATITIS

Keratitis is a severe infection of the cornea and may be caused by bacteria or fungi. If untreated, the infection can cause permanent loss of vision. The most common causes of microbial keratitis and fungal keratitis are trauma, immunodeficiency, and chronic eye surface disease. Contact lens use can also cause microbial and fungal keratitis. Soft contact lens wearers, especially those who wear their contact lenses overnight, are at greater risk for eye infection. Of the approximately 30 million soft contact lens wearers in the United States, up to 21 persons out of 10,000 will develop microbial keratitis. The incidence of fungal keratitis varies according to geographical region. The incidence is higher in the southern United States (up to 35% of microbial keratitis cases) and lowest in the northeastern United States (up to 1% of microbial keratitis cases).

STYE

A *stye* (hordeolum) is a small, painful lump located on the eyelid margin (Figure 20-4). It is caused by an acute self-limiting infection of the oil glands of the eyelid and typically resolves on its own in a few days. When more than one stye is present at the same time, the condition is called blepharitis. Styes can be self-managed and are treated by applying warm compresses to the area.

UVEITIS

Uveitis is a serious eye condition that results in inflammation of the uvea and can cause scarring of the eye and blindness if untreated. There are three kinds of uveitis, each associated with a different

TECH ALERT!

The following drugs have look-alike and sound-alike issues: Bleph-10 and Blephamide; gentamicin and tobramycin; Tobrex and Tobradex

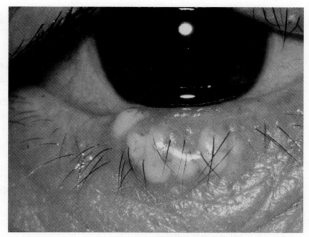

FIGURE 20-4 Stye. (Courtesy of the Cogan Collection, National Eye Institute/National Institutes of Health.)

part of the eye. Inflammation of the uvea in the area of the iris is called iritis. Inflammation in the middle of the eye is called cyclitis, and inflammation in the back of the eye is called choroiditis.

Most causes of uveitis are unknown; known causes are herpes virus, histoplasmosis (fungus), toxoplasmosis (parasite), autoimmune disease, eye trauma, and other eye disease. Other eye conditions that may cause uveitis are glaucoma, cataracts, and abnormal growth of new blood vessels in the eye.

Symptoms of uveitis include redness, blurred vision, pain, inflammation, and light sensitivity. These symptoms may develop suddenly or over a prolonged time period, as occurs with choroiditis.

Uveitis is treated with the administration of corticosteroids (to reduce inflammation); mydriatics (to reduce painful swelling); and anti-infectives, antivirals, or antifungals as appropriate. Drugs used in the treatment of uveitis are listed in the drug tables in this chapter.

Topical Ophthalmics Used to Treat Bacterial Infections

Generic Name	U.S. Brand Name(s) Canadian Brand(s)	Dosage Forms and Strengths
Aminoglycosides		
gentamicin*	Garamycin, Gentasol	Ointment, ophthalmic: 0.3%
	Diogent, Garamycin, Gentak	Solution, ophthalmic: 0.3%, 5 mg/mL (Gentak)
tobramycin*	AK-Tob, Tobrex	Ointment, ophthalmic: 0.3%
	Tobrex	Solution, ophthalmic: 0.3%
neomycin sulfate + bacitracin zinc + polymyxin B sulfate*	Generics only	Ointment, ophthalmic: 400 units/g bacitracin zinc + 3.5 mg/g neomycin + 10,000 units/g polymyxin B
	Diosporin	
neomycin sulfate + polymyxin B sulfate + gramicidin*	Neocidin, Neosporin	Solution, ophthalmic: 1.75 mg/mL neomycin + 10,000 units/mL polymyxin B + 0.025 mg/mL gramicidin
	AK Spore Liq, Optimyxin Plus Oto-Opth Gtte	
polymyxin B sulfate + gramicidin*	Not available	Solution, ophthalmic: 10,000 units/mL polymyxin B + 0.025 mg/mL gramicidin
	Optimyxin Oto-Opth Gtte, Polysporin Ear and Eye Drops [OTC]	

Continued

Topical Ophthalmics Used to Treat Bacterial Infections—cont'd

Generic Name	U.S. Brand Name(s) / Canadian Brand(s)	Dosage Forms and Strengths
polymyxin B sulfate + bacitracin*	AK-Poly Bac, Polycin-B, Polytracin	Ointment, ophthalmic: 10,000 units/g polymyxin B + 500 unit /g bacitracin
	Optimyxin Ophthalmic Ointment, Polysporin Sterile Ophthalmic Ointment	
Sulfonamides		
sulfacetamide Na⁺*	Bleph-10	Ointment, ophthalmic: 10%
	AK-Sulf Liq, Bleph-10, Sodium Sulamyd	Solution, ophthalmic: 10%
trimethoprim + polymyxin B sulfate*	Polytrim	Solution, ophthalmic: 1 mg/mL trimethoprim + 10,000 units/mL polymyxin B
	Polytrim	
Quinolones		
besifloxacin	Besivance	Suspension, ophthalmic: 0.6%
	Besivance	
ciprofloxacin*	Ciloxan	Ointment, ophthalmic: 0.3%
	Ciloxan	Solution, ophthalmic: 0.3%
gatifloxacin	Zymaxid	Solution, ophthalmic: 0.3% (Zymar), 0.5% (Zymaxid)
	Zymar	
levofloxacin	Iquix, Quixin	Solution, ophthalmic: 1.5% (Iquixin), 0.5% (Quixin)
	Not available	
moxifloxacin	Moxeza, Vigamox	Solution, ophthalmic: 0.5%
	Vigamox	
ofloxacin*	Ocuflox	Solution, ophthalmic: 0.3%
	Ocuflox	
Macrolides		
azithromycin	Azasite	Solution, ophthalmic: 1%
	Not available	
erythromycin*	Ilotycin, Romycin	Ointment, ophthalmic: 0.5%
	AK Mycin	
Anti-infective + Corticosteroid		
neomycin + bacitracin + polymyxin B + hydrocortisone*	Generics	Ointment, ophthalmic: 3.5 mg/g neomycin + 400 units/g bacitracin + 10,000 units/g polymyxin B + 1% hydrocortisone
	Cortimyxin	
neomycin + polymyxin B + dexamethasone*	Maxitrol, Poly-Dex	Ointment, ophthalmic: 0.35% neomycin + 10,000 units/g polymyxin B + 0.1% dexamethasone
	AK Trol, Maxitrolⁱⁱ	Suspension, ophthalmic: 0.35% neomycin + 10,000 units/mL polymyxin B + 0.1% dexamethasone
neomycin + polymyxin B + hydrocortisone*	Generics	Suspension, ophthalmic: 0.35% neomycin + 10,000 units/mL polymyxin B + 1% hydrocortisone
	Not available	

Topical Ophthalmics Used to Treat Bacterial Infections—cont'd

Generic Name	U.S. Brand Name(s) Canadian Brand(s)	Dosage Forms and Strengths
neomycin + polymyxin B + prednisolone	Poly-Pred Not available	Suspension, ophthalmic: 0.35% neomycin + 10,000 units/mL polymyxin B + 0.5% prednisolone
gentamicin + prednisolone*	Pred-G Not available	Suspension, ophthalmic: 0.3% gentamicin + 1% prednisolone Ointment, ophthalmic: 0.3% gentamicin + 0.6% prednisolone
sulfacetamide + prednisolone acetate*	Blephamide Blephamide	Ointment, ophthalmic: 10% sulfacetamine + 0.2% prednisolone Solution, ophthalmic: 10% sulfacetamine + 0.2% prednisolone
neomycin + fluorometholone	Not available FML Neo	Suspension, ophthalmic: 0.5% neomycin + 0.1% fluorometholone
sulfacetamide + fluorometholone	FML S Not available	Solution, ophthalmic: 10% sulfacetamide + 0.1% fluorometholone
tobramycin + dexamethasone	Tobradex Tobradex	Ointment, ophthalmic: 0.3% tobramycin + 0.1% dexamethasone Suspension, ophthalmic: 0.3% tobramycin + 0.1% dexamethasone
tobramycin + loteprednol	Zylet Not available	Suspension, ophthalmic: 0.3% tobramycin + 0.5% loteprednol

*Generic available.
║The product formulations for Maxitrol (United States) and Maxitrol (Canada) are different. The formulation in Canada contains only 6000 units of polymyxin B sulfate.

Viral Infections of the Eye

CYTOMEGALOVIRUS RETINITIS

Most adults throughout the world have been exposed to cytomegalovirus (CMV). It is estimated that 50% to 80% of adults in the United States harbor anti-CMV antibodies. In healthy individuals, exposure to CMV does not cause active disease. The virus remains dormant unless the immune system becomes depressed, and then infections of the eyes, gastrointestinal tract, lungs, and central nervous system may develop.

Cytomegalovirus retinitis is an opportunistic infection in the eye that occurs in patients who have HIV infection/AIDS or take immunosuppressive drugs. The infection can lead to hemorrhage, cell death, and blindness. The most common symptoms of CMV retinitis are decreased vision, eye pain, floaters, and photopsia. *Vitreous floaters* are particles that cast shadows on the retina and appear as spots, cobwebs, or spiders. *Photopsia* is a condition similar to floaters and is associated with flashes of light.

Cytomegalovirus retinitis is treated by administration of antivirals such as ganciclovir, valganciclovir, foscarnet, and cidofovir. Valganciclovir is the only drug that can be taken orally for the induction phase of therapy (initial therapy). Oral ganciclovir is only approved for maintenance therapy.

HERPETIC EYE DISEASE

The herpes virus is the cause of many infections throughout the body. Herpetic corneal disease is the cause of more than 500,000 cases of blindness annually. Two strains of the virus are responsible for infections of the eye. *Herpes zoster ophthalmicus* is caused by the virus that is responsible for chickenpox and shingles (varicella-zoster). *Herpes simplex keratitis* is caused by the same virus that produces cold sores on the lips and mouth (herpes simplex 1).

Herpes simplex virus (HSV) can cause blepharitis, conjunctivitis, dendritic epithelial keratitis, corneal ulceration, stromal keratitis, endothelialitis, trabeculitis, scleritis, iridocyclitis, acute retinal necrosis syndrome, and other conditions (Figure 20-5).

Both herpes zoster ophthalmicus and herpes simplex keratitis produce eye pain, redness, and cloudiness of the cornea. The virus lives around nerve fibers and, when activated, produces painful symptoms. Symptoms associated with herpes zoster ophthalmicus are swelling and rash or sores around the eye, eyelids, or forehead. Symptoms of herpes simplex keratitis are excessive tearing, decreased vision, a gritty feeling in the eye, and pain when looking at bright light.

Antivirals, administered in the eye or by mouth, are used to treat herpes zoster ophthalmicus and herpes simplex keratitis. Acyclovir is used to prevent and suppress recurrent herpetic eye disease, but its use for herpes simplex ocular infection prophylaxis is not approved by the U.S. Food and Drug Administration (FDA). Corticosteroids are used to reduce inflammatory cells that can block the trabecular meshwork, impede the outflow of eye fluids, and may lead to increased intraocular pressure and pain. Use of corticosteroids must be carefully monitored because the drugs can also increase intraocular pressure. Mydriatics may be administered to maintain the normal flow of eye fluids and prevent buildup of intraocular pressure. Drugs used in the treatment of herpetic eye disease are listed the following table. A detailed discussion of antivirals is found in Chapter 36.

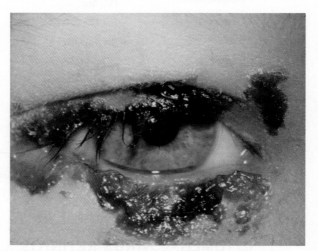

FIGURE 20-5 Herpetic blepharitis. (Courtesy of David G. Cogan Ophthalmic Pathology Collection, http://cogancollection.nei.nih.gov.)

Drugs Used to Treat Viral Infections in the Eye

Generic Name	U.S. Brand Name(s) Canadian Brand(s)	Dosage Forms and Strengths
cidofovir	Vistide Not available	Solution, for injection: 75 mg/mL
foscarnet*	Generics Not available	Solution, for injection: 24 mg/mL
ganciclovir*	Cytovene, Vitrasert, Zirgan Cytovene	Capsules: 250 mg, 500 mg Gel, ophthalmic (Zirgan): 0.15% Intravitreal implant (Vitrasert): 4.5 mg Powder, for injection (Cytovene): 500 mg
trifluridine*	Viroptic Viroptic	Solution, ophthalmic: 1%
valganciclovir	Valcyte Valcyte	Powder, for injection: 50 mg/mL Tablet: 450 mg

*Generic available.

Fungal and Protozoal Infections of the Eye

FUSARIUM KERATITIS

Fusarium keratitis is a rare fungal infection of the eye that occasionally occurs in people who wear soft contact lenses. If untreated, it can lead to blindness. See the discussion of keratitis for more information. Fusarium keratitis and other fungal infections of the eye are treated with antifungals such as natamycin.

TOXOPLASMOSIS

Ocular toxoplasmosis is caused by protozoa and is transmitted by handling or eating raw and under-cooked meat or by handling cat feces. According to the Centers for Disease Control and Prevention, there may be as many as 1.26 million people in the United States with ocular toxoplasmosis. Exposure to the protozoa causes the development of antigens that can cause ocular inflammation, vasculitis, uveitis, and retinal edema.

Drugs used in the treatment and management of toxoplasmosis are pyrimethamine and sulfonamides (sulfadiazine and trimethoprim + sulfamethoxazole).

TECH ALERT!
Natacyn and Naprosyn have look-alike and sound-alike issues.

Ophthalmic Antifungals

Generic Name	U.S. Brand Name(s) / Canadian Brand(s)	Dosage Form and Strength
natamycin	Natacyn / Not available	Suspension, ophthalmic: 5%

Helminthic Infections

Helminthes are parasitic worms that can cause eye infections and blindness. Three species can cause infection in the human eye.

ONCHOCERCIASIS

Onchocerciasis is caused by the nematode (roundworm) *Onchocerca volvulus*. The disease is also known as river blindness. Onchocerciasis is the second leading cause of infectious blindness in the world, according the World Health Organization. Most cases of onchocerciasis occur in Africa, Yemen, and Central and South America, where the flies that carry the disease live.

Onchocerciasis is treated by administering a single dose of ivermectin yearly. This anthelminthic kills living worms and prevents the inflammatory reaction and scarring in the eye that is triggered by the worms.

CYSTICERCOSIS

Cysticercosis is caused by the cestode (flat worm) *Taenia solium*. It is transmitted to humans who eat undercooked pork. Cysticercosis is most common in Andean South America, Brazil, Central America, Mexico, China, India, Southeast Asia, and sub-Saharan Africa. It is treated with praziquantel (not FDA approved), corticosteroids, and surgical removal of the living worms.

TOXOCARIASIS

Dogs, cats, wolves, and foxes are carriers of the worm that causes toxocariasis. The infection is contracted by eating soil that is infested with feces containing the worm eggs and is most common in children. Toxocariasis is the fifth leading cause of uveitis worldwide. Infections can cause loss of vision in the affected eye and strabismus. It is treated by the administration of topical corticosteroids and systemic anthelminthics such as albendazole and thiabendazole.

The dog is also the carrier of another roundworm (*Ancylostoma caninum*) that can cause diffuse unilateral subacute neuroretinitis (DUSN). The worms produce inflammation in the retina that progresses to atrophy of the optic nerve and blindness. The infection is treated with topical corticosteroids and systemic anthelminthics such as thiabendazole.

TECH NOTE!
Ophthalmic drugs can be used in the ear, but otic drugs cannot be used in the eye.

Drugs Used to Treat Parasitic Infections of the Eye

Generic Name	U.S. Brand Name(s) Canadian Brand(s)	Dosage Forms and Strengths
albendazole*	Albenza	Tablet: 200 mg
	Not available for human use	
ivermectin	Stromectol	Tablet: 3 mg
	Not available for human use	
praziquantel**	Biltricide	Tablet: 600 mg
	Biltricide	

*Generic available.
**Not FDA approved.

Summary of Treatments of Bacterial, Fungal, and Viral Infections of the Eye

Usual Dosage for Drugs Used to Treat Infections of the Eye

Generic Name	Brand Name	Usual Dosage
Aminoglycosides		
gentamicin 0.3%	Garamycin	Instill 1-2 drops every 4 hours while awake until resolved (solution) *or* Apply ½-inch ribbon of ointment 2-3 times a day to eyelid margin
tobramycin 0.3%	Tobrex	Instill 1-2 drops in eye(s) every 4 hours *or* Apply ointment 2-3 times a day (every 3-4 hours for severe infection)
neomycin + bacitracin + polymyxin B	Neosporin Ophthalmic ointment	Apply small amount to conjunctival sac every 3-4 hours for 7-10 days
neomycin + polymyxin B + gramicidin	Neosporin Ophthalmic solution	Instill 1-2 drops in eye(s) every 4 hours (or up to 2 drops every hour for severe infection)
Sulfonamides		
sulfacetamide Na+ 10%	Sodium Sulamyd, Bleph-10	Instill 1-2 drops every 1 hour while awake until resolved (solution) *or* Apply a thin ribbon of ointment 4 times a day and at bedtime to eyelid margin
trimethoprim 1 mg + polymyxin B 10,000 units	Polytrim	Instill 1 drop into eye(s) every 3 hours up to 6 doses/day for 7-10 days
Quinolones		
besifloxacin	Besivance	Instill 1 drop in the affected eye(s) 3 times daily, 4-12 hours apart, for 7 days
ciprofloxacin 0.3%	Ciloxan	Instill 1-2 drops in eye(s) every 2 hours while awake for 2 days; then 1-2 drops every 4 hours for 5 days *or* Apply ½-inch ribbon to conjunctival sac 3 times a day for 2 days; then twice daily for 5 days

Usual Dosage for Drugs Used to Treat Infections of the Eye—cont'd

Generic Name	Brand Name	Usual Dosage
gatifloxacin	Zymaxid, Zymar	1.1 On day 1, instill 1 drop in each affected eye every 2 hours while awake up to 8 times daily; on days 2-7, instill 1 drop in each affected eye 2-4 times daily while awake (Zymaxid); on first 2 days, instill 1 drop in each affected eye every 2 hours while awake up to 8 times daily; on days 3-7, instill one drop in each affected eye 4 times daily while awake
levofloxacin	Iquixin, Quixin	Instill 1-2 drops in eye(s) every 2 hours while awake days 1 to 2; then instill every 4 hours days 3-7 (up to 4 times a day)
moxifloxacin	Vigamox, Moxeza	Instill 1 drop in affected eye(s) 3 times a day for 7 days (Vigamox); instill 1 drop in affected eye(s) 2 times a day for 7 days (Moxeza)
ofloxacin	Ocuflox	Instill 1 drop in affected eye every 2-4 hours for 2 days; then use 1-2 drops 4 times a day for 5 days more
Macrolides		
azithromycin	Azasite	Instill 1 drop in the affected eye(s) twice daily (8-12 hours apart) for the first 2 days followed by 1 drop in the affected eye(s) once daily for the next 5 days
erythromycin	Generics	Apply ½-inch (1.25 cm) 2-6 times a day until resolved
Anti-infective + Corticosteroid		
neomycin + bacitracin + polymyxin B + hydrocortisone	Cortisporin Ointment	Apply a ½-inch ribbon of ointment every 3 to 4 hours to lower eyelid margin until improvement
neomycin + dexamethasone	NeoDecadron	Instill 1-2 drops into eye(s) every 3-4 hours
neomycin + polymyxin B + dexamethasone	Maxitrol	Apply a ½-inch ribbon of ointment 3-4 times a day or at bedtime *or* Instill 1-2 drops into eye(s) every 4-6 hours (up to every 1 hour if severe disease)
neomycin + polymyxin B + prednisolone	Poly-Pred	Instill 1-2 drops into eye(s) every 3-4 hours
gentamicin + prednisolone	Pred-G	Instill 1 drops into eye(s) 2-4 times a day (up to every 1 hour during 1st 24-48 hours) *or* Apply a ½-inch ribbon of ointment 1-3 times a day
sulfacetamide + prednisolone acetate	Blephamide	Apply to lower conjunctival sac up to 6 times a day
sulfacetamide + prednisolone phosphate	Generics	*or* Instill 1-3 drops into eye(s) every 2-3 hours while awake (12 drops/day)
sulfacetamide + fluorometholone	FML-S	Instill 1 drops into eye(s) 4 times a day
tobramycin + dexamethasone	Tobradex	Instill 1-2 drops in eye(s) every 4-6 hours *or* Apply ointment every 6-8 hours (every 3-4 hours for severe infection)

Continued

Usual Dosage for Drugs Used to Treat Infections of the Eye—cont'd

Generic Name	Brand Name	Usual Dosage
tobramycin + loteprednol	Zylet	Instill 1-2 drops into the conjunctival sac of the affected eye(s) every 4-6 hours
Antivirals		
cidofovir	Vistide	Infuse 5 mg/kg IV over 1 hour once weekly for 2 weeks, then once every other week
ganciclovir	Cytovene, Vitrasert, Zirgan	Infuse 5 mg/kg IV every 12 hours for 14-21 days; then once daily 7 days/week (or 6 mg/kg/day for 5 days/week) *or* 1000 mg orally 3 times a day (or 500 mg 6 times/day) *or* One implant every 5-8 months (Vitrasert) *or* 1 drop in the affected eye(s) 5 times per day until corneal ulcer heals; then 1 drop in the affected eye(s) 3 times per day for 7 days
foscarnet	Foscavir	Infuse 60 mg/kg/dose every 8 hours or 90 mg every 12 hours for 14-21 days; then 90-120 mg/kg/day as a single dose
trifluridine	Viroptic	Instill 1 drop in eye(s) every 2 hours while awake up to 9 drops/day until corneal ulcer heals; then 1 drop every 4 hours for 7 days
valganciclovir	Valcyte	900 mg twice a day for 21 days; then take once daily thereafter
Antifungal		
natamycin	Natacyn	**Keratitis:** Instill 1 drop into conjunctival sac every 1-2 hours for 3-4 days; then 1 drop every 3-4 hours for 14-21 days or until resolved. **Blepharitis & conjunctivitis:** 1 drop every 4-6 hours until resolved.

Bacterial Infections of the Ear

OTITIS EXTERNA

Otitis externa, also known as swimmer's ear, is an inflammation of the external auditory canal. It may be caused by bacterial infection, fungal infection, seborrheic dermatitis, psoriasis, and lupus erythematosus. The most common cause is bacterial infection. Fungi (*Candida* spp.) account for only 10% of the cases of otitis externa. Risk factors for development of otitis externa are (1) exposure to excessive moisture (swimming, humidity, sweating), (2) high environmental temperature, (3) irritation caused by earwax removal, (4) insertion of objects into the ear, and (5) chronic dermatologic disease. Treatments for swimmer's ear are discussed in Chapter 19.

The most common symptoms of otitis externa are ear discomfort or pain, itchiness, and discharge (*otorrhea*). Topical and systemic drugs are used to treat and control the symptoms of otitis externa. Anti-infectives used in treatment are listed in the drug tables in this chapter.

Treatment of Otitis Externa

Topical Anti-infectives Used to Treat Otitis Externa		
Generic Name	**U.S. Brand Name(s)**	**Usual Dosage**
	Canadian brand name(s)	
Aminoglycosides		
gentamicin sulfate 0.3%*	Generic	Apply 3-4 drops in ear(s) 3 times a day
	Garamycin Otic	
Quinolones		
ofloxacin 0.3%*	Floxin Otic	Instill 10 drops in affected ear(s) daily for 7 days
	Not available	
Anti-infective + Corticosteroid		
ciprofloxacin 0.3% + dexamethasone 1%	Ciprodex	Instill 4 drops in ear(s) 2-4 times a day for 7 days.
	Ciprodex	
ciprofloxacin 0.2% + hydrocortisone 1%	Cipro HC otic suspension	Instill 3 drops in affected ear(s) 2 times a day for 7 days
	Not available	
neomycin 0.35% + polymyxin B 10,000 units + hydrocortisone 1%*	Aural Otic, Cortisporin Otic, Oticin, Otimar, Otocidin	Instill 4 drops into ear(s) 3-4 times a day
	Cortisporin Otic, Cortimyxin	
acetic acid 2% + hydrocortisone 1%*	Acetasol HC, Otomycet, Vosol HC	Instill 3-5 drops in ear(s) 3-4 times a day
	Not available	

*Generic available.

OTITIS MEDIA

Otitis media is an inflammation in the middle ear. It may accompany an upper respiratory infection. Children are more susceptible to otitis media than adults because their eustachian tubes are shorter and straighter. When the eustachian tube is blocked by swelling or mucus from a cold, fluids accumulate and collect in the normally air-filled middle ear. Bacteria may collect in the fluid along with white blood cells released by the body to fight the infection. Hearing becomes impaired because the eardrum and middle ear bones are unable to move as freely. Pain and pressure builds, and finally the eardrum may tear to release the pressure.

Historically, otitis media has been treated aggressively with orally administered anti-infective drugs; however, new evidence shows that the infection is self-limiting in many cases and will resolve on its own without treatment. Excessive use of anti-infective agents may increase the risk of the development of bacterial resistance. Watchful waiting rather than antimicrobial treatment was endorsed by the American Academy of Pediatrics and American Family Physicians in 2004 in children 6 to 23 months with nonsevere illness. The non-use of antimicrobial therapy continues to be controversial, and a 2011 study has shown that amoxicillin–clavulanate may reduce the time to resolution of symptoms.

Furthermore, evidence shows that prophylactic use of antihistamines and decongestants is ineffective in preventing or treating acute otitis media and is not recommended and can be harmful in children younger than 2 years of age. Anti-infective agents used in the treatment of otitis media are listed in the following table along with usual dosages for children. These agents are described fully in Unit 10.

TECH ALERT!
The following drugs have look-alike and sound-alike issues: Pediazole and Pediapred; cefixime, cefuroxime, cefpodoxime, and cephalexin; amoxicillin, ampicillin, and Augmentin

Treatment

Selected Anti-infectives Used to Treat Otitis Media

Generic Name	U.S. Brand Name(s) Canadian Brand Name(s)	Usual Child Dosage
Penicillins		
amoxicillin*	Generics	30-90 mg/kg/day every 8-12 hours for 10 days (depending on age and severity)
	Generics	
amoxicillin + clavulanate*	Augmentin	40 mg/kg/day every 12 hours for 10 days (<40 kg); 250-500 mg every 8 hours or 875 mg every 12 hours (>40 kg)
	Clavulin	
Macrolides		
azithromycin*	Zithromax	10 mg/kg PO on the first day; then 5 mg/kg PO daily on days 2-5 or 30 mg/kg as a single dose
	Zithromax	
clarithromycin*	Biaxin	7.5 mg/kg/day in 2 divided doses for 10 days
	Biaxin	
Cephalosporins		
cefaclor*	Generics	20-40 mg/kg/day every 8-12 hours
	Ceclor	
cefdinir*	Omnicef	7 mg/kg (up to 300 mg) every 12 hours for 5-10 days or 14 mg/kg (up to 600 mg) once daily for 10 days
	Not available	
cefixime	Suprax	8 mg/kg/day in 1-2 doses/day (maximum, 400 mg/day)
	Suprax	
cefpodoxime*	Generics	5 mg/kg (maximum 200 mg/dose) every 12 hours for 5-7 days
	Not available	
cefprozil*	Cefzil	15 mg/kg every 12 hours for 10 days (>6 months old)
	Cefzil	
ceftibuten	Cedax	9 mg/kg/day for 10 days (up to maximum of 400 mg/day)
	Not available	
cefuroxime*	Ceftin	30 mg/kg/day (maximum 1000 mg/day) divided in 2 doses for 10 days
	Ceftin	
cephalexin*	Keflex, Panixine	75-100 mg/kg/day in 4 divided doses (maximum, 4 g/day)
	Keflex	
Sulfonamides		
sulfisoxazole + erythromycin ethylsuccinate*	Generics	120-150 mg/kg/day sulfisoxazole + 40-50 mg/kg/day erythromycin divided in 4 doses for 10 days
	Pediazole	
sulfamethoxazole (SMX) + trimethoprim (TMP)*	Bactrim, Bactrim DS, Septra DS	40 mg SMX + 8 mg TMP/kg/day in 2 divided doses for 10 days
	Generics	

*Generic available.

Chapter Summary

- Blepharitis is a chronic eye disease that produces distinctive flaky scales on the eyelids and eyelashes and is self-treated by applying clean warm compresses. In some cases, anti-infective ointments, corticosteroid eye drops, and artificial tears may be administered to manage the symptoms.
- Conjunctivitis (pink eye) may be caused by a virus or bacteria.
- Uveitis is treated with the administration of corticosteroids (to reduce inflammation), mydriatics (to reduce painful swelling), and anti-infectives or antivirals as appropriate.
- Microbial keratitis and fungal keratitis are most commonly caused by trauma, immunodeficiency, and chronic eye surface diseases.
- Soft contact lens wearers, especially those who wear their contact lenses overnight, are at risk for fungal keratitis.
- A stye is a small, painful lump on the eyelid that is caused by an acute self-limiting infection of the oil glands of the eyelid.
- CMV retinitis is an opportunistic infection in the eye that occurs in patients who have HIV infection/AIDS or take immunosuppressive drugs and if untreated can cause blindness.
- CMV retinitis is treated by administration of antivirals such as ganciclovir, valganciclovir, foscarnet, and cidofovir.
- Herpetic corneal disease is the cause of more than 500,000 cases of blindness annually.
- Herpes virus lives around nerve fibers and, when activated, produces painful symptoms.
- Symptoms of herpes zoster ophthalmicus are swelling and rash or sores around the eye, eyelids, or forehead.
- Symptoms of herpes simplex keratitis are excessive tearing, decreased vision, a gritty feeling in the eye, and pain when looking at bright light.
- Herpes zoster ophthalmicus and herpes simplex keratitis are treated by administering antiviral eye drops, orally administered drugs, or both.
- Ocular toxoplasmosis is caused by protozoa and is transmitted by handling or eating raw and undercooked meat or by handling cat feces.
- Toxoplasmosis can cause ocular inflammation, vasculitis, uveitis, and retinal edema and is treated by administering pyrimethamine and sulfonamides (sulfadiazine and trimethoprim + sulfamethoxazole).
- Helminthes are parasitic worms that can cause eye infections and blindness.
- Onchocerciasis (river blindness) is caused by a roundworm and is the second leading cause of infectious blindness in the world.
- Onchocerciasis is treated by administering a single dose of ivermectin yearly.
- Cysticercosis is transmitted to humans who eat undercooked pork.
- Cysticercosis is treated with praziquantel, corticosteroids, and surgical removal of the living worms.
- Toxocariasis is the fifth leading cause of uveitis worldwide.
- Toxocariasis is treated by administering topical corticosteroids and systemic anthelminthics such as thiabendazole.
- Otitis externa is inflammation of the external auditory canal and is most commonly caused by a bacterial infection.
- Risk factors for development of otitis externa are (1) exposure to excessive moisture (swimming, humidity, sweating), (2) high environmental temperature, (3) irritation caused by earwax removal, (4) insertion of objects into the ear, and (5) chronic dermatological disease.
- Otitis media is an inflammation in the middle ear.
- Excessive use of anti-infective agents to treat otitis media may increase the risk of development of bacterial resistance.
- Decongestants and antihistamines are not recommended for prophylaxis or treatment of otitis media in children.

REVIEW QUESTIONS

1. A common, self-limiting ailment that causes itching, burning, and teary outflow is
   a. blepharitis
   b. conjunctivitis
   c. iritis
   d. keratitis

2. Otitis media is an inflammation in the _____ ear.
   a. inner
   b. outer
   c. middle
   d. cochlea

3. Keratitis is a severe infection of the iris and may be caused by bacteria or fungi.
   a. true
   b. false

4. The medical term for "granulated eyelids" is
   a. uveitis
   b. keratitis
   c. blepharitis
   d. iritis

5. Aminoglycoside anti-infectives are used in the treatment of blepharitis and include
   a. gentamicin
   b. neomycin
   c. tobramycin
   d. all of the above

6. A stye (hordeolum) is a small, painful lump located on the
   a. eyelid
   b. iris
   c. conjunctiva
   d. pupil

7. Prophylactic use of _____ is ineffective in preventing otitis media.
   a. antihistamines
   b. decongestants
   c. both a and b
   d. none of the above

8. Cytomegalovirus retinitis is treated by administration of antifungals.
   a. true
   b. false

9. The most common cause of otitis externa is _____
   a. viral infection
   b. bacterial infection
   c. psoriasis
   d. lupus

10. Children are more susceptible to otitis media than adults because their eustachian tubes are longer and straighter than those of adults.
   a. true
   b. false

TECHNICIAN'S CORNER

1. How can putting a baby to bed with a bottle of milk contribute to otitis media?
2. How can nonsterile colored contact lenses cause eye infections?

Bibliography

Alberta Medical Association. Guideline for the Diagnosis and Management of Acute Otitis Media: Alberta Medical Association, 2008.

Ament C, Young L: Ocular manifestations of helminthic infections: onchocerciasis, cysticercosis, toxocariasis, and diffuse unilateral subacute neuroretinitis, *Int Ophthalmol Clin* 46:1-10, 2006.

Centers for Disease Control and Prevention: Conjunctivitis Treatment. Retrieved May 15, 2011, from http://www.cdc.gov/conjunctivitis/about/treatment.html, 2010.

Centers for Disease Control and Prevention: Pink Eye: Usually Mild and Easy to Treat. Retrieved May 15, 2011, from http://www.cdc.gov/Features/Conjunctivitis/, 2010.

Centers for Disease Control and Prevention: Fusarium keratitis—multiple states, *MMWR Morb Mortal Wkly Rep* 55:1-2, 2006. Retrieved from http://www.cdc.gov/mmwr/preview/mmwrhtml/mm55d410a1.htm.

Green L, Pavan-Langston D: Herpes simplex ocular inflammatory disease, *Int Ophthalmol Clin* 46:27-37, 2006.

Health Information Center at the Cleveland Clinic: Herpetic eye disease. Retrieved from http://www.clevelandclinic.org/health/health-info/docs/3400/3433.asp?index8861.

Hoberman A, Paradise JL, Rockette HE, et al: Treatment of acute otitis media in children under 2 years of age, *New England Journal of Medicine* 364(2): 2011.

Koo L, Young L: Management of ocular toxoplasmosis, *Int Ophthalmol Clin* 46:183-193, 2006.

MayoClinic.com: Iritis. Retrieved May 15, 2011, from http://www.mayoclinic.com/health/iritis/HQ00940, 2010.

MayoClinic.com: Sty. Retrieved May 15, 2011, from http://www.mayoclinic.com/health/sty/DS00257, 2010.

National Eye Institute: *Blepharitis resource guide*, Bethesda, MD, National Institutes of Health, US Department of Health and Human Services. Retrieved from http://www.nei.nih.gov/health/blepharitis, 2006.

National Institute on Deafness and Other Communication Disorders: *Otitis media*, Bethesda, MD, NIDCD, National Institutes of Health, US Department of Health and Human Services. Retrieved from http://www.nidcd.nih.gov/health/hearing/otitism.asp, 2002.

Sander R: Otitis externa: a practical guide to treatment and prevention, *Am Fam Phys* 63:927-936, 941-942, 2001.

US Food and Drug Administration, US Department of Health and Human Services: *Contact lenses and eye infections*. Retrieved from http://www.fda.gov/oc/opacom/hottopics/contacts.html.

Weigland T, Young L: Cytomegalovirus retinitis, *Int Ophthalmol Clin* 46:91-110, 2006.

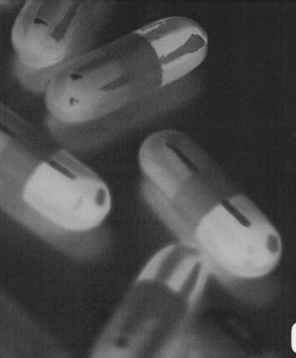

UNIT V

Drugs Affecting the Cardiovascular System

LEARNING OBJECTIVES	1 List and describe the composition of blood and properties of blood cells.
	2 Identify the different types of white blood cells and their functions.
	3 Classify the different blood groups.
	4 Explain the Rh factor and its properties.
	5 Learn the terminology associated with the hematological system.
	6 Demonstrate a basic knowledge of the physical structure of the heart.
	7 Learn and describe the circulation of blood through the heart and the different types of blood vessels
	8 Describe the conduction system of the heart.

KEY TERMS

Arteriosclerosis: Loss of elasticity (hardening) of the arteries.

Atria: Two upper chambers of the heart that receive blood from the veins.

Cardiomyopathy: Heart disease that causes abnormal enlargement of the heart.

Coronary arteries: Small blood vessels that encircle the heart.

Erythrocytes: Red blood cells.

Erythropoiesis: Formation of red blood cells.

Hemoglobin: Red pigment made up of iron atoms; transports oxygen and carbon dioxide in the body.

Hemostasis: Stoppage of blood flow.

Leukocytes: White blood cells (WBCs).

Leukocytosis: Abnormally high WBC count.

Leukopenia: Abnormally low WBC count.

Peripheral vascular disease: A condition that decreases circulation to peripheral tissues such as the hands, lower legs, or feet and results in ischemia.

Rh factor: Antigen present on the red blood cells of Rh-positive individuals.

Thrombocytes: Platelets.

Thrombocytopenia: Results from a deficiency in the platelet count.

Thrombopoeisis: Formation of platelets.

Ventricles: Two lower chambers of the heart that pump blood out of the heart to the rest of the body.

317

Anatomy and Physiology of the Hematologic System

Homeostasis of the internal environment depends on the continual transport of oxygen, nutrients, and biochemical messengers among the body's cells. Blood is a complex transport medium that performs vital pickup and delivery services for the body. It picks up food and oxygen from the digestive and respiratory systems and delivers them to the cells while picking up waste from the cells for delivery to the excretory organs. Blood also transports hormones, enzymes, buffers, and other biochemical substances that serve important functions. Blood is the keystone of the body's heat-regulating mechanism and is able to absorb large quantities of heat without an appreciable increase in its own temperature, transferring it from the body's core to the surface to be dissipated.

COMPOSITION OF BLOOD

The components of blood are plasma (fluid), *erythrocytes* (red blood cells), *leukocytes* (white blood cells), and *thrombocytes* (platelets).

Plasma is a clear straw-colored liquid that consists of approximately 90% water and 10% solutes. It contains many proteins such as factor VIII, which regulates blood clotting, gamma globulin, which helps a weakened immune system, and albumin, a blood volume expander. Other solutes present in smaller amounts are food substances (e.g., glucose, amino acids, lipids), compounds formed by metabolism (e.g., urea, uric acid, creatinine, lactic acid), respiratory gases (e.g., oxygen, carbon dioxide), and regulatory substances (e.g., hormones, enzymes).

Red Blood Cells

Red blood cells (RBCs) are formed from stem cells in the red bone marrow in a process called *erythropoiesis*. Normal mature RBCs have no nucleus and are shaped like biconcave discs. The primary component of each RBC is the red pigment hemoglobin, which is made up of iron atoms. RBCs are the most numerous of the formed elements and play a critical role in the transportation of oxygen and carbon dioxide in the body. The life span of the RBC averages 105 to 120 days.

TECH NOTE!
Whole blood contains formed elements; plasma does not contain any formed elements.

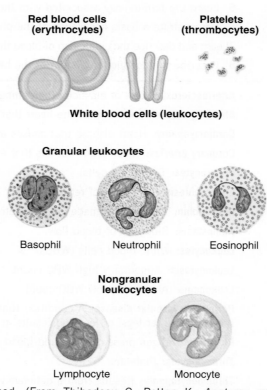

Composition of blood. (From Thibodeau G, Patton K: *Anatomy and physiology*, ed 6, St. Louis, 2007, Mosby.)

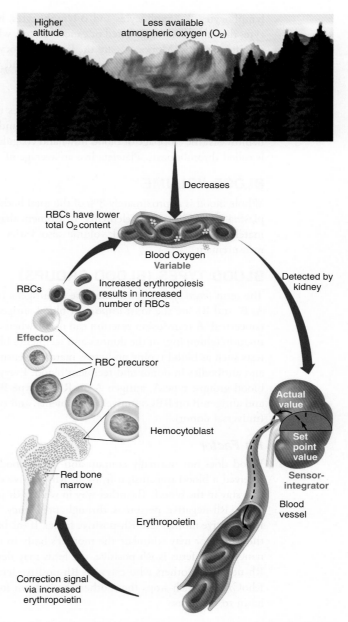

Red blood cells. (From Thibodeau G, Patton K: *Anatomy and physiology*, ed 6, St. Louis, 2007, Mosby.)

White Blood Cells

White blood cells (WBCs), or leukocytes, are differentiated into five different types. They all have nuclei and are generally larger than RBCs. They originate in red bone marrow. WBCs containing granulocytes are called neutrophils, eosinophils, and basophils. Neutrophils are very active phagocytic cells that can migrate out of blood vessels into tissue spaces and help fight off bacterial infections. Eosinophils are numerous in body areas such as the lining of the respiratory and digestive tracts and help protect against infections caused by parasitic worms and allergic reactions. Basophils are the least numerous of the WBCs and are capable of migrating out of blood vessels into tissue spaces. They contain histamine (an inflammatory biochemical) and heparin (an anticoagulant).

Lymphocytes and monocytes are categorized as agranulocytes and do not contain granules. Lymphocytes are the smallest of the leukocytes and are the most numerous. The two types of lymphocytes, T lymphocytes and B lymphocytes, have an important role in immunity. T lympho-cytes directly attack an infected or cancerous cell, whereas B lymphocytes produce antibodies against specific antigens. Monocytes are the largest leukocytes. They are motile and highly phagocytic cells capable of engulfing large bacterial organisms and virus-infected cells.

Platelets (Thrombocytes)

Blood platelets are small, almost colorless bodies that have three important physical properties—agglutination (clumping of cells), adhesiveness, and aggregation. Platelets play an important role in hemostasis (the stoppage of blood flow) and coagulation (blood clotting). The formation of platelets is called thromboposis. Platelets live an average of 7 days.

BLOOD VOLUME

Whole blood is approximately 8% of the total body weight. Total blood volume is made up of 55% plasma and 45% formed elements. In women, that amounts to 4 to 5 liters and in men, approxi-mately 5 to 6 liters. Blood volume also varies with age, body composition, and method of measurement.

BLOOD TYPES (BLOOD GROUPS)

The term *blood type* refers to the type of antigens (markers) present on RBC membranes. Antigens A, B, and Rh are the most important blood antigens as far as transfusions and newborn survival is concerned. A transfusion reaction can occur when antigens and antibodies mix. The result is agglu-tination (clumping) of the donor's and recipient's blood, a potentially fatal event. Clinical laboratory tests such as blood typing and cross matching ensure proper identification of blood group antigens and antibodies in donor and recipient blood. Every person's blood belongs to one of the four ABO blood groups: type A, antigen A on RBCs; type B, antigen B on RBCs; type AB, both antigen A and antigen B on RBCs (universal recipient); and type O, neither antigen A nor antigen B on RBCs (universal donor).

Rh Factor

Blood does not normally contain anti-Rh antibodies. It can appear if an Rh-negative person has received a blood transfusion from an Rh-positive donor. The body then makes anti-Rh antibodies that stay in the blood. The other way in which Rh-positive red blood cells can enter the bloodstream of an Rh-negative person is through pregnancy. This presents danger to the baby born to an Rh-negative mother and Rh-positive father. If the baby inherits the Rh-positive trait from the father, the Rh factor may stimulate the mother's body to make anti-Rh antibodies. During a second preg-nancy, if the fetus is Rh-positive, the fetus may develop a disease called erythroblastosis fetalis. All Rh-negative mothers who carry an Rh-positive fetus should be treated with a protein marketed as RhoGAM, which stops the mother's body from forming anti-Rh antibodies and prevents possible harm to the fetus.

BLOOD DISORDERS
Red Blood Cell Disorders

Polycythemia occurs when the bone marrow produces too many RBCs and blood becomes too thick to flow properly. Many types of anemia also affect RBCs. Anemia describes different disease condi-tions caused by the inability of the blood to carry sufficient oxygen to the body cells. Aplastic anemia causes an abnormally low number of RBCs; most cases result from destruction of bone marrow by drugs, toxic chemicals, or radiation, and perhaps even cancer. Pernicious anemia is characterized by a low number of RBCs and sometimes results from a dietary deficiency of vitamin B_{12}. Folate defi-ciency anemia results from a folic acid vitamin deficiency.

Blood loss anemia often occurs after a hemorrhage associated with trauma, extensive surgery, or some other situation involving a sudden loss of blood. Iron deficiency anemia results from an inad-equate amount of iron in the diet that causes the body not to manufacture enough hemoglobin. Hemolytic anemia applies to a variety of inherited blood disorders characterized by an abnormal amount of hemoglobin (e.g., sickle cell anemia, thalassemia).

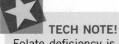

TECH NOTE!
Folate deficiency is linked to neural tube disorders in the fetus (e.g., spina bifida), so folic acid supplements are added to prenatal vitamins.

White Blood Cell Disorders

Leukopenia is an abnormally low WBC count. The opposite of leukopenia is *leukocytosis*, an abnormally high WBC count. Blood-related cancers or malignant neoplasms constitute most of the WBC disorders. Some examples are multiple myeloma and leukemia. Infectious mononuceosis is a common, noncancerous WBC disorder that appears most often in adolescents and young adults between 15 to 25 years of age. It is caused by a virus found in the saliva of infected individuals.

Bone Marrow Disorders

Most blood disorders are disorders of the formed elements. If the bone marrow is severely damaged, a bone marrow transplant may be offered to the patient.

Clotting Disorders

Hemophilia is an X-linked inherited disorder that affects 1 in every 10,000 males worldwide. It results from a failure to produce one or more plasma proteins responsible for blood clotting; it is characterized by the inability to form blood clots. The most common form is hemophilia A, caused by an absence of factor VIII protein. Hemophiliacs can receive monthly transfusions of factor VIII to aid in blood clotting. *Thrombocytopenia* results from a deficiency in the platelet count and is characterized by bleeding from many small blood vessels throughout the body, most visibly in the skin and mucous membranes. The cause is bone marrow destruction as a result of an immune system disease, or cancer. Drugs may also cause thrombocytopenia as a side effect.

Cardiovascular System

The cardiovascular system consists of the heart and a closed system of blood vessels called the arteries, veins, and capillaries. Blood contained in the circulatory system is continuously pumped by the heart around a closed circuit of vessels.

HEART

The human heart is a four-chambered muscular organ that lies in the mediastinum just behind the sternum. The heart has its own special covering. A loose-fitting sac (pericardium) is made up of two layers, the fibrous pericardium and serous pericardium. The serous pericardium consists of two sublayers, the parietal layer and visceral layer (epicardium). Between the parietal and visceral layer is a space that contains serous or pericardial fluid that helps prevent friction as the heart beats.

Structure of the Heart

The heart wall has three distinct layers, the epicardium (outer layer), the myocardium (middle muscular layer) and bulk of the heart wall, and the endocardium (the lining of the interior of the myocardial wall made up of a delicate layer of endothelial tissue). All cardiac muscle cells can contract and produce their own slow, steady rhythm.

The interior of the heart is divided into four chambers, two upper chambers (*atria*) that receive blood from the veins and two lower chambers (*ventricles*) that receive blood from the atria. The walls of the ventricles are thicker than the walls of the atria because they pump blood out of the heart to the rest of the body. The heart wall is separated by a wall of muscles known as the interatrial septum and the interventricular septum. Before birth, an opening is present in this wall, but it closes immediately after birth when the infant takes the first breath. If this opening does not close, the infant will experience a mixing of deoxygenated and oxygenated blood. This condition is commonly called blue baby syndrome because the infant has too little oxygen in the blood. Infants with this condition will need surgery to correct the problem.

Heart Valves

The heart valves are mechanical devices that permit the flow of blood in one direction only. The heart contains two sets of valves, the atrioventricular valves (bicuspid and tricuspid) and semilunar valves (pulmonary and aortic). The bicuspid and tricuspid valves guard the opening between the atria and ventricles and prevent the backflow of blood from the ventricle into the atria. The

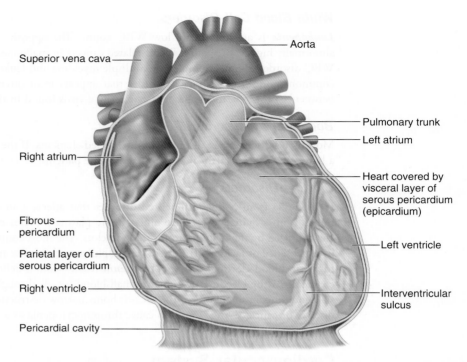

The heart. (From Thibodeau G, Patton K: *Anatomy and physiology*, ed 6, St. Louis, 2007, Mosby.)

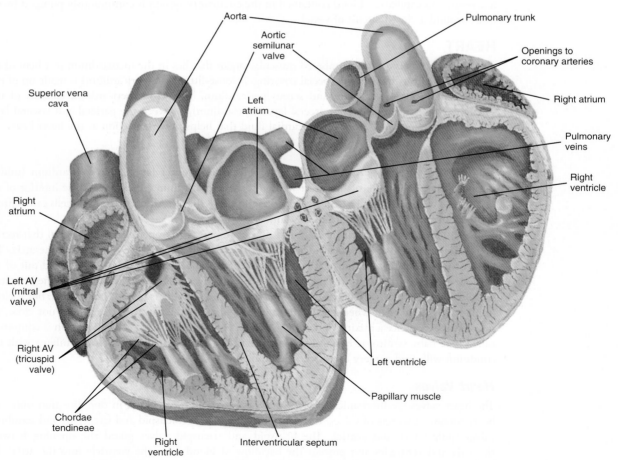

Inner chambers of the heart. (From Thibodeau G, Patton K: *Anatomy and physiology*, ed 6, St. Louis, 2007, Mosby.)

pulmonary and aortic semilunar valves are located where the pulmonary artery and the aorta arise from the right and left ventricle, respectively. Their function is to prevent the flow of blood from the aorta back into the left ventricle or from the pulmonary artery back into the right ventricle.

BLOOD VESSELS

There are three major types of blood vessels in the cardiovascular system—arteries, capillaries, and veins. Arteries are larger blood vessels and carry blood away from the heart. Almost all arteries carry oxygenated blood. The pulmonary artery is the one exception. Arterioles are smaller arteries that are important because they regulate blood flow throughout the body. Capillaries are microscopic vessels that carry blood from arterioles to venules (small veins) and transfer nutrients and other vital substances between blood and tissue cells. This is the site of gas exchange in the body. Veins are blood vessels that carry blood toward the heart and contain one-way valves that prevent its potential backflow. All the veins except the pulmonary vein contain deoxygenated blood.

BLOOD SUPPLY TO THE HEART AND BODY SYSTEMS
Pathway of Blood Flow

The flow of blood through the right and left sides of the heart occurs simultaneously by the two-sided pumping action of the heart muscle, thereby providing a constant supply of blood to the heart and its accessory structures. One can trace the flow of blood on the right side (deoxygenated; indicated by the blue arrows in figure) and the left side (oxygenated; indicated by the red arrows in figure).

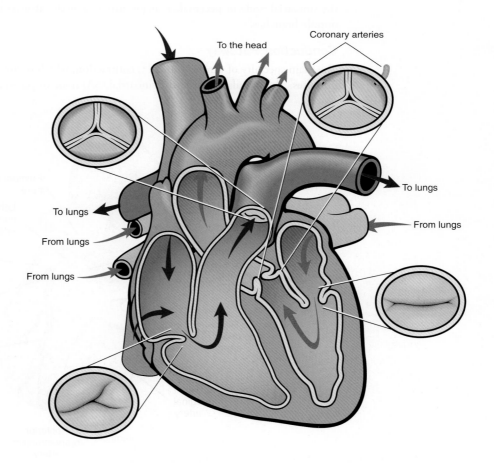

RIGHT SIDE OF THE HEART   LEFT SIDE OF THE HEART

Blood flow through the heart. (Adapted from Damjanov I: *Pathology for the health professions*, ed 3, St. Louis, 2006, WB Saunders.)

Major Circulatory Routes in the Body

Blood follows a specific pathway as it travels throughout the body. In systemic circulation, blood flows from the heart (left ventricle) through blood vessels to all parts of the body, except the lungs, and back to the heart. There are two subdivisions of systemic circulation, the hepatic portal and fetal circulations. In the hepatic portal circulation, blood flows through the systemic circulation in the abdominal cavity and then passes through the hepatic portal vein to the liver before returning to the heart. The liver detoxifies and metabolizes impurities, harmful substances, and drugs before returning the blood to systemic circulation. In the fetal circulation, fetal blood secures oxygen and food from maternal blood instead of from fetal lungs and digestive organs.

The Heart's Blood Supply

The heart itself needs a constant supply of oxygen to do its work of supplying blood to the rest of the body. This is done by the ***coronary arteries***, small blood vessels that encircle the heart. Both ventricles receive their blood supply from branches of the right and left coronary arteries. Each atrium receives blood from a small branch of the coronary artery. The most abundant blood supply goes to the myocardium of the left ventricle because the left ventricle does the most work and therefore needs the most oxygen and nutrients.

CONDUCTION SYSTEM OF THE HEART

The conduction system of the heart is responsible for ensuring that blood is ejected out of the heart chambers in a coordinated manner that permits an effective volume of distribution of blood to be pumped from the heart to the rest of the body. Four structures make up this conduction system—the sinoatrial node or pacemaker, atrioventricular node, atrioventricular bundle, and right and left bundle branches.

Conduction Pathway

The main specialty of cardiac muscle is contraction, which occurs as a result of conduction of nerve impulses. The impulse starts at the sinoatrial (SA) node or pacemaker, which sets the rhythm of the

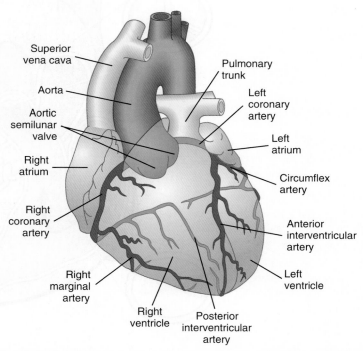

Blood supply of the heart. (From Thibodeau G, Patton K: *Anatomy and physiology*, ed 6, St. Louis, 2007, Mosby.)

heart. Next, it passes to the atrioventricular (AV) node, which lies in the right atrium along the lower part of the interatrial septum. Impulses travel down the middle of the heart through the AV bundle (bundle of His), which branches into right and left bundle branches. The bundle of His extends out to the lateral walls of the ventricles and papillary muscles and innervates the whole heart.

DISORDERS OF THE HEART LINING, MUSCLE, AND VALVES

Rheumatic heart disease results from a delayed inflammatory response to streptococcal infection and occurs most often in children. Endocarditis is inflammation of the inner lining of the heart caused by a bacterial infection; pericarditis is inflammation of the pericardium surrounding the heart. Mitral valve prolapse is a condition affecting the bicuspid or mitral valve that causes the valves not to close properly. Backflow of blood occurs from the left ventricle into the left atrium and results in turbulence, causing an extra heartbeat termed a *heart murmur*. Cardiomyopathy is literally translated as heart muscle pathology. It is an abnormal enlargement of the heart and may be caused by a number of diseases, such as heart failure, untreated hypertension, or viral infection.

DISORDERS OF BLOOD VESSELS

Arteriosclerosis results from a loss of elasticity of blood vessels. ***Peripheral vascular disease*** decreases circulation to peripheral tissues such as the hands, lower legs, or feet and results in ischemia. Damage to the arterial wall can lead to the formation of an aneurysm. An aneurysm is a section of an artery that has become abnormally widened because of the weakening in the wall. Aneurysms can be dangerous because they can rupture and cause hemorrhaging that may result in death. Varicose veins are a disorder in which the veins become enlarged and cause the blood to pool in them rather than continue toward the heart. Varicose veins of the anal canal are called hemorrhoids and may be caused by excessive straining during defecation. Several factors can cause phlebitis, or vein inflammation. An example is irritation caused by an intravenous catheter. Thrombophlebitis is caused by blood clots in the veins. A clot that is formed in a deep vein is known as deep vein thrombosis (DVT) and usually occurs in the lower legs. Raynaud disease is marked by intense constriction and vasospasm of arterioles and may be secondary to some other, more serious disorder.

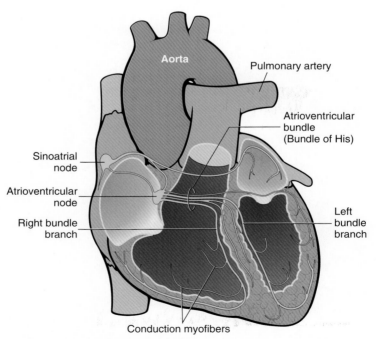

Conduction system of the heart. (From Chabner E: *The language of medicine*, ed 9, St. Louis, 2009, Saunders.)

Summary

Numerous classes of drugs are used in the treatment of heart disease. Anticoagulants prevent clot formations, beta-adrenergic drugs reduce the workload of the heart, calcium channel blockers reduce vascular contractions and improve coronary blood flow, digitalis slows and increases the strength of cardiac contractions, nitroglycerin dilates coronary blood vessels, and tissue plasminogen activator (t-PA) helps dissolve clots. The heart is strengthened by exercise so lifestyle changes that include moderate to strenuous exercise may be recommended for heart health.

Bibliography

Chabner E: *The language of medicine*, ed 9, St. Louis, 2010, Saunders.
Patton K: *Survival guide for anatomy and physiology*, St. Louis, 2010, Mosby.
Thibodeau G, Patton K: *Anatomy and physiology*, ed 7, St. Louis, 2010, Mosby.

21

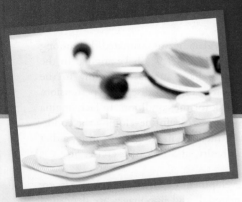

Treatment of Angina

LEARNING OBJECTIVES

1 Learn the terminology associated with the treatment of angina.
2 List the symptoms of and risk factors for angina.
3 Explain the role of coronary artery disease in the development of angina.
4 Identify lifestyle changes that reduce the risk for angina.
5 List and categorize medications used to treat angina.
6 Describe mechanism of action for each classification of drugs used to treat angina.
7 Identify significant drug look-alike and sound-alike issues.
8 List common endings for drug classes used in the treatment of angina.
9 Identify warning labels and precautionary messages associated with medications used to treat angina.

KEY TERMS

Angina pectoris: Symptomatic manifestation of ischemic heart disease characterized by a severe squeezing or pressure-like chest pain and brought on by exertion or stress.

Arteriosclerosis: Thickening and loss of elasticity of arterial walls; sometimes called "hardening of the arteries."

Atheromas: Hard plaque formed within an artery.

Atherosclerosis: Process in which plaques (atheromas) containing cholesterol, lipid material, and lipophages are formed within arteries.

Coronary artery disease: Condition that occurs when the arteries that supply blood to the heart muscle become hardened and narrowed.

Embolus: A moving blood clot.

Hyperlipidemia: Increased concentration of cholesterol and triglycerides in the blood that is associated with the development of atherosclerosis.

Ischemia: Deficient blood supply to an area of the body. Myocardial ischemia results in angina and myocardial infarction.

Ischemic heart disease: Any condition in which heart muscle is damaged or works inefficiently because of an absence or relative deficiency of its blood supply.

Necrosis: Cell death that may be caused by lack of blood and oxygen to the affected areas.

Myocardial infarction: Also referred to as a "heart attack." Results in heart muscle tissue death and is caused by the occlusion (blockage) of a coronary artery.

Thrombus: Stationary blood clot.

Vasospasm: Spasms that constrict blood vessels and reduce the flow of blood and oxygen.

Overview

The word "angina" is derived from the Latin word *ango,* which means "to choke." The symptoms of angina are described as severe squeezing or pressure-like chest pain, sometimes radiating to the arms, shoulders, neck, or jaw. The pain is sometimes described as severe heartburn or indigestion. Angina is a symptom of ***ischemic heart disease.*** *Ischemia* is caused by loss of blood supply to a region of the body.

Based on the 2000/2001 Canadian Community Health Survey data, it was estimated that among the 5% of Canadians 12 years of age and older who have heart disease, 1.9% have angina. In the United States, more than 10.2 million people are estimated to have angina, according to the American Heart Association (2010). Although people with a history of heart disease, hypertension, and diabetes are at risk for angina, lifestyle is also a significant risk for the condition. In fact, angina is often classified as a chronic disease of lifestyle because many of the risks for developing the condition are related to lifestyle. Risk factors associated with lifestyle include smoking, overeating, a diet high in cholesterol and salt, excessive alcohol consumption, obesity, and lack of exercise. Stress is also a risk factor for angina.

High dietary cholesterol is a contributing factor for the development of ***coronary artery disease*** (CAD) and causes myocardial ischemia. Cholesterol, lipid material, and lipophages are deposited within arteries. The lipid streaks harden into plaques (atheromas); this process is called ***atherosclerosis.*** An ***atheroma*** can increase in size and reduce blood flow and has the potential to result in thrombus formation (Figure 21-1). Thrombi can further occlude the artery in which it was formed. A thrombus that breaks off is called an embolus; it can travel to a smaller artery, where it completely occludes the blood vessel, causing ischemia. Prolonged ischemia can result in tissue necrosis (death),

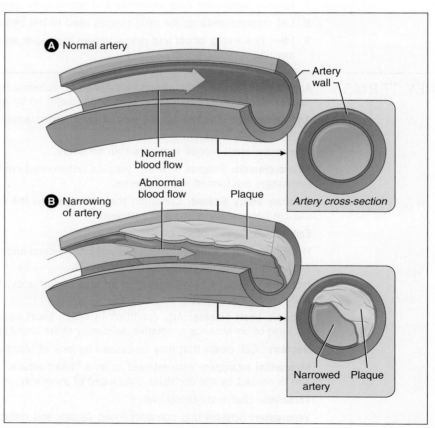

FIGURE 21-1 Plaque buildup in an artery. (Courtesy of National Institutes of Health Bethesda, MD.)

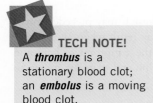

TECH NOTE!
A ***thrombus*** is a stationary blood clot; an ***embolus*** is a moving blood clot.

leading to ***myocardial infarction*** (heart attack) or stroke. ***Arteriosclerosis***, sometimes called "hardening of the arteries" is a condition where arterial walls thicken and lose elasticity. When arteriosclerosis occurs in the coronary arteries, the arteries becomes less able to dilate and increase the heart's blood supply when needed.

TYPES OF ANGINA

There are three types of angina, which vary according to their pattern and ability to be relieved by medication. They are called stable angina, unstable angina, and variant angina, also known as Prinzmetal's or vasospastic angina. In all types of angina, there is an imbalance between blood supplied to the heart muscle and the need for blood and oxygen. The symptoms of angina occur when the blood supplied to the heart is insufficient to meet the heart's need for oxygen (Figure 21-2).

STABLE (EXERTIONAL) ANGINA

Symptoms of stable angina are predictable and are typically brought on by physical exertion, smoking, eating heavy meals, exposure to extreme changes in temperature (hot or cold), and emotional stress. Physical exertion is the most common reason for the onset of angina. Whereas the amount of blood and oxygen that is supplied to the heart meets its needs under typical conditions, it is insufficient during periods of physical exertion. Rest and antianginal medications such as nitroglycerin adequately treat the acute symptoms of stable angina. Symptoms often subside within 5 minutes.

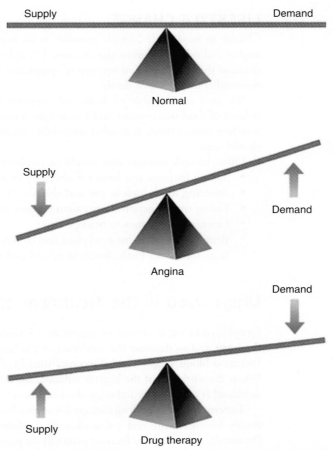

FIGURE 21-2 Imbalance between oxygen (O_2) need and blood supply. (From Lilley LL, Harrington S, Snyder JS: *Pharmacology and the nursing process,* ed 5, St Louis, 2007, Mosby.)

UNSTABLE ANGINA

Unstable angina is a serious condition requiring medical evaluation because it may precede a myocardial infarction. It may occur at rest without physical exertion and may result when an embolus partially or completely occludes an artery. Myocardial ischemia causes the symptoms of pain and chest pressure. Symptoms are not relieved by rest or antianginal medicine and may last for up to 30 minutes.

VARIANT ANGINA

Variant (Prinzmetal's) angina is also known as vasospastic angina because it is caused by *vasospasm* of the coronary arteries. Spasms reduce the opening of the artery, decreasing the blood supply and oxygen to the heart. Similar to unstable angina, the pain typically occurs at rest and during the night or early morning. Unlike unstable angina, it is relieved by medications that include nitrates and calcium channel blockers. Symptoms often persist longer than stable angina and may exceed 5 minutes.

MICROVASCULAR ANGINA

Microvascular angina or cardiac syndrome X is a form of stable effort angina that may produce greater chest pain and last longer than other types of angina. This type of angina may be a symptom of coronary microvascular disorder and results from poor functioning of the tiny blood vessels that nourish the heart. It differs from other forms of angina because some patients have no CAD risk factors. Microvascular angina most often occurs during exercise but can occur at rest.

Nonpharmacological Treatment of Angina

LIFESTYLE CHANGE

Change in modifiable lifestyle practices is an important part of the treatment and prevention of angina and other cardiovascular diseases. Lifestyle changes can reduce the risk for angina as well as decrease the frequency and severity of symptoms and prevent or slow the progression of angina to myocardial infarction or death.

We may not be able to limit our exposure to stressful situations, but we can control the volume of food we consume and lose weight if necessary. Increasing our level of daily activity, while avoiding overexertion, is another modifiable lifestyle change that we can make. If you smoke, you should quit.

Other lifestyle changes that should be implemented if possible include:
- Taking frequent rest breaks if necessary to avoid angina that is caused by exertion
- Avoiding foods high in salt and cholesterol
- Eating small portions rather than a heavy meal
- Learning techniques to manage stress
- Being an advocate for workplace and community-wide changes that facilitate lifestyle change (e.g., nutritious food choices in school and workplace cafeterias)

Drugs Used in the Treatment of Angina

Drugs used in the treatment of angina are administered to increase the blood and oxygen supply to the heart and to decrease the workload of the heart. The mechanisms of action of the drugs vary. Increased blood supply can be accomplished by dilating blood vessels or by reducing vasospasms. When the workload of the heart is reduced, the demand for oxygen decreases. Reduction in cardiac workload is achieved by reducing the heart rate.

The current focus of drug therapy for angina has shifted to emphasize reduction in cardiovascular events by treatment and prevention of cardiovascular diseases that often accompany angina. Previously, treatment was focused primarily on prevention of acute symptoms. Drugs may be administered to persons who have angina to treat comorbid conditions such as hypertension (see Chapter 22), *hyperlipidemia*, atherosclerosis, atherothrombosis, and myocardial infarction (see Chapter 24) (Table 21-1).

TABLE 21-1   **Summary of Drug Categories Used in the Treatment of Angina and Comorbid Conditions**

Drug Classification	Acute Use	Prevent Angina	Comorbid Conditions
Nitrates	√	√	Hypertension, myocardial infarction
β-Adrenergic blockers		√	Hypertension
Calcium channel blockers		√	Hypertension
ACE inhibitors		√	Hypertension, myocardial infarction
Anticoagulants, antiplatelet, glycoprotein IIb/IIIa		√	Myocardial infarction
Antihyperlipidemics		√	Myocardial infarction

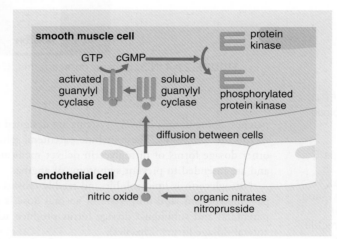

FIGURE 21-3 Mechanism of action of nitrates. (From Page C, Curtis M, Sutter M, et al. *Integrated pharmacology*, ed 3, Philadelphia, 2005, Mosby.)

TECH NOTE!
Sublingual nitroglycerin is packaged by manufacturers in amber glass bottles and should be dispensed in the manufacturer's original container. Dispense without a safety cap for easy access. It is one of the few drugs exempted from the Poison Prevention Packaging Act.

TECH NOTE!
Isosorbide dinitrate is also available in unit dose packaging.

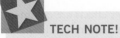

TECH NOTE!
It is important for the patients using patches to rotate the sites on the skin to prevent skin irritation.

NITRATES

The organic nitrates are the oldest class of drugs used to treat acute symptoms of angina. They dilate blood vessels (arteries and veins) and increase supply of oxygen to the heart. Nitrates that are commonly used in the treatment and prevention of angina are nitroglycerin, isosorbide dinitrate, and isosorbide mononitrate. Nitrates are also indicated for the treatment of congestive heart failure (intravenous), pulmonary hypertension, and hypertensive emergencies.

Mechanism of Action

Nitrates act to dilate veins, reduce heart muscle tension, and decrease oxygen demand (Figure 21-3). Most nitrates are prodrugs. They are converted in the body to nitric oxide. Nitric oxide acts at the cellular level to activate the enzyme guanylyl cyclase (cGMP) and inhibit protein kinases (PKs). Inhibition of cGMP PKs blocks the opening of voltage-gated calcium channels. Reduced intracellular calcium causes decreased actin–myosin combining and results in blockade of muscle contraction, relaxing blood vessels.

Nitrates relax and dilate medium- to large-size coronary arteries and veins. This increases oxygen to the heart. Nitrates also produce venodilation, which decreases cardiac preload (reduces fluid backup in the ventricles) and the work needed to pump blood out of the ventricles. In the case of obstruction of a coronary artery, nitrates may cause the dilation of adjacent arteries, shifting blood supply away for the blocked region.

Pharmacokinetics

Nitrates are formulated for a variety of dosage delivery systems. Nitroglycerin dosage forms (Figure 21-4) include parenteral, sublingual tablets, lingual spray, capsules, ointments, and transdermal

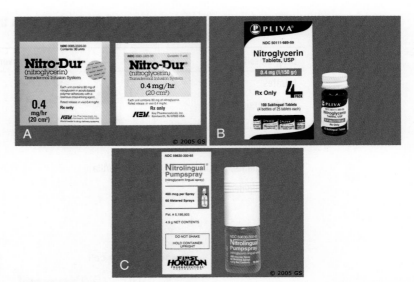

FIGURE 21-4 Nitroglycerin dosage forms. (Drug photos provided by Gold Standard.)

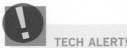

patches. Some dosage delivery systems are designed to deliver nitroglycerin quickly and are used to treat acute symptoms. These include parenteral solution, sublingual tablets, and lingual spray. The other dosage forms of nitroglycerin deliver medication over an extended period (up to 24 hours) and are intended to prevent symptoms of angina.

Nitroglycerin is lipid soluble and readily crosses cell membranes. It is subject to extensive first-pass metabolism, and only 10% of an oral dose is available to produce effects. This explains why parenteral and sublingual dosage forms produce actions more quickly and are more potent than enteral dosage forms (capsules).

Nitroglycerin is volatile and loses its potency on exposure to air, light, and moisture. Potency can also be lost if it is repackaged in plastic prescription vials. Sublingual nitroglycerin is packaged by manufacturers in amber glass bottles and should be dispensed in the manufacturer's original container.

Isosorbide dinitrate and isosorbide mononitrate are not used to treat acute symptoms. They are formulated for prevention (immediate release and extended action tablets). Isosorbide mononitrate is a long-acting metabolite of isosorbide dinitrate. Isosorbide dinitrate and isosorbide mononitrate are more stable than nitroglycerin and do not need to be dispensed in the manufacturer's original container.

Adverse Reactions

Some of the adverse reactions to nitrates are dosage form dependent, and other effects are common regardless the dosage delivery system. Adverse reactions associated with vasodilation are the most common and include hypotension, facial flushing, dizziness, and headache. Nausea and vomiting, weakness, and fatigue are additional side effects produced by nitroglycerin, isosorbide dinitrate, and isosorbide mononitrate. Sublingual dosage forms can cause stinging or burning under the tongue, and adhesives used in patches can produce allergic reactions.

Precautions

Patients who use nitrates can develop tolerance to their effects. This means the drug actions are less effective over time. Tolerance is most common with long-acting nitrates. To minimize the risk for development of tolerance, it is important to avoid continuous exposure to the drug. Transdermal patches are designed to deliver their effects for 24 hours; however, the patch should never be worn for the entire 24-hour period. Patient should be instructed to remove the patch after 10 to 12 hours. The patient must be nitrate free for at least 10 to 12 hours per day (Table 21-2).

TABLE 21-2   **Comparative Pharmacokinetics of Nitrates**

Drug Name	Dosage Form	Acute Use	Prevent Angina	Additional Use	Onset (min)	Duration (hr)
Isosorbide Dinitrate						
Dilatrate SR	Capsules, extended release		√		60	12
Isordil	Tablets, immediate acting		√	CHF, MI (adjunct)	15-40	4-6
Isosorbide Mononitrate						
Monoket	Tablets, long acting		√		30-60	6-12
Nitroglycerin						
nitroglycerin	Injection	√		High blood pressure	Instant	Minutes (dose dependent)
Nitrostat,	Sublingual	√		CHF, MI (adjunct)	1-3	½-1
Nitrolingual, Nitromist	Translingual spray	√		CHF, MI (adjunct)	2-4	3-5
Nitrol	Ointment		√	CHF, MI (adjunct)	30-0	7-12
Minitran, Nitro-Dur	Patch		√	MI (adjunct)	30-60	24

Dosage Forms and Strengths of Nitrates Used in the Treatment of Angina

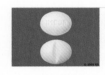

Generic Name	U.S. Brand Name(s) Canadian Brand(s)	Dosage Forms and Strengths
isosorbide dinitrate*	Dilatrate-SR, Isordil Generics	**Capsule, sustained release (Dilatrate-SR):** 40 mg **Tablets, immediate release:** 5 mg, 10 mg, 20 mg†, 30 mg, 40 mg†
isosorbide mononitrate*	Monoket Imdur	**Tablets (Monoket):** 10 mg, 20 mg **Tablets, extended release (Imdur):** 60 mg
nitroglycerin*	Minitran, Nitro-Dur, Nitrolingual, Nitromist, Nitrostat, RECTIV Minitran, Nitro-Dur, Nitrol, Nitrolingual, Nitrostat, Rho-Nitro Pumpspray, Trinipatch, Transderm- Nitro, Nitroject	**Infusion (premixed in D₅W):** 0.1 mg/mL, 0.2 mg/mL, and 0.4 mg/mL **Injection, solution (Nitroject):** 1 mg/mL‡, 5 mg/mL **Ointment (Nitrol):** 2%, RECTIV (0.4%) **Tablets, sublingual (Nitrostat):** 0.3 mg (gr1/200), 0.4 mg (gr1/150), 0.6 mg (gr1/100) **Transdermal patch (Minitran, Nitro-Dur):** 0.1 mg/hr (5 cm²), 0.2 mg/hr (10 cm²), 0.3 mg/hr (15 cm²), 0.4 mg/hr (20 cm²), 0.6 mg/hr, 0.8 mg (40 cm²) **Translingual spray (Nitrolingual, Rho-Nitro Pumpspray):** 0.4 mg/spray (200 sprays/canister)

*Generic available.
†Strength available in the United States only.
‡Strength available in Canada only.

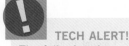

TECH ALERT!
The following drugs have look-alike and sound-alike issues: atenolol, albuterol, and timolol;
Tenormin, Norpramin, and thiamine;
metoprolol, metolazone, metaproterenol, and misoprostol;
Toprol-XL and Topamax;
Corgard, Coreg, and Cognex;
Inderal, Isordil, Toradol, Imdur, Adderall, Enduron, Enduronyl, Inderal LA, and Inderide

β-ADRENERGIC BLOCKERS

Angina pectoris occurs when there is an imbalance between the heart's demand for oxygen and the oxygen supply (see Figure 21-2). β-Adrenergic blockers are administered to reduce the heart's demand for oxygen. This is achieved by decreasing the heart rate and thereby reducing the workload of the heart. β-Adrenergic blockers are also indicated for the management of hypertension and post myocardial infarction (see Chapters 22 and 24) and for the prevention of migraine headache (see Chapter 10).

TECH NOTE!
β-Adrenergic blockers are easily identified because their generic name ends in "-lol."

TECH NOTE!
Hyperlipidemia is a risk factor for angina. Caduet is a combination drug that combines the calcium channel blocker amlodipine with the lipid-lowering drug atorvastatin.

TECH ALERT!
The following drugs have look-alike and sound-alike issues: Norvasc, Norvir, and Vasocor; amlodipine and amiloride; Cardizem, Cardura, Cardene, Cardizem SR, Cardene SR, and Cardizem CD; Tiazac, Tigan, and Ziac; nicardipine, nifedipine, and nimodipine; Procardia, Procardia XL, and Cartia XT; Covera HS and Provera; Veralan, verapamil, and Voltaren

Mechanism of Action

β-Adrenergic blockers decrease the frequency and severity of stable (exertional) angina. They bind to β-receptor sites and block activity of the sympathetic nervous system on cardiac muscle. Heart contractility is reduced and the heart rate is slowed, thereby reducing the workload of the heart. When the heart works less, its need for oxygen and blood supply is reduced.

β-Adrenergic blocking drugs, used to treat stable angina, include cardioselective β₁-adrenergic blockers and nonselective mixed beta₁/beta₂ blockers. (More discussion is found in Chapter 22.)

Pharmacokinetics

β-Adrenergic blockers are formulated in immediate- and long-acting dosage forms. The elimination half-life varies for specific agents and ranges from as short as 3 to 4 hours (propranolol) to as long as 24 hours (nadolol). Most agents are dosed once to twice a day except short-acting propranolol, which is dosed two to four times a day.

Adverse Reactions

β-Adrenergic blockers can produce dizziness, fatigue, bradycardia, hypotension, impotence, heart block, and occasionally insomnia. β-Adrenergic blockers can produce bronchospasm, so their use is cautioned in persons with asthma. The use of β-adrenergic blockers should be used cautiously in persons with diabetes because their action to decrease heart rate masks one of the principal signs of hypoglycemia. Patients with diabetes using beta blockers should be educated about other symptoms of hypoglycemia to be aware of. Abrupt discontinuation of β-adrenergic blockers should be avoided because it can produce tachycardia and a sudden increase in the workload of the heart.

CALCIUM CHANNEL BLOCKERS

Calcium channel blockers are used in the treatment of variant and stable angina. They are effective in the treatment of variant angina because of their ability to reduce vasospasms that restrict the flow of blood and oxygen. Calcium channel blockers improve exercise tolerance by decreasing the workload of the heart. Calcium channel blockers are effective in the treatment of stable angina alone and in combination with nitrates or beta blockers.

β-Adrenergic Blockers

Generic Name	U.S. Brand Name(s) / Canadian Brand(s)	Dosage Forms and Strengths
atenolol*	Tenormin	Tablets: 25 mg, 50 mg, 100 mg
	Tenormin	
metoprolol tartrate*	Lopressor	Injection, solution (Betaloc, Lopressor): 1 mg/mL (5 mL)
	Betaloc, Lopressor, Lopressor SR	Tablets: 25 mg, 50 mg, 100 mg Tablets, extended release (Lopressor SR): 100 mg, 200 mg
metoprolol succinate ER*	Toprol XL	Tablets, extended release (Lopressor SR): 25 mg and 50 mg, 100 mg, 200 mg
	Not available	
nadolol*	Corgard	Tablets: 20 mg†, 40 mg, 80 mg, 160 mg‡
	Generics	
propranolol*	Inderal, Inderal-LA, InnoPran XL	Capsules, extended release (InnoPran XL): 80 mg, 120 mg Capsules, sustained release (Inderal LA): 60 mg, 80 mg, 120 mg, 160 mg
	Inderal-LA	Injection, solution (Inderal): 1 mg/mL Solution, oral (United States only): 20 mg/5 mL Tablet: 10 mg, 20 mg, 40 mg, 60 mg†, 80 mg

*Generic available.
†Strength available in US only.
‡Strength available in Canada only.

Mechanism of Action

Calcium channel blockers block L-type voltage-dependent calcium channels, suppress depolarization, and reduce contraction of the heart muscle. There are two classes of Ca^{2+} channel blockers, dihydropyridines (amlodipine, nifedipine, nicardipine, nimodipine, nisoldipine), and nondihydropyridines, which include phenylalkylamines (verapamil) and benzothiazepines (diltiazem).

The phenylalkylamines and benzothiazepines reduce heart oxygen consumption during exercise by decreasing heart rate and heart contractions. The dihydropyridines are selective for blood vessels, so they are able to increase blood and oxygen supply without slowing heart rate or contractions or increasing the risk of heart block.

Adverse Reactions

Some adverse drug reactions are common to all calcium channel blockers; other side effects are specific to drug classification. All calcium channel blockers produce hypotension. The dihydropyridines (e.g., nifedipine) cause adverse effects associated with vasodilation, including dizziness, flushing, and headache. Peripheral edema is caused by venodilation. The phenylalkylamines and benzothiazepines (e.g., diltiazem) can produce heart failure, bradycardia, and constipation. Diltiazem and verapamil slow conduction through the atrioventricular node and can cause heart block.

Calcium Channel Blockers

Generic Name	U.S. Brand Name(s) / Canadian Brand(s)	Dosage Forms and Strengths
amlodipine*	Norvasc / Norvasc	**Tablets:** 2.5 mg, 5 mg, 10 mg
diltiazem*	Cardizem, Cardizem CD, Cardizem LA, Cardizem SR, Cartia XT, Dilacor XR, Dilt CD, Taztia XT, Tiazac / Cardizem CD, Tiazac, Tiazac XC	**Capsules, extended release:** 120 mg, 180 mg, 240 mg (Cardizem CD, Cartia XT, Dilt-CD, Dilacor XR, Taztia XT, Tiazac, Tiazac XC), 300 mg (Cardizem CD, Cartia XT, Dilt-CD, Taztia XT, Tiazac), 360 mg (Cardizem CD, Tiazac, Taztia XT only), 420 mg (Tiazac only) **Capsules, sustained release (Cardizem SR):** 60 mg, 90 mg, 120 mg, 180 mg **Injection, solution:** 5 mg/mL (5 mL, 10 mL) **Injection, powder for reconstitution:** 100 mg **Tablets, immediate release (Cardizem):** 30 mg, 60 mg, 90 mg, 120 mg **Tablets, extended release (Cardizem LA):** 120 mg, 180 mg, 240 mg, 300 mg, 360 mg, 420 mg (Cardizem LA only)
nicardipine*	Cardene, Cardene SR / Not available	**Capsules:** 20 mg, 30 mg **Capsules, sustained release (Cardene SR):** 30 mg, 60 mg **Injection, solution (Cardene):** 2.5 mg/mL **Injection, solution (Premixed Cardene):** 20 mg/200 mL in Dextrose 4.8%, 40 mg/200 mL in Dextrose 5%, 20 mg/200 mL in NaCl 0.86%, 40 mg/200 mL in NaCl 0.83%
nifedipine*	Adalat CC, Afeditab CR, Procardia, Procardia XL / Adalat XL SRT	**Capsule:** 5 mg‡, 10 mg **Capsule, liquid filled (Procardia):** 10 mg **Tablets, extended release (Adalat CC, Adalat XL SRT, Afeditab CR, Procardia XL):** 20 mg‡, 30 mg, 60 mg, 90 mg (not available as Afeditab CR)

Continued

Calcium Channel Blockers—cont'd

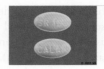

Generic Name	U.S. Brand Name(s) Canadian Brand(s)	Dosage Forms and Strengths
verapamil*	Calan, Calan SR, Covera HS, Verelan, Verelan PM Covera HS, Isoptin SR, Verelan	Capsules, extended release (Verelan PM): 100 mg, 200 mg, 300 mg Capsules, sustained release (Verelan): 120 mg, 180 mg, 240 mg, 360 mg† Injection, solution: 2.5 mg/mL (2 mL, 4 mL) Tablets, immediate release (Calan): 40 mg, 80 mg, 120 mg Tablets, extended release (Covera HS): 180 mg, 240 mg Tablets, sustained release (Calan SR, Isoptin SR): 120 mg, 180 mg, 240 mg

Calcium Channel Blocker Combinations (only combinations approved for the treatment of angina are listed)

amlodipine + atorvastatin	Caduet Caduet	Tablets: amlodipine 2.5 mg + atorvastatin 10 mg†, amlodipine 2.5 mg + atorvastatin 20 mg†, amlodipine 2.5 mg + atorvastatin 40 mg†, amlodipine 5 mg + atorvastatin 10 mg, amlodipine 5 mg + atorvastatin 20 mg, amlodipine 5 mg + atorvastatin 40 mg, amlodipine 5 mg + atorvastatin 80 mg, amlodipine 10 mg + atorvastatin 10 mg, amlodipine 10 mg + atorvastatin 20 mg, amlodipine 10 mg + atorvastatin 40 mg, amlodipine 10 mg + atorvastatin 80 mg
nifedipine + aspirin	Not available Adalat XL Plus	Tablet kit: nifedipine 20 mg + ASA 81 mg, nifedipine 30 mg + ASA 81 mg, nifedipine 60 mg + ASA 81 mg

*Generic available.
†Strength available in the United States only.
‡Strength available in Canada only.

Summary of Drugs Used in the Treatment of Angina

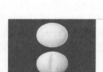

Generic	Brand	Usual Dose	Warning Labels
Nitrates			
isosorbide dinitrate	Isordil	**Angina:** 5-40 mg 4 times a day or 40 mg SR every 8-12 hours	TAKE ON AN EMPTY STOMACH—isosorbide dinitrate. SWALLOW WHOLE; DO NOT CRUSH OR CHEW—sustained and extended release. AVOID ALCOHOL. STORE IN MANUFACTURER'S ORIGINAL CONTAINER—sublingual, capsules. REPLACE VIALS 3-6 MONTHS AFTER OPENING—sublingual. ROTATE SITE OF APPLICATION—transdermal patch. HOLD SPRAY IN MOUTH FOR UP TO 10 SECONDS BEFORE SWALLOWING—translingual spray. IF NO RELIEF OF SYMPTOMS AFTER 3 DOSES OF SUBLINGUAL TABS OR LINGUAL SPRAY (OR 15 MINUTES), CALL 911—all immediate-release dosage forms. SWALLOW WHOLE; DO NOT CRUSH OR CHEW—sustained and extended release.
isosorbide mononitrate	Imdur	**Angina:** 5 mg–10 mg twice a day (7 hours apart), 30-60 mg/day (extended release) up to maximum, 240 mg/day	
nitroglycerin	Nitrostat	**Buccal:** 1-3 mg every 3-5 hours while awake **IV:** Infuse 5-10 mcg/min every 3-5 minutes **Oral:** 2.5-9 mg 2-4 times a day (maximum, 26 mg 4 times a day) **Ointment:** ½ inch (1.25 cm) twice a day (6 hours apart) **Transdermal patch:** Wear 1 patch (0.2-0.8 mg/hr) for 12-14 hr/day; patch off for 10-12 hr/day **Sublingual:** Dissolve 1 tablet sublingually as needed for chest pain; may repeat 1 tablet every 5 minutes if no relief up to 3 tablets (15 minutes) or dissolve 1 tablet sublingually 5 minutes before strenuous activity **Translingual spray:** Place 1-2 sprays in mouth as needed for chest pain; may repeat every 5 minutes if no relief up to 3 doses (15 minutes) or use 5-10 minutes before strenuous activity	

Summary of Drugs Used in the Treatment of Angina—cont'd

Generic	Brand	Usual Dose	Warning Labels
β-Adrenergic Blockers			
atenolol	Tenormin	**Angina:** 50 mg/day (may increase to 100-200 mg once daily)	MAY CAUSE DIZZINESS; USE CAUTION WHEN DRIVING OR PERFORMING TASKS REQUIRING ALERTNESS. AVOID ABRUPT DISCONTINUATION. TAKE WITH FOOD—metoprolol (immediate release). SWALLOW WHOLE; DO NOT CRUSH OR CHEW—sustained release.
metoprolol tartrate	Lopressor, Lopressor SR	**Angina (immediate release):** Start with 50 mg twice daily increasing to 100-400 mg/day in 2-3 divided doses **Angina (sustained release):** 100-400 mg/day in 2-3 divided doses	
metoprolol succinate	Toprol XL	**Angina (sustained release):** 100-400 mg/day as a single dose	
nadolol	Corgard	**Angina:** Begin at 40 mg/day; increase to 160-240 mg once daily	
propranolol	Generics, Inderal LA	**Angina:** 80-320 mg/day in 2-4 divided doses or 80-320 mg once daily (extended release)	
Calcium Channel Blockers			
amlodipine	Norvasc	**Angina:** 5-10 mg/day	MAY CAUSE DIZZINESS; USE CAUTION WHEN DRIVING OR PERFORMING TASKS REQUIRING ALERTNESS. AVOID ABRUPT DISCONTINUATION. LIMIT CAFFEINE AND ALCOHOL. SWALLOW WHOLE; DO NOT CRUSH OR CHEW—extended and sustained release. TAKE WITH FOOD—nicardipine (sustained release).
diltiazem	Cardizem, Cardizem CD, Cardizem LA	**Extended release, caps:** 120-180 mg once daily (maximum, 480 mg/day) **Extended release, tablet:** 180 mg once daily (maximum, 360 mg/day) **Immediate release, tablet:** 30 mg 4 times a day (maximum, 180-360 mg/day) **Sustained release, caps:** 60-120 mg twice a day	
nicardipine	Generics, Cardene SR	**Immediate release:** 20-40 mg 3 times a day **Sustained release:** 30-60 mg twice daily	
nifedipine	Procardia, Procardia XL	**Immediate release:** 10-30 mg 3 times a day **Sustained release:** 30-60 mg once daily (maximum, 120-180 mg per day)	
verapamil	Calan, Calan SR, Verelan, Isoptin SR, Covera HS	**Angina (immediate release):** **Calan, Verelan, Isoptin SR:** Begin 80-120 mg 3 times a day; may increase to 240-480 mg/day **Covera HS:** 180 mg/day at bedtime	
Calcium Channel Blocker Combinations			
amlodipine + atorvastatin	Caduet	5-10 mg amlodipine once daily	MAY CAUSE DIZZINESS. AVOID GRAPEFRUIT JUICE.

OTHER DRUG CLASSIFICATIONS

Angiotensin-converting enzyme (ACE) inhibitors, anticoagulants, antiplatelet drugs, glycoprotein IIb/IIIa drugs, and antihyperlipidemics may be administered to patients who have angina, especially when comorbid conditions (hypertension or myocardial infarction) are present. These drug classifications are discussed in Chapters 22 and 24.

Chapter Summary

- Angina is a symptom of ischemic heart disease.
- The symptoms of angina are described as severe squeezing or pressure-like chest pain; sometimes radiating to the arms, shoulders, neck, or jaw.
- Angina pain is sometimes described as severe heartburn or indigestion.
- People with a history of heart disease, hypertension, and diabetes are at risk for angina; however, lifestyle is a significant risk for the condition.
- Risk factors associated with lifestyle include smoking, overeating, a diet high in cholesterol and salt, excessive alcohol consumption, obesity, lack of exercise, and stress.
- Coronary artery disease causes myocardial ischemia.
- Atherosclerosis is a disease of the coronary arteries that results in the buildup of lipid streaks in arteries.
- Atherosclerosis can block the flow of blood through the artery, producing ischemia and cell death (*necrosis*).
- There are three types of angina, stable, unstable, and variant.
- In all types of angina, there is an imbalance between blood supplied to the heart muscle and the need for blood and oxygen.
- Symptoms of stable angina are typically brought on by physical exertion, smoking, eating heavy meals, exposure to extreme changes in temperature (hot or cold), and emotional stress.
- Unstable angina may occur at rest without physical exertion and results when an embolus partially or completely occludes an artery.
- Variant angina is also known as vasospastic angina because it is caused by vasospasm of the coronary arteries.
- Variant angina may occur at rest similar to unstable angina.
- Microvascular angina or cardiac syndrome X may produce greater chest pain and last longer than other types of angina; medicine may not relieve it.
- Lifestyle changes can reduce the risk, frequency, and severity of symptoms and prevent or slow the progression of angina to myocardial infarction or death.
- Recommended lifestyle changes are to (1) take frequent rest breaks, (2) avoid eating foods high in salt and cholesterol, (3) eat smaller portions, (4) learn techniques to manage stress, and (5) become an advocate for workplace and community-wide changes that facilitate lifestyle change.
- Drugs used in the treatment of angina are administered to increase the blood and oxygen supply to the heart and to decrease the workload of the heart.
- Drug therapy for angina is focused on treatment and prevention of symptoms and treatment and prevention of cardiovascular diseases that often accompany angina.
- The organic nitrates are the oldest class of drugs used to treat acute symptoms of angina. They dilate blood vessels (arteries and veins) and increase the supply of oxygen to the heart.
- Nitrates that are commonly used in the treatment and prevention of angina are nitroglycerin, isosorbide dinitrate, and isosorbide mononitrate.
- Nitroglycerin is formulated for parenteral, oral, sublingual, and topical use.
- Dosage delivery systems that are designed to deliver nitroglycerin quickly are used to treat acute symptoms; they include parenteral solution, sublingual tablets, and lingual spray.
- Nitroglycerin in the form of extended release capsules, patches, and ointments delivers medication over an extended period (up to 24 hours) and is intended to prevent symptoms of angina.
- Sublingual nitroglycerin is volatile and loses its potency when exposed to air, light, and moisture. It must be dispensed in the manufacturer's original container.
- Isosorbide dinitrate and isosorbide mononitrate are administered for prevention.
- Adverse reactions of nitrates include hypotension, facial flushing, dizziness, headache, nausea and vomiting, weakness, and fatigue.

- Sublingual dosage forms can cause stinging or burning under the tongue, and adhesives used in patches can produce allergic reactions.
- To minimize the risk for development of tolerance to nitrates, it is important to have a 10- to 12-hour drug-free period each day.
- A fatal drop in blood pressure can occur when drugs used to treat erectile dysfunction (sildenafil [Viagra], vardenafil [Cialis], and tadalafil [Levitra]) are administered to patients who are taking nitroglycerin.
- The β-adrenergic blockers are easily identified because their generic name ends in "-lol."
- The β-adrenergic blockers decrease the heart rate and workload of the heart, thereby reducing the heart's demand for oxygen.
- The β-adrenergic blockers decrease the frequency and severity of stable (exertional) angina.
- Adverse reactions of the β-adrenergic blockers are dizziness, fatigue, bradycardia, hypotension, impotence, heart block, and occasionally insomnia.
- The β-adrenergic blockers should be used cautiously in patients with asthma and diabetes because they can produce bronchospasm and mask the signs of hypoglycemia.
- Abrupt discontinuation of β-adrenergic blockers should be avoided because it could produce tachycardia and a sudden increase in the workload of the heart.
- Calcium channel blockers classified as dihydropyridines are easily identified because their generic name ends in "-dipine."
- Calcium channel blockers are used in treatment of variant and stable angina.
- Calcium channel blockers reduce vasospasms and improve exercise tolerance by decreasing the workload of the heart and improving blood flow.
- There are two classes of Ca^{2+} channel blockers, dihydropyridines (amlodipine, nifedipine, nicardipine, nimodipine, and nisoldipine) and nondihydropyridines (verapamil and diltiazem).
- The dihydropyridines are selective for peripheral blood vessels, so they are able to increase blood and oxygen supply without slowing heart rate or contractions or increasing the risk of heart block.

REVIEW QUESTIONS

1. Thickening and loss of elasticity of arterial walls that is sometimes called "hardening of the arteries" characterizes _____.
   a. atherosclerosis
   b. arteriosclerosis
   c. angiosclerosis
   d. vasosclerosis

2. People with what kind of health history are at risk for angina?
   a. heart disease
   b. hypertension
   c. diabetes
   d. all of the above

3. There are two types of angina, stable and unstable.
   a. true
   b. false

4. Which of the following is *not* true of drugs used in the treatment of angina?
   a. They are administered to increase the blood supply to the heart.
   b. They are administered to increase oxygen supply to the heart.
   c. They are administered to increase the workload of the heart.
   d. They are administered to decrease the workload of the heart.

5. The organic nitrates are the oldest class of drugs used to treat acute symptoms of angina.
   a. true
   b. false

6. Nitrates act to _____ the vein.
   a. constrict
   b. occlude
   c. dilate
   d. none of the above

7. Calcium channel blockers are used in treatment of what types of angina?
   a. variant
   b. stable
   c. unstable
   d. a and b

8. Stable angina may occur at rest without physical exertion and results when an embolus partially or completely occludes an artery.
   a. true
   b. false

9. The generic name for Tenormin is _____.
   a. atenolol
   b. nifedipine
   c. nadolol
   d. amlodipine

10. Which drug must be dispensed in the manufacturer's original container?
   a. isosorbide dinitrate
   b. isosorbide mononitrate
   c. sublingual nitroglycerin
   d. diltiazem

TECHNICIAN'S CORNER

1. What is the major difference between arteriosclerosis and atherosclerosis?
2. Both nitroglycerin and sildenafil have vasodilating effects on blood vessels. Why is it so important not to use these drugs at the same time?

Bibliography

American Heart Association: *Heart Disease and Stroke Statistics—2010 Update*, Dallas, Texas, 2010, American Heart Association. Retrieved from http://www.americanheart.org/downloadable/heart/1265665152970DS-3241%20HeartStrokeUpdate_2010.pdf.

Chow CM, Donovan L, Manuel D, et al: Canadian Cardiovascular Outcomes Research Team, regional variation in self-reported heart disease prevalence in Canada, *Can J Cardiol* 21:1265-1271, 2005.

Drug information online: Nitroglycerin drug information, professional. Retrieved from http://www.drugs.com/MMX/Nitroglycerin.html.

FDA. FDA Approved Drug Products. Retrieved May 14, 2012, from http://www.accessdata.fda.gov/scripts/cder/drugsatfda/index.cfm?fuseaction=Search.Search_Drug_Name, 2012.

Fougera: *Nitro-Bid package insert*. Retrieved from http://www.fougera.com/products/documents/1114.PI.pdf#search=%22Nitro-Bid%20ointment%20duration%20of%20action%22.

Fulcher E, Soto C, Fulcher R: *Pharmacology: principles and applications: a worktext for allied health professionals*, Philadelphia, 2003, Elsevier Saunders, pp 586-590.

Health Canada. Drug Product Database. Retrieved May 14,2012 from http://www.hc-sc.gc.ca/dhp-mps/prod-pharma/databasdon/index-eng.php, 2010.

Kalant H, Grant D, Mitchell J: *Principles of medical pharmacology*, ed 7, Toronto, Ontario, Canada, 2007, Elsevier Canada, A Division of Reed Elsevier Canada, pp 451-453, 458-460.

Lance L, Lacy C, Armstrong L, et al: *Drug information handbook for the allied health professional*, ed 12, Hudson, OH, 2005, APhA Lexi-Comp.

Lanza, GA, Cardiac syndrome X: a critical overview and future perspectives, *Heart* 93:159-166, 2007. Retrieved from http://heart.bmj.com/content/93/2/159.full.pdf.

National Heart, Lung, and Blood Institute: *Angina*, Bethesda, MD, 2006, National Heart and Blood Institute, National Institutes of Health, US Department of Health and Human Services. Retrieved from http://www.nhlbi.nih.gov/health/dci/Diseases/Angina/Angina_All.html.

Page C, Curtis M, Sutter M, et al: *Integrated pharmacology*, Philadelphia, 2005, Mosby, pp 377-383.

USP Center for Advancement of Patient Safety: *Use caution–avoid confusion*, USP Quality Review No. 79, Rockville, MD, April 2004, USP Center for Advancement of Patient Safety.

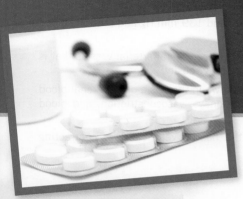

22

Treatment of Hypertension

KEY TERMS

Aldosterone: Hormone that promotes sodium and fluid reabsorption.

Angiotension II: Potent vasoconstrictor that is produced when the renin–aldosterone–angiotensin system is activated.

Angiotensin-converting enzyme: Enzyme that catalyzes the conversion of angiotensin I to angiotensin II.

Cardiac output: Volume of blood ejected from the left ventricle in 1 minute.

Diastolic blood pressure: Measure of blood pressure when the heart is at rest (diastole).

Diuretic: Drug that produces diuresis (urination).

Gynecomastia: Painful breast enlargement in men.

Hirsutism: Excessive hair growth in women.

Hyperkalemia: Excessive serum potassium levels.

Hypertension: High blood pressure. Elevated diastolic, systolic blood pressure or both.

Hypokalemia: Deficient serum potassium levels.

Isolated systolic hypertension: Elevated systolic blood pressure only. Diastolic blood pressure is within the normal range.

Metabolic syndrome: Important risk factor of hypertension that promotes the development of atherosclerosis and cardiovascular disease.

Nocturia: Nighttime urination.

Orthostatic hypotension: Sudden drop in blood pressure that occurs when arising from lying down or sitting to standing.

Photosensitivity: Increased sensitivity to sun exposure that can result in sunburn.

Preeclampsia: Sudden rise in blood pressure, excessive weight gain, generalized edema, proteinuria, severe headache, and visual disturbances occurring in late pregnancy.

Prehypertension: Systolic blood pressure ranging between 120 and 139 mm Hg and diastolic blood pressure ranging between 80 and 89 mm Hg.

Peripheral vascular resistance: Resistance to the flow of blood in peripheral arterial vessels that is associated with blood vessel diameter, vessel length, and blood viscosity.

Renin–aldosterone–angiotensin system: System that is activated when there is a drop in renal blood flow. Activation increases blood volume, blood flow to the kidneys, vasoconstriction, and blood pressure.

Systolic blood pressure: Measure of the pressure when the heart's ventricles are contracting (systole).

Blood Pressure

Blood pressure is necessary to circulate blood, oxygen (O_2), and nutrients to body organs and to remove carbon dioxide (CO_2) and waste products. Without blood pressure shock, circulatory collapse and death would result.

Blood pressure is measured using a sphygmomanometer (aneroid or mercury), or an electronic blood pressure measuring device. Two pressures are measured. They are the systolic pressure and the diastolic pressure.

$$BP = \frac{Systole}{Diastole}$$

The *systolic blood pressure* (SBP) is a measure of the pressure when the heart's ventricles are contracting (systole). The *diastolic blood pressure* (DBP) is a measure of the heart at rest (diastole).

$$\text{Average normal blood pressure is } \frac{120 \text{ (systole)}}{80 \text{ (diastole)}}$$

The formula for determining blood pressure is:

$$BP = CO \times PR$$

where CO is the *cardiac output* and PR is the peripheral resistance. Cardiac output is determined by measuring the heart rate (HR) and multiplying it by the stroke volume (volume of blood ejected by the ventricles).

Blood Pressure Control

Sensors in the body monitor blood flow, and when decreases are detected, regulatory mechanisms are "switched on." Sites that play a role in blood pressure control are the kidneys, heart, blood vessels, central nervous system (CNS), and sympathetic nerves. When the kidney detects a drop in renal blood supply, the *renin–aldosterone–angiotensin–system* (RAAS) is activated (Figure 22-1). This causes levels of *aldosterone* (endocrine hormone) and angiotensin to rise. Aldosterone and angiotensin act to increase blood volume, blood flow to the kidney, vasoconstriction, and blood pressure.

The heart controls the cardiac output (the amount of blood ejected from the ventricles) by increasing or decreasing the rate of contractions (Figure 22-2). When the CNS senses a drop in blood pressure, it signals sympathetic nerves to release neurotransmitters that control heart rate and blood flow through the arteries. Sympathetic nerves release norepinephrine, which causes vasoconstriction and increased *peripheral vascular resistance*. When peripheral vascular resistance

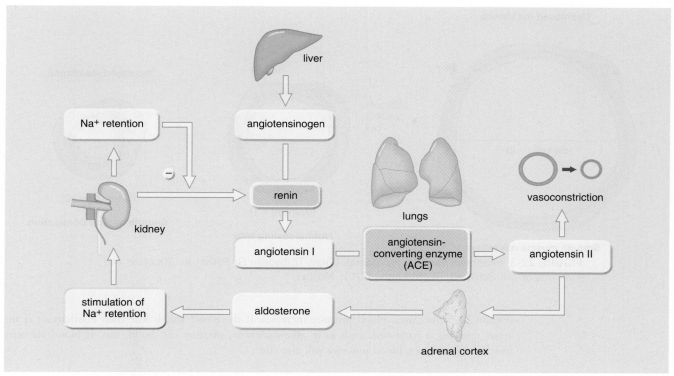

FIGURE 22-1 The renin–aldosterone–angiotensin system. (From Page C, et al: *Integrated pharmacology*, 3rd ed Philadelphia, 2006, Mosby.)

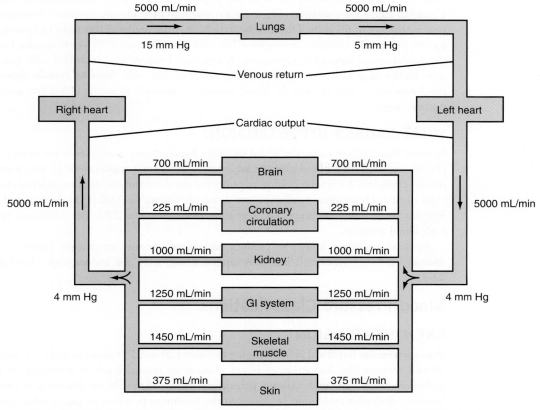

FIGURE 22-2 Diagram of cardiac output. (From Thibodeau G, PattonK: *Anatomy and Physiology*, ed 6, St Louis, 2006, Mosby)

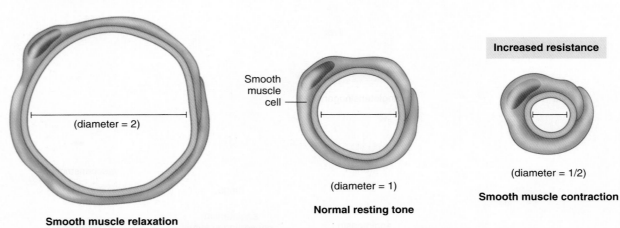

Decreased resistance

(diameter = 2)

Smooth muscle relaxation

Smooth muscle cell

(diameter = 1)

Normal resting tone

Increased resistance

(diameter = 1/2)

Smooth muscle contraction

FIGURE 22-3 Peripheral vascular resistance. (From Thibodeau G. Patton K: *Structure and Function of the Body*, ed 14, St Louis, 2011, Mosby)

(Figure 22-3) increases, blood pressure increases. If the blood vessels lose their elasticity or if the vessel opening is narrowed, such as in atherosclerosis, pressure can build, too. If blood viscosity (thickness) increases, blood pressure will also rise.

Hypertension

Hypertension is the most diagnosed medical condition in the United States, affecting more than 90 million Americans (nearly 29% of the adult population). According to Statistics Canada, more than 5.7 million Canadians (17% of the population) have high blood pressure. Up to 90% of Canadian adults are estimated to have hypertension in their lifetime with half developing hypertension by the age of 60 years. Diastolic hypertension is the predominant form of hypertension before age 50 years. SBP increases throughout life, and after the age of 50 years, systolic hypertension is the predominant form of hypertension. It was once believed that increased SBP was benign. It is now known that SBP poses an important cardiovascular risk. *Isolated systolic hypertension* is a condition where only the systolic blood pressure is elevated. Diastolic blood pressure is within the normal range.

WHAT CAUSES HYPERTENSION?

In more than 90% of cases, the actual cause for hypertension is unknown, yet some risk factors for chronic elevated high blood pressure are known. *Metabolic syndrome* is an important risk factor for hypertension. Metabolic syndrome promotes the development of atherosclerosis and cardiovascular disease. Dyslipidemia, whereby low-density lipoproteins (LDLs) are elevated and high-density lipoproteins (HDLs) are decreased, is another risk factor. Box 22-1 lists additional risk factors for high blood pressure.

Medical conditions known to produce high blood pressure are chronic kidney disease, thyroid disease, Cushing's syndrome, and sleep apnea. Drugs may also induce high blood pressure (Box 22-2).

Blood Pressure Classifications

PREHYPERTENSION

Prehypertension is defined as SBP ranging between 120 and 139 mm Hg and DBP ranging between 80 and 89 mm Hg. Reduction of blood pressure to normal levels is beneficial for persons with prehypertension with and without preexisting disease. Lifestyle modification is often sufficient; however, drug therapy should be added to the treatment program in people who have diabetes or kidney disease if lifestyle changes do not bring blood pressure down to the normal range.

BOX 22-1   **Hypertension Risk Factors**

- Age (men older than 55 years; women older than 65 years)
- Diabetes mellitus
- Family history of heart disease
- Metabolic syndrome
- Obesity
- Tobacco usage
- Decreased physical activity
- Dyslipidemia
- Diet high in salt and saturated fats
- Excessive alcohol consumption

BOX 22-2   **Select Drugs That Can Increase Blood Pressure**

- Nonsteroidal anti-inflammatory drugs (cyclooxygenase-2 inhibitors)
- Cocaine, amphetamines
- Decongestants
- Diet pills
- Oral contraceptives
- Glucocorticosteroids (e.g., prednisone, hydrocortisone, methylprednisolone)
- Mineralocorticoids (aldosterone)
- Cyclosporine and tacrolimus
- Erythropoietin
- Licorice
- Herbals (ma huang, ephedra, bitter orange)

STAGE 1 HYPERTENSION

Stage 1 hypertension is classified as SBP ranging between 140 and 159 mm Hg and DBP ranging between 90 and 99 mm Hg. It should be managed with lifestyle modification and drug therapy.

STAGE 2 HYPERTENSION AND GRADE 3 HYPERTENSION

In the United States, stage 2 hypertension is classified as SBP 160 mm Hg or greater and DBP of 100 mm Hg or greater. It is the most severe stage of hypertension and should be managed with lifestyle modification and drug therapy. In Canada, a 3-stage classification is used. Grade 2 hypertension is classified as SBP of 160 to 179 mm Hg and DBP of 100 to 110 mm Hg. Grade 3 hypertension is classified as SBP of 180 mm Hg or greater and DBP of 110 mm Hg or greater. Combination therapy with two or more drugs is necessary to reduce blood pressure in most patients. Blood pressure greater than 180/110 mm Hg is a medical emergency and should be treated immediately.

PREECLAMPSIA AND GESTATIONAL HYPERTENSION

Hypertension during pregnancy is dangerous to the pregnant woman and the fetus. Gestational hypertension typically occurs after 20 weeks of pregnancy in susceptible women. It can progress to ***preeclampsia*** and cause premature delivery and fetal growth retardation. Approximately 25% of pregnant women who have chronic hypertension for more than 4 years will develop preeclampsia during pregnancy. Preeclampsia can progress to eclampsia and cause seizures.

WHITE COAT HYPERTENSION

Some people have a condition that is known as "white coat hypertension." They have abnormally high blood pressure when the measurement is taken by a health care professional, but blood pressure measurements taken in a nonclinic setting are within normal range (Table 22-1).

Complications Associated with Untreated or Poorly Controlled Hypertension

Hypertension is sometimes called the "silent killer" because it can cause damage to the body without any obvious symptoms. Hypertension can cause damage to the kidneys, heart, brain, arteries, and eyes. Hypertension can weaken arteries and cause aneurysms that can bleed and cause death if they occur in the brain, aorta, or abdomen. Hypertension can cause blindness when blood vessels to the retina are damaged and scarred. For each 20–mm Hg increase in SBP and 10–mm Hg increase in

DBP, there is a twofold increase in risk of death from ischemic heart disease (IHD) and stroke. This is because hypertension can damage arteries and make them stiff and thick.

Nonpharmacological Management of Hypertension

Hypertension poses a serious public health challenge because of the risks for death and long-term disability. It is categorized as a chronic disease of lifestyle because it is associated with obesity, excess dietary sodium intake, physical inactivity, excessive alcohol consumption, and inadequate consumption of fruits and vegetables. More than 122 million Americans are overweight, and fewer than 20% engage in regular physical activity or consume adequate fruits and vegetables (five servings per day).

Lifestyle modification is an important strategy for prevention and management of hypertension and can reduce SBP between 4 and 20 mm Hg. A reduction of as little as 5 mm Hg can lower the risk of death from stroke by 14% and death from coronary heart disease (CHD) by 9%. The U.S. Joint National Committee on the Prevention, Detection, Evaluation, and Treatment of High Blood Pressure recommendations for lifestyle changes are listed in Table 22-2.

Drugs Used in the Treatment of Hypertension

Lifestyle modification is the first step in prevention and management of hypertension in people with normal blood pressure or who have prehypertension; however, most people with hypertension

TABLE 22-1   **Summary of Blood Pressure Classifications and Target Blood Pressure Goals**

Classification	Blood Pressure Range (mm Hg)	Blood Pressure Target (mm Hg)
Normal	<120/80	<120/80
Prehypertension	120-139/80-89	<120/80
Hypertension Stage 1 Stage 2 or Grade 2‡ Stage 3‡	≥140/90 140-159/90-99 160-179/100-109 ≥180/110	<140/90
Isolated systolic hypertension	Systolic ≥140 Diastolic ≤90	Systolic <140
Diabetes or chronic kidney disease	—	<130/80

‡Grade scale is used in Canada.

TECH NOTE!
Natural licorice may aggravate hypertension and interfere with the effects of antihypertensive drugs. It increases sodium and water retention and potassium depletion.

TECH NOTE!
Processed foods contain "hidden sodium" and account for nearly 80% of the daily sodium consumed.

TABLE 22-2   **Lifestyle Modifications for Management and Prevention of Hypertension**

Modification	Recommendation
Weight loss	Maintain normal body weight Body mass index (18.5-24.9 kg/m²)
Diet	Reduce salt (sodium) intake (≤2.4 g sodium) Reduce saturated and total fats Eat five or more servings of fruits and vegetables/day
Physical activity	Engage in 30-60 minutes of aerobic physical activity daily
Alcohol consumption	Drink no more than 2 alcoholic beverages* per day—men (women and lightweight persons, 1 drink/day)
Tobacco usage	Stop smoking cigarettes and cigars

*Alcoholic beverage = 24 oz of beer, 10 oz of wine, or 3 oz of whiskey (80 proof).
Adapted from 7th Report of the Joint National Committee on Prevention, Detection, Evaluation, and Treatment of High Blood Pressure and 2010 Canadian Hypertension Education Program (CHEP) guidelines.
http://www.cfp.ca/content/56/7/649.full
http://www.cfp.ca/content/57/12/1393.full

will require drug therapy with one or more drugs and lifestyle modification. Pharmaceutical management of hypertension can be challenging because medications prescribed to reduce blood pressure can sometimes produce more symptoms than the disease, resulting in poor adherence to drug therapy.

Drugs used in the treatment of hypertension work at the sites for blood pressure regulation, which are the kidneys, heart, blood vessels, brain, and sympathetic nerves.

DIURETICS

The kidneys play a major role in regulating blood pressure, and diuretics exert their effects on the kidneys. The *diuretics* increase the elimination of water, sodium, and selected electrolytes (K^+, Cl^-, HCO_3^-), depending on their location of action in the kidney, especially in the nephrons (Figure 22-4).

The diuretics lower blood pressure by decreasing peripheral resistance and cardiac output. They lower peripheral resistance by decreasing the blood volume. The effect of diuretics on lowering the blood volume also reduces cardiac output. When cardiac output is reduced, blood pressure decreases. Recall the formula $BP = CO \times PR$.

There are several classifications of diuretics. They are thiazide, loop, and potassium (K^+) sparing. Aldosterone antagonists are K^+ sparing and are sometimes classified as diuretics because their site of action is the kidney.

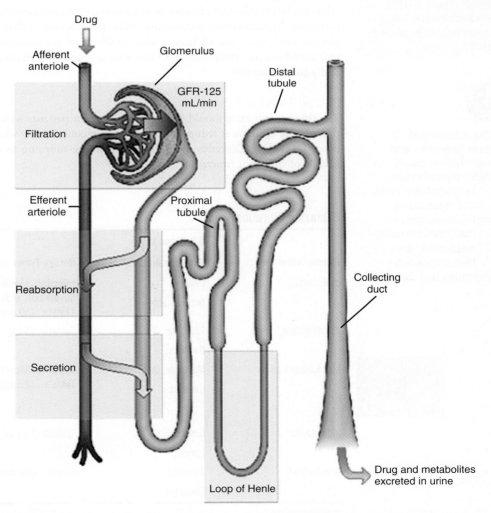

FIGURE 22-4 Nephron. (From Lilley LL, Harrington S, Snyder JS: *Pharmacology and the nursing process,* ed 5, St Louis, 2007, Mosby.)

TECH NOTE!
Most thiazide diuretics share the common ending "-thiazide."

TECH NOTE!
Patients taking thiazides may be advised to eat potassium-rich foods because of potassium depletion in the body.

TECH NOTE!
Hydrochlorothiazide is commonly abbreviated HCTZ.

TECH ALERT!
The following drugs have look-alike and sound-alike issues: hydrochlorothiazide, hydroxychloroquine, and hydralazine; metolazone, metaxalone, methimazole, metoprolol, and metoclopramide; Zaroxolyn and Zarontin

Thiazide Diuretics

Thiazide diuretics are a first-line therapy for hypertension. They promote the elimination of water, sodium, potassium, magnesium, and chloride ions. Fluid loss decreases blood volume, yet this is not the primary mechanism of action for their effectiveness in decreasing blood pressure.

Thiazides act at the distal convoluted tubule, where they block the sodium–chloride cotransporter (see Figure 22-4). This interferes with calcium transport into arterioles, decreasing vasoconstriction. Peripheral resistance is lowered along with blood pressure. Thiazides indirectly stimulate aldosterone secretion, causing potassium excretion. They stimulate calcium reabsorption, which makes them useful for the treatment of kidney stones that are caused by increased calcium in the urine (hypercalciuria) but at the expense of increasing blood calcium levels (hypercalcemia).

PHARMACOKINETICS

Thiazide diuretics are readily absorbed by oral administration. They are weak acids and are highly protein bound. After being transported into the proximal tubule of the nephron, tubular secretion is decreased. Their lipid solubility permits reabsorption along the distal nephron. Their duration of effect varies from as little as 6 hours to as long as 48 hours depending on the drug. Most thiazide diuretics are dosed once a day.

ADVERSE REACTIONS

Thiazide diuretics can cause dehydration, hyponatremia (sodium loss), and electrolyte deficiency including *hypokalemia* (potassium loss), hypomagnesemia (magnesium loss), and hypochloremia (chloride loss). Thiazides can also decrease urinary calcium excretion, resulting in hypercalcemia and can cause hyperuricemia (excess uric acid), precipitating a flare-up of gout. Hyperglycemia and glucose intolerance are additional adverse effects of the thiazides. The thiazides have direct and indirect effects on insulin release. Other adverse drug reactions are gastrointestinal upset, impotence, and *photosensitivity*.

PRECAUTIONS

The thiazide diuretics should be used cautiously in patients with gout and diabetes. The effect of the thiazide diuretics is reduced if they are taken concurrently with nonsteroidal anti-inflammatory drugs (NSAIDs). Diuretics should be taken in the morning to avoid the need to urinate in the middle of the night (*nocturia*).

Thiazide Diuretics

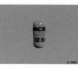

Generic Name	U.S. Brand Name / Canadian Brand(s)	Dosage Forms and Strengths
chlorothiazide*	Diuril	Injection, powder for reconstitution: 500 mg vial
	Not available	Suspension, oral: 250 mg/5 mL (237 mL) Tablets: 250 mg, 500 mg (generic only)
chlorthalidone*	Thalitone	Tablets: 15 mg† (Thalitone), 25 mg†, 50 mg†, 100 mg‡
	Generics	
hydrochlorothiazide*	Microzide. Oretic	Capsules (Microzide): 12.5 mg
	Generics	Tablets: 12.5 mg, 25 mg, 50 mg, 100 mg‡
indapamide*	Generics	Tablets: 1.25 mg, 2.5 mg
	Lozide	
metolazone*	Zaroxolyn	Tablets, slow acting (Zaroxolyn): 2.5 mg, 5 mg†, 10 mg†
	Zaroxolyn	

*Generic available.
†Strength available in the United States only.
‡Strength available in Canada only.

Loop Diuretics

The loop diuretics also block the sodium–potassium cotransporter in the ascending loop of Henle. They are the most potent diuretics because they inhibit the reabsorption of 20% to 30% of sodium load; the thiazides inhibit only 5% to 10%, and the potassium-sparing diuretics inhibit only 1% to 3% of the sodium load. Loop diuretics increase potassium excretion and are often administered with a potassium supplement because of risk of hypokalemia. They also stimulate aldosterone secretion, similar to the thiazides, and increase calcium excretion.

PHARMACOKINETICS

The loop diuretics are readily absorbed from the gastrointestinal tract. They are up to 98% protein bound. Differences among the loop diuretics are associated with their degree of metabolism in the liver and the extent to which they are eliminated unchanged in the urine. Whereas bumetanide is partially metabolized in the liver, and 50% is excreted unchanged in the urine, torsemide's metabolism in the liver is greater and 20% is excreted unchanged. Torsemide's long half-life permits once-daily dosing.

ADVERSE REACTIONS

The loop diuretics can cause dehydration, severe hypotension, hypokalemia, hyperuricemia, and photosensitivity. Deafness has occurred when large doses are infused rapidly.

PRECAUTIONS

The effect of loop diuretics is reduced if they are taken concurrently with NSAIDs. Patients taking loop diuretics should take the last dose of the day in early evening to avoid the need to urinate in the middle of the night.

Potassium-Sparing Diuretics

The potassium-sparing diuretics inhibit sodium reabsorption while avoiding potassium loss. They are less effective than loop and thiazide diuretics. Combining K^+ sparing diuretics with a thiazide diuretic increases their effectiveness. Fixed dose potassium-sparing diuretic combinations currently available are amiloride–hydrochlorothiazide and triamterene–hydrochlorothiazide.

Triamterene is readily absorbed in the gastrointestinal tract, and amiloride is 50% absorbed. The duration of effect ranges from 7 to 9 hours (triamterene) and 24 hours (amiloride).

ADVERSE REACTIONS

Hyperkalemia is the most serious adverse reaction of the potassium-sparing diuretics, and the risk is increased if they are prescribed along with angiotensin-converting enzyme (ACE) inhibitors. They may also cause nausea or vomiting.

Loop Diuretics

Generic Name	U.S. Brand Name Canadian Brand(s)	Dosage Forms and Strengths
bumetanide*	Generics Burinex	Injection, solution: 0.25 mg/mL Tablets: 0.5 mg†, 1 mg, 2 mg†, 5 mg‡
furosemide*	Lasix Lasix	Injection, solution: 10 mg/mL Solution, oral: 10 mg/mL, 40 mg/5 mL Tablets: 20 mg, 40 mg, 80 mg
torsemide*	Demadex Not available	Injection, solution: 10 mg/mL Tablets: 5 mg, 10 mg, 20 mg, 100 mg

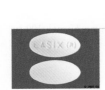

*Generic available.
†Strength available in the United States only.
‡Strength available in Canada only.

PRECAUTIONS

The potassium-sparing diuretics should be used cautiously in patients with heart failure who are taking digoxin. Patients should be advised to avoid salt substitutes because they contain potassium chloride (KCl).

ALDOSTERONE RECEPTOR ANTAGONISTS

Aldosterone is a hormone that is released when the kidney perceives a drop in blood flow and blood pressure. Aldosterone causes sodium and water reabsorption. Spironolactone is a competitive antagonist of aldosterone. It blocks the effect of aldosterone on sodium channels, decreases sodium reabsorption, and inhibits potassium elimination. Spironolactone is sometimes classified as a potassium-sparing diuretic and is also available in combination with hydrochlorothiazide. In addition to its use in treating hypertension, spironolactone is used to treat primary aldosteronism, hypokalemia, heart failure, and liver disease. It can take several weeks to see maximal effect, which differs from loop diuretics, which work immediately.

Spironolactone is about as effective as triamterene and amiloride (sodium reabsorption is approximately 1%–3%). It is readily absorbed orally and is eliminated in urine. It has a long half-life and is dosed once daily.

Eplerenone is a selective aldosterone receptor antagonist (SARA). It is indicated for the treatment of hypertension as monotherapy or used with other antihypertensive drugs. It is also indicated for the treatment of heart failure. Eplerenone decreases renin and aldosterone levels by increasing urinary excretion of the hormones. It has fewer endocrine side effects than spironolactone.

Adverse Reactions and Precautions

Hyperkalemia is a serious adverse drug reaction caused by eplerenone and spironolactone. Other adverse reactions are nausea, an unpleasant aftertaste, **gynecomastia** (breast enlargement in males), **hirsutism** (excessive hair growth in women), impotence, and menstrual irregularities. Salt substitutes should be avoided when eplerenone and spironolactone are administered.

ANGIOTENSION-CONVERTING ENZYME INHIBITORS

The ACE inhibitors lower SBP and DBP by blocking the action of **angiotensin-converting enzyme**. ACE converts angiotensin I to angiotensin II. When angiotensin II levels rise, blood pressure increases because **angiotensin II** is a potent vasoconstrictor, stimulates the release of aldosterone, and promotes the release of norepinephrine from sympathetic neurons. The ACE inhibitors are first-line therapy for treatment of hypertension in patients with chronic kidney disease (CKD), diabetes, and coronary artery disease, according the Canadian Hypertension Education Program guidelines. The Joint National Committee 7 recommends thiazides or ACE inhibitors for most patients with and without compelling indications.

★ TECH NOTE!
The ACE inhibitors share the common ending "-pril."

Aldosterone Receptor Antagonists

Generic Name	U.S. Brand Name Canadian Brand(s)	Dosage Forms and Strengths
eplerenone	Inspra	Tablets: 25 mg, 50 mg
	Inspra	
spironolactone*	Aldactone	Tablets: 25 mg, 50 mg†, 100 mg
	Aldactone	

Combination Aldosterone Receptor Antagonists

spironolactone + hydrochlorothiazide*	Aldactazide	Tablets: 25 mg spironolactone + 25 mg HCTZ
	Aldactazide	50 mg spironolactone + 50 mg HCTZ

*Generic available.
†Strength available in the United States only.

Angiotension-Converting Enzyme Inhibitors

Generic Name	U.S. Brand Name Canadian Brand(s)	Dosage Forms and Strengths
benazepril*	Lotensin Lotensin	Tablets: 5 mg, 10 mg, 20 mg, 40 mg[†]
captopril*	Capoten Generics	Tablets: 6.25 mg[‡], 12.5 mg, 25 mg, 50 mg, 100 mg
enalapril maleate*	Vasotec Generics	Injection, solution (as enalaprilat): 1.25 mg/mL Tablets: 2.5 mg, 5 mg, 10 mg, 20 mg
enalapril sodium*	Not available Vasotec	Tablets: 2 mg, 4 mg, 8 mg, 16 mg
fosinopril*	Generics Monopril	Tablets: 10 mg, 20 mg, 40 mg[†]
lisinopril*	Prinivil, Zestril Prinivil, Zestril	Tablets: 2.5 mg[†], 5 mg, 10 mg, 20 mg, 30 mg[†], 40 mg
moexipril*	Univasc Not available	Tablet, film-coated: 7.5 mg, 15 mg
perindopril*[†]	Aceon Coversyl	Tablets: 2 mg, 4 mg, 8 mg
quinapril*[†]	Accupril Accupril	Tablets: 5 mg, 10 mg, 20 mg, 40 mg
ramipril*	Altace Altace	Capsules: 1.25 mg, 2.5 mg, 5 mg, 10 mg, 15 mg[‡]
trandolapril*[†]	Mavik Mavik	Tablets: 0.5 mg[‡], 1 mg, 2 mg, 4 mg

Combination Angiotensin-Converting Enzyme Inhibitors and Diuretics

benazepril + hydrochlorothiazide*	Lotensin HCT Not available	Tablets: benazepril 5 mg + hydrochlorothiazide 6.25 mg benazepril 10 mg + hydrochlorothiazide 12.5 mg benazepril 20 mg + hydrochlorothiazide 12.5 mg benazepril 20 mg + hydrochlorothiazide 25 mg
captopril + hydrochlorothiazide*	Capozide Not available	Tablets: captopril 25 mg + hydrochlorothiazide 15 mg captopril 25 mg + hydrochlorothiazide 25 mg captopril 50 mg + hydrochlorothiazide 15 mg captopril 50 mg + hydrochlorothiazide 25 mg
enalapril + hydrochlorothiazide*	Vaseretic Vaseretic	Tablets: enalapril 5 mg + hydrochlorothiazide 12.5 mg enalapril 10 mg + hydrochlorothiazide 25 mg enalapril 4 mg + hydrochlorothiazide 12.5 mg[‡] enalapril 8 mg + hydrochlorothiazide 25 mg[‡]
fosinopril + hydrochlorothiazide*	Generics Not available	Tablets: fosinopril 10 mg + hydrochlorothiazide 12.5 mg fosinopril 20 mg + hydrochlorothiazide 12.5 mg

Angiotension-Converting Enzyme Inhibitors—cont'd

Generic Name	U.S. Brand Name / Canadian Brand(s)	Dosage Forms and Strengths
lisinopril + hydrochlorothiazide*	Prinizide, Zestoretic / Zestoretic	Tablets: lisinopril 10 mg + hydrochlorothiazide 12.5 mg; lisinopril 20 mg + hydrochlorothiazide 12.5 mg; lisinopril 20 mg + hydrochlorothiazide 25 mg
moexipril + hydrochlorothiazide*	Uniretic / Not available	Tablets: moexipril 7.5 mg + hydrochlorothiazide 12.5 mg; moexipril 15 mg + hydrochlorothiazide 12.5 mg; moexipril 15 mg + hydrochlorothiazide 25 mg
quinapril + hydrochlorothiazide*†	Accuretic / Accuretic	Tablets: quinapril 10 mg + hydrochlorothiazide 12.5 mg; quinapril 20 mg + hydrochlorothiazide 12.5 mg; quinapril 20 mg + hydrochlorothiazide 25 mg
ramipril + hydrochlorothiazide	Not available / Altace HCT	Tablets: ramipril 2.5 mg + hydrochlorothiazide 12.5 mg; ramipril 5 mg + hydrochlorothiazide 12.5 mg; ramipril 10 mg + hydrochlorothiazide 12.5 mg; ramipril 5 mg + hydrochlorothiazide 25 mg; ramipril 10 mg + hydrochlorothiazide 25 mg

Combination Angiotensin-Converting Enzyme Inhibitor and Calcium Channel Blocker

Generic Name	U.S. Brand Name / Canadian Brand(s)	Dosage Forms and Strengths
benazepril + amlodipine*	Lotrel / Not available	Capsules: benazepril 10 mg + amlodipine 2.5 mg; benazepril 10 mg + amlodipine 5 mg; benazepril 20 mg + amlodipine 5 mg; benazepril 40 mg + amlodipine 5 mg; benazepril 20 mg + amlodipine 10 mg; benazepril 40 mg + amlodipine 10 mg
ramipril + felodipine	Not available / Altace Plus Felodipine	Tablets: ramipril 2.5 mg + felodipine 2.5 mg; ramipril 5 mg + felodipine 5 mg
trandolapril + verapamil*†	Tarka / Tarka	Tablets, extended release: trandolapril 1 mg + verapamil 240 mg†; trandolapril 2 m g + verapamil 180 mg†; trandolapril 2 mg + verapamil 240 mg; trandolapril 4 mg + verapamil 240 mg

*Generic available.
*†Generic in the United States only.
†Strength available in the United States only.
‡Strength available in Canada only.

TECH ALERT!
The following drugs have look-alike and sound-alike issues: benazepril and Benadryl; Lotensin, Loniten, Lioresal, and lovastatin; Capoten and Catapres; captopril and carvedilol; Vasotec and Norvasc; enalapril and Eldepryl; Univasc and Uniretic; Accupril, Accolate, Aciphex, Accutane, Altace, and Aricept; Altace, Accupril, Amerge, and Artane; ramipril and rifampin; trandolapril and tramadol

Mechanism of Action

The ACE inhibitors inhibit the activity of ACE, reducing angiotensin II and aldosterone levels. They decrease reabsorption of sodium in the renal tubules. In addition, they cause the accumulation of bradykinins (peptides that produce dilation of arteries). This reduces peripheral resistance, further lowering blood pressure.

Pharmacokinetics

The ACE inhibitors differ in activity, metabolism, and elimination, which may influence which ACE is prescribed. For example, enalapril, perindopril, quinapril, ramipril, and trandolapril are prodrugs. They would not be drugs of first choice for patients with decreased liver function because prodrugs have limited activity until they undergo metabolism. Enalaprilat, perindoprilat, quinaprilat, ramiprilat, and trandolaprilat are their active metabolites. Captopril and lisinopril are already active compounds. Fosinopril is a good choice for patients with decreased kidney function because 50% is eliminated by the kidney and 50% by the liver. All other ACE inhibitors are 90% eliminated by the kidney and can accumulate if kidney disease is present.

Adverse Reactions

Accumulation of bradykinins by ACE inhibitors is responsible for the dry cough that is a characteristic side effect. Other adverse drug reactions are hyperkalemia, lightheadedness, hypotension, diarrhea, and skin rashes. Angioedema is a rare but potentially lethal allergic reaction associated with ACE inhibitors that may involve swelling of throat or airways.

Precautions

The ACE inhibitors are contraindicated in pregnancy because they can interfere with fetal development of the kidneys, and fetal death has been reported. Salt substitutes should be avoided to reduce risks for hyperkalemia.

ANGIOTENSIN II RECEPTOR ANTAGONISTS

The angiotensin II receptor blockers (ARBs) are competitive antagonists at the angiotensin II receptor site. They lower blood pressure by blocking the binding of angiotensin II. ARBs also inhibit angiotensin II–stimulated growth of smooth muscle, reducing ventricular and arterial hypertrophy that is associated with chronic hypertension. They do not inhibit angiotensin II–stimulated tissue growth and repair.

The ARBs are similar to ACE inhibitors in effectiveness but produce less dry cough, perhaps because they do not increase bradykinin levels like the ACE inhibitors. The ARBs are first-line therapy for treatment of hypertension, especially in patients with diabetes and coronary artery disease who cannot tolerate ACE inhibitors.

Pharmacokinetics

The plasma half-life of individual ARBs vary. Losartan, one of the first ARBs to be marketed, has a relatively short half-life (only 2 hours), but it has an active metabolite with a plasma half-life of up to 6 to 9 hours. Losartan has an active metabolite that is 10 to 40 times more potent than the parent compound. The duration of action for irbesartan, candesartan, and telmisartan is longer (12-18 hours). The drugs are administered as a single daily dose.

Adverse Reactions

Adverse drug reactions associated with the ARBs are fatigue, abdominal pain, dizziness, dry mouth, constipation, impotence, and muscle cramps.

Precautions

The ARBs are contraindicated in the second and third trimesters of pregnancy because they can interfere with fetal development of the kidneys, and fetal death has been reported.

TECH NOTE!
The contents of Altace capsules may be sprinkled on food or dissolved in liquid.

TECH NOTE!
Angiotensin II antagonists share the common ending "-sartan."

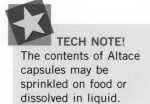

TECH ALERT!
The following drugs have look-alike and / sound-alike issues:
Atacand and Avandia;
Cozaar, Hyzaar, and
   Zocor;
Diovan, Darvon, and
   Zyban;
valsartan and losartan

Angiotension II Receptor Antagonists		
Generic Name	**U.S. Brand Name** **Canadian Brand(s)**	**Dosage Forms and Strengths**
candesartan	Atacand	**Tablets:** 4 mg, 8 mg, 16 mg, 32 mg
	Atacand	
eprosartan	Teveten	**Tablets:** 400 mg, 600 mg
	Teveten	
irbesartan	Avapro	**Tablets:** 75 mg, 150 mg, 300 mg
	Avapro	
losartan	Cozaar	**Tablets:** 25 mg, 50 mg, 100 mg
	Cozaar	

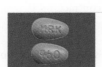

Continued

Angiotension II Receptor Antagonists—cont'd

Generic Name	U.S. Brand Name Canadian Brand(s)	Dosage Forms and Strengths
olmesartan	Benicar Not available	**Tablets:** 5 mg, 20 mg, 40 mg
telmisartan	Micardis Micardis	**Tablets:** 20 mg, 40 mg, 80 mg
valsartan	Diovan Diovan	**Tablets:** 40 mg, 80 mg, 160 mg, 320 mg

Combination Angiotension II Receptor Antagonists and Diuretics

candesartan + HCTZ	Atacand HCT Atacand Plus	**Tablets:** candesartan 16 mg + hydrochlorothiazide 12.5 mg candesartan 32 mg + hydrochlorothiazide 12.5 mg candesartan 32 mg + hydrochlorothiazide 25 mg
eprosartan + HCTZ	Teveten HCT Teveten Plus	**Tablets:** eprosartan 600 mg + hydrochlorothiazide 12.5 mg eprosartan 600 mg + hydrochlorothiazide 25 mg
irbesartan + HCTZ*	Avalide Avalide	**Tablets:** irbesartan 150 mg + hydrochlorothiazide 12.5 mg irbesartan 300 mg + hydrochlorothiazide 12.5 mg irbertan 300 mg + hydrochlorothiazide 25 mg
losartan + HCTZ	Hyzaar Hyzaar, Hyzaar DS	**Tablets:** losartan 50 mg + hydrochlorothiazide 12.5 mg losartan 100 mg + hydrochlorothiazide 12.5 mg losartan 100 mg + hydrochlorothiazide 25 mg
olmesartan + HCTZ	Benicar HCT Olmetec Plus	**Tablets:** olmesartan 20 mg + hydrochlorothiazide 12.5 mg olmesartan 40 mg + hydrochlorothiazide 12.5 mg olmesartan 40 mg + hydrochlorothiazide 25 mg
telmisartan + HCTZ*‡	Micardis HCT Micardis Plus	**Tablets:** telmisartan 40 mg + hydrochlorothiazide 12.5 mg telmisartan 80 mg + hydrochlorothiazide 12.5 mg telmisartan 80 mg + hydrochlorothiazide 25 mg
valsartan + HCTZ*	Diovan HCT Diovan HCT	**Tablets:** valsartan 80 mg + hydrochlorothiazide 12.5 mg valsartan 160 mg + hydrochlorothiazide 12.5 mg valsartan 160 mg + hydrochlorothiazide 25 mg valsartan 320 mg + hydrochlorothiazide 12.5 mg valsartan 320 mg + hydrochlorothiazide 25 mg

*Generic available.
*‡Generic available in Canada only.

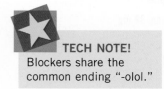

TECH NOTE!
Blockers share the common ending "-olol."

β-ADRENERGIC BLOCKERS (BETA BLOCKERS)

There are three specific β-receptors. Beta blockers used in the treatment of hypertension primarily block β_1 and β_2 receptors. β_1-Receptor binding produces cardiac stimulation, and β_2-receptor binding causes bronchial relaxation. By blocking the effect of norepinephrine and epinephrine, beta blockers reduce heart rate, reduce blood pressure by dilating blood vessels, and may constrict air passages by stimulating the muscles that surround the air passages to contract.

Mechanism of Action

β-Adrenergic blockers used in the treatment of hypertension may be selective (β_1) or nonselective (β_1, β_2). All beta blockers decrease blood pressure, but selective β_1-adrenergic blockers are less likely to produce bronchospasm. β-Selectivity is lost when higher doses are prescribed. β_1-Selective

β-Adrenergic Blockers

Generic Name	U.S. Brand Name / Canadian Brand(s)	Dosage Forms and Strengths
Beta Blockers: Non-Selective		
nadolol*	Corgard	**Tablets:** 20 mg†, 40 mg, 80 mg
	Generics	
penbutolol	Levatol	**Tablets:** 20 mg
	Not available	
pindolol*	Generics	**Tablets:** 5 mg, 10 mg, 15 mg‡
	Visken	
propranolol*	Inderal, Inderal LA, InnoPran XL,	**Capsules, extended release (InnoPran XL):** 80 mg, 120 mg
	Inderal LA	**Capsules, sustained release (Inderal LA):** 60 mg, 80 mg, 120 mg, 160 mg
		Injection, solution: 1 mg/mL
		Solution, oral: 4 mg/mL and 8 mg/mL
		Tablets: 10 mg, 20 mg, 40 mg, 60 mg, 80 mg, 120 mg‡
timolol*	Generics	**Tablets:** 5 mg, 10 mg, 20 mg
	Generics	
Beta Blockers: β-1 Selective		
acebutolol*	Sectral	**Capsules:** 100 mg‡, 200 mg, 400 mg
	Sectral	
atenolol*	Tenormin	**Tablets:** 25 mg, 50 mg, 100 mg
	Tenormin	
betaxolol*	Generics	**Tablets:** 10 mg, 20 mg
	Not available	
bisoprolol*	Zebeta	**Tablets:** 5 mg, 10 mg
	Generics	
metoprolol*	Lopressor, Toprol XL	**Injection, solution (Betaloc, Lopressor):** 1 mg/mL (5 mL)
	Betaloc, Lopressor, Lopressor SR	**Tablets, immediate release (Betaloc, Lopressor):** 25 mg, 50 mg, 100 mg
		Tablets, extended release (Toprol XL): 25 mg, 50 mg, 100 mg, 200 mg
		Tablets, extended release (Lopressor SR): 100 mg, 200 mg
Combination Beta Blockers and Diuretics		
nadolol + bendroflumethiazide*	Corzide	**Tablets:** nadolol 40 mg + bendroflumethiazide 5 mg
	Not available	nadolol 80 mg + bendroflumethiazide 5 mg
pindolol + hydrochlorothiazide	Not available	**Tablets:** pindolol 10 mg + hydrochlorothiazide 25 mg
	Viskazide	pindolol 10 mg + hydrochlorothiazide 50 mg
propranolol + hydrochlorothiazide*	Inderide	**Tablets:** propranolol 40 mg + hydrochlorothiazide 25 mg
	Not available	propranolol 80 mg + hydrochlorothiazide 25 mg
atenolol + chlorthalidone	Tenoretic	**Tablets:** atenolol 50 mg + chlorthalidone 25 mg
	Tenoretic	atenolol 100 mg + chlorthalidone 25 mg
bisoprolol + hydrochlorothiazide*	Ziac	**Tablets:** bisoprolol 2.5 mg + hydrochlorothiazide 6.25 mg
	Not available	bisoprolol 5 mg + hydrochlorothiazide 6.25 mg
		bisoprolol 10 mg + hydrochlorothiazide 6.25 mg
metoprolol + hydrochlorothiazide*	Lopressor HCT	**Tablets:** Metoprolol 50 mg + hydrochlorothiazide 25 mg
	Not available	metoprolol 100 mg + hydrochlorothiazide 25 mg
		metoprolol 100 mg + hydrochlorothiazide 50 mg

*Generic available.
†Strength available in the United States only.
‡Strength available in Canada only.

TECH ALERT!
The following drugs
have look-alike and
sound-alike issues:
Corgard and Cognex;
Inderal, Inderide,
    Adderall, Isordil,
    Toradol, and Imdur;
propranolol and
    Pravachol

TECH ALERT!
The following drugs
have look-alike and
sound-alike issues:
Sectral, Seconal, and
    Septra;
Tenormin, Imuran, and
    thiamine;
Zebeta and Diabeta;
metoprolol, metoclo-
    pramide, metola-
    zone, metronidazole,
    and misoprostol;
Toprol Xl, Topimax, And
    Tegretol Xr

agents are first-line therapy for patients who have hypertension and angina or after myocardial infarction.

All beta blockers decrease the heart rate, especially during exercise, and decrease the force of contractions in the heart. This lowers the cardiac output. Chronic use produces vasodilation. This may be caused by decreased renin release. Renin acts to convert the hormone angiotensinogen to angiotensin I, a precursor to angiotensin II.

Adverse Reactions

Adverse drug reactions associated with β-adrenergic blockers are dizziness, lethargy, nausea, palpitations, impotence, bradycardia, bronchoconstriction, hypoglycemia, cardiac rhythm disturbance, congestive heart failure, and depression.

Precautions

Beta blockers should not be discontinued abruptly because this may cause the onset of arrhythmias or angina. Important drug interactions exist between beta blockers and cimetidine (inhibits metabolic enzymes in the liver, which increases the antihypertensive effects of drugs such as propranolol and metoprolol) and salicylates (decrease the effectiveness of β_1-blockers such as atenolol and metoprolol). β-Adrenergic blockers should be used with caution in patients more than 60 years old and in patients with diabetes. Nonselective beta blockers should be avoided in patients with asthma.

α_1-BLOCKERS

The arteries have an abundance of α_1 receptors that mediate vasoconstriction. Administration of α_1-blockers produces vascular relaxation, which reduces peripheral resistance and lowers blood pressure. The α_1-adrenergic antagonists also reduce low-density lipoprotein cholesterol levels, making them useful in

Combination β_1- and α_1-Blockers

Generic Name	U.S. Brand Name / Canadian Brand(s)	Dosage Forms and Strengths
carvedilol*	Coreg, Coreg CR	**Tablets:** 3.125 mg, 6.25 mg, 12.5 mg, 25 mg
	Generics	**Capsules, extended release (Coreg CR):** 10 mg[†], 20 mg[†], 40 mg[†], 80 mg[†]
labetalol*	Trandate	**Injection, solution, and prefilled syringe:** 5 mg/mL (4 mL, 20 mL, 40 mL)
	Trandate	**Tablets:** 100 mg, 200 mg, 300 mg

*Generic available.
[†]Strength available in the United States only.

α_1-Blockers

Generic Name	U.S. Brand Name / Canadian Brand(s)	Dosage Forms and Strengths
doxazosin*	Cardura, Cardura XL	**Tablets:** 1 mg, 2 mg, 4 mg, 8 mg[†]
	Cardura-1, Cardura-2, Cardura-4	**Tablets, extended release (Cardura XL):** 4 mg[†], 8 mg[†]
prazosin*	Minipress	**Capsules:** 1 mg, 2 mg, 5 mg
	Minipress	
terazosin*	Hytrin	**Capsules:** 1 mg, 2 mg, 5 mg, 10 mg
	Hytrin	**Tablets:** 1 mg, 2 mg, 5 mg, 10 mg

*Generic available.
[†]Strength available in the United States only.

the treatment of IHD. Finally, doxazosin and terazosin have the ability to reduce urethral resistance and increase urine flow, making them effective in the treatment of benign prostatic hyperplasia.

Adverse Reactions

Adverse drug effects are postural hypotension, dizziness, reflex tachycardia, headache, weakness, and fatigue.

CALCIUM CHANNEL BLOCKERS

There are two classes of calcium channel blockers. The dihydropyridines are selective for blood vessels and are effective at lowering blood pressure because of their ability to relax blood vessels. This decreases peripheral resistance. Examples of drugs in this class are amlodipine, felodipine, isradipine, nicardipine, nifedipine, and nisoldipine. The phenylalkylamines (e.g., verapamil) and benzothiazepines (e.g., diltiazem) decrease cardiac workload, heart rate, and heart contractions. Verapamil is more selective for the myocardium than blood vessels. Diltiazem's action is intermediate between verapamil and dihydropyridines.

Adverse Effects

Dihydropyridines (e.g., nifedipine) may produce dizziness, flushing, and headache. Phenylalkylamines and benzothiazepines (e.g., diltiazem) can produce bradycardia and constipation. The exact mechanism of action, pharmacokinetics, and more adverse reactions are discussed in Chapter 21.

Calcium Channel Blockers

Generic Name	U.S. Brand Name Canadian Brand(s)	Dosage Forms and Strengths
amlodipine*	Norvasc	Tablets: 2.5 mg, 5 mg, 10 mg
	Norvasc	
diltiazem*	Cardizem, Cardizem CD, Cardizem LA, Cartia XT, Tiamate, Tiazac	Capsules, extended release (Cardizem CD, Cartia XT): 120 mg, 180 mg, 240 mg, 300 mg, 360 mg, 420 mg† (Tiazac only)
		Injection, powder for reconstitution: 100 mg
		Solution for injection: 5 mg/mL
	Cardizem CD, Tiazac, Tiazac XC	Tablets: 30 mg, 60 mg, 90 mg, 120 mg
		Tablets, extended release (Cardizem LA, Tiamate, Tiazac XC): 120 mg, 180 mg, 240 mg, 300 mg, 360 mg, 420 mg†
felodipine*	Generics	Tablets, extended release: 2.5 mg, 5 mg, 10 mg
	Plendil	
isradipine*	Dynacirc CR	Capsules: 2.5 mg, 5 mg
	Not available	Tablets, CR (Dynacirc): 5 mg, 10 mg
nicardipine*	Cardene SR	Capsules: 20 mg, 30 mg
	Not available	Capsules, extended release (Cardene SR): 30 mg, 60 mg
		Solution for injection: 2.5 mg/mL
		Solution for injection, premixed:
		1 mg/10 mL in dextrose 4.8%
		1 mg/10 mL in NaCl 0.86%
		2 mg/10 mL in dextrose 5%
		2 mg/10 mL in NaCl 0.83%
nifedipine*	Afeditab CR, Adalat CC, Procardia, Procardia XL	Capsules (Procardia): 5 mg‡, 10 mg, 20 mg
		Tablets, extended release (Adalat XL): 20 mg, 30 mg, 60 mg
	Adalat XL	Tablets, extended release (Adalat CC): 30 mg, 60 mg, 90 mg
nisoldipine*	Sular ER	Tablets, extended release: 8.5 mg, 17 mg, 20 mg, 25.5 mg, 30 mg, 34 mg, 40 mg
	Not available	

Continued

Calcium Channel Blockers—cont'd

Generic Name	U.S. Brand Name / Canadian Brand(s)	Dosage Forms and Strengths
verapamil*	Calan SR, Covera HS, Verelan Covera HS, Isoptin SR, Verelan	Capsules, extended release (Verelan): 120 mg, 180 mg, 240 mg, 360 mg Capsules, extended release (Verelan PM): 100 mg, 200 mg, 300 mg Solution for injection: 2.5 mg/mL Tablets: 40 mg, 80 mg, 120 mg Tablets, extended release (Calan SR, Covera HS, Isoptin SR): 120 mg, 180 mg, 240 mg
Combination Calcium Channel Blocker and Angiotensin II Receptor Blockers		
amlodipine + olmesartan	Azor Not available	Tablets: amlodipine 5 mg + olmesartan 20 mg amlodipine 5 mg + olmesartan 40 mg amlodipine 10 mg + olmesartan 20 mg amlodipine 10 mg + olmesartan 40 mg
amlodipine + telmisartan	Twynsta Twynsta	Tablets: amlodipine 5 mg + telmisartan 40 mg amlodipine 5 mg + telmisartan 80 mg amlodipine 10 mg + telmisartan 40 mg amlodipine 10 mg + telmisartan 80 mg
amlodipine + valsartan	Exforge Not available	Tablets: amlodipine 5 mg + valsartan 160 mg amlodipine 5 mg + valsartan 320 mg amlodipine 10 mg + valsartan 160 mg amlodipine 10 mg + valsartan 320 mg
Combination Calcium Channel Blocker + Anticholesterol		
amlodipine + atorvastatin	Caduet Caduet	Tablets: amlodipine 2.5 mg + atorvastatin 10 mg[†] amlodipine 2.5 mg + atorvastatin 20 mg[†] amlodipine 2.5 mg + atorvastatin 40 mg[†] amlodipine 5 mg + atorvastatin 10 mg amlodipine 5 mg + atorvastatin 20 mg amlodipine 5 mg + atorvastatin 40 mg amlodipine 5 mg + atorvastatin 80 mg amlodipine 10 mg + atorvastatin 10 mg amlodipine 10 mg + atorvastatin 20 mg amlodipine 10 mg + atorvastatin 40 mg amlodipine 10 mg + atorvastatin 80 mg

*Generic available.
[†]Strength available in the United States only.
[‡]Strength available in Canada only.

TECH NOTE!
Tribenzor is a new combination drug that contains amlodipine (calcium channel blocker), hydrochlorothiazide (diuretic), and olmesartan (ARB).

TECH NOTE!
The β₁-blockers share the common ending "-zosin."

TECH ALERT!
The following drugs have look-alike and sound-alike issues: clonidine, quinidine, colchicine, clomiphene, and Klonopin; Catapres and Cataflam; guanfacine and guaifenesin; methyldopa and levodopa; reserpine, risperidone, and Risperdal

CENTRAL-ACTING α₂-AGONISTS

Blood pressure is controlled by a complex feedback mechanism. Increased adrenergic stimulation in the brain results in decreased sympathetic nervous system messages flowing from the CNS. Methyldopa is a prodrug that acts like a false neurotransmitter. It is metabolized to α-methylnorepinephrine, which the body thinks is norepinephrine; however, it is selective in mimicking the autoinhibitory effects of norepinephrine. When methyldopa binds to receptors, efferent sympathetic activity is reduced, blood vessels dilate, and peripheral resistance is decreased. Clonidine inhibits norepinephrine release from the CNS and peripheral sites.

Adverse Reactions

Adverse drug effects of centrally acting α₂-agonists include sedation, dry mouth, *orthostatic hypotension*, impotence, and constipation. Methyldopa can also cause depression, nasal stuffiness, and gastrointestinal upset. Methyldopa may produce galactorrhea, hemolytic anemia, and liver dysfunction.

α₂-Agonists

Generic Name	U.S. Brand Name / Canadian Brand(s)	Dosage Forms and Strengths
clonidine*	Catapres, Catapres-TTS, Duraclon, Kapvay Catapres, Dixarit	Injection, epidural solution (Duraclon): 100 mcg/mL, 500 mcg/mL Patch, transdermal: 0.1 mg/24 hr (Catapres TTS-1) 0.2 mg/24 hr (Catapres TTS-2) 0.3 mg/24 hr (Catapres TTS-3) Tablets: 0.1 mg, 0.2 mg, 0.3 mg[†] Tablet (Dixarit): 0.025 mg Tablet, extended release (Kapvay): 0.1 mg
guanfacine*	Tenex, Intuniv Not available	Tablets (Tenex): 1 mg, 2 mg Tablets, extended release (Intuniv): 1 mg, 2 mg, 3 mg, 4 mg
methyldopa*	Generics Generics	Injection, solution: 50 mg/mL[†] Tablets: 125 mg[‡], 250 mg, 500 mg
Rauwolfia Alkaloid		
reserpine*	Generics Not available	Tablets: 0.1 mg, 0.25 mg
Combination α₂-Agonist and Diuretic		
clonidine + chlorthalidone	Clorpres Not available	Tablets: clonidine 0.1 mg + chlorthalidone 15 mg clonidine 0.2 mg + chlorthalidone 15 mg clonidine 0.3 mg + chlorthalidone 15 mg
methyldopa + hydrochlorothiazide*	Generics Generics	Tablets: methyldopa 250 mg + hydrochlorothiazide 15 mg methyldopa 250 mg + hydrochlorothiazide 25 mg

*Generic available.
[†]Strength available in the United States only.
[‡]Strength available in Canada only.

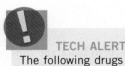

TECH ALERT!
The following drugs have look-alike and sound-alike issues: Cardura, Ridaura, Cardene, Cordarone, Coumadin, and K-Dur; Prazosin, Doxazosin, and Terazosin

RAUWOLFIA ALKALOIDS

Reserpine is a rauwolfia alkaloid and is derived from the root of a shrub native to India, *Rauwolfia serpentina*. Reserpine was one the first drugs identified to reduce blood pressure. Reserpine depletes neuronal stores of norepinephrine at CNS and peripheral sites. Prolonged use results in decreased heart rate and cardiac output, further reducing blood pressure. It may take 2 to 6 weeks before the maximum antihypertensive effects are observed. The use of reserpine has declined now that newer antihypertensive drugs that are better tolerated are available. Adverse effects include sedation, stuffy nose, and depression.

DIRECT VASODILATORS

Hydralazine and minoxidil decrease peripheral resistance and reduce blood pressure by relaxing vascular smooth muscle. Minoxidil works by activating adenosine triphosphate–sensitive K^+ channels, setting in motion a chain of events that decrease calcium influx through L-type calcium channels in vascular smooth muscle. This decreases arterial blood vessel contractions.

Neither hydralazine nor minoxidil is a first-line drug for the treatment of hypertension. Hydralazine is recommended for hypertensive emergencies (parenteral use) and is safe for the treatment of preeclampsia in pregnant women.

Adverse Reactions

The adverse drug reactions for hydralazine and minoxidil include orthostatic hypotension, headache, gastrointestinal upset, sodium and fluid retention, palpitations, and arrhythmia. Hydralazine can cause a lupus-like syndrome, and minoxidil causes facial hair growth. The discovery that minoxidil increases hair growth resulted in the drug being formulated for topical use for the treatment of baldness.

Vasodilators

Generic Name	U.S. Brand Name / Canadian Brand(s)	Dosage Forms and Strengths
hydralazine*	Generics	Injection, solution (Apresoline): 20 mg/mL (1 mL)
	Apresoline	Tablets: 10 mg, 25 mg, 50 mg, 100 mg†
minoxidil*	Generics	Tablets: 2.5 mg, 10 mg
	Loniten	

*Generic available.
†Strength available in the United States only.

Renin Inhibitors

Generic Name	U.S. Brand Name / Canadian Brand(s)	Dosage Forms and Strengths
aliskiren	Tekturna	Tablets: 150 mg, 300 mg
	Rasilez	
Combination Renin Inhibitors (New)		
aliskiren + hydrochlorothiazide	Tekturna HCT	Tablets: aliskiren 150 mg + hydrochlorothiazide 12.5 mg
	Rasilez HCT	aliskiren 150 mg + hydrochlorothiazide 25 mg
		aliskiren 300 mg + hydrochlorothiazide 12.5 mg
		aliskiren 300 mg + hydrochlorothiazide 25 mg
aliskiren + valsartan	Valturna	Tablets: aliskiren 150 mg + valsartan 160 mg
	Not available	aliskiren 300 mg + valsartan 320 mg
aliskiren + amlodipine	Tekamlo	Tablet: aliskiren 150 mg + amlodipine 5 mg
	Not available	aliskiren 150 mg + amlodipine 10 mg
		aliskiren 300 mg + amlodipine 5 mg
		aliskiren 300 mg + amlodipine 10 mg

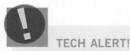

TECH ALERT!
The following drugs have look-alike and sound-alike issues: hydralazine, hydroxyzine, and hydrochlorothiazide; minoxidil and Monopril; Loniten and Lotensin

TECH NOTE!
Clonidine is also prescribed to manage heroin, nicotine, and ethanol withdrawal; glaucoma; and attention-deficit hyperactivity disorder and to prevent migraine headaches.

DIRECT RENIN INHIBITORS

Aliskiren is the first of a new class of drugs called direct renin inhibitors. It acts to block the conversion of angiotensinogen to angiotensin I, the first step in the RAAS system cascade (see Figure 22-1). The ability of aliskiren to act on this highly specific rate-limiting step may present an advantage over ACE inhibitors and ARBs. When ACE inhibitors are administered, angiotensin I may be converted to angiotensin II by alternative pathways. Renin inhibitors block the formation of both angiotensin I and angiotensin II (vasoconstrictor) and aldosterone release by interrupting the RAAS system at the beginning. Aliskiren may be used as monotherapy or in combination with other antihypertensive agents.

Precautions

Concurrent use of ACE inhibitors and ARBs with Aliskiren is contraindicated. Aliskiren is also in patients with diabetes. The FDA added a boxed warning to the package labeling in 2012 regarding the risk for fetal toxicity when aliskiren is taken during pregnancy.

Adverse Reactions

Renin inhibitors do not affect bradykinin metabolism and have a lower incidence of dry cough and angioedema than ACE inhibitors. The most common side effect is diarrhea (2.3%). Dizziness, headache, hyperkalemia, aggravation of gout and acute renal failure are other adverse reactions that may occur with aliskiren use.

Triple Combination Drugs for Hypertension

Generic Name	U.S. Brand Name Canadian Brand (s)	Dosage Forms and Strengths
olmesartan + amlodipine + hydrochlorothiazide	Tribenzor Not available	**Tablets:** olmesartan 20 mg + amlodipine 5 mg + HCTZ 12.5 mg olmesartan 40 mg + amlodipine 5 mg + HCTZ 12.5 mg olmesartan 40 mg + amlodipine 5 mg + HCTZ 25 mg olmesartan 40 mg + amlodipine 10 mg + HCTZ 12.5 mg olmesartan 40 mg + amlodipine 10 mg + HCTZ 25 mg
amlodipine + valsartan + hydrochlorothiazide	Exforge HCT Not available	**Tablets:** amlodipine 5 mg + valsartan 160 mg + HCTZ 12.5 mg amlodipine 5 mg + valsartan 160 mg + HCTZ 25 mg amlodipine 10 mg + valsartan 160 mg + HCTZ 12.5 mg amlodipine 10 mg + valsartan 160 mg + HCTZ 25 mg amlodipine 10 mg + valsartan 320 mg + HCTZ 25 mg

Summary of Drugs Used in the Treatment and Management of Hypertension[1]

Drug Name	Usual Dose and Dosing Schedule	Warning Label(s)
Diuretics		
Thiazides		
chlorothiazide	125-500 mg 1-2 times a day	TAKE WITH FOOD. MAY BE ADVISABLE TO EAT BANANAS OR DRINK ORANGE JUICE. AVOID PROLONGED EXPOSURE TO SUNLIGHT. SOME OTC DRUGS CAN AGGRAVATE YOUR CONDITION.
chlorthalidone	12.5-25 mg once daily	
hydrochlorothiazide (HCTZ)	12.5-50 mg once daily	
indapamide	1.25-2.5 mg once daily	
metolazone	0.5-5 mg once daily	
Loop		
bumetanide	0.5-2 mg twice daily	MAY BE ADVISABLE TO EAT BANANAS OR DRINK ORANGE JUICE. MAY CAUSE DIZZINESS OR LIGHTHEADEDNESS. AVOID PROLONGED EXPOSURE TO SUNLIGHT. SOME OTC DRUGS CAN AGGRAVATE YOUR CONDITION.
furosemide	20-80 mg twice a day	
torsemide	2.5-10 mg/day	
Aldosterone Receptor Antagonists		
spironolactone	25-50 mg once daily	TAKE WITH FOOD. MAY CAUSE DIZZINESS OR LIGHTHEADEDNESS. SOME OTC DRUGS CAN AGGRAVATE YOUR CONDITION. AVOID SALT SUBSTITUTES. AVOID GRAPEFRUIT JUICE.
eplerenone	50-100 mg once daily	

Continued

Summary of Drugs Used in the Treatment and Management of Hypertension—cont'd

Drug Name	Usual Dose and Dosing Schedule	Warning Label(s)
Aldosterone Receptor Antagonist Combination		
spironolactone + HCTZ	1-4 tablets daily in 1-2 divided doses 25-100 mg spironolactone + 25-100 mg HCTZ once daily	AVOID SALT SUBSTITUTES AND POTASSIUM-RICH DIETS. MAY CAUSE DIZZINESS OR LIGHTHEADEDNESS. AVOID PROLONGED EXPOSURE TO SUNLIGHT.
Potassium-Sparing Combination		
amiloride + HCTZ	10 mg amiloride + 100 mg HCTZ once daily	AVOID SALT SUBSTITUTES AND POTASSIUM-RICH DIETS. MAY CAUSE DIZZINESS OR LIGHTHEADEDNESS. AVOID PROLONGED EXPOSURE TO SUNLIGHT.
triamterene + HCTZ	37.5-75 mg triamterene + 25-50 mg HCTZ once daily	
Beta Blockers		
atenolol	25-100 mg once daily	DO NOT DISCONTINUE WITHOUT MEDICAL SUPERVISION. MAY CAUSE DIZZINESS OR LIGHTHEADEDNESS. TAKE WITH FOOD—immediate-release metoprolol. SWALLOW WHOLE; DO NOT CRUSH OR CHEW—sustained release.
acebutolol	200-600 mg twice daily	
betaxolol	5-20 mg once daily	
bisoprolol	2.5-10 mg once daily	
metoprolol	50-100 mg 1-2 times a day	
metoprolol extended release	50-100 mg once daily	
nadolol	40-120 mg once daily	
propranolol	40-160 mg twice daily	
propranolol long acting	60-180 mg once daily	
timolol	20-40 mg twice daily	
esmolol	250-500 mcg/kg/min IV bolus; then 50-100 mcg/kg/min IV infusion	FOR HYPERTENSIVE EMERGENCY.
Combined Alpha and Beta Blockers		
carvedilol	12.5-50 mg twice daily	TAKE WITH FOOD. DO NOT DISCONTINUE WITHOUT MEDICAL SUPERVISION. MAY CAUSE DIZZINESS OR LIGHTHEADEDNESS.
carvedilol CR	20-80 mg once daily	
labetalol	200-800 mg twice daily	
Beta Blockers + Diuretic Combination		
atenolol + chlorthalidone	50-100 mg atenolol + 25 mg chlorthalidone once daily	Same warnings for thiazides plus beta blockers.
bisoprolol + HCTZ	2.5-20 mg bisoprolol + 6.25-12.5 mg once daily	
metoprolol + HCTZ	100-200 mg metoprolol + 25-50 mg HCTZ once daily	
nadolol + bendroflumethiazide	40-80 mg nadolol + 5 mg bendroflumethiazide once daily	

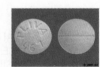

Summary of Drugs Used in the Treatment and Management of Hypertension—cont'd

Drug Name	Usual Dose and Dosing Schedule	Warning Label(s)
pindolol + HCTZ	1-2 tablets once daily	
propranolol-LA + HCTZ	80-160 mg propranolol + HCTZ 50 mg once daily	
timolol + HCTZ	1 tablet twice daily or 2 tablets once daily 10 mg timolol + 25 mg HCTZ twice daily or 20 mg timolol + 50 mg HCTZ once daily	
Angiotensin-Converting Enzyme Inhibitors		
benazepril	10-40 mg once a day	DO NOT DISCONTINUE WITHOUT MEDICAL SUPERVISION.
captopril	25-100 mg twice a day	
enalapril	5-40 mg 1-2 times a day	MAY CAUSE DIZZINESS OR LIGHTHEADEDNESS. AVOID SALT SUBSTITUTES AND POTASSIUM-RICH DIETS.
fosinopril	10-40 mg once a day	DO NOT TAKE THIS DRUG IF YOU BECOME PREGNANT.
lisinopril	10-40 mg once a day	MAY CAUSE A DRY COUGH; IF IT PERSISTS, REPORT IT TO YOUR DOCTOR.
moexipril	7.5-30 mg once a day	TAKE ON AN EMPTY STOMACH—moexipril.
perindopril	4-8 mg once a day	TAKE WITH FOOD—perindopril.
quinapril	10-80 mg once a day	
ramipril	2.5-20 mg once a day	
trandolapril	1-4 mg once a day	
Angiotensin-Converting Enzyme Inhibitor + Diuretic Combination		
benazepril + HCTZ	10-40 mg benazepril + 12.5-50 mg HCTZ once daily	Same warnings for thiazides plus ACE inhibitors.
captopril + HCTZ	25-50 mg captopril + 15-50 mg HCTZ 2-3 time a day	
enalapril + HCTZ	5-20 mg enalapril + 12.5-50 mg HCTZ once daily	
fosinopril + HCTZ	10-80 mg/12.5-50 mg/day	
lisinopril + HCTZ	10-80 mg lisinopril + 12.5-50 mg HCTZ once daily	
moexipril + HCTZ	7.5-30 mg/12.5-50 mg/day	
quinapril + HCTZ	10-40 mg quinapril + 12.5-25 mg HCTZ once daily	

Continued

Summary of Drugs Used in the Treatment and Management of Hypertension—cont'd

Drug Name	Usual Dose and Dosing Schedule	Warning Label(s)
Angiotensin II Antagonists		
candesartan	8-32 mg once daily	DO NOT DISCONTINUE WITHOUT MEDICAL SUPERVISION.
eprosartan	400-800 mg 1-2 times a day	MAY CAUSE DIZZINESS OR LIGHTHEADEDNESS.
irbesartan	150-300 mg once daily	
losartan	25-100 mg 1-2 times a day	DO NOT TAKE THIS DRUG IF YOU BECOME PREGNANT. AVOID SALT SUBSTITUTES.
olmesartan	20-40 mg once daily	
telmisartan	20-80 mg once daily	
valsartan	80-320 mg 1-2 times a day	
Angiotensin II Antagonist + Diuretic Combination		
candesartan + HCTZ	16-32 mg/12.5-25 mg once daily	Same warnings as for ARBs and thiazide diuretics.
eprosartan + HCTZ	600 mg/12.5 mg once daily	
irbesartan + HCTZ	150-300 mg/12.5 mg once daily	
losartan + HCTZ	50-100 mg/12.5-25 mg/day	
olmesartan + HCTZ	20-40 mg/12.5-25 mg once daily	
telmisartan + HCTZ	80 mg/12.5-25 mg once daily	
valsartan + HCTZ	80-160 mg/12.5-25 mg/day	
Calcium Channel Blockers		
diltiazem extended release	240-360 mg once daily	MAY CAUSE DIZZINESS.
diltiazem long acting	120-540 mg once a day	USE CAUTION WHEN DRIVING OR PERFORMING TASKS REQUIRING ALERTNESS.
verapamil immediate release	80-320 mg twice daily	AVOID ABRUPT DISCONTINUATION. LIMIT CAFFEINE AND ALCOHOL.
verapamil long acting	120-480 mg 1-2 times a day	SWALLOW WHOLE; DO NOT CRUSH OR CHEW—sustained release.
verapamil extended release	120-360 mg once daily	AVOID GRAPEFRUIT JUICE
amlodipine	2.5-10 mg once a day	
felodipine	2.5-20 mg once a day	
isradipine	2.5-10 mg twice a day	
nicardipine sustained release	60-120 mg twice a day	
nicardipine IV	5-15 mg/hr IV	
nifedipine long acting	30-60 mg once daily	
nisoldipine	17-34 mg once daily	

Summary of Drugs Used in the Treatment and Management of Hypertension—cont'd

Drug Name	Usual Dose and Dosing Schedule	Warning Label(s)
Calcium Channel Blockers + Angiotensin-Converting Enzyme Inhibitor Combination		
amlodipine + benazepril	2.5-10 mg amlodipine + 10-40 mg benazepril once daily	Same warnings as CCBs plus ACE inhibitors.
felodipine + enalapril	5-20 mg enalapril + 2.5-10 mg felodipine once daily	
verapamil + trandolapril	2-8 mg trandolapril + 180-240 mg verapamil daily in 1 or 2 divided doses	
Centrally Acting α_2-Agonist and Other Central-Acting Drugs		
clonidine	0.1-0.6 mg twice a day	ROTATE SITE OF APPLICATION—patch.
clonidine patch	0.1-0.3 mg once a week	DO NOT DISCONTINUE WITHOUT MEDICAL SUPERVISION.
methyldopa	250-1000 mg twice daily	MAY CAUSE DIZZINESS OR LIGHTHEADEDNESS.
guanfacine	0.5-2 mg once daily	
Rauwolfia Alkaloid		
reserpine	0.1-0.25 mg once a day	DO NOT DISCONTINUE WITHOUT MEDICAL SUPERVISION. MAY CAUSE DIZZINESS OR DROWSINESS.
Central-Acting Drug + Diuretic Combination		
250 mg methyldopa + 15 mg HCTZ	1 tablet 2-3 times daily	Same warnings as α_2-agonist and thiazide diuretics.
250 mg methyldopa + 25 mg HCTZ	1 tablet twice daily	
500 mg methyldopa + 50 mg HCTZ	1 tablet daily	
α_1-Antagonists		
doxazosin	1-16 mg once a day	DO NOT DISCONTINUE WITHOUT MEDICAL SUPERVISION.
prazosin	2-20 mg 2-3 times a day	MAY CAUSE DIZZINESS OR LIGHTHEADEDNESS.
terazosin	1-20 mg 1-2 times a day	
Direct Vasodilators		
hydralazine	25-100 mg twice daily 10-20 mg IV or 10-40 mg IM	DO NOT DISCONTINUE WITHOUT MEDICAL SUPERVISION. TAKE WITH FOOD. MAY CAUSE DIZZINESS OR LIGHTHEADEDNESS.
minoxidil	2.5-80 mg 1-2 times a day	
enalaprilat	1.25-5 mg every 6 hours IV	FOR HYPERTENSIVE EMERGENCIES.
fenoldopam mesylate	0.1-0.3 mcg/kg/min IV infusion	
nitroglycerin	5-100 mcg/min IV infusion	
sodium nitroprusside	0.25-10 mcg/kg/min IV infusion	
Adrenergic Inhibitor		
phentolamine	5-15 mg IV bolus	FOR HYPERTENSIVE EMERGENCIES.

Continued

Summary of Drugs Used in the Treatment and Management of Hypertension—cont'd

Drug Name	Usual Dose and Dosing Schedule	Warning Label(s)
Renin Inhibitors		
aliskiren	150-300 mg once daily	MAY CAUSE DIZZINESS.
aliskiren + HCTZ	1 tablet once daily; begin with 150 mg aliskiren/ HCTZ 12.5 mg and increase to 300 mg aliskiren/25 mg HCTZ as needed	AVOID SALT SUBSTITUTES. AVOID PROLONGED EXPOSURE TO SUNLIGHT—Tekturna HCT.
aliskiren + valsartan	1 tablet once daily; begin with 150 mg aliskiren/160 mg valsartan; titrate up to a maximum of 300 mg aliskiren/320 mg valsartan	MAY CAUSE PERSISTENT COUGH. MAY UPSET STOMACH.
aliskiren + amlodipine	1 tablet once daily; begin with 150 mg aliskiren/5 mg amlodipine; titrate up to a maximum of 300 mg aliskiren/10 mg amlodipine	

[1]7th Joint National Committee on the Prevention, Detection, Evaluation, and Treatment of High Blood Pressure recommendations.
National Heart Lung and Blood Institute. (2004). The Seventh Report of the Joint National Committee on Prevention, Detection, Evaluation, and Treatment of High Blood Pressure (No. 04-5230). Bethesda: National Institutes of Health, U.S. Department of Health and Human Services.

Chapter Summary

- Blood pressure is a ratio of the pressure when the heart's ventricles are contracting (systole) and the pressure measured when the heart is at rest (diastole).
- The average normal blood pressure is <120 mm Hg (systolic)/<80 mm Hg (diastolic).
- The formula for determining blood pressure is $BP = CO \times PR$.
- Sites for blood pressure control are the kidneys, heart, blood vessels, CNS, and sympathetic nerves.
- The RAAS responds to a drop in renal blood flow by increasing blood volume, blood flow to the kidney, vasoconstriction, and blood pressure.
- The CNS senses changes in blood pressure and signals sympathetic nerves to release neurotransmitters that control heart rate and blood flow through the arteries.
- When peripheral vascular resistance increases, blood pressure increases.
- Diastolic hypertension is the predominant form of hypertension before age 50 years.
- Risk factors for high blood pressure are age (older than 55 years in men and 65 years in women), diabetes mellitus, family history of heart disease, metabolic syndrome, obesity, tobacco usage, decreased physical activity, increased total low-density lipoprotein or low high-density lipoprotein, diet high in salt and saturated fats, and excessive alcohol consumption.
- Metabolic syndrome promotes the development of atherosclerosis and cardiovascular disease.
- Reduction of blood pressure to normal levels is beneficial for persons with prehypertension with and without preexisting disease.
- Stage 1 hypertension is classified as SBP ranging between 140 and 159 mm Hg and DPB ranging between 90 and 99 mm Hg.
- Stage 2 hypertension is classified as SBP of 160 mm Hg or greater and DPB of 100 mm Hg or greater.
- Isolated systolic hypertension is a condition whereby SBP is elevated and DBP is within the normal range.
- Hypertension during pregnancy is dangerous to the pregnant woman and the fetus.
- White coat hypertension is an abnormally high blood pressure when the measurement is taken by a health care professional.

- Hypertension is sometimes called the "silent killer" because it can cause damage to the body without any obvious symptoms. Hypertension can weaken arteries and cause aneurysms in the brain, aorta, or abdomen; blindness; kidney disease; and IHD.
- Adoption of a healthy lifestyle is often sufficient to reduce blood pressure in patients with pre-hypertension. Drug therapy should be added to the treatment program in people who have diabetes, kidney disease, or other disease.
- Lifestyle modifications include weight loss, a diet low in salt and cholesterol, increased physical activity, and decreased alcohol and tobacco consumption.
- The diuretics lower blood pressure by decreasing peripheral resistance and cardiac output.
- The diuretics are classified as thiazide, loop, and potassium sparing. Aldosterone antagonists may also be classified as diuretics.
- The thiazide diuretics promote water, sodium, potassium, and chloride ion elimination; decrease blood volume; and lower peripheral resistance.
- The thiazide diuretics should be used cautiously in patients with gout and diabetes.
- The diuretics should be taken in the morning to avoid the need to urinate in the middle of the night (nocturia).
- The loop diuretics block the sodium–potassium cotransporter in the ascending loop of Henle and are the most potent diuretics.
- The loop diuretics can cause dehydration, severe hypotension, hypokalemia, hyperuricemia, photosensitivity, and deafness.
- The effect of the loop diuretics and thiazides is reduced if they are taken concurrently with NSAIDs.
- The potassium-sparing diuretics inhibit sodium reabsorption while avoiding potassium loss. They are less effective than the loop and thiazide diuretics.
- Patients taking potassium-sparing diuretics should be advised to avoid salt substitutes because they contain potassium chloride.
- Spironolactone and eplerenone are aldosterone receptor antagonists. Spirolactone is sometimes classified as a potassium-sparing diuretic.
- The ACE inhibitors block the conversion of angiotensin I to angiotensin II by inhibiting the activity of ACE. Angiotensin II is a potent vasoconstrictor and stimulates the release of aldosterone.
- Dry cough is a common side effect of the ACE inhibitors.
- The ACE inhibitors are contraindicated in pregnancy because they can interfere with fetal development of the kidneys.
- The ARBs are competitive antagonists at the angiotensin II receptor site.
- The ARBs are similar to ACE inhibitors in effectiveness but have fewer side effects. They do not produce dry cough.
- The β-adrenergic blockers (β-blockers) lower blood pressure by decreasing heart rate and peripheral resistance.
- The beta blockers used in the treatment of hypertension may be selective (β_1) or nonselective (β_1, β_2).
- The α_1-blockers lower blood pressure by producing vascular relaxation, which reduces peripheral resistance.
- The calcium channel blockers are effective at lowering blood pressure because of their ability to relax blood vessels. They also decrease heart rate and force of contractions, lowering the cardiac output.
- Methyldopa is a prodrug that mimics the autoinhibitory effects of norepinephrine.
- When methyldopa binds to receptors, efferent sympathetic activity is reduced, blood vessels dilate, and peripheral resistance is decreased.
- Clonidine inhibits norepinephrine release from the CNS and peripheral sites, and reserpine depletes neuronal stores of norepinephrine at CNS and peripheral sites.
- Hydralazine and minoxidil decrease peripheral resistance and reduce blood pressure by relaxing vascular smooth muscle.
- Hydralazine is recommended for hypertensive emergencies (parenteral use) and is safe for use in pregnant women.

- Reserpine is derived from the root of a shrub native to India and is one of the first drugs identified to reduce blood pressure.
- The direct renin inhibitors prevent the formation of both angiotensin I and angiotensin II without affecting bradykinin metabolism; thus, the risk for dry cough and angioedema is lower than for ACE inhibitors.
- Contraindications for the use of the direct renin inhibitors are: concurrent treatment with ACE inhibitors or ARBs, in patients with diabetes and pregnancy.

REVIEW QUESTIONS

1. _____ is the most often diagnosed medical condition in the United States.
   a. Myocardial infarction
   b. Hypertension
   c. Diabetes
   d. Cancer

2. Lifestyle modification is not an important strategy for the prevention and management of hypertension.
   a. true
   b. false

3. The _____ play(s) a major role in regulating blood pressure and is (are) the site of action for diuretics.
   a. liver
   b. brain
   c. heart
   d. kidneys

4. There are several classifications of diuretics. Which of the following is not a class of diuretics?
   a. thiazide
   b. loop
   c. sodium sparing
   d. potassium sparing

5. Diuretics should be taken in the _____ to avoid the need to urinate in the middle of the night (nocturia).
   a. evening
   b. morning
   c. afternoon
   d. night

6. Spironolactone blocks the effect of _____.
   a. aldosterone
   b. antidiuretic hormone
   c. epinephrine
   d. norepinephrine

7. A common ending for ACE inhibitors is
   a. -pine
   b. -statin
   c. -pril
   d. -olol

8. Doxazosin and terazosin are examples of what class of drugs?
   a. ACE inhibitors
   b. β-blocker
   c. α_1-blocker
   d. calcium channel blocker

9. Calcium channel blockers are effective at lowering blood pressure because of their ability to constrict blood vessels.
   a. true
   b. false

10. _____ is recommended for hypertensive emergencies (parenteral use) and is safe for use in pregnant women.
    a. Hydralazine
    b. Hydroxyzine
    c. Hydrodiuril
    d. Hydrocodone

TECHNICIAN'S CORNER

1. Patients with hypertension are often advised to "cut your salt intake in half" as part of their treatment. How much salt is too much, and what is the daily healthy limit?
2. When a patient has been prescribed antihypertensive medications, can he or she ever be released from taking them?

Bibliography

Campbell N, Kwong MML: 2010 Canadian Hypertension Education Program Recommendations: The Short Clinical Summary—An Annual Update: Canadian Hypertension Education Program. Retrieved Jan 9, 2011, http://hypertension.ca/chep/wp-content/uploads/2010/02/ShortClinicalSummary_2010.pdf, 2010.

Elsevier. Gold Standard Clinical Pharmacology. Retrieved March 11, 2011, from https://www.clinicalpharmacology.com/, 2010.

FDA. FDA Approved Drug Products. Retrieved May 25, 2012, from http://www.accessdata.fda.gov/scripts/cder/drugsatfda/index.cfm?fuseaction=Search.Search_Drug_Name, 2012.

Grundy S, Cleeman J, Daniels S, et al: Diagnosis and management of the metabolic syndrome: an American Heart Association/National Heart, Lung, and Blood Institute scientific statement, 2005, American Heart Association. Available at: http://www.circulationaha.org. DOI: 10.1161/CIRCULATIONAHA.105.169404.

Health Canada: Drug Product Database. Retrieved Jan 9, 2011, from http://www.hc-sc.gc.ca/dhp-mps/prodpharma/databasdon/index-eng.php, 2010.

Kalant H, Grant D, Mitchell J: *Principles of medical pharmacology*, ed 7, Toronto, 2007, Elsevier Canada, A Division of Reed Elsevier Canada, pp 157-169, 449-464.

Khan N, McAlister F, Rabkin S, et al: The 2006 Canadian Hypertension Education Program recommendations for the management of hypertension: Part II—Therapy, *Can J Cardiol* 15:583-593, 2006.

Lance L, Lacy C, Armstrong L, et al: *Drug information handbook for the allied health professional*, ed 12, Hudson, OH, 2005, APhA Lexi-Comp.

National Heart, Lung, and Blood Institute: The Seventh Report of the Joint National Committee on Prevention, Detection, Evaluation and Treatment of High Blood Pressure. US Department of Health and Human Services, Bethesda, MD, National Heart, Lung, and Blood Institute, National Institutes of Health, National Blood Pressure Education Program, August 2004. NIH publication No. 04-5290. Available at: http://www.nhlbi.nih.gov/guidelines/hypertension/index.htm.

Page C, Curtis M, Sutter M, et al: *Integrated pharmacology*, Philadelphia, 2005, Mosby, pp 395-408.

USP Center for Advancement of Patient Safety: *Use caution–avoid confusion*, USP Quality Review No. 79, Rockville, MD, April 2004, USP Center for Advancement of Patient Safety.

http://www.ncbi.nlm.nih.gov/pubmed/2233075 ACEI's Adverse reactions—Angioedema from angiotensin converting enzyme inhibitors: a cause of upper airway obstruction; Gannon TH, Eby TL.

Department of Surgery, University of Alabama, Birmingham 35233.

http://www.medicinenet.com/beta_blockers/article.htm- Beta Blockers, Pharmacy Author: Omudhome Ogbru, PharmD Medical and Pharmacy Editor: Jay W. Marks, MD.

http://www.cvpharmacology.com/vasodilator/CCB.htm, Calcium-Channel Blockers (CCBs)Cardiovascular Pharmacology Concepts, Richard E. Klabunde, PhD.

http://www.clinicalpharmacology.com/Forms/Monograph/monograph.aspx?cpnum=539&sec=mondesc-reserpine

23

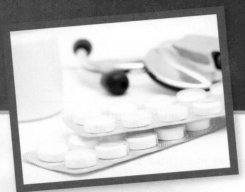

Treatment of Heart Failure

LEARNING OBJECTIVES

1 Learn the terminology associated with heart failure.
2 List the risk factors for heart failure.
3 List the symptoms of heart failure.
4 List and categorize medications used to treat heart failure.
5 Describe mechanism of action for each class of drugs used to treat heart failure.
6 Identify warning labels and precautionary messages associated with medications used to treat heart failure.

KEY TERMS

Automaticity: Spontaneous depolarization (contraction) of heart cells.

Cardioglycosides: Class of drugs, most commonly derived from the foxglove plant, that have the ability to alter cardiovascular function. Digitalis is representative of this class of drugs.

Digitalization: Process of rapidly increasing the initial dose of digoxin until the therapeutic dose is achieved.

Ejection fraction: Percentage of blood ejected from the left ventricle with each heartbeat.

Heart failure: Clinical syndrome in which the heart is unable to pump blood at a rate necessary to meet the body's metabolic needs.

Natriuretic peptides: Hormones that play a role in cardiac homeostasis.

Positive inotropic effect: Increase in the force of myocardial contractions.

Stroke volume: Equal to the volume of blood ejected by the left ventricle during each cardiac contraction minus the volume of blood in the ventricle at the end of systole. The following formula is used to calculate stroke volume.

$$\text{Stroke volume} = (\text{Cardiac output}) \times (\text{Heart rate}) \text{ or } SV = CO \times HR$$

Overview

Heart failure is a clinical syndrome in which the heart is unable to pump blood at a rate necessary to meet the body's metabolic needs. Heart failure affects more than 5 million people in the United States and is responsible for nearly 300,000 deaths each year. More than 500,000 new cases are diagnosed annually. The syndrome primarily affects the elderly, affecting more than 10% of the population older than 50 years old compared with 1% of persons younger than the age of 50 years.

Up to age 75 years, the prevalence of heart failure is higher in men, but after age 75 years, the prevalence is higher in women.

Disease, lifestyle, and drugs can contribute to the onset or aggravation of heart failure. Kidney dysfunction, diabetes, ischemic heart disease, hypertension, hypothyroidism, hyperthyroidism, bradyarrhythmia, tachyarrhythmia, pulmonary embolism, HIV/AIDS, and myocardial infarction can contribute to heart failure. Excessive salt and alcohol consumption as well of lack of physical activity can worsen heart failure. Nonsteroidal anti-inflammatory drugs, for example, worsen edema and interfere with the effect of drugs used to treat heart failure (e.g., angiotensin-converting enzyme [ACE] inhibitors). Many other medications associated with causing edema can likewise contribute to the development or exacerbation of heart failure.

Pathophysiology of Heart Failure

Heart failure may affect the left side of the heart, the right side of the heart, or both sides. Left-sided heart failure reduces the volume of oxygen and nutrient-rich blood pumped from the left ventricle to the rest of the body. The ***ejection fraction***, the percentage of blood ejected from the left ventricle with each heartbeat, is reduced. Persons with left-sided heart failure may have swelling in the legs and ankles and feel fatigued. Fluid accumulation can result in weight gain and increased urination. Right-sided heart failure reduces the capacity of the heart to pump blood to the lungs. Fluids back up (venous congestion) and cause pulmonary edema and shortness of breath. Blood pressure increases.

Heart failure may be classified as systolic heart failure (SHF) or diastolic heart failure (DHF). In SHF, left ventricular contractions are reduced causing a decrease in the volume of blood ejected from the ventricles (***stroke volume***). The result is reduced cardiac output. In DHF, stroke volume is reduced because the left ventricle is unable to accept a sufficient volume of blood during diastole. Cardiac output is reduced, causing fatigue, dyspnea, and pulmonary hypertension.

Compensatory mechanisms are "switched on" when heart function fails (Figure 23-1). In an attempt to satisfy the metabolic needs of the body, the renin–aldosterone–angiotensin system

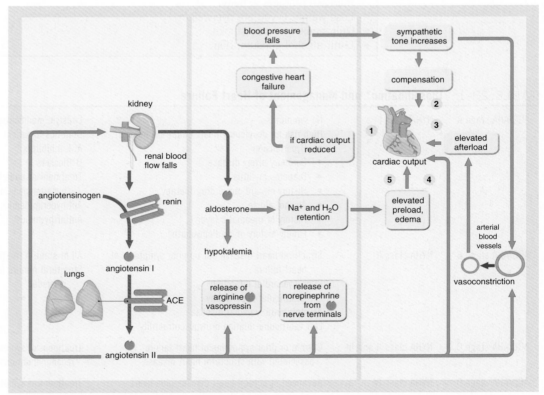

FIGURE 23-1 Compensatory mechanisms in congestive heart failure. (From Page C, Curtis M, Sutter M, et al: *Integrated pharmacology*, ed 3 Philadelphia, 2005, Mosby.)

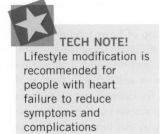

TECH NOTE!
Lifestyle modification is recommended for people with heart failure to reduce symptoms and complications (Box 23-1).

(RAAS) is activated. RAAS activation increases blood volume and cardiac output because RAAS activation produces sodium and fluid retention. Chronic sympathetic nervous system (SNS) stimulation is also linked to heart failure.

Natriuretic peptides are hormones that also play a role in cardiac physiology. Atrial natriuretic peptide (ANP) and brain natriuretic peptide (BNP) are both found in cardiac tissue and are released in response to excessive stretching of heart muscle cells. Atrial stretching causes ANP release. Fluid accumulation and filling pressure in the left ventricle stimulates BNP release. Elevated BNP levels may be used to confirm a diagnosis of heart failure.

Stages of Heart Failure

There are four stages of heart failure. Heart failure may also be described by functional class. American College of Cardiology/American Heart Association (ACC/AHA) descriptions and New York Heart Association (NYHA) functional classifications are compared in Table 23-1.

Drugs Used to Treat Heart Failure

Most of the treatments used in heart failure focus on treating symptoms, underlying causes, and factors that worsen heart failure. Many of the same drugs administered in the treatment of hypertension are also used in the treatment of heart failure. They include diuretics, aldosterone antagonists, beta blockers, ACE inhibitors, and angiotensin II receptor blockers (ARBs). These drugs are covered in detail in Chapter 22. The *cardioglycosides* are the oldest class of drugs used in the treatment of heart failure.

BOX 23-1   Lifestyle Modifications Recommended for People with Heart Failure

- Follow a diet low in salt.
- Fluid restriction if needed for management of edema.
- Increase physical activity.
- Lose weight if you are overweight.
- Quit smoking if you smoke.
- Limit alcohol consumption.

TABLE 23-1   Classification* and Management of Heart Failure

ACC/AHA stage A	NYHA class I	No symptoms High risk for developing heart failure because of: • Hypertension • Coronary artery disease • Diabetes mellitus • History of cardiotoxic drug therapy • Alcohol abuse • History of rheumatic fever • Family history of cardiomyopathy	Lifestyle modification Diuretics if patient has fluid retention ACE inhibitors β-Blockers Treatment of underlying disease (diabetes, hypertension, etc.) Antihyperlipidemics Antiarrhythmics
ACC/AHA stage B	NYHA class II	Structural heart disease but no prior symptoms of heart failure Prior myocardial infarction Left ventricular hypertrophy Asymptomatic valvular disease Left ventricular dilation or hypocontractility	All of stage A treatment options, plus Structural repairs (e.g., heart valve replacement) if needed
ACC/AHA stage C	NYHA class II and III	Current or prior symptoms of heart failure associated with structural heart disease	Treatment of symptoms as per stage A and B recommendations plus digoxin
ACC/AHA stage D	NYHA class IV	Advanced structural heart disease plus heart failure symptoms at rest despite medical therapy	Treatment of symptoms as per stage A and B recommendations plus digoxin

*American College of Cardiology/American Heart Association guidelines for evaluation and management and NHYA functional classes.

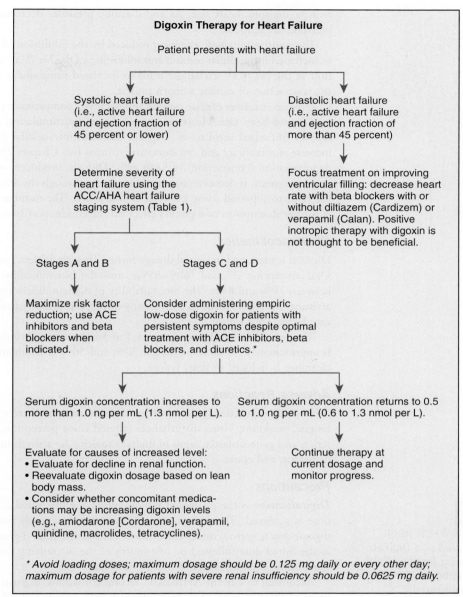

Digoxin Therapy for Heart Failure

Patient presents with heart failure

Systolic heart failure (i.e., active heart failure and ejection fraction of 45 percent or lower)

Diastolic heart failure (i.e., active heart failure and ejection fraction of more than 45 percent)

Determine severity of heart failure using the ACC/AHA heart failure staging system (Table 1).

Focus treatment on improving ventricular filling: decrease heart rate with beta blockers with or without diltiazem (Cardizem) or verapamil (Calan). Positive inotropic therapy with digoxin is not thought to be beneficial.

Stages A and B

Stages C and D

Maximize risk factor reduction; use ACE inhibitors and beta blockers when indicated.

Consider administering empiric low-dose digoxin for patients with persistent symptoms despite optimal treatment with ACE inhibitors, beta blockers, and diuretics.*

Serum digoxin concentration increases to more than 1.0 ng per mL (1.3 nmol per L).

Serum digoxin concentration returns to 0.5 to 1.0 ng per mL (0.6 to 1.3 nmol per L).

Evaluate for causes of increased level:
• Evaluate for decline in renal function.
• Reevaluate digoxin dosage based on lean body mass.
• Consider whether concomitant medications may be increasing digoxin levels (e.g., amiodarone [Cordarone], verapamil, quinidine, macrolides, tetracyclines).

Continue therapy at current dosage and monitor progress.

Avoid loading doses; maximum dosage should be 0.125 mg daily or every other day; maximum dosage for patients with severe renal insufficiency should be 0.0625 mg daily.

FIGURE 23-2 Algorithm for digoxin therapy for heart failure. (Modified from Morris S, Hatcher HF: Digoxin therapy for heart failure: An update, *Am Family Phys* 74(4):613-618, 2006.)

CARDIOGLYCOSIDES

Digitalis is a cardioglycoside derived from the foxglove plant. Digoxin is the only commercially available cardioglycoside in the United States and Canada. Despite its historical use, studies by the Digitalis Investigation Group (DIG) trial show that although digoxin reduces hospitalization and improves exercise tolerance in symptomatic patients, it fails to increase survival in patients with heart failure. In fact, digoxin may actually increase mortality in women. Digoxin is typically administered in combination with ACE inhibitors, diuretics, or beta blockers (Figure 23-2).

Mechanism of Action

Cardioglycosides such as digoxin have a ***positive inotropic effect*** on the heart; they increase the force of myocardial contractions. The greater force of contractions increases the cardiac output and reduces diastolic heart size. As end-diastolic pressures decrease, pulmonary and systemic venous pressures are reduced.

The positive inotropic effect is produced by the inhibition of the Na^+/K^+ ATPase pump, leading to increased intracellular sodium and inhibition of the Na^+/Ca^{2+} exchanger. Digoxin-induced inhibition of the Na^+/Ca^{2+} exchanger leads to increased intracellular calcium, an electrolyte involved in the contraction of cardiac smooth muscle.

Digoxin increases cardiac output and decreases compensatory sympathetic activity, which results in a slowed heart rate. Heart rate is also slowed by stimulation of parasympathetic nervous system activity (increased vagal tone). Digoxin decreases intracellular potassium. Potassium depletion can increase automaticity and can cause arrhythmias (see Chapter 25). *Automaticity* is the spontaneous depolarization (contraction) of heart cells. Digoxin produces significant effects on the heart's conduction system. It decreases conduction velocity through the atrioventricular (AV) node, prolonging the refractory period (time between contractions). The number of depolarizations is reduced, too. A further description of digoxin's effect on the conduction system is described in Chapter 25.

Pharmacokinetics

Digoxin is marketed in several dosage forms. They are tablets, oral solution, and parenteral solution. Oral absorption is good (60%-85%), and the bioavailability of orally administered digoxin is between 70% and 85%. The bioavailability of digoxin differs among commercial manufacturers, so attempts should be made to consistently dispense the same manufacturer's product each time. Food can decrease absorption.

The peak effect of digoxin occurs 1.5 to 5 hours after administration, and the half-life of digoxin is approximately 36 hours. Between 30% and 50% is eliminated unchanged by the kidneys, and clearance is reduced in heart failure.

Adverse Reactions

Adverse drug reactions produced by digoxin include diarrhea, constipation, nausea, vomiting, fatigue, weakness, visual disturbances (altered color perception, hazy vision), photophobia, impotence, and gynecomastia. Signs of digitalis toxicity are arrhythmia, dizziness, headache, convulsions, delusions, and coma.

Precautions

Digitalization is the process of rapidly increasing the initial dose of digoxin until the therapeutic dose is achieved. The patient must be monitored carefully for signs of digitalis toxicity because digoxin has a narrow therapeutic index. Half of the total digitalizing dose should be administered as the initial dose followed by one-fourth of the digitalizing dose in 8 to 12 hours. The final one-fourth dose is administered 8 to 12 hours later.

According to current AHA/ACC recommendations, digoxin is not recommended for the treatment of DHF in men or women who also have sinoatrial or AV block.

TECH ALERT!
Digibind and DigiFab (digoxin immune Fab) are antidotes for digoxin toxicity.

Cardioglycosides

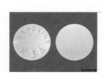

Generic Name	U.S. Brand Name(s) Canadian Brand(s)	Dosage Forms and Strengths
digoxin*	Lanoxin	Solution, oral: 0.05 mg/mL
	Lanoxin	Solution for Injection (Lanoxin): 0.25 mg/mL Lanoxin Pediatric: 0.05 mg/mL‡, 0.1 mg/mL† Tablets (Lanoxin): 0.0625 mg‡, 0.125 mg, 0.25 mg, 0.5 mg
Digoxin Antidote		
digoxin immune Fab	Not available	Injection: 38 mg (Digibind), 40 mg (Digifab) lyophilized powder for reconstitution
	Digibind, DigiFab	

*Generic available.
†Strength available in the United States only.
‡Strength available in Canada only.

Usual Dose, Dosing Schedule, and Warnings for Digoxin

Drug Name	Usual Dose and Dosing Schedule	Warning Labels
Cardioglycosides		
digoxin	0.125-0.5 mg once daily	TAKE AS DIRECTED; DO NOT SKIP OR EXCEED DOSAGE. IF YOU MISS A DOSE, TAKE IT AS SOON AS YOU REMEMBER UNLESS THE NEXT DOSE IS SCHEDULED TO BE TAKEN IN LESS THAN 12 HOURS.
Digoxin Antidote		
Digibind DigiFab	Varies according to the amount of digoxin to be neutralized	

DIURETICS

The diuretics are administered to treat volume overload. They also lower blood pressure. Elevated blood pressure can aggravate existing heart failure or precipitate its onset. The diuretics also reduce pulmonary edema and swelling in the ankles, legs, and feet (peripheral edema). When diuretics are administered, potassium levels should be monitored because loop and thiazide diuretics can cause hypokalemia (see Chapter 22). Hypokalemia can increase the effects of digoxin leading to toxicity. The diuretics drug table provides doses used for the treatment of heart failure.

ALDOSTERONE ANTAGONISTS

Aldosterone is a hormone that promotes Na^+ retention and water accumulation, leading to edema. Spironolactone and eplerenone are aldosterone antagonists. They are used as adjunctive therapy, together with other drugs, in the treatment of hypertension and management of congestive heart failure. Administration leads to decreased Na^+ and water levels and increased K^+ levels in the body. Potassium levels should be monitored for hyperkalemia, which may produce arrhythmias. Spironolactone is recommended to treat moderate to severe heart failure when the ability to pump blood out of the left ventricle is compromised. Eplerenone is specifically marketed for reducing cardiovascular risk in patients after myocardial infarction.

BETA BLOCKERS

The beta blockers reduce the heart rate, lower peripheral arterial resistance, lower blood pressure, and decrease the workload of the heart. They also reduce left ventricular hypertrophy. Studies show that beta blockers can lower the risk of mortality associated with heart failure. The mechanism of action for beta blockers use in the treatment of heart failure is to block excess sympathetic stimulation induced by heart failure. Recall that increased sympathetic tone is a compensatory mechanism commonly seen with heart failure. The beta blockers drug table in Chapter 22 shows doses used for the treatment of heart failure.

ANGIOTENSIN-CONVERTING ENZYME INHIBITORS AND ANGIOTENSIN II RECEPTOR BLOCKERS

The ACE inhibitors are one of the few classes of drugs used in the treatment of heart failure that have been shown to reduce mortality (prolong life). They reduce left ventricular hypertrophy, improve diastolic filling, increase cardiac output, and reduce peripheral vascular resistance. When angiotensin II levels are decreased, sympathetic tone and aldosterone-mediated sodium increase and blood volume expansion are also reduced. The ARBs are also administered for the treatment of heart failure. The ARBs improve exercise tolerance and diastolic filling in patients with DHF. The ACE inhibitors drug table in Chapter 22 shows doses used for the treatment of patients with heart failure.

HMG COA REDUCTASE INHIBITORS

Administration of an HMG CoA reductase inhibitor, also called "statins" (e.g., atorvastatin), in patients with heart failure may be considered to treat existing coronary artery disease or to reduce the risk for its development. Heart failure is also linked to inflammation, and statins have been shown to reduce inflammation. Statins are discussed in depth in Chapter 24.

VASODILATORS

Isosorbide dinitrate and hydralazine are used in combination for the treatment of heart failure for their vasodilating effects. This reduces peripheral resistance along with cardiac preload and afterload. Moreover, hydralazine has been shown to indirectly increase the force of myocardial contractions (positive inotropic effect). When combined with nitrates such as isosorbide dinitrate, hydralazine can decrease mortality and effectively reduce cardiac congestion.

Usual Dose and Dosing Schedule for Other Drugs Used in the Treatment of Heart Failure

Drug Name	Usual Dose and Dosing Schedule
Diuretics	
Thiazides	
chlorothiazide	500-1000 mg 1-2 times a day
chlorthalidone	50-100 mg/day or 100 mg every other day
hydrochlorothiazide (HCTZ)	25-100 mg/day
indapamide	2.5-5 mg/day
Loop	
bumetanide	0.5-2 mg/day
furosemide	40-120 mg PO or IV per day (maximum, 600 mg/day PO)
torsemide	10-20 mg PO or IV daily (maximum, 200 mg/day)
Aldosterone Receptor Antagonists	
eplerenone	50 mg once daily
spironolactone	25-200 mg/day
Beta Blockers	
bisoprolol	1.25-10 mg/day
metoprolol extended release	Begin 25 mg/day; increase up to 200 mg/day
Combined Alpha and Beta Blockers	
carvedilol	**Immediate release:** Begin 3.125 mg twice daily; increase to 25-50 mg twice daily **Controlled release:** Begin 10 mg/day; increase up to 80 mg/day as needed for clinical effect
Angiotensin-Converting Enzyme inhibitors	
benazepril	2-20 mg/day

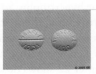

Usual Dose and Dosing Schedule for Other Drugs Used in the Treatment of Heart Failure—cont'd

Drug Name	Usual Dose and Dosing Schedule
captopril	25-50 mg 2-3 times a day
enalapril	2.5-20 mg PO twice daily
lisinopril	5-40 mg/day
quinapril	10-20 mg twice daily
ramipril	2.5-5 mg/day
trandolapril	1-4 mg/day
Angiotensin II Antagonists	
candesartan	Begin 4 mg/day; increase to 32 mg/day
losartan	50 mg/day
valsartan	40-160 mg twice daily
Vasodilators (Hydralazine + Isosorbide in Combination)	
hydralazine + isosorbide (BiDil)	1-2 tablets 3 times a day
hydralazine	Initiate at 10-25 mg 3 times a day; maintenance 200 mg/day in 2-4 divided doses (maximum, 300 mg/day) for SHF
isosorbide dinitrate	10-40 mg 3 times a day

Chapter Summary

- Heart failure is a clinical syndrome in which the heart is unable to pump blood at a rate necessary to meet the body's metabolic needs.
- Kidney dysfunction, diabetes, ischemic heart disease, hypertension, hypothyroidism, hyperthyroidism, bradyarrhythmia, tachyarrhythmia, pulmonary embolism, HIV/AIDS, and myocardial infarction can contribute to heart failure.
- Lifestyle factors such as excessive salt and alcohol consumption and lack of physical activity can worsen heart failure.
- Nonsteroidal anti-inflammatory drugs, as well as other medication classes, can worsen edema and interfere with the effect of drugs used to treat heart failure such as ACE inhibitors.
- Heart failure may affect the left side of the heart, the right side of the heart, or both sides. Left-sided heart failure reduces the volume of oxygen and nutrient blood pumped from the left ventricle to the rest of the body. Right-sided heart failure reduces the capacity of the heart to pump blood to the lungs.
- Heart failure may be classified as SHF or DHF. The choice of drug therapy is influenced by whether the patient has SHF or DHF.

- Compensatory mechanisms are "switched on" when the heart function fails. Compensatory mechanisms attempt to satisfy the metabolic needs of the body.
- RAAS activation increases blood volume and cardiac output because RAAS activation produces sodium and fluid retention.
- There are four stages of heart failure: stage A, high risk for developing heart failure; stage B, structural changes without symptoms; stage C, symptomatic; and stage D, advanced structural heart disease plus heart failure symptoms.
- Lifestyle modification is recommended for patients in all stages of heart failure.
- Drugs used in the treatment of heart failure include the cardioglycosides, diuretics, aldosterone antagonists, beta blockers, ACE inhibitors, ARBs, and vasodilators.
- Digoxin is the only cardioglycoside currently marketed in the United States and Canada.
- Digoxin reduces hospitalization and improves exercise tolerance in symptomatic patients but fails to increase survival in patients with heart failure.
- Digoxin has a positive inotropic effect on the heart; the result is an increase in the force of myocardial contractions.
- Digoxin increases cardiac output and decreases compensatory sympathetic activity.
- Available digoxin dosage forms are tablets, oral solution, and parenteral solution.
- The bioavailability of digoxin differs among commercial manufacturers, and food can decrease absorption.
- Digitalization is the process of rapidly increasing the initial dose of digoxin until the therapeutic dose is achieved. The patient must be monitored carefully for signs of toxicity because digoxin has a narrow therapeutic index.
- The diuretics are administered in heart failure to reduce edema. Diuretics that produce hypokalemia can increase the effects of digoxin leading to toxicity.
- Spironolactone and eplerenone are aldosterone antagonists.
- Spironolactone is recommended for moderate to severe heart failure to reduce water and Na^+ accumulation. Eplerenone may reduce cardiovascular risk in patients after myocardial infarction.
- Potassium levels should be monitored when spironolactone is administered because the drug may cause hyperkalemia and arrhythmias
- Studies show the beta blockers can lower the risk of mortality associated with congestive heart failure. Beta blockers reduce excess sympathetic stimulation induced by heart failure.
- ACE inhibitors and ARBs may reduce mortality. They reduce left ventricular hypertrophy, improve diastolic filling, increase cardiac output, and reduce peripheral vascular resistance.
- Isosorbide dinitrate and hydralazine are used in combination for the treatment of heart failure to decrease mortality and effectively reduce cardiac congestion.

REVIEW QUESTIONS

1. Heart failure affects only the left side of the heart.
   a. true
   b. false

2. Heart failure may be classified as _____.
   a. systolic heart failure
   b. diastolic heart failure
   c. ventricular heart failure
   d. a and b

3. The _____ are the oldest class of drugs used in the treatment of heart failure.
   a. aminoglycosides
   b. cardioglycosides
   c. diuretics
   d. antibiotics

4. Digitalis is a cardioglycoside derived from the foxglove plant.
   a. true
   b. false

5. Digitalization is the process of rapidly _____ the initial dose of digoxin until the therapeutic dose is achieved.
   a. increasing
   b. decreasing
   c. stabilizing
   d. titrating

6. Thiazide diuretics can cause
   a. hyperkalemia
   b. hypernatremia
   c. hypokalemia
   d. hypocalcemia

7. The mechanism of action for beta blockers used in the treatment of heart failure is to block excess _____ stimulation induced by heart failure.
   a. sympathetic
   b. parasympathetic

8. Spironolactone may be used in the treatment of moderate to severe heart failure to _____.
   a. reduce water and K^+ accumulation
   b. reduce water and Ca^{++} accumulation
   c. reduce water and Na^+ accumulation
   d. reduce water and Cl^- accumulation

9. ACE inhibitors are one of the few classes of drugs used in the treatment of heart failure that have been shown to _____.
   a. increase mortality
   b. reduce mortality
   c. have no effect on mortality
   d. all of the above

10. Isosorbide dinitrate and hydralazine are used in combination for the treatment of heart failure for their _____ effects.
   a. vasodilating
   b. vasoconstricting
   c. sympathetic
   d. parasympathetic

TECHNICIAN'S CORNER

1. Research and make a list of over-the-counter medications that should be avoided by patients taking digoxin for heart failure.
2. Patients with heart failure are always advised to make lifestyle modifications as part of their treatment. Why is that process so important and so difficult to do?

Bibliography

Aronow W: Epidemiology, pathophysiology, prognosis, and treatment of systolic and diastolic heart failure, *Cardiol Rev* 14:108-124, 2006.

Davies M, Gibbs C, Lip G: ABC of heart failure management: diuretics, ACE inhibitors, and nitrates, *BMJ* 320:428-431, 2000.

Felker M, Petersen J, Mark D: Natriuretic peptides in the diagnosis and management of heart failure, *CMAJ* 175:611-617, 2006.

Kalant H, Grant D, Mitchell J: *Principles of medical pharmacology*, ed 7, Toronto, 2007, Elsevier Canada, A Division of Reed Elsevier Canada, pp 22-27, 451, 453-454, 503-504.

Lance L, Lacy C, Armstrong L, et al: *Drug information handbook for the allied health professional*, ed 12, Hudson, OH, 2005, APhA Lexi-Comp.

May H, Muhlestein J, Carlquist J, et al: Relation of serum total cholesterol, C-reactive protein levels, and statin therapy to survival in heart failure, *Am J Cardiol* 98:653-658, 2006.

National Heart, Lung, and Blood Institute: *What is heart failure? Diseases and conditions index*, Bethesda, MD, July 2006, National Heart, Lung, and Blood Institute, National Institutes of Health, US Department of Health and Human Services, Available at: http://www.nhlbi.nih.gov/health/dci/Diseases/Hf/HF_WhatIs.html.

Page C, Curtis M, Sutter M, et al: *Integrated pharmacology*, Philadelphia, 2005, Mosby, pp 386-391, 393-395.

Shammas R, Khan N, Nekkanti R, et al: Diastolic heart failure and left ventricular diastolic dysfunction: What we know, and what we don't know! *Int J Cardiol* 2006;115(3):284-292.

USP Center for Advancement of Patient Safety: Use caution–avoid confusion, USP Quality Review No. 79, Rockville, MD, April 2004, USP Center for Advancement of Patient Safety.

24

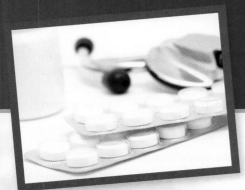

Treatment of Myocardial Infarction and Stroke

LEARNING OBJECTIVES

1 Learn the terminology associated with myocardial infarction and stroke.

2 List the symptoms of myocardial infarction and stroke.

3 List risk factors for myocardial infarction and stroke.

4 List and categorize medications used to treat myocardial infarction, stroke, and hyperlipidemia.

5 Describe the mechanism of action for each class of drugs used to treat myocardial infarction and stroke.

6 Identify significant drug look-alike and sound-alike issues.

7 List common endings for drug classes used in the treatment of myocardial infarction, stroke, and hyperlipidemia.

8 Identify warning labels and precautionary messages associated with medications used to treat myocardial infarction, stroke, and hyperlipidemia.

KEY TERMS

Aneurysm: Weakened spot of the artery wall that has stretched or burst filling the area with blood and causing damage. If in the brain, damage to nerves results.

Anoxia: Absence of oxygen supply to cells that results in cell damage or death.

Anticoagulant: Drug that prolongs coagulation time and is used to prevent clot formation.

Antiplatelet drug: Drug that prevents accumulation of platelets, thereby blocking an important step in the clot formation process.

Antithrombotic: Drug that inhibits clot formation by reducing the coagulation action of the blood protein thrombin.

Atherosclerosis: Buildup of lipids and plaque inside artery walls; impeding the flow of blood and oxygen.

Atherothrombosis: Formation of a blood clot in an artery.

Cholesterol: Naturally occurring, waxy substance produced by the liver and found in foods that maintains cell membranes and is needed for vitamin D production. Excess cholesterol can cause atherosclerosis.

Embolic stroke: Stroke caused by an emboli obstructing the flow of blood through an artery.

Hemorrhagic stroke: Sudden bleeding into or around the brain.

Hemostasis: Process of stopping the flow of blood.

High-density lipoprotein: "Good cholesterol"; lipoproteins that transport cholesterol, triglycerides, and other lipids from blood to body tissues.

Hyperlipidemia: Excess lipids or fatty substances in the blood.

Infarction: Sudden loss of blood supply to an area that results in cell death. A myocardial infarction is known as a heart attack. A cerebral infarction is also known as a stroke.

Ischemia: Reduction of blood supplied to tissues that is typically caused by blood vessel obstruction due to atherosclerosis, stenosis, or plaque.

Ischemic stroke: Ischemia in the brain.

Lipoprotein: Small globules of cholesterol covered by a layer of protein.

Low-density lipoprotein: Compound consisting of a lipid and a protein that carries the majority of the total cholesterol in the blood and deposits the excess along the inside of arterial walls; also known as "bad cholesterol."

Mitral valve stenosis: Disease of the mitral valve involving buildup of plaquelike material around the valve.

Plaque: Fatty cholesterol deposits.

Platelets: Structures found in the blood that are involved in the coagulation process.

Partial thromboplastin time: Test given to determine effectiveness of heparin in reducing antithrombotic activity.

Prothrombin time: Test given to determine the effectiveness of warfarin in reducing clotting time.

Rhabdomyolysis: Breakdown of muscle fibers and release of muscle fiber contents into the circulation. These muscle fibers are toxic to the kidneys.

Thrombolytic: Drug used to dissolve blood clots.

Thrombosis: Formation of a blood clot.

Thrombotic stroke: Stroke caused by thrombosis.

Tissue plasminogen activator: Naturally occurring thrombolytic substance.

Transient ischemic attack: Stroke that typically lasts for a few minutes; also known as a mini-stroke.

Triglycerides: Storage form of energy found in fat tissue muscle; metabolize to very low-density lipoproteins.

Overview

Americans have more than 1.2 million heart attacks annually, and up to 40% of patients die from it. That makes myocardial *infarction* the leading cause of death in the United States, accounting for nearly 500,000 deaths. More than 600,000 Americans each year will have a stroke. Stroke is the third leading cause of death in the United States. Approximately 50,000 will have a mini-stroke (*transient ischemic attack* [TIA]). Persons who have had one stroke and recover are more likely to have another. Nearly 25% of patients will have a second stroke within 5 years of the first stroke. Cardiovascular disease is the number one cause of death in Canada, accounting for 36% of deaths from all causes. Acute myocardial infarction (27%), cerebrovascular disease (20%), and ischemic heart disease (27%) are the primary causes of death from all cardiovascular disease in Canada.

Types of Strokes

Strokes occur when brain cells are deprived of oxygen or are damaged by sudden bleeding into the brain. *Ischemic strokes* account for 80% of all strokes and are caused by oxygen deprivation. *Anoxia* (absence of oxygen) occurs when arteries are obstructed and causes brain infarcts. *Thrombotic stroke* is caused by an enlarged thrombus or blood clot. *Embolic stroke* is caused by an embolus (traveling clot) or *plaque* that has been dislodged. Blood clots (thrombi, emboli) are the most common cause of strokes.

    Hemorrhagic strokes account for the remaining 20% of all strokes and are caused by bleeding in the brain. It may be the result of an *aneurysm*, a weakened spot of the artery wall that has stretched or burst, filling the area with blood and causing damage.

TABLE 24-1   **Symptoms of Stroke**

Limbs	Numbness or weakness of arms or legs Difficulty walking Loss of balance or coordination
Ears, eyes, nose, and throat	Facial numbness or weakness Impaired speech Impaired vision
Cognitive	Confusion Difficulty understanding speech
Other	Dizziness Severe headache

TABLE 24-2   **Characteristics of Myocardial Infarction versus Stroke**

Characteristics	Myocardial Infarction	Angina
Timing	Sudden onset Lasts longer than 30 minutes May occur at rest	Often occurs after exercise Lasts 1-5 minutes Rest may relieve symptoms
Location	Mid-chest radiating to jaw, neck, arms, and epigastric area	Mid-chest radiating to jaw, neck, arms, and epigastric area
Quality	Severe squeezing or heaviness in chest area	Heaviness, chest tightness, indigestion

Transient ischemic attacks are also known as mini-strokes. They typically last only a few minutes and symptoms usually resolve within 1 hour.

Symptoms of Stroke

Regardless of the cause, strokes produce similar symptoms. Symptoms (Table 24-1) appear suddenly.

Symptoms of Myocardial Infarction

Myocardial infarction produces symptoms that are similar to those of angina. Prompt treatment of myocardial infarction is essential to persons experiencing the symptoms listed in Table 24-2. If symptoms persist beyond 15 minutes, emergency assistance (dialing 911) should be sought.

Pathophysiology of Stroke and Myocardial Infarction

Stroke and myocardial infarction occur when the blood supply to the brain (stroke) or heart (myocardial infarction) is interrupted. Cells become damaged from *ischemia* (reduction of blood supplied to tissues) or die when they are deprived of oxygen and nutrients. Vascular inflammation is a cause of atherosclerosis and chronic inflammation of the arteries that supply the heart and brain can also lead to stroke and myocardial infarction. The risk for chronic vascular inflammation increases with age. *Atherosclerosis* (a buildup of lipids and plaque inside of artery walls) can block blood flow through arteries. *Atherothrombosis* (the formation of a blood clot in the artery) can also clog arteries and is triggered by atherosclerosis.

Risk Factors for Stroke and Myocardial Infarction

Risk factors for stroke and myocardial infarction are categorized as modifiable and nonmodifiable. Nonmodifiable risk factors are age, gender, and family history. In addition, chronic diseases such as hypertension, ischemic heart disease, and diabetes place patients at increased risk for stroke.

NONMODIFIABLE RISK FACTORS

Age

Age is a significant risk factor for stroke and myocardial infarction. Although stroke can occur at any age, the risk increases exponentially with each increasing decade. Approximately 66% of strokes occur in persons older than 65 years. Strokes that occur in persons older than 65 years old are more likely to be fatal.

Gender

Gender is also an important risk factor for stroke. Men are 1.25 times more likely to have a stroke than are women, yet strokes in men are less likely to be fatal. This is probably because men are often younger than women when they have a stroke. As with stroke, men have a greater risk for heart attack than do women; however, older women are more likely to die within 3 weeks of a heart attack than are men.

MODIFIABLE RISK FACTORS

Modifiable risk factors for stroke and myocardial infarction are smoking, alcohol consumption, and diet. Smoking promotes atherosclerosis, increases clotting factors in the blood (fibrinogen), stimulates vasoconstriction, and weakens the endothelial wall. These factors contribute to the risk for ischemic stroke and hemorrhagic stroke. Excessive alcohol consumption and binge drinking lead to an increase in blood pressure and can reduce *platelets*, which increase the risk for hemorrhagic stroke. After heavy drinking, a rebound effect occurs that increases platelets and thickens the blood significantly, increasing the risk of ischemic stroke. A diet high in *cholesterol* may increase the risk for atherosclerosis, and a diet high in salt can aggravate hypertension.

Hypertension

Hypertension increases the risk for stroke four to six times above that of persons without hypertension, and 90% of persons who have had a stroke have hypertension.

Atrial Fibrillation

Atrial fibrillation (see Chapter 25), a rapid and irregular beating of the atrium chamber of the heart, can increase the risk for clots. If the clots are dislodged, they can occlude an artery, leading to stroke or myocardial infarction. Malformations of the heart valves (*mitral valve stenosis*) can also lead to clot formation, increasing the risk of stroke or myocardial infarction.

High Cholesterol

High cholesterol levels are a risk factor for stroke and myocardial infarction. Cholesterol may be in the form of *high-density lipoproteins* (HDLs) and *low-density lipoproteins* (LDLs). LDLs can build up within artery walls and harden. This hardened material is called plaque, and it can impede blood supply to the heart and brain. During surgery, plaque can become dislodged, interrupting blood supply and causing stroke or myocardial infarction. Diabetes also increases the development of atherosclerosis and therefore is a risk factor for stroke and myocardial infarction.

Infection

Infection is a risk factor for stroke and myocardial infarction. The immune system response to bacterial and viral infections is to release cytokines, leukotrienes, macrophages, and other infection-fighting substances that also increase inflammation. These substances can increase the risk for ischemic and embolic stroke.

Lifestyle Modification

Lifestyle modifications are recommended to reduce risk for stroke and myocardial infarction and are listed in Box 24-1.

Drugs Used in the Treatment of Stroke and Myocardial Infarction

Atherosclerosis and atherothrombosis are important risk factors for stroke and myocardial infarction. Drugs that control the buildup of lipids and plaque and drugs that reduce the formation of blood clots are administered to prevent stroke, myocardial infarction, and acute coronary syndrome.

DRUGS THAT CONTROL HEMOSTASIS

Drugs that control **hemostasis** (the process of stopping the flow of blood) can prevent **thrombosis** and complications associated with the formation of blood clots in arteries. Clotting is a normal process without which one would bleed to death if an injury occurs (Figure 24-1). If clots form in an artery and obstruct the supply of blood and oxygen to the brain and heart, a stroke and myocardial infarction may occur. Drugs that control the rate of clot formation and clot dissolution are classified as **antithrombotics** and can prevent stroke and myocardial infarction. Antithrombotic

---

BOX 24-1   **Lifestyle Modifications Recommended for People with Heart Failure**

- Follow a diet low in salt.
- Limit the amount of fluids that you drink.
- Increase physical activity.
- Lose weight if you are overweight.
- Quit smoking if you smoke.
- Limit alcohol consumption.

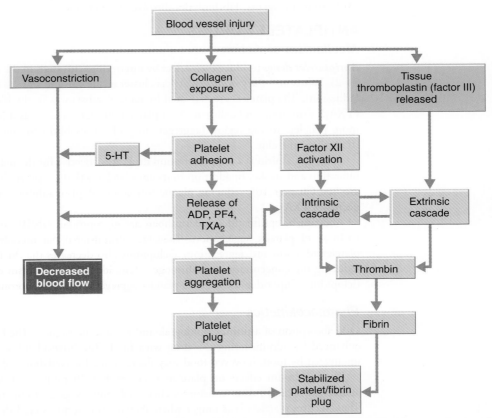

FIGURE 24-1 Clot formation. (From Lilley LL, Harrington S, Snyder JS: *Pharmacology and the nursing process*, ed 5. St. Louis, 2007, Mosby.)

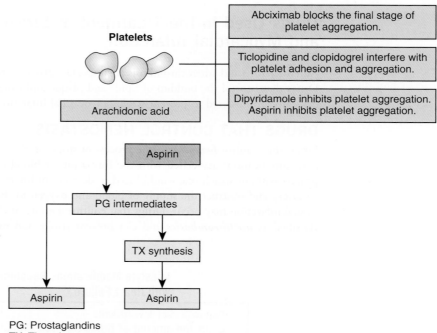

FIGURE 24-2 Action for antiplatelet drugs. (Modified from Lilley LL, Harrington S, Snyder JS: *Pharmacology and the nursing process*, ed 5. St. Louis, 2007, Mosby.)

drugs include (1) agents that inhibit platelets; (2) *anticoagulants*, which lessen coagulation; and (3) fibrinolytic agents. Fibrinolytics dissolve existing clots.

ANTIPLATELET DRUGS

Mechanism of Action

Antiplatelet drugs produce their effect by interfering with steps in the clot formation process (Figure 24-2). When an injury occurs, platelets cluster at the site and start to stick to the damaged cell wall (adhesion). The platelets are activated by natural substances in the blood such as thromboxane A2 (TXA_2), thrombin, and collagen. After platelets are activated, a cascade of events occurs that attracts more platelets to the region (aggregation) and causes fibrin to combine with the platelets. This strengthens the clot.

Although aspirin is a nonprescription drug, it is effective for the management of post–myocardial infarction and stroke. In addition to its antiplatelet activity, aspirin blocks the enzyme cyclooxygenase (see Chapter 10), reducing plaque formation. Aspirin inhibits prostaglandin synthesis, which decreases TXA_2.

Abciximab, eptifibatide, and tirofiban are glycoprotein IIb/IIIa inhibitors that block the final pathway of platelet aggregation. They are administered parenterally. Ticlopidine interferes with platelet adhesion and aggregation. Ticlopidine also decreases the thickness or viscosity of blood by reducing the concentration of fibrinogen. Clopidogrel's mechanism of action is similar to that of ticlopidine. Dipyridamole inhibits platelet aggregation and is a coronary vasodilator.

Pharmacokinetics

Oral absorption of aspirin, clopidogrel, and ticlopidine is good. The bioavailability of ticlopidine is enhanced by administering the drug with food. The bioavailability of clopidogrel and aspirin is unaffected by food; however, food may decrease the bioavailability of dipyridamole.

The maximum effects on platelets occur within 30 minutes of administration of aspirin and abciximab. A continuous infusion of abciximab must be given to maintain therapeutic blood levels. The effect on platelets lasts longer when abciximab is administered than tirofiban. Tirofiban has an elimination half-life of 2 hours. The peak effect of clopidogrel and ticlopidine is delayed and may take up to 4 days to be reached.

Adverse Reactions

Bleeding is a common side effect of antiplatelet drugs. Black, tarry stools; blood in vomit, urine, or stools; nosebleeds; and red or purple spots on the skin may indicate bleeding. Other side effects associated with antiplatelet drugs are skin rash or itching, stomach pain, and pain at the injection site (abciximab). Less commonly, patients may experience difficulty breathing, dizziness, weakness, joint pain, and bone marrow toxicity. Eptifibatide is contraindicated in patients undergoing renal dialysis.

Precautions

Many drugs can enhance the effects of antiplatelet drugs and increase the potential for bleeding or hemorrhage. Antiplatelet drugs should not be combined with anticoagulants without medical supervision. Nonprescription drugs such as nonsteroidal anti-inflammatory drugs (NSAIDs, e.g., ibuprofen), vitamin supplements (fish oil), and herbs (feverfew, garlic, ginger) can also cause interactions.

Antiplatelet Drugs

Generic Name	U.S. Brand Name(s) Canadian Brand(s)	Dosage Forms and Strengths
aspirin*	Aspirin, Bayer Low Strength, Norwich Aspirin, St. Joseph Aspirin Adult Chewable	Tablets: 81 mg, 325 mg, 500 mg
	Ascriptin Enteric, Bayer Adult Low Strength EC Aspirin, Bayer Ecotrin, Ecotrin Maximum-Strength, Halfprin, St. Joseph Aspirin Adult EC	Tablets, delayed release: 81 mg, 325 mg
	Asaphen, Entrophen, Novasen	
clopidogrel*	Plavix	Tablets: 75 mg, 300 mg
	Plavix	
dipyridamole*	Persantine	Injection: 5 mg/mL
	Persantine	Tablets: 25 mg, 50 mg, 75 mg
ticlopidine*	Generics	Tablets: 250 mg
	Generics	
dipyridamole + aspirin*†	Aggrenox	Tablets: 200 mg dipyridamole + 25 mg aspirin
	Aggrenox	

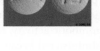

*Generic available.
*†Generic available in the United States only.

Glycoprotein IIb/IIIa Inhibitors

Generic Name	U.S. Brand Name(s) Canadian Brand(s)	Dosage Forms and Strengths
abciximab	Reopro	Injection: 2 mg/mL
	Reopro	
eptifibatide	Integrilin	Injection: 0.75 mg/mL, 2 mg/mL
	Integrilin	
tirofiban	Aggrastat	Injection: 50 mcg/mL premixed solution
	Aggrastat	

ANTICOAGULANTS

PARENTERALLY ADMINISTERED ANTICOAGULANTS

Heparin is an anticoagulant that is derived from pig intestines or cow lungs. The extraction process results in a mixture of fragments of varied molecular weights. Low-molecular-weight heparins (LMWHs) are produced by separating the heparin fragments.

Heparin and LMWH are administered parenterally to prevent the formation blood clots. Their uses include:

- Treatment of deep venous thrombosis
- Early treatment of acute myocardial infarction and unstable angina
- Prevention of pulmonary embolism
- Prevention of secondary myocardial infarction
- Prevention of clotting in indwelling catheters
- Prevention of clotting in devices used in cardiac surgery (e.g., stents or prosthetic valves)
- Bridge therapy with warfarin

ORALLY ADMINISTERED ANTICOAGULANTS

Warfarin and dabigatran are orally administered anticoagulants. Warfarin is used to prevent pulmonary embolism, thrombotic and embolic stroke, acute myocardial infarction, and atrial fibrillation. Dabigatran is the first oral anticoagulant to become available since the approval of warfarin more than 50 years ago. It is indicated to reduce the risk of stroke and systemic embolism in patients with nonvalvular atrial fibrillation. It is also approved in Canada and Europe to prevent clots in patients that have undergone hip and knee replacement surgeries.

Mechanism of Action of Anticoagulants

Heparin and LMWH increase the activity of antithrombin III (ATIII). This causes the inhibition of clotting factors of the common pathway, Xa and IIa (thrombin), and prevents clot formation (Figure 24-3). Fondaparinux and tinzaparin also inhibit Xa activity. Dabigatran is an oral direct thrombin inhibitor. To test the effectiveness of heparin and to determine whether dosage adjustments are necessary, an activated *partial thromboplastin time* (aPTT) test is performed. This test measures antithrombic activity. The aPTT is a test of the intrinsic anticoagulation pathway. It tests the time it takes for the blood to clot. If heparin is effective in reducing antithrombotic activity, the clotting time will be prolonged. The test is not performed when LMWH is administered because increases in the aPPT may occur even when antithrombotic activity has not increased. Anti-Xa activity is monitored when tinzaparin or fondaparinux are administered.

Warfarin interferes with the formation of vitamin K–dependent clotting factors. *Prothrombin time* (PT) is a test to determine how well warfarin is working to prevent clotting and to determine whether dosage adjustments are necessary. This test is also called an international normalized ratio (INR) test. The effectiveness of warfarin may be decreased by consumption of foods rich in vitamin K and nutritional supplements with vitamin K. Foods and beverages rich in vitamin K are chickpeas, kale, turnip greens, broccoli, beef and pork liver, parsley, spinach, and green tea.

Pharmacokinetics

Heparin and LMWH are administered by intravenous or subcutaneous injection. Oral absorption is poor. LMWH differs from heparin in a variety of ways. LMWH can be dosed less frequently than heparin, yet they are equally effective. Heparin is dosed two or three times a day, and LMWH is dosed once daily. LMWH has higher bioavailability, increased half-life, fewer side effects (lower risk of thrombocytopenia and osteoporosis), and less protein binding. Higher doses of heparin must be administered because of protein binding.

Warfarin has good oral absorption and bioavailability. The maximum effects of warfarin are not achieved until 4 to 5 days after initiating therapy because warfarin does not block the activity of existing coagulation factors. Stores of existing clotting factors must be depleted before the maximum effect of warfarin on clotting is achieved. Warfarin is highly protein bound, so it interacts with many other drugs. Pharmacy technicians should alert a pharmacist whenever a drug interaction is reported.

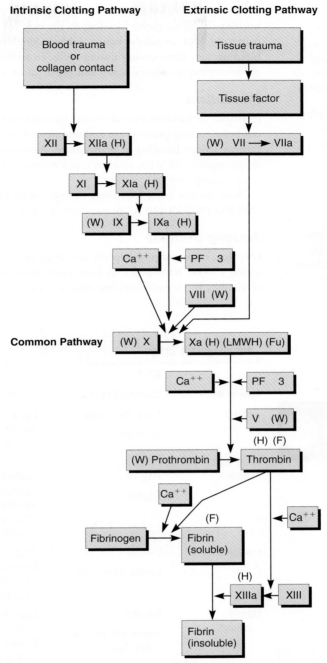

FIGURE 24-3 Clotting pathways. (From Clayton BD, Stock YN, Harroun RD: *Basic pharmacology for nurses*, ed 14. St. Louis, 2007, Mosby.)

BRIDGE THERAPY WITH LOW-MOLECULAR-WEIGHT HEPARIN AND WARFARIN

Patients transitioning between LMWH injections and oral therapy with warfarin may take both drugs for a brief time. This is called bridge therapy. Bridge therapy is continued until warfarin therapeutic level is achieved. INR level is between 2.0 and 3.0 (typically 2-3 days); then heparin is discontinued.

Adverse Reactions

Warfarin has an unpredictable and variable effect, a narrow therapeutic window requiring frequent INR monitoring, and numerous food and drug interactions. Adverse drug reactions to administered

TECH ALERT!
Warfarin can cause fetal abnormalities, so pharmacy technicians should apply the warning label "AVOID PREGNANCY" to prescription vials.

TECH NOTE!
Warfarin tablets are color coded to reduce medication errors.

anticoagulants include skin rash; itching; fever; pain; irritation or bleeding at the injection site; bruising; bleeding gums; bleeding in the eye; red spots on the skin; nosebleeds; back or stomach pain; cold, blue, or painful hands and feet; coughing up blood; difficulty breathing; heavy menstrual bleeding; and dizziness or fainting spells. In addition to bleeding, dabigatran may cause dyspepsia, gastroesophageal reflux disease, and peptic ulcer. Heparin and LMWH can cause osteoporosis.

Precautions

Pharmacy technicians should remind patients taking anticoagulants to seek the advice of a pharmacist before taking prescription and nonprescription drugs. Many drugs interact with anticoagulants, causing serious bleeding or hemorrhage. Anticoagulants should not be combined with antiplatelet drugs, aspirin, NSAIDs, vitamin supplements, and herbs (e.g., feverfew, fish oil supplements, garlic, ginger, ginkgo biloba).

Warfarin can cause fetal abnormalities, so pharmacy technicians should apply the warning label "AVOID PREGNANCY" to prescription vials.

Treating Overdose

Overdose of warfarin or heparin can result in hemorrhage and death. Overdose may be treated by giving a blood transfusion. In some cases, warfarin overdose can be reversed by the administration of vitamin K. Heparin overdose may be treated by the administration of protamine sulfate.

Anticoagulant Drugs

Generic Name	U.S. Brand Name(s) / Canadian Brand(s)	Dosage Forms and Strengths
warfarin*	Coumadin, Jantoven	**Powder, for injection:** 5 mg/vial[†]
	Coumadin	**Tablets:** 1 mg, 2 mg, 2.5 mg, 3 mg, 4 mg, 5 mg, 6 mg, 7.5 mg, 10 mg
dalteparin	Fragmin	**Solution, for injection:** 10,000, 12,500, 25,000 international units/mL
	Fragmin	**Injection, prefilled syringe:** 2500 units/0.2 mL, 5000 units/0.2 mL 7500 units/0.3 mL, 10,000 units/0.4 mL, 12,500 units/0.5 mL, 15,000 units/0.6 mL, 18,000 units/0.72 mL
enoxaparin*[†]	Lovenox	**Solution, for injection:** 100 mg/mL, 300 mg/3 mL
	Lovenox, Lovenox HP	**Injection, prefilled syringe:** 30 mg/0.3 mL, 40 mg/0.4 mL, 60 mg/0.6 mL[†], 80 mg/0.8 mL[†], 100 mg/1 mL, 120 mg/0.8 mL, 150 mg/mL[†]
heparin sodium*	Generics	**Solution, for injection (Heparin Lock Flush):** 10 units/mL, 100 units/mL
	Heparin Leo, Heparin Lock Flush	**Solution, for injection:** 1000 units/mL, 5000 units/mL, 10,000 units/mL, 20,000 units/mL
tinzaparin	Innohep	**Solution, for injection:** 10,000 units/mL[‡], 20,000 units/mL
	Innohep	
fondaparinux*[†]	Arixtra	**Solution, for injection:** 2.5 mg/0.5 mL, 5 mg/0.4 mL[†], 7.5 mg/0.6 mL[†], 10 mg/0.8 mL[†], 12.5 mg/mL[‡]
	Arixtra	
argatroban	Argatroban	**Solution, for injection:** 100 mg/mL
	Argatroban	**Solution, for injection (sodium chloride 0.9%):** 1 mg/mL (50 mL, 125 mL)
dabigatran	Pradaxa	**Capsule:** 75 mg, 110 mg[‡], 150 mg

*Generic available.
*[†]Generic available in the United States only.
[†]Strength available in the United States only.
[‡]Strength available in Canada only.

TABLE 24-3   **Sources of Thrombolytics**

Thrombolytic	Source
Alteplase (t-PA), reteplase (r-PA)	Recombinant DNA
Streptokinase	β-Hemolytic streptococci
Anistreplase (APSAC) (not marketed)	Synthetic streptococcal culture
Tenecteplase	Human tissue plasminogen activator
Urokinase	Human kidney cell extracts

THROMBOLYTICS

Just as the body has a mechanism to form clots at the site of injury to prevent hemorrhage, the body also has a system to stop excessive clot formation, thereby avoiding obstructions to blood flow in blood vessels. *Thrombolytics*, also called fibrinolytics, are drugs that can dissolve blood clots. The drugs are administered in the early stage of stroke to open blood vessels in the brain. They are also used in the treatment of acute myocardial infarction. They are derived from a variety of sources (Table 24-3).

Mechanism of Action

Thrombolytic agents currently in use in the United States and Canada are alteplase, tenecteplase, and reteplase. Streptokinase is also marketed in the United States only. All activate the fibrinolytic system, the body's normal system for preventing excess clotting. Alteplase is a tissue plasminogen activator produced by recombinant DNA technology. Tissue plasminogen activator is a naturally occurring thrombolytic substance. Thrombolytics dissolve blood clots that have formed in blood vessels. They increase the activity of plasmin, an enzyme that digests fibrin and other clotting factors. Without fibrin, the structure of the thrombin clot is weakened, and the clot dissolves.

Pharmacokinetics

Thrombolytics work rapidly. They can reopen an obstructed blood vessel within 90 minutes of administration. Alteplase, streptokinase, and tenecteplase differ in specificity and half-life. The half-life for alteplase is 30 to 45 minutes; it is 20 to 24 minutes for tenecteplase. All thrombolytics lose shelf life rapidly after reconstitution. They must be stored in the refrigerator and used within 24 hours.

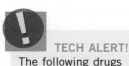

TECH ALERT!
The following drugs have look-alike and sound-alike issues: Lovenox, Lanoxin, Avonex, Luvox, Levaquin, and Lotronex; Coumadin, Cardura, Cordarone, Kemadrin, and Ambien

Thrombolytic Agents

Generic Name	U.S. Brand Name(s) / Canadian Brand(s)	Dosage Forms and Strengths
alteplase (t-PA)	Activase, Cathflo Activase powder	Injection, powder for reconstitution (Activase): 50 mg (29 million international units), 100 mg (58 million international units); 2 mg (Cathflo Activase)
	Activase, Cathflo Activase	
reteplase (r-PA)	Retavase	Injection, powder for reconstitution: 10.4 unit vial
	Retavase	
streptokinase##	Streptase	Injection, powder for reconstitution: 250,000 units/vial, 750,000 units/vial, 1,500,000 units/vial
	Not available	
tenecteplase	TNKase	Injection, powder for reconstitution: 50 mg
	TNKase	

##Available in the United States only.

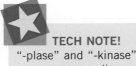

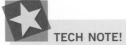

Adverse Reactions

The thrombolytics must be administered within the first 1 to 3 hours after a stroke occurs. Thereafter, the risk of hemorrhage exceeds the benefit of administering clot-dissolving drugs. The risk of intracranial hemorrhage, leading to irreversible damage or death, increases exponentially over time. Thrombolytics can cause bruising and bleeding in the gastrointestinal tract, genitourinary tract, and mouth (gums) in addition to bleeding in the brain. Other adverse reactions are nausea, vomiting, hypotension, transient arrhythmia, allergic reaction, and fever.

Drugs That Treat Hyperlipidemia

Hyperlipidemia is a disorder associated with dysfunctional fat metabolism. While fats are necessary to form steroid hormones, bile, prostaglandins, and cell membranes, excessive buildup in the blood (hyperlipidemia) is a significant risk factor for stroke and myocardial infarction. A principal focus for prevention of cardiovascular disease and stroke is treatment of hyperlipidemia. The emphasis is on reducing LDLs and raising HDL levels.

Low-density lipoprotein is known as "bad cholesterol" because elevated LDL cholesterol levels promote plaque buildup in arteries, atherothrombosis, and vasoconstriction. All increase the risk of cardiovascular disease and stroke. Recent evidence has shown that increasing HDL ("good cholesterol") in addition to reducing LDL cholesterol can further lower the risk for cardiovascular disease even in persons who have normal HDL levels before starting HDL drug therapy. HDL controls excessive levels of LDL by transporting cholesterol from cells in the artery wall back to the liver for removal. Atherosclerosis is a chronic inflammatory disorder, and HDL has protective anti-inflammatory properties. HDL acts as an antioxidant, diminishing LDL oxidation and reducing inflammation and oxidative stress. HDL also has antithrombotic, vasodilatory, and anti-infectious properties, all of which protect against cardiovascular disease.

Lipid-lowering drugs interfere with steps in the lipid metabolism pathway (Figure 24-4). They may affect cholesterol synthesis or elimination in bile or act on LDL metabolism. Although the mechanisms of action may vary, all lipid-lowering drugs reduce LDL and *triglyceride* levels.

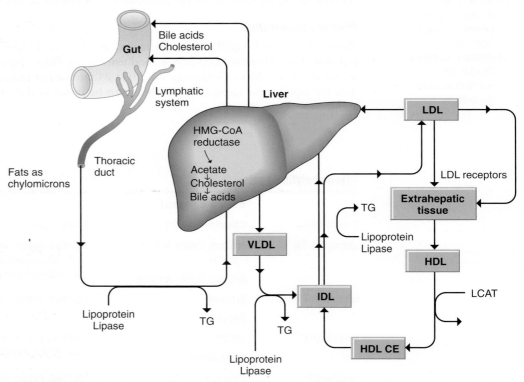

FIGURE 24-4 Lipid metabolism pathways. VLDL, Very low density liproprotein; HDL, high density liproprotein; LD, low density liprotein. (From Lilley LL, Harrington S, Snyder JS: *Pharmacology and the nursing process*, ed 5. St. Louis, 2007, Mosby.)

HMG COA REDUCTASE INHIBITORS

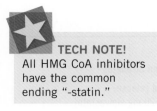

Hydroxymethylglutaryl (HMG) CoA reductase inhibitors are also called "statins." Statins are more effective than other classes of lipid-lowering drugs at lowering LDL (up to 60%). They have been shown to only minimally elevate HDL (up to 16%) above pre-drug levels.

Mechanism of Action

HMG CoA reductase is an enzyme that is involved in the final step of cholesterol synthesis. Statins also increase LDL clearance. Simvastatin and lovastatin are prodrugs and must undergo metabolic changes before they are pharmacologically active.

Adverse Reactions

Myositis (inflammation of muscle) and **rhabdomyolysis** (breakdown of muscle fibers and release of contents into the circulation) are serious, life-threatening muscle disorders that may be caused by statins. Statins can also elevate liver enzymes, resulting in liver dysfunction. More common and less serious side effects include diarrhea, gas, headache, joint pain, nausea, vomiting, stomach upset or pain, and tiredness.

Statins (HMG CoA Inhibitors)

	Generic Name	U.S. Brand Name(s) / Canadian Brand(s)	Dosage Forms and Strengths
	atorvastatin*	Lipitor	**Tablets:** 10 mg, 20 mg, 40 mg, 80 mg
		Lipitor	
	fluvastatin*†	Lescol, Lescol XL	**Capsules (Lescol):** 20 mg, 40 mg
		Lescol, Lescol XL	**Tablets (Lescol XL):** 80 mg
	lovastatin*	Altocor, Altoprev, Mevacor	**Tablets (Mevacor):** 10 mg†, 20 mg, 40 mg
		Mevacor	**Tablets, extended release (Altocor, Altoprev):** 20 mg, 40 mg, 60 mg
	pravastatin*	Pravachol	**Tablets:** 10 mg, 20 mg, 40 mg, 80 mg†
		Pravachol	
	rosuvastatin*‡	Crestor	**Tablets:** 5 mg, 10 mg, 20 mg, 40 mg
		Crestor	
	simvastatin*	Zocor	**Tablets:** 5 mg, 10 mg, 20 mg, 40 mg, 80 mg
		Zocor	
	pitavastatin	Livalo	**Tablets:** 1 mg, 2 mg, 4 mg
		Not available	
	ezetimibe + simvastatin*	Vytorin	**Tablets:** 10 mg ezetimibe + 10 mg simvastatin
		Not available	10 mg ezetimibe + 20 mg simvastatin
			10 mg ezetimibe + 40 mg simvastatin
			10 mg ezetimibe + 80 mg simvastatin

Continued

Statins (HMG CoA Inhibitors)—cont'd

Generic Name	U.S. Brand Name(s) Canadian Brand(s)	Dosage Forms and Strengths
niacin (extended release) + simvastatin	Simcor Not available	**Tablets, extended release:** niacin 500 mg + 20 mg simvastatin niacin 500 mg + 40 mg simvastatin niacin 750 mg + 20 mg simvastatin niacin 1000 mg + 20 mg simvastatin niacin 1000 mg + 40 mg simvastatin
niacin (extended release) + lovastatin	Advicor Advicor	**Tablets:** 500 mg niacin + 20 mg lovastatin 750 mg niacin + 20 mg lovastatin[†] 1000 mg niacin + 20 mg lovastatin 1000 mg niacin + 40 mg lovastatin[†]
atorvastatin + amlodipine	Caduet Caduet	**Tablets:** atorvastatin 10 mg + amlodipine 2.5 mg atorvastatin 10 mg + amlodipine 5 mg atorvastatin 10 mg + amlodipine 10 mg atorvastatin 20 mg + amlodipine 2.5 mg atorvastatin 20 mg + amlodipine 5 mg atorvastatin 20 mg + amlodipine 10 mg atorvastatin 40 mg + amlodipine 2.5 mg atorvastatin 40 mg + amlodipine 5 mg atorvastatin 40 mg + amlodipine 10 mg atorvastatin 80 mg + amlodipine 5 mg atorvastatin 80 mg + amlodipine 10 mg

*Generic available.
*[†]Generic available in the United States only.
*[‡]Generic available Canada only.
[†]Strength available in the United States only.

TECH ALERT!
The following drugs have look-alike and sound-alike issues: atorvastatin and pravastatin; Lipitor and Zocor; fluvastatin and fluoxetine; lovastatin and lotensin

TECH ALERT!
Lopid, Levbid, Lorabid, and Slo-bid have look-alike and sound-alike issues.

FIBRIC ACID DERIVATIVES

Fibric acid derivatives or fibrates are regarded as broad-spectrum lipid-lowering drugs. Fibrates increase the clearance of very low-density lipoprotein (VLDL). Fibrates are less effective than statins at reducing LDL (≈10%) and in elevating HDL (up to 10% above pretherapy levels).

Mechanism of Action

Fibrates appear to activate a protein called peroxisome proliferator-activated receptor α(PPAR-α). PPAR-α activates the enzyme lipoprotein lipase and ultimately results in decreased formation of very low-density lipoprotein (VLDL) cholesterol (which is converted into LDL cholesterol) and triglycerides and an increase in HDL cholesterol.

Precautions

If administered together, statins and fibrates produce a drug interaction that may increase the likelihood of development of myopathies.

BILE ACID SEQUESTRANTS

Bile acid sequestrants promote intestinal clearance of cholesterol. They are administered to reduce LDL levels. They are not absorbed and therefore are the drugs of choice for use in pregnancy.

Mechanism of Action

Bile acid sequestrants bind to cholesterol-containing bile acids in the intestine. The bound complex is insoluble and is excreted in the feces rather than reabsorbed. Cholesterol depletion increases LDL receptor activity, which increases removal of LDLs from the blood.

Fibric Acid Derivatives

Generic Name	U.S. Brand Name(s) Canadian Brand(s)	Dosage Forms and Strengths
gemfibrozil*	Lopid	Tablets: 300 mg‡, 600 mg
	Lopid	
fenofibric acid*	Fibricor	Tablets: 35 mg, 105 mg
	Not available	
fenofibrate*	Antara, Fenoglide, Lipofen, Tricor, Triglide	Capsules: 50 mg, 150 mg (Lipofen) Capsules (micronized): 43 mg, 130 mg (Antara); 67 mg, 134 mg, 200 mg (Tricor), Lipidil micro (200 mg only) Tablets: 50 mg, 160 mg (Triglide); 40 mg, 120 mg (Fenoglide), 48 mg, 145 mg (Tricor, Lipidil EZ) Tablets, micronized: 54 mg, 160 mg (Tricor), 100 mg, 160 mg (Lipidil Supra)
	Lipidil EZ, Lipidil Micro, Lipidil Supra	

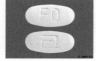

*Generic available.
‡Strength available in Canada only.

Bile Acid Sequestrants

Generic Name	U.S. Brand Name(s) Canadian Brand(s)	Dosage Forms and Strengths
cholestyramine*	Prevalite	Powder, for reconstitution (regular and sugar free): 4 g/packet or scoop
	Olestyr	
colesevelam	Welchol	Tablets: 625 mg Powder, for suspension##: 1.875 g, 3.75 g
	Lodalis	
colestipol*†	Colestid	Granules, for reconstitution: 5 g/packet or scoop Tablets: 1 g
	Colestid	
ezetimibe	Zetia	Tablets: 10 mg
	Ezetrol	

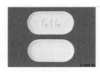

*Generic available.
*†Generic available in the United States only.
##Available in the United States only.

Adverse Effects and Precautions

Bile acid sequestrants produce bloating and gas and must be administered at least 1 hour before or 4 hours after other medications to avoid decreasing the absorption of other drugs. Bile acid sequestrants can lower body levels of fat-soluble vitamins such as vitamins A, D, E, and K. Unfortunately, the resins can increase triglyceride levels.

NICOTINIC ACID DERIVATIVES

Niacin is vitamin B_3. It is less effective at decreasing LDL than statins, but it is the most effective lipid-lowering agent for increasing HDL (up to 35%). Niacin produces vasodilation, causing flushing, pruritus, headaches, or pain, which some find intolerable. Niacinamide does not produce vasodilation, but it is not effective in lowering lipid levels. Sustained release preparations may minimize vasodilation and gastrointestinal upset. Glucose intolerance and abnormal liver function may limit the use of niacin.

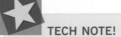

Mechanism of Action

The mechanism of niacin's antilipemic action is unknown. It is thought that effects may be linked to decreased VLDL synthesis and clearance in the liver; decreased VLDL triglyceride transport; and actions on free fatty acid release, lipoprotein lipase activity, and triglyceride synthesis. Nicotinic acid elevation of HDL is possibly associated with an increase in serum levels of Apo A-I and lipoprotein A-I, and a decrease in serum levels of Apo-B.

Nicotinic Acid

Generic Name	U.S. Brand Name(s) Canadian Brand(s)	Dosage Forms and Strengths
niacin*	Niaspan, Niacor Niaspan, Niaspan FCT	Capsules, time released: 125 mg, 250 mg, 400 mg, 500 mg (various generic) Tablets: 50 mg, 100 mg, 250 mg, 500 mg (Niacor, various) Tablets, time released: 500 mg, 750 mg, 1000 mg (Niaspan, Niaspan FCT)

*Generic available.

Summary of Drugs Used in the Treatment and Prevention of Myocardial Infarction and Stroke

Generic Name	U.S. Brand Name	Dosage Form(s)	Usual Dose and Dosing Schedule	Warning Labels
Drugs to Control Hemostasis				
Antiplatelet Drugs				
abciximab	ReoPro	Injection, IV infusion	0.25 mg/kg bolus followed by 0.125 mcg/kg/min infusion for up to 12 hours	DO NOT SHAKE. AVOID ASPIRIN, NSAIDs, AND OTHER OTC DRUGS WITHOUT SUPERVISION. REFRIGERATE AT 2° TO 8° C; DO NOT FREEZE.
aspirin	Various	Tablet, enteric-coated tablet	81-325 mg once daily	TAKE WITH FOOD. AVOID PREGNANCY (THIRD TRIMESTER).
eptifibatide	Integrilin	Injection	180 mcg/kg IV bolus (maximum, 22.6 mg); 2 mcg/kg/min continuous IV infusion (maximum, 15 mg/hr)	REFRIGERATE AT 2° TO 8° C; DO NOT FREEZE—eptifibatide. PROTECT FROM LIGHT. DISCARD DILUTED SOLUTIONS WITHIN 24 HOURS.
tirofiban	Aggrastat	Injection	0.4 mcg/kg/min IV for 30 minutes followed by 0.1 mcg/kg/min IV	STABLE AT ROOM TEMP. FOR 24 HOURS—tirofiban.
clopidogrel	Plavix	Tablet	75 mg once daily	TAKE ON AN EMPTY STOMACH—dipyridamole. AVOID ASPIRIN, NSAIDs, AND OTHER OTC DRUGS. TAKE WITH FOOD—ticlopidine. REPORT SIGNS OF BLEEDING.
dipyridamole	Persantine	Tablet	75 mg 3 times/day up to 400 mg/day	
ticlopidine	Ticlid	Tablet	250 mg twice daily	

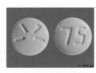

Summary of Drugs Used in the Treatment and Prevention of Myocardial Infarction and Stroke—cont'd

Generic Name	U.S. Brand Name	Dosage Form(s)	Usual Dose and Dosing Schedule	Warning Labels
Anticoagulants				
dalteparin	Fragmin	Injection SC	150 international units/kg/day	AVOID OTC WITHOUT MEDICAL SUPERVISION—vitamins, herbals, analgesics
enoxaparin	Lovenox	Injection IV and SC	30 mg IV bolus followed by 1 mg/kg SC every 12 hours for up to 7 days	AVOID ASA AND NSAIDs WITHOUT MEDICAL SUPERVISION—all. REPORT SIGNS OF BLEEDING—all.
heparin Na$^+$	Generics	Injection IV	60 international units/kg IV bolus with initial dose of thrombolytic therapy; then 12 international units/kg per hour IV	AVOID PREGNANCY—warfarin. SWALLOW WHOLE; DO NOT CRUSH OR CHEW—dabigatran. PROTECT FROM MOISTURE—dabigatran.
tinzaparin	Innohep	SC injection	175 units/kg (or 0.00875 mL/kg) SC once daily	STORE IN MANUFACTURER'S ORIGINAL PACKAGING—dabigatran.
dabigatran	Pradaxa	Capsule	150 mg orally twice daily	AVOID ABRUPT DISCONTINUATION
warfarin	Coumadin	Injection, Tablet	2-5 mg/day for 2-4 days; then adjust as required	
Thrombolytics				
alteplase (t-PA)	Activase	IV	15 mg IV bolus followed by 50 mg infused over 30 minutes; then 35 mg infused over 60 minutes	REFRIGERATE RECONSTITUTED SOLUTION (2°-8° C). STABLE FOR 24 HOURS AFTER RECONSTITUTION (UNDER REFRIGERATION).
streptokinase	Streptase	IV	1,500,000 units by IV infusion over 60 min or 20,000 units intracoronary followed by 2000 units administered over 1 hour	REFRIGERATE RECONSTITUTED SOLUTION (2°-8° C). STABLE FOR 24 HOURS AFTER RECONSTITUTION (under refrigeration). DO NOT SHAKE.
tenecteplase	TNKase	IV	30-50 mg bolus over 5 seconds	STABLE FOR 8 HOURS AFTER RECONSTITUTION (2°-8° C). REFRIGERATE RECONSTITUTED SOLUTION (2°-8° C). DO NOT SHAKE.
reteplase (r-PA)	Retavase	IV	10 units IV bolus over 2 minutes followed by another 10-unit bolus	STABLE FOR 4 HOURS AFTER RECONSTITUTION (2°-30° C).

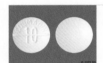

Continued

Summary of Drugs Used in the Treatment and Prevention of Myocardial Infarction and Stroke—cont'd

Generic Name	U.S. Brand Name	Dosage Form(s)	Usual Dose and Dosing Schedule	Warning Labels
Combination Drugs				
aspirin + dipyridamole	Aggrenox	Capsule	Take 1 capsule twice daily	SWALLOW WHOLE; DO NOT CRUSH OR CHEW.
Drugs to Control Hyperlipidemia				
HMG CoA reductase inhibitors (statins)				
atorvastatin	Lipitor	Tablet	10-80 mg once daily	AVOID GRAPEFRUIT JUICE—atorvastatin, lovastatin, simvastatin. AVOID ALCOHOL.
lovastatin	Mevacor	Tablet	10-80 mg once daily	AVOID PREGNANCY—all. SWALLOW WHOLE; DO NOT CHEW—extended release.
fluvastatin	Lescol	Capsule	20-80 mg once daily	
pravastatin	Pravachol	Tablet	10-40 mg once daily	
rosuvastatin	Crestor	Tablet	10-40 mg once daily	
simvastatin	Zocor	Tablet	5-80 mg once daily; usually 40 mg daily	
pitavastatin	Livalo	Tablet	1-4 mg once daily	
Fibric Acid Derivatives				
fenofibrate	Tricor	Capsule	200 mg once daily	MAY CAUSE DROWSINESS—fenofibrate, fenofibric acid. AVOID PROLONGED EXPOSURE TO SUNLIGHT—fenofibrate, fenofibric acid.
fenofibric acid	Fibricor, Trilipix	Capsule	45-135 mg once daily (Trilipix); 35-105 mg once daily (Fibricor)	TAKE ON AN EMPTY STOMACH—gemfibrozil.
gemfibrozil	Lopid	Capsule	600 mg twice daily	
Bile Acid Sequestrants				
cholestyramine	Questran	Powder	4-8 g 2-3 times/day	TAKE 1 HOUR BEFORE OR 4 HOURS AFTER OTHER DRUGS.
colestipol	Colestid	Granule Tablet	5-15 g twice/day	RECONSTITUTE WITH 2 to 6 OZ OF LIQUID; SHAKE WELL.
colesevelam	Welchol	Tablet	1.9-4.4 g daily in 1-2 doses	SWALLOW WHOLE, TAKE WITH HALF GLASS WATER AND FOOD.

Summary of Drugs Used in the Treatment and Prevention of Myocardial Infarction and Stroke—cont'd

Generic Name	U.S. Brand Name	Dosage Form(s)	Usual Dose and Dosing Schedule	Warning Labels
Miscellaneous				
ezetimibe	Zetia	Tablet	10 mg once daily	AVOID ALCOHOL.
niacin (vit. B$_3$)	Various	Tablet	0.5-2 g 3 times/day	AVOID ALCOHOL.
	Niaspan	Capsule	1-2 g once daily	TAKE WITH FOOD.
Combination				
ezetimibe + simvastatin	Vytorin	Tablet	1 tablet once daily in the evening	AVOID GRAPEFRUIT JUICE. TAKE WITH FOOD. AVOID ALCOHOL. AVOID PREGNANCY AND BREASTFEEDING.
niacin + lovastatin	Advicor	Tablet	1-2 tablets at bedtime (maximum, 40 mg lovastatin + 2000 mg niacin/day)	
niacin + simvastatin	Simcor	Tablet	1-2 tablets daily at bedtime	

Chapter Summary

- Myocardial infarction is the leading cause of death in the United States.
- Stroke is the third leading cause of death in the United States.
- Strokes occur when brain cells are deprived of oxygen or are damaged by sudden bleeding into the brain.
- There are four major types of strokes: ischemic stroke, thrombotic stroke, embolic stroke, and hemorrhagic stroke.
- Transient ischemic attacks are also known as mini-strokes and last only a few minutes.
- Myocardial infarction produces symptoms that are similar to those of angina.
- Chronic inflammation of arteries that supply the heart and brain can also lead to stroke and myocardial infarction because vascular inflammation is a cause of atherosclerosis.
- Atherosclerosis (a buildup of lipids and plaque inside of artery walls) can block blood flow through arteries.
- Atherothrombosis (the formation of a blood clot in the artery) is triggered by atherosclerosis and can also cause clogged arteries.
- The risk for stroke and myocardial infarction is increased by nonmodifiable risk factors, modifiable risk factors, and chronic disease.
- Nonmodifiable risk factors are age, gender, and family history of stroke and myocardial infarction.
- Modifiable risk factors are smoking, heavy alcohol consumption, and diet high in cholesterol.
- Diseases that can increase risk for stroke and myocardial infarction are diabetes, hypertension, hyperlipidemia, atrial fibrillation, and infection.
- Drugs administered to prevent stroke and myocardial infarction control the buildup of lipids and plaque and reduce the formation of blood clots.

- Drugs that control hemostasis (the process of stopping the flow of blood) prevent the formation of clots that can obstruct the supply of blood to the brain and heart.
- Antithrombotic drugs include (1) agents that inhibit platelets; (2) anticoagulants, which attenuate coagulation; and (3) fibrinolytic agents. Fibrinolytics dissolve existing clots.
- Antiplatelet drugs interfere with early steps in the clot formation process.
- Aspirin is a nonprescription drug that has antiplatelet activity.
- Dabigatran is an oral direct thrombin inhibitor indicated to reduce the risk of stroke and systemic embolism in patients with nonvalvular atrial fibrillation.
- Abciximab, eptifibatide, and tirofiban are parenteral antiplatelet drugs. They block the final pathway for platelet aggregation
- Ticlopidine, clopidogrel, and dipyridamole are orally administered antiplatelet drugs.
- Bleeding is a common side effect of all antiplatelet drugs. Other side effects associated with antiplatelet drugs are skin rash or itching, stomach pain, and pain at the injection site (abciximab).
- Nonprescription drugs, vitamin supplements, and herbs can enhance the effects of antiplatelet drugs. These drugs include NSAIDs (e.g., ibuprofen), feverfew, fish oil supplements, garlic, and ginger.
- Heparin and LMWH are anticoagulants that are administered to prevent the formation of blood clots.
- LMWHs are not substitutable.
- To test the effectiveness of heparin and to determine whether dosage adjustments are necessary, an aPTT test is performed.
- Warfarin interferes with the formation of vitamin K–dependent clotting factors. PT is a test to determine how well warfarin is working to reduce clotting.
- Maximum effects of warfarin are not achieved until 4 to 5 days after initiating therapy.
- Warfarin can cause fetal abnormalities, so pharmacy technicians should apply the warning label "AVOID PREGNANCY" to prescription vials.
- Warfarin overdose is reversed by the administration of vitamin K. Heparin overdose is treated with protamine sulfate.
- Thrombolytics, also called fibrinolytics, are drugs that can dissolve blood clots and must be administered within the first few hours of a stroke.
- A principal focus for prevention of cardiovascular disease and stroke is treatment of hyperlipidemia.
- LDL is known as "bad cholesterol" because elevated LDL cholesterol levels promote plaque buildup in arteries, atherothrombosis, and vasoconstriction.
- Increasing HDL ("good cholesterol"), in addition to reducing LDL cholesterol, can further lower the risk for cardiovascular disease.
- Statins are HMG CoA reductase inhibitors and block the final step of cholesterol synthesis and promote LDL elimination.
- Fibrates increase clearance of VLDL. Fibrates are less effective than statins.
- Bile acid sequestrants promote intestinal clearance of cholesterol.
- Niacin is vitamin B_3. It is less effective at decreasing LDL than statins, but it is the most effective lipid-lowering agent for increasing HDL.

REVIEW
QUESTIONS

1. Strokes occur when brain cells are deprived of _____ or are damaged by sudden bleeding into the brain.
   a. carbon dioxide
   b. oxygen
   c. both a and b
   d. none of the above

2. _____ last only a few minutes and symptoms usually resolve within 1 hour.
   a. Embolic strokes
   b. Hemorrhagic strokes
   c. Transient ischemic attacks
   d. Aneurysms

3. Age does not pose a significant risk factor for stroke or myocardial infarction.
   a. true
   b. false

4. Drugs that control the rate of clot formation and clot dissolution are classified as _____ and can prevent stroke and myocardial infarction.
   a. antihyperlipidemics
   b. antifibrinolytics
   c. antithrombotics
   d. antihemorrhagics

5. Aspirin is not effective for the management of post–myocardial infarction and stroke.
   a. true
   b. false

6. _____ is a parenteral antiplatelet drug.
   a. Ticlopidine
   b. Dipyridamole
   c. Abciximab
   d. Simvastatin

7. Warfarin interferes with the formation of vitamin _____–dependent clotting factors.
   a. A
   b. D
   c. E
   d. K

8. Heparin and LMWH are administered to prevent the formation blood clots.
   a. true
   b. false

9. Thrombolytics must be administered within the first _____ hours after a stroke has occured.
   a. 1 to 3
   b. 2 to 4
   c. 3 to 5
   d. 4 to 6

10. Statin drugs primarily lower what kind of cholesterol?
    a. LDL
    b. bile
    c. HDL
    d. all of the above

TECHNICIAN'S
CORNER

1. What kind of reaction happens if aspirin and warfarin are used at the same time?
2. What kind of diet helps to lower cholesterol levels?

Bibliography

Chapman J: Therapeutic elevation of HDL-cholesterol to prevent atherosclerosis and coronary heart disease, *Pharmacol Ther* 111:893-908, 2006.

Hoffman R, Benz E, Shattil S, et al: *Hematology: Basic principles and practice*, ed 4, 2005, Figure 130-1, Chapter 130.

Kalant H, Grant D, Mitchell J: *Principles of medical pharmacology*, ed 7, Toronto, 2007, Elsevier Canada, A Division of Reed Elsevier Canada, pp 472-482.

Lance L, Lacy C, Armstrong L, et al: *Drug information handbook for the allied health professional*, ed 12, Hudson, OH, 2005, APhA Lexi-Comp.

National Heart, Lung, and Blood Institute: Heart attack. Bethesda, MD, National Institutes of Health, US Department of Health and Human Services. Available at: http://www.nhlbi.nih.gov/health/dci/Diseases/HeartAttack/HeartAttack_All.html.

National Heart, Lung, and Blood Institute: High blood cholesterol. Bethesda, MD, National Institutes of Health, US Department of Health and Human Services. Available at: http://www.nhlbi.nih.gov/health/dci/Diseases/Hbc/HBC_all.html.

National Institute of Neurological Disorders and Stroke: Stroke: Hope through research. Bethesda, MD, National Institute of Mental Health, National Institutes of Health, US Department of Health and Human Services, July 2004. Last updated December 20, 2006; NIH publication No. 99-2222. Available at: http://www.ninds.nih.gov/disorders/stroke/detail_stroke.htm.

Otto M, Hochadel M: Thrombolytic agents—Overview, *Clin Pharmacol*, 2000. Available at: http://www.clinicalpharmacology.com/apps/default.asp?entry=11andrNum=791.

Ringleb, P: Thrombolytics, anticoagulants, and antiplatelet agents, *Stroke* 37:312-313, 2006. Available at: http://stroke.ahajournals.org/cgi/content/full/37/2/312.

USP Center for Advancement of Patient Safety: *Use caution–avoid confusion,* USP Quality Review No. 79, Rockville, MD, April 2004, USP Center for Advancement of Patient Safety.

Vieson, K: Low-molecular weight heparins (LMWHs), *Clin Pharmacol*, 2001. Available at: http://www.clinicalpharmacology.com/apps/default.asp?entry=11andrNum=206.

Pradaxa- http://www.clinicalpharmacology.com/Forms/Monograph/monograph.aspx?cpnum=3547&sec=mondesc.

http://www.drugs.com/drug-class/fibric-acid-derivatives.html.

http://www.drugs.com/drug-class/bile-acid-sequestrants.html.

25

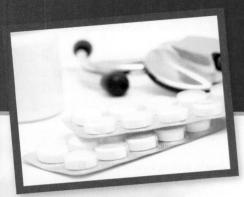

Treatment of Arrhythmia

Overview

The heart normally beats at a rate between 60 and 100 beats/min or approximately 100,000 beats per day. With each beat or contraction, blood is pumped throughout the body, supplying oxygen and nutrients to cells and organs, including the heart. An arrhythmia is defined as an irregular heart rhythm or a heart rate that is too rapid or too slow. Arrhythmias can produce heart rates that exceed 600 beats/min. An arrhythmia can impair the heart's ability to distribute blood. Symptoms of arrhythmia are listed in Box 25-1.

Atrial fibrillation is the most common arrhythmia, and although not usually life threatening, it is a risk factor for stroke. It affects approximately 1% of the population and it is estimated that it will affect nearly 15 million Americans by 2050. Risk factors for atrial fibrillation are similar to risk factors for coronary heart disease (CHD) and are similarly categorized as nonmodifiable risk factors, modifiable risk factors, and disease risk factors (Table 25-1). A description of these risk factors is found in chapters on hypertension, heart failure, myocardial infarction, and stroke (see Chapters 22 through 24).

Ventricular fibrillation is the leading cause of sudden cardiac death, killing nearly 600,000 people in the United States and Europe each year.

How Arrhythmias Are Formed

Heart contractions occur when cardiac cells "fire." This is known as ***depolarization***. During depolarization, positively charged ions enter the cells through specialized exchange channels, and an action potential is formed (Figure 25-1). Sodium entry initiates depolarization of the atria and ventricles, and calcium entry results in depolarization of the sinoatrial (SA) and atrioventricular (AV) nodes. When the heart cells have fired, another contraction cannot occur until repolarization occurs. ***Repolarization*** is the process of returning the cells to their resting state. The time it takes for repolarization to occur is called the ***refractory period***.

Arrhythmias occur when the cardiac ion exchange channels function improperly. This can result in excessive firing, extra currents during the refractory period, and establishment of sinus rhythm by nonpacemaker cells. These conditions may occur after a heart attack because fibrous scar tissue may develop in the healing process. Conduction is poor across fibrous tissue. Inflammation and oxidative stress (see Chapter 24) can cause arrhythmias, too. In addition, after arrhythmias have occurred, they may stimulate the formation of other arrhythmias. Moreover, treatment of arrhythmia can result in secondary arrhythmias.

BOX 25-1   **Symptoms of Arrhythmia**

- Palpitations or fluttering in the chest
- Rapid heart rate
- Slow heart rate
- Chest pain
- Shortness of breath
- Lightheadedness or dizziness
- Fainting

TABLE 25-1   **Risk Factors for Atrial Fibrillation**

Nonmodifiable	Age, gender, low heart rate, emotional stress
Modifiable	Obesity, smoking, excessive alcohol consumption, stimulant use
Disease	Hypertension, heart failure, CHD, stroke, infection, diabetes, thyroid disease, obstructive sleep apnea

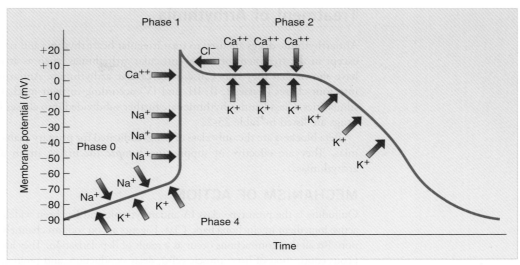

FIGURE 25-1 Action potential. (From Lilley LL, Harrington S, Snyder JS: *Pharmacology and the nursing process*, ed 5. St Louis, 2007, Mosby.)

Types of Arrhythmias

ATRIAL FLUTTER

Atrial flutter refers to an irregular heartbeat in which contractions in the atrium exceed the number of contractions in the ventricle. The heart rate may be between 160 and 350 beats/minute. It usually occurs in the right atrium and is treated by inserting a catheter into the atrium (catheter ablation) rather than drug therapy.

ATRIAL FIBRILLATION

Atrial fibrillation is defined as rapid and uncoordinated contractions of the atria. The heart may beat between 300 to 400 beats/minute. Atrial fibrillation is the most common arrhythmia and occurs with increasing frequency as people age, affecting approximately 10% of the population after age 80 years. Atrial fibrillation often accompanies other cardiac diseases such as coronary artery disease, heart failure, and hypertension.

SUPRAVENTRICULAR TACHYCARDIA

Supraventricular tachycardia (SVT) occurs in areas of the heart that lay above the ventricles. SVT may occur intermittently (paroxysmal) or frequently. The heartbeat may increase up to 200 beats/minute and last several seconds to a few hours.

VENTRICULAR TACHYCARDIA

Ventricular tachycardia causes the ventricles to beat faster than 200 beats/minute. It may occur when the spread of electrical impulses between heart chambers is "short circuited" across scar tissue caused by a heart attack.

VENTRICULAR FIBRILLATION

Ventricular fibrillation may cause the ventricles to beat faster than 600 beats/minute. Ventricular fibrillation is life threatening because the ventricles are unable to fill with blood and blood is not effectively pumped throughout the body. Ventricular fibrillation is typically reversed only after electrical cardioversion. *Electrical cardioversion* is the process of applying an electrical shock to the heart with a defibrillator to return the heart to a normal rhythm.

The mechanism for ventricular fibrillation is thought to be complex, and multiple mechanisms are involved, including self-generated reentry of unstable wavelets and rapid, intermittent excitation alternating with conduction block.

Treatment of Arrhythmia

Antiarrhythmic drugs are used to treat irregular heart rhythms and rate. Their use has been declining except in the treatment of supraventricular arrhythmias, such as atrial fibrillation, because studies have shown that they may cause other cardiac arrhythmias. Antiarrhythmic drugs are categorized into four classes (classes I, II, III, and IV) according to their mechanisms of action and structural similarities. Class I antiarrhythmics are further subdivided into classes IA, IB and IC. Antiarrhythmic drugs are listed in Table 25-2.

Beta blockers are the only class of drugs indicated for primary management of ventricular arrhythmias. They are effective in suppressing *ectopic* (occurring in an abnormal location) beats and arrhythmias.

MECHANISM OF ACTION

Quinidine is the prototype class IA antiarrhythmic and has been widely used since the 1920s. It is the active ingredient in cinchona bark. Class I agents act on sodium channels and slow the rate of depolarization. Recall that contractions occur as a result of depolarization. They also reduce *automaticity* (spontaneous contraction of heart muscle cells), delay conduction, and prolong the time between contractions (refractory period). Class IA agents have a moderate effect on depolarization and intermediate effects on the sodium channel. Class IB agents have a minimal effect on depolarization, and their effect on the sodium channel is rapid. The effect of class IC antiarrhythmic drugs on sodium channels is very slow, and they produce marked effects on depolarization. They are 80% to 90% effective at suppressing arrhythmias. All class I antiarrhythmic agents may be administered orally except lidocaine.

Class II antiarrhythmic agents are β-adrenergic antagonists. Beta blockers antagonize stimulation of the AV and SA nodes. They increase the refractory period, decrease automaticity, and slow conduction velocity.

Amiodarone, dofetilide, dronedarone, ibutilide, and sotalol are class III antiarrhythmic agents. Class III antiarrhythmic agents block potassium channels except for ibutilide, which promotes the influx of sodium through slow inward sodium channels. Dronedarone also inhibits sodium and calcium ion channels. Class III antiarrhythmics prolong depolarization and prolong the refractory period. Amiodarone's effectiveness is achieved through multiple mechanisms of action, and it can suppress both supraventricular and ventricular arrhythmias, notably by increasing reentry time. Dofetilide, ibutilide, and sotalol are indicated for the treatment of atrial fibrillation and atrial flutter. Dronedarone is only indicated for the treatment of atrial fibrillation. Sotalol is also indicated for ventricular tachycardia. Class IV antiarrhythmic agents are calcium channel blockers, although only verapamil and diltiazem are effective in treating supraventricular arrhythmias, atrial fibrillation, and atrial flutter.

ADVERSE REACTIONS

All antiarrhythmic agents are proarrhythmic (can cause other arrhythmias). They all can cause bradycardia, hypotension, and dizziness. Most antiarrhythmic agents cause nausea and vomiting, diarrhea, or constipation. Class I antiarrhythmic agents can produce local anesthesia and itchy, flaky rashes. Class II antiarrhythmics can contribute to depression in addition to the general side effects listed. Amiodarone has many adverse effects, and up to 20% of patients discontinue the drug because of side

TECH NOTE!
Unlike other commercially available class III antiarrhythmic agents that block outward potassium currents, ibutilide exerts its actions by promoting the influx of sodium through slow inward sodium channels.

TABLE 25-2   **Antiarrhythmic Drugs**

Class	Category	Generic Name	Site of Action
Class IA	Na⁺ channel blocker	quinidine sulfate, quinidine gluconate, procainamide, disopyramide	Na⁺ channels
Class IB	Na⁺ channel blocker	lidocaine, mexiletine, tocainide	Na⁺ channels
Class IC	Na⁺ channel blocker	flecainide, propafenone	Na⁺ channels
Class II	β-Blockers	propranolol, esmolol, acebutolol	β-Adrenergic receptors
Class III	K⁺ channel blocker	amiodarone, sotalol, dofetilide, dronedarone, ibutilide	K⁺ channels
Class IV	Ca²⁺ channel blockers	verapamil	Ca²⁺ channels

effects. Common side effects are photosensitivity, skin discoloration, stomach upset, visual disturbances (sun sensitivity, blurred vision, dry eyes), and corneal deposits. Calcium channel blockers (class IV) produce headache, flushing, and peripheral edema in addition to the adverse reactions listed earlier.

PRECAUTIONS

Tinnitus is a sign of quinidine toxicity. Quinidine and procainamide can also produce a lupus-like syndrome, causing arthritis and chest pain. Class II antiarrhythmics (beta blockers) should be used with caution in patients with asthma, diabetes, and heart failure. They can cause bronchospasm and mask the signs of hypoglycemia and may increase or decrease blood sugar levels. Amiodarone may induce thyroid disease and fatal hepatotoxicity. Dofetilide is contraindicated in renal failure (creatine clearance <20 mL/min), and ibutilide should be avoided in women who are pregnant or breast-feeding.

MISCELLANEOUS

Digoxin and phenytoin are miscellaneous drugs used in the treatment of arrhythmias. Phenytoin administration for arrhythmia is uncommon; and not approved by the U.S. Food and Drug Administration. Digoxin, on the other hand, is approved for the treatment of atrial fibrillation. It reduces arrhythmias by slowing the conduction velocity and prolonging the refractory period in the Purkinje fibers and AV node. In the atria and ventricles, digoxin shortens the refractory period. Digoxin also reduces electrical discharges from the SA node. It may be administered intravenously or orally. Digoxin has a narrow therapeutic index, so it is important to avoid excessive doses. It is administered so the first dose equals approximately half the total daily dose. The remainder is divided in half and given every 6 hours for two doses. The adverse effects of digoxin are described in Chapter 23.

TECH ALERT!
The following drugs have look-alike and sound-alike issues: Procan SR and Proscar; Procardia and Provera; quinidine and quinine

Class IA Antiarrhythmic Drugs

Generic Name	U.S. Brand Name(s) Canadian Brand(s)	Dosage Forms and Strengths
disopyramide*	Norpace, Norpace CR	Capsules: 100 mg, 150 mg
	Rythmodan	Capsules, extended release (Norpace CR): 100 mg†, 150 mg†
procainamide*	Generics	Solution, injection: 100 mg/mL, 500 mg/mL
	Procan SR	Tablets, extended release: 250 mg, 500 mg, 1000 mg‡
quinidine gluconate*	Generics	Solution, injection: 80 mg/mL
	Not available	Tablets, extended release: 324 mg
quinidine sulfate*	Generics	Solution, injection (Canada only): 190 mg/mL
	Generics	Tablet: 200 mg, 300 mg
		Tablet, extended release: 300 mg

*Generic available.
†Strength available in the United States only.
‡Strength available in Canada only.

Class IB Antiarrhythmic Drugs

Generic Name	U.S. Brand Name(s) Canadian Brand(s)	Dosage Forms and Strengths
lidocaine*	Xylocaine	Solution, injection: 20% (Xylocard)
	Xylocard	Solution, in dextrose 5%: 0.2%, 0.4%, 0.5%, 0.8%
mexiletine*	Generic	Capsules: 100 mg‡, 200 mg, 150 mg†, 250 mg†
	Generic	

*Generic available.
†Strength available in the United States only.
‡Strength available in Canada only.

Class IC Antiarrhythmic Drugs

Generic Name	U.S. Brand Name(s) / Canadian Brand(s)	Dosage Forms and Strengths
flecainide*	Tambocor	Tablets: 50 mg, 100 mg, 150 mg[†]
	Tambocor	
propafenone*	Rhythmol, Rhythmol SR	Capsules, extended release (Rhythmol) SR: 225 mg[†], 325 mg[†], 425 mg[†] Tablets: 150 mg, 225 mg[†], 300 mg
	Rhythmol	

*Generic available.
[†]Strength available in the United States only.

Class II Antiarrhythmic Drugs

Generic Name	U.S. Brand Name(s) / Canadian Brand(s)	Dosage Forms and Strengths
acebutolol*	Sectral	Capsules: 100 mg[‡], 200 mg, 400 mg
	Sectral	
esmolol*	Brevibloc, Brevibloc Double Strength	Solution, injection: 10 mg/mL (Brevibloc), 20 mg/mL (Brevibloc Double Strength)
	Brevibloc	
propranolol*	Inderal LA, InnoPran XL	Capsules, extended release (Inderal LA): 60 mg, 80 mg, 120 mg, 160 mg, 160 mg Solution, injection: 1 mg/mL Solution, oral: 20 mg/5 mL; 40 mg/5 mL Tablets: 10 mg, 20 mg, 40 mg, 60 mg, 80 mg
	Inderal LA	

*Generic available.
[‡]Strength available in Canada only.

Class III Antiarrhythmic Drugs

Generic Name	U.S. Brand Name(s) / Canadian Brand(s)	Dosage Forms and Strengths
amiodarone*	Cordarone, Pacerone	Solution, injection: 50 mg/mL Tablets: 100 mg, 200 mg, 400 mg[†]
	Cordarone	
dofetilide	Tikosyn	Capsules: 0.125 mg, 0.25 mg, 0.5 mg
	Not available	
dronedarone	Multaq Tablet/ Multaq	Tablets: 400 mg
ibutilide*	Corvert	Solution: Injection: 0.1 mg/mL
	Corvert	
sotalol* sotalol AF*	Betapace, Betapace AF, Sorine	Tablets: 80 mg, 120 mg[†], 160 mg, 240 mg Tablets (AF): 80 mg, 120 mg, 160 mg Solution, injection: 150 mg/10 mL
	Generics	

*Generic available.
[†]Strength available in the United States only.

Class IV Antiarrhythmic Drugs

Generic Name	U.S. Brand Name(s) / Canadian Brand(s)	Dosage Forms and Strengths
verapamil*	Calan SR, Isoptin SR, Verelan, Verelan PM Covera HS Covera HS, Isoptin SR, Verelan	Capsules, extended release: 120 mg, 180 mg, 240 mg, 360 mg Capsules, extended release (Verelan PM): 100 mg, 200 mg, 300 mg Solution, injection: 2.5 mg/mL Tablets: 40 mg, 80 mg, 120 mg, Tablets, extended release (Calan SR, Covera HS, Isoptin SR): 120 mg, 180 mg, 240 mg

*Generic available.

TECH ALERT!
The following drugs have look-alike and sound-alike issues: acebutolol and albuterol; esmolol and Osmitrol; Brevibloc and Brevital; propranolol and Pravachol; Inderal, Adderall, Isordil, and Toradol

TECH ALERT!
The following drugs have look-alike and sound-alike issues: amiodarone, amantadine, and trazodone; Cordarone, Cardura, and Coumadin; Betapace AF and Betapace

TECH ALERT!
The following drugs have look-alike and sound-alike issues: verapamil and Verelan; Calan SR and Calan

Drug Used to Prevent Arrhythmias

Arrhythmia management is currently focused on prevention. Prevention is important because atrial fibrillation is a risk factor for stroke (see Chapter 24). Hypertension doubles the risk for atrial fibrillation; therefore, hypertension should be treated to reduce the risk. Angiotensin-converting enzyme (ACE) inhibitors and angiotensin II type 1 receptor blockers (ARBs) can significantly reduce the risk for first-time atrial fibrillation in patients with hypertension or heart failure and post–myocardial infarction. The use of these drugs to treat hypertension is discussed in Chapter 22.

MECHANISM OF ACTION

The ACE inhibitors lengthen the refractory period and shorten conduction time. The ACE inhibitors also decrease dilatation of coronary arteries, reducing blood pressure. The ARBs have a similar mechanism but also reduce inflammation and structural changes in the atria that can activate atrial fibrillation.

Summary of Drugs Used in the Treatment of Arrhythmia

Generic Name	Usual Dose and Dosing Schedule	Warning Labels
Antiarrhythmic Drugs		
Class IA		
disopyramide*	150-200 mg every 6 hours (immediate release) 300 mg every 12 hours (extended release)	MAY CAUSE DIZZINESS OR DROWSINESS. SWALLOW WHOLE; DO NOT CRUSH OR CHEW—extended release. TAKE ON AN EMPTY STOMACH—procainamide. AVOID GRAPEFRUIT JUICE—quinidine sulfate. REFRIGERATE; DO NOT FREEZE—Diluted quinidine gluconate solution may be stored for up to 48 hours at 4° C (39° F) or 24 hours at room temperature.
procainamide*	Atrial arrhythmias and ventricular arrhythmias: Oral loading dose: 1000-1250 mg PO. After 1 hour, may give an additional 750 mg PO if arrhythmia persists. Oral maintenance dose: 750-1500 mg every 6 hours (extended release) 50 mg/kg every 3-4 hours	
quinidine gluconate*	324-648 mg PO every 8-12 hours 600 mg IM followed by 400 mg IM repeat every 2 hours; 800 mg IV in 50 mL of D5W infused 1 mL/min	
quinidine sulfate*	200-300 mg every 6-8 hours (immediate release); 300-600 mg every 8-12 hours (extended release)	

Continued

Summary of Drugs Used in the Treatment of Arrhythmia—cont'd

Generic Name	Usual Dose and Dosing Schedule	Warning Labels
Class IB		
lidocaine*	50-100 mg IV infused 25-50 mg/min; repeat in 5 minutes (Loading dose) **Continuous infusion:** 1 mg-4 mg/min (Maintenance dose) **IM:** 300 mg (Loading dose)	MAY CAUSE DIZZINESS OR DROWSINESS. TAKE WITH FOOD—mexiletine.
mexiletine*	200-300 mg every 8 hours	
Class IC		
flecainide*	50-300 mg every 12 hours	DO NOT SKIP OR EXCEED DOSE.
propafenone*	150-300 mg every 8 hours 225-425 mg every 12 hours (extended release)	WEAR SUNGLASSES—propafenone. AVOID GRAPEFRUIT JUICE. SWALLOW WHOLE; DO NOT CRUSH OR CHEW—extended release.
Class II		
acebutolol*	600-1200 mg/day in 2 divided doses	MAY CAUSE DIZZINESS OR DROWSINESS. CONCENTRATE; MUST BE DILUTED—esmolol. ORAL CONCENTRATE; MUST BE DILUTED—propranolol. SWALLOW WHOLE; DO NOT CRUSH OR CHEW—extended release. DO NOT SKIP DOSES.
esmolol*	500 mcg/kg IV loading dose over 1 minute **Maintenance infusion rate:** 50 mcg/kg/min IV for 4 minutes; repeat prn increasing maintenance infusion in 50 mcg/kg/min increments	
propranolol*	160-320 mg/day in 3-4 divided doses.	
Class III		
amiodarone*	800-1600 mg/day PO in single or divided doses; maintenance dose, 400 mg/day **IV:** rapid infusion of 150 mg over first 10 minutes; then slow IV infusion of 1 mg/min for next 6 hours (total = 360 mg); then 0.5 mg/min for the next 18 hours (total dose infused = 540 mg); after 24 hours, a maintenance IV infusion of 0.5 mg/min (720 mg/day)	AVOID PROLONGED EXPOSURE TO SUNLIGHT—amiodarone. MAY CAUSE DIZZINESS OR DROWSINESS. AVOID GRAPEFRUIT JUICE—amiodarone, dofetilide, dronedarone. SHOULD NOT BE ADMINISTERED DURING PREGNANCY—ibutilide. TAKE ON AN EMPTY STOMACH—sotalol. AVOID SALT SUBSTITUTES—sotalol PROTECT FROM MOISTURE—dofetilide.
ibutilide	1 mg/IV infused over at least 10 minutes; Repeat prn	
dofetilide	1000 mcg/day PO; initiation of dofetilide in a hospitalized setting for a minimum of 3 days	
dronedarone	400 mg two times a day with meals	
sotalol*	80-160 mg two times a day; Betapace is usually taken twice a day, and Betapace AF is taken once or twice a day	
Class IV		
verapamil*	Paroxysmal supraventricular tachycardia: 240-480 mg/day PO in 3-4 divided doses (immediate release) 2.5-5 mg IV over 2-4 minutes; may repeat 5-10 mg every 15-30 minutes up to 20 mg IV Atrial fib/flutter: 120-360 mg/day	TAKE WITH FOOD. SWALLOW WHOLE; DO NOT CRUSH OR CHEW—extended release.
Angiotensin-Converting Enzyme Inhibitors—see Chapter 22		
Angiotensin II type 1 Receptor Antagonists—see Chapter 22		
Miscellaneous		
digoxin*	**Loading dose:** 10-15 mcg/kg PO or IV given in 3 divided doses every 6-8 hours **Maintenance:** 125-500 mcg PO or IV once a day	TAKE ON AN EMPTY STOMACH. AVOID HIGH-FIBER DIET. ASK PHARMACIST BEFORE TAKING OTC MEDICINES.

*Generic available.

Chapter Summary

- An arrhythmia is defined as an irregular heart rhythm or a heart rate that is too rapid or too slow.
- An arrhythmia can impair the heart's ability to distribute blood.
- Atrial fibrillation is the most common arrhythmia; it affects approximately 1% of the population and can increase the risk for stroke.
- Nonmodifiable risk factors for arrhythmia are age, gender, low heart rate, and emotional stress.
- Modifiable risk factors for arrhythmia are obesity, smoking, excessive alcohol consumption, and stimulant use.
- Disease risk factors for arrhythmia are hypertension, heart failure, CHD, stroke, infection, diabetes, thyroid disease, and obstructive sleep apnea.
- Ventricular fibrillation is the leading cause of sudden cardiac death.
- Arrhythmias occur when the cardiac ion exchange channels function improperly. This can result in excessive firing, extra currents during the refractory period, and establishment of sinus rhythm by nonpacemaker cells.
- When arrhythmias form, they may stimulate the formation of other arrhythmias.
- Atrial flutter refers to a heart rate of 160 to 350 beats/min.
- Atrial fibrillation is defined as a rapid heart rate between 300 and 400 beats/min.
- Ventricular tachycardia causes the ventricles to beat faster than 200 beats/min.
- Ventricular fibrillation may cause the ventricles to beat faster than 600 beats/min.
- Antiarrhythmic drugs are categorized into four classes (classes I, II, III, and IV) according to their mechanisms of action and structural similarities.
- Class I antiarrhythmic drugs produce a sodium channel blockade.
- Class I antiarrhythmic drugs reduce automaticity (spontaneous contraction of heart muscle cells), delay conduction, and prolong the time between contractions (refractory period).
- Class II antiarrhythmic drugs are β-adrenergic blockers.
- Beta blockers antagonize stimulation at the AV and SA nodes. They increase the refractory period, decrease automaticity, and slow conduction velocity.
- Class III antiarrhythmic drugs produce potassium channel blockade.
- Class III antiarrhythmic drugs prolong depolarization and prolong the refractory period.
- Class IV antiarrhythmic drugs produce calcium channel blockade.
- Beta blockers are the only class of drugs indicated for primary management of ventricular arrhythmias.
- All antiarrhythmic agents are proarrhythmic (can cause other arrhythmias).
- Digoxin is approved for the treatment of atrial fibrillation. It reduces arrhythmias by slowing the conduction velocity and prolonging the refractory period in the Purkinje fibers and AV node.
- In the atria and ventricles, digoxin shortens the refractory period. Digoxin also reduces electrical discharges from the SA node.
- The ACE inhibitors and ARBs can significantly reduce the risk for first-time atrial fibrillation in patients with hypertension or heart failure and post–myocardial infarction.
- The ACE enzyme inhibitors lengthen the refractory period and shorten conduction time.
- The ARBs also reduce inflammation and structural changes in the atria that can activate atrial fibrillation.

1. Arrhythmias can produce heart rates that exceed _____ beats/min.
   a. 200
   b. 400
   c. 600
   d. 800

2. _____fibrillation is the most common arrhythmia.
   a. Atrial
   b. Ventricular
   c. Aortic
   d. Pulmonary

3. What kind of fibrillation is life threatening?
   a. atrial
   b. ventricular
   c. aortic
   d. a and b

4. Beta blockers are the only class of drugs indicated for primary management of atrial arrhythmias.
   a. true
   b. false

5. All antiarrhythmic agents are proarrhythmic (can cause other arrhythmias). They also can cause all of the following symptoms except _____.
   a. bradycardia
   b. hypotension
   c. hypertension
   d. dizziness

6. Digoxin has a narrow therapeutic index, so it is important to avoid excessive doses.
   a. true
   b. false

7. Arrhythmia management is currently focused on _____.
   a. cure
   b. prevention
   c. medication
   d. all of the above

8. A sign of quinidine toxicity is _____.
   a. fibrillation
   b. tinnitus
   c. clot formation
   d. numbness

9. Dofetilide is placed in which class of drugs for arrhythmias?
   a. class I
   b. class II
   c. class III
   d. class IV

10. The brand name for verapamil is _____.
    a. Covera HS
    b. Calan
    c. Isoptin
    d. all of the above

TECHNICIAN'S
CORNER

1. What is the difference between a palpitation and an arrhythmia?
2. How is an arrhythmia diagnosed?

Bibliography

Aksnes T, Flaa A, Strand A, Kjeldsen SE. Prevention of new-onset atrial fibrillation and its predictors with angiotensin II-receptor blockers in the treatment of hypertension and heart failure, *J Hypertens* 25(1):15-23, 2007.

Elsevier. Gold Standard Clinical Pharmacology. Retrieved April 2, 2011, from https://www.clinicalpharmacology.com/, 2010.

FDA. FDA Approved Drug Products. Retrieved May 14, 2012, from http://www.accessdata.fda.gov/scripts/cder/drugsatfda/index.cfm?fuseaction=Search.Search_Drug_Name, 2012.

Health Canada. Drug Product Database. Retrieved May 14,2012 from http://www.hc-sc.gc.ca/dhp-mps/prod-pharma/databasdon/index-eng.php, 2010.

Kalant H, Grant D, Mitchell J: *Principles of medical pharmacology*, ed 7, Toronto, 2007, Elsevier Canada, A Division of Reed Elsevier Canada, pp 366-376.

Lance L, Lacy C, Armstrong L, et al: *Drug information handbook for the allied health professional*, ed 12, Hudson, OH, 2005, APhA Lexi-Comp.

Nash M, Mourad A, Clayton R, et al: Evidence for multiple mechanism in human ventricular fibrillation, *Circulation* 114:536-542, 2006. Available at: http://circ.ahajournals.org/cgi/content/full/114/6/536.

Page C, Curtis M, Sutter M, et al: *Integrated pharmacology*, Philadelphia, 2005, Mosby, pp 432-446.

Tveit A, et al: Candesartan in the prevention of relapsing atrial fibrillation, *Int J Cardiol* 1-7, 2006.

Zipes DP, et al: ACC/AHA/ESC practice guidelines, *J Am Coll Cardiol* 48:e268–e270, 2006.

UNIT VI

Drugs Affecting the Gastrointestinal System

KEY TERMS

Alimentary canal: A tube all the way through the ventral cavities of the body and is open at both ends.

Deglutition: Swallowing.

Digestion: Complete process of altering the physical and chemical composition of ingested food materials so that it can be absorbed and used by the body cells.

Mastication: Chewing.

Role of the Digestive System

The organs of the digestive system work together to perform a vital function, preparing food for absorption and for use by the millions of body cells. Food that is eaten must be modified in its chemical composition and physical state so that nutrients can be absorbed and used by the body's cells. The complete process of altering the physical and chemical composition of ingested food materials so that it can be absorbed and used by the body's cells is called *digestion*. The first step in the digestive process is called mechanical digestion; this involves the physical breaking down of ingested food material into smaller pieces. It begins in the mouth and continues with the churning and mixing of food as it passes through the digestive system. The second phase of digestion, called chemical digestion, completes the breakdown process. It results in the release of nutrient end products such as glucose and amino acids, which can be absorbed and that enter cells for use as an energy source or for other metabolic functions.

Organization of the Digestive System

ORGANS OF DIGESTION

The main organs of digestive system form a tube all the way through the ventral cavities of the body. It is open at both ends. The tube is commonly called the *alimentary canal* or gastrointestinal (GI)

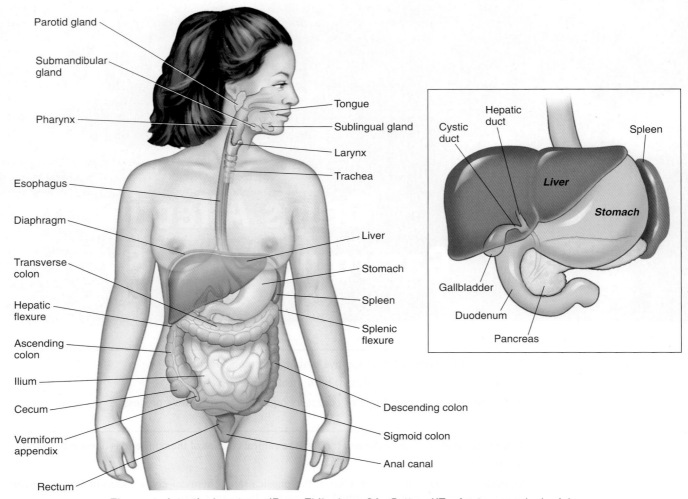

The gastrointestinal system. (From Thibodeau GA, Patton KT: *Anatomy and physiology*, ed 6, St Louis, 2007, Mosby.)

tract and, from beginning to end, it follows a specific path—oral cavity, oropharynx, esophagus, stomach, small intestine, large intestine, rectum, and anal canal. Organs not part of the alimentary tube are called accessory organs and play a support role in digestion. The accessory organs are the salivary glands, tongue, teeth, liver, gallbladder, pancreas, and appendix.

STRUCTURES OF THE ORAL CAVITY

The oral cavity is made up the mouth, lips, cheeks, tongue, and hard and soft palates. The hard palate and soft palate form a partition between the mouth and nasopharynx. Suspended from the middle of the soft palate is the uvula. The tongue is a solid mass of skeletal muscle that assists during *mastication* (chewing), *deglutition* (swallowing), and speech. The surface of the tongue contains papillae; embedded in these papillae are the taste buds. Three pairs of salivary glands—the parotid, submandibular, and sublingual glands—secrete most of the saliva that is produced each day and contains enzymes and mucus, which facilitate the breakdown of food.

The pharynx serves as a passageway for air and food, which pass from the mouth to the pharynx and then to the esophagus.

The esophagus is a collapsible, muscular, mucus-lined tube that extends from the pharynx to the stomach and pierces the diaphragm. It serves as a dynamic passageway for food, pushing the food toward the stomach. Each end of the esophagus is guarded by a muscular sphincter. The upper esophageal sphincter helps prevent air from entering during respiration. The lower esophageal sphincter opens into the diaphragm.

STOMACH

Just below the diaphragm is an elongated pouchlike structure, the stomach. The stomach is divided into the fundus, body, and pylorus. Sphincter muscles guard the openings between the upper and lower ends of the stomach. The lower esophageal sphincter controls the entry of contents between the esophagus and stomach. The pyloric sphincter controls the opening from the pyloric portion of the stomach into the duodenum, the first part of the small intestine.

The epithelial lining of the stomach is composed of folds called rugae and is marked by depressions called gastric pits. Gastric glands are found below the gastric pits and secrete most of the gastric juice, a mucous fluid containing digestive enzymes and hydrochloric acid. The gastric glands also contain three major secretory cells—chief cells, parietal cells, and endocrine cells.

The stomach performs the following functions:
- Serves as a reservoir for food
- Secretes gastric juice (chief cells) and hydrochloric acid (parietal cells) to break down food chemically; secretes the intrinsic factor (binds to vitamin B_{12})
- Produces the hormone gastrin to regulate digestion and ghrelin (endocrine cells) to increase appetite
- Helps protect the body by destroying pathogenic bacteria swallowed with food or mucus

SMALL AND LARGE INTESTINES

The small intestine consists of three divisions, the duodenum (uppermost), jejunum (middle), and ileum (lowest). The lining of the intestines contain circular plicae (folds) that have many tiny projections called villi. The presence of villi and microvilli increases the surface area of the small intestine and makes this organ the main site of digestion and absorption. The large intestine is divided into the cecum, colon, rectum, and anal canal.

APPENDIX

The appendix is found just behind the cecum or over the pelvic rim. Its functions are not certain; and it is thought to serve as a so-called breeding ground for some of the nonpathogenic intestinal bacteria believed to aid in the digestion or absorption of nutrients.

LIVER

The liver is the largest gland in the body and lies immediately under the diaphragm. It consists of two lobes. The functions of the liver are as follows:
- Detoxification
- Secretion of bile
- Metabolism of foods: proteins, fats, and carbohydrates
- Kupffer cells (phagocytic cells) that remove bacteria, worn red blood cells, and other particles from the bloodstream
- Storage—iron, vitamins A, B_{12}, and D
- Production of plasma proteins
- Serves as a site of hematopoiesis during fetal development

GALLBLADDER

The gallbladder lies on the undersurface of the liver. Functions of the gallbladder are to store and concentrate bile and to contract and eject concentrated bile into the duodenum.

PANCREAS

The pancreas is composed of two different types of glandular tissues, one endocrine (alpha and beta cells) and one exocrine (acinar cells). The beta cells secrete insulin and alpha cells secrete glucagon. These hormones control carbohydrate metabolism. Acinar cells secrete digestive enzymes found in pancreatic juice.

Summary

The organs of the digestive system together perform a vital function, that of preparing food for absorption and for use by the millions of body cells. The process involves physical and chemical alteration of ingested food. To protect itself from self-erosion (autodigestion) by digestive juices, epithelial cells in the stomach produce then secrete a bicarbonate-rich solution that coats the mucosa. Bicarbonate is alkaline, a base, and neutralizes the hydrochloric acid secreted by the parietal cells, producing water in the process. Bicarbonate secretions that neutralize the acid from the stomach are also produced in the intestines and pancreas.

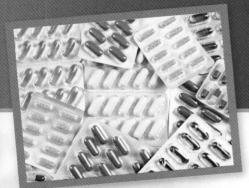

26

Treatment of Gastroesophageal Reflux Disease, Laryngopharyngeal Reflux, and Peptic Ulcer Disease

KEY TERMS

Duodenal ulcer: Ulcer located in the upper portion of the small intestine or duodenum.

Endoscopy: Test used to look for ulcers inside the stomach and small intestine using an endoscope. An endoscope is a thin flexible tube with a small video camera and light attached to one end.

Gastric ulcer: Ulcer located in the stomach.

Gastroesophageal reflux disease: Motility disorder associated with impaired peristalsis that results in the backflow of gastric contents into the esophagus.

Hiatal hernia: Condition in which the lower esophageal sphincter shifts above the diaphragm.

Laryngopharyngeal reflux: Reflux of gastric contents into the larynx and pharynx.

Lower esophageal sphincter: Sphincter separating the esophagus and the stomach.

Peptic ulcer disease: Term used to describe ulcers located in the duodenum or stomach.

Peristalsis: Forceful wave of contractions in the esophagus that moves food and liquids from the mouth to the stomach.

Reflux: Backflow of gastric contents into esophagus or laryngopharyngeal region.

Ulcer: Open wound or sore.

Upper esophageal sphincter: Sphincter separating the pharynx and esophagus. It relaxes to permit passage of food and liquids during swallowing, prevent air from entering the esophagus during breathing, and prevent gastric secretions from entering the pharynx.

Overview

Gastroesophageal reflux disease, peptic ulcer disease, and *laryngopharyngeal reflux* are diseases that affect millions of Americans and Canadians. It is estimated that 33% of Americans have GERD and 1 of 5 Americans has been diagnosed with PUD. As of 2010, annual health care costs attributed to PUD were estimated to be greater than $10 billion. In addition, nearly 500,000 new cases of ulcers are diagnosed and 4 million ulcer recurrences are reported each year in the United States.

Although these diseases initially produce minor discomfort, they may progress to life threatening hemorrhage or stomach cancer. GERD may increase the risk for development of chronic disease such as asthma.

Gastroesophageal Reflux Disease

GERD is a motility disorder associated with impaired peristalsis. *Peristalsis* is a forceful wave of contractions in the esophagus that moves food and other orally ingested contents from the mouth to the stomach. The *lower esophageal sphincter* (LES) is a muscle located at the junction between the esophagus and upper stomach that relaxes to permit food and liquids to pass from the esophagus into the stomach and then contracts to prevent stomach contents from returning to the esophagus. Heartburn is experienced when natural body processes fail to prevent backflow (*reflux*) of acidic stomach contents and digestive enzymes up into the esophagus. Excessive or chronic exposure to gastric acid and pepsin can lead to inflammation, ulceration, and changes to the epithelial cells that can lead to esophageal cancer.

WHAT CAUSES REFLUX?

Stomach contents back up into the esophagus when there is a buildup of pressure in the stomach that causes the LES to open and leak stomach contents back up into the esophagus. Delayed gastric emptying or transient relaxation of the LES, especially after eating, may also cause gastroesophageal reflux.

Persons of any age can develop GERD. Infants may have GERD because their digestive system is immature. Many children will outgrow GERD by their first birthday. Obesity, smoking, and pregnancy are additional risk factors. Normally, the LES lies below the diaphragm, which helps keep the stomach contents from flowing back into the esophagus. *Hiatal hernia* is a significant risk factor for GERD in persons older than 50 years. When a hiatal hernia occurs, the diaphragm muscle is unable to hold the LES in normal position and the sphincter shifts above the diaphragm. Larger hiatal hernias are linked to more severe esophagitis (Figure 26-1).

FACTORS CONTRIBUTING TO GASTROESOPHAGEAL REFLUX DISEASE

Many factors can aggravate GERD; these include foods, lifestyle, prescription and over-the-counter (OTC) medicines, and even body position. Foods that can aggravate GERD are citrus fruits, chocolate, caffeinated beverages, fried and fatty foods, mint flavoring, spicy foods, tomato-based foods and sauces, garlic, and onions. Lifestyle factors that aggravate GERD include alcohol consumption and cigarette smoking. GERD symptoms are made worse when the body is in a prone position (lying down). Raising the head of the bed 6 to 8 inches can reduce symptoms. Pregnancy and obesity can also aggravate GERD. Many prescription and OTC medicines can worsen GERD. Prescription medicines that worsen gastroesophageal reflux are anticholinergics (e.g., hyoscyamine), opioids (e.g., codeine), calcium channel blockers (e.g., verapamil), nonsteroidal anti-inflammatory drugs (e.g., naproxen), hormones (e.g., progesterone), benzodiazepines (e.g., diazepam), antiarrhythmics (e.g., quinidine), bisphosphonates (e.g., alendronate), and xanthines (e.g., theophylline). These drugs impair peristalsis, delay gastric emptying, decrease esophageal sphincter tone, decrease the protective mucosal lining, and/or increase gastric acid levels. OTC iron and potassium supplements, and NSAIDs irritate the esophagus and may cause heartburn.

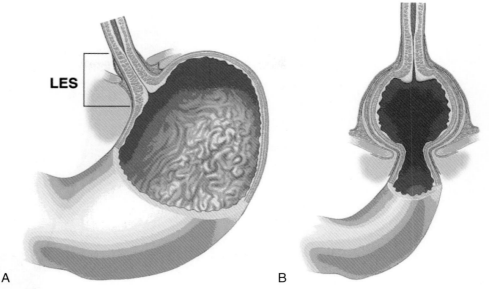

FIGURE 26-1 Gastroesophageal junction. **A,** Location of the lower esophageal sphincter (LES). **B,** Hiatal hernia. (Courtesy Dr. J.T. Laitman, Mount Sinai School of Medicine, Center for Anatomy and Functional Morphology, New York.)

Laryngopharyngeal Reflux

Laryngopharyngeal reflux is closely related to GERD and can occur simultaneously. When gastric contents reflux into the larynx and pharynx, located in the head and neck region, inflammation occurs that may cause hoarseness, voice fatigue, laryngitis, sore throat, chronic cough, bad breath, sinusitis, wheezing, aggravation of asthma, and even middle ear infections.

As in GERD, LPR occurs when the normal reflux barriers fail. Anatomic barriers that protect against LPR are the gastroesophageal junction (includes the LES), esophageal motor function and acid clearance, and ***upper esophageal sphincter*** (UES). Laryngeal mucosal resistance also protects the larynx from damage caused by reflux.

The UES separates the pharynx and esophagus and relaxes to permit the passage of food and liquids during swallowing, prevent air from entering the esophagus during breathing, and prevent gastric secretions entering the pharynx via the esophagus. If the UES is damaged by exposure to stomach contents, it can become less sensitive and lose its ability to function properly. This increases the likelihood of reflux and more damage (Figure 26-2).

Peptic Ulcer Disease

An ***ulcer*** is an open wound or sore. Ulcers can occur anywhere on the body. Examples are ***gastric ulcers*** form in the stomach (Figure 26-3), ***duodenal ulcers*** form in the upper region of the small intestines, and peptic ulcers form in the stomach or duodenum.

RISK FACTORS FOR PEPTIC ULCER DISEASE

Almost two thirds of the global population is infected with *Helicobacter pylori (H. pylori),* the primary cause of peptic ulcer disease (PUD). More than 90% of people who have duodenal ulcers and 80% of people who have gastric ulcers are infected with *H. pylori. H. pylori* infection is also a risk factor for the development of stomach cancer. Worldwide, most people infected with *H. pylori* develop the infection in childhood. Infections are transmitted person to person by the gastric-oral route. Once the bacteria are ingested, they release buffers that enable the bacteria to survive in the acidic contents of the stomach. The bacteria also release virulence factors that are responsible for inflammation and tissue damage. Fortunately, most people who are infected with *H. pylori* will not develop

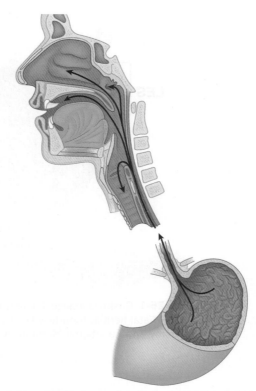

FIGURE 26-2 Laryngopharyngeal reflux—direction of backflow into head and neck regions. (Courtesy Dr. J.T. Laitman, Mount Sinai School of Medicine, Center for Anatomy and Functional Morphology, New York.)

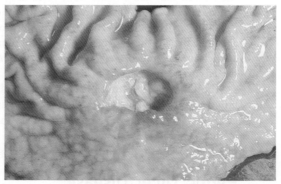

FIGURE 26-3 Gastric ulcer. (From Rosai J: *Rosai and Ackerman's surgical pathology*, ed 9, Philadelphia, 2004, Mosby.)

chronic gastritis or PUD. Researchers are working to develop a vaccine to prevent *H. pylori* infection that can be administered in childhood.

When a person exhibits symptoms of an ulcer, several simple tests can be performed to see whether the person has an *H. pylori* infection. A sample of blood may be drawn to look for antibodies and other evidence of past or current infection or a breath test may be done to check for evidence of urease, an enzyme released by *H. pylori*. An **endoscopy** may be performed to look for ulcers inside the stomach and small intestine using an endoscope, a thin flexible tube with a small video camera and light attached to one end that is passed down the esophagus into the stomach.

Risk factors for the development of ulcers are family history of ulcers or living with close relatives who have PUD; age (those >50 years are at increased risk); and use of medicines such as salicylates (e.g., aspirin), NSAIDs (e.g., naproxen), and corticosteroids (e.g., prednisone). NSAIDs and salicylates are irritants and reduce the protective mucous lining of the stomach and/or duodenum.

Symptoms of Gastroesophageal Reflux Disease, Laryngopharyngeal Reflux, and Peptic Ulcer Disease

Some of the symptoms of GERD, LPR, and PUD are common to all three conditions, whereas others are disease-specific. Symptoms associated with GERD, LPR, and PUD are categorized in Table 26-1.

Lifestyle Modification

Cigarette smoking and alcohol consumption can increase the risk for PUD and aggravate existing disease. Cigarette smoking interferes with the healing of an ulcer by constricting blood vessels to the ulcerated area. Alcohol is a gastric irritant. See Box 26-1 for lifestyle modifications recommended for people with GERD and PUD.

TABLE 26-1   **Symptoms of Gastroesophageal Reflux Disease, Laryngopharyngeal Reflux, and Peptic Ulcer Disease**

Disease	Unique Symptoms	Common Symptoms
Gastroesophageal reflux disease	Difficulty swallowing Dry cough Bad breath Bloated stomach Rumbling noise in stomach Belching or burping Respiratory problems Hoarseness	Heartburn Stomachache Hunger pains Nausea or vomiting Chest pain
Laryngopharyngeal reflux	Hoarseness Voice fatigue or breaks Sore throat Excessive phlegm or saliva Chronic cough Bad breath Middle ear infection Wheezing Chronic sinusitis	
Peptic ulcer disease	Burning pain in the gut beginning 2 to 3 hr after a meal Weight loss Loss of appetite	

BOX 26-1   **Lifestyle Modifications Recommended for People With Gastroesophageal Reflux Disease or Peptic Ulcer Disease**

- Avoid lying down after eating (wait at least 3 hr).
- Elevate the head of the bed 6 to 8 inches.
- Eat small meals.
- Lose weight if you are overweight.
- Quit smoking if you smoke.
- Do not drink alcohol.
- Limit use of aspirin and NSAIDs.

TABLE 26-2   **Natural Alternatives for Gastroesophageal Reflux Disease**

Safe Foods	Food to Avoid	Natural Alternative
Fruits—apples, bananas	Fruits—tomatoes, lemon	Magnesium oxide— increases lower esophageal sphincter tone
Vegetables—broccoli, carrots, cabbage, peas, green beans, baked potato	Juices—orange juice, cranberry juice, grapefruit juice, lemonade	Almonds—chew on a few almonds after each meal
Meat products—skinless chicken breast, extra lean ground beef, London broil, egg whites and substitutes, non fatty fish	Meat products—ground beef, chicken nuggets, buffalo wings, marbled sirloin Vegetables—raw onion, french fries, mashed potatoes	Fennel tea or chamomile tea— soothing effect, sip slowly
Dairy—fat-free cream cheese, goat cheese, low-fat soy cheese, fat-free sour cream	Dairy products—regular cottage cheese, sour cream, ice cream, milk shake	Ginger (any form)—reduces acid in stomach
Grains—brown or white rice, multigrain or white bread, cereal (e.g., bran, oatmeal), corn bread, graham crackers, pretzels, rice cakes	Grains—spaghetti (pasta) with tomato sauce, macaroni and cheese	Organic apple cider—shake well; pulp contains enzymes to reduce acid
Salad—low-fat salad dressing	Salad—creamy and oil and vinegar salad dressings	Chewing gum—produces saliva, which dilutes stomach acid
Sweets—fat-free cookies, jelly beans, red licorice, baked potato chips	Sweets—high-fat butter cookies, chocolate, doughnuts, corn chips, brownies	
Beverage—mineral water	Beverages—wine, liquor, decaffeinated or regular coffee or tea	

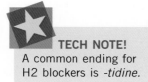

TECH NOTE!
It is a myth that stress and spicy foods can cause ulcers; however, some foods can aggravate existing GERD (Table 26-2).

TECH NOTE!
A common ending for H2 blockers is *-tidine*.

Drugs Used in the Treatment of Gastroesophageal Reflux Disease, Laryngopharyngeal Reflux, and Peptic Ulcer Disease

The treatment of GERD, LPR, and PUD is aimed at reducing gastrointestinal (GI) irritants (e.g., volume of gastric acid, digestive enzymes such as pepsin) and increasing protective factors (e.g., mucus secretion by epithelial cells). Drugs used in the treatment of PUD, GERD, and LPR are classified according to their pharmacologic effects: (1) acid-neutralizing drugs (e.g., antacids); (2) acid-suppressing drugs (e.g., histamine 2 [H2] receptor antagonists, proton pump inhibitors [PPIs]); (3) mucosal protectants (e.g., prostaglandins, sucralfate); (4) drugs that eliminate *H. pylori* (e.g., anti-infectives); and (5) prokinetic drugs (e.g., metoclopramide).

There are some major differences in treatment strategies for GERD, LPR, and PUD. Treatment of PUD also involves eliminating *H. pylori* infection. Patients who have GERD and LPR may be prescribed drugs that increase GI motility (prokinetic drugs).

HISTAMINE 2 RECEPTOR ANTAGONIST DRUGS

There are four H2 receptor antagonists marketed in the United States and Canada—cimetidine, famotidine, nizatidine, and ranitidine. H2 receptor antagonists are used for the treatment of GERD, LPR, and PUD. All H2 receptor antagonists are available in prescription and nonprescription strengths.

Mechanism of Action

Histamine stimulates acid secretion by gastric parietal cells. H2 receptor antagonists competitively and reversibly bind to H2 receptors, blocking histamine-mediated acid secretion. The secretion of pepsin, a digestive enzyme released when the volume of acid in the stomach is high, occurs when food is present in the stomach and decreases as gastric acid levels decrease. Chronic exposure to pepsin can cause inflammation and peptic ulcers.

Pharmacokinetics

The H2 receptor antagonists have a similar time to peak plasma levels, half-life ($t_{1/2}$), and duration of action. The time required to reach maximum effect ranges from 0.5 hour (nizatidine) to 2 to 3

Histamine 2 Receptor Antagonists (H2 Blockers)

Generic Name	U.S. Brand Name(s) Canadian Brand Name(s)	Dosage Forms and Strengths
cimetidine*	Tagamet, Tagamet HB Tagamet	Tablet: 200 mg$, 300 mg, 400 mg, 800 mg Solution, oral: 300 mg/5 mL Injection, solution: 300 mg/2 mL†, 300 mg/5 mL† Injection, 0.9% NaCl solution: 300 mg/50 mL†
famotidine*	Pepcid, Pepcid AC$, Pepcid AC Maximum Strength$ Maalox H2 Acid Controller$, Pepcid, Pepcid AC$, Maximum Strength Pepcid AC$	Tablet: 10 mg$, 20 mg$, 40 mg Tablet, chewable: 20 mg$ Tablet, geltab: 10 mg$ Injection, solution: 10 mg/mL Injection, preservative free: 0.4 mg/mL; 10 mg/mL Powder for oral suspension: 40 mg/5 mL†
nizatidine*	Axid$, Axid AR$ Axid, Axid AR$	Capsule: 150 mg, 300 mg Tablet: 75 mg$ (Axid AR) Oral solution: 15 mg/mL
ranitidine*	Zantac Zantac	Capsule: 150 mg, 300 mg Tablet: 75 mg$, 150 mg‖, 300 mg Injection, solution: 25 mg/mL Oral solution/syrup: 15 mg/mL Effervescent tablet: 25 mg†
H2 Receptor Antagonist Combinations		
famotidine + calcium carbonate + magnesium hydroxide	Pepcid Complete$ Pepcid Complete$	10 mg famotidine + 800 mg calcium carbonate + 165 mg magnesium hydroxide

*Generic available.
†Strength available in the United States only.
$OTC in Canada and the United States.
‖OTC Canada only.

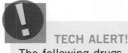

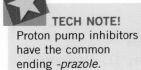

TECH ALERT!
The following drugs have look-alike and sound-alike issues:
cimetidine and simethicone
Axid and Ansaid
ranitidine, rimantadine, and amantidine
Zantac, Xanax, Zyrtec, and Zarontin

TECH NOTE!
Proton pump inhibitors have the common ending -*prazole*.

hours (ranitidine). The elimination $t_{1/2}$ is approximately 2 hours for all H2 receptor antagonists. The effect of H2 receptor antagonists on nocturnal acid secretion is significantly greater than on acid secretion after meals. The duration of effect on nocturnal secretion ranges from 8 hours (cimetidine) to 13 hours (ranitidine). The duration of effect on secretion after meals is reduced to 3 to 5 hours. There are differences in potency between the H2 receptor antagonists. Ranitidine is the most potent and is up to 10 times more effective than cimetidine.

Adverse Reactions

H2 receptor antagonists can produce dizziness or drowsiness, constipation or diarrhea, bloating, headache, and confusion when taken at therapeutic doses. Older adults are more susceptible to these adverse effects than other patient populations. Other less common adverse effects include skin rash, agitation, depression, hepatitis, decreased libido, and gynecomastia (caused by high-dose cimetidine). Males who develop gynecomastia have symptoms of breast swelling and tenderness.

Precautions

Cimetidine inhibits several cytochrome P-450 (CYP450) metabolic enzymes and is responsible for increasing the elimination of more than 25 different drugs. The pharmacist should be alerted to all drug interactions that are flagged by prescription-filling software.

PROTON PUMP INHIBITOR DRUGS

There are six PPIs currently marketed in the United States and Canada—dexlansoprazole, esomeprazole, lansoprazole, omeprazole, pantoprazole, and rabeprazole. PPIs are effective in treating

GERD, LPR, and PUD because they decrease gastric acid levels. They are more potent than H2 receptor antagonists. Omeprazole and lansoprazole are available for OTC use in the United States. All other PPIs are only commercially available in prescription strengths. OTC PPIs are marketed for the treatment of heartburn.

Mechanism of Action

PPIs decrease gastric acids by interfering with the final step in gastric acid production. PPIs interfere with hydrogen and potassium ion exchange via the H^+/K^+-ATPase proton pump located on parietal cells in the stomach (Figure 26-4).

Pharmacokinetics

PPIs are acid-labile; therefore, they can be destroyed in gastric acids. It is recommended they be taken on an empty stomach when gastric acid volume is lowest. Zegerid is a formulation combining an antacid with omeprazole to reduce omeprazole degradation by gastric acids. PPIs are delayed release formulations. They must not be crushed or chewed. Esomeprazole is an S isomer (mirror image) of omeprazole. Delayed-release tablets (lansoprazole) disintegrate in less than 1 minute.

Adverse Reactions

All the PPIs have a similar side effect profile. More common side effects are abdominal pain, headache, diarrhea or constipation, flatulence (gas), and nausea. Less common side effects are: jaundice, skin rash, unusual tiredness or fatigue, agitation, vitamin B_{12} deficiency, dark yellow or brown urine, and vomiting.

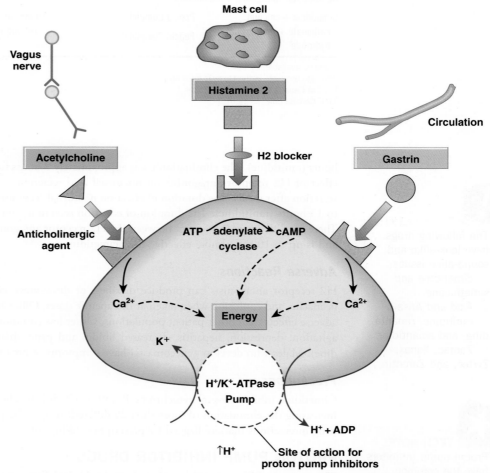

FIGURE 26-4 Mediators of gastric acid production. (From Lilley LL, Harrington S, Snyder JS: *Pharmacology and the nursing process*, ed 5, St Louis, 2007, Mosby.)

Proton Pump Inhibitors

Generic Name	U.S. Brand Name(s) Canadian Brand Name(s)	Dosage Forms and Strengths
dexlansoprazole	Dexilant	Capsules, delayed release: 30 mg, 60 mg
	Dexilant	
esomeprazole	Nexium	Capsules, delayed release: 20 mg[†], 40 mg[†]
	Nexium	Powder for oral suspension: 10 mg, 20 mg[†], 40 mg/packet[†]
		Powder for injection: 20 mg/vial[†], 40 mg/vial[†]
		Tablet, delayed-release: 20 mg[‡], 40 mg[‡]
lansoprazole*	Prevacid, Prevacid 24 HR▲	Capsules, delayed-release (Prevacid, Prevacid 24 HR): 15 mg▲, 30 mg
	Prevacid, Prevacid FasTab	Disintegrating tablets (Prevacid FasTab): 15 mg, 30 mg
omeprazole*	Prilosec, Prilosec OTC▲	Capsules, delayed-release: 10 mg, 20 mg, 40 mg
	Losec	Granules for suspension: 2.5 mg, 10 mg
		Tablets, delayed-release: 10 mg, 20 mg▲
pantoprazole sodium*, pantoprazole magnesium	Protonix	Granules, for oral suspension: 40 mg
	Pantoloc, Tecta	Powder for injection: 40 mg
		Tablet, delayed release, as sodium salt (Protonix, Pantoloc): 20 mg, 40 mg
		Tablet, enteric-coated, as magnesium salt (Tecta): 40 mg
rabeprazole*‡	Aciphex	Tablet, delayed-release: 10 mg[‡], 20 mg
	Pariet	

PPI Combination Products

esomeprazole + naproxen	Vimovo	Tablet: 20 mg esomeprazole + 375 mg naproxen
	Vimovo	20 mg esomeprazole + 500 mg naproxen[†]
lansoprazole + amoxicillin + clarithromycin	Prevpac	Combo pack: 30 mg lansoprazole capsule + 500 mg amoxicillin capsule + 500 mg clarithromycin tablet
	HP-PAC	
omeprazole + sodium bicarbonate	Zegerid, Zegerid OTC▲	Capsule: 20 mg omeprazole + 1100 mg sodium bicarbonate capsule▲
	Not available	40 mg omeprazole + 1100 mg sodium bicarbonate capsule
		Powder, for oral suspension: 20 mg omeprazole + 1680 mg sodium bicarbonate
		40 mg omeprazole + 1680 mg sodium bicarbonate

*Generic available.
*‡Generic available in Canada only.
[†]Strength available in the United States only.
[‡]Strength available in Canada only.
▲OTC in the United States only.

MUCOSAL PROTECTANTS

Mucosal protectants decrease the susceptibility of epithelial cells that line the stomach and small intestine to damage by gastric acids, pepsin, and *H. pylori*. Misoprostol is approved for the prevention of NSAID-induced peptic ulcers. Sucralfate is approved for the treatment and maintenance therapy of duodenal ulcers.

Mucosal Protectant Drugs

Generic Name	U.S. Brand Name(s) Canadian Brand Name(s)	Dosage Forms and Strengths
misoprostol*	Cytotec	Tablet: 0.1 mg; 0.2 mg
	Generic	
sucralfate*	Carafate	Suspension, oral: 1 g/5 mL‡, 1 g/10 mL†
	Sulcrate	Tablet: 1 g
Combination Products		
misoprostol + diclofenac	Arthrotec-50, Arthrotec-75	Tablet, delayed-release:
	Arthrotec-50, Arthrotec-75	0.2 mg misoprostol + 50 mg diclofenac 0.2 mg misoprostol + 75 mg diclofenac

*Generic available.
†Strength available in the United States only.
‡Strength available in Canada only.

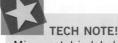

TECH NOTE!
Misoprostol is labeled with a boxed warning that the drug should not be taken by pregnant women. The drug may stimulate uterine contractions. Misoprostol must be dispensed in the manufacturer's original container.

TECH ALERT!
The following drugs have look-alike and sound-alike issues:
Prevacid, Prevpac, Prilosec, Pravachol, and Prinivil
Prilosec, Plendil, Prozac, and prilocaine
Protonix, Lotronex, Lovenox, and protamine
rabeprazole and aripiprazole
Aciphex, Aricept, and Accupril

Mechanism of Action

Misoprostol is a synthetic prostaglandin E (PGE). It stimulates the production of protective mucus and bicarbonate in the stomach. Misoprostol also increases the regeneration of gastric epithelial cells and enhances blood flow to the stomach.

Sucralfate binds to the ulcerated area and forms a protective barrier, much like a bandage protects a sore. It also promotes the regeneration of stomach epithelial cells. It is a weak inhibitor of *H. pylori*.

Adverse Reactions

Misoprostol may produce abdominal cramps, diarrhea, menstrual irregularities, headache, and dizziness. Sucralfate may produce constipation, gas, dry mouth, and headache.

Precautions

Misoprostol is contraindicated in pregnancy because it stimulates uterine contractions. Sucralfate blocks the absorption of several drugs including H2 receptor antagonists, PPIs, and several antibiotics. To avoid drug interactions, the drugs should not be taken at the same time as sucralfate.

PROKINETIC DRUGS

Prokinetic drugs are used for the treatment of GERD and LPR. They increase peristalsis, the wave-like movement throughout the GI tract, speed gastric emptying, and improve LES tone.

Mechanism of Action

Metoclopramide increased peristalsis by stimulating the release of acetylcholine in the periphery and increasing cholinergic activity. Domperidone blocks peripheral dopamine receptors to increase peristalsis. Both drugs enhance gastroduodenal coordination. Centrally, metoclopramide and domperidone block dopamine receptors, which decreases nausea. Metoclopramide is currently the only prokinetic drug approved by the U.S. Food and Drug Administration (FDA). Domperidone is approved in Canada for the symptomatic management of motility disorders associated with chronic gastritis and diabetic gastroparesis.

Adverse Reactions

More common adverse effects associated with metoclopramide and domperidone include diarrhea, abdominal pain, constipation, restlessness, dizziness and headache. Metoclopramide may cause drowsiness. Less common effects are leg cramps, skin rash, irregular heartbeat, and breast enlargement in men and women.

Prokinetic Drugs

Generic Name	U.S. Brand Name(s) / Canadian Brand Name(s)	Dosage Forms and Strengths
metoclopramide*	Metozolv ODT, Reglan / Generics	Tablet, oral disintegrating tablet (Metozolv ODT): 5 mg[†], 10 mg[†] Tablet (Reglan): 5 mg, 10 mg Solution, for injection: 5 mg/mL Solution, oral: 1 mg/mL
domperidone*	Not available / Generics	Tablet: 10 mg

*Generic available.
[†]Strength available in the United States only.

Examples of Selected Antacids

Generic Name	U.S. Brand Name(s) / Canadian Brand Name(s)
aluminum hydroxide*	Alternagel
	Not available
aluminum hydroxide + magnesium hydroxide*	Mag-Al, Mylanta Ultimate
	Gelusil
aluminum hydroxide + magnesium hydroxide + simethicone	Almacone, Maalox Max, Mintox, Mylanta Maximum Strength, Mylanta Regular Strength, Rulox
	Diovol Plus, Maalox with Anti-gas, Maalox with Anti-gas Extra Strength
calcium carbonate*	Caltrate, Alka-Mints, Maalox Antacid Barrier, Pepto Bismol Children's Chewable, Rolaids Extra Strength, TUMS, TUMS EX, TUMS Ultra
	Caltrate, TUMS, TUMS Ultra, TUMS Extra Strength
calcium carbonate + magnesium hydroxide*	Rolaids Chewable, Rolaids Extra Strength Chewable, Mylanta Supreme Suspension, Mylanta Ultra Chewable
	Not available
calcium carbonate + simethicone	Titralac Plus, Tums Plus
	Maalox Extra Strength with Anti-gas, Rolaids Extra Strength Plus Gas
alginic acid + magnesium carbonate	Gaviscon
	Gaviscon, Gaviscon Max Relief

*Generic available.

ANTACIDS

Antacids are the oldest drugs used for the treatment of GERD and PUD. Antacid use has declined since more potent drugs, requiring fewer daily doses, have been developed. Antacids can be obtained without prescription.

Mechanism of Action

Antacids neutralize gastric acids and decrease pepsin secretion. The acid-neutralizing capacity (ANC) is a standard used to evaluate the potency of antacids. The ANC is a measure of the ability of an antacid to do the following: (1) neutralize approximately 1 to 2 ounces hydrochloric acid (i.e., the volume of acid normally present between meals); and (2) raise the pH of the stomach to 3.5 within 10 minutes.

TECH ALERT!

The following drugs have look-alike and sound-alike issues:
    misoprostol and metoprolol;
    Cytotec and Cytoxan;
    sucralfate and salsalate;
    Carafate and Cafergot

Adverse Reactions

The side effects of antacids are related to their active ingredient and are dose-related. Magnesium-containing antacids cause diarrhea; aluminum-containing antacids cause constipation and, in high doses, deplete phosphates levels in blood (hypophosphatemia). Calcium-containing antacids cause constipation and, in high doses, produce hypercalcemia and kidney stones. Sodium bicarbonate (baking soda) has been associated with rebound hyperacidity, metabolic alkalosis, edema, and hypertension.

ANTIMICROBIALS

Antimicrobials are prescribed for the treatment of PUD to eradicate *H. pylori* infection. Clarithromycin, metronidazole, amoxicillin, and tetracycline are effective for eradicating *H. pylori*. They are prescribed in combination with drugs that decrease gastric acids and protect the gastric mucosa. Antimicrobials will be described in detail in Chapter 35.

Summary of Drugs Used for Treatment of Gastroesophageal Reflux Disease, Laryngopharyngeal Reflux, and Peptic Ulcer Disease

Generic Name	U.S. Brand Name	Usual Adult Oral Dosage and Dosing Schedule	Warning Labels
H2 Receptor Antagonists			
cimetidine	Tagamet	PUD: 800 mg daily at bedtime, or 400 mg bid or 300 mg qid for 8-12 wk GERD: 800 mg bid or 400 mg qid for 12 wk	AVOID ANTACIDS WITHIN 2 HR OF DOSE (CIMETIDINE, NIZATIDINE). AVOID ALCOHOL—ALL. SHAKE SUSPENSION WELL. DISCARD FAMOTIDINE ORAL SUSPENSION 30 DAYS AFTER MIXING. STORE INJECTION IN THE REFRIGERATOR (FAMOTIDINE, RANITIDINE). STORE CIMETIDINE INJECTION AT ROOM TEMPERATURE.
famotidine	Pepcid	PUD: 40 mg once daily at bedtime for 4 to 8 wk GERD: 20-40 mg bid for 6-12 wk	
nizatidine	Axid	PUD: 150 mg every 12 hr or 300 mg at bedtime for up to 8 wk GERD: 150 mg every 12 hr for up to 12 wk	
ranitidine	Zantac	PUD: 150 mg bid or 300 mg once daily at bedtime for 4-6 wk GERD: 150 mg bid for 4-8 wk	
Proton Pump Inhibitors			
esomeprazole	Nexium	PUD: 40 mg once daily GERD: 20-40 mg once daily for up to 4-8 wk	SWALLOW WHOLE; DO NOT CRUSH OR CHEW (CAPSULES CAN BE SPRINKLED ONTO FOOD BUT DO NOT CRUSH THE CONTENTS INTO THE FOOD). DELAYED RELEASE—TAKE 30 MIN BEFORE A MEAL (LANSOPRAZOLE). TAKE 60 MIN BEFORE A MEAL (ESOMEPRAZOLE). GRANULES FOR ORAL SUSPENSION MUST BE MIXED WITH 1 TO 2 TABLESPOONFULS OF LIQUID. ALLOW MIXTURE TO STAND FOR 2-3 MIN, THEN IMMEDIATELY DRINK ENTIRE MIXTURE. DISSOLVE DISINTEGRATING TABLETS ON TONGUE.
lansoprazole	Prevacid	PUD: 15 mg once daily in the morning for up to 4 wk GERD: 15-30 mg once daily in the morning for up to 8 wk	
omeprazole	Prilosec	PUD: 40 mg once daily for 4-8 wk GERD: 20 mg once daily for 4-8 wk	
pantoprazole	Protonix	PUD: 40 mg once daily after the morning meal for 2-4 wk GERD: 40 mg once daily for up to 8 wk	

Summary of Drugs Used for Treatment of Gastroesophageal Reflux Disease, Laryngopharyngeal Reflux, and Peptic Ulcer Disease—cont'd

Generic Name	U.S. Brand Name	Usual Adult Oral Dosage and Dosing Schedule	Warning Labels
rabeprazole	Aciphex	PUD: 20 mg once daily after the morning meal for 3-6 wk GERD: 20 mg once daily for 4 wk; repeat course of treatment if necessary.	
Prokinetic Drugs			
metoclopramide	Reglan	GERD: 10-15 mg, up to qid	MAY CAUSE DROWSINESS. AVOID ALCOHOL. TAKE 15-30 MIN BEFORE MEALS.
domperidone	Generics	10 mg tid to qid	
Mucosal Protectants			
misoprostol	Cytotec	NSAID-induced PUD prevention: 100-200 mcg qid for 4-8 wk	AVOID PREGNANCY.
sucralfate	Carafate	Duodenal ulcer: 1 g qid for 4-8 wk	TAKE ON AN EMPTY STOMACH. SHAKE SUSPENSION WELL.
Antimicrobial Combinations for *H. pylori* Eradication			
metronidazole + tetracycline + bismuth	Helidac: 14-day kit	*H. pylori*–associated ulcer: 1 metronidazole tablet + 1 tetracycline cap + 2 bismuth tablets qid for 14 days, with an H2 receptor antagonist or proton pump inhibitor	AVOID ALCOHOL. MAY CAUSE DISCOLORATION OF URINE OR FECES. AVOID PROLONGED EXPOSURE TO SUNLIGHT. AVOID DAIRY PRODUCTS, ANTACIDS, AND IRON PRODUCTS.
lansoprazole + amoxicillin + clarithromycin	PrevPAC	*H. pylori*–associated ulcer: 2 amoxicillin caps + 1 lansoprazole cap + 1 clarithromycin tablet bid for 10-14 days	SWALLOW WHOLE; DON'T CRUSH OR CHEW. MAY DECREASE EFFECTIVENESS OF ORAL CONTRACEPTIVES

TECH ALERT!
The following drugs have look-alike and sound-alike issues:
metoclopramide and metolazone;
Reglan, Regonol, and Renagel

Chapter Summary

- Gastroesophageal reflux disease, peptic ulcer disease, and laryngopharyngeal reflux are diseases that affect millions of Americans and Canadians.
- Persons of any age can develop GERD.
- Although these diseases initially produce minor discomfort, they may progress to life-threatening hemorrhage or stomach cancer.
- GERD causes a chronic backflow (reflux) of acidic stomach contents and digestive enzymes up into the esophagus.
- Stomach contents back up into the esophagus when there is a buildup of pressure in the stomach. Pressure buildup causes the lower esophageal sphincter, a muscle located at the junction between the esophagus and the upper stomach, to open and leak.
- Excessive or chronic exposure to gastric acids can lead to inflammation, ulceration, and changes to the epithelial cells that can cause stomach cancers.
- GERD may also increase the risk for development of chronic disease, such as asthma.
- Hiatal hernia is a significant risk factor for GERD in persons older than 50 years.
- Fried food, mint flavoring, spicy foods, tomato-based foods, and citrus fruits are some foods that can aggravate GERD.
- Consumption of caffeinated beverages and alcohol and cigarette smoking are lifestyle factors that make GERD symptoms worse.
- Prescription and OTC medicines can aggravate GERD.

- Laryngopharyngeal reflux is closely related to GERD; it occurs when gastric contents reflux into the larynx and pharynx.
- LPR causes hoarseness, voice fatigue, laryngitis, sore throat, chronic cough, bad breath, sinusitis, wheezing, aggravation of asthma, and even middle ear infections.
- An ulcer is an open wound or sore. A peptic ulcer may be located in the stomach or duodenum.
- Almost two thirds of the world's population is infected with *H. pylori*, the primary cause of peptic ulcer disease.
- *H. pylori* releases buffers that enable the bacteria to survive in the acidic contents of the stomach. These bacteria also release virulence factors that are responsible for inflammation and tissue damage.
- Age, medicines, and family history or living with close relatives who have PUD are risk factors for developing an ulcer.
- Medicines that can cause the development of ulcers are salicylates (e.g., aspirin), nonsteroidal anti-inflammatory drugs (e.g., naproxen), and corticosteroids (e.g., prednisone).
- The treatment of GERD, LPR, and PUD is aimed at reducing gastrointestinal irritants (e.g., gastric acid, digestive enzymes such as pepsin) and increasing protective factors (e.g., mucus secretion by epithelial cells).
- Acid-neutralizing drugs (antacids), acid-suppressing drugs (proton pump inhibitors and H2 receptor antagonists), and mucosal protectants (e.g., misoprostol, sucralfate) are used to treat GERD, LPR, and PUD.
- Treatment of PUD also involves eliminating *H. pylori* infection with antimicrobials.
- Patients who have GERD and LPR may be prescribed prokinetic drugs (e.g., metoclopramide) to increase GI motility.
- The four H2 receptor antagonists marketed in the United States and Canada are cimetidine, famotidine, nizatidine, and ranitidine.
- H2 receptor antagonists competitively and reversibly bind to H2 receptors, blocking histamine-mediated acid secretion.
- H2 receptor antagonists can produce dizziness or drowsiness, constipation or diarrhea, bloating, headache, and confusion when taken at therapeutic doses.
- The six proton pump inhibitors currently marketed in the United States and Canada are dexlansoprazole, esomeprazole, lansoprazole, omeprazole, pantoprazole, and rabeprazole.
- PPIs decrease gastric acids by interfering with the final step in gastric acid production.
- PPIs are delayed-release formulations and must not be crushed or chewed.
- The most common side effects linked to PPIs are abdominal pain, headache, diarrhea or constipation, flatulence (gas), and nausea.
- Misoprostol is synthetic prostaglandin E. It stimulates the production of protective mucus and bicarbonate in the stomach.
- Misoprostol may produce abdominal cramps, diarrhea, menstrual irregularities, headache, and dizziness. It is contraindicated in pregnancy.
- Sucralfate binds to the ulcerated area and forms a protective barrier, much like a bandage protects a sore.
- Sucralfate may produce constipation, gas, dry mouth, and headache.
- Prokinetic drugs (e.g., metoclopramide, domperidone) increase peristalsis, speed gastric emptying, and improve lower esophageal sphincter tone.
- Common adverse effects associated with domperidone and metoclopramide include dizziness, diarrhea, abdominal pain, constipation, restlessness, and headache.
- Antacids neutralize gastric acids and decrease pepsin secretion.
- Antimicrobials are prescribed for the treatment of PUD to eradicate *H. pylori* infection. Clarithromycin, metronidazole, amoxicillin, and tetracycline are effective for eradicating *H. pylori*.

REVIEW QUESTIONS

1. Which sphincter in the digestive system is affected by GERD?
   a. Cardiac sphincter
   b. Pyloric sphincter
   c. Lower esophageal sphincter
   d. Laryngeal sphincter

2. What bacteria contribute to peptic ulcer disease?
   a. *Streptococcus*
   b. *Helicobacter pylori*
   c. *Staphylococcus*
   d. *Helicobacter spirella*

3. Name two H2 receptor antagonist drugs:
   a. Prilosec and cimetidine
   b. Prevacid and ranitidine
   c. Famotidine and diphenhydramine
   d. Ranitidine and famotidine

4. Proton pump inhibitors are effective in treating GERD, LPR, and PUD because they _____.
   a. Decrease gastric acid
   b. Block histamine
   c. Decrease respiratory mucus
   d. Do none of the above

5. Name two proton pump inhibitor drugs.
   a. Omeprazole and ketoconazole
   b. Esomeprazole and lansoprazole
   c. Pantoprazole and miconazole
   d. Omeprazole and nizatidine

6. _____ is currently the only prokinetic drug approved by the FDA.
   a. Pantoprazole
   b. Misoprostol
   c. Metoclopramide
   d. Sucralfate

7. _____-containing antacids cause diarrhea; _____-containing antacids cause constipation.
   a. Calcium; aluminum
   b. Magnesium; sodium
   c. Calcium; magnesium
   d. Magnesium; calcium

8. Antacids are the oldest drugs used in the treatment of GERD and PUD. Is this statement true or false?
   a. True
   b. False

9. What is the brand name for esomeprazole?
   a. Aciphex
   b. Protonix
   c. Pepcid
   d. Nexium

10. Which drug binds to the ulcerated area and forms a protective barrier, much like a bandage protects a sore?
    a. Sucralfate
    b. Misoprostol
    c. Axid
    d. Nexium

TECHNICIAN'S
CORNER

1. Describe the function of the lower esophageal sphincter and how it is affected by GERD.
2. Consumption of which two products increases the risk for peptic ulcer disease and can aggravate existing disease? How does it interfere with the healing of an ulcer?

Bibliography

FDA: FDA Approved Drug Products. 2012. Retrieved May 26, 2012, from http://www.accessdata.fda.gov/scripts/cder/drugsatfda/index.cfm?fuseaction=Search.Search_Drug_Name.

Guimarães E, Marguet C, Moreira Camargos P: Treatment of gastroesophageal reflux disease, *J Pediatr* 82(Suppl):S133-S145, 2006.

Health Canada: Drug Product Database. 2010. Retrieved May 26, 2012, form http://www.hc-sc.gc.ca/dhp-mps/prodpharma/databasdon/index-eng.php

Howden C, Blume S, de Lissovoy G: Practice patterns for managing *Helicobacter pylori* infection and upper gastrointestinal symptoms, *Am J Manag Care* 13:37-44, 2007.

Lance L, Lacy C, Armstrong L, et al: *Drug information handbook for the allied health professional*, ed 12, Hudson, OH, 2005, APhA Lexi-Comp.

Kabir S: The current status of *Helicobacter pylori* vaccines: a review, *Helicobacter* 12:89-102, 2007.

Kalant H, Grant D, Mitchell J: *Principles of medical pharmacology*, ed 7, Toronto, 2007, Elsevier Canada, pp 557-571.

Lipan M, Reidenberg J, Laitman J: *Anatomy of reflux: a growing health problem affecting structures of the head and neck, the anatomical record. Part B: new anatomy*, New York, 2006, Wiley-Liss, pp 261-270.

Mayo Clinic: GERD: Can certain medications increase severity? 2012 (http://www.mayoclinic.com/health/heartburn-gerd/AN00720/METHOD=print).

National Digestive Diseases Information Clearinghouse: *Heartburn, hiatal hernia, and gastroesophageal reflux disease (GERD) (NIH Publ. No. 03-0882)*, Bethesda, MD, 2003, National Institute of Diabetes and Digestive and Kidney Diseases (http://www.digestive.niddk.nih.gov).

Pilotto A, Franceschi M, Leandro G, et al. Clinical features of reflux esophagitis in older people: a study of 840 consecutive patients, *J Am Geriatr Soc* 54:1537-1542, 2006.

Melissa Archer, PharmD, Clinical Pharmacist, Gary Oderda, PharmD, MPH, Professor, University of Utah College of Pharmacy, Copyright © 2012 by University of Utah College of Pharmacy, Salt Lake City, Utah. All rights reserved. Drug Class review: Histamine H2 Receptor Antagonists March 2012

U.S. Pharmacopeia Center for Advancement of Patient Safety: *Use caution–avoid confusion (USP Quality Review No. 79)*, Rockville, MD, 2004, USP Center for Advancement of Patient Safety.

Web MD: Heartburn/GERD health center, 2012 (http://www.webmd.com/heartburn-gerd/guide).

27

Treatment of Irritable Bowel Syndrome, Ulcerative Colitis, and Crohn's Disease

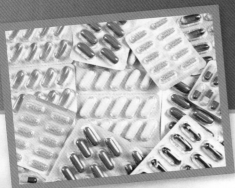

LEARNING
OBJECTIVES

1   Learn the terminology associated with irritable bowel syndrome (IBS), ulcerative colitis, and Crohn's disease.

2   List the symptoms of and risk factors for IBS, ulcerative colitis, and Crohn's disease.

3   List and categorize medications used to treat IBS, ulcerative colitis, and Crohn's disease.

4   Describe mechanism of action for drugs used to treat IBS, ulcerative colitis, and Crohn's disease.

5   Identify significant drug look-alike and sound-alike issues.

6   List common endings for drug classes used for the treatment of IBS, ulcerative colitis, and Crohn's disease.

7   Identify warning labels and precautionary messages associated with medications used to treat IBS, ulcerative colitis, and Crohn's disease.

KEY TERMS

Antidiarrheals: Drugs that prevent or relieve diarrhea.

Colonoscopy: Examination of the colon for signs of inflammation and damage performed by inserting a thin tube with a small light and camera at the end (i.e., an endoscope) into the anus.

Constipation: Abnormally delayed or infrequent passage of dry hardened feces.

Crohn's disease: Irritable bowel disease that produces inflammation and damage anywhere along the gastrointestinal tract.

Diarrhea: Abnormally frequent passage of loose and watery stools.

Fistula: Ulcer that tunnels from the site of origin to surrounding tissues.

Gastroenteritis: Inflammation of the lining membrane of the stomach and the intestines.

Inflammatory bowel disease: Chronic disorder of the gastrointestinal tract characterized by inflammation of the intestine and resulting in abdominal cramping and persistent diarrhea.

Irritable bowel syndrome: Condition that causes abdominal distress and erratic movement of the contents of the large bowel resulting in diarrhea and/or constipation.

Laxative: Medicine that induces evacuation of the bowel.

Toxic megacolon: Life-threatening condition characterized by a very inflated colon, abdominal distention, and sometimes fever, abdominal pain, or shock.

Ulcer: Crater-like wound or sore.

Ulcerative colitis: Irritable bowel disease that produces inflammation, ulcers, and damage to the colon.

Overview

Irritable bowel syndrome (IBS) and *inflammatory bowel disease* (IBD) are conditions of the GI tract. The similar names sometimes cause confusion but the root causes are not the same. The two major types of IBD are *ulcerative colitis* (UC) and *Crohn's disease* (CD). Both conditions are linked to inflammation of the gastrointestinal (GI) tract, unlike IBS. Based on symptoms, a diagnosis of IBS may be made after diagnostic tests have been performed to rule out other diseases (e.g., ulcerative colitis, CD). Diagnostic tests that may be performed to diagnose ulcerative colitis and CD include testing stool samples, taking x-rays, and performing a *colonoscopy*. A colonoscopy enables the physician to examine the colon for inflammation and damage (Figure 27-1).

Irritable Bowel Syndrome

Irritable bowel syndrome (IBS) is a condition that causes abdominal distress and erratic movement of the large bowel. An estimated 10% to 15% of people in North America have IBS (5% to 20% of men and 15% to 25% of women), which can involve abdominal pain, bloating, and other discomfort, including constipation and diarrhea. IBS affects quality of life and productivity for millions of people. Symptoms commonly occur before the age of 35 years. When an individual has IBS, movement of waste through the colon (large bowel) may occur too slowly and *constipation* results, or it occurs too rapidly, causing *diarrhea*. IBS is sometimes called colitis, but it is not the same condition as ulcerative colitis.

WHAT CAUSES IRRITABLE BOWEL SYNDROME?

There is no one specific cause for IBS. Persons with IBS have an overly sensitive colon. Food allergies, stress, antibiotic use, chronic alcohol use, and bile acid malabsorption are possible causes of IBS. *Gastroenteritis*, a stomach and intestinal inflammation, may be triggered by infection. Postinfectious IBS may follow an acute bout of gastroenteritis. IBS may also be associated with abnormally low levels of the neurotransmitter serotonin. Up to 95% of the body's serotonin (5-HT) is found in the stomach epithelium. The remaining 5% is found in neurons in the brain (see Chapter 6). Low levels of serotonin can cause GI motility problems and increase the sensitivity of pain receptors in the GI tract.

Inflammatory Bowel Disease

IBD is thought to be an autoimmune disorder, whereby the body reacts to its own intestinal tract. The four inflammatory diseases of the bowel are ulcerative colitis, Crohn's disease, ulcerative proctitis,

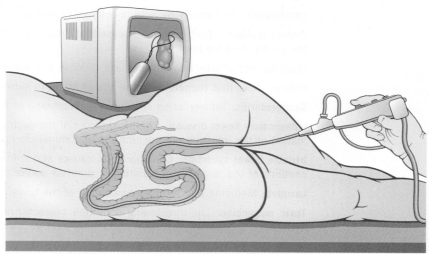

FIGURE 27-1 Colonoscopy and sigmoidoscopy. (From Chabner DE: *The language of medicine*, ed 8, St Louis, 2008, Saunders.)

and pouchitis. UC and CD are the most common and will be discussed in this chapter. UC only affects the colon and CD can involve any segment of the GI tract. CD may also cause inflammation in the eye, mouth, or some joints.

Ulcerative Colitis

Ulcerative colitis is one of several irritable bowel diseases that produce inflammation and damage to the colon. Ultimately, *ulcers* (or sores) form in the lining of the colon and rectum. UC can occur at any age, but most commonly occurs between the ages of 15 and 30 years and affects men and women equally.

Ulcerative colitis differs from Crohn's disease in two important ways. Ulcerative colitis produces inflammation in the upper layers of the lining of the small intestine and colon, whereas Crohn's disease produces inflammation deep in the intestinal wall. Moreover, the inflammation is limited to the small intestine and colon rather than other areas of the GI tract.

WHAT CAUSES ULCERATIVE COLITIS?

The exact cause of ulcerative colitis is unknown, but it is believed to be linked to abnormal functioning of the immune system. When a person has ulcerative colitis, the body's immune system recognizes the bacteria that normally inhabit the GI tract as harmful invaders. Tumor necrosis factor (TNF) and other substances that are released to fight the so-called infection cause pain and inflammation.

Crohn's Disease

Crohn's disease is one of several irritable bowel diseases. Like ulcerative colitis, it causes chronic inflammation of the entire GI tract. Inflammation can occur anywhere along the entire length of the GI tube, from the mouth to the anus, although typically it affects the ileum (the lower part of the small intestine). The inflammation is formed deep within the intestinal wall causing abdominal pain.

CAUSES

The root cause for Crohn's disease is not known. The body's immune system is thought to target the bacteria that normally inhabit the GI tract, foods and other substances, thinking they are harmful invaders. This produces an inflammatory response, which if chronic can lead to ulceration. It is not known whether genes, environmental antigens, microbes, or the body's own immune system triggers the onset of the disease. As with ulcerative colitis, high levels of TNF and other substances that are released to fight the infection are present in those with Crohn's disease.

SYMPTOMS OF IRRITABLE BOWEL SYNDROME, ULCERATIVE COLITIS, AND CROHN'S DISEASE

Many of the symptoms of IBS, ulcerative colitis, and Crohn's disease are similar; however, there are some symptoms that are disease-specific. Table 27-1 compares symptoms common to IBS, ulcerative colitis, and Crohn's disease.

Lifestyle Modification

People who have IBS, ulcerative colitis, or Crohn's disease can reduce their symptoms by making changes in their lifestyle. Food and beverages that aggravate diarrhea, bloating, and gas should be avoided. Stress management may reduce the frequency of symptoms even where it is not the direct cause of the disease, as with ulcerative colitis. A list of lifestyle modifications is given in Box 27-1.

Drugs Used for the Treatment of Irritable Bowel Syndrome

IBS is treated by administering a serotonin receptor antagonist (5-HT$_3$), prostaglandin E1 derivative, antidiarrheal, *laxative*, fiber supplement, or anticholinergic.

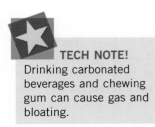

TECH NOTE!
Drinking carbonated beverages and chewing gum can cause gas and bloating.

TABLE 27-1   **Symptoms of Irritable Bowel Syndrome, Ulcerative Colitis, and Crohn's Disease**

	Irritable Bowel Syndrome	Ulcerative Colitis	Crohn's Disease
Similar symptoms	Abdominal pain Diarrhea (mucus, pus) Cramping	Abdominal pain Diarrhea (bloody) Cramping	Abdominal pain Diarrhea Cramping
Disease-specific symptoms	Erratic bowel movements (diarrhea alternating with constipation) Abdominal pain relieved by having a bowel movement Bloating Constipation	Rectal bleeding Anemia Weight loss, loss of appetite Fatigue Loss of vitamins and minerals Skin lesions Joint pain (arthritis) Decreased growth in children Fever	Rectal bleeding Anemia Weight loss, loss of appetite Loss of vitamins and minerals Skin lesions Joint pain (arthritis) Decreased growth in children Fever

BOX 27-1   **Lifestyle Modification to Reduce Symptoms of Irritable Bowel Syndrome, Ulcerative Colitis, and Crohn's Disease**

- Eat small meals.
- Drink at least six to eight glasses of water daily.
- Avoid alcohol.
- Avoid caffeinated beverages (e.g., coffee, tea, cola drinks).
- Limit carbonated beverages.
- Avoid foods that worsen symptoms.*
- Engage in stress reduction activities.

*Following a diet for celiac disease may reduce symptoms of irritable bowel syndrome. Avoid wheat, rye, barley, dairy, and chocolate.

SEROTONIN RECEPTOR ANTAGONIST

New medications have been developed that selectively target the serotonin receptors. The neurotransmitter serotonin controls GI motility. There are a number of types of serotonin receptors. Stimulation of 5-HT$_3$ receptors can cause diarrhea. Stimulation of 5-HT$_4$ receptors produces constipation.

Mechanism of Action

Serotonin receptor antagonists used to treat IBS act at the 5-HT$_3$ receptor. Antagonism of the 5-HT$_3$ receptors by alosetron in the terminal of the vagus nerve (extends from brain to the abdomen) in the intestines and periphery decreases gastric motility and regulates transit through the colon, GI secretion, and visceral pain. Antagonism of 5-HT$_3$ receptors in the chemoreceptor trigger zone, such as with ondansetron (Zofran), prevents and controls nausea and vomiting produced by cancer chemotherapy.

Adverse Reactions

The most common side effects of alosetron are constipation, anxiety, difficulty sleeping or drowsiness, dry mouth, frequent urination, gas, headache, nausea, and restlessness. Alosetron's side effects limit its use. Alosetron may cause severe GI obstruction or impaction, leading to *toxic megacolon*.

Precautions

Alosetron is approved for women with severe IBS when other therapies have failed. The drug was withdrawn from the market shortly after its introduction. The U.S. Food and Drug Administration (FDA) permitted alosetron to be reintroduced, but with restricted access. Refills are not permitted until the patient has a follow-up examination by her prescribing physician. Patients and physicians must agree to adhere to therapeutic plans. The drug must be used cautiously because it can significantly decrease blood flow to the colon, causing ischemic colitis, toxic megacolon, and death.

TECH NOTE!
Alosetron is available only from health care providers who participate in a special prescribing program.

Serotonin Receptor Antagonist

Generic Name	U.S. Brand Name(s)	Dosage Forms and Strengths
	Canadian Brand Name(s)	
alosetron	Lotronex	Tablet: 0.5 mg, 1 mg
	Not available	

TECH ALERT!
Lotronex and Lovenox have look-alike and sound-alike issues.

PROSTAGLANDIN E1 DERIVATIVE

Lubiprostone (Amitiza) is FDA-approved for the treatment of IBS in women when constipation is the predominant symptom. Lubiprostone increases intestinal fluid secretion, improving the consistency of the stool, and reduces straining.

Mechanism of Action

Numerous chloride ion channels are found in the GI tract; their role is to secrete and transport fluids. Lubiprostone activates type 2 chloride channels (CIC-2) in the gut, increasing the flow of chloride ions into the intestines; this is followed by sodium and water. The increased intestinal fluid volume softens the stool, increases motility in the intestine, and promotes spontaneous bowel movements.

Adverse Reactions

Up to one third of the patients treated with lubiprostone experience nausea. Other side effects are abdominal pain and diarrhea.

Prostaglandin E1 (PGE1) Derivative

Generic Name	U.S. Brand Name(s)	Dosage Forms and Strengths
	Canadian Brand Name(s)	
lubiprostone	Amitiza	Capsule: 8 mcg, 24 mcg
	Not available	

BULK-FORMING LAXATIVES AND FIBER SUPPLEMENTS

Bulk-forming laxative and fiber supplements are administered to relieve constipation and diarrhea. They are the laxative of choice for treating the symptoms of IBS. Bulk-forming laxatives swell in the presence of liquid. Bacteria normally live in the colon and digest cellulose and polysaccharide fibers. As the bacteria colony grows, colonic bulk increases. This causes the bowel to feel full and stimulates evacuation. Polycarbophil is the only bulk-forming laxative that is FDA-approved for the treatment of IBS. It can be obtained without prescription.

Mechanism of Action

Polycarbophil is a polyacrylic resin that can absorb 60 to 100 times its weight in water to form a gel that expands and increases bulk and moisture in the stool. The increased bulk stimulates peristalsis and promotes the transit of contents through the bowel. This bulk-forming laxative also promotes fluid accumulation in the colon.

Adverse Reactions

Bulk-forming laxatives can cause bloating, gas, abdominal cramps, nausea, diarrhea, or constipation.

Bulk-Forming Laxatives

Generic Name	U.S. Brand Name(s)	Dosage Forms and Strengths	Over the Counter or Prescription
	Canadian Brand Name(s)		
polycarbophil*	Equalactin, Fiberall, Fibercon, Fibertab, Konsyl Fiber Tablet	Tablet: 500 mg, 625 mg, 1250 mg chewable	OTC
	Equalactin, Prodiem Bulk Fiber Therapy		

*Generic available.

OPIOID ANTIDIARRHEALS

Opioid *antidiarrheals* are administered to control watery and frequent stools. Those prescribed for the treatment of diarrhea are difenoxin, diphenoxylate, and loperamide. Difenoxin and loperamide are more potent than diphenoxylate. Difenoxin and diphenoxylate are controlled substances and may produce dependence at high doses,

Mechanism of Action

Opioid antidiarrheals such as difenoxin bind to opioid receptors on smooth muscle cells of the GI tract. They induce spasms that interfere with effective peristalsis. They decrease propulsive contractions by inhibiting the release of acetylcholine. Difenoxin is an active metabolite of diphenoxylate.

Adverse Reactions

Sedation and dizziness are the most common side effects of opioid antidiarrheals. They may also produce constipation. Diphenoxylate and its metabolite difenoxin are controlled substances and may cause tolerance and dependence. Loperamide is not habit-forming and is available without a prescription. Antidiarrheals should be used cautiously for patients with ulcerative colitis because they can cause toxic megacolon.

ANTICHOLINERGICS

Anticholinergic drugs are used for the treatment of IBS when diarrhea is the primary symptom. Atropine and dicyclomine are FDA-approved agents for the treatment of IBS. Atropine and dicyclomine decrease GI muscular tone and motility by producing a nonspecific, direct spasmolytic action on GI smooth muscle.

TECH ALERT!
The following drugs have look-alike and sound-alike issues:
difenoxin + atropine
diphenoxylate + atropine

Antidiarrheals

Generic Name	U.S. Brand Name(s)	Dosage Forms and Strengths	U.S. Controlled Substance Schedule
	Canadian Brand Name(s)		
difenoxin + atropine	Motofen	Tablet: 1 mg difenoxin + 0.025 mg atropine	C-IV
	Not available		
diphenoxylate + atropine*	Lomotil, Lonox	Tablet: 2.5 mg diphenoxylate + 0.025 mg atropine	C-V
	Lomotil		
loperamide*	Imodium-AD	Capsule: 2 mg Tablet, chewable: 2 mg Tablet: 2 mg Solution, oral: 1 mg/5 mL Suspension, oral: 1 mg/7.5 mL	Not scheduled
	Imodium, Diarr-Eze, Imodium Quick Dissolve		
loperamide + simethicone	Imodium Multi-Symptom Relief	Tablet, chewable: 2 mg loperamide + 125 mg simethicone	Not scheduled
	Imodium Advanced Multi-Symptom chewable tablets		

*Generic available.

Anticholinergics

Generic Name	U.S. Brand Name(s)	Dosage Forms and Strengths
	Canadian Brand Name(s)	
dicyclomine*	Bentyl	Capsule: 10 mg
	Bentylol, Formulex	Solution, for injection: 10 mg/mL
		Tablet: 10 mg‡, 20 mg
		Syrup: 10 mg/5 mL

*Generic available.
‡Strength available in Canada only.

Adverse Reactions

Anticholinergic agents may produce constipation, difficulty sleeping, dry mouth, change in taste, headache, photophobia (increased sensitivity of the eyes to light), nausea, sexual difficulty (e.g., impotence), fast or slow heartbeat, urinary retention, dizziness, or drowsiness. At higher doses, hallucinations may occur.

Aminosalicylates

Generic Name	U.S. Brand Name(s)	Dosage Forms and Strengths
	Canadian Brand Name(s)	
balsalazide*	Colazal, Giazo	Capsule: 750 mg, 1.1 Gm
	Not available	
mesalamine* (known as mesalazine in Canada; 5-aminosalicylic acid [5-ASA])	Apriso, Asacol, Asacol HD, Lialda, Canasa, Pentasa, Rowasa, SFRowasa	Capsule, biphasic, extended-release (Apriso): 0.375 g†
		Capsule, extended-release (Pentasa): 250 mg†, 500 mg†
		Suppository (Canasa, Salofalk): 500 mg‡, 1 g
	Asacol, Asacol-800, Mesasal, Mezavant, Pentasa, Salofalk	Suspension, rectal (Pentasa): 1 g/100 mL‡, 4 g/100 mL‡
		Suspension, rectal: 2 g/60 mL‡ (Salofalk); 4 g/60 mL (Rowasa, SFRowasa, Salofalk)
		Tablet, delayed-release (Asacol, Asacol HD, Asacol-800): 400 mg, 800 mg
		Tablet, delayed- and extended-release (Lialda, Mezavant): 1.2 g
		Tablet, enteric-coated (Mesasal, Salofalk): 500 mg‡
		Tablet, extended-release (Pentasa): 500 mg‡
olsalazine	Dipentum	Capsule: 250 mg
	Dipentum	
sulfasalazine*	Azulfadine, Azulfadine EN tablets	Suspension, oral: 250 mg/5 mL†
		Tablet: 500 mg
	Salazopyrin, Salazopyrin EN tablets	Tablet, enteric-coated: 500 mg

*Generic available.
†Strength available in the United States only.
‡Strength available in Canada only.

Drugs Used for the Treatment of Ulcerative Colitis

Medicines administered for the management of ulcerative colitis are used to reduce symptoms and induce remission.

AMINOSALICYLATES

Aminosalicylates are administered to patients with ulcerative colitis and Crohn's disease to reduce inflammation. The four aminosalicylate anti-inflammatory agents available in the United States and Canada are sulfasalazine, olsalazine, mesalamine (mesalazine in Canada), and balsalazide.

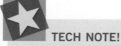

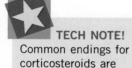
Mechanism of Action

The mechanism of anti-inflammatory action produced by aminosalicylates is not completely known. Sulfasalazine inhibits substances released by the body that produce the symptoms of inflammation (e.g., leukotrienes, prostaglandins, cytokines). It also decreases cytokine production.

Pharmacokinetics

Sulfasalazine, olsalazine, mesalamine (mesalazine in Canada) are all formulations that contain 5-aminosalicylic acid (5-ASA). Balsalazide is a prodrug of mesalamine. Sulfasalazine (sulfapyridine+5-ASA) and olsalazine (two 5-ASA molecules) are also prodrugs. Bacteria in the colon metabolize the drugs and release the active metabolite (5-ASA). The effectiveness of sulfasalazine and olsalazine is reduced by factors that decrease the bacteria in the colon (e.g., antibiotics) and decrease the gut pH. Delayed release formulations of 5-ASA coated with a pH-dependent resin, release their active moiety in a less acidic environment. The optimal activity of 5-ASA depends on a rise in the pH of pH > 7 in the distal ileum. Pentasa is a time-release formulation.

Adverse Reactions

The most common adverse effects of sulfasalazine, olsalazine, mesalamine (mesalazine), and balsalazide are nausea, vomiting, heartburn, headache, and watery diarrhea. Side effects that occur less frequently are inflammation of the heart muscle and pericardium, pancreatitis, and pneumonitis. Sulfasalazine may also cause sunburn, impaired folic acid absorption, crystalluria, and damage to white blood cells (cytopenias).

CORTICOSTEROIDS

Glucocorticosteroids are commonly prescribed to suppress inflammation, reduce flare-ups, and treat pain associated with ulcerative colitis and Crohn's disease. Glucocorticosteroids are potent anti-inflammatory drugs. They decrease the synthesis of proinflammatory substances such as prostaglandins (see Chapter 10), leukotrienes, cytokines, arachidonic acid, and macrophages that are released as part of the inflammatory response. Glucocorticosteroids have immunosuppressive actions that may inhibit the abnormal immune system activity associated with Crohn's disease and ulcerative colitis.

Adverse Reactions

Corticosteroids prescribed to treat ulcerative colitis and Crohn's disease may be administered by mouth or rectally in the form of an enema or suppository. Oral administration produces systemic

Corticosteroids

Generic Name	U.S. Brand Name(s) / Canadian Brand Name(s)	Dosage Forms and Strengths
hydrocortisone*	Colocort, Cortenema, Cortifoam, Cortef	Foam, rectal (Cortifoam): 10% Suspension, rectal (Colocort, Cortenema, Hycort): 100 mg/60 mL Tablet (Cortef): 5 mg, 10 mg, 20 mg
	Cortef, Cortenema, Cortifoam, Hycort	
prednisone*	Generics	Tablet: 1 mg, 2.5 mg†, 5 mg, 10 mg†, 20 mg†, 50 mg Oral concentrate: 5 mg/mL Oral solution: 5 mg/5 mL
	Winpred	
dexamethasone*	Generics	Tablet: 0.5 mg, 0.75 mg, 1 mg, 1.5 mg, 2 mg, 4 mg, 6 mg Oral concentrate: 0.5 mg/5 mL solution†; 1 mg/mL†
	Dexasone	
methylprednisolone*	Medrol	Tablet: 4 mg, 8 mg†, 16 mg, 32 mg†
	Medrol	

*Generic available.
†Strength available in the United States only.

effects, described in Chapter 15. Adverse effects caused by rectal administration may be local (e.g., burning, itching) or systemic (e.g., nausea, constipation or diarrhea, appetite changes, headache).

Drugs Used for the Treatment of Crohn's Disease

Given the similarity of symptoms and the similar mechanism of disease progression of Crohn's disease and ulcerative colitis, many agents used for the treatment of the two diseases are the same. Aminosalicylates, corticosteroids, immunosuppressants, antidiarrheals, and nutritional supplements are used for the treatment of Crohn's disease and ulcerative colitis. Additional medications used for the treatment of Crohn's disease are immunomodulators and antibiotics.

IMMUNOSUPPRESSANTS

Azathioprine, 6-mercaptopurine, and methotrexate are classified as antimetabolites. They are used for the treatment of Crohn's disease to induce remission. Azathioprine suppresses T cell–mediated immune system response. Methotrexate decreases cytokine and immunoglobulin production and cyclooxygenase-2 (COX-2) activity, reducing inflammation and immune system activity (see Chapter 15).

IMMUNOMODULATORS

Infliximab and natalizumab are immunomodulators that have been approved for the treatment of moderate to severe Crohn's disease. They are administered to induce remission of active disease and then are continued as maintenance therapy in patients who have had unsuccessful results with other therapies.

Mechanism of Action

Infliximab (Remicade) is a genetically engineered TNF-α inhibitor. Infliximab blocks the inflammatory process triggered by high concentrations of tumor necrosis factor. TNF levels are increased in Crohn's disease. Infliximab prevents cell lysis (destruction) and the release of substances that cause

TECH ALERT!
Prednisone and prednisolone have look-alike and sound-alike issues.

TECH ALERT!
The following drugs have look-alike and sound-alike issues:
azathioprine and Azulfidine;
Imuran and Imdur

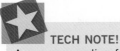

TECH NOTE!
A common ending for immunomodulators is -mab.

Immunosuppressants

Generic Name	U.S. Brand Name(s) / Canadian Brand Name(s)	Dosage Forms and Strengths
azathioprine*,†	Azasan, Imuran	Powder, for injection: 50 mg/vial‡, 100 mg/vial†
	Imuran	Tablet: 25 mg†, 50 mg, 75 mg†, 100 mg†
6-mercaptopurine*,†	Purinethol	Tablet: 50 mg
	Purinethol	
methotrexate*	Trexall	Tablet: 2.5 mg, 5 mg†, 7.5 mg†, 10 mg, 15 mg†
	Generics	Solution, injection: 25 mg/mL
		Powder, injection: 1 g

*Generic available.
†Strength available in the United States only.
‡Strength available in Canada only.

Immunomodulators

Generic Name	U.S. Brand Name(S) / Canadian Brand Name(s)	Dosage Forms and Strengths
infliximab	Remicade	Powder for injection: 100 mg/vial
	Remicade	
natalizumab	Tysabri	Solution for injection: 300 mg/15 mL
	Tysabri	

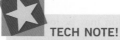

TECH NOTE!
Infliximab package labeling contains an FDA-required boxed warning that teenage or young adult males with Crohn's disease or ulcerative colitis taking infliximab and azathioprine or 6-mercaptopurine may develop a rare form of fatal lymphoma.

TECH NOTE!
Natalizumab should not be used in combination with TNF-α inhibitors or immunosuppressants such as 6-mercaptopurine, azathioprine, cyclosporine, or methotrexate. Reauthorization of treatment is needed every 6 months.

inflammation. A detailed description of the mechanism of action for TNF-α inhibitors is given in Chapter 15. Natalizumab is an α₄ integrin inhibitor. It reduces T cell–mediated intestinal inflammation by interfering with counterreceptors in the intestines and vascular endothelium, needed for lymphocytes to enter the intestine and central nervous system (CNS).

Adverse Reactions

Nausea, stomach pain, headache, redness, itching at the site of infusion, chest pain, hypertension, dyspnea, increased susceptibility to opportunistic infections, reactivation of dormant infections (e.g., tuberculosis), and worsening of existing infection are adverse reactions produced by infliximab.

ANTI-INFECTIVES

Patients who have Crohn's disease may develop fistulas. A fistula forms when an ulcer tunnels from the site of origin to surrounding tissues. Fistulas may be located in the bladder, vagina, and skin surrounding the anus and rectum. Anti-infective agents may be prescribed to treat infections that develop in the fistula. Anti-infectives prescribed to treat fistulas include ampicillin, sulfonamides, cephalosporins, tetracycline, or metronidazole; these are described in Chapter 35.

Summary of Drugs Used for the Treatment of Irritable Bowel Disease, Ulcerative Colitis, and Crohn's Disease

Generic Name	U.S. Brand Name	Usual Adult Oral Dose and Dosing Schedule	Warning Labels
Serotonin Receptor Antagonist			
alosetron	Lotronex	IBS: 0.5-1 mg twice daily for 4 wk###	MAY CAUSE DIZZINESS OR DROWSINESS; AVOID DRIVING. AVOID ALCOHOL. TAKE WITH A FULL GLASS OF WATER.
Prostaglandin E1 Derivative			
lubiprostone	Amitiza	IBS: 8-16 mcg twice per day	TAKE WITH A FULL GLASS OF WATER. TAKE WITH FOOD.
Bulk-Forming Laxatives			
polycarbophil	Equalactin, Fiberall, Fibercon, Fibertab	IBS: 1 g 1-4 times per day	TAKE WITH A FULL GLASS OF WATER.
Antidiarrheals			
difenoxin + atropine**	Motofen	Acute diarrhea: 2 tablets immediately; then 1 tablet after each loose stool	MAY CAUSE DIZZINESS OR DROWSINESS; AVOID DRIVING. AVOID ALCOHOL. DRINK LOTS OF FLUIDS.
diphenoxylate + atropine**	Lomotil	Acute diarrhea: 2 tablets immediately; then 1 tablet 2-3 times a day	
loperamide**	Imodium	Acute diarrhea: 2 tablets immediately; then 1 tablet after each loose stool	
Anticholinergics			
atropine	Atreza	IBS: 0.3 mg to 1.2 mg every 4 to 6 hr	MAY CAUSE DIZZINESS OR DROWSINESS; AVOID DRIVING. AVOID ALCOHOL. DRINK LOTS OF FLUIDS. TAKE ON AN EMPTY STOMACH. AVOID ANTACIDS WITHIN 1-2 HR OF DOSE (DICYCLOMINE).
dicyclomine	Bentyl	IBS: 20 mg to 40 mg 4 times a day	

Summary of Drugs Used for the Treatment of Irritable Bowel Disease, Ulcerative Colitis, and Crohn's Disease—cont'd

Generic Name	U.S. Brand Name	Usual Adult Oral Dose and Dosing Schedule	Warning Labels
Aminosalicylates			
balsalazide	Colazal	Ulcerative colitis: 3 caps (2250 mg) 3 times a day	SWALLOW WHOLE; DON'T CRUSH OR CHEW. CAPSULE CONTENTS MAY BE SPRINKLED ON APPLESAUCE.
mesalamine (5-ASA)	Canasa	Ulcerative colitis: Insert one suppository rectally twice a day	REMOVE FOIL AND INSERT (SUPPOSITORY). MAY DISCOLOR CLOTHING OR SKIN (ORANGE-YELLOW, SUPPOSITORY). SHAKE WELL (RECTAL SUSPENSION). SWALLOW WHOLE; DON'T CRUSH OR CHEW (DELAYED RELEASE). TAKE WITH FOOD (DELAYED RELEASE).
	Rowasa	Ulcerative colitis: 4 g enema nightly	
	Asacol	Ulcerative colitis: 1 tablet 3 times a day	
	Lialda	Ulcerative colitis: 1 tablet daily	
	Pentasa, Mesasal, Salofalk	Ulcerative colitis: 1 g qid	
olsalazine	Dipentum	Ulcerative colitis: 1 g daily in two divided doses	SWALLOW WHOLE; DON'T CRUSH OR CHEW. TAKE WITH FOOD.
sulfasalazine	Azulfidine	Ulcerative colitis: 1 g tid or qid	SWALLOW WHOLE; DON'T CRUSH OR CHEW (ENTERIC-COATED TABLETS). AVOID PROLONGED EXPOSURE TO SUNLIGHT. DRINK LOTS OF FLUIDS.
Corticosteroids			
hydrocortisone	Cortema	Ulcerative colitis: 100 mg rectal enema nightly for 21 days	SHAKE WELL.
	Anucort	Ulcerative colitis: 1 suppository rectally 2 to 3 times a day for 2 wk	REMOVE FOIL AND INSERT.
	Cortifoam	Ulcerative colitis: 1 applicatorful 1 to 2 times a day for 2 to 3 wk; then every other day	SHAKE WELL.
	Hydrocortone, Cortef	Crohn's or ulcerative colitis: 20 mg to 240 mg daily in 2 to 4 divided doses	TAKE WITH FOOD. DON'T DISCONTINUE ABRUPTLY.
dexamethasone	Generic	Crohn's or ulcerative colitis: 0.75 mg/day to 9 mg/day in 2 to 4 divided doses	TAKE WITH FOOD. DON'T DISCONTINUE ABRUPTLY.
prednisone	Generic	Crohn's or ulcerative colitis: 40 mg to 60 mg daily; taper over 2 to 3 months	
methylprednisolone	Medrol	Crohn's or ulcerative colitis: 4 mg to 48 mg daily in 4 divided doses	

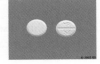

Continued

Summary of Drugs Used for the Treatment of Irritable Bowel Disease, Ulcerative Colitis, and Crohn's Disease—cont'd

Generic Name	U.S. Brand Name	Usual Adult Oral Dose and Dosing Schedule	Warning Labels
Immunosuppressants			
azathioprine**	Azasan, Imuran	Crohn's or ulcerative colitis: 1.5-2 mg/kg/day	TAKE WITH FOOD.
6-mecaptopurine**	Purinethol	1.5-2 mg/kg/day	AVOID ALCOHOL. AVOID PREGNANCY.
methotrexate**	Trexall	Crohn's or ulcerative colitis: 25 mg IM weekly for at least 3 months or 15 mg SC weekly for 16 wk	AVOID ALCOHOL. AVOID PREGNANCY.
Immunomodulators			
infliximab	Remicade	Crohn's or ulcerative colitis: 5 mg/kg IV at week 0, 2, and 6; then every 8 wk	
natalizumab	Tysabri	Crohn's: 300 mg IV infusion given over 1 hour every 4 wk. Revaluate every 6 months	MAY DISCOLOR URINE OR FECES. AVOID PREGNANCY AND DO NOT BREAST-FEED. MAY INCREASE RISK FOR INFECTION.

###Alosetron is only approved for 4-wk course of therapy and should be discontinued if symptoms are not controlled after 4 wk of therapy.
**Not FDA-approved for IBS, Crohn's disease or ulcerative colitis.

Chapter Summary

- Irritable bowel syndrome, ulcerative colitis, and Crohn's disease are conditions that are linked to inflammation of the gastrointestinal tract.
- IBS is a condition that causes abdominal distress and erratic movement of the large bowel.
- Persons with IBS may have diarrhea or constipation.
- IBS may also be associated with abnormally low levels of the neurotransmitter serotonin.
- Low levels of serotonin can cause GI motility problems and increase the sensitivity of pain receptors in the GI tract.
- Ulcerative colitis and Crohn's disease are irritable bowel diseases.
- In ulcerative colitis and Crohn's disease, the body's immune system recognizes the bacteria that normally inhabit the GI tract as harmful invaders and releases tumor necrosis factor.
- Ulcerative colitis produces inflammation in the upper layers of the lining of the small intestine and colon.
- Crohn's disease may produce inflammation and can occur anywhere along the entire length of the GI tube, from the mouth to the anus, although typically it affects the ileum (the lower part of the small intestine). Inflammation occurs deep in the intestinal wall.
- Abdominal pain, diarrhea, and cramping are common symptoms of IBS, ulcerative colitis, and Crohn's disease.
- Lifestyle modification can reduce symptoms of IBS, ulcerative colitis, and Crohn's disease.
- Stress management, eating small meals, and avoiding alcohol and caffeinated and carbonated beverages are recommended lifestyle changes.
- IBS may be treated by administering a serotonin receptor antagonist, antidiarrheal, laxative, fiber supplement, or anticholinergic agent.

- Alosetron is a 5-HT$_3$ receptor antagonist used to control diarrhea in women caused by severe IBS when other types of treatments have failed.
- Alosetron must be used cautiously because it can significantly decrease blood flow to the colon, causing ischemic colitis, toxic megacolon, and death.
- Alosetron prescriptions may not be refilled without a follow-up examination by the physician.
- Lubiprostone is a prostaglandin derivative approved for the treatment of IBS with constipation.
- Bulk-forming laxative and fiber supplements are given to relieve constipation and diarrhea.
- Antidiarrheals control watery and frequent stools.
- Diphenoxylate and difenoxin are controlled substances and may cause tolerance and dependence. Loperamide is not habit-forming and is sold over the counter (OTC).
- Antidiarrheals should be used cautiously in patients with ulcerative colitis because they can cause toxic megacolon.
- Atropine and dicyclomine decrease diarrhea by reducing GI muscular tone and motility.
- The aminosalicylates sulfasalazine, olsalazine, balsalazide, and mesalamine (mesalazine) are administered to patients with ulcerative colitis and Crohn's disease to reduce inflammation.
- All commercially available aminosalicylates are formulated as delayed-release products.
- Glucocorticosteroids are prescribed commonly to suppress inflammation, reduce flare-ups, and treat pain associated with ulcerative colitis and Crohn's disease.
- Glucocorticosteroids also have immunosuppressive actions that may inhibit the abnormal immune system activity that is associated with Crohn's disease and ulcerative colitis.
- Azathioprine, 6-mercaptopurine, and methotrexate are prescribed for the treatment of Crohn's disease to induce remission.
- Infliximab is an immunomodulator that has been approved for the treatment of Crohn's disease and is administered to induce remission.
- Infliximab is a TNF-α inhibitor that is genetically engineered to block the inflammatory process.
- Patients who have Crohn's disease may develop fistulas. Anti-infective agents may be prescribed to treat fistula infections.

REVIEW QUESTIONS

1. Which disease(s) is/are conditions linked to inflammation of the entire gastrointestinal tract?
   a. Irritable bowel syndrome
   b. Ulcerative colitis
   c. Crohn's disease
   d. All of the above

2. Which tests may be performed to diagnose ulcerative colitis and Crohn's disease?
   a. Sigmoidoscopy and proctoscopy
   b. Proctoscopy and colonoscopy
   c. Colonoscopy and sigmoidoscopy
   d. Jejunoscopy and stool sample

3. Which disease affects men and women equally?
   a. Ulcerative colitis
   b. Diverticulitis
   c. Crohn's disease
   d. Proctitis

4. Name three common symptoms of irritable bowel syndrome, ulcerative colitis, and Crohn's disease:
   a. Bloating, constipation, cramping
   b. Abdominal pain, diarrhea, cramping
   c. Rectal bleeding, bloating, diarrhea
   d. Cramping, abdominal pain, bloating

5. Which of the following drugs is used to treat IBS in which constipation is the primary symptom?
   a. Amitiza
   b. Lotronex
   c. Lovenox
   d. Alosetron

6. The laxatives of choice for treating the symptoms of irritable bowel syndrome are_____.
   a. Bulk-forming laxatives
   b. Fiber supplements
   c. Bile acid sequestrants
   d. a and b

7. An immunomodulator that has been approved for the treatment of Crohn's disease is _____.
   a. Infliximab
   b. Methotrexate
   c. Lomotil
   d. Dexamethasone

8. Patients who have Crohn's disease may develop _____, which form when an ulcer tunnels from the site of origin to surrounding tissues.
   a. Ulcers
   b. Fistulas
   c. Diverticuli
   d. None of the above

9. Give the trade name for the rectally administered corticosteroid.
   a. Dexacortef
   b. Medrol
   c. Imuran
   d. Cortenema

10. These warning labels should be applied to prescription vials for which class of drugs used for IBS? "May cause dizziness or drowsiness; avoid driving, avoid alcohol, drink lots of fluids, take on an empty stomach."
    a. Anticholinergics
    b. Bulk-forming laxatives
    c. Serotonin antagonists
    d. Corticosteroids

TECHNICIAN'S CORNER

1. Why might bulk-forming laxatives be useful for treating IBS with diarrhea or constipation?
2. Which lifestyle modifications can be made to lessen the symptoms of irritable bowel syndrome?

Bibliography

American College of Gastroenterology Task Force on Irritable Bowel Syndrome, Brandt LJ, Chey WD, Foxx-Orenstein AE, et al: An evidence-based position statement on the management of irritable bowel syndrome, *Am J Gastroenterol* 104(Suppl 1):S1-S35, 2009.

Behavioural Neurotherapy Clinic: IBS—diagnostic criteria and prevalence, 2006 (http://www.ibs-irritable-bowel-syndrome.com.au/IBS_Criteria.htm).

Chang J, Talley N: Current and emerging therapies in irritable bowel syndrome: from pathophysiology to treatment, *Trends Pharmacol Sci* 31:326-328, 2010.

FDA: *FDA-Approved Drug Products*, 2012. Retrieved May 26, 2012, from http://www.accessdata.fda.gov/scripts/cder/drugsatfda/index.cfm?fuseaction=Search.Search_Drug_Name.

Health Canada: Drug product database, 2010 (http://www.hc-sc.gc.ca/dhp-mps/prodpharma/databasdon/index-eng.php).

Kalant H, Grant D, Mitchell J: *Pharmacotherapy of intestinal Motility Disorders and Inflammatory Bowel Disease Principles of medical pharmacology*, ed 7, Toronto, 2007, Elsevier Canada, pp 572-583.

Lance L, Lacy C, Armstrong L, et al: *Drug information handbook for the allied health professional*, ed 12, Hudson, OH, 2005, APhA Lexi-Comp.

National Digestive Diseases Information Clearinghouse: Crohn's disease (NIH Publ. No. 06-3410), 2011 (http://www.digestive.niddk.nih.gov/ddiseases/pubs/crohns/index.aspx).

National Digestive Diseases Information Clearinghouse: Irritable bowel syndrome (NIH Publ. No. 06-693), 2007 (http://www.digestive.niddk.nih.gov/ddiseases/pubs/ibs/index.aspx).

National Digestive Diseases Information Clearinghouse: Ulcerative colitis (NIH Publ. No. 06-1597), 2011 (http://www.digestive.niddk.nih.gov/ddiseases/pubs/colitis/index.aspx).

USP Center for Advancement of Patient Safety: *Use caution–avoid confusion, USP Quality Review No. 79*, Rockville, MD, 2004, USP Center for Advancement of Patient Safety.

http://en.wikipedia.org/wiki/5-HT3_antagonist – King, Frank D, Jones Brian J, Sanger Gareth J: *5-Hydroxytryptamine-3 receptor antagonists*, 1993, CRC Press. pp. 2-3. ISBN 978-0-8493-5463-2.

www.accessdata.fda.gov/drugsatfda_docs/label/2008/021908s005lbl.pdf – Xia H: Post-infectious irritable bowel syndrome, *World J Gastroenterol* 15(29):3591-3596, 2009 August 7.

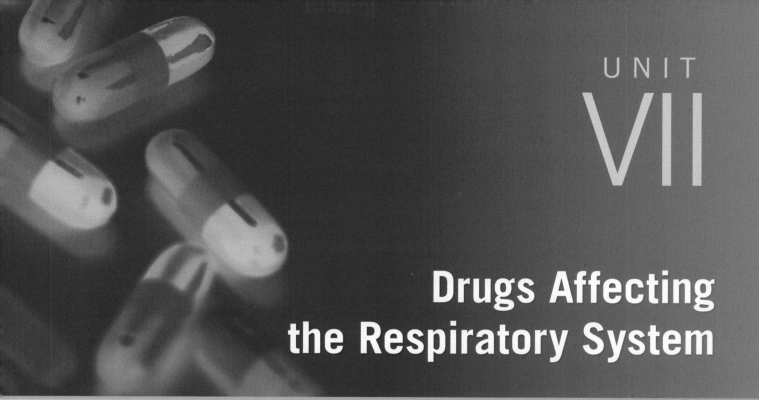

UNIT VII

Drugs Affecting the Respiratory System

<table>
<tr><td>LEARNING OBJECTIVES</td><td>1   Identify and describe the functions of the parts of the respiratory system.
2   Describe the alveoli and their function in gas exchange.
3   Describe the role of the thorax cavity in respiration.</td></tr>
<tr><td>KEY TERMS</td><td>**Expiration:** Moving air out of the lungs.
Inspiration: Moving air into the lungs.
Olfaction: Sense of smell.
Phonation: Speech Production.
Surfactant: Fluid in alveolus that helps reduce surface tension.</td></tr>
</table>

Functions of the Respiratory System

The respiratory system functions as an air distributor and gas exchanger so that oxygen may be supplied to and carbon dioxide removed from the body's cells. In addition, the respiratory system effectively filters, warms, and humidifies the air we breathe. Respiratory organs also influence sound reproduction, including speech used in communicating oral language. Specialized epithelia in the respiratory tract make the sense of smell (*olfaction*) possible. The respiratory system also plays an important role in the regulation, or homeostasis, of pH (acid-base balance) in the body.

Structural Plan of the Respiratory System

The respiratory system is divided into upper and lower tracts, or divisions. The ***upper respiratory tract*** is composed of the nose, nasopharynx, oropharynx, laryngopharynx, and pharynx. The ***lower respiratory tract*** consists of the trachea, all segments of the ***bronchial tree***, and the lungs.

Functionally, the respiratory system also includes accessory structures such as the oral cavity, rib cage, and respiratory muscles, including the diaphragm.

UPPER RESPIRATORY TRACT

Nose Structure

The nose consists of an internal portion, the **nasal cavity**, and external portion. The internal portion lies over the roof of the mouth where the palatine bones separate the nasal cavities from the mouth cavity. The hollow nasal cavity is separated into a right and left cavity by a midline partition called the **septum**. The external openings into the nasal cavities (nostrils) are named the anterior **nares** and open into an area called the **vestibule**. Once air passes over the vestibule, it enters the respiratory portion of each nasal passage, and then air passes into the **pharynx**.

Respiratory Mucosa (Nose)

Once air has passed over the skin of the vestibule and enters the respiratory portion of the nasal passage, it passes over the **respiratory mucosa**. The respiratory mucosa of the nose possesses a rich blood supply and contains many olfactory nerve cells and a rich lymphatic plexus. A ciliated mucous membrane lines the rest of the respiratory tract as far down as the smaller bronchioles.

Paranasal Sinuses

The four pairs of paranasal sinuses are air-containing spaces that open, or drain, into the nasal cavity. These paranasal sinuses are the frontal, maxillary, ethmoid, and sphenoid sinuses. Like the nasal cavity, each paranasal cavity is lined by respiratory mucosa.

FUNCTION OF THE NOSE

The nose serves as a passageway for air going to and from the lungs. Air is filtered of impurities and chemically examined for substances that might prove irritating to the lining of the respiratory tract. The **respiratory membrane** produces mucus and possesses a rich blood supply, which permits rapid warming and moistening of the dry inspired air. Mucous secretions, fluid from the lacrimal glands (tear ducts), and mucus produced in the paranasal sinuses help trap particulate matter and moisten air passing through the nasal passages. In addition, the hollow sinuses act to lighten the bones of the skull and serve as resonating chambers for speech.

Pharynx Structure and Function

Another name for the **pharynx** is the throat. The **nasopharynx** lies behind the nose, the **oropharynx** lies behind the mouth, and the **laryngopharynx** extends from the hyoid bone to its termination in the esophagus. The **pharyngeal tonsils** are located in the nasopharynx on its posterior wall. Two pairs of organs are found in the oropharynx, the palatine tonsils and **linguine tonsils**. The pharynx serves as a common pathway for the respiratory and digestive tracts. It also affects **phonation** (speech production).

Larynx Structure and Function

The **larynx**, or voice box, consists largely of cartilages that are attached to one another and to surrounding structures by muscles; it is lined by a ciliated mucous membrane. The mucous membrane of the larynx forms two pairs of folds, the upper pair, or vestibular, and the lower pair, which serve as the true vocal cords. The true vocal cords and the space between them are together designated as the glottis. Nine cartilages form the framework of the larynx. The **thyroid cartilage** is the largest cartilage of the larynx. The **epiglottis** is attached below the thyroid cartilage and moves up and down during swallowing to prevent food or liquids from entering the trachea.

The larynx functions in respiration as part of the vital airway of the lungs. It helps in the removal dust particles and in warming and humidification of inspired air. It also protects the airway against the entrance of solids and liquids during swallowing and serves as the instrument of voice production—hence, the name voice box. Air expired through the glottis and narrowed by partial adduction of the true vocal cords causes them to vibrate. Their vibration produces sound, and the size and shape of the nose, mouth, pharynx, and bony sinuses help determine the quality of the sound or voice.

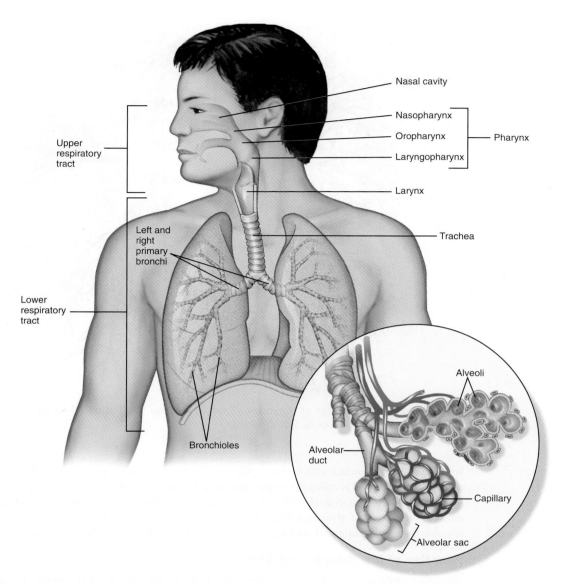

Structure of the respiratory system-inset shows alveolar sacs where O_2 and CO_2 exchange takes place. (From Thibodeau GA, Patton KT: *Anatomy and physiology*, ed 6, St. Louis, 2007, Mosby.)

LOWER RESPIRATORY TRACT

Trachea Structure and Function

The **trachea**, or windpipe, is a tube that extends from the larynx in the neck to the primary bronchi in the thoracic cavity. Its walls consist of C-shaped cartilages that provide firmness to the wall and tend to prevent it from collapsing and shutting off the vital airway. The trachea furnishes part of the open passageway through which air can reach the lungs from the outside.

Bronchi Structure

The trachea divides at its lower end into two **primary bronchi**. The bronchi and trachea are lined by ciliated mucosa. The primary bronchus divides into smaller branches called **secondary bronchi**, which continue to branch to form **tertiary bronchi** and small **bronchioles**. The bronchioles subdivide into smaller tubes, eventually terminating in microscopic branches that divide into alveolar ducts, which terminate in several alveolar sacs, the walls of which consist of numerous alveoli.

Alveoli Structure

The alveoli are the primary gas exchange structures of the respiratory tract. Alveoli are effective in the exchange of carbon dioxide (CO_2) and oxygen (O_2) because each alveolus is extremely thin-

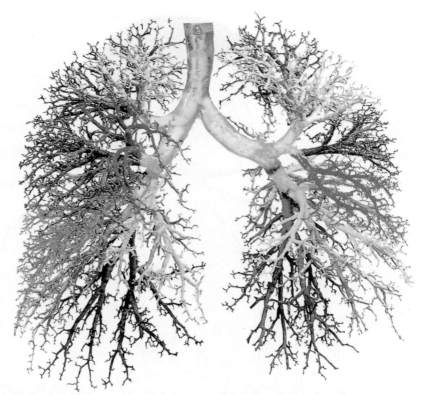

Plastic cast of air spaces of the lungs. (From Thibodeau GA, Patton KT: *Anatomy and physiology*, ed 6, St. Louis, 2007, Mosby.)

walled and lies in contact with blood capillaries. The barrier at which gases are exchanged between alveolar air and blood is called the ***respiratory membrane***. The surface of the respiratory membrane inside each alveolus is coated with a fluid containing ***surfactant***. Surfactant helps reduce surface tension—the force of attraction between water molecules—of the fluid. This helps prevent each alveolus from collapsing and sticking shut as air moves in and out during respiration.

Function of the Bronchi and Alveoli

The tubes composing the bronchial tree distribute air to the interior of the lungs. The alveoli are responsible for the main and vital function of the lungs, gas exchange between air and blood. The layer of protective mucus that covers a large portion of the membrane that lines the respiratory tree serves as the most important air purification mechanism.

Structure and Function of the Lungs

The lungs extend from the diaphragm to slightly above the clavicles and lie against the ribs anteriorly and posteriorly. The primary bronchi and pulmonary blood vessels enter each lung through a slit on its medial surface called the ***hilum***. Each lung is divided into lobes by fissures. The left lobe is divided into two lobes (superior and inferior) and the right lung into three lobes (superior, middle, and inferior). ***Visceral pleura*** cover the outer surfaces of the lungs and adhere to them. The lungs perform two functions, air distribution and gas exchange. Gas exchange between the air and blood is the joint function of the alveoli and the networks of blood capillaries that envelop them.

Structure and Function of the Thoracic Cavity

The thoracic cavity has three divisions, separated from each other by a partition of ***pleura***. The ***parietal pleura*** lines the entire thoracic cavity. A separate pleural sac encases each lung. The outer surface of each lung is covered by the ***visceral pleura***, which lies against the parietal pleura and is separated by a potential space (***pleural space***) that contains just enough pleural fluid for lubrication. Thus, when the lungs inflate with air, the smooth, moist visceral pleura coheres (sticks together) to the smooth, moist parietal pleura. The **thorax** plays a major role in respiration. It becomes larger when the chest is raised and smaller when it is lowered. An even greater change in the thorax occurs when the diaphragm contracts and relaxes. When the diaphragm contracts, it flattens out and thus pulls the floor of the thoracic cavity downward, thereby enlarging the volume of the thorax. When the diaphragm relaxes, it returns to its resting, domelike shape, reducing the volume of the thoracic cavity.

Respiratory Physiology

The proper functioning of the respiratory system ensures that the tissues of the body receive an adequate oxygen supply and carbon dioxide is promptly removed. This complex function would not be possible without integration between numerous physiological control systems, including acid-base balance, water, electrolyte balance, circulation, and metabolism. Functionally, the respiratory system is composed of an integrated set of regulated processes that include the following: external respiration—pulmonary respiration (breathing) and gas exchange in the pulmonary capillaries of the lungs; transport of gases by blood; and internal respiration—gas exchange in the systemic blood capillaries and cellular respiration and overall regulation of respiration.

PULMONARY VENTILATION

Pulmonary ventilation is the technical term for breathing. One phase of it, *inspiration*, moves air into the lungs, and the other phase, *expiration*, moves air out of the lungs.

PULMONARY VOLUME AND CAPACITY

Pulmonary Volume

A *spirometer* is a device that is used to measure pulmonary volume and to create a *spirogram*, a graphic recording of the volume of air exchanged during breathing. Tidal volume (TV), volume of air exhaled after each inspiration, expiratory reserved volume (ERV), air forcibly expelled after the TV, and inspiratory reserve volume (IRV), air forcibly inspired after a normal inspiration, can all be measured. The volume of air moved in and out of the lungs and remaining in them is of great importance. The sum of TV + ERV + IRV is called the vital capacity and is maximum volume of air that a person can move in and out of their lungs. Forced expiratory volume (FEV_1) is another important measure of the volume of air forcibly expired in the first second. The FEV_1 test is used to detect respiratory obstruction as occurs in asthma and chronic pulmonary obstruction disease (COPD).

REGULATION OF PULMONARY FUNCTION

Respiratory Control Centers

Various mechanisms operate to maintain the relative constancy of the blood percentage of oxygen (PO_2) of carbon dioxide (PCO_2). Control of the nerves that affect inspiratory and expiratory muscles is in the brainstem (medulla, pons) in the respiratory centers. The apneustic and pneumotaxic centers located in the pons prevent overinflation of the lungs and permit a normal rhythm of breathing.

Summary

Respiration involves the exchange of O_2 and CO_2 between the organ and its environment (air in lungs to blood, then blood with every body cell). Premature birth can cause potentially fatal respiratory problems. Other diseases like cystic fibrosis and asthma occur in children and emphysema occur in older adults. Respiratory functions are dependent on the organization of its system parts and its interrelationships with other body systems.

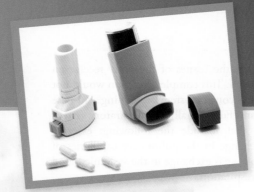

28

Treatment of Asthma and Chronic Obstructive Pulmonary Disease

1 Learn the terminology associated with asthma and chronic obstructive pulmonary disease (COPD).
2 List risk factors for asthma and COPD.
3 List the symptoms of asthma and COPD.
4 List and categorize medications used in the treatment of asthma and COPD.
5 Describe the mechanism of action for drugs used to treat asthma and COPD.
6 Identify significant drug look-alike and sound-alike issues.
7 List common endings for drug classes used for the treatment of asthma and COPD.
8 Identify warning labels and precautionary messages associated with medications used to treat asthma and COPD.

KEY TERMS

Allergic asthma: Asthma symptoms induced by a hypersensitivity reaction caused by overexpression of immunoglobulin E antibodies on exposure to environmental allergens.

Asthma: Chronic disease that affects the airways producing irritation, inflammation, and difficulty breathing.

Bronchodilator: Drug that relaxes tightened airway muscles and improves air flow through the airways.

Chronic obstructive pulmonary disease: Progressive disease of the airways that produces gradual loss of pulmonary function.

Forced expiratory volume: The maximum volume of air that can be breathed out in 1 second; also called forced vital capacity.

Metered-dose inhaler: A device used for delivering a dose of inhaled medication. A solution or powder is delivered as a mist and inhaled.

Nebulizer: Device that creates a mist out of a liquid inhalant solution, making drug delivery easier.

Peak flow meter: Handheld device used to measure the volume of air exhaled and how rapidly the air is moved out.

Spacer: Device attached to the end of a metered-dose inhaler that facilitates drug delivery into the lungs (rather than to the back of the throat).

Spirometry: Test that measures the volume of air that is expired (blown out of the lungs) after taking a deep breath and how rapidly the volume of air is expired.

Asthma

OVERVIEW

Asthma is a chronic disease that affects the airways, producing irritation, inflammation, and difficulty breathing. According to 2010 Centers for Disease Control and Prevention (CDC) statistics, approximately 7.7% of U.S. adults (17.5 million) and as many as 7.1 million U.S. children (9.6%) have been diagnosed with asthma, making it the number one chronic disease of childhood. In 2009, 8.1% of Canadians 12 years of age and older and 9.8% of children were reported as having been diagnosed with asthma by a health professional. Females were more likely than males to report that they had asthma, 9.4% compared with 6.7% in 2009.

The burden of disease attributed to asthma is great; the disease is responsible for missed days at school and work and increased health care system use (e.g., outpatient office visits, emergency department visits, hospitalization), more than for those without asthma. The number of visits to physicians' offices and hospital outpatient and emergency departments with asthma as the primary diagnosis is 13.3 million.

Asthma is classified according to frequency and severity of symptoms. The four classifications for asthma are mild intermittent, mild persistent, moderate persistent, and severe persistent asthma (Box 28-1).

It is not known exactly why some people develop asthma and others do not; however, there are factors that can increase the risk for asthma. A prime example is a positive family history of asthma and exposure to tobacco smoke. Research has suggested that second-hand smoke exposure during pregnancy may be just as damaging to the unborn baby as to the mother. Chronic exposure to other sources of air pollution and exposure to some allergens and infections early in life may also be risk factors.

PATHOPHYSIOLOGY

Symptoms of asthma are linked to a progression of physiological changes in the airways. Initially, the airways (bronchial tube and bronchioles) become irritated. This causes airway constriction, which impedes the passage of air. Airways also become inflamed and swollen, further restricting the flow of air through the bronchial passages. Mucus production is increased above normal levels, which can also obstruct breathing passages (Figure 28-1).

SYMPTOMS

Airway constriction, inflammation, and mucus produce characteristic asthma symptoms (Box 28-2) that include coughing, wheezing, shortness of breath, and chest tightness. Symptoms may be mild or severe (i.e., life-threatening) and vary for each individual. During an asthma episode, or attack, breathing may be noisy and labored. A whistling or creaking sound may be heard with inspiration and expiration. Patients describe chest tightness that feels as if something or someone is "squeezing or sitting on your chest." and they describe feeling that they cannot get enough air into the lungs. Actually, shortness of breath (SOB) is associated with reduced expiration rather than decreased inspiration. Breathing may become faster and shallow. Nocturnal asthma is a condition characterized by decreased FEV1 (*forced expiratory volume* in 1 second). The maximum volume of air that can be breathed out in 1 second is reduced. Increased airway inflammation is present, along with exaggerated bronchial constriction (hyperresponsiveness). Cough at night may disrupt sleep. In one study of patients with asthma, as many as 74% reported nocturnal asthma symptoms at least once weekly. In nocturnal asthma, lung function and anti-inflammatory hormones (e.g., cortisol) decrease and the release of proinflammatory mediators (e.g., leukotrienes, cytokines) increases in the middle of the night, according to circadian rhythm (biological clock).

ASTHMA TRIGGERS

Asthma triggers are events or circumstances that can precipitate an asthma episode in those with asthma (Box 28-3). An asthma episode is also called an asthma attack. Examples of triggers are exposure to allergens such as animal dander, environmental pollutants, cleaning fluid, mold, tobacco smoke, and even cold air. Exposure to cockroach droppings and air pollution are linked to the rise of asthma in inner city youth. Other triggers are upper respiratory infection and strenuous exercise. The risks for exercise-induced asthma can be minimized by taking prescribed medicines prior to exercise.

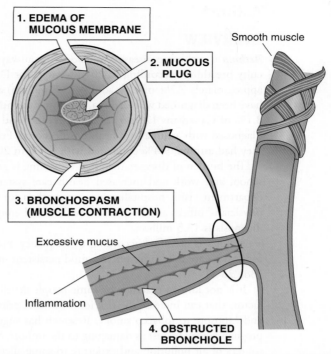

FIGURE 28-1 Airway changes during an asthma episode. (From Gould BE: *Pathophysiology for the heart professions*, ed 3, St. Louis, 2007, Saunders.)

BOX 28-1   **Classification of Asthma***

- Mild intermittent: Symptoms occur twice a week or less, nighttime symptoms are bothersome twice a month or less, and, between episodes, there are no symptoms and lung function is normal.
- Mild persistent asthma: Symptoms occur more than twice a week, but not more than once in a single day. Nighttime symptoms are bothersome more than twice a month and symptoms affect normal activity levels.
- Moderate persistent asthma: Symptoms occur daily and nighttime symptoms are bothersome more than once a week. Asthma attacks may affect normal activity levels.
- Severe persistent asthma: Symptoms occur throughout the day on most days and nighttime symptoms occur frequently. Physical activity is typically limited.

*A severe asthma attack may occur with all classifications of asthma.

BOX 28-2   **Common Symptoms of Asthma**

- Cough
- Wheezing
- Shortness of breath
- Chest tightness

MANAGING ASTHMA SYMPTOMS

Asthma symptoms can be managed with a combination of medication, lifestyle modification, and home monitoring of breathing using a peak flow meter and medication. Asthma has two main components, airway inflammation and acute bronchoconstriction (constriction of the airways). The drugs administered for asthma treatment and management of asthma are divided into two classes. Rescue medicines are for the treatment of acute symptoms and include short-acting β_2-adrenergic agonists such as albuterol (salbutamol in Canada). Maintenance therapy is used to prevent asthma episodes; this includes long-acting β_2-adrenergic agonists (e.g., salmeterol), inhaled corticosteroids

BOX 28-3   **Asthma Triggers**

ALLERGENS
- Animal dander (from the skin, hair, or feathers of animals)
- Dust mites (contained in house dust)
- Cockroaches
- Pollen from trees and grass
- Mold (indoor and outdoor)

IRRITANTS
- Cigarette smoke
- Air pollution
- Cold air or changes in weather
- Strong odors from painting or cooking
- Scented products
- Strong emotional expression (including crying or laughing hard) and stress

OTHERS
- Medicines such as aspirin and beta blockers
- Sulfites in food (dried fruit) or beverages (wine)
- Gastroesophageal reflux disease and laryngopharyngeal reflux can worsen asthma symptoms.
- Irritants or allergens that you may be exposed to at work, such as special chemicals or dusts

---

TECH NOTE!
To comply with the U.S. Food and Drug Administration (FDA) ruling that by December 31, 2008, the propellant used in metered-dose inhalers must no longer contain chlorofluorocarbons (CFCs), a compound known to deplete the ozone layer, manufacturers have begun to replace CFCs with hydrofluoroalkanes (HFAs).

TECH NOTE!
To determine whether the contents of the metered-dose inhaler canister are low, patients may suspend the canister in a glass of water. A canister that floats to the top is empty and a canister that sinks to the bottom is full.

(e.g., budesonide), leukotriene modifiers (e.g., montelukast), mast cell stabilizers (e.g., ipratropium bromide), and xanthine derivatives (e.g., aminophylline). The key goal to preventing asthma attacks, hospitalizations, and death from asthma is reducing and preventing further inflammation.

A *peak flow meter* is a handheld device used to measure the volume of air exhaled and how fast the air is exhaled. Regular measurements can enable a person with asthma to spot trends that signal an impending asthma attack. A peak flow meter permits self-management of asthma, similar to how monitoring blood glucose levels enables self-management of diabetes. Low peak flow numbers signal that asthma is not controlled. Another test (spirometry) is performed to measure the volume of air that is expired (blown out of the lungs) after taking a deep breath and how rapidly the volume of air is expired.

Drugs Used for Treatment of Acute Symptoms: Relievers

Rescue medicines, also known as relievers, provide rapid and short-term relief of asthma symptoms. They reverse bronchospasm and open airways. Albuterol, also known as salbutamol, is a short-acting β_2-adrenergic agonist, and the most frequently prescribed *bronchodilator*. Other β_2-adrenergic agonists currently prescribed for the treatment of asthma include levalbuterol, metaproterenol, and terbutaline. Inhaled anticholinergic ipratropium bromide may also be administered in combination with a β_2-adrenergic agonist for the relief of acute symptoms.

MECHANISM OF ACTION

Bronchial airways are composed of smooth muscle that is innervated by β_2, α_1, α_2, and muscarinic (M1 and M3) receptors. When short-acting β_2-adrenergic agonists bind to β_2 receptors, bronchial smooth muscle relaxes and bronchospasm is reversed. Stimulation of β_2 receptors activates adenyl cyclase on bronchial smooth muscle, increasing the intracellular cyclic AMP (cAMP) level, which, in turn, produces bronchodilation. Levalbuterol is an isomer of albuterol and is a moderately selective β_2-adrenergic receptor agonist.

PHARMACOKINETICS

Short-acting β_2-adrenergic agonists have a rapid onset of action and short duration of action. The onset of action for albuterol is within 15 minutes and the peak effect occurs within 30 minutes to 2 hours. The duration of action of albuterol is 2 to 6 hours compared with its isomer, levalbuterol, which has a duration of action of approximately 3 to 6 hours. β_2-Adrenergic agonists are commonly administered by oral inhalation using a *metered-dose inhaler* (MDI) or *nebulizer*.

Ipratropium bromide is also administered by the inhalation route. Bioavailability is low, which accounts for the low incidence of adverse reactions.

ADVERSE REACTIONS

Drugs such as albuterol can produce nervousness, difficulty sleeping, dry mouth, mild headache, and throat irritation (inhalants only). Beta receptors are also located on the heart and skeletal muscle, so the use of β_2-adrenergic agonists can increase the heart rate and can lead to arrhythmias, hypertension, palpitations, tachycardia, and tremors. β_2-adrenergic stimulation may also produce hyperglycemia, hypokalemia, and increased insulin secretion. Ipratropium bromide can also cause difficulty urinating and blurred vision.

PRECAUTIONS

Store the canister at room temperature. Exposure to excessive heat can cause the canister to explode. Excessive cold can reduce the effectiveness of albuterol. Keep albuterol (DuoNeb) nebulizer solution in its foil package until time of use; protect from light.

TECH NOTE!
Excessive use of reliever medication is a sign that the asthma is not well controlled.

Short-Acting β_2-Adrenergic Agonists

Generic Name	U.S. Brand Name(s) / Canadian Brand Name(s)	Dosage Forms and Strengths
albuterol* (salbutamol)	AccuNeb, Proair HFA, Proventil HFA, Ventolin HFA, VoSpire ER Airomir, Ventolin Diskus, Ventolin HFA	Inhaler, metered-dose (Proventil, Proair, Ventolin): 90 mcg/actuation, 100 mcg/actuation (Airomir) Solution, for inhalation: 0.083%[†], 0.5%[†], 0.63 mg/3 mL (0.021%)[†], 1.25 mg/3mL (0.042%)[†], 0.5 mg/mL[‡], 1 mg/mL[‡], 2 mg/mL[‡] Powder, for inhalation (Ventolin Diskus): 200 mcg/dose Solution, for I.V. use: 1 mg/mL[‡] Syrup: 2 mg/5 mL Tablet, immediate-release: 2 mg, 4 mg Tablet, extended-release (United States only): 4 mg, 8 mg
levalbuterol*	Xopenex, Xopenex HFA Not available	Inhaler (Xopenex HFA): 45 mcg/actuation Inhalant solution (Xopenex): 0.31 mg/3 mL (0.0103%), 0.63 mg/3 mL (0.021%), 1.25 mg/3 mL (0.042%), 1.25 mg/0.5 mL (0.25%)
metaproterenol*	Generics only Not available	Inhalant solution: 0.4%, 0.6% Solution, oral: 10 mg/5 mL Tablet: 10 mg, 20 mg
pirbuterol	Maxair Autohaler Not available	Inhaler MDI: 0.2 mg/actuation
terbutaline*	Generics Bricanyl inhaler	Inhaler (Canada only): 0.5 mg/actuation[‡] Tablet: 2.5 mg[†], 5 mg[†] Solution, for injection: 1 mg/mL[†]
Combinations		
albuterol + ipratropium bromide* (salbutamol + ipratropium bromide in Canada)	Combivent, Combivent Respimat, DuoNeb Combivent	Inhaler MDI: albuterol 103 mcg/actuation + ipratropium bromide 18 mcg/actuation (Combivent[†]); albuterol 0.1 mg/actuation + ipratropium bromide 0.02 mg/actuation (Combivent Respimat) Inhalant solution: albuterol 3 mg/3 mL + ipratropium bromide 0.5 mg/3 mL (DuoNeb); salbutamol 1 mg/1 mL + ipratropium bromide 0.5 mg/2.5 mL (Combivent[‡])
fenoterol hydrobromide + ipratropium bromide	Not available DuoVent	Inhaler (MDI): fenoterol hydrobromide 0.3125 mg + ipratropium bromide 0.125 mg

*Generic available.
[†]Strength available in the United States only.
[‡]Strength available in Canada only.

TECH NOTE!
The FDA has announced that CFC-containing inhalers, including Combivent, will be removed from the U.S. market; December 31, 2013, is the last date that Combivent will be manufactured, sold, or dispensed in the United States.

TECH ALERT!
The following drugs have look-alike and sound-alike issues:
   albuterol and atenolol;
   metoproterenol and metoprolol;
   Combivent and Combivir;
   terbutaline and terbinafine

TECH NOTE!
The FDA has advised that "long-acting β₂-adrenergic agonists, such as salmeterol, the active ingredient in Serevent Diskus, have been associated with an increased risk of severe asthma exacerbations and asthma-related death."

MAINTENANCE THERAPY TO PREVENT ASTHMA FLARE-UPS

Drugs that are intended for long-term use and taken daily to prevent asthma symptoms are called controllers. The five classes of drugs used for asthma prophylaxis are: long-acting β₂-adrenergic agonists, inhaled corticosteroids, leukotriene modifiers, mast cell stabilizers, and xanthine derivatives.

Long-Acting β₂-Adrenergic Agonists

The FDA and Health Canada have updated the indications for the use of long-acting beta agonists (LABAs) in the treatment of asthma because of safety concerns. To ensure the safe use of these products, the following guidelines are recommended:

- LABAs are contraindicated without the use of an inhaled corticosteroid. Single-ingredient LABAs should not be used alone.
- LABA use should be limited to the shortest duration of time required to achieve control of asthma symptoms, and then discontinued.

Long-term use of LABAs should be restricted to patients whose asthma cannot be adequately controlled with controller medications:

- Combination inhaled corticosteroid and an LABA are recommended for pediatric and adolescent patients when the addition of an LABA is required.

Glucocorticosteroids

Glucocorticosteroids are anti-inflammatory drugs. They reduce the infiltration of mediators of the inflammatory response into airway cells, thus reducing the mucus and swelling that make breathing difficult (see Figure 28-1). Glucocorticosteroids decrease the synthesis of proinflammatory substances—prostaglandins, leukotrienes, cytokines, arachidonic acid, and macrophages—that are released as part of the inflammatory response (see Figure 15-6).

Anticholinergics

Generic Name	U.S. Brand Name(s) Canadian Brand Name(s)	Dosage Forms and Strengths
ipratropium bromide	Atrovent HFA	Inhaler (MDI): 20 mcg/spray‡, 21 mcg/spray†
	Atrovent HFA	Solution, for inhalation: 0.02%†, 0.0125%‡, 0.025%‡, 0.03%‡
tiotropium bromide	Spiriva	Powder, for inhalation: 18 mcg
	Spiriva	

†Strength available in the United States only.
‡Strength available in Canada only.

Long-Acting β₂-Adrenergic Agonists

Generic Name	U.S. Brand Name(s) Canadian Brand Name(s)	Dosage Forms and Strengths
arformoterol	Brovana	Solution, for inhalation: 15 mcg/2 mL
	Not available	
formoterol	Foradil Aerolizer, Foradil Certihaler Perforomist	Powder, for inhalation: 8.5 mcg (Foradil Certihaler); 12 mcg (Foradil)
	Foradil, Oxeze Turbuhaler	Inhaler (Oxeze): 6 mcg, 12 mcg Solution, for inhalation (Perforomist): 20 mcg/2 mL
salmeterol	Serevent Diskus	Inhalation, powder: 50 mcg/actuation
	Serevent Diskhaler, Serevent Diskus	

MECHANISM OF ACTION AND PHARMACOKINETICS

The mechanism of action and pharmacokinetics of glucocorticosteroids are discussed in detail in Chapter 15. The primary route of administration for corticosteroids used for the treatment of asthma is inhalation; however, they may be administered orally for more severe symptoms. Inhaled corticosteroids include fluticasone (Flovent), budesonide (Pulmicort), beclomethasone (Qvar), and mometasone (Asmanex).

ADVERSE REACTIONS

Adverse reactions to inhaled corticosteroids are primarily local and include coughing, hoarseness, throat irritation, dry mouth, flushing, loss of taste, or unpleasant taste. Some patients may develop an infection in the mouth or throat, called thrush. Risks can be minimized by gargling or rinsing the mouth after administering the prescribed dose of medicine. Systemic effects are dose-dependent

Inhaled Corticosteroids

Generic Name	U.S. Brand Name(s) / Canadian Brand Name(s)	Dosage Forms and Strengths
beclomethasone	Qvar 40, Qvar 80 / Qvar	**Inhaler:** 40 mcg/actuation[†], 50 mcg/actuation[‡], 80 mcg/actuation[†], and 100 mcg/actuation[‡]
budesonide	Pulmicort Flexhaler, Pulmicort Respules / Pulmicort Nebuamp, Pulmicort Turbuhaler	**Inhalant powder (Pulmicort Flexhaler):** 80 mcg, 160 mcg/actuation; **Inhaler, metered-dose (Pulmicort Turbuhaler):** 100 mcg, 200 mcg, 400 mcg/actuation **Inhalant suspension (Pulmicort Nebuamp, Pulmicort Respules):** 0.25 mg/2 mL, 0.5 mg/2 mL, 1 mg/2 mL
ciclesonide	Alves / Alvesco	**Inhalation solution:** 80 mcg/actuation[†], 100 mcg/actuation[‡], 160mcg/actuation[†], and 200 mcg/actuation[‡]
fluticasone	Flovent Diskus, Flovent HFA / Flovent Diskus, Flovent HFA	**Inhalant powder (Flovent Diskus):** 50 mcg, 100 mcg, 250 mcg/actuation **Inhaler, MDI (Flovent HFA):** 44 mcg/actuation[†], 50 mcg/actuation[‡], 110 mcg/actuation[†], 125 mcg/actuation[‡], 220 mcg/actuation[†], 250 mcg/actuation[‡]
mometasone	Asmanex / Asmanex	**Inhalation powder:** 110 mcg[†], 200 mcg[‡], 220 mcg[†], 400 mcg[‡]

Long-Acting β₂-Adrenergic Agonist + Corticosteroid

Generic Name	U.S. Brand Name(s) / Canadian Brand Name(s)	Dosage Forms and Strengths
formoterol + mometasone	Dulera / Zenhale	**Inhalation powder:** 5 mcg formoterol + 50 mcg mometasone[‡], 5 mcg formoterol + 100 mcg mometasone, 5 mcg formoterol + 200 mcg mometasone/actuation
formoterol + budesonide	Symbicort / Symbicort	**Inhaler, MDI:** 4.5 mcg formoterol + 80 mcg budesonide/actuation[†]; 4.5 mcg formoterol + 160 mcg budesonide/actuation[†]; 6 mcg formoterol + 100 mcg budesonide/actuation[‡], 6 mcg formoterol + 200 mcg budesonide/actuation[‡]
salmeterol + fluticasone	Advair Diskus, Advair HFA / Advair, Advair Diskus	**Inhalant, powder (Advair Diskus):** 50 mcg salmeterol + 100 mcg fluticasone, 50 mcg salmeterol + 250 mcg fluticasone, 50 mcg salmeterol + 500 mcg fluticasone **Inhaler (Advair, Advair HFA):** 21 mcg salmeterol + 45 mcg fluticasone[†], 21 mcg salmeterol + 115 mcg fluticasone[†], 21 mcg salmeterol + 230 mcg fluticasone[†]; 25 mcg salmeterol + 125 mcg fluticasone[‡], 25 mcg salmeterol + 250 mcg fluticasone[‡]

[†]Strength available in the United States only.
[‡]Strength available in Canada only.

and more likely to occur at higher doses. Flovent HFA is contraindicated in children younger than 4 years and budesonide, beclomethasone, and triamcinolone inhalers are contraindicated in children younger than 6 years. Symbicort and Advair HFA are contraindicated in children younger than 12 years.

Leukotriene Modifiers

Leukotrienes are proinflammatory substances that are released as part of the inflammatory response. Leukotriene modifiers are administered to patients with mild asthma to reduce inflammation.

MECHANISM OF ACTION

Zileuton inhibits the action of 5-lipoxygenase, the enzyme responsible for converting arachidonic acid to leukotriene A4. This is the first step in the leukotriene pathway.

Montelukast and zafirlukast interfere with the binding of cysteinyl leukotrienes C_4, D_4, and E_4 to their receptor on airway smooth muscle. They act as antagonists and drug-receptor binding reduces allergen-induced airway inflammation, produces airway relaxation, and reduces edema.

PHARMACOKINETICS

Montelukast is readily absorbed when administered orally. The maximum concentration of oral tablets is reached within 3 to 4 hours. Chewable tablets work faster, reaching a maximum concentration within approximately 2.5 hours. Food does not decrease the bioavailability of montelukast, unlike zafirlukast, which must be taken on an empty stomach. Montelukast, zafirlukast, and zileuton are metabolized in the liver by cytochrome P-450 (CYP450) isozymes and can interfere with the metabolism of other drugs using the same metabolic pathway.

ADVERSE REACTIONS

Montelukast and zafirlukast may produce cough, hoarseness or sore throat, headache, indigestion, heartburn or stomach upset, and runny nose. Montelukast may also produce difficulty sleeping, dizziness, drowsiness, muscle aches or cramps, or unusual dreams. Zileuton extended-release tablets may produce abdominal pain in addition to the adverse reactions listed for montelukast and zafirlukast.

PRECAUTIONS

The packet of montelukast granules should not be opened until ready for use. Once opened, packet contents (with or without mixing with food) must be administered within 15 minutes. Zileuton may cause abnormal liver function and jaundice, so liver function tests should be conducted every 2 to 3 months.

TECH ALERT!

The following drugs have look-alike and sound-alike issues:
   Foradil and Toradol; salmeterol and salbutamol;
   Serevent and Serentil

TECH NOTE!

A common ending for leukotriene modifiers is -lukast.

TECH ALERT!

The following drugs have look-alike and sound-alike issues:
   Singulair and Sinequan;
   Accolate, Accutane, and Aclovate

Leukotriene Modifiers

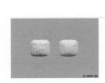

Generic Name	U.S. Brand Name(s) / Canadian Brand Name(s)	Dosage Forms and Strengths
montelukast∞	Singulair	Oral granules: 4 mg Tablet: 10 mg
	Singulair	Tablet, chewable: 4 mg, 5 mg
zafirlukast*†	Accolate	Tablet: 10 mg†, 20 mg
	Accolate	
zileuton	Zyflo, Zyflo CR	Tablet (Zyflo): 600 mg
	Not available	Tablet, controlled-release (Zyflo CR): 600 mg

*Generic available.
∞Generic available in Canada.
†Strength available in the United States only.

Mast Cell Stabilizers

Mast cells are released as part of the immune system response to allergens. Mast cell degranulation results in the release of histamine and mediators of inflammation (e.g., leukotrienes, eosinophils, basophils, cytokines, prostaglandins). Cromolyn sodium is an example of a mast cell stabilizer. Cromolyn is administered for prophylaxis and does not control acute symptoms.

MECHANISM OF ACTION

Cromolyn sodium reduces the release of inflammatory substances responsible for producing the symptoms of asthma by making mast cells less reactive to antigens. It inhibits the degranulation of mast cells and prevents the release of histamine and the slow-reacting substance of anaphylaxis (SRS-A). Cromolyn sodium improves exercise tolerance and reaction to cold air and environmental pollutants by reducing hyperactivity of the bronchi.

PHARMACOKINETICS

Cromolyn sodium is not used to treat acute symptoms. Several weeks of therapy are required before maximum response to the drug is achieved. Cromolyn produces a local effect on cell membranes. Only 1% of the drug is absorbed systemically.

ADVERSE REACTIONS

Cromolyn sodium may be administered using a metered-dose inhaler or nebulizer. Systemic absorption of cromolyn sodium is minimal, so side effects are generally localized. The most common adverse reactions are a bad taste in the mouth, irritated dry throat, and coughing or wheezing.

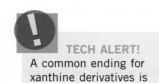

TECH ALERT!
A common ending for xanthine derivatives is -phylline.

Xanthine Derivatives

The xanthines are one of the oldest classes of drug used for the treatment of asthma. Theophylline occurs naturally in tea and is chemically similar to caffeine. Xanthines have bronchodilator and anti-inflammatory properties.

MECHANISM OF ACTION

The exact mechanism of action of xanthines is unknown. They are believed to have a number of possible mechanisms of action, including the following: (1) prostaglandin antagonism; (2) inhibition of calcium ion influx into smooth muscle; (3) stimulation of endogenous catecholamine; (4) inhibition of release of mediators from mast cells and leukocytes; and (5) adenosine receptor antagonism. Actions 1 and 4 are responsible for reducing airway inflammation, 2 for reducing bronchospasm, and 3 and 5 for producing bronchodilation.

PHARMACOKINETICS

The half-life ($t_{1/2}$) of theophylline and aminophylline varies with patient age, liver function, smoking status, and use of concurrent drugs. Smoking decreases $t_{1/2}$ by nearly 50%. In children ages 1 to 9 years, $t_{1/2}$ can be as much as 50% shorter than that in adults. Liver disease and pulmonary edema can prolong $t_{1/2}$ up to 24 hours. Theophylline is extensively metabolized by the CYP450 enzyme

Mast Cell Stabilizers

Generic Name	U.S. Brand Name(s) Canadian Name Brand(s)	Dosage Forms and Strengths
cromolyn sodium*	Generics	Solution, for inhalation: 20 mg/2 mL
	Generics	
tiotropium	Spiriva	Powder, for inhalation: 18 mcg
	Spiriva	

*Generic available.

system and is involved in numerous drug interactions (Box 28-4). The bioavailability of theophylline varies by manufacturer. It is recommended that patients receive the same manufacturer's product each time that their prescription is refilled.

ADVERSE REACTIONS

Xanthine derivatives (e.g., theophylline) may produce insomnia, dizziness, headache, irritability, decreased appetite, stomach cramps, and urinary retention.

Monoclonal Antibodies

Omalizumab is a recombinant human monoclonal antibody (anti-IgE) and is indicated for the treatment of moderate to severe allergic asthma. In patients with *allergic asthma*, symptoms occur as a result of a hypersensitivity reaction caused by the overexpression of immunoglobulin E (IgE) antibodies on exposure to environmental allergens. Omalizumab is indicated as add-on therapy for patients whose asthma is not controlled with inhaled corticosteroids and β_2-adrenergic agonists.

MECHANISM OF ACTION AND PHARMACOKINETICS

The action of omalizumab is specifically directed toward IgE. Omalizumab prohibits the binding of IgE to mast cells and prevents binding of the IgE-anti-IgE complex to $F_{cepsilon}RI$ receptors on monocytes, eosinophils, dendritic cells, epithelial cells, and platelets. The result is prevention of early- and late-stage allergic responses and the release of inflammatory mediators (e.g., cytokines).

TECH NOTE!
A common ending for monoclonal antibody drugs is -*mab*.

BOX 28-4   Modifiers of Serum Blood Levels of Theophylline

DRUGS AND FOODS THAT INCREASE LEVELS
- Oral contraceptives
- Erythromycin
- Calcium channel blockers
- Cimetidine
- Caffeine
- Chocolate

DRUGS THAT DECREASE LEVELS
- Phenobarbital
- Phenytoin
- Carbamazepine

Xanthine Derivatives

Generic Name	U.S. Brand Name(s) / Canadian Name Brand(s)	Dosage Forms and Strengths
aminophylline*	Generics	Solution, for injection: 25 mg/mL, 50 mg/mL‡
	Generics	Tablets: 100 mg, 200 mg†
theophylline*	Elixophyllin, Theo-24, Theochron, Theolair	Capsule, extended-release (Theo-24): 100 mg, 200 mg, 300 mg, 400 mg
	Theo ER, Theolair, Uniphyl	Elixir (Elixophyllin): 80 mg/15 mL
		Solution, for injection (in dextrose 5% 100 mL): 40 mg†, 80 mg†, 160 mg†, 200 mg†, 320 mg†, 400 mg†
		Tablet (Theolair): 125 mg, 250 mg
		Tablet, extended–release (Theochron, Uniphyl): 100 mg, 200 mg, 300 mg, 400 mg, 450 mg‡, 600 mg

*Generic available.
†Strength available in the United States only.
‡Strength available in Canada only.

Monoclonal Antibodies

Generic name	U.S. Brand Name(s) Canadian Brand Name(s)	Dosage Forms and Strengths
omalizumab	Xolair	Powder, injection: 75 mg, 150 mg
	Xolair	

Omalizumab is administered by subcutaneous injection. Maximum serum concentration is reached within 7 to 8 hours of the administered dose; however, maximum effects from omalizumab are not achieved for several weeks after administration.

ADVERSE REACTIONS

Adverse reactions caused by omalizumab injections include mild redness, itching, swelling, or bruising at the injection site, headache, and nausea. Difficulty breathing, hives or skin rash, and unusual bleeding are more serious adverse effects and may be a prelude to anaphylaxis.

PRECAUTIONS

The package insert for omalizumab carries a boxed warning indicating that patients should be instructed to watch for signs and symptoms of anaphylaxis and provided with instructions for self-treatment in the event of an emergency.

Chronic Obstructive Pulmonary Disease

OVERVIEW

Chronic obstructive pulmonary disease (COPD) is a progressive disease of the airways that produces gradual loss of pulmonary function. Emphysema, chronic bronchitis, and chronic obstructive bronchitis are all classified under the heading of COPD. For the past 5 years, COPD has been ranked as the third or fourth leading cause of death in the United States and Canada. In COPD, the lungs are chronically inflamed. Inflammatory cells such as $CD8^+$ T lymphocytes are recruited to the lung, where they infiltrate the airways. Interleukin-6 is also present (see Chapter 15).

RISK FACTORS

Various lifestyle and environmental factors contribute to the risk for developing COPD. Cigarette smoking or exposure to second-hand smoke, occupational irritants to the lungs such as asbestos, industrial chemicals, dust, and air pollution may all contribute to or worsen existing COPD. Viral infections also aggravate COPD—in particular, respiratory syncytial virus (RSV) and adenovirus.

SYMPTOMS

Air flow obstruction produces shortness of breath. Persons with COPD may also exhibit a chronic persistent cough, wheezing, and increased sputum production.

TREATMENT

The aim for COPD management is to (1) relieve symptoms and airway obstruction, (2) correct hypoxia, and (3) treat any precipitating factors and/or comorbidities. Pharmacological treatment of COPD involves the administration of bronchodilators, glucocorticosteroids, and antibiotics, when infections are present. Nonpharmacological treatments include oxygen therapy and mechanical ventilation.

Pharmacological Treatment

The use of bronchodilators and glucocorticosteroids in reducing inflammation and opening airways has been described earlier (see "Maintenance Therapy to Prevent Asthma Flare-Ups"). Usual doses administered for the treatment of COPD are listed in the drug table at the end of this chapter. Additional drugs specifically indicated for the treatment of COPD are the anticholinergics (tiotropium) and antimucolytics (acetylcysteine). Inhaled anticholinergics are first-line maintenance therapy for COPD in patients with persistent symptoms.

MECHANISM OF ACTION

Tiotropium bromide and ipratropium bromide are antimuscarinic anticholinergic bronchodilators. Tiotropium is dosed once daily and is indicated for the treatment of COPD. Ipratropium bromide prescribed for short-term relief of asthma symptoms must be given three or four times daily. Anticholinergics bind to muscarinic receptors and block the effects of acetylcholine (released by the vagus nerve), resulting in the relaxation of bronchial smooth muscle. Antagonism of cholinergic receptors relaxes bronchial smooth muscle, producing bronchodilation. Recall that parasympathetic nervous system stimulation produces increased mucus and bronchoconstriction. Review the Unit II opener.

ADVERSE REACTIONS

Dry mouth is the most common side effect of tiotropium use. Diarrhea, nausea, hoarseness, dizziness, headache, and cardiac arrhythmias have also been reported.

Drug Delivery Devices for Use with Asthma and Chronic Obstructive Pulmonary Disease Medicines

Delivery of the prescribed dose of medication using an MDI is fast but may be challenging for some individuals and is inappropriate for small children. It is not uncommon for a substantial amount of the drug to be delivered to the back of the throat rather than into the lungs when an MDI is used. A dry powder inhaler (DPI) is similar to an MDI, but the medication is in powder form rather than in liquid form. You inhale a puff of the powder rather than a mist of liquid. A nebulizer is a device that converts a liquid dose of medicine into an aerosolized mist that can be inhaled by normal breathing when used with a mask (Figure 28-2). A mouthpiece may also be attached to the end of the nebulizer and the mist inhaled using slow deep breaths.

A *spacer* is a device that is attached to the end of the MDI (Figure 28-3). The drug is sprayed into the device's chamber and then slowly inhaled into the lungs. Some devices produce a whistling sound to alert the patient when inhalation is too rapid or is not controlled.

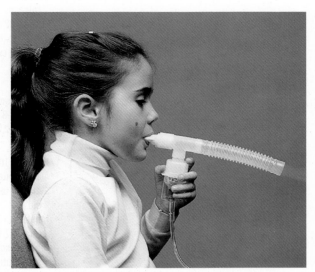

FIGURE 28-2 Nebulizer. (From Hopper T: *Mosby's pharmacy technician*, ed 2, St Louis, 2007, WB Saunders.)

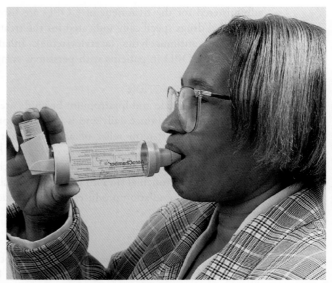

FIGURE 28-3 Spacer. (From Hopper T: *Mosby's pharmacy technician*, ed 2, St Louis, 2007, WB Saunders.)

Summary of Drugs Used for the Treatment of Asthma and Chronic Obstructive Pulmonary Disease

Generic Name	U.S. Brand Name	Usual Adult Oral Dose and Dosing Schedule[a]	Warning Labels
Short-Acting β₂-Adrenergic Agonists			
albuterol (salbutamol)	Ventolin HFA	**Asthma** **Inhaler:** 1-2 puffs every 4-6 hr as needed **Inhalant solution:** 2.5 mg every 6-8 hr prn delivered over 5-15 min, *or* **AccuNeb:** 0.63-1.25 mg tid or qid; deliver over 5-15 min as needed **Solution or tablet, immediate-release:** 2-4 mg every 6-8 hr (max, 32 mg/day) **Tablet, extended-release:** 4-8 mg every 12 hr (max, 32 mg/day)	SHAKE WELL (INHALER).
levalbuterol	Xopenex	**Asthma** **Inhalant solution:** 0.63-1.25 mg every 6-8 hr **Inhaler:** 2 puffs every 4-6 hr	DO NOT EXCEED RECOMMENDED DOSE.
metoproterenol	Generics	**COPD** **Inhaler:** 100-200 mcg tid or qid **Asthma and COPD** **Syrup or tablets:** 20 mg 3 tid or qid **Inhaler:** 2-3 puffs every 3-4 hr (max, 12 puffs/day) **Inhalant solution:** 0.2-0.3 mL of 5% solution, diluted in 2.5-3 mL normal saline, tid or qid	

Summary of Drugs Used for the Treatment of Asthma and Chronic Obstructive Pulmonary Disease—cont'd

Generic Name	U.S. Brand Name	Usual Adult Oral Dose and Dosing Schedule[a]	Warning Labels
pirbuterol	Maxair	**Asthma and COPD** **Inhaler:** 1-2 puffs every 4-6 hr (max: 12 puffs/day)	
terbutaline	Generics	**Asthma and COPD** **Injection:** 0.25 mg SC; repeat in 15-30 min if needed **Tablet:** 2.5-5 mg tid **Asthma Inhaler:** 2 puffs (400 mcg) every 4 hr	
Long-Acting β₂-Adrenergic Agonists			
formoterol	Foradil	**Asthma and COPD:** Inhale contents of 1 capsule every 12 hr	DO NOT SWALLOW CAPSULES (FOR INHALATION DEVICE USE ONLY).
salmeterol	Serevent Diskus	**Asthma and COPD:** 1 inhalation every 12 hr	
β₂-Adrenergic Agonists + Anticholinergics			
albuterol + ipratropium bromide	Combivent, DuoNeb	**COPD:** Inhale 2 puffs 4 times a day (Combivent) or 3 mL qid (DuoNeb)	SHAKE WELL (INHALER).
fenoterol hydrobromide + ipratropium bromide	DuoVent	**COPD:** Inhale 4 mL every 4-6 hr	
Anticholinergics			
ipratropium bromide	Atrovent HFA	**COPD:** Inhale 2 sprays tid or qid (MDI) or inhale 1 vial of nebulizer solution (500 mcg) every 6-8 hr	SHAKE WELL.
tiotropium	Spiriva	**COPD:** Inhale contents of 1 capsule once daily.	DO NOT SWALLOW CAPSULES (FOR INHALATION DEVICE USE ONLY).
Inhaled Corticosteroids			
beclomethasone	Q-Var	**Asthma:** 1-4 puffs twice daily (max, 320 mcg/day)	SHAKE WELL (INHALER).
budesonide	Pulmicort	**Asthma:** 1-2 puffs bid	
ciclesonide	Alvesco	**Asthma:** 1-2 puffs bid	
fluticasone	Flovent HFA	**Asthma:** 2 sprays up to bid (max, 440 mcg/day)	
mometasone	Asmanex	**Asthma:** 1-2 sprays once or twice daily (max, 440 mcg/day)	
β₂-Adrenergic Agonists + Inhaled Corticosteroids			
formoterol + budesonide	Symbicort	**Asthma:** 2 puffs bid	SHAKE WELL (INHALER).
formoterol + mometasone	Dulera	**Asthma:** 2 puffs bid	
salmeterol + fluticasone	Advair HFA	**Asthma:** 2 puffs every 12 hr	
	Advair Diskus	**Asthma and COPD:** 1 puff every 12 hr	

Continued

Summary of Drugs Used for the Treatment of Asthma and Chronic Obstructive Pulmonary Disease—cont'd

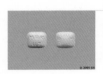

Generic Name	U.S. Brand Name	Usual Adult Oral Dose and Dosing Schedule[a]	Warning Labels
Leukotriene Modifiers			
montelukast	Singulair	**Asthma:** 1 tablet daily	TAKE WITH A LARGE GLASS OF WATER (CHEWABLE TABLETS). DISCARD UNUSED PORTION OF GRANULES WITHIN 15 MIN.
zafirlukast	Accolate	**Asthma:** 20 mg (1-2 tablets) bid	TAKE ON AN EMPTY STOMACH (1-2 HR AFTER EATING).
zileuton	Zyflo	**Asthma:** 2 tablets bid	TAKE WITH FOOD. SWALLOW WHOLE; DON'T CRUSH OR CHEW.
Mast Cell Stabilizers			
cromolyn sodium	Generics	**Asthma** **Inhaler:** 2 sprays qid **Nebulizer:** 20 mg (2 mL) qid	SHAKE WELL (INHALER).
Xanthine Derivatives			
aminophylline[b]	Generics	**Asthma and COPD:** 10 mg/kg/day PO or IV in divided doses every 6-8 hr (max, 800 mg/day)	SWALLOW WHOLE; DON'T CRUSH OR CHEW (EXTENDED-RELEASE).
theophylline	Theolair Theo-24	**Asthma and COPD:** **Immediate-release:** 10 mg/kg/day (max, 300-800 mg/day) PO or IV in divided doses every 6-8 hr **Extended-release:** 10 mg/kg/day (max, 300-800 mg/day) PO or IV in divided doses every 12-24 hr (Theo-24)	TAKE 30-60 MIN BEFORE MEALS WITH A FULL GLASS OF WATER.
Monoclonal Antibody			
omalizumab	Xolair	**Asthma:** 150-375 mg SC every 2 or 4 wk (based on baseline IgE levels)	REFRIGERATE POWDER AND RECONSTITUTED SOLUTION BETWEEN 2° AND 8° C (36°-46° F). DISCARD RECONSTITUTED SOLUTION AFTER 24 HR.

[a]Adult dose for asthma and COPD unless specified.
[b]Aminophylline dose expressed as theophylline.

Chapter Summary

- Asthma is a chronic disease that affects the airways, producing irritation, inflammation, and difficulty breathing.
- Asthma is classified according to the frequency and severity of symptoms. The four classifications for asthma are mild intermittent, mild persistent, moderate persistent, and severe persistent asthma.
- Family history of asthma, smoking, including exposure to second-hand smoke, chronic exposure to air pollution, exposure to some allergens, and infections early in life are risk factors for developing asthma.

- Symptoms of asthma are caused by airway irritation that result in bronchial constriction and impedes the passage of air. Airways also become inflamed, which produces swelling and further restricts the flow of air. Mucus production is increased, which further obstructs breathing passages.
- Symptoms of asthma include coughing, wheezing, shortness of breath, and chest tightness.
- Nocturnal asthma is a condition characterized by decreased FEV1 and by increased airway inflammation and hyperresponsiveness that occurs in the middle of the night.
- Asthma triggers can precipitate an asthma attack. Examples are animal dander, cockroach droppings, environmental pollutants, cleaning fluids, mold, tobacco smoke, air pollution, upper respiratory infection, vigorous exercise, and even cold air.
- Asthma symptoms can be managed with a combination of medication, lifestyle modification, and home monitoring of breathing using a peak flow meter and medication.
- Chronic obstructive pulmonary disease is a progressive disease of the airways that produces gradual loss of pulmonary function.
- Cigarette smoking or exposure to second-hand smoke, occupational irritants, industrial chemicals, or dust can increase the risk of developing COPD.
- Air pollution and viral infections may contribute to and worsen existing COPD.
- Shortness of breath, chronic persistent cough, wheezing, and increased sputum production are symptoms of COPD.
- A peak flow meter permits self-management of asthma, similar to how monitoring blood glucose levels enables self-management of diabetes.
- Low peak flow numbers signal that asthma is not controlled.
- Pharmacological treatment of COPD involves the administration of bronchodilators, glucocorticosteroids, and antibiotics when infection is present.
- Nonpharmacological treatments include oxygen therapy and mechanical ventilation.
- Drugs used for the treatment and management of asthma are divided into two classes. Drugs for the treatment of acute symptoms are classified as rescue or reliever medicines. Drugs administered to prevent asthma episodes are classified as maintenance therapies.
- Short-acting β_2-adrenergic agonists provide short-term relief of acute symptoms. Reliever medicines currently prescribed for the treatment of asthma include albuterol, levalbuterol, metaproterenol, and terbutaline.
- Because of safety concerns, the FDA and Health Canada have required changes to how long-acting beta-agonists are used in the treatment of asthma.
- The inhaled anticholinergic ipratropium bromide is administered for the relief of acute asthma symptoms; tiotropium is used to treat COPD.
- Anticholinergics bind to muscarinic receptors and block the effects of acetylcholine, resulting in relaxation of bronchial smooth muscle.
- Levalbuterol is an isomer of albuterol and is a moderately selective β_2-adrenergic receptor agonist.
- Drugs such as albuterol can produce nervousness, difficulty sleeping, dry mouth, mild headache, and throat irritation (by inhalants).
- Salmeterol and formoterol should not be administered as primary therapy.
- Long-acting β_2-adrenergic agonists have been associated with an increased risk of severe asthma exacerbations and asthma-related death.
- Glucocorticosteroids decrease the synthesis of proinflammatory substances such as prostaglandins, leukotrienes, cytokines, arachidonic acid, and macrophages.
- Inhaled corticosteroids include fluticasone (Flovent), budesonide (Pulmicort), mometasone (Asmanex), and beclomethasone (Qvar).
- Adverse reactions to inhaled corticosteroids are primarily local and include coughing, hoarseness, throat irritation, dry mouth, flushing, loss of taste, and/or unpleasant taste.
- Risks for thrush can be minimized by gargling or rinsing the mouth after administering the prescribed dose of glucocorticosteroid.
- Leukotriene modifiers are administered to patients with mild asthma to reduce inflammation.
- Leukotriene modifiers inhibit the release of proinflammatory leukotrienes, substances that are released as part of the inflammatory response.
- The packet of montelukast granules should not be opened until ready for use. Once opened, packet contents (with or without mixing with food) must be administered within 15 minutes.

- Cromolyn sodium is an example of a mast cell stabilizer; it makes mast cells less reactive to antigens and reduces the release of inflammatory substances responsible for producing the symptoms of asthma.
- Xanthines have bronchodilator and anti-inflammatory properties.
- Smoking cigarettes decreases the $t_{1/2}$ of theophylline by almost 50%.
- It is recommended that patients receive the same manufacturer's product each time their prescription for theophylline is refilled.
- Omalizumab is recombinant human monoclonal antibody (anti-IgE) and is indicated for the treatment of moderate to severe allergic asthma.
- Omalizumab is indicated as add-on therapy for patients whose asthma is not controlled with inhaled corticosteroids and β_2-adrenergic agonists.
- Omalizumab carries a boxed warning that patients should be instructed to watch for signs and symptoms of anaphylaxis.
- A nebulizer is a device that converts a liquid dose of medicine into an aerosolized mist.
- A spacer is a device attached to the end of the metered-dose inhaler that is used to control the delivery of an inhaled medicine.

1. A drug that relaxes tightened airway muscles and improves airflow through the airways is known as a _____.
   a. Bronchodilator
   b. Bronchoconstrictor

2. Asthma is classified according to _____ and _____ of symptoms.
   a. Frequency, duration
   b. Duration, presentation
   c. Frequency, severity
   d. Timing, duration

3. All of the following are risk factors for developing asthma *except*_____.
   a. Family history
   b. Exposure to cigarette smoke
   c. Vigorous exercise
   d. Chronic exposure to air pollutants

4. A peak flow meter is a device _____.
   a. That is attached to the end of the metered-dose inhaler
   b. That aids in self-management of asthma
   c. Used to administer asthma medication
   d. Used to diagnose and treat COPD

5. Emphysema, chronic bronchitis, and chronic obstructive bronchitis are all classified under the heading of _____.
   a. Asthma
   b. COPD
   c. Cystic fibrosis
   d. RSV

6. Persons with _____ may also exhibit a chronic persistent cough, wheezing, and increased sputum production.
   a. Smoking habit
   b. COPD
   c. Bronchitis
   d. None of the above

7. Nonpharmacological treatments for COPD include which of the following?
   a. Oxygen therapy
   b. Mechanical ventilation
   c. Inhalers
   d. a and b

8. Pharmacological treatment of COPD, when infections are present, involves the administration of _____.
   a. Bronchodilators
   b. Glucocorticosteroids
   c. Anti-infectives
   d. All of the above

9. Ipratropium bromide is administered by the _____ route.
   a. Oral
   b. Inhalation
   c. Transdermal
   d. Intravenous

10. A _____ is a device that converts a liquid dose of medicine into an aerosolized mist that can be inhaled by normal breathing when used with a mask.
    a. Aerosolizer
    b. Nebulizer
    c. Spacer
    d. Inhaler

TECHNICIAN'S
CORNER

1. Can lung damage be reversed when a smoker stops smoking?
2. What are some lifestyle modifications that can be implemented to manage asthma?

Bibliography

Centers for Disease Control and Prevention: Asthma (data are for the U.S.), 2012 (http://www.cdc.gov/nchs/fastats/asthma.htm).

Centers for Disease Control and Prevention: Latex allergy: A prevention guide (NIOSH Publ. No. 98-113), 1998 (http://www.cdc.gov/niosh/docs/98-113/).

Centers for Disease Control and Prevention: Occupational latex allergies (NIOSH Alert No. 97-135), 2010 (http://www.cdc.gov/niosh/docs/97-135).

FDA. FDA-Approved Drug Products, 2012. Retrieved May 29, 2012, from http://www.accessdata.fda.gov/scripts/cder/drugsatfda/index.cfm?fuseaction=Search.Search_Drug_Name.

Health Canada: Drug product database, 2010 (http://www.hc-sc.gc.ca/dhp-mps/prodpharma/databasdon/index-eng.php).

Health Canada: Safety information about a class of asthma drugs known as long-acting beta-2 agonists, 2005 (http://www.hc-sc.gc.ca/ahc-asc/media/advisories-avis/_2005/2005_107-eng.php).

Asthma in the US— http://www.cdc.gov/vitalsigns/Asthma/.

National Heart, Lung, and Blood Institute: Asthma, 2006 (http://www.cdc.gov/nchs/products/pubs/pubd/hestats/ashtma03-05/asthma03-05.htm).

National Heart, Lung, and Blood Institute: What is asthma? 2011 (http://www.nhlbi.nih.gov/health/dci/Diseases/Asthma/Asthma_WhatIs.html).

National Heart, Lung, and Blood Institute: What is COPD? 2010 (http://www.nhlbi.nih.gov/health/health-topics/topics/copd/).

National Institute of Environmental Health Sciences: Asthma and its environmental triggers, 2006 (http://www.niehs.nih.gov/health/materials/asthma_and_its_environmental_triggers.pdf).

Page C, Curtis M, Sutter M, et al: *Integrated pharmacology*, Philadelphia, 2005, Mosby, pp 415-423.

Papi A, Contoli M, Gaetano C, et al: Models of infection and exacerbations in COPD, *Curr Opin Pharmacol* 7:259-265, 2007.

Pleis JR, Lethbridge-Çejku M: Summary health statistics for U.S. adults: National health interview survey, 2005 (http://www.cdc.gov/nchs/data/series/sr_10/sr10_232.pdf).

Shigemitsu H, Afshar K: Nocturnal asthma, *Curr Opin Pulm Med* 13:49-55, 2007.

Statistics Canada: Asthma, 2009 (http://www.statcan.gc.ca/pub/82-625-x/2010002/article/11256-eng.htm).

U.S. Food and Drug Administration: FDA drug safety communication: New safety requirements for long-acting inhaled asthma medications called long-acting beta-agonists (LABAs), 2010 (http://www.fda.gov/Drugs/DrugSafety/PostmarketDrugSafetyInformationforPatientsandProviders/ucm200776.htm).

Web MD: Secondhand smoke may harm fetus like smoking, 2012 (http://www.webmd.com/baby/news/20050727/secondhand-smoke-may-harm-fetus-like-smoking).

29

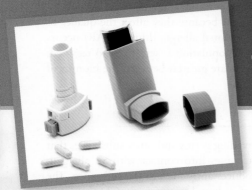

Treatment of Allergies

LEARNING OBJECTIVES

1 Learn the terminology associated with allergies.

2 Describe the causes and list the symptoms of allergic reactions.

3 List and categorize medications used for the treatment of allergies.

4 Describe the mechanism of action for drugs used to treat allergies.

5 Identify significant drug look-alike and sound-alike issues.

6 Identify warning labels and precautionary messages associated with medications used for the treatment of allergies.

KEY TERMS

Allergen: Substance that produces an allergic reaction.

Allergic conjunctivitis: Inflammation of the tissue lining the eyelids caused by the reaction to an allergy-causing substance.

Allergic rhinitis: Seasonal condition characterized by inflammation and swelling of the nasal passageways (rhinitis) accompanied by runny nose (rhinorrhea).

Allergy: Hypersensitivity reaction by the immune system on exposure to an allergen.

Anaphylaxis: Life-threatening allergic reaction.

Angioedema: Allergic skin disease characterized by patches of circumscribed swelling involving the skin and its subcutaneous layers, the mucous membranes, and sometimes the viscera.

Histamine: An organic nitrogen compound involved in local immune responses as well as regulating physiological function in the gut and acting as a neurotransmitter.

Immunoglobulin E: An antibody associated with allergies.

Leukotriene: A proinflammatory mediator released as part of the allergic inflammatory response. Leukotrienes also trigger contractions in the smooth muscles of airways.

Mast cells: Granule-containing cells found in connective tissue. They contain many granules rich in histamine, which are released during allergic reactions.

Urticaria: Hives.

Wheal: Raised blister-like area on the skin.

Overview

An *allergy* is a hypersensitivity reaction by the immune system on exposure to an allergen. An *allergen* is a substance that produces an allergic reaction. It is not known why some individuals are more likely than others to develop allergies; however, exposure to allergens in the environment is a major determinant for the development of allergies. Allergic conditions affect between 40 and 50 million people in the United States and are a public health issue because they affect the quality of life, productivity, and performance of sensitive individuals. Seasonal allergic rhinitis (SAR) occurs on exposure to seasonal pollens. Up to 20% of the total U.S. population is sensitized to ragweed; symptoms of seasonal allergic rhinitis and allergic conjunctivitis are greatest between the months of August and October, when ragweed pollen levels are high.

What Triggers an Allergic Response?

The immune system functions to defend the body against invading germs and other substances that it believes are harmful. When a person with allergies first comes into contact with an allergen, the immune system treats the allergen as an invader and produces antibodies to the substance. The human allergic response is engineered by different types of T lymphocytes (e.g., CD4+, CD8+, natural killer T [NKT] cells). Their ability to respond to allergens varies. CD4+ T cells are the predominant T lymphocytes responsible for producing allergies, although CD8+ T cells are involved in allergic asthma. CD4+ T cells exert their effects through the production of interleukins (e.g., IL-4, IL-5, and IL-13) and secretion of cytokines when activated by allergens (Figure 29-1). IL-4 is involved in *immunoglobulin E* (IgE) synthesis, a major risk factor for the development of allergic asthma (see Chapter 28). IL-5 orchestrates eosinophil recruitment. Eosinophils are cells linked to the control of mechanisms associated with allergy and asthma.

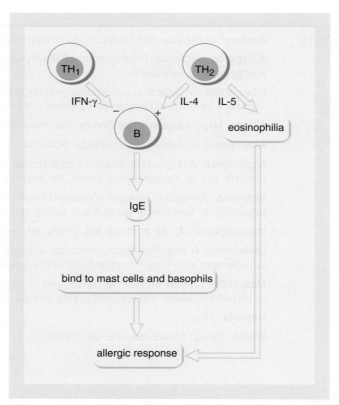

FIGURE 29-1 CD4+-mediated allergic response. TH₁, TH₂, T helper cells; IFN-γ, interferon gamma; IL, interleukin. (From Page C, Hoffman B, Curtis M, et al: *Integrated pharmacology*, ed 3, Philadelphia, 2006, Mosby.)

The production of allergen-specific IgE antibodies and T cell responses directed against allergens develops within the first few years of life. It is now known that exposure early in life to high levels of multiple endotoxins, as occurs when children live with multiple pets, may reduce the risks for development of asthma and allergies. The degree of IgE antibody response varies, and allergens from some sources (e.g., dust mites, cat) are more potent than others.

ALLERGIC REACTION SEQUENCE

The allergic reaction sequence is a cascade of events that begins with the ingestion or inhalation of allergen. Exposure to the allergen triggers an immune system reaction and the production of specialized antibodies (IgE). Antibodies attach to **mast cells** containing **histamine**, which when released produces allergic reaction symptoms such as itching, runny nose, hives, and wheezing.

ALLERGIC CONJUNCTIVITIS

Allergic conjunctivitis produces red, watering, itchy or burning eyes. Sufferers may also have ocular puffiness and a stringy discharge from the eyes. Symptoms occur on exposure to an allergen. Seasonal allergic conjunctivitis may worsen during allergy and hay fever season. Overuse of decongestants to treat red eyes may result in conjunctivitis medicamentosa or rebound eye redness and congestion. More information about conjunctivitis is found in Chapter 20.

ALLERGIC RHINITIS

Allergic rhinitis is a condition characterized by nasal itching (rhinitis), runny nose (rhinorrhea), nasal congestion (stuffiness), and sneezing. Allergic rhinitis is typically self-limiting and will resolve without treatment with anti-infective agents. Symptoms are caused by inflammation and swelling of the nasal passageways and may occur throughout the year or seasonally. With seasonal allergic rhinitis, allergy symptoms appear after a period of absence from allergen exposure. Symptoms are produced by T lymphocytes and eosinophil infiltration of the nasal epithelium, which occurs as a result of stimulation of mast cells by allergens. The recurrence of allergic symptoms seasonally is

Drugs for Allergic Conjunctivitis

Generic Name	Selected U.S. and Canadian Brand Name(s)	Dosage Forms and Strengths	Status and Warnings
Decongestant			
naphazoline*	Albalon[†], All-Clear AR[¶], Clear Eyes[§]	1-2 drops in affected eye(s), up to qid	Should only be used for short periods of time; overuse can lead to conjunctivitis medicamentosa
Decongestant, Antihistamine			
naphazoline, pheniramine**	Visine-A[¶], Naphcon-A[¶], Opcon-A[¶]	1-2 drops in affected eye(s) up to qid	Should only be used for short periods of time; overuse can lead to conjunctivitis medicamentosa
Antihistamine			
azelastine[†]	**Optivar** 0.05%	Instill 1 drop in affected eye(s) twice daily	Discard 30 after removing from foil pouch
ketotifen	Alaway, Claritin Eye, Zaditor, Zyrtec Itchy Eye	Instill 1 drop every 8-12 hr in each affected eye.	Wait 10 min before applying any other eye drops or contact lenses
Mast Cell Stabilizer			
cromolyn na+	Opticrom[‡] 2%[§], 4%[†]	1-2 drops in affected eye(s) 4 times a day	Remove soft contact lenses during treatment

*Generic available.
[†]Strength available in the United States only.
[‡]Strength available in Canada only.
[§]OTC in Canada.
[¶]OTC in the United States.
**Not FDA-approved.

believed to be caused by the presence of memory CD4⁺ T cells. There are two types of memory CD4⁺ T cells. Central memory T cells (TCMs) multiply on exposure to antigens. Effector memory T cells (TEMs) travel to inflamed tissues, secreting cytokines, mediators of the immune system response (and inflammation). Memory CD4⁺ T cells are allergen-specific (e.g., tree, grass, weed pollen).

URTICARIA

Urticaria (also known as hives) is a condition characterized by itching and *angioedema* (swelling). Redness, swelling, and *wheals* (blister-like vesicles) appear on the skin. Urticaria may be caused by an insect bite, drug or food allergy, or injection of allergen extracts (allergy shots). The condition usually subsides within a few days but, if severe, may need to be managed by the administration of H_1 receptor antagonists and glucocorticosteroids. Acute pharyngeal or laryngeal angioedema must be managed by the administration of drugs that rapidly reduce swelling in the throat and restore breathing capacity (e.g., short-acting β_2-adrenergic agonists).

OCCUPATIONAL ALLERGENS

Pharmacy technicians are at risk for developing latex allergy. Allergic reactions occur when latex-sensitive individuals breathe in or come into physical contact with latex proteins. Latex proteins in disposable gloves may form a complex with the lubricant powder used in some gloves. When the pharmacy technician changes gloves, the protein–powder particle complex may become airborne and then inhaled.

Latex allergy may produce mild reactions such as skin redness, rash, hives, or itching. Respiratory symptoms such as runny nose, sneezing, itchy eyes, and scratchy throat may occur. More severe reactions involve asthma (difficult breathing, coughing spells, and wheezing) and, rarely, *anaphylaxis*, which is life-threatening.

The National Institute for Occupational Safety and Health recommends taking the following steps to protect oneself from latex exposure and allergy in the workplace.

1. Avoid contact with latex gloves and products. Select nonlatex gloves when possible. Appropriate barrier protection is necessary when handling infectious materials.
2. If you choose latex gloves, use powder-free gloves with reduced protein content.
3. Use appropriate work practices to reduce the chance of reactions to latex.
4. Do not use oil-based hand creams or lotions when wearing latex gloves because they can cause glove deterioration.
5. After removing latex gloves, wash hands with a mild soap and dry thoroughly.
6. Practice good housekeeping by frequently cleaning areas and equipment contaminated with latex-containing dust.
7. Avoid areas where you might inhale the powder from latex gloves worn by other workers.
8. Tell your employer and health care providers (e.g., physician, nurse, dentist) that you have latex allergy.

Pharmacy technicians may come into contact with a wide variety of products containing latex in the workplace. Box 29-1 provides examples of products that may contain latex.

Symptoms of Allergies

Symptoms associated with an allergic reaction may be localized to a specific area of contact, as with contact dermatitis, or may be more generalized. Persons with chronic airborne allergies may develop

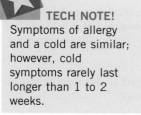

TECH NOTE!
Symptoms of allergy and a cold are similar; however, cold symptoms rarely last longer than 1 to 2 weeks.

BOX 29-1   **Products Containing Latex**

- Disposable gloves
- Intravenous tubing
- Intravenous bag ports
- Syringes
- Catheters
- Injection ports
- Rubber tops of multidose vials

BOX 29-2   **Common Allergy Symptoms**

DERMAL	RESPIRATORY
• Redness	• Itchy eyes, nose, and throat
• Swelling	• Runny nose
• Urticaria	• Stuffy nose
• Wheal	• Sneezing
	• Coughing and postnasal drip
	• Watery eyes
	• Conjuctivitis
	• Allergic shiners
	• Allergic salute

allergic shiners (dark circles under the eyes caused by increased blood flow near the sinuses) and an allergic salute (a crease across the bridge of the nose caused by persistent upward rubbing of the nose). Common allergy symptoms are listed in Box 29-2.

Drugs Used for the Treatment of Allergies

The pharmacological treatment of allergies is aimed at reducing swelling and inflammation and at suppression of the release of cells that mediate immune system and inflammatory responses, as well as blocking receptor sites of the mediators. Drugs used to treat allergic symptoms include antihistamines, inhaled corticosteroids and mast cell stabilizers, leukotriene receptor antagonists, and vasoconstrictors.

H_1 RECEPTOR ANTAGONISTS

Allergic reactions associated with the binding of histamine to H_1 receptor sites can be reduced by the administration of antihistamines. Recall that when allergens bind to specific IgE antibodies on mast cells, mast cell degranulation occurs, resulting in the release of histamine, prostaglandins, and *leukotrienes*. Histamine release causes vasodilation and swelling, itchiness, runny nose, watery eyes, and other allergic symptoms. It also produces smooth muscle contraction in the bronchial airways and gastrointestinal tract.

There are several classes of antihistamines—ethylenediamines, ethanolamines, alkylamines, piperazines, phenothiazines, phthalazinones, and piperidines. Most are available without prescription. An additional use for piperazine antihistamines (e.g., meclizine, cyclizine) is the treatment of nausea and vomiting. Phenothiazines are also administered for their antiemetic properties and for the treatment of schizophrenia (see Chapter 7).

Mechanism of Action and Pharmacokinetics

Administration of antihistamines prevents histamine binding to H_1 receptor sites. The drugs compete with free histamine for binding at H_1 receptor sites. All H_1 receptor antagonists have good oral absorption and reach maximum serum levels within 1 to 2 hours. The half-life ($t_{1/2}$) of the antihistamines varies, ranging from as short as 4 to 6 hours (e.g., diphenhydramine) to 24 hours (fexofenadine). Hydroxyzine is metabolized to the active metabolite cetirizine (Zyrtec). Desloratadine and loratadine are formulated as disintegrating tablets for rapid dissolution and onset of action.

Adverse Reactions

Antihistamines that cross the blood-brain barrier decrease alertness and/or produce sedation. Sedation, dizziness, decreased alertness, dry mouth, blurred vision, lack of coordination, and urinary retention are the most common adverse reactions of antihistamines. Antihistamines that are classified as ethanolamines (e.g., diphenhydramine) and phenothiazines (e.g., promethazine) produce the most sedation and have the greatest anticholinergic effects. Ethylenediamines (e.g., pyrilamine) and piperazines (e.g., cetirizine) produce fewer sedative effects, and newer agents produce the least sedation. Piperidines (e.g., loratadine, fexofenadine) are relatively nonsedating.

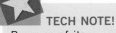

TECH NOTE!
The Centers for Disease Control and Prevention (CDC) and the U.S. Food and Drug Administration (FDA) have issued public health warnings recommending that cold and cough products containing antihistamines,* decongestants, and expectorants not to be used in children younger than 2 years. The FDA nonprescription Drug Advisory Committee and Pediatric Advisory Committee recommendations extend to children younger than 6 years.

*Chlorpheniramine, diphenhydramine, brompheniramine, clemastine.

TECH NOTE!
Because of its sedating effects, diphenhydramine is also administered for the treatment of insomnia.

Precautions

Antihistamines should be used cautiously in men with prostate disease, persons with asthma, and women who are breast-feeding. Antihistamine use in children younger than 2 years is not recommended. These drugs can decrease urination, thicken bronchial secretions, and decrease milk production.

GLUCOCORTICOSTEROIDS

Glucocorticosteroids are anti-inflammatory drugs that are administered intranasally to control symptoms of rhinitis. When administered intranasally, they inhibit the onset of the inflammatory response by reducing the permeability of the nasal mucosa cells to T lymphocytes and eosinophils, thereby decreasing the release of mediators of the inflammatory response (e.g., cytokines). They also reduce the number of inflammatory cells. The result is a reduction in mucus and swelling that make

Selected Antihistamines (H1 Receptor Antagonists)

Generic Name	U.S. Brand Name(s) Canadian Brand Name(s)	Dosage Forms and Strengths	Prescription Status
Alkylamines			
brompheniramine*	Generics	Tablet: 4 mg	RX
	Not available		
chlorpheniramine*	Chlor-Trimeton,	Tablet: 4‡ mg	OTC
	Chlor-Tripolon, Chlor-Tripolon 12 mg Long Acting, Chlor-Tripolon Day and Night	Tablet, extended-release: 12 mg	
dexchlorpheniramine*	Generics	Solution: 2 mg/5 mL	RX
	Not available		
Ethanolamines			
diphenhydramine*	Benadryl Children's Allergy, Benadryl Children's Allergy Fastmelt, Benadryl Allergy, Benadryl Allergy Quick Dissolve Strip, Benadryl Itch Stopping Extra Strength, PediaCare Children's Allergy	Capsule (Allerdryl, Benadryl): 25 mg, 50 mg Capsule, liquid-filled (Benadryl Allergy Liquigel): 25 mg Cream (Benadryl): 2% Elixir (Allernix, Benadryl): 12.5 mg/5 mL Gel (Benadryl Itch Stopping Extra Strength): 2% Film, oral dissolving: 12.5 mg (Triaminic Thin Strips Cough and Runny Nose), 25 mg (Benadryl Allergy Quick Dissolve Strip)	OTC
	Aller-Aide, Allerdryl, Allernix, Benadryl, Benadryl Elixir, Benadryl Allergy Liquigel, Dimetane Allergy, Triaminic Thin Strips Cough and Runny Nose	Solution (Benadryl Children's Allergy): 12.5 mg/5 mL Solution, for injection§: 50 mg/mL Spray (Benadryl): 2% Suspension: 25 mg/5 mL Syrup: 6.25 mg/5 mL Tablet (Aller-Aide, Benadryl Allergy): 25 mg, 50 mg Tablet, oral disintegrating (Benadryl Children's Allergy Fastmelt): 12.5 mg Tablet, as citrate (Dimetane Allergy): 38 mg	

Selected Antihistamines (H1 Receptor Antagonists)—cont'd

Generic Name	U.S. Brand Name(s) / Canadian Brand Name(s)	Dosage Forms and Strengths	Prescription Status
clemastine*	Tavist-1 / Tavist	Syrup: 0.5 mg/5 mL Tablet: 1 mg‡, 1.34 mg†, 2.68 mg† (RX only)	OTC, Prescription
Piperazines			
cetirizine*	Zyrtec, Children's Zyrtec Allergy, Children's Zyrtec Hives Relief, Zyrtec Allergy, Zyrtecc Hives Relief / Reactine	Capsule: 5 mg†, 10 mg Syrup: 1 mg/mL Tablet, chewable (Reactine, Zyrtec): 5 mg, 10 mg Tablet: 5 mg, 10 mg, 20 mg‡ (RX only) Tablet, ODT (Reactine Fast Melt): 10 mg	OTC, Prescription
levocetirizine*	Xyzal / Not available	Solution, oral: 2.5 mg/5 mL Tablet: 5 mg	Prescription (US)
Piperidines			
desloratadine*	Clarinex, Clarinex RediTab / Aerius*, Aerius Kids	Syrup: 0.5 mg/mL Tablet: 5 mg Tablet, oral disintegrating (Clarinex RediTab): 2.5 mg, 5 mg	Prescription (US) OTC (Canada)
loratadine*	Alavert 24-Hour Allergy, Claritin, Children's Claritin, Claritin Hives Relief, Claritin RediTab, Claritin Liqui-gel, / Claritin, Claritin Kids, Claritin Rapid Dissolve	Capsule, liquid-filled (Claritin Liqui-gel): 10 mg Syrup (Claritin, Claritin Kids, Dimetapp Children's Non-Drowsy Allergy): 1 mg/mL Tablet (Claritin, Tavist ND): 10 mg Tablet, chewable: 5 mg Tablet, extended-release (Alavert 24 hr): 10 mg Tablet, oral disintegrating (Alavert 24 Hour), Claritin Rapid Dissolve, Claritin RediTab: 10 mg	OTC
fexofenadine*	Allegra, Children's Allegra Allergy, Allegra ODT / Allegra 12 Hour, Allegra 24 Hour	Suspension: 30 mg/5 mL Tablet: 30 mg, 60 mg (Allegra 12 Hour), 120 mg (Allegra 24 Hour, Canada), 180 mg (Allegra 24 Hour, United States) Tablet, oral disintegrating (Allegra Children's Allergy, Allegra ODT): 30 mg	OTC
Phthalazinone			
azelastine*	Astelin, Astepro, Optivar / Not available	Nasal spray solution: 137 mcg/actuation (Astelin); 187.6 mcg/actuation (Astepro) Ophthalmic solution (Optivar): 0.05%	Prescription

*Generic available.
†Strength available in the United States only.
‡Strength available in Canada only.
§Prescription in the United States

breathing difficult. Additional mechanisms of action and pharmacokinetics of glucocorticosteroids are discussed in detail in Chapters 15 and 28. Glucocorticosteroids for intranasal use include fluticasone (Flonase), budesonide (Rhinocort), triamcinolone (Nasacort AQ), flunisolide (Nasarel), mometasone (Nasonex), and beclomethasone (Beconase AQ).

Adverse Reactions

Adverse reactions to corticosteroids administered intranasally are primarily local and include nasal irritation, throat irritation, and nosebleed. Some patients may develop a *Candida* infection in the nostril that may present as burning or stinging in the nostril(s).

MAST CELL STABILIZERS

Cromolyn sodium is a mast cell stabilizer available for intranasal and ophthalmic use. It is administered to reduce the reactivity to allergens; therefore, they cause decreased mast cell degranulation and release of inflammatory substances.

Cromolyn sodium is not used to treat acute symptoms and therapy should be initiated 1 week before coming into contact with allergens and continued for the duration of allergen exposure. Mechanisms of action, pharmacokinetics, and adverse reactions for cromolyn sodium are described in Chapter 28. Adverse effects include bad taste in the mouth, cough, dry throat, or difficulty breathing, headache, nosebleeds, runny nose, sneezing, and stinging, burning, or irritation inside

Inhaled Corticosteroids for Allergic Rhinitis (Nasal Spray)

Generic Name	U.S. Brand Name(s) Canadian Brand Name(s)	Dosage Forms and Strengths	Prescription Status
beclomethasone	Beconase AQ, QNASL Generics	Pump spray: 42 mcg/actuation (Beconase AQ), 50 mcg/actuation[‡], 80 mcg/actuation (QNASL)	Prescription only
budesonide*	Rhinocort Aqua Rhinocort Aqua	Pump spray (suspension): 32 mcg/actuation[†], 64mcg/actuation[‡], 100 mcg/actuation[‡]	Prescription only
flunisolide*	Generics Rhinalar	Pump spray: 25 mcg/actuation, 29 mcg/actuation	Prescription only
fluticasone*	Flonase, Veramyst Avamys, Flonase	Pump spray, as furoate (Avamys, Veramyst): 27.5 mcg/actuation Pump spray, as propionate (Flonase): 50 mcg/actuation	Prescription only
mometasone	Nasonex Nasonex	Pump spray: 50 mcg/actuation	Prescription only
triamcinolone	Nasacort AQ Nasacort, Nasacort AQ	Pump spray (Nasacort AQ): 55 mcg/actuation Spray (Nasacort): 100 mcg/actuation	Prescription only

*Generic available.
[†]Strength available in the United States only.
[‡]Strength available in Canada only.

Mast Cell Stabilizer for Allergic Rhinitis

Generic Name	U.S. Brand Name(s) Canadian Brand Name(s)	Dosage Forms and Strengths	Prescription Status
cromolyn sodium*	NasalCrom Rhinaris-CS Anti-Allergic Nasal Mist	Pump Spray (Nasalcrom): 5.2 mg/actuation, 2% (Rhinaris-CS Anti-Allergic Nasal)	OTC

*Generic available.

the nose. Cromolyn sodium for nasal (Nasalcrom) and ophthalmic (Opticrom) use is available without prescription.

LEUKOTRIENE RECEPTOR ANTAGONISTS

The leukotriene receptor antagonist montelukast is used to control allergic rhinitis symptoms. Montelukast is a selective antagonist of the cysteinyl leukotriene D_4 receptor found in the human airway. Montelukast may produce cough, hoarseness or sore throat, headache, indigestion, heartburn or stomach upset, and runny nose. Montelukast may also produce difficulty sleeping, dizziness, drowsiness, muscle aches or cramps, or unusual dreams. More information about leukotrienes antagonists is presented in Chapter 28.

Leukotriene Receptor Antagonist for Allergic Rhinitis

Generic Name	U.S. Brand Name(s) / Canadian Brand Name(s)	Dosage Forms and Strengths	Prescription Status
montelukast	Singulair / Singulair	Oral granules (United States only): 4 mg Tablet: 10 mg Tablet, chewable: 4 mg, 5 mg	Prescription only

Summary of Drugs Used in the Treatment of Allergic Conditions

Generic Name	U.S. Brand Name(s)	Usual Adult Oral Dose and Dosing Schedule	Warning Labels
Antihistamine (H1 Receptor Antagonist)			
brompheniramine	Generic	Allergic rhinitis, pruritus, and urticaria Immediate-release: 4-8 mg every 6-8 hr Extended-release: 1-2 tablets every 12 hr	MAY CAUSE DIZZINESS OR DROWSINESS; ALCOHOL MAY INCREASE THIS EFFECT: BROMPHENIRAMINE, CHLORPHENIRAMINE, DIPHENHYDRAMINE, CLEMASTINE, CETIRIZINE, DESLORATADINE, LORATADINE, LEVOCETIRIZINE.
chlorpheniramine	Chlor-Trimeton	Allergic rhinitis Immediate-release: 4 mg every 4-6 hr up to 24 mg/day Extended-release: 8 mg-12 mg bid or tid	SWALLOW WHOLE; DON'T CRUSH OR CHEW—EXTENDED-RELEASE.
diphenhydramine	Benadryl	Allergic rhinitis, pruritus, and urticaria: 25-50 mg tid or qid	PROTECT FROM MOISTURE; LEAVE IN FOIL PACKET UNTIL READY FOR USE—DISINTEGRATING TABLETS.
clemastine	Tavist	Allergic rhinitis and urticaria: 1.34-2.68 mg bid or tid Pruritus and angioedema: 2.68 mg 1-3 times daily	DISSOLVE REDITAB UNDER THE TONGUE—DISINTEGRATING TABLETS.
cetirizine	Zyrtec	Allergic rhinitis and urticaria: 5-10 mg once daily	MAY CAUSE DIZZINESS OR DROWSINESS
desloratadine	Clarinex	Allergic rhinitis, pruritus, and urticaria: 5 mg once daily	AVOID ORANGE, GRAPEFRUIT, AND APPLE JUICE—FEXOFENADINE.
fexofenadine	Allegra	Allergic rhinitis and urticaria: 60 mg bid or 180 mg once daily	
levocetirizine	Xyzal	Allergic rhinitis and urticaria: 5 mg once daily in the evening	
loratadine	Alavert, Claritin	Allergic rhinitis and urticaria: 10 mg once daily	

Summary of Drugs Used in the Treatment of Allergic Conditions—cont'd

Generic Name	U.S. Brand Name(s)	Usual Adult Oral Dose and Dosing Schedule	Warning Labels
Phthalazinone H1 Antagonist			
azelastine	Astelin, Optivar	Allergic conjunctivitis: 1 drop in affected eye(s) bid Allergic rhinitis: 1-2 sprays each nostril bid	PRIME INHALER BEFORE USE. MAY CAUSE SEDATION; DO NOT DRIVE OR OPERATE MACHINERY.
Intranasal Corticosteroids			
beclomethasone	Beconase AQ	Allergic rhinitis: 1-2 sprays each nostril bid	SHAKE WELL. RINSE AND DRY TIP AFTER EACH USE (NASAL INHALERS).
budesonide	Rhinocort Aqua	Allergic rhinitis: 1-2 sprays each nostril once daily	
flunisolide	Nasarel	Allergic rhinitis: 2-3 sprays each nostril bid	
fluticasone propionate	Flonase	Allergic rhinitis: 1 spray each nostril bid or 2 sprays in each nostril daily	
fluticasone furoate	Veramyst, Avamys	Allergic rhinitis: 2 sprays each nostril once daily or 1 spray each nostril bid	
mometasone	Nasonex	Allergic rhinitis: 2 sprays each nostril once daily	
triamcinolone	Nasacort	Allergic rhinitis: 1-2 sprays each nostril bid	
Mast Cell Stabilizer			
cromolyn sodium	Nasalcrom,	Allergic rhinitis: 1 spray each nostril tid or qid (up to 6 times daily)	RINSE AND DRY TIP AFTER EACH USE (NASALCROM).
Leukotriene Receptor Antagonist			
montelukast	Singulair	Allergic rhinitis: 10 mg PO once daily Adults, chewable tablets: Chew 1 tablet (4 or 5 mg) once daily. Children and infants, 6 mo–2 yr: 4 mg PO once daily Children, 2-5 yr, oral granules: dissolve and consume 1 packet once daily	TAKE WITH A LARGE GLASS OF WATER (CHEWABLE TABLET). DISCARD UNUSED PORTION OF SOLUTION WITHIN 15 MIN.

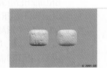

Immunotherapy

Allergy shots represent a form of immunotherapy. They may be administered to persons with perennial (symptoms all year round) or seasonal allergies. The rationale for immunotherapy is to reduce the level of IgE antibodies in the blood while at the same time stimulating the production of IgG, a protective antibody. Allergy shots are administered by SC injection as a series of shots; each injection has an increased concentration of the allergen that produces sensitivity. Allergy shots can reduce allergy symptoms over a longer period of time than all other treatments.

Chapter Summary

- An allergy is a hypersensitivity reaction by the immune system on exposure to an allergen.
- Allergic conditions affect the quality of life, productivity, and performance of sensitive individuals.

- Seasonal allergic rhinitis occurs on exposure to seasonal pollens.
- When a person with allergies first comes into contact with an allergen, the immune system treats the allergen as an invader and produces antibodies to the substance.
- CD4$^+$ T cells are the predominant T lymphocytes responsible for producing allergies, although CD8$^+$ is involved in allergic asthma. CD4$^+$ T cells exert their effects through the production of interleukins (e.g., IL-4, IL-5, IL-13) and secretion of cytokines when activated by allergens.
- IL-4 is involved in immunoglobulin E synthesis.
- The production of allergen-specific IgE antibodies and T cell responses directed against allergens develop within the first few years of life.
- The degree of IgE antibody response varies; allergens from some sources (e.g., dust mites, cat) are more potent than others.
- Allergic rhinitis is a condition characterized by nasal itching (rhinitis), runny nose (rhinorrhea), nasal congestion (stuffiness), and sneezing. Allergic conjunctivitis produces itchy and watering eyes.
- The recurrence of allergic symptoms seasonally is caused by the presence of memory CD4$^+$ T cells. There are two types of memory CD4$^+$ T cells. Central memory T cells multiply on exposure to antigens. Effector memory T cells travel to inflamed tissues, secreting cytokines, mediators of immune system response (and inflammation).
- Urticaria (also known as hives) is condition characterized by itching and angioedema (swelling).
- Pharmacy technicians are at risk for developing latex allergy. Allergic reactions occur when latex-sensitive individuals breathe in or come into physical contact with latex proteins.
- Latex allergy may produce mild reactions such as skin redness, rash, hives, or itching. Respiratory symptoms such as runny nose, sneezing, itchy eyes, and scratchy throat may occur.
- Pharmacological treatment of allergies is aimed at reducing swelling and inflammation and suppressing the release of cells that mediate immune system and inflammatory responses, as well as blocking receptor sites of the mediators.
- Drugs used to treat allergic symptoms include antihistamines, inhaled corticosteroids and mast cell stabilizers, leukotriene modifiers, and vasoconstrictors.
- Antihistamines compete with free histamine for binding at histamine 1 receptor sites.
- There are seven classes of antihistamines—ethylenediamines, ethanolamines, alkylamines, piperazines, phenothiazines, phthalazinones, and piperidines.
- Sedation, dizziness, decreased alertness, dry mouth, blurred vision, lack of coordination, and urinary retention are the most common adverse reactions of antihistamines.
- Antihistamines that are classified as ethanolamines (e.g., diphenhydramine) and phenothiazines (e.g., promethazine) produce the most sedation and have the greatest anticholinergic effects.
- Piperidines (e.g., loratadine, desloratadine, fexofenadine) are relatively nonsedating.
- Antihistamines should be used cautiously in men with prostate disease, persons with asthma, and women who are breast-feeding. They are not recommended for use in children younger than 2 years old.
- Glucocorticosteroids are administered intranasally to control symptoms of allergic rhinitis.
- Glucocorticosteroids for intranasal use include fluticasone (Flonase), budesonide (Rhinocort), triamcinolone (Nasacort), flunisolide (Nasalide), mometasone (Nasonex), and beclomethasone (Beconase AQ).
- Adverse reactions to corticosteroids administered intranasally are primarily local and include: nasal irritation, throat irritation, and nose bleed.
- Cromolyn sodium is a mast cell stabilizer available for intranasal and ophthalmic use.
- Therapy with cromolyn sodium should be initiated 1 week before coming into contact with allergens and continued for the duration of allergen exposure.
- Montelukast is a leukotriene receptor antagonist used to treat allergic rhinitis.
- Allergy shots are a form of immunotherapy.
- Allergy shots are administered as a series of SC injections; they can reduce allergy symptoms over a longer period of time than all other treatments.

1. Which of the following is a life-threatening allergic reaction?
    a. Urticaria
    b. Pruritus
    c. Anaphylaxis
    d. Wheal

2. An allergy is a hypersensitivity reaction that occurs on exposure to an allergen.
    a. True
    b. False

3. A condition characterized by nasal itching (rhinitis), runny nose (rhinorrhea), nasal congestion (stuffiness), and sneezing is called _____.
    a. Urticaria
    b. Allergic rhinitis
    c. Wheals
    d. Angioedema

4. Symptoms associated with an allergic reaction are always localized.
    a. True
    b. False

5. Some antihistamines are available without a prescription.
    a. True
    b. False

6. Glucocorticosteroids are administered intraorally to control symptoms of rhinitis.
    a. True
    b. False

7. Cromolyn sodium is a (an) _____ available for intranasal use.
    a. Mast cell stabilizer
    b. Glucocorticoid
    c. Antihistamine
    d. Leukotriene

8. Diphenhydramine has a side effect of _____.
    a. Insomnia
    b. Sedation
    c. Burning
    d. None of the above

9. Loratadine is the generic name for Clarinex.
    a. True
    b. False

10. Cetirizine is available in which of the following dosage forms?
    a. Tablet
    b. Chewable tablet
    c. Syrup
    d. All of the above

1. What is the best way to identify what is causing an allergy?
2. Should all antihistamines be available as OTC drugs?

Bibliography

Elsevier: Gold Standard Clinical Pharmacology, 2010. Retrieved April 2, 2011, from https://www.clinicalpharmacology.com/

Health Canada: Drug product database, 2010 (http://www.hc-sc.gc.ca/dhp-mps/prodpharma/databasdon/index-eng.php).

Kaiser H, Naclerio R, Given J, et al: Fluticasone furoate nasal spray: A single treatment option for the symptoms of seasonal allergic rhinitis, *J Allergy Clin Immunol* 119:1430-1437, 2007.

Kalant H, Grant D, Mitchell J: *Principles of medical pharmacology*, ed 7, Toronto, 2007, Elsevier Canada, pp 22-27, 397-400, 451, 453-454.

National Institute of Allergy and Infectious Disease: Airborne allergens: Something in the air (NIH Publ. No. 03-7045), 2003 (http://www.allergywatch.org/basic/airborne_allergens.pdf).

National Library of Medicine. Allergic conjunctivitis. Retrieved April 10, 2011, from http://www.ncbi.nlm.nih.gov/pubmedhealth/, 2008.

Page C, Curtis M, Sutter M, et al: *Integrated pharmacology*, Philadelphia, 2005, Mosby, pp 330-336, 428-430.

UT Southwestern Medical Center: Allergic cascade, 2007 (http://www.utsouthwestern.edu/vgn/images/portal/cit_56417/13/18/415119Education-_Allergic_Cascade.pdf).

Växa: Ragweed allergy affects up to 20 percent of Americans, (http://www.vaxa.com/ragweed-allergy.cfm).

Woodfolk J: T-cell responses to allergens, molecular mechanisms in allergy and clinical immunology, *J Allergy Clin Immunol* 119:280-294, 2007.

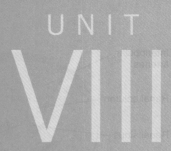

Drugs Affecting the Urinary System

LEARNING
OBJECTIVES

1 Identify the organs of the urinary system.

2 Understand the function of each part of the urinary system.

3 Explain the process of the formation and elimination of urine.

4 Understand the importance of the kidney in maintaining homeostasis.

KEY TERMS

Incontinence: Involuntary micturition, or voiding of urine.

Micturition: Urination.

Tubular reabsorption: Movement of molecules such as water, sodium, and electrolytes out of the kidney tubules into the blood stream.

Overview of the Urinary System

The principal organs of the urinary system are the *kidneys*, which process blood and form urine as a waste to be excreted. The excreted urine travels from the kidneys to the outside of the body via accessory organs—the *ureters, urinary bladder,* and *urethra*.

The urinary system is primarily thought of as a urine producer but a better concept is that of blood plasma balancer. The water content is adjusted to maintain constancy of the internal environment. Similarly, the blood content of sodium and potassium and the pH of blood can be altered to match normal levels.

Anatomy of the Urinary System

KIDNEY

The kidneys lie in a retroperitoneal position against the posterior wall of the abdomen and are located on either side of the vertebral column. Each kidney is roughly oval with a medial indentation. The medial surface has a concave notch called the *hilum*; it is here that the ureters and blood vessels enter and leave the kidney. The main internal structures of the kidney are the renal cortex (outer region), renal medulla (inner region), and renal pyramids (medullary tissue). Each point of a pyramid

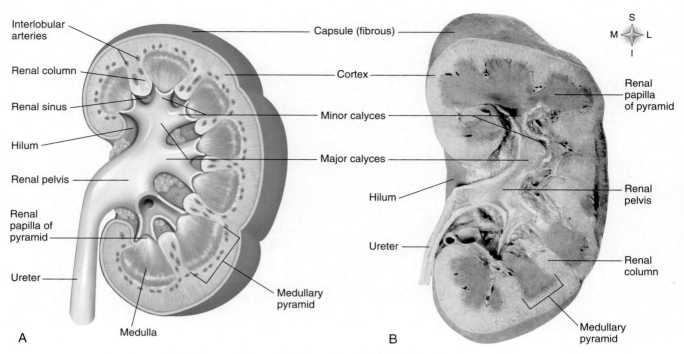

Structure of the Kidney. (**A** from Brundage DJ: *Renal disorders*. St. Louis, Mosby, 1992; **B** from Abrahams P, Hutchings RT, Marks SC: *McMinn's color atlas of human anatomy*, ed 4, St Louis, 1999, Mosby.)

(papilla) juts into a cuplike structure called a *calyx*. Urine leaving the renal papilla is collected for transport out of the body. The calyces join together to form a large collection reservoir called the renal pelvis, which narrows as it exits the hilum to become the ureter.

Blood Vessels of the Kidney

The renal artery, a branch of the aorta, brings blood to each kidney. The renal artery branches into smaller arteries and then into the afferent arteriole, which branches into a tuftlike grouping of five to eight capillaries (glomerular capillaries) called the *glomerulus*. Blood leaving the glomerular capillaries flows from efferent arterioles into the peritubular capillaries, then into venules, and finally into the renal vein.

The Nephron

The microscopic functional units and working unit of the kidney are called nephrons; there are approximately 1.25 million/kidney. Each nephron contains the following structures—renal corpuscle, Bowman's capsule, proximal convoluted tubule, loop of Henle, distal convoluted tubule, and collecting duct.

BOWMAN'S CAPSULE

Bowman's capsule is the cup-shaped mouth of the nephron and is formed by two layers of epithelial cells with a space, called Bowman's space. Fluids, waste products, and electrolytes constitute the glomerular filtrate, which will be processed in the nephron to form urine. The *glomerulus* is made up of a fine network of capillaries that fits neatly into the Bowman's capsule. The *proximal tubule*, *loop of Henle*, and *distal tubule* extend out from the glomerulus; it is here that secretion of waste products and resorption of nutrients take place. The *juxtaglomerular apparatus* is found at the point at which the afferent arteriole brushes past the distal tubule. This structure is important in maintaining homeostasis of blood flow because it secretes renin when blood pressure in the afferent arteriole drops. The *collecting duct* is a straight tubule joined by the distal tubules of several nephrons. Collecting ducts join larger ducts and converge to form one tube that opens at a renal papilla into one of the small calyces. See Figure 22-2 for the anatomy of the nephron.

Ureters

The ureters are the two tubes that actively transport urine from the kidneys to the urinary bladder. Each ureter is composed of three layers of tissue, a mucous lining, a muscular middle layer, and fibrous outer layer. The muscular layer is composed of smooth muscle and propels the urine by peristalsis.

Urinary Bladder

The urinary bladder is located directly behind the symphysis pubis and in front of the rectum. In women, it is anterior of the vagina and in front of the uterus, whereas in men it rests on the prostate. The wall of the bladder is made of mostly smooth muscle tissue, often called the detrusor muscle. The bladder is lined with mucous transitional epithelium that forms folds called *rugae*, which enable it to distend considerably when full. There are three openings on the floor of the bladder, two from the ureters and one into the urethra. The bladder performs two major functions, as a reservoir for urine and for expelling urine from the body aided by the urethra.

Urethra

The urethra is a small tube that leads from the floor of the bladder (trigone) to the exterior of the body. In females, it lies directly behind the symphysis pubis and anterior to the vagina as it passes through the muscular floor of the pelvis. It then extends down from the bladder and ends at the *external urinary meatus*. The male urethra passes through the center of the prostate gland just after leaving the bladder. Within the prostate, it is joined by two ejaculatory ducts. After leaving the prostate, the urethra extends down into the penis and ends as a urinary meatus at the tip of the penis.

Overview of Kidney Function

The chief functions of the kidney are to process blood plasma and excrete urine. These vital functions maintain the homeostatic balance of the body, such as electrolyte and acid-balance. Sodium, potassium, chloride, and nitrogenous wastes (especially urea) are blood constituents that need to be held within their normal concentration range to prevent kidney failure. Nitrogenous wastes from protein metabolism, notably urea, leave the blood by way of the kidneys.

The kidney also performs other functions such as influencing the rate of secretion of antidiuretic hormone (ADH) and aldosterone. The nephrons of the kidney function to resorb fluids and electrolytes, filter blood, and eliminate waste in urine.

1. Filtration is the movement of water and protein-free solutes from plasma in the glomerulus, across the glomerular membrane, and into the capsular space of Bowman's capsule. The result is approximately 180 liters of glomerular filtrate being formed each day.
2. Tubular reabsorption is the process of movement of molecules such as water, sodium, and electrolytes out of the various segments of the tubule and into the blood.
3. Tubular secretion is the process of movement of molecules out of blood and into the tubule for excretion. The distal tubules and collecting tubules secrete potassium, hydrogen, and ammonium ions. Tubule cells also secrete certain drugs like penicillin.

REGULATION OF URINE VOLUME

ADH has a central role in the regulation of urine volume by reducing water loss by the body. Another hormone that tends to decrease urine volume and conserves water is aldosterone. It reabsorbs sodium, which in turn causes an osmotic imbalance that drives the resorption of water from the tubule. Atrial natriuretic hormone (ANH) also influences water resorption in the kidneys. ANH is secreted by specialized muscle fibers in the atrial wall of the heart. ANH promotes natriuresis (loss of sodium in urine).

Micturition

The mechanism of voiding urine begins with voluntary relaxation of the external sphincter muscle of the bladder. Injury to any of these nerves, by a cerebral hemorrhage or a spinal cord injury, for example, results in involuntary micturition, or *incontinence*. Various medical conditions and changes in aging can also contribute to incontinence.

URINE COMPOSITION

Urine is approximately 95% water, in which are dissolved several different types of substances:

- Nitrogenous wastes: Urea, uric acid, ammonia, and creatinine.
- Electrolytes: Sodium, potassium, ammonium, chloride, bicarbonate, phosphate, and sulfate (amounts vary with diet and other factors). Electrolytes are present in the human body and are essential for normal function of our cells and our organs.
- Toxins: During disease, bacterial poisons leave the body in urine.
- Pigments: Yellowish pigments (urochromes) from the breakdown of old red blood cells in the liver and elsewhere (e.g., food, drugs).
- Hormones: High hormone levels sometimes result in significant amounts of hormones in the filtrate, and therefore in the urine.
- Abnormal constituents: Blood, glucose, and albumin (a plasma protein) or calculi (kidney stones) are substances that if found in the urine could signal disease or an infection.

Electrolytes and Minerals Influencing Body Function

Electrolyte	Function
Calcium (Ca)	Most abundant mineral in body Basic structural building block of bones and teeth Essential for maintenance of normal heartbeat, functioning of nerve and muscles Plays a role in metabolism, blood coagulation
Magnesium (Mg)	50% of total body magnesium found in bone, 50% found predominantly inside cells of body tissues and organs Maintains normal muscle and nerve function, keeps heart rhythm steady, supports a healthy immune system, keeps bones strong Magnesium also helps regulate blood sugar levels, promotes normal blood pressure, and known to be involved in energy metabolism and protein synthesis
Sodium (Na)	Major positive ion (cation) in fluid outside of cells Regulates the total amount of water in the body and transmission of sodium into and out of individual cells; plays a role in critical body functions Brain, nervous system, and muscles require electrical signals for communication; the movement of sodium is critical in generation of these electrical signals
Chloride (Cl)	Major anion (negatively charged ion) found in the fluid outside of cells and in the blood Plays a role in helping the body maintain a normal fluidbalance
Potassium (K)	Major positive ion (cation) found inside of cells Proper level essential for normal cell function Responsible for regulation of heartbeat and muscle function
Phosphorus (P)	Builds and repairs bones and teeth Helps nerves function, makes muscles contract Most (≈85%) of phosphorus contained in phosphate is found in bones; the rest is stored in tissues throughout the body
Sulfur (S)	Component of amino acids Major source of sulfates is degradation of sulfur-containing amino acids
Bicarbonate (HCO₃)	Acts as a buffer to maintain normal levels of acidity (pH) in blood and other body fluids Levels are measured to monitor acidity of blood and body fluids Chemical notation on most laboratory reports is shown as HCO_3^- or concentration of carbon dioxide (CO_2)

Adapted from MedicineNet: Stöppler M, Shiel W: Electrolytes, 1996-2012 (http://www.medicinenet.com/electrolytes/page2.htm); and Office of Dietary Supplements: Magnesium, 2009 retrieved Aug 13, 2012 (http://ods.od.nih.gov/factsheets/magnesium).

Summary

Homeostasis of water and electrolytes in body fluids depends largely on proper functioning of the kidneys. Both endocrine and nervous systems must operate properly to ensure proper kidney function and without the blood pressure generated by the cardiovascular system, the kidneys could not filter blood plasma. The urinary system interacts with many of the other body systems and tissues.

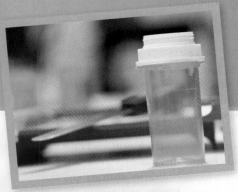

30

Treatment of Prostate Disease and Erectile Dysfunction

KEY TERMS

Benign prostatic hyperplasia: Noncancerous growth of cells in the prostate gland.

Digital rectal examination: Screening examination involving palpation of the prostate gland; conducted by insertion of a gloved, lubricated finger into the rectum.

Ejaculation: Release of semen from the penis during orgasm.

Erectile dysfunction: Persistent inability to achieve and/or maintain an erection sufficient for satisfactory sexual intercourse.

Hyperplasia: Abnormal increase in the number of cells in an organ or tissue.

Incontinence: Loss of bladder or bowel control.

Phosphodiesterase type 5 inhibitor: Drug used to relax smooth muscle and blood vessels that supply the corpus cavernosum and control penile engorgement.

Prostate gland: Gland in the male reproductive system just below the bladder surrounding the urethra.

Prostate-specific antigen: Protein produced by the prostate gland. Levels are elevated in men who have prostate cancer, infection, or inflammation and *tumors* of the prostate gland and benign prostate hyperplasia.

Prostate-specific antigen test: Blood test to measure prostate-specific antigen. A free prostate-specific antigen test result reports the percentage of prostate-specific antigen that is not attached to another chemical compared with the total amount in a man's blood. Free prostate-specific antigen is linked to benign prostate hyperplasia but not to cancer.

Prostatitis: Inflammation of the prostate gland.

Semen: Fluid containing sperm and secretions from glands of the male reproductive tract.

Tumor: Abnormal mass of tissue that results from excessive cell division. Tumors may be benign (not cancerous) or malignant (cancerous).

Urinary frequency: Need to urinate more often than is normal.

Urinalysis: Microscopic and chemical examination of a fresh urine sample.

Benign Prostatic Hyperplasia

The *prostate gland* is a part of the male reproductive system located just below the bladder that surrounds the urethra. The gland produces *semen*, the fluid that contains sperm. *Prostatitis* is an inflamed or infected prostate gland. Symptoms may be burning on urination, fever, body ache, groin, rectal, or low back pain, difficulty urinating, urge *incontinence*, painful *ejaculation*, and decreased libido. Although some of the symptoms are similar, prostatitis is usually an acute condition, unlike *benign prostatic hyperplasia* (BPH). This is a condition in which noncancerous cells in the prostate grow and increase the size of the prostate gland (Figure 30-1). It may grow from the size of a walnut to the size of a small lemon. As the gland grows, it begins to obstruct the flow of urine through the urethra. The urethra is a small tube that carries urine and semen through the penis.

The risk for developing BPH increases with age. More than 50% of adult males will have BPH by age 60 years and, by age 85, approximately 90% will have BPH. Not all men with BPH have symptoms. Almost 70% are asymptomatic.

DIAGNOSIS

Several tests are available to check the health of the prostate. A *digital rectal examination* (DRE) is the first step for examining the prostate. This examination involves the insertion of a gloved finger into the rectum and palpating the prostate to determine whether it is enlarged. A *prostate-specific antigen* (PSA) *test* may be performed to determine whether levels of the PSA protein are elevated. A higher than normal level is a sign of BPH, infection, inflammation, or prostate cancer. A free PSA test, the percentage of PSA that is not attached to another chemical, may be conducted to differentiate between BPH and cancer. Free PSA is linked to BPH but not to cancer. *Urinalysis* and a biopsy of prostate tissue may also be taken.

SYMPTOMS OF BENIGN PROSTATIC HYPERPLASIA

The first symptom of an enlarged prostate gland is a weak or slow stream of urine (Box 30-1). There may also be a delayed start in the flow of urine or straining to urinate. As the disease progresses,

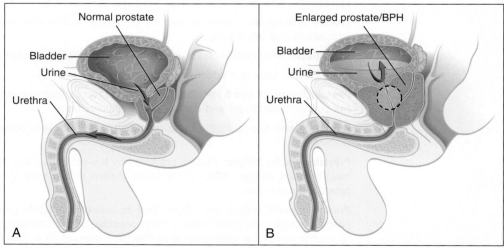

FIGURE 30-1 A, Normal prostate. **B,** Enlarged prostate. (Courtesy National Institutes of Health, Bethesda, MD.)

the bladder becomes hypersensitive and the need to urinate becomes more frequent (***urinary frequency***). Some men may develop urinary infection(s) from the condition. BPH may also produce bladder stones, sudden inability to urinate, or kidney damage.

TREATMENT OF BENIGN PROSTATIC HYPERPLASIA

Pharmacotherapy for BPH is initiated when symptoms are uncomfortable enough to warrant treatment (Figure 30-2). Watchful waiting is recommended when patients are asymptomatic or symptoms do not produce much discomfort. Two classes of drugs are administered to manage symptoms, alpha blockers and 5α-reductase inhibitors.

BOX 30-1   **Symptoms of Benign Prostatic Hyperplasia**

- Weak or slow stream of urine
- Delay in starting urination
- Urinary stream that starts and stops
- Frequent urination
- Urinary urgency
- Nighttime awakening to urinate
- Need to strain to urinate

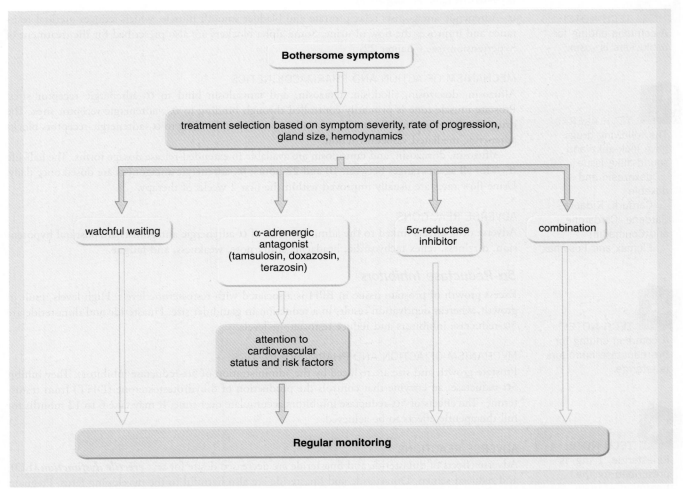

FIGURE 30-2 Summary of treatment options for BPH. (From Page C, Hoffman B, Curtis M, et al: *Integrated pharmacology*, ed 3, Philadelphia, 2006, Mosby.)

α₁-Adrenergic Antagonists

Generic Name	U.S. Brand Name(s) / Canadian Brand Names(s)	Dosage Forms and Strengths
alfuzosin*	Uroxatral	Tablet, extended-release: 10 mg
	Xatral	
doxazosin*	Cardura	Tablet: 1 mg, 2 mg, 4 mg, 8 mg†
	Cardura	Tablet, extended release (Cardura XL): 4 mg, 8 mg
terazosin*	Generics only	Capsule: 1 mg†, 2 mg†, 5 mg†, 10 mg†
	Hytrin	Tablet: 1 mg, 2 mg, 5 mg, 10 mg
tamsulosin*	Flomax	Capsule: 0.4 mg
	Flomax, Flomax CR	Capsule, extended release: 0.4 mg
silodosin	Rapaflo	Capsule: 4 mg, 8 mg
	Rapaflo	

*Generic available.
†Strength available in the United States only.

TECH NOTE!
A common ending for α-blockers is -osin.

TECH ALERT!
The following drugs have look-alike and sound-alike issues:
doxazosin and doxepin;
Cardura, Ridaura, Cardene, Cordarone, and Coumadin;
Flomax and Fosamax

TECH NOTE!
A common ending for 5α-reductase inhibitors is -steride.

TECH NOTE!
Finasteride, 1 mg, is prescribed for the treatment of male pattern baldness.

α₁-Adrenergic Antagonists

α₁-Adrenergic antagonists relax prostate and bladder smooth muscle, which reduces urethral resistance and improves the flow of urine. Some alpha blockers are also prescribed for the treatment of hypertension (see Chapter 22).

MECHANISM OF ACTION AND PHARMACOKINETICS

Alfuzosin, doxazosin, silodosin, terazosin, and tamsulosin bind to α₁-adrenergic receptor sites. Prostate muscle tone is primarily controlled through binding to α₁A-adrenergic receptor sites. The drugs also have varying affinity for α₁B and α₁D subtypes. Binding to α₁-adrenergic receptors blocks adrenergic-mediated vasoconstriction.

Alfuzosin, doxazosin, and tamsulosin are available in extended-release dosage forms. The half-life ($t_{1/2}$) for all agents ranges between 10 and 22 hours; α₁-adrenergic antagonists are dosed once daily. Urine flow rates are usually improved within the first 2 weeks of therapy.

ADVERSE REACTIONS

Adverse drug effects linked to the administration of α-adrenergic antagonists are postural hypotension, dizziness, reflex tachycardia, headache, stuffy nose, weakness, and fatigue.

5α-Reductase Inhibitors

Excess growth of prostate tissue in BPH is associated with testosterone levels. High levels result in growth, whereas deprivation results in a reduction in glandular size. Finasteride and dutasteride are 5α-reductase inhibitors and reduce testosterone levels.

MECHANISM OF ACTION AND PHARMACOKINETICS

Prostate growth and size are reduced by the administration of 5α-reductase inhibitors. They inhibit 5α-reductase, an enzyme that controls the production of dihydrotestosterone (DHT) from testosterone. The effects of 5α-reductase inhibitors accumulate over time. It may take 6 to 12 months for full therapeutic effects to be achieved.

ADVERSE REACTIONS

Adverse effects of dutasteride and finasteride are decreased desire for sex, *erectile dysfunction* (ED), and reduced semen. Dutasteride and finasteride are also harmful to the developing fetus. Pregnant women and women of childbearing age should be advised to avoid contact with broken or crushed tablets. The use of a barrier contraceptive, such as condoms, is recommended.

5α-Reductase Inhibitors

Generic Name	U.S. Brand Name(s) Canadian Brand Names(s)	Dosage Forms and Strengths
dutasteride*†	Avodart	Capsule: 0.5 mg
	Avodart	
finasteride*	Proscar, Propecia	Tablet (Proscar): 5 mg
	Proscar, Propecia	Tablet (Propecia)**: 1 mg

*Generic available.
*†Generic available in the United States only.
**Propecia is used for hair loss.

Combination: 5α-Reductase Inhibitor and Alpha Blocker

Generic Name	U.S. Brand Name(s) Canadian Brand Names(s)	Dosage Forms and Strengths
dutasteride + tamsulosin	Jalyn	Capsule: 0.5 mg dutasteride + 0.4 mg tamsulosin
	Jalyn	

Summary of Drugs Used in the Treatment of Benign Prostatic Hyperplasia

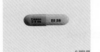

Generic Name	U.S. Brand Name	Usual Adult Oral Dose and Dosing Schedule	Warning Labels
α₁-Adrenergic Antagonist			
alfuzosin	Uroxatral	10 mg once daily	DO NOT DISCONTINUE WITHOUT MEDICAL SUPERVISION.
doxazosin	Cardura	4-8 mg once daily	MAY CAUSE DIZZINESS OR LIGHTHEADEDNESS.
terazosin	Hytrin	5-10 mg at bedtime	AVOID DRIVING OR OPERATING HAZARDOUS MACHINERY.
silodosin	Rapaflo	8 mg daily	SWALLOW WHOLE; DO NOT CRUSH OR CHEW (TAMSULOSIN).
tamsulosin	Flomax	0.4 mg once daily	TAKE 30 MIN AFTER THE SAME MEAL EACH DAY (TAMSULOSIN). TAKE WITH MEAL (SILODOSIN).
5α-Reductase Inhibitors			
dutasteride	Avodart	0.5 mg once daily	SWALLOW CAPSULES WHOLE; DO NOT CHEW (DUTASTERIDE).
finasteride	Proscar	5 mg once daily	SWALLOW THE TABLETS WITH A DRINK OF WATER (FINASTERIDE). PREGNANT WOMEN SHOULD AVOID CONTACT WITH BROKEN OR CRUSHED TABLETS.
Combination: 5α-Reductase Inhibitor and Alpha Blocker			
dutasteride + tamsulosin	Jalyn	1 capsule daily	MAY CAUSE DIZZINESS. SWALLOW CAPSULES WHOLE; DO NOT CHEW. PREGNANT WOMEN SHOULD AVOID CONTACT WITH BROKEN OR CRUSHED TABLETS.

TECH ALERT!
Proscar, Prozac, Propecia, and Psorcon have look-alike and sound-alike issues.

Nonpharmacological Treatment Options

When symptoms of BPH are severe, surgery is indicated. There are several surgical options. Some procedures are more invasive than others. Following are brief definitions of surgical procedures for BPH:

HoELP (holmium laser enucleation of prostate): Excess prostate tissue is vaporized using a holmium laser.

Prostatic stent: A stent (scaffolding) is inserted into the urethra to open a passage and improve urine flow.

Prostiva RF therapy: Delivers a low-level radiofrequency signal directly into the prostate and destroys the prostate tissue, improving the symptoms of BPH.

TURP (transurethral resection of the prostate): Excess prostate tissue is trimmed away.

TUIP (transurethral incision of the prostate): One or two slits are made in the prostate to relieve the pressure and improve urine flow.

TUMT (transurethral microwave thermal therapy of the prostate): Computer-regulated microwaves are sent through a catheter to heat portions of the prostate.

Erectile Dysfunction

ED is defined as the total inability to achieve erection, an inconsistent ability to achieve erection, or difficulty maintaining erection long enough to sustain sexual intercourse. It is also known as impotence. Up to 30 million American men have reported symptoms of ED. ED appears to increase with age; however, it is not an inevitable part of the aging process. By age 40 years, approximately 5% of men experience ED. By age 65, approximately 15% to 25% of men have ED.

WHAT CAUSES ERECTILE DYSFUNCTION?

An erection is produced pursuant to vascular changes that are orchestrated to enhance penile rigidity and enable effective intercourse. The smooth muscle of the corpus cavernosum of the penis relaxes (Figure 30-3). Arteries and sinusoids in the corpus cavernosum fill with blood. Intracorporal blood pressure increases while at the same time venous outflow decreases.

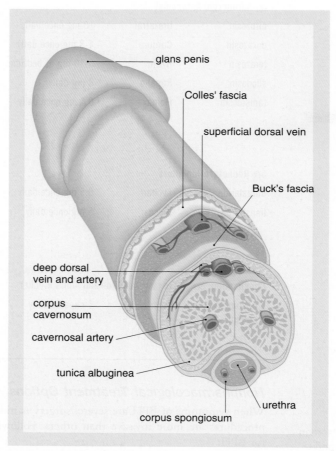

FIGURE 30-3 Structure of the penis. (From Page C, Hoffman B, Curtis M, et al: *Integrated pharmacology*, ed 3, Philadelphia, 2006, Mosby.)

BOX 30-2   **Neurotransmitters That Relax Smooth Muscle in the Penis**

- Acetylcholine (ACh)
- Nitric oxide (NO)
- Prostaglandin E1 (PGE1)
- Vasoactive intestinal polypeptide (VIP)
- Calcitonin gene-related peptide (CGRP)

ED may have physiological, psychological, neurological, or endocrinological causes. Physiological causes include age-related changes and chronic disease (e.g., hypertension, hyperlipidemia, multiple sclerosis). Diabetes is a disease of the endocrine system (see Chapter 33) that can cause vascular and nerve changes that affect erectile function. Depression may produce ED, too. ED may also be caused by lifestyle factors such as smoking, obesity, and alcoholism.

DRUGS USED FOR THE TREATMENT OF ERECTILE DYSFUNCTION

ED is managed by the administration of drugs that promote penile engorgement and slow loss of erection. This control is orchestrated by relaxation and contraction of the smooth muscle in the corpus cavernosum. Neurotransmitters of the autonomic nervous system and nonadrenergic, non-cholinergic system control relaxation and contractions. Neurotransmitters that promote relaxation produce an erection. They are listed in Box 30-2.

Nitric oxide is a mediator of smooth muscle relaxation that is released by the nonadrenergic noncholinergic system as a response to sexual stimulation. It activates several intracellular enzymes; **phosphodiesterase type 5** (PDE5), an enzyme involved in the reversal of an erection, is an example. Drugs currently marketed for the treatment of ED are PDE5 inhibitors and prostaglandin E analogues.

Phosphodiesterase Inhibitors

Sildenafil, tadalafil, and vardenafil are PDE5 inhibitors, the most commonly prescribed drugs for the treatment of erectile dysfunction. They are taken prior to intercourse to produce an erection. Sildenafil and tadalafil are taken 30 minutes prior to intercourse. Vardenafil is taken up to 60 minutes before sexual activity.

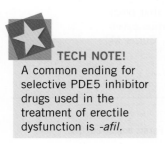

TECH NOTE!
A common ending for selective PDE5 inhibitor drugs used in the treatment of erectile dysfunction is -afil.

MECHANISM OF ACTION

Avanafil, sildenafil, tadalafil, and vardenafil are selective inhibitors of cyclic guanosine monophosphate (cGMP)–specific PDE5. They relax smooth muscle and blood vessels that supply the corpus cavernosum and control penile engorgement (Figure 30-4). At the cellular level, the drugs increase levels of nitric oxide (NO) in the corpus cavernosum, which blocks the opening of calcium voltage-gated channels and reduces calcium-mediated vascular contractions.

PHARMACOKINETICS

The oral absorption of sildenafil, vardenafil, and tadalafil is good and maximum concentration (C_{max}) and onset of action of vardenafil are reached between 30 minutes and 2 hours after a dose of drug is administered. C_{max} for tadalafil and sildenafil is similar, averaging approximately 2 hours. The C_{max} may be reduced if the drugs are taken with a meal that is high in fat. Bioavailability can be reduced by up to 50%. Protein binding is approximately 94% to 95% for all PDE5s.

ADVERSE REACTIONS

Many of the adverse reactions associated with the use of phosphodiesterase inhibitors are a result of vasodilation. These side effects include dizziness, flushing, headache, and nasal congestion. Gastrointestinal side effects are diarrhea and indigestion. Sildenafil, tadalafil, and vardenafil may also produce visual effects that range from light sensitivity and difficulty distinguishing between green and blue to loss of vision. The incidence of visual disturbances is greater with sildenafil than with vardenafil and tadalafil. In 2007, the U.S. Food and Drug Administration (FDA) approved labeling changes for Cialis, Levitra, and Viagra to display the potential risk of sudden hearing loss more prominently.

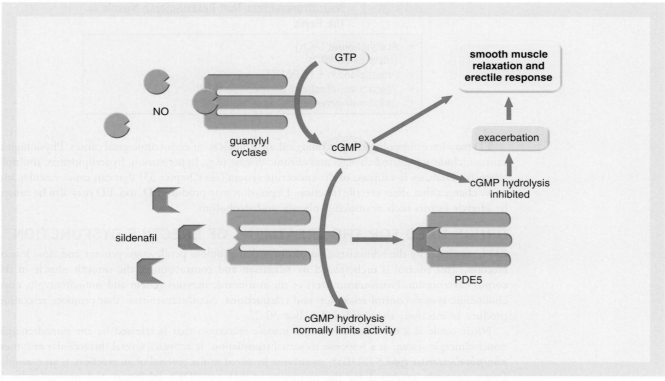

FIGURE 30-4 Mechanism of action for sildenafil. Sildenafil binds to receptors that block the degradation of cGMP and increase the effects of nitric oxide (NO) on the corpus cavernosum (relaxation and increased erectile response). (From Page C, Hoffman B, Curtis M, et al: *Integrated pharmacology*, ed 3, Philadelphia, 2006, Mosby.)

Phosphodiesterase Inhibitors

| | U.S. Brand Name(s) | |
Generic Name	Canadian Brand Names(s)	Dosage Forms and Strengths
sildenafil*‡	Viagra, Revatio	Tablet (Viagra): 25 mg, 50 mg, 100 mg
	Viagra, Revatio	Tablet (Revatio): 20 mg
		IV solution (Revatio): 0.8 mg/mL
tadalafil	Cialis, Adcirca	Tablet: 2.5 mg, 5 mg, 10 mg, 20 mg
	Cialis, Adcirca	Adcirca-20 mg
vardenafil*†	Levitra, Staxyn	Tablet: 2.5 mg*, 5 mg, 10 mg, 20 mg
	Levitra, Staxyn	Tablet, oral disintegrating (Staxyn): 10 mg
avanafil	Stendra	Tablet: 50 mg, 100 mg, 200 mg (drug not avaiable in Canada)

*Generic available.
*†Generic available in the United States only.
*‡Generic available in Canada only.

PRECAUTIONS

PDE5 inhibitors are involved in numerous drug interactions. A life-threatening drop in blood pressure has occurred in men who have taken nitrates such as nitroglycerin (for angina), so the use of nitrates, in all dosage forms, is contraindicated while taking PDE5 inhibitors. Concurrent administration of α-adrenergic agonists (e.g., alfuzosin, terazosin, doxazosin) used for the treatment of BPH requires caution. Other important drug interactions to avoid are concurrent administration

BOX 30-3　Instructions for Administration of Intraurethral Pellets

1. Gently and slowly stretch the penis upward to its full length.
2. Slowly insert the stem of the applicator into the urethra up to the collar; then gently and completely push down the button at the top of the applicator until it stops (and medicated pellet is released).
3. Hold the applicator in this position for 5 seconds; then remove applicator while keeping the penis upright. Roll the penis firmly between the hands for at least 10 seconds to ensure that the medication is adequately distributed along the walls of the urethra.
4. An erection should begin to form within 10 minutes of application.

BOX 30-4　Instructions for Administration of Intracavernosal Injection

1. Gently and slowly stretch the penis upward to its full length.
2. Insert the needle into the corpus cavernosum at 90 degrees until the metal portion of the needle is almost completely into the penis. Avoid visible veins, urethra, and corpus spongiosum.
3. Slowly inject the contents of the syringe over 5 to 10 seconds.
4. Withdraw syringe and apply pressure to injection site for 5 minutes or until bleeding stops.

Prostaglandins

Generic Name	U.S. Brand Name(s) Canadian Brand Names(s)	Dosage Forms and Strengths
alprostadil$^\alpha$	Caverject, Caverject Impulse, Muse, Prostin VR, Edex cartridge	Powder, for injection, (Caverject): 5 mcg[†], 10 mcg[†], 20 mcg[†], 23.2 mcg[‡], 40 mcg[†]
	Caverject, Muse, Prostin VR$^\alpha$	Urethral insert (Muse): 125 mcg[†], 250 mcg, 500 mcg, 1000 mcg
		Injection, solution (Prostin VR): 500 mcg /mL

$^\alpha$Prostin VR is administered as a continuous infusion to neonates with congenital heart disease such as ductus arteriosus, pulmonary stenosis, or interruption of the aortic arch until corrective surgery can be performed.
[†]Strength available in the United States only.
[‡]Strength available in Canada only.

of PDE5 inhibitors with antifungals *(-azoles),* cimetidine, grapefruit juice, and macrolide antiinfectives (e.g., erythromycin, clarithromycin). Drug interactions also occur with the coadministration of selective serotonin reuptake inhibitor and monoamine oxidase inhibitor antidepressants.

Prostaglandins

Alprostadil is naturally occurring prostaglandin E_1 (PGE_1) present in the seminal vesicles and cavernous tissues of males. It can also be found in the placenta of the fetus. PGE_1 mediates the relaxation of penile smooth muscle.

MECHANISM OF ACTION AND PHARMACOKINETICS
PGE_1 mobilizes intracellular calcium in the corpus cavernosum, resulting in smooth muscle contraction; however, in the endothelium, PGE_1 mediates the release of nitric oxide, which relaxes cavernosal smooth muscle, causing an erection.

Oral absorption of alprostadil is poor; therefore, the drug is formulated for intraurethral insertion and intracavernosal injection. The intracavernosal route of administration is more effective than the intraurethral route. Instructions for inserting alprostadil intraurethral inserts are provided in Box 30-3. Instructions for using the alprostadil intracavernosal injection is provided in Box 30-4.

ADVERSE REACTIONS
Adverse reactions are specific to the route of administration. Side effects caused by intracavernosal administration include hypotension, dizziness, bleeding, bruising, or pain at the site of injection and painful erection. Adverse effects associated with intraurethral administration of alprostadil are itching in the penis, testicles, legs, and perineum, redness of the penis, warmth or burning sensation

Summary of Drugs Used in the Treatment of Erectile Dysfunction

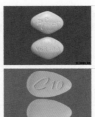

Generic Name	U.S. Brand Name	Usual Adult Oral Dose and Dosing Schedule	Warning Labels
Phosphodiesterase Inhibitors (PDE5)			
sildenafil	Viagra	25-100 mg ½-4 hr prior to sexual intercourse; not more than once daily	DO NOT DRINK ALCOHOL TO EXCESS (E.G., FIVE GLASSES WINE OR FIVE SHOTS OF WHISKEY). MAY CAUSE DIZZINESS.
tadalafil	Cialis	2.5-20 mg prior to sexual intercourse; not more than once daily or 2.5-5 mg once daily	DO NOT TAKE WITHIN 4 HR OF TAKING ALPHA BLOCKERS (ALFUZOSIN, DOXAZOSIN, TERAZOSIN). AVOID GRAPEFRUIT JUICE (TADALAFIL).
vardenafil	Levitra	2.5-20 mg up to 60 minutes prior up to sexual intercourse; not more than once daily	DISSOLVE ORAL DISINTEGRATING TABLETS UNDER TONGUE. TAKE 30 MIN BEFORE SEXUAL ACTIVITY (SILDENAFIL, TADALAFIL). TAKE 1 HR BEFORE SEXUAL ACTIVITY (VARDENAFIL, SILDENAFIL).
Prostaglandins			
alprostadil	Muse	Insert 1 pellet 30-60 min prior to sexual intercourse; not more than once daily	REFRIGERATE (MAY BE STORED AT ROOM TEMPERATURE FOR 14 DAYS).
	Caverject	Inject individualized dose not more than once in 24 hr or >3 times/wk	ROTATE SITE OF INJECTION. MAY STORE AT ROOM TEMPERATURE FOR UP TO 3 MO. AVOID DRUG EXPOSURE TO EXTREMES IN HEAT OR COLD.

in the urethra, and leg swelling. Urethral bleeding or spotting may occur when the drug is administered improperly. Both dosage forms may produce prolonged erection (lasting >4 hours).

Nonpharmacological Management of Erectile Dysfunction

ED may also be treated by attaching a mechanical vacuum device to the penis, which uses suction to produce engorgement. An alternative approach is to surgically implant a device with inflatable tubes that can cause the penis to become erect. Vascular surgery may be performed to reconstruct arteries that supply the penis and to block off veins that allow blood to leak from penile tissue.

Herbal Remedies for Benign Prostatic Hyperplasia and Erectile Dysfunction

The ripened fruit of saw palmetto contains fatty acids and plant sterols that inhibit 5α-reductase and cystolic androgen binding, producing anti-inflammatory and antiestrogenic effects. Saw palmetto may reduce urinary symptoms of BPH. The usual dose is 160 to 320 mg once daily. Prostate cancer should be ruled out prior to taking saw palmetto. Yohimbe is an α₂-adrenergic blocker, related to reserpine, that may improve erectile dysfunction. Clinical trials have not been conducted and evidence to support yohimbe's effectiveness is lacking. The usual dose is 5.4 mg three times daily. Adverse effects include increased blood pressure and heart rate, headache, insomnia, anxiety, nausea and vomiting. Drug interactions may occur if yohimbe is taken concurrently with monoamine oxidase inhibitors (MAOIs), tricyclic antidepressants (TCAs), and phenothiazines.

Chapter Summary

- The prostate gland is part of the male reproductive system.
- Prostatitis is an inflamed or infected prostate gland.

- Benign prostatic hyperplasia is a condition in which noncancerous cells in the prostate grow and increase the size of the prostate gland.
- The risk for developing benign prostatic hyperplasia increases with age; by age 85 years, approximately 90% of men will have BPH.
- A prostate-specific antigen test may be performed to determine whether levels of the PSA protein are elevated. Higher than normal levels are a sign of BPH, infection, inflammation, or prostate cancer.
- Pharmacotherapy for BPH is initiated only when symptoms are uncomfortable enough to warrant treatment.
- Watchful waiting is recommended when patients are asymptomatic or symptoms do not produce much discomfort.
- Two classes of drugs are administered to manage symptoms of BPH, alpha blockers and 5α-reductase inhibitors.
- A common ending for alpha blockers is *-osin*.
- α_1-Adrenergic antagonists relax prostate and bladder smooth muscle, which reduces urethral resistance and improves the flow of urine.
- Alfuzosin, doxazosin, silodosin, terazosin, and tamsulosin bind to α_1-adrenergic receptor sites. Prostate muscle tone is primarily controlled by binding to α_{1A}-adrenergic receptor sites.
- Alfuzosin, doxazosin, and tamsulosin are available in extended-release dosage forms.
- Adverse drug effects linked to the administration of α-adrenergic antagonists are postural hypotension, dizziness, reflex tachycardia, headache, stuffy nose, weakness, and fatigue.
- A common ending for 5α-reductase inhibitors is *-steride*.
- Finasteride and dutasteride are antiandrogens, capable of reducing testosterone levels.
- The effects of 5α-reductase inhibitors accumulate over time. It may take 6 to 12 months for therapeutic effects to be achieved.
- Dutasteride and finasteride are also harmful to the developing fetus. Pregnant women and women of childbearing age should be advised to avoid contact with broken or crushed tablets. The use of barrier contraceptive is also recommended.
- Several surgical procedures are available for the management of prostate disease.
- Erectile dysfunction is defined as a total inability to achieve erection, an inconsistent ability to achieve erection, or difficulty maintaining erection long enough to sustain sexual intercourse.
- By age 65 years, approximately 15% to 25% of men have erectile dysfunction.
- Erectile dysfunction may have physiological, psychological, neurological, or endocrinological causes.
- Lifestyle factors, smoking, obesity, and alcoholism may cause erectile dysfunction.
- Erectile dysfunction is managed by the administration of drugs that promote penile engorgement and slow the loss of erection.
- Drugs currently marketed for the treatment of erectile dysfunction are phosphodiesterase inhibitors and prostaglandin E analogues.
- A common ending for selective phosphodiesterase type 5 inhibitor drugs used for the treatment of erectile dysfunction is *-afil*. Sildenafil, tadalafil, and vardenafil are selective inhibitors of cyclic guanosine monophosphate–specific PDE5.
- PDE5 inhibitors relax smooth muscle and blood vessels that supply the corpus cavernosum and control penile engorgement by increasing levels of nitric oxide.
- Side effects of PDE5 inhibitors are dizziness, flushing, headache, nasal congestion, diarrhea, indigestion, and visual disturbances.
- The administration of nitrates, such as nitroglycerin, in all dosage forms, is contraindicated in patients taking PDE5 inhibitors.
- Concurrent administration of α-adrenergic agonists (e.g., alfuzosin, terazosin, doxazosin) used for the treatment of BHP in patients taking PDE5 inhibitors should be done with caution.
- Alprostadil is a naturally occurring prostaglandin E_1 present in male seminal vesicles and cavernous tissues.
- Prostaglandin E_1 mediates the relaxation of penile smooth muscle.
- Oral absorption of alprostadil is poor; therefore, the drug is formulated for intraurethral insertion and intracavernosal injection.
- Both dosage forms may produce prolonged erection (lasting >4 hours).

- Erectile dysfunction may also be treated by attaching a mechanical vacuum device to the penis, which uses suction to produce engorgement.
- An alternative approach to the treatment of erectile dysfunction is to implant an inflatable device surgically that can produce an erection.

REVIEW QUESTIONS

1. Benign prostatic hyperplasia is a condition that is cancerous.
   a. True
   b. False

2. The first symptom(s) of an enlarged prostate gland is(are) _____.
   a. A weak or slow urine stream
   b. A delayed start in the flow of urine
   c. Straining to urinate
   d. All of the above

3. Class(es) of drugs administered to manage the symptoms of benign prostatic hyperplasia are
   _____.
   a. Alpha blockers and beta blockers
   b. α-Reductase inhibitors and beta blockers
   c. Alpha blockers and α-reductase inhibitors
   d. All of the above

4. A common ending for alpha blockers is -osin.
   a. True
   b. False

5. The generic name for Hytrin is _____.
   a. Doxazosin
   b. Tamsulosin
   c. Alfuzosin
   d. Terazosin

6. Which of the following is not an adverse effect of dutasteride and finasteride?
   a. Decreased desire for sex
   b. Erectile dysfunction
   c. Increased desire for sex
   d. Reduced semen

7. Which of the following drugs is not used for erectile dysfunction?
   a. Sildenafil
   b. Penadafil
   c. Tadalafil
   d. Vardenafil

8. Higher than normal levels of PSA may be a sign of _____.
   a. BPH
   b. Infection and inflammation
   c. Prostate cancer
   d. All of the above

9. Finasteride and dutasteride are androgens, capable of reducing testosterone levels.
   a. True
   b. False

10. _____ are currently marketed for the treatment of erectile dysfunction.
   a. Phosphodiesterase inhibitors
   b. Prostaglandin E analogues
   c. Testosterone therapy
   d. All of the above

TECHNICIAN'S
CORNER

1. What is the active ingredient in saw palmetto that promotes a healthy prostate gland?
2. What lifestyle changes can be made to prevent erectile dysfunction?

Bibliography

American Urological Foundation: Benign prostatic hyperplasia: Treatment choices, 2005. (http://www.urologyhealth.org/content/moreinfo/bphtreatment.pdf).

http://www.umm.edu/altmed/articles/benign-prostatic-000018.htm

Read more:

http://www.umm.edu/md_prostate/treatment_bph.htm, 2007, University of Maryland Medical Center (UMMC), Michael J. Naslund, M.D.

www.umm.edu/prostate/bph.htm

Elsevier: Gold Standard Clinical Pharmacology, 2010. Retrieved April 2, 2011, from https://www.clinicalpharmacology.com/

FDA. FDA Approved Drug Products, 2012. Retrieved June 8, 2012, from http://www.accessdata.fda.gov/scripts/cder/drugsatfda/index.cfm?fuseaction=Search.Search_Drug_Name

Health Canada: Drug product database, 2010 (http://www.hc-sc.gc.ca/dhp-mps/prodpharma/databasdon/index-eng.php).

Knapp-Dlugosz C: *OTC advisor: Popular herbal and dietary supplements*, Washington, DC, 2010, American Pharmacists Association.

Lance L, Lacy C, Armstrong L, et al: *Drug information handbook for the allied health professional*, ed 12, Hudson, OH, 2005, APhA Lexi-Comp.

Medtronic: Prostiva: RF ablation system for symptomatic BPH, 2012 (http://www.medtronic.com/for-healthcare-professionals/products-therapies/urological/rf-ablation-system-for-symptomatic-bph/index.htm).

National Cancer Institute: Understanding prostate changes: A health guide for men, 2011 (http://www.cancer.gov/cancertopics/screening/understanding-prostate-changes/prostate_booklet.pdf).

National Kidney & Urologic Diseases Information Clearinghouse: Erectile dsyfunction, 2010 (http://kidney.niddk.nih.gov/kudiseases/pubs/ED/index.aspx).

National Center for Complementary and Alternative Medicine: Herbs at a glance: Yohimbe, 2010 (http://nccam.nih.gov/sites/nccam.nih.gov/files/herbs/NIH_Herbs_at_a_Glance.pdf).

Page C, Curtis M, Sutter M, et al: *Integrated pharmacology*, Philadelphia, 2005, Mosby, pp 495-500.

U.S. Food and Drug Administration: Questions and answers about Viagra, Levitra, Cialis, and Revatio: Possible sudden hearing loss, 2011 (http://www.fda.gov/Drugs/DrugSafety/PostmarketDrugSafetyInformationforPatientsandProviders/ucm106525.htm).

USP Center for Advancement of Patient Safety: Use caution–avoid confusion (USP Quality Review No. 79), Rockville, MD, 2004, USP Center for Advancement of Patient Safety.

31

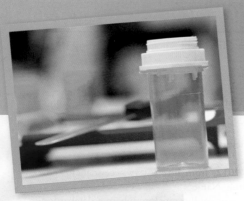

Treatment of Fluid and Electrolyte Disorders

LEARNING OBJECTIVES

1 Learn terminology associated with fluid and electrolyte imbalances.

2 Learn the properties of electrolytes.

3 Know the symptoms of and identify treatments for electrolyte imbalances.

4 Describe mechanism of action for drugs used for the treatment of fluid and electrolyte disorders.

5 Identify significant drug look-alike and sound-alike issues.

6 Identify warning and precautionary messages associated with medications used for the treatment of fluid and electrolyte disorders.

KEY TERMS

Anion: Negatively charged particle.

Bicarbonate: Substance used as a buffer to maintain the normal levels of acidity (pH) in blood and other fluids in the body.

Cation: Positively charged electrolyte.

Chloride: Major anion (negatively charged ion) found in the fluid outside of cells and in blood.

Colloids: Proteins or other large molecules that remain suspended in the blood for a long period of time and are too large to cross membranes.

Crystalloids: Intravenous solutions that contain electrolytes in concentrations similar to those of plasma.

Dehydration: Condition that results from excessive loss of body water.

Edema: Presence of abnormally large amounts of fluid in the intercellular tissue spaces of the body.

Electrolytes: Small charged molecules essential for homeostasis that play an important role in body chemistry.

Extracellular fluid: Type of fluid that surrounds the cells; consists mainly of the plasma found in blood vessels.

Homeostasis: Constancy or balance that is maintained by the body despite constant changes.

Hypercalcemia: Condition in which the total serum calcium level is higher than 5.16 mEq/liter(2.56 mEq/liter ionized).

Hyperchloremia: Condition in which the serum chloride level is higher than 107 mEq/liter.

Hyperkalemia: Condition in which the serum potassium level is higher than 5.5 mEq/liter.

Hypermagnesemia: Condition in which the serum level of magnesium is higher than 2.5 mEq/liter.

Hypernatremia: Elevation of the serum sodium concentration higher than 145 mEq/liter.

Hypertonic: Fluids with a higher osmolarity than serum.

Hypocalcemia: Condition in which the total serum calcium level is lower than 4.3 mEq/liter (2.26 mEq/liter ionized).

Hypochloremia: Condition in which the serum chloride level is lower than 97 mEq/liter.

Hypokalemia: Condition in which potassium is lost from the body, resulting in a serum potassium level lower than 3.5 mEq/liter.

Hypomagnesemia: Condition in which the serum level of magnesium is lower than 1.5 mEq/liter.

Hyponatremia: Condition of decreased serum sodium concentration below the normal range (<136 mEq/liter).

Hypophosphatemia: Condition in which the serum phosphate level is defined as mild (2 to 2.5 mg/dL, or 0.65 to 0.81 mmol/liter), moderate (1 to 2 mg/dL, or 0.32 to 0.65 mmol/liter), or severe (<1 mg/dL, or 0.32 mmol/liter).

Hypotonic: Refers to fluid with less osmolarity than serum.

Intracellular fluid: Fluid inside cells.

Ions: Charged particles.

Isotonic: Refers to fluid close to the same osmolarity as serum.

Magnesium: Fourth most common cation in the body.

Milliequivalent: Unit used to measure the number of ionic charges or electrovalent bonds (electrolytes) in a solution.

Osmolarity: Osmotic pressure of a solution expressed as milliosmoles per liter (mOsm/L) or millimoles per liter (mmol/liter) of the solution.

Osmosis: the movement of water across a semipermeable membrane from a higher to lower concentration.

Potassium: Main electrolyte in extracellular fluid.

Sodium: Chief electrolyte in interstitial fluid.

Overview of Fluid and Electrolyte Disorders

A fluid and electrolyte disorder is defined as an imbalance of electrolytes or fluids above or below the normal levels of serum concentrations in the body. The term *fluid and electrolyte balance* implies **homeostasis**, or constancy of body fluid and electrolyte levels. The volume of fluid and the electrolyte levels inside the cells, in the interstitial spaces, and in the blood vessels all remain relatively constant. For homeostasis to be maintained, body input of water and electrolytes must be balanced by output. Fluid and electrolyte imbalance, then, means that both the total volume of water and the level of electrolytes in the body or the amounts in one or more of the compartments have increased or decreased outside of normal limits.

Electrolytes

The chemical bond(s) between molecules of certain chemical compounds break-up or dissociate when in solution. For example, sodium chloride (NaCl) dissociates into separate charged particles (Na^+ and Cl^-) called **electrolytes**. Positively charged electrolytes are called **cations**; negatively charged **ions** are called **anions** (Table 31-1).

The number of ionic charges or electrovalent bonds (electrolytes) in a solution is measured in **milliequivalents** (mEq). Common electrolytes that are measured by clinicians using blood testing include sodium, potassium, chloride, and bicarbonate. The normal range values for these electrolytes are described in Table 31-2.

Electrolytes are essential for homeostasis and play an important role in body chemistry. They circulate in the blood at specific levels where they are available when needed by the cells. An imbalance of electrolytes, such as when levels are too high or too low, can cause serious disease that requires treatment to restore balance in the body. Electrolytes are essential to many body functions such as nerve conduction, muscle contraction, and bone growth.

TABLE 31-1   **Important Cations and Anions**

Ions	Examples
Anions	Bicarbonate (HCO_3^-)
	Chloride (Cl^-)
	Phosphate (PO_4^-)
	Sulfate (SO_4^{-2})
Cations	Calcium (Ca^{2+})
	Magnesium (Mg^{2+})
	Potassium (K^+)
	Sodium (Na^+)

TABLE 31-2   **Electrolyte Values**

Electrolyte	Normal Adult Values (mEq/liter)
Calcium	4.3-5.16 (ionized 2.26-2.56)
Chloride	97-107
Potassium	3.5-5.3
Magnesium	1.5-2
Sodium	135-145

Sodium is the major positive ion (cation) in fluid outside of cells. Sodium regulates the total amount of water in the body and the transmission of sodium into and out of individual cells also plays a role in critical body functions. Many processes in the body, especially in the brain, nervous system, and muscles, require electrical signals for communication. The movement of sodium is critical for the generation of these electrical signals. Too much or too little sodium, therefore, can cause cells to malfunction, and extremes (too much or too little) can be fatal. Although excess sodium (e.g., from eating fast food hamburgers and French fries) is excreted in the urine, sodium accumulation is implicated in hypertension and cardiovascular disease.

Potassium is the other major cation found inside of cells. The proper level of potassium is essential for normal cell function. Regulation of the heartbeat and muscle are two important functions of potassium. A seriously abnormal increase of potassium (hyperkalemia) or decrease of potassium (hypokalemia) can profoundly affect the nervous system and increases the chance of irregular heartbeats (arrhythmias), which, when extreme, can be fatal.

Chloride is the major anion (negatively charged ion) found in the fluid outside of cells and in blood. Seawater has almost the same concentration of chloride ion as human fluids. The balance of the chloride ion (Cl^-) is closely regulated by the body. Significant increases or decreases in chloride can have deleterious or even fatal consequences. Chloride plays a role in helping the body maintain a normal fluid balance.

The *bicarbonate* anion acts as a buffer to maintain the normal levels of acidity (pH) in blood and other fluids in the body. The pH is affected by foods or medications that we ingest and the function of the kidneys and lungs. The chemical notation for bicarbonate on most laboratory reports is HCO_3^- but may be represented as the concentration of carbon dioxide (CO_2). The normal serum range for bicarbonate is 22 to 30 mmol/liter.

Magnesium, the fourth most common cation in the body, has been the focus of much clinical and scholarly interest. Previously underappreciated, this ion is now established as a central electrolyte in a large number of cellular metabolic reactions, including DNA and protein synthesis, neurotransmission, and hormone-receptor binding. It is a component of GTPase and a cofactor for Na^+/K^+-ATPase, adenylate cyclase, and phosphofructokinase. Phosphofructokinase's enzymatic action results in maintaining steady adenosine triphosphate (ATP) levels, the energy carrier for our cells. Magnesium also is necessary for the production of parathyroid hormone. Accordingly, magnesium deficiency has an effect on a number of body functions. Magnesium is present in greatest concentration within the cell and is the second most abundant intracellular cation after potassium. The total body content of magnesium is 2000 mEq. The intracellular concentration of magnesium is 40 mEq/liter; the serum concentration is 1.5 to 2 mEq/liter. Most of the body's magnesium is found in bone. Only 1% of the total body magnesium is extracellular; of this amount, 50% is ionized and 25% to 30% is protein-bound.

Phosphorus is essential for membrane structure, energy storage, and transport in all cells. In particular, phosphate is necessary to produce ATP, which provides energy for almost all cell functions. Phosphate is an essential component of DNA and RNA and is also necessary in red blood cells for the production of 2,3-diphosphoglycerate (2,3-DPG), which facilitates the release of oxygen from hemoglobin. Approximately 85% of the body's phosphorus is in bone as hydroxyapatite; most of the remainder (15%) is present in soft tissue. Only 0.1% of phosphorus is present in extracellular fluid, and it is this fraction that is measured by a serum phosphorus level.

Body Fluid Compartments

Functionally, the total body water can be divided into two major fluid compartments, the extracellular and intracellular fluid compartments. **Extracellular fluid** consists mainly of the plasma found in the blood vessels and the interstitial fluid that surrounds the cells. **Intracellular fluid** refers to the water inside the cells. When compared to all sources of fluid volume in the body, intracellular fluid is the largest amount (25 liters), plasma is the smallest amount (3 liters), and interstitial fluid falls in between (12 liters). The cardinal principal of fluid balance is that it can be maintained only if intake equals output.

Regulation of Water and Electrolyte Levels in Intracellular Fluid

The cellular membrane separates the intracellular and extracellular fluid compartments. Most of the body sodium is outside of the cells. Sodium is the chief electrolyte in interstitial fluid. The main electrolyte of intracellular fluid is potassium. A change in the sodium or potassium concentration of either of these fluids causes the exchange of fluid between them to be unbalanced. Fluid balance depends on electrolyte balance. Conversely, electrolyte balance depends on fluid balance.

TABLE 31-3   **Location of Body Fluids**

Body Fluid	Location in Body
Cerebrospinal fluid	Surrounding the brain and spinal cord
Synovial fluid	Surrounding bone joints
Intracellular fluid	Fluids inside cells
Blood	Connective tissue found all through the body, mainly in blood vessels
Aqueous humor and vitreous humor	Fluids found in the eyeballs

Fluid and Electrolyte Disorders

Fluids and electrolytes are generally in equilibrium in the body. Internal body fluids, which are not leaked or excreted to the outside world, include those identified in Table 31-3. When fluid levels drop lower or go higher than normal, disorders result. This chapter will center on intracellular, interstitial, and plasma fluids.

FLUID DISORDERS
Dehydration

The term **dehydration** is used to describe a condition that results from excessive loss of body fluids. Water deprivation or loss triggers a complex series of protective responses designed to maintain homeostasis of water and electrolyte levels. If water intake is reduced to the point of dehydration, a corresponding quantity of electrolytes must be removed to maintain the normal ionic content of the body fluids. The same is true in the case of electrolyte loss. An accompanying loss of water must occur to maintain homeostasis of fluid and electrolyte levels. Understanding the close interrelationships of water and electrolyte loss in dehydration provides the rationale for effective treatment. Signs and symptoms of dehydration include thirst, dry mucous membranes, weakness, dizziness, fever, low urine output, and poor skin turgor. Skin that is well hydrated will be elastic and quickly return to shape after being gently pinched.

Management of dehydration requires appropriate replacement therapy with oral electrolyte solutions, intravenous fluids with added electrolytes such as 0.9% sodium chloride, or normal saline. Water alone is inadequate (Boxes 31-1 and 31-2).

BOX 31-1   Management and Treatment of Dehydration

- Oral electrolyte solutions (mild diarrhea or vomiting)
- 2.0%–2.5% glucose
- 0.9% sodium chloride, 75-90 mEq/liter (parenteral)

BOX 31-2   Management of Fluid and Electrolyte Depletion

ORAL REHYDRATION SOLUTIONS
Electrolyte (freezer pops): Infalyte, Oralyte
Pedialyte (solution, freezer pops)
Pedia-Pop Palsicles (freezer pops)
Rehydralyte

PARENTERAL SOLUTIONS
Inosol B, Inosol MB, and Inosol T in 5% dextrose
Isolyte H, Isolyte P, and Isolyte S in 5% dextrose
Normosol R
Plasmalyte A and Plasmalyte R
Plasmalyte M and Plasmalyte T in 5% dextrose
Travert with 5% electrolytes and 10% electrolytes

Edema

Edema is a classic example of fluid imbalance; it may be described as the presence of abnormally large amounts of fluid in the intercellular tissue spaces of the body. Edema may occur in any organ or tissue of the body; however, the lungs, brain, the legs and lower part of the back are affected most often. One of the most common areas for swelling to occur is in the subcutaneous tissue of the ankle and foot. The following are causes of edema:

- Retention of electrolytes (especially Na^+) in the extracellular fluid.
- An increase in capillary blood pressure. The general venous congestion of heart failure is the most common cause of widespread edema.
- A decrease in the concentration of plasma proteins normally retained in the blood. This can be caused by burns, infection, or shock.
  Box 31-3 describes the management and treatment of edema.

BOX 31-3   Management and Treatment of Edema

- Treat underlying disease.
- Decrease sodium and water intake.
- Administer loop diuretics (see Chapters 22 and 23).*

*Loop diuretics (furosemide, bumetanide, and torsemide).

ELECTROLYTE DISORDERS
Hyponatremia

Hyponatremia is a condition in which the serum sodium concentration falls below the normal range (<136 mEq/liter). Causes of hyponatremia include profuse perspiration (sweating), overzealous use of salt-wasting diuretics, adrenal insufficiency, renal or liver failure, low salt intake, and excessive water intake. Signs and symptoms of hyponatremia include muscle cramps, nausea and vomiting, cold and clammy skin, postural blood pressure changes, poor skin turgor, fatigue, and difficulty breathing, hypotension, irritability, and tachycardia. Cerebral swelling can occur in severe cases, causing confusion, hemiparesis (motor weakness on one side of the body), seizures, and coma.

- Pseudohyponatremia occurs when too much water is drawn into the blood; it is commonly seen in people with hypoglycemia (low blood sugar level).
- Psychogenic polydipsia occurs in people who compulsively drink more than 4 gallons of water a day.
- Hypovolemic hyponatremia (with low blood volume caused by fluid loss) occurs in dehydrated people who rehydrate (drink a lot of water) too quickly, in patients taking thiazide diuretics, and after severe vomiting or diarrhea.
- Hypervolemic hyponatremia (high blood volume caused by fluid retention) occurs in people with liver cirrhosis, heart disease, or nephrotic syndrome. Edema (swelling) often develops with fluid retention.
- Euvolemic hyponatremia (decrease in total body water) occurs in people with hypothyroidism, adrenal gland disorder, and disorders that increase the release of the antidiuretic hormone (ADH), such as tuberculosis, pneumonia, and brain trauma.

CAN YOU REALLY DRINK TOO MUCH WATER?

In a word, yes. Drinking too much water can lead to a condition known as water intoxication and to a related problem resulting from the dilution of sodium in the body, hyponatremia. Water intoxication is most commonly seen in infants younger than 6 months and sometimes in athletes. A baby can get water intoxication as a result of drinking several bottles of water a day or from drinking infant formula that has been diluted too much. Athletes can also suffer from water intoxication. Athletes sweat heavily, losing both water and electrolytes. Rapid rehydration may result in water intoxication.

WHAT HAPPENS DURING WATER INTOXICATION?

When too much water enters the body's cells, the tissues swell with the excess fluid. Your cells maintain a specific concentration gradient, so excess water outside the cells (the serum) draws sodium from within the cells out into the serum in an attempt to re-establish the necessary concentration. As more water accumulates, the serum sodium concentration drops—a condition known as hyponatremia. The other way cells try to regain the electrolyte balance is for water outside the cells to rush into the cells via osmosis. *Osmosis* is the movement of water across a semipermeable membrane from a higher to lower concentration. Electrolytes are more concentrated inside than outside the cells and the water outside the cells is less concentrated, or dilute, because it contains fewer electrolytes. Electrolytes and water movement across the cell membrane is orchestrated to maintain homeostasis, the body's normal balance of electrolytes; however, theoretically, cells could swell to the point of bursting.

From the cell's point of view, water intoxication produces the same effects as would result from drowning in fresh water. Electrolyte imbalance and tissue swelling can cause an irregular heartbeat, allow fluid to enter the lungs, and may cause fluttering eyelids. Swelling puts pressure on the brain and nerves, which can cause behaviors resembling those of alcohol intoxication. Swelling of brain tissues can cause seizures, coma, and ultimately death unless water intake is restricted and a hypertonic saline (salt) solution is administered. If treatment is given before tissue swelling causes too much cellular damage, a complete recovery can be expected within a few days.

Hypernatremia

Hypernatremia is elevation of the serum sodium concentration to higher than 145 mEq/liter. Causes of hypernatremia include lack of fluid intake, diarrhea, diabetes insipidus, loss of water via the respiratory tract, heart disease or congestive heart failure, renal failure, and ingestion of salt in abnormally high amounts. Signs and symptoms are similar to those of dehydration and include thirst, disorientation, lethargy, and seizures. The neurological symptoms are thought to be caused by cerebral cellular dehydration. Administration of hypotonic solution helps lower the sodium level slowly, thereby reducing the risk of cerebral edema (Box 31-4).

TECH NOTE!
Water follows sodium ions when they are moved through the cell membrane. Lots of sodium in the body means that water stays inside (instead of leaving through kidney cells and then the bladder), which means that there is more blood volume and blood pressure is higher.

BOX 31-4   **Management of Hypernatremia and Hyponatremia**

HYPERNATREMIA
- Administration of hypotonic solution such as 0.45% NaCl (half-normal saline)

HYPONATREMIA
- Administration of sodium orally (salt tablets)
- Intravenous saline solution, 3% sodium
- Water restriction

BOX 31-5   **Management of Hyperkalemia**

- Restrict dietary intake of potassium in mild cases.
- Emergency intravenous administration of calcium gluconate may be required to correct cardiac symptoms.
- Administer a cation exchange resin (e.g., sodium polystyrene sulfonate) to exchange sodium and hydrogen ions for potassium ions in the large intestine and eliminate the potassium resin in feces.
- Dialysis to remove the excess potassium can be instituted to correct severe hyperkalemia.

Hypokalemia

Hypokalemia is a condition in which potassium is lost from the body, resulting in a serum potassium level lower than 3.5 mEq/liter. Hypokalemia may be caused by overuse of potassium-wasting diuretics, increased urine output with loss of potassium, and vomiting or gastric suctioning without potassium replacement. Signs and symptoms include anorexia, nausea, vomiting, depression, confusion, impaired thought processes, drowsiness, muscle weakness, decreased reflexes, low blood pressure, and cardiac arrhythmias.

Hyperkalemia

Hyperkalemia is a condition in which the serum potassium level is higher than 5.5 mEq/liter. This can be even more dangerous than hypokalemia because myocardial muscle can be profoundly affected. Hyperkalemia can induce ventricular dysrrhythmias, thereby possibly leading to cardiac arrest. Possible causes of hyperkalemia are kidney disease (most common), vomiting, diarrhea, potassium-conserving diuretics and other medications, extensive tissue damage as in burn or trauma victims, severe infections, and Cushing's syndrome. Signs and symptoms can include muscle weakness or failure of the respiratory muscles, intermittent diarrhea, nausea, vomiting, intestinal colic, irritability, anxiety, confusion, abdominal distress, and cardiac arrhythmias (Box 31-5).

Hypochloremia

Chloride is normally lost in the urine, sweat, and stomach secretions. Excessive loss—*hypochloremia*—can occur from heavy sweating, vomiting, and adrenal gland and kidney disease. Symptoms include dehydration, fluid loss, or high levels of blood sodium.

Hyperchloremia

Elevations in chloride (*hyperchloremia*) may be associated with diarrhea, certain kidney diseases, and overactivity of the parathyroid glands. Hyperchloremia is often comorbid with diabetes or hyponatremia. Certain drugs, especially diuretics such as carbonic anhydrase inhibitors and hormonal treatments, may contribute to this disorder.

Hypocalcemia

Hypocalcemia is a condition in which the serum calcium level is lower than 4.3 mEq/liter (2.26 mEq/liter ionized). Causes of hypocalcemia can be dietary deficiency, parathyroid disease, or accidental removal of the parathyroid glands during surgery of the thyroid gland. Signs and symptoms include tetany, muscle spasms, lethargy, and seizures.

Hypercalcemia

Hypercalcemia is a condition in which the serum calcium level is higher than 5.16 mEq/liter (2.56 mEq/liter ionized). It may occur in patients with an overactive parathyroid gland, lung and breast cancer, or even osteoporosis. Thiazide diuretics, lithium, and excessive doses of calcium, vitamin D supplements, or alkaline antacids may produce hypercalcemia. Dehydration may also produce hypercalcemia. Hypercalcemia may lead to kidney stones, renal failure, arrhythmia, and coma.

Hypomagnesemia

Hypomagnesemia is a condition in which the serum level of magnesium is lower than 1.5 mEq/ liter. Hypomagnesemia may be caused by pregnancy-induced hypertension. Signs and symptoms include confusion, leg and foot cramps, hypertension, tachycardia, arrhythmias, weakness, nystagmus, neuromuscular irritability, tremor, hyperactive deep tendon reflexes, visual and auditory hallucinations, paresthesias, and seizures. Magnesium sulfate is used as replacement therapy for the prevention and control of seizures in obstetric patients with pregnancy-induced hypertension.

Hypermagnesemia

Hypermagnesemia is a condition in which the serum level of magnesium is higher than 2.5 mEq/ liter. Excessive levels of magnesium rarely occur in the absence of kidney failure but have been reported in patients overusing magnesium laxatives, such as epsom salts. Hyperkalemia may produce cardiac arrest, decreased tendon reflexes, muscle weakness, nausea, and sedation.

Hypophosphatemia

Hypophosphatemia is a condition in which the serum phosphorus or phosphate level in adults is defined as mild (2 to 2.5 mg/dL, or 0.65 to 0.81 mmol/liter), moderate (1 to 2 mg/dL, or 0.32 to 0.65 mmol/liter), or severe (<1 mg/dL, or 0.32 mmol/liter). Decreased dietary intake is a rare cause of hypophosphatemia because of the ubiquity of phosphate in foods. Certain conditions such as anorexia nervosa or chronic alcoholism may lead to hypophosphatemia. Signs and symptoms of hypophosphatemia are anorexia, bone or muscle weakness, respiratory failure, congestive heart failure, hemolysis, and rhabdomyolysis. Respiratory insufficiency may occur in some patients with severe hypophosphatemia, particularly when the underlying cause is malnourishment. Phosphate deficiency may compromise a single organ or the entire body system. The critical role that phosphate plays in every cell, tissue, and organ explains the systemic nature of injury caused by phosphate deficiency. As for other intracellular ions (e.g., potassium, magnesium), a decrease in the level of serum phosphate (hypophosphatemia) should be distinguished from a decrease in total body storage of phosphate (phosphate deficiency).

Hyperphosphatemia

Hyperphosphatemia is a condition in which the serum phosphorus or phosphate level in adults is higher than 5 mg/dL. Hyperphosphatemia is most common in patients with end-stage renal disease but may also be caused by muscle cell destruction (rhabdomyolysis), excessive use of phosphate-containing laxatives, calcium or magnesium deficiency, or vitamin D excess. It may produce muscle cramping, tetany, delirium, and seizures.

An electrolyte imbalance is diagnosed based on information gained from the following:
- History of symptoms
- Physical examination
- Urine and blood test results
- Electrocardiogram
- Ultrasound or radiography (if imbalance is caused by kidney problems)

Treatment of Fluid and Electrolyte Disorders

The goal of treatment is to restore electrolyte balance and proper hydration. Electrolyte imbalances may be treated by the following means:
- Identification of the underlying problem
- Intravenous fluids
- Electrolyte replacement

TECH NOTE!
0.9% sodium chloride (NaCl) is also known as normal saline (NS) because it is the same concentration (isotonic) as in the body.

TECH ALERT!
The following drugs have look-alike and sound-alike issues:
Os-cal and Asacol; Citracal and Citrucel

- Diet changes
- Restriction of water
- Fluid replacement

Electrolytes may be replaced via dietary or pharmacological therapy (Box 31-6).

PHARMACOLOGICAL TREATMENT

Table 31-4 lists the phosphate, sodium, and potassium content of selected preparations of sodium phosphate and potassium phosphate.

BOX 31-6   Management of Electrolyte Depletion

- Diet rich in depleted electrolyte(s)
- Dietary supplements
- Parenteral administration of depleted electrolyte(s), as necessary

TABLE 31-4   Phosphate, Sodium, and Potassium Content of Selected Preparations of Sodium Phosphate and Potassium Phosphate

Preparations of Sodium Phosphate and Potassium Phosphate	Dosage Forms and Strengths	Content	
		Sodium Phosphate	Potassium Phosphate
Oral Preparations			
Skim cow's milk	1 g/liter	28 mEq/liter	38 mEq/liter
Neutra-Phos	250 mg/packet	7.1 mEq/packet	7.1 mEq/packet
Neutra-Phos K	250 mg/capsule	0	14.25 mEq/capsule
K-Phos Original	150 mg/capsule	0	3.65 mEq/capsule
K-Phos Neutral	250 mg/tablet	13 mEq/tablet	1.1 mEq/tablet
Intravenous Preparations			
Neutral sodium-potassium PO_4	1.1 mmol/mL	0.2 mEq/mL	0.02 mEq/mL
Neutral sodium-potassium PO_4	0.09 mmol/liter	0.2 mEq/mL	0
$NaPO_4$	3.0 mmol/mL	4.0 mEq/mL	0
KPO_4	3.0 mmol/mL	0	4.4 mEq/mL

Electrolyte Replacement Therapy: Sodium

Generic Name	U.S. Brand Name(s) Canadian Brand Name(s)	Dosage Forms and Strengths
sodium chloride*	Generics / Generics	Intravenous solution: 0.45% NaCl (½ NS), 0.9% NaCl (NS), 3%, 5% Solution for injection: 2.5 mEq/mL, 4 mEq/mL Tablet: 1 g

*Generic available.

Electrolyte Replacement Therapy: Chloride

Generic Name	U.S. Brand Name(s) Canadian Brand Name(s)	Dosage Forms and Strengths
ammonium chloride*	Generics / Generics	Solution, injection: 5 mEq/ml

*Generic available.

Electrolyte Replacement Therapy: Calcium

Generic Name	U.S. Brand Name(s) Canadian Brand Name(s)	Dosage Forms and Strengths
calcium carbonate* (oyster shell calcium)	Calci-Mix, Caltrate, Os Cal 500, Os Cal 1250, Tums, Tums Ex, Tums Ultra, Rolaids Extra Strength, TUMS, TUMS EX, TUMS Ultra	Tablets: 200 mg, 500 mg, 600 mg, 750 mg, 1250 mg Chewable tablets: 1250 mg, 1000 mg, 750 mg, 500 mg Soft chew (Rolaids Extra Strength): 1177 mg Capsule (Calci-Mix): 1250 mg Suspension: 500 mg/5 mL, 1250 mg/5 mL
	Caltrate-600, Os Cal, Tums, TUMS Ultra, TUMS Extra Strength	
calcium citrate*	Cal-Citrate	Tablet (Cal-Citrate): 250 mg, 400 mg, 630 mg, 950 mg
	—	
calcium gluconate*^	Generics	Injection: 10% Tablet: 500 mg, 648 mg
	Generics	
calcium chloride*+	Generics	Injection: 1 g/10 mL
	Generics	
calcium lactate*	Generics	Tablet: 650 mg, 648 mg
	Generics	

*Generic available.
^Calcium is also used as an adjunctive therapy for insect bites and stings to reduce muscle cramping (e.g., black widow spider bites).
+Calcium chloride should not be given IM or SC because severe tissue necrosis can occur.

Electrolyte Replacement Therapy: Potassium

Generic Name	U.S. Brand Name(s) Canadian Brand Name(s)	Dosage Forms and Strengths
potassium bicarbonate*	Klor Con EF	Powder, effervescent: 25 mEq/pkt
	Not available	
potassium bicarbonate, citrate*	Effer-K	Powder, effervescent: 10 mEq/pkt , 20 mEq/pkt
	Not available	
potassium chloride*	Klor Con, Klor Con M10, Klor Con M15, Klor Con M20, K-Tab, Micro-K	Capsule (Micro-K): 8 mEq, 10 mEq Tablet, wax matrix (K-Tab, Klor Con, K-Dur, Slow K): 8 mEq, 10 mEq Tablet, microdispersed (Klor Con M): 10 mEq (750 mg), 15 mEq (1125 mg), 20 mEq (1500 mg)
	K-10, K-Dur, K-Lor, K-Lyte, Slow K	Tablet, long-acting (K-Dur): 1500 mg (20 mEq) Liquid (Kaon, K-10): 20 mEq/15 mL Solution: 10%, 20% Effervescent powder (K-Lyte, Klor Con EF, Kay Ciel): 25 mEq/pkt, 1.5 g/pkt Effervescent tablet (Effer K): 25 mEq Powder (K-Lor): 20 mEq/pkt IV (in D_5W): 20 mEq/mL, 30 mEq, 40 mEq
potassium gluconate*	Generics	Tablet: 550 mg, 595 mg Time release: 95 mg
	Kaon	
potassium acetate*	Generics	Solution, injection: 2 mEq/mL, 4 mEq/mL
	Not available	

*Generic available.

Electrolyte Replacement Therapy: Phosphorus

Generic Name	U.S. Brand Name(s)	Dosage Forms and Strengths
phosphorus salts*	K-Phos Original, Neutra Phos K, K-Phos MF, K-Phos Neutral, K-Phos No. 2	**Tablet (K-Phos Original):** 500 mg; K-Phos MF, 155-350 mg; K-Phos Neutral, 155-852-130 mg; K-Phos No. 2, 700-305 mg **Powder for solution (Neutra Phos K):** 14.25 mEq phosphate + 14.25 mEq potassium; potassium 280 mg, sodium 160 mg, phosphorus 250 mg (Phos-NaK) **Solution, injection (potassium phosphate):** 236 mg potassium phosphate (dibasic) + 224 mg potassium phosphate (monobasic) **Solution, injection (sodium phosphate):** 268 mg/mL sodium phosphate (dibasic) + 76 mg/mL sodium phosphate (monobasic); 142 mg sodium phosphate (dibasic) + 76 mg sodium phosphate (monobasic)

*Generic available.

Electrolyte Replacement Therapy: Magnesium

Generic Name	U.S. Brand Name(s)	Dosage Forms and Strengths
magnesium sulfate*	Mag-200	**Solution, injection:** 50%, 40 mg/mL, 80 mg/mL
		Tablet (Mag-200): 200 mg, 400 mg
magnesium oxide*	Mag-Ox 400, Mag-gel 600, Uro-Mag	**Tablet (Mag-Ox):** 400 mg
		Capsule: 140 mg (Uro-Mag); 600 mg (Mag-gel)
magnesium gluconate*	Mag-G, Magonate, Magtrate	**Liquid, oral (Magonate):** 54 mg/5 mL
		Tablet (Mag-G, Magtrate): 500 mg
magnesium chloride*	Chloromag	**Solution, injection:** 200 mg/mL
magnesium lactate*	Mag-Tab	**Tablet, extended-release:** 84 mg

*Generic available.

Loop Diuretics

Generic Name	U.S. Brand Name(s) Canadian Brand Name(s)	Dosage Forms and Strengths
bumetanide*	Bumex	**Solution, for injection:** 0.25 mg/mL
	Burinex	**Tablet:** 0.5 mg, 1 mg‡, 2 mg, 5 mg‡
furosemide*	Lasix	**Solution, for injection:** 10 mg/mL
	Lasix, Lasix Special	**Solution, oral:** 10 mg/mL; 40 mg/5 mL **Tablet:** 20 mg, 40 mg, 80 mg, 500 mg (Lasix Special)
torsemide*	Demadex	**Solution, for injection:** 10 mg/mL
	Not available	**Tablet:** 5 mg, 10 mg, 20 mg, 100 mg

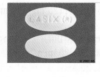

*Generic available.
‡Strength available in Canada only.

TECH ALERT!
Rapid infusion of potassium chloride may cause cardiac arrest; KCl should never be administered by IV push or IM injection.

TREATMENT WITH INTRAVENOUS FLUIDS

More than 200 types of commercially prepared IV fluids are available to treat fluid and electrolyte imbalances. IV solutions are used to replace fluids and electrolytes that have been lost or provide volume replacement that has been lost through hemorrhage, severe burns, diarrhea, vomiting, or inadequate fluid intake, to administer medication, to provide electrolyte balance, for amino acid utilization, and to monitor cardiac functions.

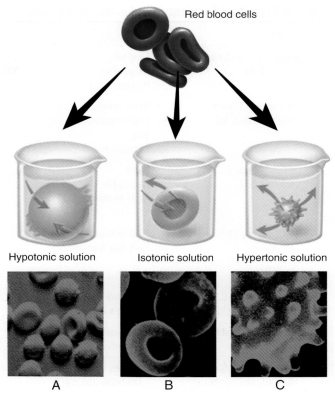

FIGURE 31-1 Beakers filled with hypotonic, isotonic, and hypertonic solutions. (From Thibodeau GA, Patton KT: *Anatomy and physiology*, ed 6, St Louis, 2007, Mosby.)

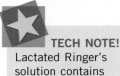

TECH NOTE!
Lactated Ringer's solution contains 28 mmol/liter of lactate, 4 mmol/liter of potassium (K^+), and 3 mmol/liter of calcium (Ca^{2+}).

TECH ALERT!
K-Phos-Neutral and Neutra-Phos-K have look-alike and sound-alike issues.

TECH ALERT!
The following drugs have look-alike and sound-alike issues:
    magnesium sulfate, morphine sulfate, and manganese sulfate;
    Magonate and Magtrate

TECH ALERT!
$MgSO_4$ is on the Joint Commission's list of dangerous abbreviations. It can easily be confused with MSO_4 (morphine sulfate).

IV electrolyte solutions may be classified as isotonic, hypotonic, or hypertonic according to their osmolality (tonicity), the concentration of ions in a solution (Figure 31-1). The osmolality of blood plasma is approximately 290 mOsm/liter. Fluids in the range of 240 to 340 mOsm/liter are considered isotonic. Fluids with tonicities higher than 340 mOsm/liter are hypertonic, and those with tonicities lower than 240 mOsm/liter are hypotonic.

Isotonic fluids are close to the same *osmolarity* as serum. They remain inside the intravascular compartment, thus expanding it. They can be helpful in hypotensive or hypovolemic patients; however, their use may cause overloading, especially in patients with congestive heart failure (CHF) and hypertension.

Hypotonic fluids have less osmolarity than serum. They dilute the serum and pull fluids into cells, decreasing serum osmolarity. Water is then pulled from the vascular compartment into the interstitial fluid compartment. As the interstitial compartment is diluted, its osmolarity decreases, which draws water into adjacent cells. Hypotonic solutions can be helpful when cells are dehydrated, such as in a dialysis patient who is on diuretic therapy. They may also be used for hyperglycemic conditions such as diabetic ketoacidosis, in which high serum glucose levels draw fluid out of the cells and into the vascular and interstitial compartments. Hypotonic fluids can worsen hypotension in a patient with low blood pressure. They can cause a dangerous shift in fluid from the intravascular space to the cells, resulting in cardiovascular collapse and increased intracranial pressure.

Hypertonic fluids have a higher osmolarity than serum. They pull fluid and electrolytes from the intracellular and interstitial compartments into the intravascular compartment and can help stabilize blood pressure, increase urine output, and reduce edema.

IV fluids may be grouped into categories called colloids and crystalloids.

Colloids are proteins or other large molecules that remain suspended in the blood for a long period of time because they are too large to cross membranes. While circulating, they draw water molecules from the cells to the tissues into blood vessels through their ability to increase osmotic pressure. These agents are sometimes called plasma or volume expanders. Examples of colloids include plasma protein fraction, albumin, dextran 40, and hetastarch. Blood itself is a colloid.

TABLE 31-5   **Common Crystalloid Solutions Used for Intravenous Administration**

Type of Solution	Solution	Uses	Adverse Effects
Isotonic	Dextrose 5% in sterile water (D₅W)	Fluid loss Dehydration Hypernatremia	Can cause fluid overload Use cautiously in renal and cardiac patients.
Isotonic	0.9% sodium chloride (normal saline, NS)	Hyponatremia Blood transfusion Shock Resuscitation	Can lead to fluid overload Use cautiously in patients with heart failure (HF) or edema.
Isotonic crystalloid	Lactated Ringer's solution (LR)	Burns Dehydration Acute hemorrhage	Use cautiously in renal patients because of potassium content. Use cautiously in liver patients (cannot metabolize lactate).
Hypotonic crystalloid	0.45% sodium chloride (½ NS)	Fluid (water) replacement Fluid loss from vomiting	May cause cardiovascular collapse or increase intracranial pressure Do not use in patients with liver disease, burns, or trauma.
Hypertonic	Dextrose 5% and 0.9% sodium chloride (D₅ NS)	Temporary treatment for shock, Addison's disease crisis	Do not use in cardiac or renal patients.
Hypertonic	Dextrose 10% in sterile water or D₁₀W	Water replacement Malnutrition	Monitor blood glucose levels.
Hypertonic	Dextrose 5% and 0.45% NaCl (D₅ and ½ NS)	Use when blood glucose levels fall below 250 mg/dL	Use cautiously in surgical patients and those with circulatory insufficiency and in pregnancy.

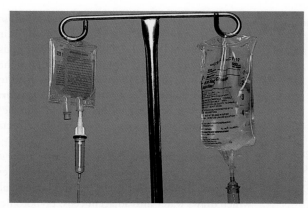

FIGURE 31-2 Piggyback method. (From Hopper T: *Mosby's pharmacy technician*, ed 2, St Louis, 2007, WB Saunders.)

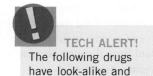

TECH ALERT!
The following drugs have look-alike and sound-alike issues:
   Bumex, Buprenex, Nimbex, and Permax;
   Lasix, Luvox, and Lanoxin;
   furosemide, torsemide, fluoxetine, famotidine, and fosinopril

Crystalloids are IV solutions that contain electrolytes in concentrations resembling those of plasma. Unlike colloids, crystalloid solutions leave the blood and enter cells. They are used to replace fluids that have been lost and promote urine output. Common crystalloids include normal saline (NS), lactated Ringer's solution, Plasma-Lyte, hypertonic saline (3% sodium chloride), and 5% dextrose in water (D₅W) (Table 31-5).

If additional medications need to be administered to a patient placed on an IV electrolyte solution, the piggyback method provides an intermittent IV drip of a second solution through the venipuncture site of an established primary IV system (Figure 31-2). The piggyback technique eliminates the need for another venipuncture and dilutes the medication to reduce irritation.

Summary of Drugs Used in the Treatment of Fluid and Electrolyte Disorders

Drug Name	Usual Dose and Dosing Schedule	Warning Labels
Loop Diuretics		
bumetanide	0.5-2 mg bid	MAY BE ADVISABLE TO EAT BANANAS OR DRINK ORANGE JUICE.
furosemide	20-80 mg bid	MAY CAUSE DIZZINESS OR LIGHTHEADEDNESS. AVOID PROLONGED EXPOSURE TO SUNLIGHT. SOME OVER-THE-COUNTER (OTC) DRUGS CAN AGGRAVATE YOUR CONDITION.
torsemide	2.5-10 mg daily	
Electrolyte Replacement		
sodium chloride	**Hyponatremia and dehydration** IV: Individualized Oral: 650 mg-2.25 g as directed for specific product (max, 4.8 g/day)	TAKE WITH A FULL GLASS OF WATER (ORAL).
calcium carbonate	**Hypocalcemia** 2-4 g/day of elemental calcium (5-10 g calcium carbonate), given in three or four divided doses	TAKE WITH FOOD (CALCIUM CARBONATE). AVOID FERROUS PRODUCTS WITHIN 1-2 HR OF DOSE (MAY DECREASE IRON ABSORPTION).
calcium chloride	500 mg-1 g at 1- to 3-day intervals	DO NOT INJECT CALCIUM CHLORIDE IM OR SEVERE SLOUGHING OR NECROSIS MAY OCCUR.
potassium chloride	20 mEq/day given in one or two divided doses	TAKE WITH WATER. SWALLOW WHOLE; DON'T CRUSH OR CHEW (EXTENDED-RELEASE FORMULATIONS). DILUTE EFFERVESCENT POWDERS AND TABLETS IN WATER OR JUICE.
magnesium sulfate	25 mg/kg-50 mg/kg/dose every 4-6 hr	MONITOR ARRHYTHMIAS AND HYPOTENSION. MAY CAUSE RESPIRATORY AND CENTRAL NERVOUS SYSTEM DEPRESSION.
magnesium oxide	250 mg-1.5 g qid	
potassium phosphate	**Hypophosphatemia** IV: 0.5-0.25 mmol/kg IV over 4-6 hr	MONITOR FOR DIARRHEA AND SIGNS OF HYPERMAGNESEMIA.
K-Phos Neutral	Oral: 700 mg per day	

Chapter Summary

- The term *fluid and electrolyte balance* implies homeostasis, or constancy, of body fluid and electrolyte levels. For homeostasis to be maintained, body input of water and electrolytes must be balanced by output.
- Electrolytes are essential to many body functions such as nerve conduction, muscle contraction, and bone growth.
- Functionally, the total body water can be divided into two major fluid compartments, the extracellular and the intracellular fluid compartments. Extracellular fluid consists mainly of the plasma found in the blood vessels and the interstitial fluid that surrounds the cells. Intracellular fluid refers to the water inside the cells.
- There are many causes of electrolyte imbalances, such as hormonal or endocrine disorders, kidney disease, dehydration, inadequate diet, lack of dietary vitamins, malabsorption, and medication adverse effects.
- The goal of treatment is to restore electrolyte balance and restore the levels of body fluids to normal.
- An electrolyte imbalance is diagnosed based on information gained from the history of symptoms, physical examination, urine and blood test results, electrocardiography, ultrasonography, or radiography (if imbalance is caused by kidney problems).

- The term *dehydration* is used to describe the condition that results from excessive loss of body water.
- Edema is a classic example of fluid imbalance; it may be described as the presence of abnormally large amounts of fluid in the intercellular tissue spaces of the body.
- Intravenous solutions are used to replace fluids and electrolytes that have been lost and to provide calories through their carbonate content.
- There are three main types of IV fluids—isotonic, hypotonic, and hypertonic.
- There are two main groups of fluids, crystalloid and colloid.

REVIEW QUESTIONS

1. A cation is a negatively charged electrolyte and an anion is a positively charged particle.
   a. True
   b. False

2. Fluids close to the same osmolarity as serum are called _____.
   a. Hypotonic
   b. Isotonic
   c. Hypertonic
   d. Serotonic

3. Which of the following is not an example of an electrolyte?
   a. Calcium
   b. Magnesium
   c. Selenium
   d. Sodium

4. Electrolytes are essential to many body functions such as _____.
   a. Nerve conduction
   b. Muscle contraction
   c. Bone growth
   d. All of the above

5. Which of the following electrolytes is important for the regulation of the heartbeat and function of the muscles?
   a. Calcium
   b. Potassium
   c. Sodium
   d. Magnesium

6. The _____ ion acts as a buffer to maintain the normal levels of acidity (pH) in blood and other fluids in the body.
   a. Chlorine
   b. Magnesium
   c. Bicarbonate
   d. Phosphate

7. Which of the following is necessary to produce ATP, which provides energy for nearly all cell functions?
   a. Phosphate
   b. Bicarbonate
   c. Citrate
   d. All of the above

8. Two types of fluid disorders are _____ and _____.
   a. Edema; dehydration
   b. Dehydration; shock
   c. Hyponatremia; hypomagnesemia
   d. Water intoxication; diarrhea

9. What are two types of intravenous (IV) fluids used to treat fluid imbalances?
    a. Crystalloids and onsmolite
    b. Osmolite and colloids
    c. Colloids and crystalloids
    d. All of the above

10. Furosemide is the generic name for Bumex.
    a. True
    b. False

TECHNICIAN'S CORNER

1. Why is the intake of water so important for proper cell function?
2. What types of food provide potassium?

Bibliography

drugs.com: Electrolyte freezer pops. (http://www.drugs.com/cdi/electrolyte-freezer-pops.html). 2012.

drugs.com: Isolyte S. (http://www.drugs.com/pro/isolyte-s.html). 2011.

drugs.com: Normosol-R. (http://www.drugs.com/pro/normosol-r.html). 2012.

Fulcher EM, Fulcher RM, Soto CD: *Pharmacology: Principles and applications, ed 2, Appendix XI: Intravenous administration basics*, Philadelphia, 2005, Saunders.

Harris P, Nagy S, Vardaxis N: *Mosby's dictionary of medicine, nursing, and health professions*, ed 7, Philadelphia, 2005, Elsevier Mosby, pp 625-626, 1008-1011.

Martin S: *Intravenous therapy, business briefing, long-term health care strategies*, Fort Lauderdale, FL, 2003, College of Allied Health and Nursing, Nova Southeastern University, pp 1-4.

Phillips B: Critical care medicine: Electrolyte replacement, a review. (journal/the-internet-journal-of-internal-medicine/volume-5-number-1/electrolyte-replacement-a-review.html). 2012.

http://www.freemd.com/dehydration/treatment.htm; Authors: Stephen J. Schueler, MD; John H. Beckett, MD; D. Scott Gettings, MD, Jun 9, 2011.

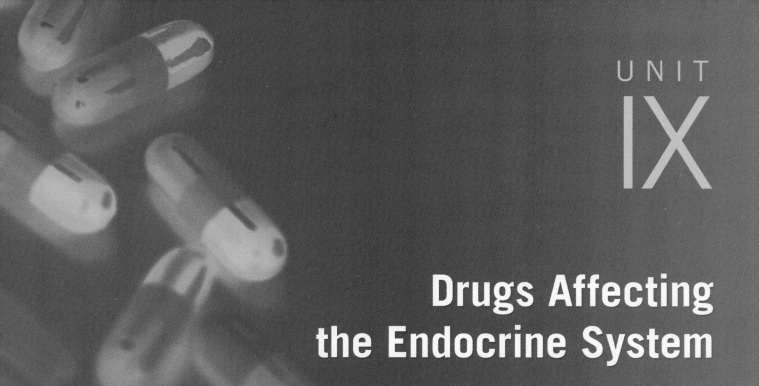

UNIT IX

Drugs Affecting the Endocrine System

LEARNING OBJECTIVES

1 Identify the target organs and understand the functions of the endocrine system.

2 Explain the process of the negative feedback system.

3 Understand the importance of hormones in maintaining homeostasis.

KEY TERMS

Androgens: Male sex hormones.

Hormones: Chemical messengers.

Prostaglandins: Group of lipid molecules known as "tissue hormones".

Organization of the Endocrine System

The endocrine system and nervous system both function to maintain stability of the internal environment. In the endocrine system, regulatory function is performed by chemical messengers called *hormones*. Unlike neurotransmitters, which are sent over short distances across synapses and rapidly produce effects, hormones diffuse into the blood to be carried to almost every point in the body and their effects appear more slowly and last longer. Endocrine glands are known as ductless glands because they secrete hormones directly into the blood.

Hormones

CLASSIFICATION OF HORMONES

Hormones are classified by their target site, their chemical composition (steroid or nonsteroid), and whether they are hydrophilic or hydrophobic. *Tropic* hormones target other endocrine glands and stimulate their growth and secretion. *Sex* hormones target reproductive tissues. *Anabolic* hormones stimulate anabolism in their target cells.

Steroid Hormones

Hormones secreted by endocrine tissues can be classified simply as steroid or nonsteroid. Examples of important steroid hormones include cortisol, aldosterone (a mineralocorticoid), and sex hormones estrogen, progesterone, and testosterone.

523

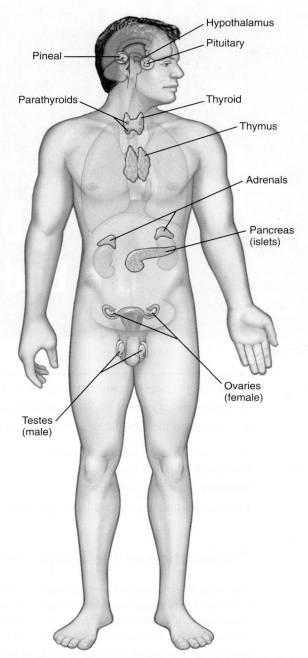

Location of Endocrine Glands. (From Thibodeau GA, Patton KT: *Anatomy and physiology*, ed 6, St. Louis, 2007, Mosby.)

Nonsteroid Hormones

Most nonsteroid hormones are proteins and are synthesized primarily from amino acids rather than from cholesterol. Insulin, parathyroid hormone (PTH), growth hormone (GH), prolactin (PRL), calcitonin (CT), glucagon, and adrenocorticotropic hormone (ACTH) are protein hormones. Protein hormones that have carbohydrate groups attached to the amino acids chains are classified as **glycoprotein hormones** and include follicle-stimulating hormone (FSH), luteinizing hormone (LH), thyroid-stimulating hormone (TSH), and human chorionic gonadotropin (hCG). **Peptide hormones** are another category of nonsteroid hormones. Examples of peptide hormones are oxytocin (OT), antidiuretic hormone (ADH), melatonin-stimulating hormone (MSH), somatostatin (SS), thyrotropin-releasing hormone (TRH), gonadotropin-releasing hormone (GnRH), and atrial natriuretic hormone (ANH). Another category of nonsteroid hormones consists of amino acid derivative

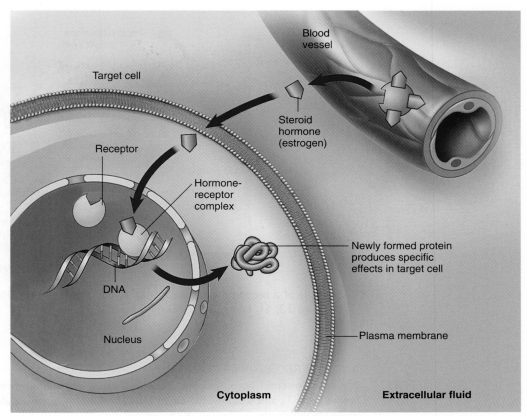

Steroid hormone mechanism. (From Thibodeau GA, Patton KT: *Structure of the body*, ed 13, St. Louis, 2007, Elsevier.)

hormones derived from a single amino acid molecule. There are two subgroups within this category—**amine hormones** (epinephrine and norepinephrine) and those produced by the thyroid gland, thyroxine (T_4) and triiodothyronine (T_3).

HOW HORMONES WORK

Hormones signal a cell by binding to a specific receptor on or in the cell. In a so-called lock-and-key mechanism, hormones will only bind to receptor molecules that fit them exactly. Any cell with more than one receptor for a particular hormone is said to be a target for that hormone. Hormones travel to their target cells by way of the circulating bloodstream. Because they only affect their target cells, the effects of a particular hormone may be limited to specific tissues in the body.

Mechanism of Action for Steroid Hormones

Steroid hormones are lipids and are not very soluble in blood plasma. They attach to soluble plasma proteins and dissociate upon approaching the target cell. After a steroid hormone diffuses into the cell, it passes into the nucleus, where it binds to a hormone-receptor complex. Steroid hormones regulate cells by controlling their production of certain critical proteins, such as enzymes.

Mechanism of Action for Nonsteroid Hormones

SECOND MESSENGER OF ACTION

Nonsteroid hormones typically operate according to a mechanism called the second messenger model. A nonsteroid hormone acts as the first messenger, delivering its chemical messenger to fixed receptors on target cell's plasma membrane. The messenger is then passed into the cell, where a second messenger triggers the appropriate cellular changes. Thus, the first messenger hormone binds to a membrane receptor, triggering the formation of an intracellular second messenger, which activates a cascade of chemical reactions that produce the target's cell response.

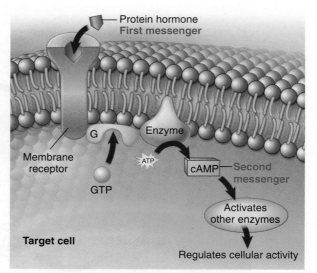

Example of a second messenger model. (From Thibodeau GA, Patton KT: *Structure of the body*, ed 13, St. Louis, 2007, Elsevier.)

NUCLEAR RECEPTOR MECHANISM

Not all nonsteroid hormones operate according to the second-messenger model. The iodinated amino acids T_4 and T_3 enter the target cells and bind to receptors already associated with a DNA molecule within the nucleus of the target cell.

Regulation of Hormone Secretion

Secretion of hormones by many endocrine glands is regulated by a hormone produced by another gland. The control of hormonal secretion is usually part of a negative feedback loop. Secretion of hormones by the anterior pituitary gland is regulated by releasing hormones or inhibiting hormones secreted by the hypothalamus. Secretion of hormones from the posterior pituitary gland is not regulated by releasing hormones but by direct nervous system input from the hypothalamus. Similarly, sympathetic nerve impulses that reach the medulla of the adrenal glands trigger the secretion of epinephrine and norepinephrine. Many other glands, including the pancreas, are also influenced to some degree by nervous system input.

Regulation of Target Cell Sensitivity

The sensitivity of a target cell to any particular hormone partly depends on how many receptors it has for that hormone. Production of too much hormone by a diseased gland is called *hypersecretion*. If too little hormone is produced, the condition is called *hyposecretion*.

Prostaglandins

The *prostaglandins* are a unique group of lipid molecules that do not meet the usual definition of a hormone. The term *tissue hormone* is appropriate because their secretion is produced in a tissue and diffuses only a short distance to other cells within the same tissue, thus integrating the activities of neighboring cells.

Secretory Glands

PITUITARY GLAND (HYPOPHYSIS)

The pituitary gland has been called the master gland. This gland has a stemlike stalk, on the *infundibulum*, which connects to the hypothalamus of the brain. The pituitary gland is divided into two parts, the *adenohypophysis* or anterior pituitary gland and the *neurohypophysis* or posterior pituitary gland. The release of hormones from the adenohypophysis is controlled by chemicals made in

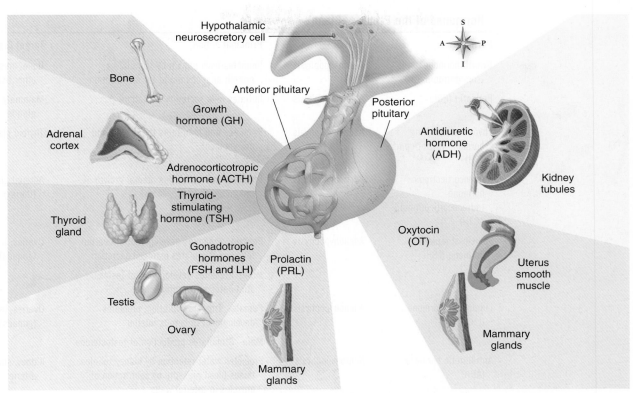

Pituitary hormones. (From Thibodeau GA, Patton KT: *Structure of the body*, ed 13, St. Louis, 2007, Elsevier.)

the hypothalamus called releasing hormones. The hypothalamus, through its releasing hormones, integrates the endocrine and nervous systems, particularly in times of stress. When survival is threatened, the hypothalamus can take over the adenohypophysis and thus gain control of every cell in the body. The neurohypophysis serves as a storage and release site for two hormones, ADH and oxytocin, which are made by the hypothalamus and controlled by nervous stimulation.

THYROID GLAND

The thyroid gland is located in the neck on the anterior and lateral surfaces of the trachea, just below the larynx and is primarily responsible for the regulation of metabolism. Iodine is an important component in the synthesis of thyroid hormones T_4 and T_3. In countries in which iodized salt is consumed in the diet, the prevalence of iodine deficiency goiter (enlarged thyroid gland) is reduced. Another thyroid hormones is calcitonin. Calcitonin helps control calcium levels in the body by increasing bone formation by osteoblasts and inhibiting bone breakdown by osteoclasts. It may slightly decrease blood calcium levels and promote conservation of hard bone matrix.

PARATHYROID GLANDS

There are four to five **parathyroid glands** embedded in the posterior surface of the thyroid's lateral lobes. They secrete PTH, which, along with calcitonin, maintains calcium homeostasis. PTH acts on bone and kidney cells to increase the release of calcium into the blood, causing less new bone to be formed and more old bone to be dissolved. PTH increases the body's absorption of calcium from food by activating vitamin D in the kidney, which then can be transported through the intestinal cells and into the blood.

ADRENAL GLANDS

The **adrenal glands** are located on top of the kidneys, fitting like a cap over these organs. The outer portion of the gland is called the **adrenal cortex** and secretes three sets of hormones—mineralocor-

Hormones of the Pituitary Gland

Hormone	Source	Principal Action	Target Organ
Growth hormone (somatotropin; GH)	Adenohypophysis	Promotes body growth by stimulating protein anabolism and fat mobilization	Bone, muscle, other tissues
Prolactin (PRL)	Adenohypophysis	Initiates milk secretion (lactation)	Mammary glands
Thyroid-stimulating hormone (thyrotropin; TSH)	Adenohypophysis	Promotes and maintains the growth and development	Thyroid gland
Adrenocorticotropic hormone (adrenocorticotropin; ACTH)	Adenohypophysis	Promotes and maintains normal growth of the adrenal cortex	Adrenal gland (Cortex)
Follicle-stimulating hormone (FSH)	Adenohypophysis	**Female:** Promotes development of ovarian follicles; stimulates estrogen secretion **Male:** Promotes development of testes; stimulates sperm production	Ovaries, testes (gonads)
Luteinizing hormone (LH)	Adenohypophysis	**Female:** Triggers ovulation; promotes development of corpus luteum **Male:** Stimulates production of testosterone	Ovaries, testes (gonads)
Antidiuretic hormone (ADH)	Neurohypophysis	Promotes water retention by kidney tubules; raises blood pressure by contraction of muscles in arterial walls	Kidney, small arteries
Oxytocin	Neurohypophysis	Stimulates the contractions of uterine muscles; stimulates ejection of milk into the ducts of lactating women	Uterus, mammary glands

ticoids, glucocorticoids, and sex hormones. The inner portion is called the **adrenal medulla** and secretes two important hormones, epinephrine and norepinephrine. Both are in the class of nonsteroid hormones called catecholamines. Epinephrine, or adrenaline, accounts for approximately 80% of the medulla's secretion. The other 20% is norepinephrine.

PANCREATIC HORMONES

The **pancreas** is an elongated gland lying at the beginning of the small intestine behind the stomach and touching the spleen. The tissue of the pancreas is made up of endocrine and exocrine tissue. The endocrine portion is made up of scattered islands of cells called pancreatic islets (islets of Langerhans). These hormone-producing cells are surrounded by cells called acini, which secrete a serous fluid containing digestive enzymes that drain into the small intestine. The pancreatic islets cells are the **alpha (α) cells**, which secrete the hormone glucagon, **beta (β) cells**, which secrete the hormone insulin, **delta cells**, which secrete the hormone somatostatin, and pancreatic **polypeptide cells**, which secrete pancreatic polypeptide.

GONADS

The **gonads** are the primary sex organs in the male (testes) and female (ovaries). Each is structured differently and each produces its own set of hormones. The testes are composed mainly of coils of sperm-producing seminiferous tubules, with a scattering of endocrine interstitial cells found in the area between the tubules. These interstitial cells produce **androgens** (male sex hormones); the principal androgen is testosterone. The ovaries are a set of paired glands in the pelvis that produce several types of sex hormones, including estrogen and progesterone. Regulation of ovarian hormone secretion basically depends on changing levels of FSH and LH from the adenohypophysis.

Hormones of the Adrenal Glands

Hormone	Source	Principal Action	Target Organ
Aldosterone (mineralocorticoid)	Adrenal cortex	Stimulates kidney tubules to conserve sodium, which triggers the release of ADH and then causes the conservation of water by the kidney	Kidney
Cortisol (glucocorticoid)	Adrenal cortex	Influences metabolism of food molecules; in large amounts, has an anti-inflammatory effect	General body
Adrenal androgens (sex hormones)	Adrenal cortex	Exact role uncertain but may support sexual function	Sex organs
Adrenal estrogens (sex hormones)	Adrenal cortex	Thought to be physiologically insignificant	Sex organs
Epinephrine	Adrenal medulla	Enhances and prolongs the effect of the sympathetic division of the autonomic nervous system	Sympathetic nervous system
Norepinephrine	Adrenal medulla	Enhances and prolongs the effects of the sympathetic division of the autonomic nervous system	Sympathetic nervous system

Hormones of the Pancreatic Islets

Hormone	Source	Principal Action	Target Organ
Glucagon	Alpha (α) cells	Promotes increase of blood glucose levels by stimulating conversion of glycogen to glucose in liver cells	General tissues in the body
Insulin	Beta (β) cells	Promotes movement of glucose, amino acids, and fatty acids out of the blood into tissue cells	General tissues in the body
Somatostatin	Delta (δ) cells	Can have general effects on the body but primary role is to regulate pancreatic hormones	Pancreatic cells and other effectors
Pancreatic polypeptide	Pancreatic islets	Exact function uncertain but seems to influence absorption in the digestive tract	Intestinal cells and effectors

Hormones of the Gonads

Hormone	Source	Principal Action	Target Organ
Testosterone	Testes	Stimulates sperm production; stimulates growth and maintenance of male sexual characteristics, promotes muscle growth	Sperm-producing tissues of the testes, muscles, and other tissues
Estrogen	Ovaries	Stimulates development of female sexual characteristics, breast development, bone and nervous system maintenance	Uterus, breasts, and other tissues
Progesterone	Ovaries	Maintains the lining of the uterus necessary for successful pregnancy	Uterus, mammary glands, other tissues

Additional Hormones of the Body

Additional Hormones

Hormone	Source	Principal Action	Target Organ
Melatonin	Pineal gland	Helps set the body's biological clock by signaling light changes during the day, month, seasons; may help induce sleep	Nervous system
Human chorionic gonadotropin (hCG)	Placenta	Stimulates secretion of estrogen and progesterone during pregnancy	Ovary
Thymosins and thymopoietins	Thymus gland	Stimulate development of T lymphocytes, which are involved in immunity	Certain lymphocytes (white blood cells)
Gastrin	Stomach mucosa	Triggers increased gastric juice	
Secretory glands	Exocrine glands of stomach	Secrete products into ducts, which lead directly into the external environment	sweat glands, salivary glands, mammary glands, stomach, liver, pancreas
Secretin	Intestinal mucosa	Increases alkaline secretions of the pancreas and slows emptying of the stomach	Stomach and pancreas
Cholecystokinin (CCK)	Intestinal mucosa	Triggers the release of bile from gallbladder and enzymes from the pancreas	Gallbladder and pancreas
Ghrelin	Stomach mucosa	Stimulates hypothalamus to boost appetite; affects energy balance in various tissues	Hypothalamus; other diverse tissues
Atrial natriuretic hormone (ANH)	Heart muscle	Promotes loss of sodium from the body into urine, thus promoting water loss and decrease in blood volume and pressure	Kidney
Glucogen-like peptide-1 (GLP-1)	Small intestine endothelial cells	Incretin hormone that increases glucose-dependent insulin secretion	Pancreas
Glucose-dependent insulinotropic peptide (GIP)	Small intestine endothelial cells	Incretin hormone that affects the pancreatic beta cells, where it stimulates insulin secretion,	Pancreas

Summary

Endocrine regulation of body processes first begins during early development in the womb. Many basic hormones are active from birth, but most of the hormones related to reproductive function are not produced or secreted until puberty. The secretion of male hormones continues from puberty until a slight tapering off in late adulthood, whereas the secretion of female reproductive hormones such as estrogen declines late in life, but more suddenly and completely, often during or just at the end of middle adulthood. It is important to recognize the partnership of two major regulatory systems, the endocrine and nervous systems. Through the secretion of hormones and autonomic nervous regulation, almost every process in the human organism is kept in balance by nervous system and endocrine regulatory chemicals.

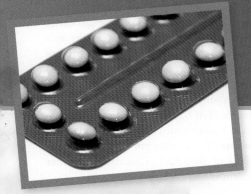

32

Treatment of Thyroid Disorders

KEY TERMS

Antithyroid drugs: Group of drugs administered to treat hyperthyroidism.

Graves' disease: Autoimmune disorder that causes hyperthyroidism.

Hashimoto's disease: Autoimmune disorder that causes hypothyroidism.

Hyperthyroidism: Condition in which there is an excessive production of thyroid hormones.

Hypothyroidism: Condition in which there is insufficient production of thyroid hormones.

Radioactive iodine uptake: Test using radioactive iodine to screen for thyroid disease.

Thyroid antibody test: Diagnostic test used to measure levels of thyroid antibodies that are diagnostic for autoimmune thyroid disease.

Thyroid-releasing factor: Hormone released by the hypothalamus that stimulates the pituitary gland to release thyroid-stimulating hormone.

Thyroid-stimulating hormone: Hormone released by the pituitary gland that stimulates the thyroid gland to produce and release thyroid hormones.

Thyroid-stimulating hormone test: Diagnostic test used to measure the level of thyroid-stimulating hormone in the blood. A low level signals hyperthyroidism.

Tetraiodothyronine: Most abundant thyroid hormone. It contains four atoms of iodine and is also known as thyroxine.

Tetraiodothyronine test: Measure of free circulating thyroid hormone.

Triiodothyronine: Hormone secreted by the thyroid gland. It contains three atoms of iodine.

Overview

More than 20 million Americans and 3 million Canadians have a thyroid disorder and up to 50% of cases are undiagnosed. The disease affects more than 200 million persons worldwide. Thyroid disorders result in overactivity or underactivity of the thyroid gland, causing hypersecretion or hyposecretion of thyroid hormones, respectively. Risk factors for thyroid disease are gender, disease (e.g., diabetes, glycogen storage disease), aging, and pregnancy. Thyroid disease is up to eight times more common in women than men. Hyperthyroidism is most common in women between the ages of 20 and 40 years. Diabetes is a risk factor for thyroid disease; a family history of type 1 diabetes increases risk. The incidence of hypothyroidism increases with age and, by age 60 years, up to 17% of women and 9% of men will have an underactive thyroid. Cigarette smoking increases the risk for developing thyroid-related eye disease. Smokers with Graves' disease are five times more likely than nonsmokers to develop thyroid-associated ophthalmopathy (TAO).

The thyroid gland secretes hormones that have an effect on almost all cells in the body. The thyroid hormones *tetraiodothyronine* (T_4) and *triiodothyronine* (T_3) regulate growth and metabolism. The physiological actions of thyroid hormone are listed in Box 32-1. Calcitonin, another hormone secreted by the thyroid gland, helps to maintain calcium homeostasis.

BOX 32-1   **Physiological Actions of Thyroid Hormones**

- Growth of skeletal tissues
- Fetal growth and development (cognitive and physical)
- Growth and development of the central nervous system
- Regulation of protein, lipid, and carbohydrate metabolism
- Regulation of hepatic metabolic enzymes
- Regulation of body temperature
- Cardiac functions (heart rate and contractility)
- Circulatory volume
- Respiratory functions
- Peripheral vasodilation
- Bone turnover

THYROID HORMONE CONTROL

Releasing and inhibiting hormones that are secreted by the hypothalamus regulate the secretion of hormones by the anterior pituitary gland in a process called negative feedback. Thyroid levels are tightly controlled by a negative feedback loop. When an increased need for thyroid hormones is required, the hypothalamus secretes *thyroid-releasing factor* (TRF), a hormone that signals the pituitary to release *thyroid-stimulating hormone* (TSH). The target site of TSH is the thyroid gland, which produces and secretes T_4 and T_3. Once desired levels are achieved, TSH release is turned off (Figure 32-1). More information about the negative feedback loop is described in the Unit IX opener.

SYNTHESIS OF THYROID HORMONES

The thyroid gland is one of the few glands that produces and stores its hormones. Thyroid hormones (T_4, T_3) are synthesized by a coupling process in which atoms of iodine are bound to the thyroid protein thyroglobulin. The process is activated by the oxidation of the enzyme peroxidase. When one atom of iodide is bound to thyroglobulin, the resultant product is monoiodotyrosine (MIT). When two atoms bind to thyroglobulin, the product formed is diiodotyrosine (DIT). MIT combines with DIT to form T_3. When two DIT molecules combine, T_4 is formed. Tetraiodothyronine is more commonly called thyroxine. In the body, T_4 is converted to T_3 by the process of deiodination.

Diagnosis of Thyroid Disorders

Diagnostic tests are available to determine the cause for excess or deficient thyroid hormone levels. The *thyroid-stimulating hormone test* measures the level of TSH in the blood. A low TSH level signals hyperthyroidism. This is to be expected because TSH levels are regulated by a negative feedback loop. TSH release is turned off when the body recognizes that T_4 levels are high and attempts to stop its further production and release. A high TSH level is a signal for hypothyroidism. A ***tetraiodothyronine test*** measures free T_4 (FT_4) and the free T_4 index (FT_4I). FT_4 and FT_4I tests measure circulating thyroid hormone. In hyperthyroidism, FT_4 levels are elevated and TSH levels are depressed. The reverse is true in the case of hypothyroidism. The presence of thyroid-stimulating antibodies can be measured by a ***thyroid antibody test***. When thyroid antibodies are present, auto-immune thyroid disease is diagnosed. A ***radioactive iodine uptake*** (RAIU) test may also be conducted to test for thyroid disease. Iodine is selectively taken up by the thyroid gland in the process of synthesizing T_4 and T_3 (Figure 32-2); thus, when a low dose of radioactive iodine (^{131}I) is administered, the amount of radioactivity in the thyroid gland can be measured. The RAIU is high when a person has hyperthyroidism and low when the person has hypothyroidism.

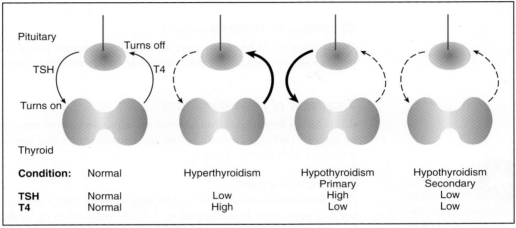

FIGURE 32-1 Comparison of TSH and T_4 levels for normal function, hyperthyroidism, and hypothyroidism. (Courtesy American Thyroid Association, www.thyroid.org.)

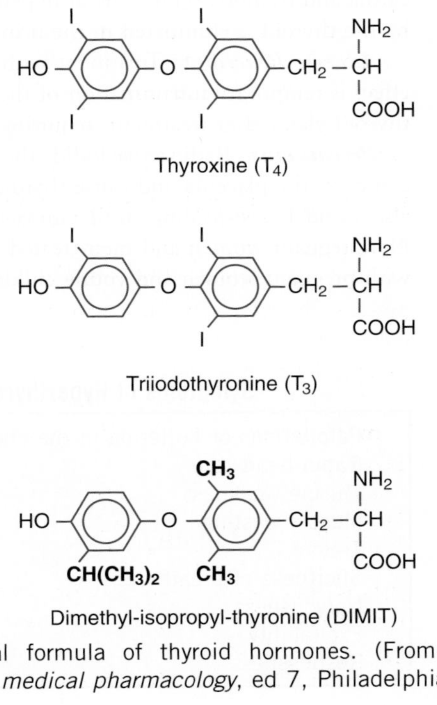

FIGURE 32-2 Structural formula of thyroid hormones. (From Kalant H, Grant DM, Mitchell J: *Principles of medical pharmacology*, ed 7, Philadelphia, 2007, WB Saunders.)

Types of Thyroid Disorders

HYPERTHYROIDISM

Hyperthyroidism is a condition in which the thyroid gland secretes excessive amounts of thyroid hormones. Conditions known to cause hyperthyroidism are the following: (1) thyroid nodules (lumps on the thyroid gland that secrete thyroid hormone); and (2) inflammation of the thyroid gland (e.g., subacute thyroiditis, postpartum thyroiditis, lymphatic thyroiditis). *Graves' disease* is an autoimmune disease and a primary cause of thyroid hyperactivity. Thyroid-stimulating antibodies called thyroid-stimulating immunoglobulins (TSIs) mimic thyroid-stimulating hormone. When TSI binds to receptors on the thyroid gland, the gland releases hormones (see Figure 32-1). Circulating TSI is not sensitive to the negative feedback loop that turns off thyroid hormone release when levels are elevated. Postpartum thyroiditis and subacute thyroiditis cause hyperthyroidism; however, both conditions may be followed by a period of temporary hypothyroidism.

Symptoms of Hyperthyroidism

Given that thyroid hormones have an effect on numerous cells throughout the body, it is not surprising that symptoms of thyroid disease are widespread. These are listed in Box 32-2.

Treatment of Hyperthyroidism

Treatment of hyperthyroidism involves the administration of *antithyroid drugs*, radioactive iodine, or surgery. There are currently no therapeutic modalities that specifically target the autoantibodies associated with Graves' disease.

RADIOACTIVE IODINE

Low-dose radioactive iodine is used for diagnosis and higher dose radioactive iodine is administered for the treatment of hyperthyroidism. It is selectively taken up by the thyroid gland, where it causes glandular destruction while minimizing damage to other tissues. The rate of cure is approximately 66%. Pretreatment with an antithyroid drug is recommended for approximately 2 weeks to block the synthesis of thyroid hormone prior to the administration of ^{131}I. The full effects of ^{131}I therapy are achieved after 2 to 3 months in most people, but sometimes a second or third course of therapy is required. Beta blockers (see Chapter 25) may be administered concurrently with ^{131}I until tachycardia and tremors, symptoms of hyperthyroidism, subside. Radioactive iodine that is not retained by the thyroid is eliminated in the urine within 2 or 3 days.

Adverse Reactions. Treatment with ^{131}I produces few adverse effects. The most common side effect is temporary inflammation of the salivary glands. Most patients also develop an underactive thyroid gland after treatment, requiring lifelong therapy for hypothyroidism.

Precautions. Radioactive iodide therapy is contraindicated in pregnant women because the drug can cross the placenta and cause thyroid damage in the developing fetus. Nursing mothers should also avoid breast-feeding until radioactive iodine can no longer be detected in the breast milk. Nonpregnant women and men treated with radioactive iodide should avoid close physical contact with pregnant women and young children for a few days after the dose is administered.

BOX 32-2   **Symptoms of Hyperthyroidism**

- Palpitations or fluttering in the chest
- Rapid heart rate
- Muscle weakness
- Muscle wasting
- Tremor
- Shortness of breath
- Nervousness
- Excitability
- Restlessness
- Enlarged thyroid (goiter)
- Amenorrhea
- Breast enlargement
- Bulging eyes
- Rapid speech
- Sweating
- Facial flushing
- Heat intolerance, warm skin

Radioactive Iodine (^{131}I)

Generic Name	U.S. Brand Name(s) Canadian Brand Name(s)	Dosage Forms and Strengths
radioactive iodine (^{131}I)*	No commercial preparations	Individualized
	No commercial preparations	

*Generic available.

Thioamides

Generic Name	U.S. Brand Name(s) Canadian Brand Name(s)	Dosage Forms and Strengths
methimazole* (thiamazole in Canada)	Tapazole	Tablet: 5 mg, 10 mg
	Tapazole	
propylthiouracil* (thiouracil in Canada)	Generics	Tablet: 50 mg, 100 mg‡
	Propyl-Thyracil	

*Generic available.
‡Strength available in Canada only.

TECH ALERT!
The following drugs have look-alike and sound-alike issues: methimazole and metolazone; propylthiouracil and Purinethol

TECH ALERT!
The abbreviation PTU (propylthiouracil) has been misread as 6-MP (6-mercaptopurine).

TECH ALERT!
The U.S. Food and Drug Administration (FDA) requires a boxed warning for PTU stating the risk for fatal hepatotoxicity. PTU should be avoided in pediatric populations unless there are no other treatment options available and the patient is allergic or intolerant to methimazole.

THIOAMIDES

Thioamides are thiourea derivatives that are classified as antithyroid drugs. They are used for the primary treatment of hyperthyroidism or to deplete excess thyroid hormone in patients awaiting treatment with radioactive iodine or thyroid surgery.

Mechanism of Action and Pharmacokinetics. Propylthiouracil (PTU), thiouracil (Canada), thiamazole (Canada), and methimazole block the synthesis of T_4 and T_3. They bind thyroid peroxidase enzyme, which is the enzyme that activates the coupling of iodine and thyroglobulin and inhibits the coupling of iodinated tyrosine (MIT and DIT). Only propylthiouracil is capable of blocking the deiodination process that converts T_4 to T_3. It takes 2 to 4 months of therapy with propylthiouracil before maximum effects are achieved because thioamides do not antagonize the activity of thyroid hormones stored in the follicles of the thyroid gland. They only stop the synthesis of new thyroid hormone.

Adverse Reactions. Methimazole and PTU may cause nausea or vomiting, muscle aches and pains, and/or minor rash or itching. Side effects requiring medical attention include fever accompanied by sore throat and hoarseness, goiter, severe redness or itching, hepatitis, arthritis, unusual bleeding, bruising, and red spots. Methimazole and PTU may also produce a dangerous decrease in the number of white blood cells (agranulocytosis), which increases the risk for serious infections. Dosages higher than 40 mg/day of methimazole may increase the risk for agranulocytosis.

Like radioactive thyroid therapy, treatment with antithyroid drugs typically induces hypothyroidism. Hypothyroidism may appear as soon as 6 months after the onset of therapy or as long as 25 years after disease remission and discontinuation of drug therapy.

HYPOTHYROIDISM

Hypothyroidism is a condition in which the thyroid gland secretes deficient amounts of thyroid hormones. The following conditions are known to cause hypothyroidism: (1) treatment for hyperthyroidism with radioactive iodine and antithyroid drugs; (2) treatment with medications for non–thyroid-related conditions (e.g., lithium, amiodarone); (3) thyroidectomy (removal of all or a portion of the thyroid gland); (4) pituitary gland damage that affects TSH secretion; (5) congenital conditions (birth defects); and (6) thyroiditis. Autoimmune thyroiditis occurs when the body produces antibodies to its own thyroid cells. The antibodies and white blood cells attack and damage the thyroid. *Hashimoto's disease* is an autoimmune disorder and is the most common cause of non–iodine deficiency hypothyroidism.

BOX 32-3   **Symptoms of Hypothyroidism**

- Slowed heart rate
- Slowed pulse
- Lethargy
- Dry coarse hair
- Deep coarse voice
- Slow speech, thick tongue
- Enlarged heart
- Hypertension
- Cold intolerance
- Facial swelling

TABLE 32-1   **Comparison between Liothyronine and Levothyroxine**

Liothyronine (T₃)	Levothyroxine (Synthetic T₄)
Rapid onset	Longer onset
Short duration	Longer duration
Half-life ($t_{1/2}$) up to 24 hr	$t_{1/2}$ > 7 days
Three to four times more potent	Less potent
Administered in divided doses	Once daily dosing

TECH NOTE!
With the exception of liotrix, the generic name of thyroid replacement hormones contains the name of the naturally occurring hormone(s) they replace. For example, levothyroxine is the replacement for naturally occurring thyroxine.

TECH NOTE!
Pharmacy technicians should attempt to dispense the same manufacturer's product each time a patient's prescription is refilled.

TECH ALERT!
The following drugs have look-alike and sound-alike issues:
   levothyroxine and liothyronine;
   Levoxyl, Luvox, and Lanoxin;
   Synthroid and Symmetrel

Symptoms

The effects of insufficient thyroid hormones can be felt throughout the body. Symptoms of hypothyroidism are listed in Box 32-3.

Treatment of Hypothyroidism

Thyroid replacement therapy is the principal treatment for hypothyroidism. Replacement can be achieved by the administration of dessicated (dried, powdered) whole-gland animal thyroid or synthetic T_4, synthetic T_3, or a combination of the two hormones. The most widely prescribed treatment for hypothyroidism is synthetic T_4, which is converted in the body to T_3.

MECHANISM OF ACTION

Exogenously administered thyroid hormones, animal gland and synthetic, bind to the same receptor sites and produce the same actions as thyroid hormones produced by the body. Synthetic T_4, known as levothyroxine (L-thyroxine), is generally the only thyroid hormone prescribed for the treatment of hypothyroidism. Additional administration of liothyronine is typically unnecessary because levothyroxine is converted to liothyronine in the body, just as naturally occurring T_4 is metabolized to T_3.

PHARMACOKINETICS

Liothyronine (T_3) and levothyroxine are dissimilar in their onset and duration of action. They also differ in potency and dosing frequency. A comparison of the two drugs is presented in Table 32-1.

Bioavailability issues exist between different manufacturer's formulations of synthetic and naturally occurring thyroid preparations.

Numerous medications interact with thyroid hormones (Box 32-4). Ferrous products, calcium supplements, cholesterol-lowering agents (e.g., colestipol, cholestyramine), and didanosine interfere with the absorption of thyroid hormones. Food delays absorption. Antiseizure medicines such as phenytoin and carbamazepine accelerate the rate of metabolism of thyroid hormones. Soy isoflavones, oral contraceptives, and raloxifene reduce the clinical response to administered thyroid hormone by altering TSH, thyroglobulin, T_4, and T_3 levels. Thyroid hormones may increase the response to warfarin and decrease the response to oral antidiabetic agents, requiring close monitoring of the international normalized ratio (INR) and blood glucose levels.

Adverse Reactions. Given that thyroid replacement therapy is achieved by administering naturally occurring or synthetic thyroid hormone, adverse effects produced are the same as symptoms of hypothyroidism (subtherapeutic doses) or symptoms of hyperthyroidism (taking too much thyroid hormone).

Precautions. Diabetic patients may require an adjustment in their dose of diabetes medicine once thyroid replacement therapy is initiated. Thyroid hormones can affect blood sugar levels.

TECH NOTE!
Sometimes, the strength of dessicated thyroid is written as the grain (gr) strength. For example, 60 mg thyroid is equivalent to 1 gr thyroid.

TECH NOTE!
The various strengths of levothyroxine are color-coded to help avoid dispensing errors.

BOX 32-4 Medications That Interact with Thyroid Hormones

- Ferrous products (iron supplements)
- Calcium supplements and dairy products
- Soy isoflavones
- Raloxifene
- Cholestyramine
- Colestipol
- Oral contraceptives
- Phenytoin
- Carbamazepine

Thyroid Replacements

Generic Name	U.S. Brand Name(s) / Canadian Brand Name(s)	Dosage Forms and Strengths
levothyroxine* (T_4)	Levothroid, Levoxyl, Levo-T, Synthroid, Tirosint, Unithroid Eltroxin, Euthrox, Synthroid	**Capsule (Tirosint):** 25 mcg, 50 mcg, 75 mcg, 88 mcg, 100 mcg, 112 mcg, 125 mcg, 137 mcg, 150 mcg **Powder, for injection:** 100 mcg†, 200 mcg†, 500 mcg **Tablet:** 25 mcg###, 50 mcg, 75 mcg###, 88 mcg###, 100 mcg, 112 mcg, 125 mcg, 137 mcg, 150 mcg, 175 mcg###, 200 mcg, 300 mcg
liothyronine* (T_3)	Cytomel, Triostat Cytomel	**Solution, injection (Triostat):** 10 mcg/mL **Tablet (Cytomel):** 5 mcg, 25 mcg, 50 mcg†
liotrix* (T_4:T_3)	Thyrolar-1/4, Thyrolar-1/2, Thyrolar-1, Thyrolar-2, Thyrolar-3 Not available	**Tablet:** levothyroxine 12.5 mcg + liothyronine 3.1 mcg (Thyrolar-1/4), levothyroxine 25 mcg + liothyronine 6.25 mcg (Thyrolar-1/2), levothyroxine 50 mcg + liothyronine 12.5 mcg (Thyrolar-1), levothyroxine 100 mc + liothyronine 25 mcg (Thyrolar-2), levothyroxine 150 mcg + liothyronine 37.5 mcg (Thyrolar-3)
dessicated thyroid*	Armour, Bio-Throid, Nature Thyroid (NT-1/4, NT-1/2, NT-3/4, NT-1, NT-2, NT-2.5, NT-3, NT-4, NT-5) Generics	**Capsule (Bio-Throid):** 15 mg, 30 mg, 60 mg, 90 mg, 120 mg, 180 mg, 240 mg **Tablet (Armour, Nature Thyroid):** 15 mg†, 16.25 mg (NT-1/4)†, 30 mg, 32.5 mg (NT-1/2)†, 48.75 mg (NT-3/4)†, 60 mg, 65 mg (NT-1)†, 90 mg†, 97.5 mg (NT-1.5)†, 120 mg†, 125 mg‡, 130 mg (NT-2)†, 162.5 mg (NT-2.5)†, 180 mg†, 195 mg (NT-3)†, 240 mg†, 260 mg (NT-4)†, 300 mg†, 325 mg (NT-5)†

*Generic available.
†Strength available in the United States only.
‡Strength available in Canada only.
###Not available as Eltroxin.

Summary of Drugs Used in the Treatment of Thyroid Disorders

Generic Name	Brand Name	Usual Dose and Dosing Schedule	Warning Labels
Hyperthyroidism			
methimazole	Tapazole	15-60 mg in one to three divided doses/day until symptoms controlled for 2 mo; then reduce to 5-30 mg in one to three divided doses every 8 hr	AVOID PREGNANCY. TAKE ON AN EMPTY STOMACH OR WITH FOOD, BUT FOR CONSISTENT EFFECTS ALWAYS TAKE IT THE SAME WAY.
propylthiouracil (thiouracil)	Generics	Begin 300-1200 mg in three divided doses/day, maintenance 100-150 mg every 8-12 hr	
radioactive iodine,[131]I	Manufactured in pharmacy	6 to 15 µCi as a single dose	AVOID PREGNANCY.
Hypothyroidism			
levothyroxine	Synthroid, Levothroid	25-150 mcg once daily	AVOID ANTACIDS, DAIRY, CALCIUM AND IRON PILLS WITHIN 4 HR OF DOSE. TAKE ON AN EMPTY STOMACH. TAKE WITH A FULL GLASS OF WATER. DON'T SKIP DOSES.
liothyronine	Cytomel	25-75 mcg once daily	
liotrix	Thyrolar	50-100 mcg T_4 + 12.5-25 mcg T_3 once daily	
desiccated thyroid	Generics	60-120 mg once daily	

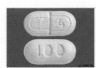

Chapter Summary

- Thyroid disorders result in overactivity of the thyroid gland or underactivity of the thyroid gland.
- Hyperthyroidism is a condition in which the thyroid gland secretes excessive amounts of thyroid hormones.
- Graves' disease is an autoimmune disease that causes hyperthyroidism.
- Thyroid-stimulating antibodies (TSAs), called thyroid-stimulating immunoglobulins, mimic TSH. When TSA binds to receptors on the thyroid gland, the gland releases hormones.
- Hypothyroidism is a condition in which the thyroid gland secretes deficient amounts of thyroid hormones.
- Hashimoto's disease is an autoimmune disorder that causes hypothyroidism.
- Hyperthyroidism and hypothyroidism are more prevalent in women than in men.
- Hyperthyroidism is most common in women between the ages of 20 and 40 years; women have a five to eight times greater prevalence of hypothyroidism than men.
- The incidence of hypothyroidism increases with age; by age 60 years, up to 17% of women and 9% of men will have an underactive thyroid.
- Patients with an autoimmune disease (e.g., type 1 diabetes) are at increased risk for developing thyroid disease.
- Cigarette smoking increases the risk for developing thyroid-related eye disease.
- The thyroid gland secretes hormones that have an affect on almost all cells in the body; they regulate growth and metabolism.
- The thyroid gland is one of the few glands that produces and stores its hormones.
- Thyroid hormones are synthesized by a coupling process that binds atoms of iodine to the thyroid protein thyroglobulin. T_4 has four atoms of iodine, and T_3 has three atoms of iodine.

- The TSH test measures the level of thyroid-stimulating hormone in the blood. A low TSH level signals hyperthyroidism.
- Free T_4 index (FT_4I) or FT_4 levels are high when hyperthyroidism is present and low if hypothyroidism is present.
- When thyroid antibodies are present, autoimmune thyroid disease is diagnosed.
- Low-dose radioactive iodine (^{131}I) is administered to measure the amount of radioactivity taken up by the thyroid gland. The RAIU is high when a person has hyperthyroidism and low when the person has hypothyroidism.
- Treatment of hyperthyroidism involves the use of antithyroid drugs, high-dose radioactive iodine (^{131}I), or surgery.
- Radioactive iodine is selectively taken up by the thyroid gland, where it causes glandular destruction without producing damage to other tissues. The rate of cure is approximately 66%. Pretreatment with an antithyroid drug is recommended.
- The full effects of ^{131}I therapy are usually achieved after 2 to 3 months.
- Most patients treated with ^{131}I develop an underactive thyroid gland after treatment, requiring lifelong therapy for hypothyroidism.
- Radioactive iodide therapy is contraindicated in pregnant women because the drug can cross the placenta and cause thyroid damage in the developing fetus.
- Radioactive iodine ^{131}I is made in nuclear pharmacies and is regulated by the Nuclear Regulatory Commission.
- Propylthiouracil and methimazole block the synthesis of T_4 and T_3. They bind thyroid peroxidase enzyme, which is the enzyme that activates the coupling of iodine and thyroglobulin and inhibits the coupling of iodinated tyrosine (MIT and DIT).
- PTU is capable of blocking the process that converts T_4 to T_3.
- It takes 2 to 4 months of therapy with PTU before maximum effects are achieved.
- Thyroid replacement therapy is the principal treatment for hypothyroidism. Replacement can be achieved by the administration of dessicated (dried, powdered) whole-gland animal thyroid or synthetic T_4, synthetic T_3, or a combination of the two hormones.
- Synthetic T_4, known as levothyroxine (L-thyroxine), is usually prescribed for the treatment of hypothyroidism.
- Levothyroxine is converted to liothyronine in the body, just as naturally occurring T_4 is metabolized to T_3.
- Liothyronine (T_3) and levothyroxine differ in their onset of action, duration of action, potency, and dosing frequency.
- Pharmacy technicians should attempt to dispense the same manufacturer's product each time a patient's prescription is refilled.
- Ferrous products, calcium supplements, and food can decrease the absorption of thyroid hormones.
- Sometimes, the strength of dessicated thyroid is written as the grain strength. For example, 60 mg thyroid is equivalent to 1 gr thyroid.
- The various strengths of levothyroxine are color-coded to help avoid dispensing errors.

REVIEW QUESTIONS

1. Tetraiodothyronine is the most abundant thyroid hormone. It contains _____ atom(s) of iodine and is also known as thyroxine.
   a. Three
   b. Four
   c. Two
   d. One

2. Hyperthyroidism and hypothyroidism are more prevalent in women than in men.
   a. True
   b. False

3. _____ is an autoimmune disease that is the primary cause of thyroid hyperactivity.
    a. Hashimoto's disease
    b. TSH disease
    c. Graves' disease
    d. All of the above

4. Treatment of hyperthyroidism involves the administration of _____.
    a. Antithyroid drugs
    b. Radioactive iodine
    c. Surgery
    d. All of the above

5. Which thyroid drug could produce a dangerous drop in the number of white blood cells (agranulocytosis), which increases the risk for serious infection?
    a. Propylthiouracil
    b. Cytomel
    c. Synthroid
    d. Thyrolar

6. It takes _____ of therapy with propylthiouracil before maximum effects are achieved.
    a. 1 to 2 months
    b. 2 to 4 months
    c. 5 to 6 months
    d. 6 to 8 months

7. A brand name for levothyroxine is _____.
    a. Cytomel
    b. Thyrolar
    c. Proloid
    d. Synthroid

8. Ferrous products, calcium supplements, and food can increase the absorption of thyroid hormones.
    a. True
    b. False

9. Hashimoto's disease is an autoimmune disorder that causes _____.
    a. Hypothyroidism
    b. Hyperthyroidism

10. Diabetes is not a risk factor for thyroid disease.
    a. True
    b. False

TECHNICIAN'S CORNER

1. What is an autoimmune disease, and what are the effects of an autoimmune disease such as Graves' disease?
2. What types of food provide iodine?

Bibliography

Becker D, Hurley J, Detres R, Thyroid Foundation of Canada: Radioactive iodine treatment of hyperthyroidism. 1992 (http://www.thyroid.ca/thyrotoxicosis.php).

Cawood T, Moriarty P, O'Farrelly C, et al: Smoking and thyroid-associated ophthalmopathy: A novel explanation of the biological link. *J Clin Endocrinol Metab* 92:59-64, 2007.

De Moraes A, Pedro A, Romaldini J: Spontaneous hypothyroidism in the follow-up of Graves' hyperthyroid patients treated with antithyroid drugs. *South Med J* 99:1068-1072, 2006.

Elsevier: Gold Standard Clinical Pharmacology. Retrieved June 12, 2011, from https://www.clinical pharmacology.com/. 2010.

FDA: FDA Approved Drug Products. Retrieved June 12, 2012, from http://www.accessdata.fda.gov/scripts/cder/drugsatfda/index.cfm?fuseaction=Search.Search_Drug_Name. 2012.

Health Canada: Drug product database. Retrieved June 12, 2012, from http://www.hc-sc.gc.ca/dhp-mps/prodpharma/databasdon/index-eng.php. 2010.

Hormone Foundation: Hormones & you: Hyperthyroidism. (http://www.hormone.org/Resources/upload/hyperthyroidism-bilingual-042810.pdf). 2010.

Hormone Foundation: Hormones & you: Hypothyroidism. (http://www.hormone.org/Resources/upload/hypothyroidism-bilingual-042810.pdf). 2010.

Kalant H, Grant D, Mitchell J: *Principles of medical pharmacology*, ed 7, Toronto, 2007, Elsevier Canada, pp 613-619.

Lance L, Lacy C, Armstrong L, et al: *Drug information handbook for the allied health professional*, ed 12, Hudson, OH, 2005, APhA Lexi-Comp.

National Institute of Diabetes and Digestive and Kidney Diseases: Graves' disease (NIH Publ. No. 08-6217). (http://endocrine.niddk.nih.gov/pubs/graves). 2008.

National Institute of Diabetes and Digestive and Kidney Diseases: Hashimoto's disease (NIH Publ. No. 09-6399). (http://endocrine.niddk.nih.gov/pubs/Hashimoto). 2009.

Page C, Curtis M, Sutter M, et al: *Integrated pharmacology*, Philadelphia, 2005, Mosby, pp 288-291.

Raffa R, Rawls S, Beyzarov E: *Netter's illustrated pharmacology*, Philadelphia, 2005, Saunders Elsevier, pp 10-11, 136-142.

Thyroid Foundation of Canada: About thyroid disease. (http://www.thyroid.ca/thyroid_disease.php). 2011.

Wang S, Baker J Jr: Targeting B cells in Graves' disease, *Endocrinology* 147:4559-4560, 2006.

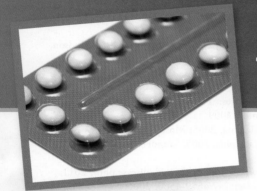

33

Treatment of Diabetes Mellitus

KEY TERMS

Diabetes mellitus: Chronic condition in which the body is unable to use glucose (sugar) as energy properly.

Diabetic neuropathy: Nerve disorder caused by uncontrolled diabetes. This disorder leads to pain or loss of feeling in the toes, feet, legs, hands, and/or arms.

Fasting blood glucose: Blood glucose level after a person has not eaten for 8 to 12 hours (usually overnight).

Gestational diabetes: Diabetes that may be caused by the hormones of pregnancy or a shortage of insulin.

Hemoglobin A1c: Blood test that measures a person's average blood glucose level over a period of 2 to 3 months.

Hyperglycemia: Elevated blood glucose levels.

Hypoglycemia: Low blood glucose levels.

Insulin resistance: Condition in which the body does not respond to insulin; contributes to the development of type 2 diabetes.

Postprandial: After eating.

Prediabetes: Condition of impaired fasting glucose and impaired glucose tolerance in which the body consistently has elevated glucose levels.

Type 1 diabetes: An autoimmune disease that results in high blood glucose levels. Pancreatic beta cells are destroyed and insufficient amounts of insulin are produced.

Type 2 diabetes: A condition that results in high blood glucose levels. People with type 2 diabetes have insulin resistance.

Overview

Diabetes mellitus is a disorder of metabolism that involves glucose utilization. It is a chronic condition in which the body cannot properly use glucose as energy. Glucose is the body's primary energy source. Under normal conditions, as glucose levels in the blood rise, hormones are released that move the glucose out of the bloodstream and into cells, where it is needed for growth and energy. In diabetes, glucose accumulates in the blood. Much like a person with sticky hands walking through a room, glucose in the bloodstream leaves a sticky residue over all the body's organs and cells in which it comes in contact and causes damage.

According to the National Institutes of Diabetes and Digestive and Kidney Diseases (NIDDK), 25.6 million people older than 20 years have diabetes in the United States and 1.9 million were newly diagnosed in 2010. According to the Centers for Disease Control and Prevention (CDC), it is estimated that by 2050 the number of people diagnosed with diabetes will jump 165% above current levels. In 2005, 5.5% (1.8 million) of the Canadian population older than 12 years were diagnosed with diabetes mellitus and it is estimated that 2.4 million will have the disease by 2016. The number of people diagnosed with prediabetes is also alarmingly high, 54 million. Almost 50% of the estimated cases of diabetes are undiagnosed.

Diabetes mellitus is one of the leading causes of disability in the United States. It is the leading cause of non–war-related amputations. In the United States, diabetes was the seventh leading cause of death in 2007 and, according to the 2005 Canadian Community Health Survey, diabetes was the seventh leading cause of death in Canada. In the United States, one of every eight federal health care dollars is spent treating people with diabetes. NIDDK National Statistics has estimated the direct and indirect cost of diabetes in the United States is $174 billion dollars. The costs in Canada were estimated to be 10% of health care dollars ($5.6 billion) in 2005.

HORMONE REGULATION OF BLOOD GLUCOSE LEVEL

Insulin is a hormone that is essential for the regulation of carbohydrates, fat, and protein metabolism. When the blood glucose level rises, as occurs after a meal, beta cells in the islets of Langerhans secrete insulin. The control of glucose levels occurs by a second-messenger reaction. Insulin binds to receptors on the cell membrane. This stimulates the docking of intracellular glucose transporters that carry glucose out of the bloodstream and into cells where it is needed. Insulin, along with glucagon, is released by the pancreas in response to the rise and fall of blood glucose, amino acid, and gut-derived hormone levels (Figure 33-1).

When glucose levels drop, glucagon is secreted by alpha cells in the islets of Langerhans. The physiological effects of insulin are primarily anabolic; for example, glucose that is not needed for energy immediately is stored in the liver as glycogen, a reservoir for future energy needs (Figure 33-2). The physiological effects of glucagon are primarily catabolic. It releases energy stores. The physiological effects of insulin are listed in Box 33-1.

TYPES OF DIABETES MELLITUS

Prediabetes, type 1 diabetes, type 2 diabetes, and gestational diabetes all produce elevated blood glucose levels. A normal *fasting blood glucose* level is 70 to 99 mg/dL, or less than 4 to 6 mmol/liter.

BOX 33-1   **Physiological Effects of Insulin**

CARBOHYDRATE METABOLISM
- Increased glycogen synthesis (liver)
- Decreased gluconeogenesis (liver)
- Increased glucose transport (muscle and fat cells)

LIPID METABOLISM
- Sets the level of triglyceride production from free fatty acids
- Decreased lipolysis

PROTEIN METABOLISM
- Increased amino acid synthesis
- Increased amino acid transport (precursors for protein synthesis)

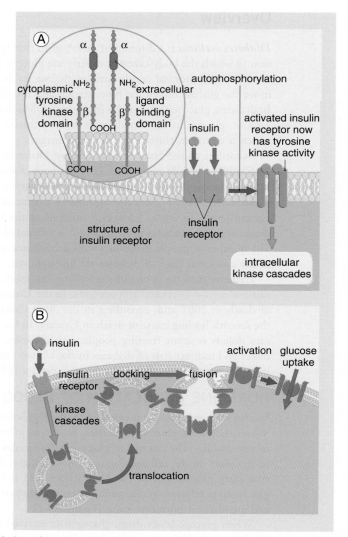

FIGURE 33-1 Insulin action. (From Page C, Curtis M, Sutter M, et al: *Integrated pharmacology*, ed 3, Philadelphia, 2006, Mosby.)

Prediabetes

Prediabetes causes impaired fasting glucose (IFG) and impaired glucose tolerance (IGT). When blood glucose levels range between 100 and 125 mg/dL (6.1 to 6.9 mmol/liter) after an overnight fast, glucose levels are said to be impaired. After a 2-hour oral glucose tolerance test, blood glucose levels are high and range from 140 to 199 mg/dL (7.8 to 11.0 mmol/liter) in those with IGT. Prediabetes increases the risk of cardiovascular disease.

Type 1 Diabetes

Type 1 diabetes is an autoimmune disease. The immune system attacks and destroys the insulin-producing beta cells in the pancreas. Hypotheses for the cause of this autoimmune disorder include exposure to environmental factors, viruses, and possibly genetics. Only 5% to 10% of all persons with diabetes have type 1 diabetes. Those with this type of diabetes must inject insulin daily. Their body can no longer produce sufficient amounts of the hormone insulin. The onset of type 1 diabetes is typically in childhood; hence, the condition was formerly called juvenile-onset diabetes mellitus. Type 1 diabetes can occur at any age. Type 1 diabetes occurs equally among males and females but is more common in whites than in nonwhites.

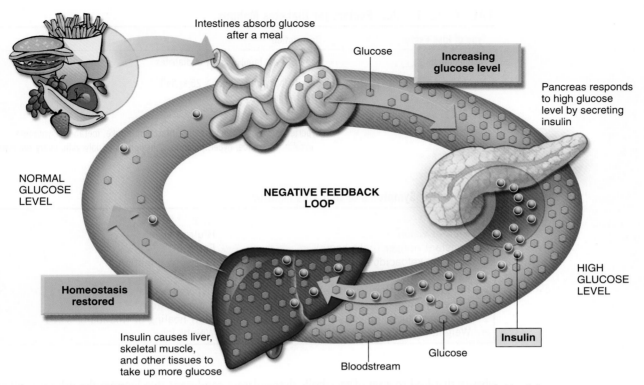

FIGURE 33-2 Role of insulin. (From Thibodeau GA, Patton KT: *Anatomy and physiology*, ed 6, St. Louis, 2007, Mosby.)

Type 2 Diabetes

Type 2 diabetes is most common, accounting for 90% to 95% of all cases of diabetes. In type 2 diabetes, the pancreas initially produces sufficient amounts of insulin, but the body is unable to use the insulin effectively. This condition is called *insulin resistance*. Insulin production eventually decreases; however, this may not occur for several years. Risk factors of type 2 diabetes are obesity, lack of physical activity, family history of diabetes, prior gestational diabetes, and increasing age. Approximately 80% of persons diagnosed with type 2 diabetes are overweight. Type 2 diabetes was formerly called non–insulin-dependent diabetes (NIDDM); however, this term has been replaced because people with type 2 diabetes may sometimes be required to manage their condition with insulin.

The prevalence of type 2 diabetes is increased in Aboriginal Canadians, Native Americans, African Americans, and Mexican Americans. Genetics is one possible explanation; however, it is also believed that the increased prevalence may be linked to internalized racism, chronic stress, and consumption of a "diabetes" diet that is high in fat and carbohydrates.

Gestational Diabetes

Gestational diabetes occurs in approximately 3% to 8% of all pregnant women. It typically occurs late in pregnancy. Because it may have no symptoms, pregnant women are routinely tested for gestational diabetes. Blood glucose levels are normally lower than normal during pregnancy so an elevated blood glucose level is a sign of gestational diabetes. Gestational diabetes may be caused by the hormones of pregnancy or by a shortage of insulin. Symptoms often disappear after delivery; however, women who have had gestational diabetes have a 20% to 50% increased risk for the development of type 2 diabetes within 5 to 10 years.

INSULIN RESISTANCE AS A CAUSE OF DIABETES

Insulin resistance is a condition in which the body does not respond to insulin. It is a precursor to type 2 diabetes. Insulin resistance is a syndrome associated with genetic factors, inactivity, diet, and

TABLE 33-1 **Risk Factors for Diabetes Mellitus**

Type of Risk Factor	Description
Nonmodifiable	Age (≥40 yr), family history of diabetes
Modifiable	Obesity (body mass index ≥ 25 kg/m^2) Physical inactivity Smoking
Disease	Hypertension, angina, myocardial infarction, stroke, metabolic syndrome, insulin resistance, hyperlipidemia, schizophrenia, polycystic ovary syndrome

BOX 33-2 **Symptoms of Diabetes Mellitus**

TYPE 1
- Blurred vision
- Constant hunger (polyphagia)
- Diabetic ketoacidosis
- Extreme fatigue
- Frequent urination (polyuria)
- Hyperglycemia
- Increased thirst (polydipsia)
- Weight loss

TYPE 2
- Blurred vision
- Fatigue
- Frequent urination
- Hunger
- Hyperglycemia
- Increased thirst
- Slow healing of wounds or sores
- Weight loss

obesity that lead to a set of metabolic dysregulatory conditions that increase the risk for cardiovascular disease, hypertension, dyslipidemia, elevated triglyceride and low-density lipoprotein (LDL) levels, decreased high-density lipoprotein (HDL) levels, microalbuminuria, and diabetes. It may also increase risk for obesity, a risk factor for type 2 diabetes, because one role of the hormone insulin is to signal the need to increase food intake. Feedback signals are proportionate to body fat (Table 33-1).

SYMPTOMS AND DIAGNOSIS OF DIABETES MELLITUS
Symptoms
Symptoms of diabetes mellitus are listed in Box 33-2.

Diagnostic Tests
Blood glucose testing for elevated glucose levels is the principal method used to diagnose diabetes. Typically, blood glucose levels are measured after fasting; however, the oral glucose tolerance test measures blood glucose levels after consumption of a dose of glucose that has been administered.
- Fasting blood glucose test: Blood glucose level 126 mg/dL or higher (≥7 mmol/liter) or more after an 8-hour fast.
- Oral glucose tolerance test (OGTT): Blood glucose level 200 mg/dL or higher (≥11 mmol/liter) 2 hours after drinking a beverage containing 75 g of glucose dissolved in water.
- Random blood glucose: Blood glucose level 200 mg/dL or higher (≥11 mmol/liter), along with the presence of diabetes symptoms.

The *hemoglobin A1c* (Hb$_{A1c}$) test is the only test that provides information about blood glucose levels over a 2- to 3-month period. The American Diabetes Association and Canadian Diabetes Association now approve the Hb$_{A1c}$ test for diagnosis of diabetes.

DIABETES COMPLICATIONS
Complications of untreated or poorly controlled diabetes mellitus occur throughout the body (Box 33-4). Diabetes mellitus causes microvascular and macrovascular damage. Microvascular damage may lead to weakened blood vessels in the eye that leak contents into the retina (retinopathy), leading to blurred vision and blindness. Nephropathy (kidney damage) and *diabetic neuropathy* also occur. Nerve damage caused by peripheral neuropathy results in numbness in the lower limbs. Patients with diabetes must frequently inspect their feet because if they develop a foot injury, they might

TECH NOTE!
Alcohol, aspirin, and decongestants can alter blood glucose levels. A list of drugs that increase and decrease blood glucose levels is provided in Box 33-3.

not feel it. Diabetes causes poor wound healing, so foot infections sometimes become serious enough to require limb amputation. Macrovascular changes can lead to hypertension, angina, and myocardial infarction. Diabetes can also cause hyperlipidemia. Individuals with untreated or poorly controlled type 1 diabetes may develop ketoacidosis, a condition in which the body breaks down fats to obtain its energy needs. Ketones are a byproduct of lipid metabolism, and their accumulation can lead to coma and death. Poorly controlled diabetes mellitus may also result in continued hyperglycemia and some drugs used for treatment may produce hypoglycemia. Symptoms of *hyperglycemia* and *hypoglycemia* and are listed in Box 33-5.

BOX 33-3   **Drugs That Increase or Decrease Blood Glucose Levels**

DRUGS ASSOCIATED WITH HYPERGLYCEMIA	DRUGS ASSOCIATED WITH HYPOGLYCEMIA
• Atypical antipsychotics • Beta blockers • Diuretics, thiazides (>25 mg hydrochlorothiazide) • Glucocorticoids • Growth hormone • Nicotinic acid • Pentamidine • Phenytoin • Protease inhibitors • Sympathomimetics	• Acetylsalicylic acid (ASA; salicylates) • Alcohol • Angiotensin-converting enzyme inhibitors; angiotensin II receptor blockers • Beta blockers

BOX 33-4   **Diabetes Complications**

• Amputation • Angina • Blindness • Blurred vision • Heart attack • Hyperlipidemia • Hypertension • Increased birth defects	• Infections • Ketoacidosis • Nephropathy • Peripheral neuropathy • Pregnancy complications • Retinopathy • Stroke

BOX 33-5   **Symptoms of Hyperglycemia and Hypoglycemia**

HYPERGLYCEMIA	HYPOGLYCEMIA
• Blurred vision • Breath that smells fruity • Decreased consciousness • Dry mouth • Elevated blood glucose level • Extreme hunger • Extreme thirst • Frequent urination • Shortness of breath • Upset stomach and vomiting • Weakness	• Anxiety, nervousness, irritability • Blurred vision • Cold sensations • Confusion • Difficulty concentrating • Fatigue, uncontrolled yawning • Headache • Hunger • Loss of consciousness • Low blood glucose level • Muscle weakness • Nausea • Numbness of the mouth • Pale skin • Palpitations, rapid heartbeat • Shallow breathing • Sweating • Tingling in the fingers • Tremors

Management of Diabetes

NONPHARMACOLOGICAL MANAGEMENT

Diabetes mellitus is sometimes classified as a disease of lifestyle because lifestyle factors can increase the risk for type 2 diabetes and all types of diabetes can be improved by weight loss, engaging in physical activity, consuming foods with a low glycemic index, quitting smoking, and other lifestyle changes. Physical activity lowers the risk of type 2 diabetes by up to 30%. For those with diabetes, increased physical activity decreases risks of mortality from the disease. A minimum of 150 minutes of exercise weekly is recommended to maintain glycemic control, of which at least 90 minutes should be vigorous aerobic exercise. Loss of 5% to 7% of body weight through diet and increased physical activity can lower the risks of diabetes (Box 33-6).

BLOOD GLUCOSE MONITORING

Blood glucose monitoring is an essential component of diabetes management (Figure 33-3). Measurement of blood glucose levels may be recommended one to four times daily, depending on the type of diabetes (type 1, type 2, or gestational) and on the antihyperglycemic drug regimen that the patient is prescribed. Knowledge of blood glucose levels enables individuals with diabetes to take control of their disease and adjust their level of diet, exercise, and insulin (Figure 33-4).

Maintenance of the blood glucose level within a normal range has been shown to minimize the risk of diabetic complications. According to the Diabetes Control and Complications Trial (DCCT), a 10-year study sponsored by the NIDDK and the United Kingdom Prospective Diabetes Study, intensive control of blood glucose and blood pressure reduces complications in types 1 and 2 diabetes.

BOX 33-6   **Recommended Lifestyle Modifications**

- Eat low glycemic index foods.
- Engage in physical activity.
- Stop smoking.
- Lose weight.

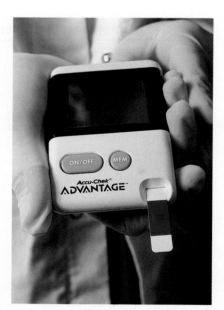

FIGURE 33-3 Blood glucose monitor. (From Bonewit-West K: *Clinical procedures for medical assistants*, ed 7, St. Louis, 2008, Saunders.)

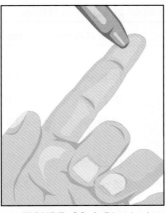
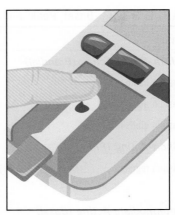
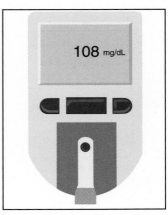

FIGURE 33-4 Blood glucose testing using a blood glucose meter (From MedlinePlus: *Diabetes.* [http://www.nlm.nih.gov/medlineplus/diabetes.html]. 2012.)

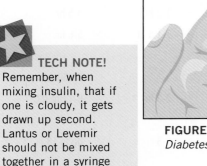

TECH NOTE!
Remember, when mixing insulin, that if one is cloudy, it gets drawn up second. Lantus or Levemir should not be mixed together in a syringe with any other form of insulin.

TECH NOTE!
Rapid-acting insulin (aspart, glulisine, lispro), regular insulin, and long-acting insulin (detemir, glargine) are clear solutions that should be discarded if they appear cloudy.

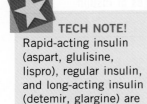

TECH NOTE!
Individuals with diabetes must eat scheduled meals. Basal bolus insulin administration mimics normal fluctuations of insulin levels throughout the day in response to preprandial and *postprandial* glucose levels.

TECH NOTE!
Insulin is the most effective agent for glycemic control and reduces the Hb$_{A1c}$ level by more than 2%.

PHARMACOLOGICAL MANAGEMENT

At present, type 1 diabetes is primarily managed with insulin. Pramlintide (Symlin) is a synthetic analogue of the hormone amylin that is also used for the treatment of type 1 diabetes. Type 2 diabetes may be treated with oral agents. Oral antidiabetic agents are only indicated as an adjunct to diet and exercise in the treatment of type 2 diabetes mellitus.

Insulin

Insulin is administered for the management of all types of diabetes. It helps the body metabolize carbohydrates, fats, and proteins from the diet. It may be the sole drug administered, as in type 1 diabetes, or may be added to oral therapy or replace oral therapy, as in type 2 diabetes. Insulin was originally manufactured from animal sources (pig and cow); however, genetically engineered insulin using recombinant DNA technology (see Chapter 1) to match human insulin has replaced animal source insulin. Pork and bovine insulins are no longer marketed in the United States or Canada but are still available in other parts of the world.

MECHANISM OF ACTION AND PHARMACOKINETICS

Insulin is a protein, so it cannot be taken orally, because it would be digested in the stomach by gastric acids. Insulin is administered subcutaneously. Regular insulin may also be administered intravenously. The insulin administered for the treatment of diabetes has the identical mechanism of action as naturally occurring human insulin. It is formulated in rapid-acting, short-acting, intermediate-acting, and long-acting form. The onset of action for rapid-acting insulin (aspart, glulisine, lispro insulin) begins within 15 minutes, whereas the onset of action for long-acting insulin (detemir, glargine insulin) is 90 minutes (Table 33-2). Rapid-acting insulin is injected 5 to 15 minutes before eating, or even after a meal for some individuals. Long-acting basal insulin, administered at bedtime, has the advantage of lower risk for nighttime hypoglycemia when compared with NPH insulin, which is also used for basal insulin needs. Basal bolus insulin administration is recommended by the Canadian Diabetes Association Clinical Guidelines for people with type 1 diabetes. Intermediate- or long-acting basal insulin is typically administered once or twice daily and rapid-acting prandial insulin is injected at mealtime.

Dosage delivery systems for the administration of insulin are the insulin pump, vial and syringe, and insulin pen (Figure 33-5).

ADVERSE REACTIONS

Insulin replacement therapy produces symptoms similar to effects produced by the naturally secreted hormone at its target site. In addition to hypoglycemia, insulin therapy may cause weight gain, pain, or irritation at the injection site and lipohypertrophy or lipoatrophy. Lipohypertrophy results in fat accumulation around the injection site. Lipoatrophy results in areas of fat loss around the site of injection, causing depressions. Patients should be advised to rotate the site of injection.

TABLE 33-2   **Onset, Peak, and Duration of Action of Insulin**

Insulin	Onset of Action	Peak Action	Duration of Action
Ultra–Rapid-Acting (Prandial)			
insulin lispro	10-15 min	1-1.5 hr	6-8 hr
insulin aspart	10-15 min	1-2 hr	3-5 hr
insulin glulisine	10-15 min	1-1.5 hr	5-6 hr
Short-Acting (Prandial)			
insulin regular	15 min (IV)	—	30-60 min (IV)
	30 min (SC)	2-3 hr	8-12 hr (SC)
Intermediate-Acting (Basal)			
Neutral protamine Hagedorn (NPH), recombinant	1-3 hr	5-8	Up to 18 hr
Long-Acting (Basal)			
insulin glargine	1.5 hr	Not applicable	Up to 24 hr
insulin detemir	1.5 hr	6-8 hr	Up to 24 hr

TABLE 33-3   **Recommended Storage for Opened Vials and Cartridges of Insulin**

Type of Insulin	Storage
insulin aspart and insulin glulisine	Vials: Room temperature or refrigerated—discard after 28 days. Cartridges: Store at room temperature; discard after 28 days.
insulin detemir	Vials: Room temperature or refrigerated—discard after 42 days. Cartridges: Store at room temperature; discard after 42 days.
insulin glargine	Vials and cartridges: Refrigerated—discard after 28 days (5 and 10 mL).
insulin lispro	Vial, cartridges, and pens: Room temperature or refrigerated—once opened, discard after 28 days. Insulin pump: Discard after 7 days.
NPH insulin	Vial: Room temperature or refrigerated—discard after 42 days. Cartridges: Room temperature or refrigerated—once opened, store at room temperature; discard after 14 days.

Insulin

Generic Name	U.S. Brand Name(s) / Canadian Brand Name(s)	Dosage Forms and Strengths
insulin aspart (rDNA origin)	Novolog, Novolog FlexPen, Novolog Penfill / Novorapid	Suspension, for injection (vial, pen, cartridge): 100 units/mL
insulin lispro	Humalog, Humalog cartridge, Humalog KwikPen / Humalog, Humalog cartridge, Humalog KwikPen	Suspension, for injection (vial, pen, cartridge): 100 units/mL
insulin glulisine	Apidra, Apidra SoloStar / Apidra, Apidra SoloStar, Apidra cartridge	Injection, solution (vial, pen, cartridge): 100 units/mL
insulin regular (rDNA origin)	Humulin R, Novolin R / Humulin R, Humulin R cartridge	Injection, solution (vial, cartridge): 100 units/mL, 500 units/mL
Neutral Protamine Hagedorn (NPH) insulin (rDNA origin)	Humulin N, Humulin N Pen, Novolin N / Humulin N, Humulin N Pen, Humulin N cartridge, Novolin GE NPH, Novolin GE NPH pen, Novolin GE Toronto‡^	Suspension, for injection (vial, pen, cartridge): 100 units/mL
insulin detemir (rDNA origin)	Levemir, Levemir FlexPen / Levemir Penfill	Solution, for injection (vial, pen, cartridge): 100 units/mL

TECH NOTE!
Insulin must be protected from extremes in heat and cold. Refrigerate unopened vials; do not freeze. Opened vials of insulin may be stored at room temperature, but this will shorten the expiry date for most insulin. Check the manufacturer's insert (Table 33-3).

Insulin—cont'd

Generic Name	U.S. Brand Name(s) Canadian Brand Name(s)	Dosage Forms and Strengths
insulin glargine (rDNA origin)	Lantus, Lantus SoloStar Lantus, Lantus SoloStar, Lantus cartridge	Solution, for injection (vial, pen, cartridge): 100 units/mL
Insulin Mixtures		
insulin regular + insulin isophane	Humulin 70/30, Novolin 70/30 Humulin 30/70, Humulin 30/70 cartridge Novolin GE Penfill 30/70 Novolin GE Penfill 40/60 Novolin GE Penfill 50/50	Suspension, for injection (vial, pen, cartridge): 30 units/mL insulin + 70 units/mL insulin isophane 50 units/mL insulin + 50 units/mL insulin isophane 40 units/mL insulin + 60 units/mL insulin isophane‡
lispro insulin + lispro protamine suspension	Humalog Mix 50/50, Humalog KwikPen 50/50, Humalog Mix 75/25, Humalog Mix 75/25 KwikPen Humalog Mix 25, Humalog (pen) 25, Humalog Mix 50, Humalog (pen) 50	Suspension, for injection (cartridge, pen): 75 units lispro protamine suspension + 25 units lispro insulin 50 units lispro insulin + 50 units lispro protamine suspension
insulin aspart + insulin aspart protamine	Novolog Mix, Novolog Mix Flexpen Novomix-30 penfill	Suspension, for injection (vial, pen, cartridge): 30 units insulin aspart + 70 units insulin aspart protamine

‡Strength available in Canada only.
^For SC, IM, or IV administration.

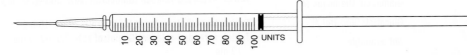

A

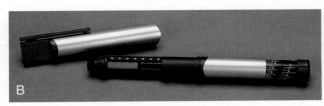

B

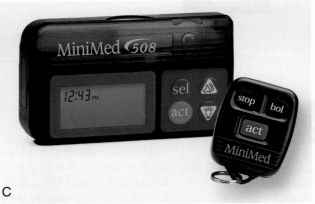

C

FIGURE 33-5 Dosage delivery systems for the administration of insulin. A. Standard insulin syringe, B. Insulin Pen, C. Insulin Pump. (A and B from Fulcher EM, Fulcher RM, Soto CD: Pharmacology Principles and Applications, ed 3, St Louis, 2012, Saunders. C Courtesy of MiniMed, Sylmar, California in Fulcher EM, Fulcher RM, Soto CD: Pharmacology Principles and Applications, ed 3, St Louis, 2012, Saunders.) (From National Institutes of Diabetes and Digestive and Kidney Diseases: *Alternative devices for taking insulin* [NIH Publ. No. 09-4643].) (http://diabetes.niddk.nih.gov/dm/pubs/insulin/ Alternative_Devices_Insulin.pdf. 2009.)

Sulfonylureas

Sulfonylureas are sometimes categorized as oral hypoglycemic agents (OHAs). They are only effective for the treatment of type 2 diabetes. They are very effective in producing glycemic control and can reduce the Hb_{A1c} level by 1% to 2%.

MECHANISM OF ACTION AND PHARMACOKINETICS

Sulfonylureas primarily stimulate insulin release from pancreatic beta cells. Sulfonylureas also decrease glycogenolysis, the process of converting glycogen (storage form of glucose) to glucose.

Sulfonylureas are classified as first- or second-generation agents. First-generation agents—chlorpropamide, tolbutamide, and tolazamide—are still marketed but are rarely prescribed. Sulfonylureas differ in pharmacokinetics, pharmacodynamics, and incidence of hypoglycemic reactions. For example, glyburide has the highest risk for hypoglycemia, followed by glicazide, and glimepiride has the lowest risk. Glyburide has active metabolites that can accumulate in patients with kidney disease.

ADVERSE REACTIONS

Sulfonylureas can produce hypoglycemia, a serious side effect. Other side effects include weight gain, abdominal pain, diarrhea, dyspepsia, nausea and vomiting, headache, and dizziness. Infrequently, sulfonylureas may produce bone marrow toxicity and cholestatic jaundice.

TECH NOTE!
Conventional and micronized dosage forms of glyburide are not substitutable.

Sulfonylureas

Generic Name	U.S. Brand Name(s)	Dosage Forms and Strengths
	Canadian Brand Name(s)	
glyburide*	Diabeta, Glynase PresTab	Tablet (Diabeta, Micronase): 1.25 mg, 2.5 mg, 5 mg
	Diabeta, Euglucon	Tablet, micronized (Glynase PresTab): 1.5 mg, 3 mg, 4.5 mg, 6 mg
glicazide*	Not available	Tablet, immediate-release (Diamicron): 80 mg
	Diamicron, Diamicron MR	Tablet, extended-release (Diamicron MR): 30 mg, 60 mg
glipizide*	Glucotrol, Glucotrol XL	Tablet, immediate-release (Glucotrol): 5 mg, 10 mg
	Not available	Tablet, extended-release (Glucotrol XL): 2.5 mg, 5 mg, 10 mg
glimepiride*	Amaryl	Tablet: 1 mg, 2 mg, 4 mg
	Amaryl	

*Generic available.

TECH ALERT!
The following drugs have look-alike and sound-alike issues:
  tolazamide and tolbutamide;
  glyburide, glipizide, and glicazide;
  Diabeta and Zebeta;
  Micronase, Micro K, and Micronor;
  Glucotrol and Glucotrol XL;
  Amaryl and Amerge

Biguanides

Metformin is classified as a biguanide antidiabetic agent. Its effects are unrelated to pancreatic islet cell function. Metformin acts to control fasting blood glucose. It is effective in producing glycemic control and reduces HbA1c levels by 1% to 2% without producing hypoglycemia. This makes metformin a first-line drug for the treatment of type 2 diabetes. Unlike most other antihyperglycemic agents, metformin does not cause weight gain, which is a benefit when treating obese patients with type 2 diabetes.

MECHANISM OF ACTION

Metformin improves glucose tolerance and insulin resistance by increasing peripheral glucose uptake and utilization in skeletal muscles and adipose tissue. It increases glucose transport across cell membranes. Metformin also lowers postprandial plasma glucose levels, decreases hepatic gluconeogenesis (new glucose) production, and decreases intestinal absorption of glucose.

PHARMACOKINETICS

Metformin may be administered in immediate-release (tablets and solution) and extended-release dosage forms. Peak blood levels are achieved in 2.5 hours for immediate-release tablets, 2.2 hours

Biguanides

Generic Name	U.S. Brand Name(s)	Dosage Forms and Strengths
	Canadian Brand Name(s)	
metformin*	Fortamet, Glucophage, Glucophage XR, Glumetza, Riomet	Solution, oral (Riomet): 100 mg/mL Tablet, immediate-release: 500 mg, 850 mg, 1000 mg† Tablet, extended-release: (Glumetza): 500 mg, 1000 mg (Fortamet): 500 mg, 1000 mg (Glucophage XR): 500 mg, 750 mg
	Glucophage, Glumetza	

Combination Biguanide + Sulfonylureas

metformin + glyburide*	Glucovance	Tablet: 250 mg metformin + 1.25 mg glyburide 500 mg metformin + 2.5 mg glyburide 500 mg metformin + 5 mg glyburide
	Not available	
metformin + glipizide*	Generic	Tablet: 250 mg metformin + 2.5 mg glipizide 500 mg metformin + 2.5 mg glipizide 500 mg metformin + 5 mg glipizide
	Not available	

*Generic available.
†Strength available in the United States only.

for oral solution, and 7 hours for extended-release tablets. Food decreases the absorption of immediate-release tablets but increases the absorption of metformin solution and extended-release tablets. Glumetza, Glucophage XR, and Fortamet are all extended-release dosage forms of metformin; however, they are not substitutable because different processes are used to make the drug into a time-release formulation.

ADVERSE REACTIONS

Gastrointestinal adverse reactions are common. They include gas, heartburn, metallic taste in the mouth, mild stomachache, nausea, and weight loss. Metformin may produce lactic acidosis, a rare but potentially fatal condition. Metformin may stimulate ovulation in infertile women that have polycystic ovary syndrome.

α-Glucosidase Inhibitors

α-Glucosidase inhibitors prolong the digestion of carbohydrates and delay their absorption in the small intestine. They reduce peak plasma glucose levels. α-Glucosidase inhibitors do not promote insulin secretion like many other antidiabetic agents, nor do they cause hypoglycemia. They produce a minimal effect on reducing Hb_{A1c} levels (< 1%) and therefore are not used as monotherapy.

MECHANISM OF ACTION AND PHARMACOKINETICS

Acarbose is an inhibitor of several α-glucosidases (e.g., glycoamylase, sucrase, maltase, dextranase). The antidiabetic agent miglitol also inhibits the α-glucosidases maltase and sucrase. α-Glucosidases are enzymes that break down carbohydrates. Acarbose and miglitol must be administered with the first bite of each meal. The drugs are oral oligosaccharides that compete for binding sites with oligosaccharides and disaccharides in foods. It is important to eat a diet rich in complex carbohydrates while taking acarbose and miglitol.

ADVERSE REACTIONS

α-Glucosidase inhibitors most commonly produce gastrointestinal side effects. Adverse reactions include a bloated feeling, diarrhea, stomach or intestinal gas, or rumbling stomach and stomach pain or discomfort.

Meglitinides

Meglitinides are oral antidiabetic agents used in the treatment and management of type 2 diabetes. Meglitinides, like the sulfonylureas, are only effective in individuals who have functioning

α-Glucosidase Inhibitors

Generic Name	U.S. Brand Name(s) Canadian Brand Name(s)	Dosage Forms and Strengths
acarbose	Precose	Tablet: 25 mg[†], 50 mg, 100 mg
	Glucobay	
miglitol	Glyset	Tablet: 25 mg, 50 mg, 100 mg
	Not available	

[†]Strength available in the United States only.

Meglitinides

Generic Name	U.S. Brand Name(s) Canadian Brand Name(s)	Dosage Forms and Strengths
nateglinide*,*[†]	Starlix	Tablet: 60 mg, 120 mg
	Starlix	
repaglinide*	Prandin	Tablet: 0.5 mg, 1 mg, 2 mg
	Gluconorm	

*Generic available.
*[†]Generic available in the United States only.

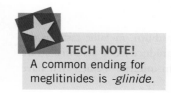

beta cells. Repaglinide is more effective in producing glycemic control than netaglinide. Repaglinide reduces Hb$_{A1c}$ levels by 1% to 2% whereas netaglinide only reduces Hb$_{A1c}$ levels by less than 1%.

MECHANISM OF ACTION AND PHARMACOKINETICS

Repaglinide and nateglinide lower postprandial blood glucose levels by stimulating insulin secretion from pancreatic beta cells, similar to sulfonylureas. Their action on basal insulin is less effective. Repaglinide is rapidly and completely absorbed from the intestinal tract. The onset of action is within 15 to 30 minutes. Peak effects of repaglinide and netaglinide are achieved in approximately 1 to 1.5 hours, and elimination is equally as rapid. The drugs must only be taken with meals to avoid hypoglycemia. Their short half-life accounts for the multiple daily dosing required. Both drugs are metabolized via the cytochrome P-450 (CYP450) system and are subject to many drug-drug interactions.

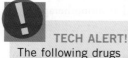

ADVERSE REACTIONS

Meglitinides may cause hypoglycemia; however, the risk is lower than with sulfonylureas if they are taken appropriately with meals. Other side effects are headache, nausea, and vomiting. Nateglinide and repaglinide should be used with caution in patients with liver dysfunction.

Thiazolidinediones

Thiazolidinediones are also called insulin sensitizers; they are used for the treatment of type 2 diabetes. They are effective in the treatment of insulin resistance. Two agents are currently marketed in the United States and Canada, pioglitazone and rosiglitazone. Both drugs reduce fasting plasma glucose (FPG) and Hb$_{A1c}$ levels by approximately 1% to 2%.

MECHANISM OF ACTION

Thiazolidinediones increase tissue sensitivity to insulin. They do not increase insulin secretion so they do not produce hypoglycemia when used as monotherapy. Insulin receptor sensitivity is most prominent in adipose tissue, skeletal muscle, and the liver. Pioglitazone and rosiglitazone increase the uptake of glucose in the liver and muscles. Pioglitazone also lowers free fatty acid and triglyceride levels; plasma glucose, insulin, and Hb$_{A1c}$ levels are all reduced.

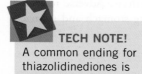

Thiazolidinediones

Generic Name	U.S. Brand Name(s) Canadian Brand Name(s)	Dosage Forms and Strengths
pioglitazone∞	Actos	**Tablet:** 15 mg, 30 mg, 45 mg
	Actos	
rosiglitazone	Avandia	**Tablet:** 2 mg, 4 mg, 8 mg
	Avandia	
Thiazolidinediones + Biguanides		
pioglitazone + metformin	Actosplus Met, Actosplus Met XR	**Tablet:** pioglitazone 15 mg + metformin 500 mg pioglitazone 15 mg + metformin 850 mg
	Not available	**Tablet, biphasic extended-release (Actosplus Met XR):** pioglitazone 15 mg + metformin 1000 mg pioglitazone 30 mg + metformin 1000 mg
rosiglitazone + metformin	Avandamet	**Tablet:** rosiglitazone 1 mg + metformin 500 mg‡ rosiglitazone 2 mg + metformin 500 mg
	Avandamet	rosiglitazone 4 mg + metformin 500 mg rosiglitazone 2 mg + metformin 1000 mg rosiglitazone 4 mg + metformin 1000 mg
Thiazolidinediones + Sulfonylureas		
pioglitazone + glimepiride	Duetact	**Tablet:** pioglitazone 30 mg + glimepiride 2 mg pioglitazone 30 mg + glimepiride 4 mg
	Not available	
rosiglitazone + glimepiride	Avandaryl	**Tablet:** rosiglitazone 4 mg + glimepiride 1 mg rosiglitazone 4 mg + glimepiride 2 mg
	Not available	rosiglitazone 4 mg + glimepiride 4 mg rosiglitazone 8 mg + glimepiride 2 mg rosiglitazone 8 mg + glimepiride 4 mg

∞Generic available in Canada.
‡Strength available in Canada only.

TECH ALERT!
The use of products containing rosiglitazone (e.g., Avandia, Avandamet, Avandaryl) is contraindicated in patients with heart failure and its use is restricted by Health Canada and the U.S. Food and Drug Administration (FDA). The FDA now requires health care providers and patients using rosiglitazone-containing drugs to be enrolled in a Medicines Access Program. Rosiglitazone-containing drugs were not to be sold in retail pharmacies in the United States after November 18, 2011.

TECH ALERT!
The following drugs have look-alike and sound-alike issues:
Actos, Actidose, and Actonel;
Avandia and Avalide

TECH NOTE!
A common ending for dipeptidyl peptidase-4 inhibitors is -gliptin.

PHARMACOKINETICS
Pioglitazone and rosiglitazone are both administered orally. The time to reach peak plasma concentration is within 1 hour for rosiglitazone and 2 hours for pioglitazone. Food doubles the time needed to reach the maximum concentration for pioglitazone but has no effect on rosiglitazone. Food does not reduce the bioavailability of either drug.

ADVERSE REACTIONS
The most common adverse reactions of therapy with pioglitazone and rosiglitazone are headache, weight gain, diarrhea, nausea, and vomiting. Patients should be instructed to report signs of muscle pain, jaundice, blurred vision, and signs of hypoglycemia or hyperglycemia. Serious side effects linked to pioglitazone and rosiglitazone are heart failure, heart attack, and liver failure.

Dipeptidyl Peptidase-4 Inhibitors
Sitagliptin, saxagliptin, and linagliptin are oral antidiabetic agents known as dipeptidyl peptidase 4 (DPP-4) inhibitors administered for the treatment of type 2 diabetes. They increase insulin release and decrease glucagon levels by potentiating the activity of peptide hormones released in response to eating a meal. Sitagliptin, saxagliptin, and linagliptin decrease fasting plasma glucose, postprandial glucose, and Hb_{A1c} levels. The decrease in Hb_{A1c} levels is 0.5% to 1%, less than that produced by sulfonylureas and biguanides.

Dipeptidyl Peptidase-4 Inhibitor

Generic Name	U.S. Brand Name(s)	Dosage Forms and Strengths
	Canadian Brand Name(s)	
linagliptin	Tradjenta	Tablet: 5 mg
	Trajenta	
saxagliptin	Onglyza	Tablet: 2.5 mg, 5 mg
	Onglyza	
sitagliptin	Januvia	Tablet: 25 mg†, 50 mg†, 100 mg
	Januvia	
Combination Dipeptidyl Peptidase-4 Inhibitor + Biguanide		
saxagliptin + metformin	Kombiglyze XR	Tablet: saxagliptin 5 mg + metformin 500 mg saxagliptin 2.5 mg + metformin 1000 mg saxagliptin 5 mg + metformin 1000 mg
	Not available	
sitagliptin + metformin	Janumet	Tablet: sitagliptin 50 mg + metformin 500 mg sitagliptin 50 mg + metformin 850 mg‡ sitagliptin 50 mg + metformin 1000 mg
	Janumet	

†Strength available in the United States only.
‡Strength available in Canada only.

MECHANISM OF ACTION AND PHARMACOKINETICS

Sitagliptin, saxagliptin, and linagliptin are DPP-4 inhibitors. DPP-4 is the enzyme responsible for the degradation of circulating glucagon-like peptide-1 (GLP-1) and glucose-dependent insulinotropic peptide (GIP). These peptide hormones are key agents in glucose homeostasis. The action of the hormones is prolonged by sitagliptin and saxagliptin. DPP-4 inhibitors also increase beta cells responsiveness to glucose in the islets of Langerhans.

Oral absorption and bioavailability of DPP-4 inhibitors are good and peak effects are reached 1 to 4 hours after administration. Sitagliptin and saxagliptin are primarily eliminated in the urine, so dosage adjustments may be required in those with kidney disease.

ADVERSE REACTIONS

The most common adverse reactions linked to the use of sitagliptin are intestinal upset, gas, heartburn, stomach pain, decreased appetite, metallic taste, and stuffy or runny nose. Pancreatitis is a rare but serious adverse reaction associated with the use of sitagliptin. The drug may also cause hypoglycemia when used in combination with sulfonylureas.

Incretin Mimetics

Exenatide (Byetta) and liraglutide (Victoza) are parenterally administered agents. Exenatide is approved as monotherapy or in combination with other antidiabetic agents. Liraglutide is not approved as monotherapy. Both drugs are administered as adjuncts to diet and exercise and may only be administered for type 2 diabetes mellitus. Exenatide is approved for use with insulin glargine but not prandial insulin.

MECHANISM OF ACTION AND PHARMACOKINETICS

Exenatide and liraglutide are GLP-1 receptor agonists. GLP-1 receptor agonists stimulate GLP-1 receptors in the alpha and beta cells in the pancreas. Beta cell stimulation mediates insulin secretion when glucose levels are elevated. Alpha cell stimulation suppresses glucagon release. GLP-1 receptor agonists also delay gastric emptying, slowing the rise of postprandial blood glucose levels and causing decreased appetite. Exenatide is administered subcutaneously within 60 minutes before the morning and evening meals. It is rapidly absorbed and has a half-life ($t_{1/2}$) of 2.5 hours. Exenatide powder for injection is a long acting formulation that is administered once per week. Liraglutide is administered subcutaneously once daily. It is absorbed slowly and the $t_{1/2}$ is 11 to 14 hours. Exenatide reduces Hb_{A1c} levels by 0.5% to 1%. Liraglutide reduces Hb_{A1c} levels by 0.8% to 1.5%.

Incretin Mimetic

Generic Name	U.S. Brand Name(s)	Dosage Forms and Strengths
	Canadian Brand Name(s)	
exenatide	Byetta	Solution, for injection: 250 mcg/mL
	Byetta	
	Bydureon	Powder, for injection: 2 mg/vial
	Not available	

Glucagon-Like Peptide Receptor Agonist

Generic Name	U.S. Brand Name(s)	Dosage Forms and Strengths
	Canadian Brand Name(s)	
liraglutide	Victoza	Solution, for injection: 18 mg/3 mL (6 mg/mL)
	Victoza	

Amylin Analogue

Generic Name	U.S. Brand Name(s)	Dosage Forms and Strengths
	Canadian Brand Name(s)	
pramlintide	Symlin, Symlin Pen 60, Symlin Pen 120	Solution, for injection: 600 mcg/mL pen cartridge (Symlin pen); 1000 mcg/mL, 1.5 mL (Symlin Pen 60); 1000 mcg/mL, 2.7 mL (Symlin Pen 120)
	Not available	

ADVERSE EFFECTS

Nausea is the most common side effect with exenatide and liraglutide, affecting up to 50% of patients. Gastrointestinal (GI) side effects are most common in the first month of therapy. Nausea associated with both drugs may be minimized by gradually increasing the dose. Other side effects include hypoglycemia, heartburn, itching, burning, swelling, or rash at the injection site, diarrhea or constipation, reduced appetite, and a slight weight loss. Exenatide may cause mild dizziness, weakness, headaches, or nausea. Pancreatitis is a rare but serious side effect of liraglutide.

Amylin Analogue

Pramlintide (Symlin) is a synthetic analogue of the hormone amylin. Amylin levels are absent in type 1 diabetes and decreased in type 2 diabetes. Pramlintide is used with mealtime insulin to control blood sugar levels in people who have type 1 or 2 diabetes mellitus.

MECHANISM OF ACTION AND PHARMACOKINETICS

Like amylin, pramlintide slows gastric emptying, reduces postprandial glucagon secretion, and reduces appetite. It should be injected subcutaneously immediately prior to each meal. The maximum concentration of pramlintide is reached within 20 minutes of administration and the therapeutic effects last approximately 3 hours.

ADVERSE REACTIONS

Adverse reactions associated with pramlintide include hypoglycemia, redness, swelling, bruising, itching at the injection site, loss of appetite, stomach pain, indigestion, upset stomach, excessive tiredness, dizziness, coughing, sore throat, and joint pain. Nausea and vomiting are dose-dependent

TECH NOTE!
Pramlintide may cause hypoglycemia. The risk is greater during the first 3 hours after pramlintide is injected.

Dopamine agonist

Generic Name	U.S. Brand Name(s)	Dosage Forms and Strengths
	Canadian Brand Name(s)	
bromocriptine	Cycloset	Tablet: 0.8 mg
	Not available	

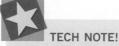

TECH NOTE!
Rotate the site of injection to minimize risk of developing an increase or a decrease in fatty tissue under the skin at the injection site.

TECH NOTE!
Do not mix pramlintide with any other injection, including insulin.

and may be reduced by gradually titrating the dose. This side effect decreases over time. To avoid lipodystrophy, patients should be advised to rotate the site of injection.

Miscellaneous Agents

Colesevelam (Welchol) is a cholesterol-lowering agent that is FDA-approved for the management of type 2 diabetes. The mechanism of action for reducing fasting plasma glucose and Hb$_{A1c}$ levels is unknown. Bromocriptine (Cycloset) is a dopamine agonist. It improves glycemic control; however, the mechanism of action for its effect on postprandial glucose levels is unknown. Bromocriptine and colesevelam are approved for the treatment of type 2 diabetes as an adjunct to diet and exercise. The most common side effects of colesevelam are heartburn or upset stomach. Nausea, drowsiness, and headache are side effects of bromocriptine.

COMPLEMENTARY AND ALTERNATIVE MEDICINES AND DIABETES

Six dietary supplements have been of particular interest in recent years as adjunct therapy for people with diabetes. They are alpha-lipoic acid (ALA), chromium, coenzyme Q10, garlic, magnesium, and omega-3 fatty acids. None has been extensively studied using randomized, double-blind studies. Of the six dietary supplements, alpha-lipoic acid, magnesium, and omega-3 fatty acids have shown the most evidence of possible usefulness.

Alpha-Lipoic Acid

Alpha-lipoic acid is an antioxidant. Antioxidants prevent cell damage caused by oxidative stress by substances called free radicals. Elevated blood glucose levels can cause oxidative stress. ALA might lower the blood sugar level too much, so blood glucose levels must be monitored closely when it is used.

Magnesium

Magnesium is a mineral found in green leafy vegetables, nuts, seeds, and some whole grains. Magnesium levels are depressed in people with diabetes. Low magnesium levels may worsen glucose control in type 2 diabetes by interrupting insulin secretion and increasing insulin resistance.

Omega-3 Fatty Acids

Omega-3 fatty acids are naturally found in fish, fish oil, canola and soybean oils, walnuts, and wheat germ. Studies have shown that supplementation with omega-3 fatty acids can reduce the incidence of cardiovascular disease (CVD) and slow the progression of atherosclerosis. Omega-3 fatty acids have been of interest because diabetes can increase the risk of CVD.

Garlic

Evidence about the value of garlic is mixed. It is believed that garlic may be involved in some biological activities associated with type 2 diabetes. The mechanism is not known.

Summary of Drugs Used in the Treatment of Diabetes

Generic Name	Brand Name	Usual Dose and Dosing Schedule	Warning Labels
Insulin			
insulin	Apidra, Detemir, Humulin, Humalog, Lantus, Levemir, Novolin, Novolog, Novolin GE Toronto	Individualized	STORE IN THE REFRIGERATOR; DO NOT FREEZE.
Sulfonylureas			
gliclazide	Generics	80 mg bid (max, 320 mg/day); gliclazide MR, 30 mg/day (max, 120 mg/day)	AVOID PROLONGED EXPOSURE TO SUNLIGHT (GLIPIZIDE, GLIMEPIRIDE). LIMIT OR AVOID ALCOHOL (ALL). TAKE 30 MIN BEFORE BREAKFAST (GLIPIZIDE, GLYBURIDE). SWALLOW WHOLE; DON'T CRUSH OR CHEW (SUSTAINED RELEASE). TAKE WITH A MEAL (GLICLAZIDE, GLIMEPIRIDE).
glipizide	Glucotrol	10-15 mg once daily	
	Glucotrol XL	5-10 mg once daily	
glyburide	Diabeta, Micronase	1.25-20 mg/day given in single or divided doses	
	Glynase PresTab	0.75-12 mg/day, given in single or divided doses	
glimepiride	Amaryl	1-4 mg once daily, (max, 8 mg/day)	
Biguanides			
metformin	Glucophage	500 mg twice daily or 850 mg PO once daily (max, 2000 mg/day)	TAKE WITH MEALS. SWALLOW WHOLE; DON'T CRUSH OR CHEW (SUSTAINED-RELEASE).
	Glumetza	1000 mg once or twice daily	
	Fortamet	500-1000 mg once daily	
α-Glucosidase Inhibitors			
acarbose	Precose	25-100 mg tid	TAKE WITH THE FIRST BITE OF A MEAL.
miglitol	Glyset	25-100 mg tid	
Dipeptidyl Peptidase-4 Inhibitors			
linagliptin	Tradjenta	5 mg once daily	TAKE AT THE SAME TIME EACH DAY, WITH OR WITHOUT FOOD.
saxagliptin	Onglyza	2.5-5 mg once daily	
sitagliptin	Januvia	100 mg once daily	
Meglitinides			
nateglinide	Starlix	120 mg tid	TAKE IMMEDIATELY PRIOR TO MEALS (SKIP DOSE IF THE MEAL IS MISSED). TAKE WITH A FULL GLASS OF WATER.
repaglinide	Prandin	1-4 mg up to qid	
Thiazolidinediones			
pioglitazone	Actos	15-45 mg once daily	LIMIT OR AVOID ALCOHOL. TAKE WITH A FULL GLASS OF WATER.
rosiglitazone	Avandia	4-8 mg daily in single or divided doses	

Continued

Summary of Drugs Used in the Treatment of Diabetes—cont'd

Generic Name	Brand Name	Usual Dose and Dosing Schedule	Warning Labels
Combinations			
metformin + glipizide	Metaglip	1 or 2 tablets once or twice daily (max, 2000 mg metformin + 20 mg glipizide per day)	TAKE WITH MEALS (ALL). LIMIT OR AVOID ALCOHOL (ALL). AVOID PROLONGED EXPOSURE TO SUNLIGHT (METAGLIP, GLUCOVANCE). SWALLOW WHOLE; DON'T CRUSH OR CHEW (ACTOPLUS MET XR, SUSTAINED-RELEASE).
metformin + glyburide	Glucovance	1 or 2 tablets once or twice daily (max, 2500 mg metformin + 20 mg glyburide/day)	
metformin + pioglitazone	Actoplus Met Actosplus Met XR	1 tablet once or twice daily (max, 2250 mg metformin + 45 mg pioglitazone/day)	
metformin + rosiglitazone	Avandamet	1 tablet once or twice daily or 1 tab once daily (Actosplus Met XR)	
metformin + saxagliptin	Kombiglyze	1 tablet once daily	
metformin + sitagliptin	Janumet	1 tablet bid	
pioglitazone + glimepiride	Duetact	1 tablet daily with the first meal of the day	
rosiglitazone + glimepiride	Avandaryl	1 tablet daily with the first meal of the day	
Glucagon-Like Peptide Receptor Agonist			
liraglutide	Victoza	Initiate with 0.6 mg subcut once daily for 1 wk; then increase to 1.2-1.8 mg subcut once daily	REFRIGERATE; DO NOT FREEZE. DISCARD PEN UNIT 30 DAYS AFTER OPENING.-Victoza, Byetta.
exenatide	Byetta	Initiate with 5 mcg subcut twice daily, increase to 10 mcg after 1 month based on response.	INJECT 60 MINUTES PRIOR TO MORNING AND EVENING MEAL-Byetta. USE IMMEDIATELY AFTER RECONSTITUTION- Bydureon. DO NOT USE DILUENT IF CLOUDY-Bydureon.
	Bydureon	Inject 2 mg subcut once every 7 days	
Dopamine Agonist			
bromocriptine	Cycloset	1.6-4.8 mg once daily within two hours after waking in the morning	TAKE WITH FOOD.

Chapter Summary

- Diabetes mellitus is a disorder of metabolism that involves glucose utilization. Glucose accumulates in the blood, leaving a sticky residue over all the body's organs and cells with which it comes into contact and causes damage.
- Diabetes mellitus is one of the leading causes of disability in the United States. It is the leading cause of non–war-related amputations.
- Diabetes is the seventh leading cause of death in Canada.

- Insulin is released by the beta cells in the islets of Langerhans of the pancreas in response to the rise of blood glucose, amino acid, and gut-derived hormone levels.
- When glucose levels drop, glucagon is secreted by alpha cells in the islets of Langerhans.
- Prediabetes causes impaired fasting glucose and impaired glucose tolerance.
- Type 1 diabetes is an autoimmune disease. The immune system attacks and destroys the insulin-producing beta cells in the pancreas.
- Type 1 diabetes is formerly known as insulin-dependent diabetes mellitus because the body can no longer produce sufficient amounts of the hormone insulin.
- Type 2 diabetes is most common, accounting for 90% to 95% of all cases of diabetes.
- In type 2 diabetes, the pancreas usually produces sufficient amounts of insulin early in the disease, but the body is unable to use the insulin effectively.
- Gestational diabetes may be caused by the hormones of pregnancy or a shortage of insulin.
- Insulin resistance is a condition in which the body does not respond to insulin. It is a precursor to type 2 diabetes.
- The hemoglobin A1c (Hb_{A1c}) test is the only test that provides information about blood glucose levels over a 2- to 3-month period.
- Blood glucose testing is the principal method used to diagnose diabetes.
- Individuals with type 1 or 2 diabetes will reduce risks for complications by weight loss, engaging in physical activity, consuming foods with a low glycemic index, quitting smoking, and other lifestyle changes.
- Insulin may be administered for the management of all types of diabetes. It is available in dosage forms to be administered by intravenous infusion, insulin pump, and subcutaneous injection.
- Insulin is formulated in rapid-acting, short-acting, intermediate-acting, and long-acting forms.
- Rapid-acting insulins (aspart, glulisine, and lispro) are typically injected 5 to 15 minutes before eating.
- Rapid-acting insulin (aspart, glulisine, lispro), regular insulin, and long-acting insulin (detemir, glargine) are clear solutions that should be discarded if they appear cloudy.
- Sulfonylureas are also known as oral hypoglycemic agents. They are only effective for the treatment of type 2 diabetes.
- Sulfonylureas stimulate insulin release from pancreatic beta cells, increase insulin binding and insulin receptor sensitivity, and decrease glycogenolysis.
- Metformin is classified as a biguanide antidiabetic agent. Metformin improves glucose tolerance and insulin resistance, lowers postprandial plasma glucose levels, decreases hepatic gluconeogenesis, and decreases the intestinal absorption of glucose.
- α-Glucosidase inhibitors (acarbose, miglitol) prolong the digestion of carbohydrates, delay their absorption in the small intestine, and are administered with the first bite of each meal.
- Meglitinides (nateglinide and repaglinide) stimulate insulin secretion from pancreatic beta cells, similar to sulfonylureas.
- A common ending for thiazolidinediones is -*glitazone.*
- Thiazolidinediones are also called insulin sensitizers and are used in the treatment of type 2 diabetes.
- Sitagliptin, saxagliptin, and linagliptin are dipeptidyl peptidase-4 inhibitors. They decrease fasting plasma glucose, postprandial glucose, and hemoglobin A1c levels.
- Exenatide and liraglutide are glucagon-like peptide receptor agonists.
- Colesevelam is a cholesterol-lowering agent that, along with diet and exercise, is approved for the treatment of type 2 diabetes.
- Bromocriptine is a dopamine agonist that, along with diet and exercise, is approved for the treatment type 2 diabetes.
- Alpha-lipoic acid, magnesium, omega-3 fatty acids, and garlic are nutritional supplements that show some evidence of effectiveness for the treatment of diabetes mellitus.

REVIEW QUESTIONS

1. The condition of elevated blood glucose levels is termed _____.
   a. Hypoglycemia
   b. Hyperglycemia

2. An autoimmune disease in which beta cells are destroyed and insufficient amounts of insulin are produced is _____.
   a. Type 1 diabetes
   b. Type 2 diabetes
   c. Gestational diabetes
   d. All of the above

3. In diabetes, _____ accumulates in the blood.
   a. Calcium
   b. Glucose
   c. Magnesium
   d. Insulin

4. A hormone that is essential for the regulation of carbohydrate, fat, and protein metabolism is _____.
   a. Aldosterone
   b. Serotonin
   c. Dopamine
   d. Insulin

5. Type 2 diabetes is most common, accounting for 90% to 95% of all cases of diabetes.
   a. True
   b. False

6. Select the common symptoms of diabetes.
   a. Polyphagia
   b. Polydipsia
   c. Polyuria
   d. All of the above

7. The risk for diabetes mellitus cannot be lowered by making lifestyle changes.
   a. True
   b. False

8. Insulin is only administered for the management of type 1 diabetes.
   a. True
   b. False

9. Glipizide and glyburide are examples of _____.
   a. Sulfonylureas
   b. Dipeptidyl peptidase-4 inhibitors
   c. Thiazolidinediones
   d. Nutritional supplements

10. Pioglitazone and rosiglitazone are both administered parenterally.
    a. True
    b. False

TECHNICIAN'S CORNER

1. If your family has a history of type 2 diabetes, which lifestyle precautions should you take to reduce your risk for developing the disease?
2. What are some basic changes in diet that can be implemented to avoid developing type 2 diabetes?

Bibliography

Berkrot B: Study finds staggering cost of treating diabetes. (http://www.nlm.nih.gov/medlineplus/news/fullstory_51076.html). 2007.

Bloomgarden Z: Insulin resistance concepts, *Diabetes Care* 30:1320-1326, 2007.

Bosi E, Camisasca R, Collober C, et al: Effects of vildagliptin on glucose control over 24 weeks in patients with type 2 diabetes inadequately controlled with metformin, *Diabetes Care* 30:890-895, 2007.

Canadian Diabetes Association Clinical Practice Guidelines Expert Committee: Canadian Diabetes Association 2008 clinical practice guidelines for the prevention and management of diabetes in Canada, *Can J Diabetes* 32(Suppl 1):S1-S201, 2008.

Elsevier: Gold Standard Clinical Pharmacology. Retrieved June 13, 2012, from https://www.clinical pharmacology.com/. 2010.

FDA: FDA Approved Drug Products. Retrieved June 13, 2012, from http://www.accessdata.fda.gov/scripts/cder/drugsatfda/index.cfm?fuseaction=Search.Search_Drug_Name. 2012.

Gangji A, Cukierman T, Gerstein H, et al: A systemic review and meta-analysis of hypoglycemia and cardio-vascular events, *Diabetes Care* 30:389-394, 2007.

Health Canada: Drug product database. (http://www.hc-sc.gc.ca/dhp-mps/prodpharma/databasdon/index-eng.php). 2010.

Kalant H, Grant D, Mitchell J: *Principles of medical pharmacology*, ed 7, Toronto, 2007, Elsevier Canada, pp 635-642.

Lance L, Lacy C, Armstrong L, et al: *Drug information handbook for the allied health professional*, ed 12, Hudson, OH, 2005, APhA Lexi-Comp.

Morrato E, Hill J, Wyatt H, et al: Physical activity in U.S. adults with diabetes and at risk for developing diabetes, 2003, *Diabetes Care* 30:203-209, 2007.

National Diabetes Information Clearinghouse: Diabetes overview (NIH Publ. No. 06-3873). http://diabetes.niddk.nih.gov/dm/pubs/overview/index.aspx. 2006.

National Diabetes Information Clearinghouse: National diabetes statistics (NIH Publ. No. 11-3892). (http://www.diabetes.niddk.nih.gov/dm/pubs/statistics). 2011.

National Center for Complementary and Alternative Medicine (NCCAM): Diabetes and CAM: A focus on dietary supplements. (http://nccam.nih.gov/health/diabetes/CAM-and-diabetes.htm). 2009.

Ottawa Health Statistics Division: *Your community, your health: Findings from the 3.1 smoking and diabetes care: Results from the Canadian Community Health Survey (CCHS) cycle*, Ottawa, 2005, Health Statistics Division, pp 49-59.

Page C, Curtis M, Sutter M, et al: *Integrated pharmacology*, ed 3, Philadelphia, 2006, Mosby, pp 293-299.

U.S. Food and Drug Administration: FDA drug safety communication: Updated risk evaluation and mitigation strategy (REMS) to restrict access to rosiglitazone-containing medicines including Avandia, Avandamet, and Avandaryl. (http://www.fda.gov/Drugs/DrugSafety/ucm255005.htm#Safety_Announcement). 2011.

34

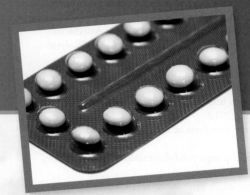

Drugs That Affect the Reproductive System

KEY TERMS

Amenorrhea: Absence of normal menstruation.

Atrophic vaginitis: Postmenopausal thinning and dryness of the vaginal epithelium related to decreased estrogen levels.

Condom: Thin, flexible, penile sheath made of synthetic or natural materials that is placed over the penis; used to prevent pregnancy and some sexually transmitted infections.

Diaphragm: Rubber or plastic cup that fits over the cervix; used for contraceptive purposes.

Dysfunctional uterine bleeding: Irregular or excessive uterine bleeding that results from a structural problem or hormonal imbalance.

Dysmenorrhea: Difficult or painful menstruation.

Endometriosis: Presence of functioning endometrial tissue outside the uterus.

Fertility: Being fertile; able to reproduce.

Hypogonadism: Inadequate production of sex hormones.

Hysterectomy: Surgical removal of the uterus.

Infertility: Inability to achieve pregnancy during 1 year or more of unprotected intercourse.

Intrauterine device: Device inserted in the uterus to prevent pregnancy.

Kallman's syndrome: Congenital disorder that causes hypogonadism and loss of the sense of smell.

Klinefelter's syndrome: A chromosomal disorder in males. People with this condition are born with at least one extra X chromosome.

Menopause: Termination of menstrual cycles; an event usually marked by the passage of at least 1 full year without menstruation.

Menorrhagia: Excessive menstrual bleeding.

Pelvic inflammatory disease: Infection of the uterus, fallopian tubes, and adjacent pelvic structures that is not associated with pregnancy or surgery.

Polycystic ovary disease: Condition characterized by ovaries twice the normal size that contain fluid-filled cysts.

Pregnancy: Condition of having a developing embryo or fetus in the body after successful conception.

Premenstrual dysphoric disorder: Disorder characterized by symptoms such as depression, anxiety, hopelessness, sad feelings, and self-deprecation.

Premenstrual syndrome: Condition involving a set of symptoms (headache, irritability, depression, fatigue, sleep changes, weight gain) that occur before the start of the menstrual cycle.

Prolactinoma: Pituitary tumor that produces excessive amount of prolactin.

Salpingitis: Inflammation of the fallopian tube, usually as a result of a sexually transmitted infection.

Supraovulation: Simultaneous rupture of multiple mature follicles.

Toxic shock syndrome: Rare disorder caused by certain *Staphylococcus* aureus strains that occurs in women using tampons.

Turner's syndrome: Congenital endocrine disorder caused by a failure of the ovaries to respond to pituitary hormone (gonadotropin) stimulation.

Vaginitis: Inflammation of the vagina.

Pregnancy and Contraception

PREGNANCY

Pregnancy is the condition of having a developing embryo or fetus in the body after successful conception. The average gestational period is 280 days, or 40 weeks. Approximately 7 million Americans become pregnant each year, and approximately two thirds of those pregnancies result in live births. Common symptoms include *amenorrhea*, nausea and vomiting, breast tenderness, urinary frequency, fatigue, and changes in skin pigmentation (chloasma). Physiological changes and disorders of pregnancy that affect body systems are outlined in Table 34-1.

CONTRACEPTION: PREVENTION OF PREGNANCY

A variety of methods exist to prevent pregnancy (Box 34-1). *Hormonal* methods of contraception alter the level of sex hormone responsible for ovulation. In addition to oral contraceptives, other types of hormonal birth control delivery mechanisms are also available. They include hormone-impregnated vaginal inserts, hormone injections, skin patches, and surgical implants. Many other methods of contraception exist. They have differing rates of effectiveness and unique advantages and disadvantages. For example, spermicidal methods involve the use of preparations (e.g., foams, jellies, creams) that act to kill sperm; mechanical barrier methods use devices such as a condom, diaphragm, cervical cap, or vaginal sponge to block sperm from entering the uterus. Surgical methods such as tubal ligation and male vasectomy result in permanent sterility. Behavioral methods involve abstaining from sexual intercourse for a specified number of days before, during, and after ovulation. The rhythm method is a natural method based on calculating the fertile period by the use of a calendar, on which the supposed infertile days are marked. The ovulation method includes keeping a temperature chart to detect a minute change in temperature at the time of ovulation or determining the time of ovulation by observing changes in cervical mucus.

BOX 34-1 **Methods of Contraception**

• Behavioral	• Mechanical barriers
• Hormonal	• Spermicidal

TABLE 34-1   **Physiological Changes during Pregnancy**

Body Systems Affected by Pregnancy	Physiological Changes	Disorders
Mammary glands	Enlarged, tender, and more nodular Areolae darken; nipples become more sensitive and erect Colostrum may leak out during the last trimester as breasts prepare for lactation	
Reproductive—uterus, cervix	Softening Change in size, shape, and consistency Increase in muscle mass	Vaginal bleeding
Vagina	Increase in secretions Lowering of pH levels Elongation; increase in vascularity, elasticity Thickening of mucus discharge	
Endocrine	Elevated levels of estrogen and progesterone Increased size and activity of thyroid gland Increased level of triiodothyronine and globulin Placental hormones prevent ovulation, development of corpus luteum	**Placenta** Abruptio placentae Placenta previa Placentitis Gestational diabetes
Cardiovascular	Increase in circulation blood volume Increase in red blood cell count Rising levels of clotting factors (VII-X) Increase in pulse rate and stroke volume	**Preeclampsia** Hypertension Edema Proteinuria **Eclampsia** Severe hypertension Convulsions Coma Varicose veins Hemorrhoids
Musculoskeletal	Softening, increased mobility of pelvic articulations Increase in lumbar curve	Cramping charley horse Back pain Pedal edema
Respiratory	Decreased airway resistance Shortness of breath	Edema Congestion of nasal mucosa (nosebleeds and stuffiness)
Gastrointestinal		Nausea and vomiting (first trimester) Heartburn Constipation
Skin	Chloasma Areolar darkening Linea nigra (pigmented line vertically bisecting abdomen)	Pruritus
Urinary	Increase in urinary frequency Increase in bladder capacity Increased voiding	
Weight	Weight gain of 25-39 lb (11.4-17.7 kg)	

Condoms

A **condom** is a device, usually made of latex or polyurethane, which is placed on a man's erect penis prior to sexual intercourse to block ejaculated semen physically from entering the body of the sexual partner. Female condoms are placed in the vagina. Condoms are used to prevent pregnancy and transmission of sexually transmitted infections (STIs) such as gonorrhea, syphilis, and HIV. Condoms are easy to use, inexpensive, have few side effects, and offer protection against STIs. Condom use is typically combined with a spermicide for greater protection. Condoms come in various sizes, from magnum to snug. Mass-produced condoms do not vary much in width but do vary significantly in length.

- Latex condoms are the most widely distributed type of condom; there are thousands of variants in regard to thickness, size, and texture.
- Polyurethane condoms are thinner than latex condoms (0.02 mm). They conduct heat better than latex, are not as sensitive to temperature and ultraviolet light, can be used with oil-based lubricants, are less allergenic than latex, and do not have an odor. They are more likely to slip or break than latex and are more expensive.
- Lambskin condoms made from lamb intestines are the oldest form of condom available. They have a greater ability to transmit body warmth and tactile sensation compared with synthetic condoms and are less allergenic than latex. Because the pores of the lambskin condoms are larger, they are considered ineffective in preventing the transmission of STIs.
- The female condom (femidom) is larger and wider than male condoms but equivalent in length. It has a flexible ring-shaped opening and is inserted into the vagina. It contains an inner ring that aids insertion and helps keep the condom from sliding out of the vagina during sexual intercourse. This condom is made from polyurethane.

Diaphragms

The **diaphragm** is a barrier type of birth control method. It is dome-shaped and made of latex or silicone. The spring-molded rim creates a seal against the wall of the vagina. The rim of the diaphragm is squeezed into an arc shape for insertion. A water-based lubricant (usually spermicide) may be applied to the rim of the diaphragm to aid insertion. One teaspoonful (5 mL) of spermicide is placed in the dome of the diaphragm before insertion or with an applicator after insertion. The diaphragm must be inserted some time before sexual intercourse and remain in the vagina for 6 to 8 hours after a male's last ejaculation. On removal, a diaphragm should be cleaned with warm soapy water before storage. The diaphragm must be removed for cleaning at least once every 24 hours. Oil-based products should not be used with latex diaphragms. Lubricants or vaginal medications that contain oil will cause the latex to degrade rapidly and greatly increase the chance of the diaphragm breaking or tearing. A latex diaphragm should be replaced every 1 to 3 years. Silicone diaphragms may last much longer, up to 10 years.

Diaphragms come in different sizes. A correctly fitting diaphragm will cover the cervix and rest snugly against the pubic bone. A diaphragm that is too small might fit inside the vagina without covering the cervix or might become dislodged from the cervix during intercourse or bowel movements. Diaphragms should be refitted after a weight change of 4.5 kg (10 lb) or more. Diaphragms should also be refitted after any pregnancy of 14 weeks or longer. In the United States and Canada, diaphragms are available by prescription only. Many European countries do not require prescriptions.

ADVERSE REACTIONS

Diaphragms are associated with an increased risk of urinary tract infection. **Toxic shock syndrome** (TSS) occurs at a rate of 2.4 cases/100,000 women using diaphragms, almost exclusively when the device is left in place longer than 24 hours.

Types of Diaphragms

Generic Name	U.S. Brand Name(s) Canadian Brand Name(s)	Dosage Forms and Strengths
arcing spring	Ortho All-Flex Milex Wide-Seal Milex Wide-Seal Arcing	50-105 mm (2-4 inches)

Cervical Cap, Cervical Shield, Contraceptive Sponge, and Vaginal Contraceptive Film

The cervical cap, cervical shield, contraceptive sponge and vaginal contraceptive film (VCF) are barrier contraceptive methods like the diaphragm. The cervical cap is placed over the cervix opening and is the size of a thimble. It is used with spermicide and has a 9% to 16% failure rate in women who have not previously been pregnant. It is less effective in women who have given birth. The cervical cap must be fitted and is obtained by prescription. The contraceptive shield (Lea's Shield) is a reusable silicone cup placed over the cervix and held in place by a one-way suction valve. It is also used with spermicide. It comes in one size and does not need to be specifically fitted to each woman. It is available by prescription in the United States, although it is obtainable over the counter in Europe and Canada. The contraceptive sponge (Today Sponge, Protectaid) is used with spermicide and has a 9% to 28% failure rate. It provides protection immediately after insertion and should remain inserted for 6 hours after intercourse. The VCF is a thin film that is impregnated with the spermicide nonoxynol-9. It is placed over the cervix 15 minutes prior to intercourse. The failure rate for VCF is approximately 6%.

Intrauterine Device

An *intrauterine device* (IUD) is a contraceptive device that is placed in the uterus and is the world's most widely used reversible birth control method. More than 70 million women currently use IUDs. The device has to be inserted or removed from the uterus by a physician or qualified medical practitioner. Depending on the type, a single IUD is approved for 5 to 10 years' use. The IUD is more than 99% effective. IUDs have a plastic T-shaped frame; the arms of the frame hold the IUD in place near the top of the uterus. There are two broad categories, copper-releasing and hormone-releasing IUDs. A copper-releasing IUD is wrapped with copper and/or has copper bands. Mirena is an IUD that releases levonorgestrel, a progestin. Progestin-releasing IUDs reduce menstrual bleeding or prevent menstruation all together and can be used as a treatment for *menorrhagia* (heavy periods).

MECHANISM OF ACTION

The presence of an object in the uterus prompts the release of leukocytes and prostaglandins by the endometrium. These substances are hostile to sperm and eggs; the presence of the copper prevents the sperm from reaching the egg and the egg from attaching to the uterus. Progestin-releasing IUDs prevent ovulation and thicken cervical mucus, thus preventing the sperm from reaching the egg. IUDs do not protect against STIs, and their use is contraindicated in women with pelvic inflammatory disease or who are pregnant.

Some physicians prefer to insert the IUD during menstruation to verify that the woman is not pregnant at the time of insertion. However, IUDs may be safely inserted at any time during the menstrual cycle.

ADVERSE REACTION

Insertion of an IUD may introduce bacteria into the uterus. The insertion carries a small transient risk of pelvic inflammatory disease (PID) in the first 20 days after insertion. If pregnancy does occur, presence of the IUD increases the risk of miscarriage, particularly during the second trimester.

Intrauterine Devices

Generic Name	U.S. Brand Name(s)
	Canadian Brand Name(s)
Copper-releasing T-shaped IUD	Paraguard
	Flex-T 300, Flex-T 380, Nova T
Hormone-releasing (levonorgestrel) T-shaped IUD	Mirena
	Mirena

TABLE 34-2   **Oral Contraceptives**

Estrogen-Progestin Combination	Description
Monophasic	Provides a fixed dose of estrogen and progestin throughout cycle of 21- or 28-day package
Biphasic	Amount of estrogen remains the same throughout cycle; less progestin in first half of cycle, increased progestin in second half of cycle
Triphasic	Amount of estrogen is the same or varies throughout cycle; progestin amount varies

Oral Contraceptives

Oral contraceptives (OCs) have been collectively called the pill. Numerous OC products are available containing different types, combinations, and dosages of estrogen and progestins (Table 34-2). The so-called minipill contains only progestin. The pill can be used to regulate menstruation and prevent pregnancy. If used correctly and consistently, the pill is an extremely effective contraceptive, with an unintended pregnancy rate estimated at between 0.1% and 3%. Only total abstinence is 100% effective in preventing pregnancy.

MECHANISM OF ACTION

Most hormonal contraceptives were developed to prevent pregnancy by initiating negative feedback inhibition of follicle-stimulating hormone (FSH) and luteinizing hormone (LH) secretion. As a result, mature follicles do not develop, and LH does not reach the level required to initiate ovulation. The next menses takes place when the progestin and estrogen dosage is stopped in time to allow blood levels to decrease as they normally do near the end of the cycle to bring on menstruation.

ADVERSE REACTIONS

Smoking increases the risk of adverse reactions, including increased risk of thromboembolic events and heart attacks. Loss of appetite and constipation can also occur. Women taking OCs should immediately report pain or muscle soreness, swelling, heat, or redness in calves, shortness of breath, sudden loss of vision, unresolved leg or foot swelling, weight gain (>5 lb [2.3 kg]), change in menstrual pattern, breast tenderness that does not go away, acute abdominal cramping, signs of vaginal infection, blurred vision, and central nervous system (CNS) symptoms (e.g., confusion, acute anxiety, unresolved depression).

Oral Contraceptives

Generic Name	U.S. Brand Name(s) Canadian Brand Name(s)	Dosage Forms and Strengths
Estrogen and Progestin Combinations		
ethinyl estradiol + desogestrel	Apri, Caziant, Cyclessa, Desogen, Emoquette, Kariva, Mircette, Ortho-Cept, Solia, Velivet	**Tablet, monophasic (Apri, Desogen, Marvelon, Ortho-Cept, Solia):** 21 days each—ethinyl estradiol 0.03 mg + desogestrel 0.15mg **Tablet, biphasic (Kariva, Mircette):** 21 days each—ethinyl estradiol 0.02 mg + desogestrel 0.15 mg; 5 days each—ethinyl estradiol 0.01 mg **Tablet, triphasic (Caziant, Cyclessa, Linessa, Velivet):** 7 days each—ethinyl estradiol 0.025 mg + desogestrel 0.125 mg; 7 days each—ethinyl estradiol 0.025 mg + desogestrel 0.15 mg; 7 days each— ethinyl estradiol 0.025 mg + desogestrel 0.1 mg
	Apri, Linessa, Marvelon, Ortho-Cept	
ethinyl estradiol + drospirenone	Angeliq, Loryna, Syeda, Yasmin, Yaz	**Tablet, monophasic:** ethinyl estradiol 0.02 mg + drospirenone 3 mg (Yaz); ethinyl estradiol 0.02 mg + drospirenone 3 mg (Yasmin)
	Yasmin, Yaz, Angeliq	

Continued

Oral Contraceptives—cont'd

Generic Name	U.S. Brand Name(s) Canadian Brand Name(s)	Dosage Forms and Strengths
ethinyl estradiol + drospirenone + levomefolate	Beyaz, Safyral Not available	**Tablet, monophasic:** 24 days each—ethinyl estradiol 0.02 mg + drospirenone 3 mg + levomefolate 0.451 mg; 4 days each—levomefolate 0.451 mg
ethinyl estradiol + ethynodiol	Zovia 1+ 35, Zovia 1+ 50 Demulen 30	**Tablet, monophasic:** 21 days each—ethinyl estradiol 0.035 mg + ethynodiol 1 mg (Zovia 1+ 35); 21 days each—ethinyl estradiol 0.05 mg + ethynodiol 1 mg (Zovia 1+ 50); 21 days each—ethinyl estradiol 0.03 mg + ethynodiol 2 mg (Demulen 30)
ethinyl estradiol + levonorgestrel*	Altavera, Aviane, Enpresse, Falmina, Introvale, Lessina, Levora, Lo-Seasonique, Marlissa, Nordette, Portia, Seasonale, Seasonique, Trivora Min-Ovral, Portia, Triquilar	**Tablet, monophasic:** 21 days each—ethinyl estradiol 0.03 mg + levonorgestrel 0.15 mg (Altavera, Levora, Min-Ovral, Nordette, Portia); 21 days each—ethinyl estradiol 0.02 mg + levonorgestrel 0.1 mg (Aviane, Lessina,) **Tablet, triphasic:** 6 days each—ethinyl estradiol 0.03 mg + levonorgestrel 0.05 mg; 10 days each—ethinyl estradiol 0.03 mg + levonorgestrel 0.125 mg; 5 days each—ethinyl estradiol 0.04 mg + levonorgestrel 0.75 mg (Enpresse, Triquilar, Trivora) **Tablet, 84-day extended cycle (Introvale, Seasonale):** 84 days each—ethinyl estradiol 0.03 mg + levonorgestrel 0.15 mg **Tablet, 84-day biphasic cycle (Lo-Seasonique, Seasonique):** 7 days each—ethinyl estradiol 0.01 mg; 84 days each—ethinyl estradiol 0.02 mg + levonorgestrel 0.1 mg **Tablet, continuous cycle (Lybrel):** ethinyl estradiol 0.02 mg + levonorgestrel 0.09 mg
ethinyl estradiol + norethindrone*	Aranelle, Brevicon, Cyclafem, Loestrin 1/20, Loestrin 1.5/30, Microgestin 1.5/30, Modicon, Norinyl 1 + 35 and 1 + 50, Nortrel 7/7/7, Ortho-Novum 1/35, Ortho-Novum 7/7/7, Ovcon 35, Ovcon 50, Tri-Norinyl Brevicon 0.5/35, Brevicon 1/35, Loestrin 1.5/30, Minestrin 1/20, Ortho 0.5/35, Ortho 1/35, Ortho 7/7/7, Select 1/35, Synphasic	**Tablet, monophasic:** 21 days each—ethinyl estradiol 0.035 mg + norethindrone 0.4 mg (Ovcon 35); 21 days each—ethinyl estradiol 0.035 mg + norethindrone 0.5 mg (Brevicon, Modicon, Ortho 0.5/35); 21 days each—ethinyl estradiol 0.035 mg + norethindrone 1 mg (Norinyl 1 + 35 and 1 + 50, Ortho 1/35); 21 days each—ethinyl estradiol 0.05 mg + norethindrone 1 mg (Ovcon 50); ethinyl estradiol 0.03 mg + norethindrone 1.5 mg (Loestrin 1.5/30); ethinyl estradiol 0.02 mg + norethindrone 1 mg (Loestrin 1/20, Minestrin 1/20) **Tablet, biphasic:** 12 days each—ethinyl estradiol 0.035 + norethindrone, 0.5 mg; 9 days each— ethinyl estradiol 0.035 mg + norethindrone 1 mg Aranelle, Synphasic, Tri-Norinyl; 10 days each—ethinyl estradiol 0.035 + norethindrone, 0.5 mg; 11 days each—ethinyl estradiol 0.035 mg + norethindrone 1 mg (generic) **Tablet, triphasic (Cyclafem 7/7/7, Ortho Novum 7/7/7):** 7 days each—ethinyl estradiol 0.035 + norethindrone, 0.5 mg; 7 days each—ethinyl estradiol 0.035 mg + norethindrone 0.75 mg, 7 days each—ethinyl estradiol 0.035 mg + norethindrone 1 mg

Oral Contraceptives—cont'd

Generic Name	U.S. Brand Name(s) / Canadian Brand Name(s)	Dosage Forms and Strengths
ethinyl estradiol + norgestimate*	Ortho-Cyclen, Ortho Tri-Cyclen, Ortho Tri-Cyclen Lo, Previfem, Sprintec, TriNessa, Tri-Prevofem, Tri-Sprintec, Tri-Lo-Sprintec Cyclen, Tri-Cyclen, Tri-Cyclen Lo	Tablet, monophasic (Cyclen, Ortho-Cyclen, Previfem, Sprintec): ethinyl estradiol 0.035 mg + norgestimate 0.25 mg Triphasic formulation: 7 days each—ethinyl estradiol 0.035 mg + norgestimate 0.18 mg, 7 days each—ethinyl estradiol 0.035 mg + norgestimate 0.215 mg, 7 days each—ethinyl estradiol 0.035 mg + norgestimate 0.25 mg (Ortho Tri-Cyclen, Tri-Cyclen, TriNessa, Tri-Sprintec); 7 days each—ethinyl estradiol 0.025 mg + norgestimate 0.18 mg, 7 days each—ethinyl estradiol 0.025 mg + norgestimate 0.215 mg, 7 days each—ethinyl estradiol 0.025 mg + norgestimate 0.25 mg (Ortho Tri-Cyclen Lo, Tri-Cyclen Lo, Tri-Lo-Sprintec)

Progestins

Generic Name	U.S./Canadian Brand Name(s)	Dosage Forms and Strengths
norethindrone* norethindrone acetate	Camila, Errin, Heather, Jolivette, Micronor, Nor QD Micronor, Norlutate	Tablet: 0.35 mg, 5 mg^ (Norlutate)

*Generic available.
^Strength not used for contraception; used for amenorrhea, abnormal uterine bleeding, and endometriosis.

Miscellaneous Contraceptive Dosage Forms

Generic Name	U.S. Brand Name(s) / Canadian Brand Name(s)s	Dosage Forms and Strengths
ethinyl estradiol + etonogestrel	NuvaRing NuvaRing	Intravaginal ring: ethinyl estradiol 0.015 mg/24 hr + etonogestrel 0.12 mg/24 hr
ethinyl estradiol + norelgestromin	Ortho Evra Ortho Evra	Patch, weekly: ethinyl estradiol 0.02 mg/24 hr + norelgestromin 0.15 mg/24 hr
etonogestrel	Implanon, Nexplanon Not available	Implantable rod: etonogestrel 68 mg
medroxyprogesterone*	Depo-Provera, Depo-subQ Depo-Provera, Depo-Provera-SC	Injection: 50 mg/mL‡, 104 mg/0.65 mL†, 150 mg/mL

*Generic available.
†Strength available in the United States only.
‡Strength available in Canada only.

Other Contraceptive Dosage Forms

Depo-Provera injection is a synthetic derivative of progesterone that induces and maintains the endometrium. It prevents ovulation and thickens cervical mucus, preventing the passage of sperm. An advantage is that the injection is administered once every 3 months, but there are many disadvantages, including sensitivity to sunlight, dizziness, anxiety, depression, changes in appetite, decreased libido, hot flashes, increased body hair (reversible when drug is discontinued), and osteoporosis.

Ortho-Evra is a transdermal patch containing a combination of estrogen and progestin. One patch is applied each week for 3 weeks followed by 1 patch-free week. Each patch should be applied on the same day each week and only one patch should be worn at a time. No more than 7 days

TECH NOTE!

In Canada, Plan B is listed as a schedule II nonprescription drug (requires pharmacist intervention) and a schedule III nonprescription drug (may be sold without pharmacist intervention). For schedule II, the manufacturer's labeled dosing is one tablet followed by a second tablet 12 hours later. For schedule III, the manufacturer's labeled dosing is two tablets as a single dose.

TECH NOTE!

In the United States, Plan B and Plan B One-Step are available without prescription to consumers 17 years and older. Women younger than16 years can obtain Plan B and Plan B One-Step by prescription only.

should pass during the patch-free interval. An advantage over other methods of contraception is that it is a weekly dose, noninvasive, and easy to use. Disadvantages are that the patch can become partially or completely detached and can irritate the skin.

Nuva-Ring is a hormonal vaginal ring inserted for 3 weeks and then removed for 1 week. A new ring is inserted 7 days after the last one was removed and should be inserted the same time as the insertion of the previous ring. Advantages are that it is easy to use and is a once-monthly dosing. Although rare, it is possible for the ring to slip outside the vagina; if this occurs, it must be replaced within 3 hours.

ADVERSE REACTIONS

Adverse reactions include increased blood pressure, loss of appetite, constipation, pain or muscle soreness, swelling, heat, shortness of breath, sudden loss of vision, weight gain, breast tenderness, acute abdominal cramping, signs of vaginal infection, and headache. Smoking increases the risk of thromboembolic events, stroke, and heart attacks.

Emergency Contraception

The emergency use of OC pills containing levonorgestrel (Plan B) reduces the risk of pregnancy after unprotected intercourse by 89%. The Yuzpe method of emergency contraception involves taking an OC containing ethinyl estradiol and norgestrel (e.g., Ovral). The risk of pregnancy is reduced by 75%. Emergency contraception (EC) should be initiated as soon as possible after unprotected intercourse. The Plan B and Yuzpe method are most effective if used within 72 hours after unprotected sexual intercourse. The EC protocol of Plan B is two tablets as a single dose or one tablet followed by a second tablet 12 hours later. The dosing for the Yuzpe method is two tablets as a single dose followed by two tablets 12 hours later. EC may be used at any time during the menstrual cycle. If conception has already occurred, EC will not terminate pregnancy. Known or suspected pregnancy is a contraindication to the provision of emergency contraception.

The emergency insertion of a copper IUD also is highly effective, reducing the risk of pregnancy by as much as 99%.

Emergency Contraceptives

Generic Name	U.S. Brand Name(s) / Canadian Brand Name(s)	Dosage Forms and Strengths
levonorgestrel	Plan B, Plan B One-Step	Tablet: 0.75 mg, 1.5 mg (One-Step)
	Plan B	

MENOPAUSE AND ATROPHIC VAGINITIS

Unlike other body systems, the female reproductive system does not begin to perform its functions until puberty and, unlike the male reproductive system, the female reproductive system ceases its principal function in middle adulthood, at approximately 35 to 58 years of age. **Menopause** is the termination of menstrual cycles; it is usually marked by the passage of at least 1 full year without menstruation. Natural menopause will occur in 25% of women by age 47, 50% by age 50, 75% by age 52, and 95% by age 55 years. After that time, a woman may continue to enjoy normal sexual activity, but she cannot produce more offspring. Menopause caused by surgical removal of the ovaries (**hysterectomy**) occurs in almost 30% of U.S. women who are 50 years or older.

Symptoms of menopause may last from a few months to years and vary from hardly noticeable to severe. Symptoms include vasomotor instability, nervousness, hot flashes (flushes), chills, excitability, fatigue, apathy, mental depression, crying episodes, insomnia, palpitation, vertigo, headache, numbness, tingling, myalgia, urinary disturbances (e.g., incontinence), atrophic vaginitis, and various disorders of the gastrointestinal system. The long-range effects of lower estrogen levels are osteoporosis and atherosclerosis.

Atrophic vaginitis is the postmenopausal thinning and dryness of the vaginal epithelium related to decreased estrogen levels. Symptoms include burning and pain during intercourse. Hormone replacement therapy or application of topical estrogen restores the integrity of the vaginal epithelium and supporting tissues and relieves symptoms.

Hormone Replacement Therapy

Hormone replacement therapy (HRT) is the administration of medication containing one or more female hormones, commonly estrogen plus progestin. Some women receive estrogen-only therapy, usually women who have had their uterus removed (Box 34-2). The medication may be taken in the form of a pill, patch, or vaginal cream. HRT has been prescribed to treat symptoms of menopause, such as hot flashes, vaginal dryness, mood swings, sleep disorders, and decreased sexual desire. Many physicians once believed that HRT might be beneficial for reducing the risk of heart disease and bone fractures caused by osteoporosis (thinning of the bones) in addition to treating menopausal symptoms. The Women's Health Initiative (WHI) HRT trials were conducted to look for evidence of these benefits. Research led to early discontinuation of the HRT trials in 2002 and led physicians to revise their recommendations regarding the use of HRT. Study results showed an increased of developing breast cancer, heart attacks, strokes, and blood clots. A component of the WHI, which studied the use of estrogen and progestin in women who had a uterus, was stopped early because the health risks exceeded the health benefits. The estrogen-progestin study showed that there was a 26% increase in the incidence of breast cancer. A second component of the WHI, which studied estrogen-only therapy in women who no longer had a uterus, was also stopped early in 2004 because it showed an increase in the risk of strokes.

Hormone replacement typically involves the administration of oral or vaginal estrogens, with or without progestins. Table 34-3 lists oral estrogen and estrogen-progestin products.

Treatment protocols vary according to whether or not the woman has a uterus or has had a hysterectomy.

The dosage form may vary according to the symptoms to be treated. For example, a vaginal estrogen ring or cream (Table 34-4) can ease vaginal dryness, urinary leakage, or vaginal or urinary infection but does not relieve hot flashes.

ADVERSE REACTIONS

HRT may increase the risk of heart disease, pulmonary embolism, and breast and endometrial cancers. Other adverse effects are nausea, vomiting, bloating, cramping, breast tenderness, return of menstruation or spotting, migraine headaches, and weight gain.

BOX 34-2   Typical Hormonal Replacement Therapy Regimens

- Continuous—combined
- Cyclic or sequential
- Estrogen and progestin daily without a break
- Estrogen every day
- Progesterone or progestin added for 10 to 14 days out of every 4 wk

Adapted from National Heart, Lung, and Blood Institute: Facts about menopausal hormone therapy (NIH Publ. No. 05-5200), 2005 (http://www.nhlbi.nih.gov/health/women/pht_facts.pdf).

Hormone Replacement Therapy

Generic Name	U.S. Brand Name(s) Canadian Brand Name(s)	Dosage Forms and Strengths
Estrogen		
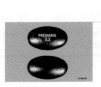 conjugated estrogens* (equine and synthetic)	Cenestin Enjuvia, Premarin C.E.S., Congest, Premarin	Vaginal cream: 0.625 mg/g Powder, for injection: 25 mg Tablet: 0.3 mg, 0.45 mg†, 0.625 mg, 0.9 mg, 1.25 mg, 2.5 mg‡

Continued

Hormone Replacement Therapy—cont'd

Generic Name	U.S. Brand Name(s) / Canadian Brand Name(s)	Dosage Forms and Strengths
estradiol*	Alora, Climara, Depo-Estradiol, Delestrogen, Divigel, Elestrin, Estrogel, Estrace, Estraderm, Estrasorb, Evamist, Femtrace, Femring, Menostar, Vivelle, Vivelle Dot	**Gel, topical:** 0.1% (Divigel), 0.06% (Elestrin, Estrogel) **Emulsion, topical (Estrasorb):** 0.25% **Solution, for injection, as cypionate (Depo-Estradiol):** 5 mg/mL **Solution, for injection, as valerate (Delestrogen):** 10 mg/mL, 20 mg/mL, 40 mg/mL **Spray, topical (Evamist):** 1.53 mg/spray **Tablet (Estrace):** 0.5 mg, 1 mg, 2 mg **Tablet, as acetate (Femtrace):** 0.45 mg, 0.9 mg, 1.8 mg
	Activelle, Activelle LD, Climara, Estrace, Estraderm, Estra Dot, Estring, Estrogel, Oesclim, Vagifem	**Transdermal patch, biweekly (Alora, Estraderm, Oesclim, Vivelle dot):** 0.025 mg/24 hr, 0.0375 mg/24 hr (Vivelle dot only), 0.5 mg/24 hr, 0.075 mg/24 hr **Transdermal patch, weekly (Climara):** 0.025 mg/24 hr, 0.0375 mg/24 hr, 0.5 mg/24 hr, 0.6 mg/24 hr, 0.075 mg/24 hr; 14 mcg/24 hr (Menostar) **Vaginal cream (Estrace):** 0.01% **Vaginal ring:** 0.5 mg/24 hr, 0.1 mg/24 hr (Femring); 2 mg (Estring) **Vaginal tablet (Vagifem):** 10 mcg/tablet
estrogen (esterified)	Menest Estragyn	**Tablet:** 0.3 mg, 0.625 mg, 1.25 mg[†], 2.5 mg[†]
estropipate*	Ogen Ogen	**Tablet:** 0.75 mg, 1.5 mg, 3 mg, 6 mg[†]

Estrogen and Progestin Combinations

Generic Name	U.S./Canadian Brand Name(s)	Dosage Forms and Strengths
estradiol + levonorgestrel	Climara Pro Climara Pro	**Transdermal patch, weekly:** 0.45 mg/24 hr estradiol + 0.15 mg/24 hr levonorgestrel
estradiol + norethindrone*	Activella, Combipatch Activella, Activelle LD, Estalis	**Tablet:** 0.5 mg estradiol + 0.1 mg norethindrone; 1 mg estradiol + 0.5 mg estradiol (Activella) **Transdermal patch, biweekly:** 0.05 mg/24 hr estradiol + 0.14 mg/hr norethindrone (Combipatch 50/140, Estalis 50/140); 0.05 mg/hr estradiol + 0.25 mg/hr norethindrone (Combipatch 50/250, Estalis 50/250)
estradiol + norgestimate	Prefest Not available	**Tablet:** estradiol 1 mg + norgestimate 0.09 mg
conjugated estrogens + medroxyprogesterone	Prempro, Premphase Premplus	**Tablet:** conjugated estrogens 0.625 mg + medroxyprogesterone 5 mg (Premphase); conjugated estrogens 0.3 mg + medroxyprogesterone 1.5 mg (Prempro); conjugated estrogens 0.45 mg + medroxyprogesterone 5 mg (Prempro); conjugated estrogens 0.625 mg + medroxyprogesterone 2.5 mg (Prempro); conjugated estrogens 0.625 mg + medroxyprogesterone 5 mg (Prempro)
ethinyl estradiol + norethindrone	FemHRT, FemHRT Lo FemHRT	**Tablet:** 5 mcg ethinyl estradiol + 1 mg norethindrone (FemHRT); 2.5 mcg ethinyl estradiol + 0.5 mg norethindrone (FemHRT)

*Generic available.
[†]Strength available in the United States only.
[‡]Strength available in Canada only.

TABLE 34-3 **Oral Estrogen and Estrogen-Progestin Products**

Brand Name	Generic Name
Estrogen Pills	
Premarin	conjugated equine estrogens
Cenestin	synthetic conjugated estrogens
Estratab	esterified estrogens
Menest	esterified estrogens
Ogen	estropipate (piperazine estrone sulfate)
Estrace	micronized 17β-estradiol
Estinyl	ethinyl estradiol
Progestin Pills	
Provera	medroxyprogesterone acetate
Aygestin	norethindrone acetate
Norlutate	norethindrone acetate
Prometrium	progesterone USP (in peanut oil)
Estrogen Plus Progestin Pills	
Premphase	conjugated equine estrogens and medroxyprogesterone acetate
Prempro	conjugated equine estrogens and medroxyprogesterone acetate
FemHRT	ethinylestradiol and norethindrone acetate
Activella	17β-estradiol and norethindrone acetate
Ortho-Prefest	17β-estradiol and norgestimate

Adapted from National Heart, Lung, and Blood Institute: Facts about menopausal hormone therapy (NIH Publ. No. 05-5200), 2005 (http://www.nhlbi.nih.gov/health/women/pht_facts.pdf).

TECH ALERT!

The following drugs have look-alike and sound-alike issues:
 fluoxetine and fluvastatin;
 Prozac, Prilosec, Proscar, Prosom, and Prostep;
 Sarafem and Serophene;
 Paroxetine and pyridoxine;
 Paxil, Plavix, and Taxol;
 sertraline, selegiline, and Serentil;
 Zoloft and Zocor

TECH ALERT!

The following drugs have look-alike and sound-alike issues:
 Aleve and Alesse;
 Anaprox, Anaspaz, and Avapro;
 Naprelan and Naprosyn;
 Naprosyn, naproxen, Natacyn, and Nebcin;
 Oruvail, Clinoril, and Elavil

Menstrual Disorders

PREMENSTRUAL SYNDROME

Premenstrual syndrome (PMS) is a condition that involves a collection of symptoms that regularly occur in women during the premenstrual phase of their reproductive cycles. Symptoms include headache, irritability fatigue, nervousness, weight gain, sleep changes, depression, and other problems that are distressing enough to limit activity and affect personal relationships. Because the causes of PMS are still unclear, current treatments focus on relieving the symptoms. A more severe form of PMS is *premenstrual dysphoric disorder* (PMDD). It is characterized by more pronounced features of PMS and occurs during the last week of the luteal phase in most menstrual cycles during the year preceding diagnosis. These symptoms begin to remit within a few days of the onset of the menses (follicular phase) and are always absent the week following menses. Five or more of the following symptoms must be present to be diagnosed with PMDD: feeling sad, hopeless, or self-deprecating; feeling tense, anxious, or on edge; marked lability of mood interspersed with frequent tearfulness; persistent irritability, anger, and increased interpersonal conflicts; decreased interest in usual activities, difficulty concentrating, feeling fatigue, lethargic, or lacking in energy; marked changes in appetite such as binge eating and cravings; hypersomnia or insomnia; a subjective feeling of being out of control; and physical symptoms such as bloating, weight gain, breast tenderness, and joint or muscle pain. The symptoms may be accompanied by suicidal thoughts. Women commonly report that their symptoms worsen with age until relieved by the onset of menopause. PMDD is treated with antidepressants such as selective serotonin reuptake inhibitors (SSRIs).

TABLE 34-4 **Gels, Creams, Patches, and Other Hormone Products**

Type	Brand Name	Generic Name
Estrogen Products		
Vaginal cream	Estrace	Micronized 17β-estradiol
	Ogen	Estropipate (piperazine estrone sulfate)
	Premarin	Conjugated equine estrogens
Vaginal tablet	Vagifem	Estradiol hemihydrate
Vaginal ring	Estring	Micronized 17β-estradiol
	Femring	Estradiol acetate
Skin patch	Alora	Micronized 17β-estradiol
	Climara	Micronized 17β-estradiol
	Esclim	Micronized 17β-estradiol
	Estraderm	Micronized 17β-estradiol
	Vivelle	Micronized 17β-estradiol
	Vivelle-Dot	Micronized 17β-estradiol
Skin gel	Estrogel	Estradiol gel
Skin cream	Estrasorb	Estradiol topical emulsion
Progestin Products		
Vaginal gel	Crinone	Progesterone
IUD	Mirena	Levonorgestrel
Estrogen Plus Progestin Products		
Skin patch	Combipatch	17β-estradiol and norethindrone acetate
	Ortho-Prefest	17β-estradiol and norgestimate

Adapted from National Heart, Lung, and Blood Institute: Facts about menopausal hormone therapy (NIH Publ. No. 05-5200).

Selective Serotonin Reuptake Inhibitors for Treatment of Premenstrual Dysphoric Disorder

Generic name	U.S. Brand Name(s) / Canadian Brand Name(s)	Dosage Forms and Strengths
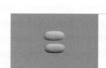 fluoxetine*	Prozac, Prozac Weekly, Sarafem / Prozac	Capsule (Prozac, Sarafem): 10 mg, 20 mg, 40 mg, 60 mg; Capsule, delayed-release (Prozac Weekly): 90 mg; Oral solution (Prozac): 20 mg/5 mL; Tablet, as HCl: 10 mg, 20 mg, 60 mg; 10 mg, 15 mg, 20 mg (Sarafem)
sertraline*	Zoloft / Zoloft	Solution, oral concentrate: 20 mg/mL†; Tablet: 25 mg, 50 mg, 100 mg
paroxetine*	Paxil, Paxil CR, Pexeva / Paxil, Paxil CR	Oral suspension (Paxil): 10 mg/5 mL; Tablet, as HCl (Paxil): 10 mg, 20 mg, 30 mg, 40 mg; Tablet, as mesylate (Pexeva): 10 mg, 20 mg, 30 mg, 40 mg; Tablet, controlled-release (Paxil CR): 12.5 mg, 25 mg, 37.5 mg†

*Generic available.
†Strength available in the United States only.

DYSMENORRHEA

Dysmenorrhea, or painful menstruation, is the term used to describe menstrual cramps. Up to 75% to 85% of all women will have painful periods sometime during their reproductive years. Severe lower abdominal cramping and back pain accompanied by headache, nausea, and vomiting will disrupt their education, work, athletic, or other activities. Primary dysmenorrhea is the most common type, occurring primarily in adolescents and young women. Symptoms, which can last from hours to days and vary in severity from cycle to cycle, are caused by an abnormally increased concentration of certain prostaglandins produced by the uterine lining. High concentrations of prostaglandin E2 (PGE2) and prostaglandin F2 (PGF2) cause painful spasms by decreasing blood flow and oxygen delivery to the uterine muscle. Fortunately, primary dysmenorrhea is not associated with pelvic disease, such as an infection or a tumor. In more severe cases, anti-inflammatory drugs or certain hormones, including OCs, are administered to alter menstrual cycle activity or reduce the level of cyclical uterine contractions. Secondary dysmenorrhea refers to menstrual-related pain caused by a pelvic pathological condition, including inflammatory conditions and cervical stenosis. Treatment involves treating the underlying disorder. Primary dysmenorrhea can generally be treated effectively with over-the-counter (OTC) drugs such as nonsteroidal anti-inflammatory drugs (NSAIDs), discussed in Chapter 10.

AMENORRHEA

Amenorrhea is the absence of normal menstruation. Primary amenorrhea is the failure of the menstrual cycles to begin, and it may be caused by various factors, such as hormone imbalances, genetic disorders, brain lesions, or structural deformities of the reproductive organs. Secondary amenorrhea occurs when a woman who has previously menstruated slows to three or fewer cycles per year.

Nonsteroidal Anti-Inflammatory Drug Treatment for Dysmenorrhea

Generic Name	U.S. Brand Name(s) / Canadian Brand Name(s)	Dosage Forms and Strengths
ibuprofen*	Advil, Motrin, Midol	Tablet: 200 mg, 300 mg, 400 mg, 600 mg, 800 mg
	Advil, Motrin	
naproxen*	Aleve, Anaprox, Anaprox DS, Naprelan, Naprosyn, Pamprin	Caplet: 220 mg Tablet: 250 mg, 375 mg, 500 mg (Anaprox DS: 550 mg) Tablet, controlled release, extended release: 375 mg, 500 mg
	Aleve, Anaprox, Anaprox DS, Naprelan, Naprosyn, Naprosyn E	
ketoprofen*	Nexcede	Caplet: 50 mg, 75 mg Capsule, extended release: 100 mg†, 150 mg†, 200 mg† Suppositories: 100 mg‡ Tablet, enteric coated: 50 mg‡, 100 mg‡ Tablet, extended release: 200 mg‡ Tablet (Nexcede): 12.5 mg (OTC)
	Generics	
meclofenamate*	Generics	Capsule: 50 mg, 100 mg
	Not available	

*Generic available.
†Strength available in the United States only.
‡Strength available in Canada only.

Pharmaceutical Treatment of Amenorrhea

Generic Name	U.S. Brand Name(s) / Canadian Brand Name(s)	Dosage Forms and Strengths
bromocriptine*,ᵃ	Parlodel	Tablet: 2.5 mg Capsule: 5 mg
	Generics	
oral contraceptives	See earlier, "Oral Contraceptives"	See earlier, "Oral Contraceptives"

*Generic available.
ªAlso available as Cycloset (used to treat diabetes).

Amenorrhea may be a symptom of excessive weight loss, pregnancy, lactation, menopause, or disease of the reproductive system. If amenorrhea occurs because of sports training, then treatment may become part of an extensive long-term strategy to address a number of complex nutritional, hormonal, and self-image issues.

DYSFUNCTIONAL UTERINE BLEEDING

Dysfunctional uterine bleeding (DUB) is defined as irregular or excessive uterine bleeding resulting from a structural problem or hormonal imbalance that causes a disruption of blood supply. Excessive uterine bleeding from any cause can result in life-threatening anemia. DUB is a significant medical problem, one that affects almost 2 million women in the United States every year. To diagnose the cause, a physician may use specialized ultrasound or x-ray studies, look directly inside the uterus, or examine tissue obtained by biopsy to exclude cancer. Symptoms may include excessive bleeding and cramping for an abnormal period of time beyond the normal menstrual cycle.

Excessive growth (hyperplasia) and the breakdown of delicate endometrial tissue result in heavy bleeding and hormonal imbalance. Treatment with NSAIDs and hormonal manipulation using low-dose birth control pills may be prescribed. If conservative treatment fails to stop the endometrial lining from hemorrhaging, hysterectomy remains one of the most curative options.

Disorders Caused by Infection or Inflammation of the Reproductive System

STIs are infections caused by communicable pathogens such as viruses (e.g., human papilloma virus), bacteria (e.g., *Neisseria gonorrhoeae*), fungi (e.g., *Candida albicans*), and protozoa (e.g., *Trichomonas vaginalis*). They can all be transmitted by sexual contact.

Treatment of Selected Sexually Transmitted Infections

Generic Name	U.S. Brand Name(s) Canadian Brand Name(s)	Dosage Forms and Strengths	Sexually Transmitted Infection
azithromycin	Zithromax	1 g, single dose	Chancroid
azithromycin*	Zithromax	1 g, single dose	Chlamydia
amoxicillin*	Amoxil	3 g, single dose, with 1 g probenecid	Gonorrhea
azithromycin*	Zithromax	1 g, single dose	
cefpodoxime*	Generics	200 mg, single dose	
ceftriaxone*	Rocephin	125 mg IM, single dose	
cefixime*	Suprax	400 mg, single dose	
cefuroxime*	Ceftin	1 g, single dose	
spiramycin (Canada only)	Rovamycine	12-13.9 million units (8-9 capsules) as a single dose	
doxycycline*	Vibramycin	100 mg every 12 hr for 7 days or 300 mg as a single dose, followed by 300 mg in 1 hr in combination with chlamydial treatment	
tetracycline*	Generics	200-500 mg every 6 hr in combination with chlamydial treatment	

*Generic available.

Pelvic inflammatory disease (PID) may be an acute or chronic inflammatory condition caused by several different pathogens, which usually spread upward from the vagina. PID is a major cause of infertility and sterility and affects more than 750,000 women each year in the United States and 1 in 10 women in Canada. It is a common complication of STIs such as chlamydia and gonorrhea. Infection involving the uterus, uterine tubes, ovaries, and other pelvic organs often results in the development of scar tissue and adhesions.

Salpingitis is a uterine tube inflammatory condition characterized by obstruction of the lumen and marked by dilation at the end of the tube. Fluids accumulate that cannot escape.

Vaginitis is inflammation or infection of the vaginal lining. Vaginitis most often results from an STI or a yeast infection. Yeast infections are opportunistic infections caused by the fungus *C. albicans*. Yeast infections are also known as candidiasis and are characterized by a whitish discharge (leukorrhea).

Diseases classified as STIs can be but do not have to be transmitted sexually. For example, acquired immunodeficiency syndrome (AIDS) is a viral condition that can be spread through sexual contact but is also spread by the transfusion of infected blood and the use of contaminated medical instruments, such as intravenous needles and syringes.

Infertility and Hypogonadism

Infertility is often defined as a failure to conceive after 1 year of regular unprotected intercourse. Infertility may be caused by a wide variety of medical, environmental, and even lifestyle factors, such as smoking or alcohol abuse. Of the causal factors, 90% may be traced to various problems in the male or female partner. For the remaining 10%, the reason is never determined. Approximately 25% of women in the overall population will experience some period of infertility during their reproductive years. In many cases, infertility results from an inability to ovulate, often caused by a medical condition such as *polycystic ovary disease,* a condition characterized by ovaries twice the normal size that contain fluid-filled cysts. Infertile women experiencing ovulatory dysfunction who desire to become pregnant may be eligible to receive fertility drugs, alone or in combination with other assisted reproductive procedures such as artificial insemination. This decision is typically made after a complex medical workup and selection process.

Hypogonadism is a condition in which the sex glands produce little or no hormones. In men, these glands (gonads) are the testes; in women, they are the ovaries. The cause of hypogonadism may be primary or central. In primary hypogonadism, the ovaries or testes themselves do not function properly. Some causes of primary hypogonadism include surgery, radiation, genetic or developmental disorders, liver or kidney disease, infection, and certain autoimmune disorders. The most common genetic disorders that cause primary hypogonadism are *Turner's syndrome* (in women) and *Klinefelter's syndrome* (in men). In central hypogonadism, the centers in the brain that control the gonads (hypothalamus, pituitary) do not function properly. A genetic cause of central hypogonadism that also causes an inability to smell is *Kallman's syndrome* (males). In girls, hypogonadism during childhood will result in lack of menstruation and breast development and short height. If hypogonadism occurs after puberty, symptoms include loss of menstruation, low libido, hot flashes, and loss of body hair. In boys, hypogonadism in childhood results in a lack of muscle and beard development and growth problems. In men, the usual complaints are sexual dysfunction, decreased beard and body hair, breast enlargement, and muscle loss. If a brain tumor is present, there may be headaches or visual loss or symptoms of other hormonal deficiencies (e.g., hypothyroidism). In *prolactinoma,* there may be a milky breast discharge. Additional causes of hypogonadism include tumors, surgery, radiation, infections, trauma, bleeding, nutritional deficiencies, iron excess (hemochromatosis), and drug therapy for prostate disease. Anorexia nervosa (excessive dieting to the point of starvation) may result in central hypogonadism.

TREATMENT OF INFERTILITY

Pharmaceutical treatment of infertility may involve the administration of antiestrogens, menotropins, human chorionic gonadotropin, and recombinant human FSH.

Antiestrogens

Clomiphene is an antiestrogen agent that competes with estrogen for estrogen-receptor binding sites. By blocking estrogen, it acts as an ovulatory stimulant. This agent works by effectively tricking the pituitary gland into producing FSH and LH.

Gonadotropins

Supraovulation, or simultaneous rupture of multiple mature follicles, is an infertility treatment option that may be used if clomiphene proves ineffective or if multiple ova are considered to be useful for assisted reproductive procedures, such as in vitro fertilization. It usually involves self-administered injections of menotropins or genetically developed (recombinant) gonadotropins. Menotropins are purified combination preparations of the human pituitary gonadotropins, FSH, and LH. Menotropins contain a small amount of human chorionic gonadotropin (hCG) and are derived from the urine of postmenopausal women; hCG may be obtained from natural or synthetic sources. The synthetic recombinant formulation is called choriogonadotropin alfa (rhCG). The natural source is the urine of pregnant females.

Follitropin is a recombinant version of human FSH (rFSH). It mimics the actions of naturally released FSH and is required for normal follicular growth, maturation, and gonadal steroid production.

MECHANISM OF ACTION

The production of FSH and LH (gonadotropins) causes normal follicle growth and subsequent ovulation. Clomiphene is given starting on day 5 of the menstrual cycle and, if treatment is successful, ovulation begins 5 to 10 days after a course of the drug.

The effects of hCG on women are essentially identical to those of LH. hCG and human menotropins (human menopausal gonadotropins [hMGs]) are peptides and are quickly destroyed in the gastrointestinal tract; therefore, they must be administered parenterally as an IM injection or, for select products, as an SC injection. Urine-derived hCG is administered IM and recombinant hCG is administered SC. The action of hMG is to mimic the action of naturally released FSH. Administration usually results in follicular growth and maturation, immediately followed by the administration of hCG to produce ovulation.

Infertility Therapy

Generic Name	U.S. Brand Name(s) Canadian Brand Name(s)	Dosage Forms and Strengths
clomiphene	Clomid, Serophene	Tablet: 50 mg
	Clomid, Serophene	
follitropin-alpha	Gonal-f, Gonal-f RFF	Powder, for injection: 75 units, (Gonal-f RFF), 75 units/vial‡, 150 units/vial‡, 450 units/vial, 1050 units/vial, 1200 units/vial‡ (Gonal-f)
	Gonal-f, Gonal-f pen	Solution, for injection-pen (Gonal-f RFF): 300 units, 450 units, 900 units
follitropin-beta	Follistim AQ	Solution, for injection: 75 units†, 150 units, 300 units, 600 units, 900 units
	Puregon	
urofollitropin	Bravelle	Solution, for injection: 75 units/vial
	Bravelle	
human chorionic gonadotropin (hCG)* (choriogonadotropin)	Ovidrel, Pregnyl	Powder for injection (Pregnyl): 10,000 units/vial
	Ovidrel, Pregnyl	Solution, prefilled syringe, for injection (Ovidrel): 250 mcg/0.5 mL
human menopausal gonadotropin (hMG)	Menopur, Repronex	Powder, for injection: 75 units/vial
	Menopur, Repronex	

*Generic available.
†Strength available in the United States only.
‡Strength available in Canada only.

ADVERSE REACTIONS

Clomiphene may cause visual disturbances, dizziness, and lightheadedness. It should not be used during pregnancy. Side effects of gonadotropin administration include headache, lightheadedness, nausea, abdominal discomfort, flushing, and local inflammation at the injection site.

The incidence of multiple births when clomiphene is administered is approximately 5% to 7% (mostly twins). This percentage is much lower than that observed following direct administration (injection) of FSH and LH, in which the intent is to produce multiple follicles before inducing ovulation.

TREATMENT OF HYPOGONADISM

Treatment of hypogonadism involves the administration of synthetic LH, estrogens, and androgens. Gonadotropin therapy works by stimulating the anterior pituitary to release the gonadotropin LH. The effect that LH produces in males differs from that in females. In females, recombinant human LH (rhLH) is indicated for the stimulation of follicular development in infertile hypogonadotropic, hypogonadal women with profound LH deficiency. In males, androgens (e.g., testosterone) play a critical role in sexual maturation throughout life.

Gonadotropin therapy is also used to evaluate functional capacity and response of the gonadotropes of the anterior pituitary and for suspected gonadotropin deficiency. It is also used to evaluate residual gonadotropic function of the pituitary gland following surgical or radiological removal of a pituitary tumor. Unlabeled uses are treatment of delayed puberty, amenorrhea, and infertility in males.

ADVERSE REACTIONS

Common adverse effects produced by rhLH are abdominal bloating, breast tenderness, diarrhea, and gas. Less common adverse reactions are fast heartbeat, skin itching, lightheadedness, headache, stomach, painful menstrual periods and heavy bleeding, and redness, pain, or swelling at the injection site.

Endometriosis

Endometriosis is the benign but painful condition that commonly affects the female reproductive tract. It is characterized by the presence of functioning endometrial tissue outside the uterus. The displaced endometrial tissue is usually attached to an ovary or to the pelvic or abdominal organs; it is occasionally found in other areas of the body. Endometriosis often causes infertility, dysmenorrhea, and severe pain. Symptoms reflect the fact that displaced endometrial tissue reacts to ovarian hormones in the same way as the normal endometrium—exhibiting a cycle of growth and sloughing off. The disorder affects approximately 10% of women; most are aged 30 to 45 years.

Treatment of Hypogonadism

Generic Name	U.S. Brand Name(s) / Canadian Brand Name(s)	Dosage Forms and Strengths
Female		
lutropin alfa	Luveris / Luveris	Injection: 75 units
estrogens	See earlier, "Oral Contraceptives" and "Hormone Replacement Therapy"	See earlier, "Oral Contraceptives" and "Hormone Replacement Therapy"
Male		
methyltestosterone	See later, "Androgen Agonists"	See later, "Androgen Agonists"
testosterone	See later, "Androgen Agonists"	See later, "Androgen Agonists"

TREATMENT OF ENDOMETRIOSIS

Danazol

Danazol, an androgen steroid derivative of testosterone, is used to treat endometriosis and fibrocystic breast disease to reduce breast pain, tenderness, and nodules. It is also used to prevent attacks of hereditary angioedema in males and females.

MECHANISM OF ACTION

Danazol works by suppressing the pituitary output of FSH and LH, resulting in anovulation and associated amenorrhea. It interrupts the progression and pain of endometriosis by causing atrophy of normal and ectopic endometrial tissue.

ADVERSE REACTIONS

Adverse reactions include masculinity effects, gastrointestinal distress, diarrhea, or jaundice, and menstrual irregularities.

Gonadotropin-Releasing Hormone Analogues

Gonadotropin-releasing hormone analogues are synthetic agonists used to treat prostate cancer, endometriosis, advanced breast cancer, and endometrial thinning. It is a synthetic form of LH-releasing hormone (LHRH, or gonadotropin-releasing hormone [GnRH]) that inhibits pituitary gonadotropin secretion. With chronic administration, serum testosterone levels fall into the range normally seen with castrated males.

Treatment of Endometriosis

Generic Name	U.S. Brand Name(s) / Canadian Brand Name(s)	Dosage Forms and Strengths
danazol*	Generics	Capsule: 50 mg, 100 mg, 200 mg
	Cyclomen	

*Generic available.

Gonadotropin-Releasing Hormone and Its Analogues

Generic Name	U.S. Brand Name(s) / Canadian Brand Name(s)	Dosage Forms and Strengths
buserelin	Not available	Implant (Suprefact Depot): 6.3 mg, 9.45 mg
	Suprefact, Suprefact Depot	Solution, injection: 1 mg/mL
goserelin	Zoladex, Zoladex LA	Injection (Zoladex), 1-month implant: 3.6 mg
	Zoledex, Zoladex LA	Injection (Zoladex LA), 3-month implant: 10.8 mg
leuprolide*	Eligard, Lupron, Lupron Depot	Solution, for injection: 5 mg/mL
	Eligard, Lupron, Lupron Depot	Suspension, for injection (Eligard, Lupron Depot): 3.75 mg, 7.5 mg (1 mo); 11.25 mg, 22.5 mg (3 mo); 30 mg (4 mo), 45 mg[†] (6 mo)
nafarelin	Synarel	Solution, nasal spray: 2 mg/mL, 60 metered doses
	Synarel	
histrelin	Supprelin LA, Vantas	Implant: 50 mg
	Vantas	

*Generic available.
[†]Strength available in the United States only.

MECHANISM OF ACTION
Goserelin acetate works by inhibiting gonadotropin secretion.

ADVERSE REACTIONS
Adverse reactions to goserelin acetate include headache, tumor flare, gynecomastia, breast swelling and tenderness, postmenopausal symptoms, vaginal spotting, breakthrough bleeding, decreased libido, impotence, bone pain, and bone loss.

Androgen Deficiency in Men

TREATMENT
Androgen Agonists

The male hormone testosterone and its derivatives are collectively called androgens. They are secreted by the anterior pituitary gland and are responsible for masculinization (development of male secondary sexual characteristics). Small amounts are produced by the adrenal gland. Anabolic steroids closely resemble the androgen testosterone. Androgen therapy is used as replacement therapy for testosterone deficiency such as hypogonadism, select cases of delayed puberty, and postpuberty testosterone deficiency. Anabolic steroids are synthetic drugs chemically related to androgens. They promote the tissue-building process and, in normal dosages, can have a minimal effect on accessory sex organs and secondary sex characteristics.

MECHANISM OF ACTION AND PHARMACOKINETICS
Androgens aid in the development and maintenance of secondary sexual characteristics such as facial hair, deepening of voice, growth of body hair, fat distribution, and muscle development, in adolescent boys. Testosterone also stimulates the growth of accessory sex organs (penis, testes, vas deferens, prostate). Androgens also promote tissue-building processes (anabolism) and tissue-depleting processes (catabolism).

Androgen Agonists

Generic Name	U.S. Brand Name(s) / Canadian Brand Name(s)	Dosage Forms and Strengths
fluoxymesterone	Generics / Not available	Tablet: 10 mg
methyltestosterone*	Android, Testred / Not available	Capsule (Testred): 10 mg / Tablet (Android): 10 mg
oxandrolone	Oxandrin / Not available	Tablet: 2.5 mg, 10 mg
testosterone*	Androderm, Axiron, Delatestryl, Fortesta, Striant, Testim, Testopel / Andriol, Androderm, Androgel, Delatestryl, Testim	Capsule, as undeconate (Andriol): 40 mg; Topical gel (Androgel, Testim): 1%, 1.62%[†]; Spray, solution (Axiron): 30 mg/actuation; Spray, gel (Fortesta): 10 mg/activation; Solution, injection: 100 mg/mL[‡], 200 mg/mL; Oil, as enanthate injection: 200 mg/mL; Tablet, buccal (Striant): 30 mg; Pellet (Testopel): 75 mg; Patch (Androderm): 2 mg/24 hr[†], 2.5 mg/24hr[‡], 4 mg/24 hr[†], 5 mg/24 hr[‡]

*Generic available.
[†]Strength available in the United States only.
[‡]Strength available in Canada only.

They are available in different dosage forms as patches, gels, tablets, capsules, mucoadhesives (buccal), injections, transdermal patches, and pellets. The mucoadhesive form produces twice the androgen activity of oral tablets, the transdermal patch is applied daily to the scrotum or other parts of the body, and the gel is applied to the shoulder, upper arm, and abdomen (it should not be applied to the genitals).

ADVERSE REACTIONS

Androgens may produce gynecomastia (breast enlargement), testicular atrophy, impotence, decreased testicular function, penis enlargement, nausea, jaundice, headache, anxiety, male pattern baldness, acne, and depression. Fluid electrolyte imbalances (e.g., sodium, chloride, potassium, calcium, phosphate, water retention) may also occur. Prolonged use of anabolic steroids can cause many of the same serious adverse effects as androgens, as well as testicular atrophy, blood-filled cysts in the liver or spleen, malignant and benign liver tumors, increased risk of atherosclerosis, and mental changes (e.g., rage). These adverse effects are why androgens (anabolic steroids) are regulated as controlled substances.

Summary of Drugs That Affect the Reproductive System

Generic Name	Brand Name	Usual Dose and Dosing Schedule	Warning Labels
Premenstrual Dysphoric Disorder: Selective Serotonin Reuptake Inhibitors			
fluoxetine	Prozac, Sarafem	20 mg/day starting 14 days prior to menstruation through first full day of menses	MAY CAUSE DIZZINESS. MAY IMPAIR ABILITY TO DRIVE. AVOID ALCOHOL.
sertraline	Zoloft	50 mg/day through luteal phase; can increase to 100 mg/day in 3-day increments	SWALLOW WHOLE; DON'T CRUSH OR CHEW (DELAYED- RELEASE).
paroxetine	Paxil, Paxil CR, Prexeva	12.5-25 mg/day through luteal phase; increase dose at 1-wk intervals if needed	
Nonsteroidal Anti-Inflammatory Drugs Used For Dysmenorrhea			
ibuprofen	Advil, Motrin, Midol	Initial dose 200 mg; then 400 mg every 4-6 hr (max daily dose, 1200 mg/24 hr)	TAKE WITH FOOD. AVOID ASPIRIN WHILE TAKING THIS PRODUCT. MAY CAUSE DROWSINESS.
naproxen	Aleve, Anaprox, Naprelan, Naprosyn, Pamprin	Initial dose, 500 mg; then 250 mg every 6-8 hr (max daily dose,1250 mg)	
ketoprofen	Generic	25-50 mg every 6-8 hr (max daily dose, 300 mg)	
meclofamate	Generic	50 mg every 6-8 hr (max daily dose, 400 mg)	
Amenorrhea			
bromocriptine	Parlodel	1.25-2.5 mg/day (max daily dose, 30 mg/day)	TAKE WITH FOOD OR MILK. MAY CAUSE DROWSINESS. LIMIT ALCOHOL USE.
oral contraceptives	See earlier, "Oral Contraceptives"	See earlier, "Oral Contraceptives"	

Summary of Drugs That Affect the Reproductive System—cont'd

Generic Name	Brand Name	Usual Dose and Dosing Schedule	Warning Labels
Oral Contraceptives			
Estrogen and Progestin Combinations			
ethinyl estradiol + desogestrel	Apri, Cyclessa, Desogen, Kariva, Mircette, Ortho-Cept, Solia, Velivet	Take 1 tablet daily at same time every day for 21 days; off 7 days (21 day cycle), or take 1 tablet daily at same time every day (28-day cycle)	MAY TAKE WITH FOOD. TAKE AT THE SAME TIME EACH DAY. AVOID PROLONGED EXPOSURE TO SUNLIGHT MAY CAUSE CONTACT LENSES TO FEEL UNCOMFORTABLE. DO NOT BREAST-FEED WHILE ON THIS DRUG. REPORT ANY OF THE FOLLOWING: SEVERE HEADACHES, VOMITING, DISTURBED VISION OR SPEECH, NUMBNESS OR WEAKNESS IN EXTREMITIES, DEPRESSION, UNUSUAL BLEEDING. USE EXACTLY AS PRESCRIBED. AVOID SMOKING.
ethinyl estradiol + drospirenone	Yasmin, Yaz		
ethinyl estradiol + etonogestrel	Nuva-Ring	Insert ring vaginally and leave in place for 3 wk. Remove for 1 wk. Insert new ring 7 days after last one was removed.	
ethinyl estradiol + levonorgestrel	Alesse, Aviane, Enpresse, Levlite, Levora, Lutera, Nordette, Portia, Seasonale, Triphasil, Trivora	Take 1 tablet at same time every day for 21 days; off 7 days (21 day cycle), or take 1 tablet daily at same time every day (28-day cycle)	
	Min-Ovral, Triquilar		
ethinyl estradiol + norethindrone	Aranelle, Brevicon, Estrostep Fe, Junel, Junel 0.5/35, Norinyl - available as 1 + 35 and 1 + 50 Norinyl 1 + 35, Nortrel, Nortrel 7/7/7, Ortho-Novum, Ovcon, Tri-Norinyl	Take 1 tablet at same time every day for 21 days; off 7 days (21 day cycle), or take 1 tablet daily at same time every day (28-day cycle)	
	Minestrin 1/20, Select 1/35, Symphasic		
ethinyl estradiol + norgestimate	Ortho-Cyclen, Ortho Tri-Cyclen, Previfem, Sprintec, Tri-Nessa, Tri-Prevofem, Tri-Sprintec	Take 1 tablet at same time every day for 21 days; off 7 days (21 day cycle), or take 1 tablet daily at same time every day (28 day cycle)	
Intrauterine Devices			
copper-releasing	ParaGard	**Intrauterine device:** Insert IUD into uterine cavity; replace 10 yr after insertion.	CALL YOUR HEALTH CARE PROVIDER IF YOU CANNOT FEEL THE IUD THREADS OR THEY FEEL LONGER. CALL IF YOU HAVE PELVIC PAIN OR PAIN DURING SEXUAL INTERCOURSE. REPORT SUDDEN LOSS OF VISION OR MIGRAINE HEADACHE (MIRENA).
levonorgestrel	Mirena	**Intrauterine device:** Insert IUD into uterine cavity; replace 5 yr after insertion.	

Continued

Summary of Drugs That Affect the Reproductive System—cont'd

Generic Name	Brand Name	Usual Dose and Dosing Schedule	Warning Labels
Contraceptive Implant			
etonogestrel	Implanon	Insert 1 rod under the skin in upper arm; replace 3 yr after insertion.	CALL YOUR DOCTOR IF YOU CANNOT FEEL THE IMPLANT.
Emergency Contraceptives			
levonorgestrel	Plan B	Take 1 tablet within 72 hr of unprotected sexual intercourse; take another tablet 12 hr later or take 2 tablets as a single dose.	AVOID SMOKING REPORT SUDDEN LOSS OF VISION OR SUDDEN ACUTE HEADACHE
Hormone Replacement Therapy			
Estrogen			
estradiol	Alora, Climara, Delestrogen, Depo-estradiol, Esclim, Estrace, Estraderm, Estrasorb, Estring, EstroGel, Femring, Gynodiol, Menostar, Vagifem, Vivelle, Vivelle-Dot, Estradot, Oesclim	**Vaginal cream:** Insert 2 g/day to 4 g/day intravaginally for 2 wk; then reduce to half the initial dose for 2 wk, followed by maintenance dose of 1 g two or three times/wk **Topical emulsion:** Apply 3.84 g once daily in the morning. **Topical gel:** 1.25 g/day applied at same time daily **Patch:** Apply 0.025 mg once/wk; 0.05 mg twice/wk. **Vaginal ring:** Insert 0.05 mg ring intravaginally: leave in for 3 mo. **Vaginal tablet:** Insert 1 tablet daily for 2 wks; maintenance, insert 1 tablet twice weekly.	ROTATE SITE OF APPLICATION (TRANSDERMAL PATCH). REPORT SUDDEN SEVERE HEADACHE, VOMITING, VISION OR SPEECH DISTURBANCE, LOSS OF VISION, NUMBNESS OR WEAKNESS IN EXTREMITIES, SHARP OR CRUSHING CHEST PAIN, SHORTNESS OF BREATH, SEVERE ABDOMINAL PAIN OR MASS, DEPRESSION, UNUSUAL BLEEDING. AVOID SMOKING.
estrogens (conjugated A) estrogens (conjugated B)	Cenestin Enjuvia	**Tablet:** 0.45-1.25 mg/day for 21 days followed by 7 days drug-free or 1 tablet daily on days 1-25 of each month coadministered with progestin the last 10-14 days of cycle; drug-free last 5 days of cycle.	TAKE WITH FOOD (TABLET)
estrogens (equine)	Premarin, C.E.S. Congest	**Vaginal cream:** Insert 0.5-2 g/day intravaginally for 3 wk, then 1 wk off (cyclically) **Tablet:** 0.3 mg/day cyclically or daily	
estrogen (esterified)	Menest, Estratab	**Tablet:** 0.3-1.25 mg/day cyclically	
estropipate	Ogen	**Tablet:** 0.75-6 mg daily	

Summary of Drugs That Affect the Reproductive System—cont'd

Generic Name	Brand Name	Usual Dose and Dosing Schedule	Warning Labels
Estrogen and Progesterone Combinations			
estradiol + levonoregestrel	ClimaraPro	**Transdermal:** apply 1 patch weekly	DO NOT EXPOSE PATCH TO SUNLIGHT FOR LONG PERIODS OF TIME.
estradiol + norethindrone	Activella, CombiPatch	**Transdermal patch:** apply new patch twice weekly during 28-day cycle	ROTATE SITE OF APPLICATION.
	Estalis, Estalis-Sequi	**Combination:** apply estradiol patch only for 14 days, followed by Estalis patch twice weekly for 14 days for 28-day cycle **Tablet:** 1 daily	TAKE WITH FOOD. AVOID PROLONGED EXPOSURE TO SUNLIGHT.
estradiol + norgestimate	Prefest	**Tablet:** 1 mg pink tablet daily for 3 days followed by 0.09 mg white tablet for 3 days: repeat sequence	
estrogens + medroxyprogesterone acetates (MPA)	Premphase, Premplus, Prempro	**Premphase:** 1 maroon tablet days 1 to 14 followed by 1 light blue tablet days 15 to 28	
	Premplus	**Prempro:** 0.3-0.625 mg/MPA; 1.5-5 mg tablet daily	
estrogen + methyl testosterone	Estratest, Estratest H.S., Syntest D.S., Syntest H.S.	**Tablet:** 1 daily; 3 wk on, 1 wk off	TAKE WITH FOOD.
Infertility Therapy			
clomiphene	Clomid, Serophene	**Male:** 25 mg/day for 25 days with 5 days rest *or* 100 mg every Monday, Wednesday, Friday **Female:** 50 mg/day for 5 days	TAKE EXACTLY AS DIRECTED; DON'T SKIP DOSES.
menotropins	Pergonal	**Pergonal: Male:** IM injection 75-150 IU 3 times/wk **Female:** 75-150 IU for 7-12 days **Repronex, female:** 150-450 IU daily for 5 to 12 days	REFRIGERATE DILUTED POWDER; DO NOT FREEZE. PROTECT FROM LIGHT.
follitropin-alpha	Gonal-f	**Infertility:** 75 IU/day SC; if no response in 5 to 7 days, may increase by 37.5 IU weekly until max 300 IU **Hypogonadism (men):** 150 IU SC 3 times/wk with hCG, 1000 units	USE IMMEDIATELY AFTER RECONSTITUTION.
human chorionic gonadotropin(recombinant)	Profasi	**Injection: Female:** 5,000- 10,000 units for 1 day **Male:** 1500-3000 units, 2 times/wk	DISCARD ANY UNUSED RECONSTITUTED SOLUTION.
Endometriosis			
danazol	Generics Cyclomen	**Capsule:** 200-400 mg/day in 2 divided doses (individualized dosage) **Maintenance dose:** 800 mg/day in 2 divided doses	TAKE WITH FOOD.

Continued

Summary of Drugs That Affect the Reproductive System—cont'd

Generic Name	Brand Name	Usual Dose and Dosing Schedule	Warning Labels
Gonadotropin-Releasing Hormone and Analogues			
goserelin	Zoladex Zoladex LA	**Injection:** Inject dose every 28 days **Implant:** Insert every 1-3 mo (1-month implant, 3.6 mg; 3-month implant, 10.8 mg)	STORE AT ROOM TEMPERATURE UNTIL READY FOR USE. DO NOT FREEZE. INJECT ACCORDING TO PRESCRIBED SCHEDULE.
leuprolide	Eligard, Lupron, Lupron Depot,	**Precocious puberty:** **Injection:** 7.5 mg, 11.25 mg, or 15 mg as single dose monthly **Anemia caused by uterine fibroids (Lupron Depot):** 3.5 mg monthly or 11.25 mg every 3 mo	RESHAKE SUSPENSION IF SETTLING OCCURS. DISCARD ANY UNUSED SUSPENSION (DEPOT SUSPENSION). STORE AT ROOM TEMPERATURE (SOLUTION). ROTATE INJECTION SITE.
nafarelin	Synarel	**Endometriosis:** 2 sprays in one nostril in the morning and 1 spray in the other nostril in the evening **Precocious puberty:** 2 sprays in each nostril every morning and evening	DO NOT USE NASAL DECONGESTANTS FOR 30 MIN AFTER USING NAFARELIN SPRAY.
Treatment for Hypogonadism			
lutropin alfa	Luveris	75-150 IU SC once daily	DISCARD ANY UNUSED PORTION OF VIAL.
Androgen Agonists			
fluoxymesterone	Halotestin	**Tablet:** 5-20 mg/day	TAKE AS DIRECTED.
methyltestosterone	Android	**Oral:** 10-50 mg/day **Buccal:** 5 mg/day to 25 mg/day	TAKE WITH FOOD. DISSOLVE BUCCAL TABLETS IN CHEEK: DO NOT EAT, DRINK, CHEW, OR SMOKE WHILE BUCCAL TABLET IS IN PLACE.
oxandrolone	Oxandrin	**Cachexia:** 2.5-20 mg daily in 2-4 divided doses for 2-4 wk	TAKE AS DIRECTED.
testosterone	Androderm, Delatestryl, Striant Testoderm	**Pellet:** SC implantation, 150-450 mg every 3-6 mo **Scrotal patch (Testoderm):** 6 mg daily to scrotum **Transdermal patch (Androderm, Testoderm TTS):** Apply daily to back, abdomen, thigh, or arm **Injection:** 50-400 mg every 2-4 wk **Gel:** 5 g daily **Oral, buccal (Striant):** 30 mg every 12 hr	ROTATE SITE OF APPLICATION (PATCH, INJECTION). APPLY TO THE UPPER GUM ABOVE THE INCISOR TOOTH (BUCCAL TABLET). APPLY TO ARM, ABDOMEN, BACK, OR THIGH (ANDRODERM). APPLY TO SCROTUM (TESTODERM).

Chapter Summary

- The average gestational period for pregnancy is 280 days, or 40 weeks. approximately 7 million American women become pregnant each year, and approximately two thirds of those pregnancies result in live births.
- Infertility may be caused by a wide variety of medical, environmental, and even lifestyle factors, such as smoking or alcohol abuse.
- Symptoms of premenstrual syndrome include headache, irritability fatigue, nervousness, weight gain, sleep changes, depression, and other problems that are distressing enough to limit activity and affect personal relationships.
- Amenorrhea may be a symptom of weight loss, pregnancy, lactation, menopause, or disease of the reproductive system.
- Dysfunctional uterine bleeding is irregular or excessive uterine bleeding that usually results from a structural problem or some type of hormonal imbalance.
- Pelvic inflammatory disease occurs as an acute or chronic inflammatory condition caused by several different pathogens, which usually spread upward from the vagina.
- Sexually transmitted infections (previously referred to as sexually transmitted diseases or venereal diseases) are infections caused by communicable pathogens such as viruses, bacteria, fungi, and protozoa. They can be transmitted by sexual contact.
- Menopause is the termination of menstrual cycles and is usually marked by the passage of at least 1 full year without menstruation.
- Endometriosis is a benign but painful condition that commonly affects the female reproductive tract and is characterized by the presence of functioning endometrial tissue outside the uterus.
- Condoms are used to prevent pregnancy and transmission of sexually transmitted infections such as gonorrhea, syphilis, and HIV.
- Most hormonal contraceptives were developed to prevent pregnancy by initiating negative feedback inhibition of follicle-stimulating hormone and luteinizing hormone secretion.
- The diaphragm must be inserted sometime before sexual intercourse and remain in the vagina for 6 to 8 hours after a male's last ejaculation.
- The presence of an intrauterine device in the uterus prompts the release of leukocytes and prostaglandins by the endometrium. These substances are hostile to sperm and eggs.
- If used correctly and consistently, the pill is an extremely effective contraceptive, with an unintended pregnancy rate estimated at between 0.1% and 3%.
- Emergency use of oral contraceptive pills containing levonorgestrel alone reduces the risk for pregnancy after unprotected intercourse by 89%.
- Hormone replacement therapy is generally used to treat symptoms of menopause such as hot flashes, vaginal dryness, mood swings, sleep disorders, and decreased sexual desire.
- The Women's Health Initiative and other studies are providing important information about the risks and benefits of long-term hormone replacement therapy and offer women some guidance on HRT use. http://www.nhlbi.nih.gov/whi/ -
- Gonadotropin-releasing hormone analogues are used to treat prostate cancer, endometriosis, advanced breast cancer, and endometrial thinning.
- The male hormone testosterone and its derivatives are called androgens, secreted by the anterior pituitary gland, and responsible for masculinization (development of male secondary sexual characteristics).

1. The average human gestational period is _____.
   a. 280 days, or 40 weeks
   b. 294 days, or 42 weeks
   c. 290 days, or 42 weeks
   d. 273 days, or 39 weeks

2. Menorrhagia is a term used for _____ menstrual bleeding.
   a. Diminished
   b. Excessive
   c. Absence of
   d. Painful

3. Bromocriptine is a drug used to treat _____.
   a. Premenstrual dysphoric disorder
   b. Dysmenorrhea
   c. Amenorrhea
   d. All of the above

4. Pelvic inflammatory disease is a common complication following infection by _____.
   a. Human immunodeficiency virus (HIV)
   b. Chlamydial organism
   c. Gonococcal organism
   d. b and c

5. Menopause is the termination of menstrual cycles that is usually marked by the passage of at least 2 full years without menstruation.
   a. True
   b. False

6. Oral contraceptives (the pill) are 100% effective in preventing pregnancy.
   a. True
   b. False

7. The WHI study on hormonal replacement therapy concluded that hormonal replacement therapy may increase the risk for _____.
   a. Heart disease and breast cancer
   b. Heart attack and blood clots
   c. Strokes
   d. All of the above

8. Clomiphene is a drug used to treat _____.
   a. Contraception
   b. Infertility
   c. Hypogonadism
   d. Amenorrhea

9. Gonadotropin therapy works by stimulating the _____ pituitary to release the gonadotropin LH.
   a. Anterior
   b. Posterior
   c. Interior
   d. Exterior

10. Testosterone and anabolic steroids are _____ controlled substances in the United States and _____ in Canada.
    a. Schedule I, C1
    b. Schedule II, C2
    c. Schedule III, C3
    d. Schedule IV, C4

TECHNICIAN'S CORNER

1. Since the WHI study, many women have turned to herbal preparations to combat menopausal symptoms. How effective are these preparations in improving these symptoms?
2. Many athletes have been using anabolic steroids to gain an edge in their sport. What are some long-term effects of these steroids on the body and mind?

Bibliography

Centers for Disease Control and Prevention, Workowski KA, Berman SM: Sexually transmitted diseases treatment guidelines, 2006, *MMWR Recomm Rep* 55(RR-11):1-94, 2006.

Cervical Barrier Advancement Society: Diaphragms, 2010 (http://www.cervical barriers.org/information/diaphragms.cfm).

Elsevier. (2010). Gold Standard Clinical Pharmacology. Retrieved June 15, 2012, from https://www.clinicalpharmacology.com/

Health Canada. (2010). Drug Product Database. Retrieved June 15, 2012, from http://www.hc-sc.gc.ca/dhp-mps/prodpharma/databasdon/index-eng.php

Hutten-Czapski P, Goertzen J: The occasional intrauterine contraceptive device insertion, *Can J Rural Med* 13:31-35, 2008.

Lance L, Lacy C, Armstrong L, et al: *Drug information handbook for the allied health professional*, ed 12, Hudson, OH, 2005, APhA Lexi-Comp.

MBC 3320 androgens (http://www.neurosci.pharm.utoledo.edu/MBC3320/androgens.htm) http://www.riwarijn.org/uploads/tx_deriwa/142_thyroid_rapport.pdf—Cached These comprise the estrogen/androgen system (Hypothalamus-pituitary-sex organ system, ... http://www.neurosci.pharm.utoledo.edu/MBC3320/thyroid.htm. [j] ...

MedLine Plus: Amenorrhea, 2012 (http://www.nlm.nih.gov/medlineplus/ ency/article/ 001218.htm).

MedLine Plus: Hormone replacement therapy, 2012 (http://www.nlm.nih.gov/medlineplus/hormonereplacementtherapy.html).

MedLine Plus: Hypogonadism, 2012 (http://www.nlm.nih.gov/medlineplus/ ency/article/001195.htm).

National Heart Lung and Blood Institute: (2002). NHLBI Stops Trial of Estrogen Plus Progestin Due to Increased Breast Cancer Risk, Lack of Overall Benefit. Retrieved June 13, 2012, from http://www.nhlbi.nih.gov/news/press-releases/2002/nhlbi-stops-trial-of-estrogen-plus-progestin-due-to-increased-breast-cancer-risk-lack-of-overall-benefit.html

National heart Lung and Blood Institute. (2004). NIH Asks Participants in Women's Health Initiative Estrogen-Alone Study to Stop Study Pills, Begin Follow-up Phase. Retrieved June 13, 2012, from http://www.nhlbi.nih.gov/news/press-releases/2004/nih-asks-participants-in-womens-health-initiative-estrogen-alone-study-to-stop-study-pills-begin-follow-up-phase.html

National Heart, Lung, and Blood Institute: Facts about menopausal hormone therapy (NIH Publ. No. 05-5200), 2005 (http://www.nhlbi.nih.gov/health/women/pht_facts.pdf).

Roach S: *Pharmacology for health professionals*, Baltimore, 2005, Lippincott, Williams & Wilkins.

Shannon M, Wilson B, Stang C: *Health professionals drug guide, 2005-2006*, Upper Saddle River, NJ, 2006, Prentice-Hall.

Kallmann's Syndrome, Tabers Medical Dictionary, ed 20, Philadelphia, 2005, FA. Davis, p 1163.

Teva Women's Health: ParaGard, 2012 (http://www.paragard.com/default.aspx).

Thibodeau G, Patton K: *Anatomy and physiology*, ed 6, St. Louis, 2007, Mosby.

U.S. Department of Health and Human Services Office on Women's Health: Birth Control Methods, 2009. Retrieved June 6, 2011, from http://www.womenshealth.gov/publications/our-publications/fact-sheet/birth-control-methods.cfm.

U.S. Food and Drug Administration: Plan B (0.75 mg levonorgestrel) and Plan B One-Step (1.5 mg levonorgestrel) tablets information, 2011 (http://www.fda.gov/Drugs/DrugSafety/PostmarketDrugSafetyInformationforPatientsandProviders/UCM109775).

Women's College Hospital: Pelvic inflammatory disease, 2012 (http://www.womenshealthmatters.ca/health-resources/pelvic-health/pelvic-inflammatory-disease).

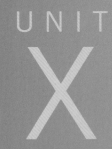

Drugs Affecting the Immune System

---

1 Identify the organs and vessels and understand the functions of the lymphatic system.
2 Understand the function of cells of the immune system.
3 Explain the process of adaptive and innate immunity.

Adaptive immunity: Involves mechanisms that recognize specific threatening agents and then adapts, or responds, by targeting their activity only against these agents. Also called specific immunity.

Antibodies: Proteins (immunoglobulins), on the surface of B cells that mount an immune response and fight disease by recognizing and attacking antigens, substances that are considered foreign or abnormal.

Innate immunity: Nonspecific immunity that is not dependent on pre-exposure to a harmful particle or condition. The primary types of cells involved in innate immunity are epithelial barrier cells, phagocytic cells (neutrophils, macrophages), and natural killer (NK) cells.

Opsonization: The process of modifying (as a bacterium) by various proteins (as complement or antibodies) that bind to foreign particles and microorganisms (as bacteria) making them more susceptible to the action of phagocytes.

Overview of the Lymphatic System

The lymphatic system serves various functions in the body. The two most important functions of this system are maintenance of fluid balance in the internal environment and immunity. A third function is absorption of fats from the small intestines by lymphatic vessels located in the intestinal wall, with transport to the bloodstream. The lymphatic system consists of moving fluid (*lymph*) derived from the blood and tissue fluid through a group of vessels (*lymphatics*) that return the lymph to the blood. In addition to the lymph and lymphatic vessels, the system includes lymphoid tissue containing lymphocytes and other specialized cells. Lymph nodes are located along the paths of collecting lymphatic vessels. Peyer's patches are in the intestinal wall. Additional lymphoid structures include the tonsils, thymus, spleen, and bone marrow.

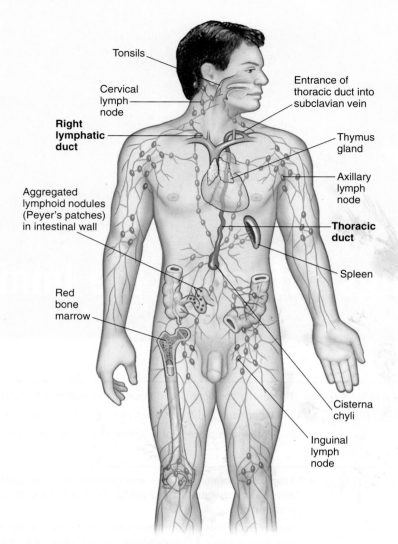

The Lymphatic System. (From Thibodeau GA, Patton KT: *Anatomy and physiology*, ed 6, St. Louis, 2007, Mosby.)

LYMPH VESSELS

Lymph capillaries are thin-walled tubes that form complex networks transporting lymph from tissue spaces to larger lymphatic vessels. The larger lymphatic vessels lead to specialized masses of tissue called *lymph nodes* located along the paths of the lymph vessels. After leaving the nodes, the vessels merge to form even larger vessels called lymphatic trunks that join one of two collecting ducts, the right lymphatic duct or thoracic duct. After leaving the collecting ducts, lymph enters the venous system through the left subclavian vein.

LYMPH NODES

Lymph nodes not only produce lymphocytes but also filter and trap inflammatory causing substances to cancerous lesions. They contain specialized cells called *macrophages* located in the lymph nodes—as well as in the spleen, liver, lungs, brain, and spinal cord—that engulf and destroy antigens (substances not recognized as self). This process is called phagocytosis. Specialized lymphocytes (*B cells*) present in the nodes produce antibodies. *T cell* lymphocytes attack bacteria and foreign cells by accurately recognizing a cell surface protein as nonself and attaching to and destroying it.

SPLEEN AND THYMUS GLAND

The spleen is located in the upper left quadrant of the abdomen, adjacent to the stomach, and has several important functions—destruction of old erythrocytes by macrophages, filtration of microorganisms and other harmful substances from the blood, activation of lymphocytes as it filters antigens from the blood, and storage of blood, especially erythrocytes and platelets. The ***thymus gland*** is a lymphatic organ located in the upper mediastinum between the lungs. During fetal life and childhood it is large, but becomes smaller with age. The thymus gland is composed of nests of lymphoid cells. The development of T lymphocytes, especially in the early years of growth, plays an important role in the body's ability to protect itself from disease.

Organization of the Immune System

The immune system is continually patrolling the body for harmful or internal enemies. To do this, the immune system must recognize unique molecules and groups of molecules on the surface of cells, viruses, and other particles that can be used to identify them. Similarly, our own cells have unique cell markers (***antigens***) embedded in our plasma membrane that identify our cells as ***self***. Foreign cells or particles have ***nonself*** molecules that serve as recognition markers for our immune system. The ability of our immune system to attack abnormal cells but spare our own normal cells is called ***self-tolerance***. All these defensive mechanisms can be categorized into two major categories, innate immunity and adaptive immunity.

INNATE IMMUNITY

Innate or nonspecific immunity is in place before a person is exposed to a particular harmful particle or condition. The primary types of cells involved in innate immunity are epithelial barrier cells, phagocytic cells (neutrophils, macrophages), and natural killer (NK) cells. ***Cytokines***, which are chemicals released from cells to trigger innate and adaptive immune responses, also participate in innate immunity. Examples of cytokines include interleukins, leukotrienes, and interferons. In addition to cytokines, other chemicals play a regulatory role in immunity, such as complements, other enzymes, and histamine, an amine.

Mechanisms of Innate Defense

Mechanism	Description
Species resistance	Phenomenon in which the genetic characteristics common to a particular type of organism, or species, provide defense against certain pathogens (disease-causing agents).
Mechanical and chemical barriers	Physical impediments to the entry of foreign cells or substances. The skin and mucosa form a continuous wall that separates the internal environment from the external environment, preventing the entry of pathogens. Secretions such as sebum, mucus, and enzymes and hydrochloric acid chemically inhibit the activity of pathogens.
Inflammatory response	Isolates the pathogens and stimulates the speedy arrival of a large number of immune cells. The inflammation mediators include histamine, kinins, prostaglandins, leukotrienes, interleukins, and related compounds. Many of these mediators are chemotactic factors. They attract white blood cells to the area in the process called chemotaxis.
Phagocytosis	Ingestion and destruction of pathogens by phagocytic cells such as neutrophils and macrophages (monocytes). The movement of phagocytes from blood vessels to inflammation sites is called diapedesis. Phagocytes have a very short life span; thus, dead cells tend to pile up at the inflammation site, forming a white substance called pus.
Natural killer cells	Group of lymphocytes that kill many different types of cancer cells and virus-infected cells. They are produced in red bone marrow and are neither T cells nor B cells.
Interferon	Protein produced by cells after they become infected by a virus; inhibits the spread or further development of a viral infection.
Complement	Group of plasma proteins ($\approx$20 inactive enzymes) that produce a cascade of chemical reactions that ultimately cause lysis (rupture) of a foreign cell.

ADAPTIVE IMMUNITY

Adaptive immunity is also called *specific immunity* and involves mechanisms that recognize specific threatening agents and then adapts, or responds, by targeting their activity only against these agents. Lymphocytes (T -cells and B -cells) are the primary leukocytes (white blood cells) involved in adaptive immunity, B cell lymphocytes do not attack pathogens themselves but instead produce molecules called *antibodies* that attack the pathogens or direct other cells, such as phagocytes, to attack them. B cell mechanisms are classified as antibody-mediated immunity, or *humoral immunity*. Because T cells attack pathogens more directly, T cell mechanisms are classified as *cell-mediated immunity*, or cellular immunity. The densest populations of lymphocytes occur in the bone marrow, thymus gland, lymph nodes, and spleen.

Antibodies (Immunoglobulins)

Antibodies are proteins called *immunoglobulins* (Ig). There are five classes of antibodies, identified by letter names as immunoglobulins M, G, A, E, and D. IgM is the antibody that immature B cells synthesize and insert into their plasma membranes. It is also the predominant class of antibody produced after initial contact with an antigen. The most abundant circulating antibody is IgG. The IgG antibodies cross the placental barrier during pregnancy to impart natural passive immunity to the offspring. IgA is present in the mucous membranes of the body, in saliva, and in tears. IgE can produce major harmful effects, such as those associated with allergies. The precise function of IgD is unknown. The function of antibody molecules is to produce antibody-mediated immunity. They fight disease first by recognizing substances that are foreign or abnormal.

Complement

Complement is a component of blood plasma that consists of approximately 20 protein compounds. They are inactive enzymes and are triggered by adaptive or innate immunity mechanisms. Ultimately, they cause the lysis (rupture) of the cell that triggered it. Complement also marks microbes for destruction by phagocytic cells in a process called *opsonization*, which promotes the inflammatory response.

Types of Adaptive Immunity

Type	Mechanism and Example
Natural Immunity	Exposure to a causative agent that is not deliberate
Active (exposure)	A child develops measles and acquires immunity to a subsequent infection
Passive (exposure)	A fetus receives protection from the mother through the placenta or an infant receives protection through the mother's milk
Artificial Immunity	Exposure to a causative agent that is deliberate
Active (exposure)	Injection of the causative agent, such as a vaccination against polio, that confers immunity
Passive (exposure)	Injection of a protective material (antibodies) that was developed by another individual's immune system

Antibody Isotypes of Mammals

Name	Isotype	Description
IgA	2	Prevents colonization by pathogens
IgD	1	Precise function is unknown; believed to stimulate B cell, basophil, and mast cell activation
IgE	1	Triggers histamine release from mast cells and basophils, producing allergic symptoms
IgG	4	In its four forms, provides most antibody-based immunity against invading pathogens
IgM	1	Inactivates pathogens in the early stages of B cell–mediated (humoral) immunity; appears early in an infection; presence signals a recent infection

T Cells and Cell-Mediated Immunity

DEVELOPMENT OF T CELLS

T cells are lymphocytes that have made a detour through the thymus gland before migrating to the lymph nodes and spleen. Each T cell, like each B cell, displays antigen receptors on its surface membrane. T cells are activated when antigen fragments from foreign proteins bind to T cell receptors. B cells, on the other hand, react mainly to antigens that are in plasma. When an antigen is present, the T cells are activated or sensitized. The T cells then divide repeatedly to form identical clones, *effector T cells* and *memory T cells*. Effector T cells include cytotoxic T cells, which are also called killer T cells because they kill the target cell. In addition to cytotoxic T cells, there are two types of effector T cells found in the body, *helper T cells* and *suppressor T cells*. Both types of cells help regulate adaptive immune function by regulating B cell and T cell function. Helper T cells help other lymphocytes by secreting cytokines that stimulate B cells and cytotoxic T cells. Suppressor T cells act to suppress B cell differentiation into plasma cells. The antagonistic action allows the immune system to fine-tune its antibody-mediated response. Suppressor T cells also regulate other T cells, helping to turn off an immune response to restore homeostasis.

Summary

The immune system, along with the nervous and endocrine systems, maintains the relative constancy of the body's internal environment. When the immune system overreacts to antigens or fails to react to antigens, the body reacts and disease may result. Autoimmune disorders such as diabetes type 1 are a result of a hyperactive immune response. The body destroys beta cells in the pancreas that the body perceives as harmful invaders. Similarly, rejection of transplanted organs is associated with an immune system response. Immune deficiencies can be congenital (improper lymphocyte development before birth) or acquired (developed after birth), and result in the body's failure to defend against pathogens.

35

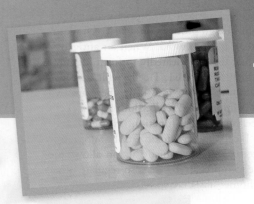

Treatment of Bacterial Infection

LEARNING OBJECTIVES

1 Learn the terminology associated with treatments for infection.
2 Compare bacteriostatic with bactericidal.
3 Describe the morphology of bacterial cells.
4 Explain microbial resistance and list several reasons for its development.
5 List and categorize anti-infective agents.
6 Describe the mechanism of action for anti-infective agents.
7 List common beginnings and endings for anti-infective agents.
8 Identify significant drug look-alike and sound-alike issues.
9 Identify warning labels and precautionary messages associated with anti-infective agents.

KEY TERMS

Antibiotic: Naturally occurring substance produced by a microorganism or semisynthetic substance derived from a microorganism that is capable of destroying or inhibiting the growth of another microorganism.

Antimicrobial: A substance capable of destroying or inhibiting the growth of a microorganism.

Bactericidal: Able to destroy bacteria.

Bacteriostatic: Able to inhibit bacterial proliferation; host defense mechanisms destroy the bacteria.

β-Lactamase: Enzyme secreted by some microbes that has the ability to destroy β-lactam antibiotics.

Broad-spectrum antibiotic: Antimicrobial that is capable of destroying a wide range of bacteria.

Deoxyribonucleic acid: DNA is the repository of hereditary characteristics; this nucleic acid contains the genetic blueprint.

Microbial resistance: Ability of bacteria to overcome the bactericidal or bacteriostatic effects of an anti-infective. Resistance traits are encoded on bacterial genes and can be transferred to other bacteria.

Ribonucleic acid: RNA is a nucleic acid involved in protein synthesis that carries and transfers genetic information and assembles proteins.

Overview

Although chronic noninfectious disease is a leading cause of disability and death in developed and industrialized countries, infectious disease is still one of the leading causes of morbidity and mortality globally. In developing countries, infectious diarrhea is a major cause of infant mortality. The incidence of infectious diseases such as malaria and tuberculosis is also high. Poverty, malnutrition, the lack of clean water, poor sanitation, and inadequate housing increase the risk for infectious disease and decrease the likelihood for adequate treatment.

Antibiotics have played a key role in improving the survival of individuals with bacterial infections. An ***antibiotic*** may be a naturally occurring substance produced by a microorganism or a semisynthetic substance derived from a microorganism that is capable of destroying or inhibiting the growth of another microorganism. Antibiotics are also referred to as ***antimicrobial*** or antibacterial agents. A specific class of antibiotics may be more effective against gram-positive or gram-negative bacteria so a Gram stain test may be performed. Gram stain is also used to detect yeast infections. Gram-positive bacteria stain purple and gram-negative bacteria stain pink. In addition to a Gram stain test, a culture and sensitivity test may also be performed. A small disk with antibiotic is placed in a culture from the infected patient and incubated in a Petri dish. The larger the zone of inhibition (area of no bacterial growth) around the disk, the more effective the antibiotic will be in treating the bacterial infection.

Mechanisms of Antimicrobial Action

Effective treatment of bacterial infections is dependent on host factors, bacterial factors, and drug factors (Figure 35-1).

BACTERICIDAL VERSUS BACTERIOSTATIC

Antibacterial agents may be classified as bactericidal or bacteriostatic. ***Bactericidal*** agents are able to destroy rapidly proliferating, bacteria. ***Bacteriostatic*** agents slow the growth of bacteria enough for the host's (our body's) defense mechanism to destroy the invading bacteria. Whether an agent is bactericidal or bacteriostatic is dependent on the drug, concentration administered, or how long the bacteria are exposed to toxic concentrations.

INHIBITORY EFFECTS
Bacterial Cell Wall Synthesis

Many bacteria have a cell wall, which is the target of antibacterial agents. Because human cells lack cell walls, antibacterial agents that target the cell wall harm the bacteria without damaging the host.

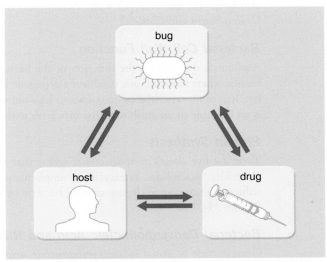

FIGURE 35-1 Factors that influence successful antimicrobial therapy. (From Page C, Curtis M, Sutter M, et al: *Integrated pharmacology*, ed 3, Philadelphia, 2006, Mosby.)

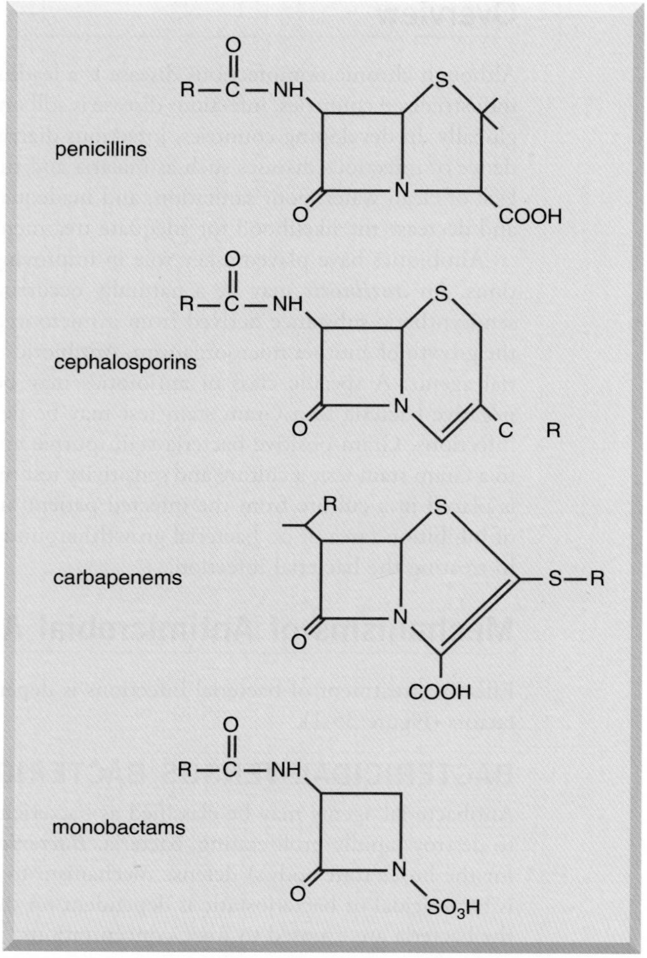

FIGURE 35-2 Basic structure of β-lactam antibiotics. (From Page C, Curtis M, Sutter M, et al: *Integrated pharmacology*, ed 3, Philadelphia, 2006, Mosby.)

β-Lactam antibiotics target the bacterial cell wall (Figure 35-2). Penicillins, cephalosporins, carbapenems, and monobactams are β-lactam antibiotics that inhibit cell wall synthesis. Glycopeptides also target the bacterial cell wall. Vancomycin is the only glycopeptide antibiotic available in the United States and Canada.

Bacterial Cell Wall Function

Antibiotics that inhibit the function of the bacterial cell wall work by binding to bacterial membranes, where the antibiotic produces a detergent-like action that increases cell membrane permeability. This causes essential cell contents to leak out of the cell and destroys the bacteria. Polymyxin B is an example of an antibiotic that interferes with cell wall function.

Protein Synthesis

There are five classes of antibacterial agents that act to inhibit bacterial protein synthesis—aminoglycosides, macrolides, tetracyclines, amphenicols, and oxazolidinone. These antibacterial agents reduce the number of disease-causing bacteria by interfering with the bacteria's ability to replicate (Figure 35-3).

Bacterial Deoxyribonucleic Acid and Ribonucleic Acid Synthesis

Genetic code is stored in **deoxyribonucleic acid** (DNA). In the replication process, a strand of **ribonucleic acid** (RNA) forms along a strand of DNA. The job of transfer RNA (tRNA) is to put the base pairs in the correct sequence. The job of messenger RNA (mRNA) is to carry the code

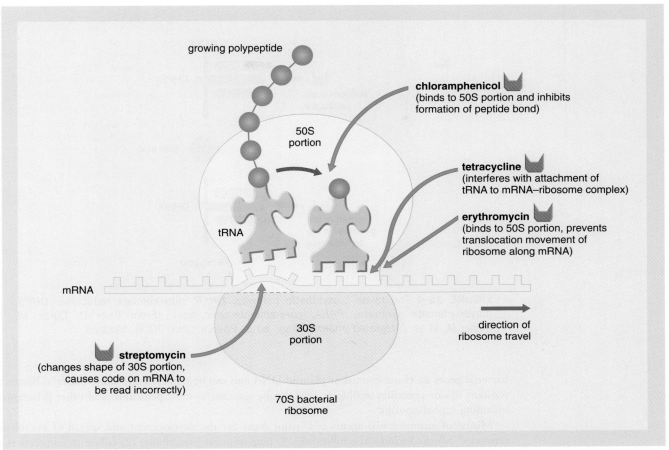

FIGURE 35-3 Antibiotics that inhibit bacterial protein synthesis. (From Page C, Curtis M, Sutter M, et al: *Integrated pharmacology*, ed 3, Philadelphia, 2006, Mosby.)

message to the ribosome. RNA also regulates specific cell functions, such as editing strands of code. Editing occurs on the ribosome by the RNA enzyme (ribozyme). Without the ability to transfer genetic codes for the synthesis of bacteria cell constituents, bacteria are unable to replicate and spread. Fluoroquinolones and nitroimidazoles are classes of antibiotics capable of inhibiting DNA synthesis. The action of fluoroquinolones (e.g., ciprofloxacin) and nitroimidazoles (e.g., metronidazole) is predominantly bactericidal. Rifampin inhibits bacterial RNA synthesis.

ANTIFOLATES

Folic acid is needed for the bacterial synthesis of DNA and, unlike humans, bacteria must synthesize their own folic acid; they cannot get it from external sources. Bacteria synthesize folic acid from para-aminobenzoic acid (PABA). Antifolate agents and dihydrofolate reductase inhibitors block the bacterial synthesis of folic acid. Sulfonamides are antifolate drugs and trimethoprim is a dihydrofolate reductase inhibitor (Figure 35-4).

Microbial Resistance

Microbes proliferate rapidly, mutate frequently, and adapt with relative ease to new environments and hosts. Unfortunately, microbes can learn how to withstand the effects of antibiotics; at present, there exist superbugs that are resistant to currently available antimicrobial agents. Multidrug resistance is a serious problem and, although previously only a risk for hospitalized patients, multidrug-resistant tuberculosis (MDR-TB), vancomycin-resistant enterococci (VRE), and methicillin-resistant *Staphylococcus aureus* (MRSA) are spreading outside of hospitals. **Microbial resistance** is the ability of bacteria to overcome the bactericidal effects of an antibiotic. Resistance traits are encoded on

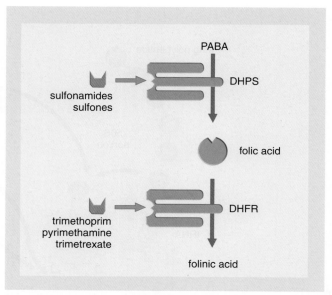

FIGURE 35-4 The folate biosynthetic pathway. *DHFR*, dihydrofolate reductase; *DHPS*, dihydropteroate synthase; *PABA*, para-aminobenzoic acid. (From Page C, Curtis M, Sutter M, et al: *Integrated pharmacology*, ed 3, Philadelphia, 2006, Mosby.)

bacterial genes on chromosomal or plasmid DNA and can be transferred to other bacteria. Bacteria resistant to one penicillin antibiotic may also be resistant to most penicillins and other β-lactams, including cephalosporins.

Misuse of antimicrobial agents is a major cause for the development and spread of microbial resistance. Misuse includes the following: (1) inappropriate prescribing; (2) failure to complete the full course of therapy; (3) administration of antibacterial agents for viral infections (e.g., the common cold); (4) antibiotics in the food chain (agriculture, animal husbandry, fish farms); and (5) lack of guidelines for preventing the spread of infections in institutional care settings.

MECHANISMS

Secretion of Enzymes That Inactivate the Antibiotic

β-Lactamase is an enzyme produced by some microbes that has the ability to destroy β-lactam antibiotics. It breaks the bonds of the β-lactam ring. β-Lactamase inhibitors have no antimicrobial activity of their own. They are added to some β-lactam antibiotics (e.g., amoxicillin plus clavulanic acid) to increase the antibiotic's resistance to microbial destruction. There are three β-lactamase inhibitors—clavulanic acid (clavulanate), sulbactam, and tazobactam. Macrolides are inactivated by bacterial production of enzymes e.g., erythromycin ribosomal methylase.

Modification of the Ribosomal Target

Microbial resistance develops when bacteria mutate to modify the site on the ribosome to which the antibiotic normally binds. This is a mechanism of microbial resistance to macrolide antibiotics.

Production of Antibiotic-Modifying Enzymes

Bacteria previously sensitive to the effects of aminoglycosides can become resistant by adding an acetyl or phosphoryl group to the antibiotic, which inhibits the antibiotic's ability to reach the bacterial binding site.

Mutations That Change Bacterial Transport Mechanisms

Bacteria that are resistant to tetracyclines have mutated to change the transport mechanism that causes the antibiotic to accumulate in the bacterial cell. Bacteria resistant to macrolides are capable of lowering the concentration of the antibiotic by transporting the antibiotic out of the cell.

Classification of Antimicrobial Agents

AMINOGLYCOSIDES

Aminoglycoside antibiotics are effective for treating aerobic gram-negative bacilli, staphylococci, and mycobacterium. They are used for the treatment of serious infections of the bone, abdomen, heart, brain, urinary tract, reproductive system, skin, and kidneys. Examples are lower respiratory infections, peritonitis, septicemia, meningitis, pelvic inflammatory disease, endocarditis, and osteomyelitis. Aminoglycosides may also be administered to sterilize the bowel prior to bowel surgery. Ophthalmic dosage forms are also prescribed for the treatment of blepharitis and conjunctivitis (see Chapter 20).

MECHANISM OF ACTION AND PHARMACOKINETICS

Aminoglycosides inhibit bacterial protein synthesis. They enter the bacterial cell via an oxygen-dependent transport system, which explains why they are effective against aerobic bacteria and not anaerobic bacteria. They bind to a site on the bacterial ribosome that causes the genetic code carried by mRNA to be read incorrectly.

Aminoglycosides are not absorbed systemically when administered by mouth. The only aminoglycoside that is administered orally (neomycin) is used to reduce the bacteria in the bowel *neo mycin* prior to colorectal surgery. Other nonparenteral use is topical application for skin, eye, and ear infections.

Aminoglycosides

Generic Name	U.S. Brand Name(s) / Canadian Brand Name(s)	Dosage Forms and Strengths
amikacin*	Generic	Solution, for injection: 50 mg/mL[†], 250 mg/mL
	Generic	
gentamicin*	Generics	Cream: 0.1%
	Diogent, Garamycin, Garasol, Gentak, Septopal	Implant (Septopal): 4.5 mg[‡] Ointment: 0.1% Solution, for injection: 1 mg/mL[‡], 1.2 mg/mL[‡], 1.4 mg/mL, 1.6 mg/mL[‡], 2 mg/mL, 10 mg/mL, 40 mg/mL Solution, in normal saline: 0.6 mg/mL[†], 0.7 mg/mL[†], 0.8 mg/mL, 0.9 mg/mL[†], 1 mg/mL[†], 1.2 mg/mL, 1.4 mg/mL, 1.6 mg/mL[†] Ointment, ophthalmic (Garamycin, Gentak): 0.3% Solution, ophthalmic (Garamycin, Gentak, Gentasol): 0.3%, 5 mg/mL
kanamycin*	Generic	Solution, for injection: 333 mg/mL
	Not available	
neomycin*	Neo-Fradin	Solution: 125 mg/5 mL
	Not available	Tablet: 500 mg
streptomycin*	Generics	Powder, for injection: 1 g
	Generics	
tobramycin*	Tobi, Tobrex	Capsule, for inhalation (Tobi Podhaler): 28 mg[‡]
	Tobi, Tobi Podhaler, Tobrex	Ointment, ophthalmic (Tobrex): 0.3% Powder, for injection: 1.2 g Solution, for inhalation (Tobi): 300 mg/5 mL Solution, for injection: 10 mg/mL, 40 mg/mL Solution, for injection in NS: 0.8 mg/mL[†], 1.2 mg/mL[†], 1.6 mg/mL[†] Solution, ophthalmic (Tobrasol, Tobrex): 0.3%

*Generic available.
[†]Strength available in the United States only.
[‡]Strength available in Canada only.

ADVERSE REACTIONS

Serious adverse reactions are linked to aminoglycoside use including hearing loss (ototoxicity) and kidney damage (nephrotoxicity). These effects limit their use to the treatment of serious infections.

CEPHALOSPORINS

Cephalosporins have a β-lactam ring structure. Like penicillins, the different side chains added to the basic β-lactam ring structure can affect the antimicrobial spectrum of activity. They are classified as first, second, third-, and fourth-generation cephalosporins. First-generation cephalosporins are most effective against gram-positive (+) aerobic bacteria. They are effective in the treatment of staphylococcal infections and streptococcal infections of the skin and soft tissue. Second-generation cephalosporins have effectiveness against gram-positive and gram-negative (−) bacteria and are effective for treating upper respiratory infections such as *Haemophilus influenzae*. Third-generation cephalosporins are the most effective against gram-negative anaerobic bacteria and are effective for treating bacterial meningitis, gonorrhea, intra-abdominal infections (e.g., peritonitis), and bone and joint infections. The fourth-generation cephalosporin cefepime has a greater ability to penetrate the bacterial cell wall of gram-negative bacteria than third-generation agents and is more resistant to destruction by β-lactamases.

MECHANISM OF ACTION

Cephalosporins inhibit the third and final stage of bacterial cell wall synthesis by binding to specific penicillin-binding proteins (PBPs) located inside the bacterial cell wall. Because PBPs vary among different bacterial species, cephalosporin spectrum of activity is dependent on the drug's ability to bind to a specified bacterial PBP.

PHARMACOKINETICS

Cephalosporins are formulated for oral, intramuscular, and intravenous use. All except one third-generation cephalosporin (cefixime) is administered parenterally and only two second-generation cephalosporins are available for oral use (cefaclor, cefuroxime). First-generation cephalosporins do not penetrate the cerebrospinal fluid (CSF) in adequate concentration to treat meningitis, whereas most third-generation agents reach a high enough level. Although fourth-generation agents penetrate the CSF when meninges are inflamed, cefepime is not used in the treatment of meningitis. It is administered to treat pneumonia (community-acquired and nosocomial) and urinary tract infections (UTIs).

Cephalosporins

Generic Name	U.S. Brand Name(s) / Canadian Brand Name(s)	Dosage Forms and Strengths
First-Generation Cephalosporins		
cefazolin*	Generics	Powder, for injection: 0.5 g, 1 g, 10 g, 20 g
	Generics	Solution, for injection (premixed): 10 mg/ mL†, 20 mg/mL†
cefadroxil*	Generics	Capsule: 500 mg
	Generics	Powder, for oral suspension: 125 mg/5 mL†, 250 mg/5 mL†, 500 mg/5 mL†
		Tablet: 1 g†
cephalexin*	Keflex	Capsule (United States): 250 mg, 500 mg, 750 mg†
	Keflex	Powder, for oral suspension: 125 mg/5 mL, 250 mg/5 mL
		Tablet (Canada): 250 mg, 500 mg
cephalothin	Not available	Powder for injection: 1 g/vial
	Ceporacin	

Cephalosporins—cont'd

Generic Name	U.S. Brand Name(s) / Canadian Brand Name(s)	Dosage Forms and Strengths
Second-Generation Cephalosporins		
cefaclor*	Generics	Capsule: 250 mg, 500 mg
	Ceclor	Powder for oral suspension: 125 mg/5 mL, 187 mg/5 mL[†], 250 mg/5 mL, 375 mg/5 mL
		Tablet, extended release: 375 mg[†], 500 mg[†]
cefotetan*	Cefotan	Powder for injection: 1 g, 2 g, 10 g
	Not available	
cefoxitin*	Mefoxin	Powder for injection: 1 g, 2 g, 10 g
	Generic	Solution for injection (Mefoxin): 20 mg/mL[†], 40 mg/mL[†]
cefuroxime*	Ceftin, Zinacef	Powder for injection: 75 mg[†], 225 mg[†], 750 mg, 1.5 g, 7.5 g/vial
	Ceftin	Powder for oral suspension (Ceftin): 125 mg/5 mL, 250 mg/5 mL[†]
		Solution, for injection (Zinacef): 15 mg/mL[†], 30 mg/mL[†], 1.5 g/20 mL[†]
		Tablet: 125 mg[†], 250 mg, 500 mg
Third-Generation Cephalosporins		
cefotaxime	Claforan	Powder for injection: 500 mg, 1 g, 2 g, 10 g[†]
	Claforan	Solution for injection: 20 mg/mL, 40 mg/mL
ceftazidime*	Fortaz, Tazicef	Powder, for injection: 500 mg[†], 1 g, 2 g, 6 g
	Fortaz	Solution, for injection (premixed): 1 g/50 mL[†], 2 g/50 mL[†]
ceftriaxone*	Rocephin	Powder for injection: 250 mg, 500 mg, 1 g, 2 g, 10 g
	Generics	Solution, for injection: 20 mg/mL[†], 40 mg/mL[†]
cefixime*	Suprax	Capsule: 400 mg[†]
	Suprax	Powder, for oral suspension: 100 mg/5 mL, 200 mg/5 mL[†]
		Tablet: 400 mg
		Tablet, Chewable: 100 mg[†], 150 mg[†], 200 mg[†]
cefpodoxime*	Generics	Powder, for oral suspension: 50 mg/5 mL, 100 mg/5 mL
	Not available	Tablet: 100 mg, 200 mg
ceftibuten	Cedax	Capsule: 400 mg
	Not available	Powder, for oral suspension: 90 mg/5 mL
Fourth-Generation Cephalosporin		
cefepime*	Maxipime	Powder, for injection: 500 mg[†], 1 g, 2 g
	Maxipime	Solution, for injection: 1 g/50 mL[†], 2 g/50 mL[†]

*Generic available.
[†]Strength available in the United States only.

ADVERSE REACTIONS

Adverse reactions produced by cephalosporins include diarrhea, headache, dizziness, nausea, vomiting, gas, abdominal pain, dry mouth, and heartburn.

FLUOROQUINOLONES

Fluoroquinolones are indicated for the treatment of urinary tract infections, sinusitis, sexually transmitted infections (see Chapter 34), bacterial conjunctivitis (see Chapter 20), infectious diarrhea, anthrax, and numerous other infections.

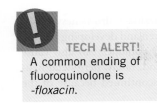

TECH ALERT!
A common ending of fluoroquinolone is
-floxacin.

Fluoroquinolones

Generic Name	U.S. Brand Name(s) / Canadian Brand Name(s)	Dosage Forms and Strengths
ciprofloxacin*	Cetraxal, Cipro, Cipro XR, Ciloxan / Ciloxan, Cipro, Cipro XL	Tablet (Cipro): 100 mg†, 250 mg, 500 mg, 750 mg Tablet, extended-release (Cipro XL, Cipro XR): 500 mg, 1000 mg Ophthalmic ointment and solution (Ciloxan): 0.3% Otic solution (Cetraxal): 0.2%† Powder, for oral suspension (Cipro): 250 mg/5mL†, 500 mg/5mL Solution, for injection (Cipro): 10 mg/mL Solution, for injection in 5% dextrose (Cipro): 2 mg/mL
gatifloxacin*†	Zymar, Zymaxid / Zymar	Ophthalmic solution: 0.3% (Zymar), 0.5% (Zymaxid)
gemifloxacin	Factive / Not available	Tablet: 320 mg
levofloxacin*	Iquix Levaquin, Quixin / Levaquin	Ophthalmic solution: 0.5% (Quixin), 1.5% (Iquix) Solution for injection: 25 mg/mL† Solution for injection in 5% dextrose (Levaquin): 5 mg/mL Solution, oral (Levaquin): 25 mg/mL† Tablet: 250 mg, 500 mg, 750 mg
moxifloxacin	Avelox, Moxeza, Vigamox / Avelox, Vigamox	Ophthalmic solution (Moxeza, Vigamox): 0.5% Tablet: 400 mg Solution for IV: 400 mg/250 mL 0.8% NaCl
ofloxacin*	Floxin Otic, Ocuflox / Ocuflox	Ophthalmic solution (Ocuflox): 0.3% Otic solution (Floxin Otic): 0.3%† Tablet: 200 mg, 300 mg, 400 mg
norfloxacin*‡	Noroxin / Generics	Tablet: 400 mg

*Generic available.
†Strength available in the United States only.
*†Generic available in the United States only.
*‡Generic available in Canada only.

TECH ALERT!
The following drugs have look-alike and sound-alike issues:
Ciloxan and Cytoxan; Avelox and Avonex; Noroxin and Norflex; Ocuflox and Ocufen

TECH ALERT!
Oral and parenteral fluoroquinolones are contraindicated in pregnant women and children younger than 16 to 18 years because of the risk for cartilage malformations and tendon rupture.

MECHANISM OF ACTION
The process of DNA replication and transcription begins with the separation of the two strands of DNA. Excessive coiling (supercoiling) occurs when the strands separate. An enzyme, DNA gyrase, is responsible for blocking the supercoiling. Fluoroquinolones inhibit the enzyme DNA gyrase. This results in the inhibition of bacterial DNA synthesis.

PHARMACOKINETICS
Fluoroquinolones are formulated for oral, ophthalmic, and parenteral use. Oral absorption is good. The half-life ($t_{1/2}$) of the newer agents such as moxifloxacin is long, permitting once-daily dosing, whereas ciprofloxacin ($t_{1/2} \cong 4$ hr) is dosed every 12 hr.

ADVERSE REACTIONS
Common adverse reactions are diarrhea, crystalluria, photosensitivity, dizziness, drowsiness, headache, nausea, and stomach upset. Cartilage deformities may occur in children and developing fetuses, so quinolones are contraindicated in children and pregnant women. Quinolones can also cause arrhythmias by prolongation of the QT interval, musculoskeletal pain, and, rarely, peripheral neuropathy. Oral gatifloxacin, grepafloxacin, and sparfloxacin have been discontinued because of the risk of fatal adverse effects.

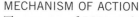

MACROLIDES AND RELATED ANTIBIOTICS

Macrolide antibiotics are primarily used for the treatment of upper respiratory infections (URIs). Azithromycin and clarithromycin are more active against the bacterium *H. influenzae* than erythromycin. Clarithromycin is a key ingredient in treatment regimens for peptic ulcer disease caused by the bacterium *Helicobacter pylori* (see Chapter 26). Erythromycin, the prototype for the macrolides, is used for the prevention of neonatal eye infections and acne in addition to URI treatment. Ketolides are structurally similar to macrolides but have greater antimicrobial effects and a lower incidence of antimicrobial resistance. Telithromycin is currently the only marketed ketolide. Because of its risk for serious side effects, telithromycin is only indicated for community-acquired pneumonia.

MECHANISM OF ACTION
Macrolides inhibit bacterial protein synthesis by binding to the 50S ribosomal unit and blocking the translocation movement along mRNA.

Macrolides and Related Anti-Infectives

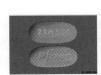

Generic Name	U.S. Brand Name(s) / Canadian Brand Name(s)	Dosage Forms and Strengths
azithromycin*	Azasite, Zithromax, Zmax / Zithromax, Zmax SR	Ophthalmic solution (Azasite): 1% Powder, for injection: 500 mg, 2.5 g[†] Powder, for oral suspension (Zithromax): 100 mg/5 mL, 200 mg/5 mL, 1 g (single dose) Powder, for oral suspension, extended-release (Zmax, Zmax SR): 2 g Tablet (Zithromax): 250 mg, 500 mg[†], 600 mg
clarithromycin*	Biaxin, Biaxin XL / Biaxin, Biaxin BID, Biaxin XL	Powder, for suspension (Biaxin): 125 mg/5 mL, 250 mg/5 mL Tablet (Biaxin, Biaxin BID): 250 mg, 500 mg Tablet, extended-release (Biaxin XL): 500 mg
erythromycin base* (immediate-release)	Akne-mycin, C-Solve-2, Ery-gel / Erysol	Gel, topical (Ery-gel): 2% Ophthalmic ointment: 0.5% Tablet (generics): 250 mg, 500 mg Solution, topical (Akne-mycin, C-Solve-2, Erysol): 2% Swab: 2%
erythromycin base* (delayed-release)	Ery-tab, ERYC, PCE / Erybid, ERYC, PCE	Capsule (PCE): 250 mg, 333 mg, 500 mg Tablet: 250 mg, 333 mg, 500 mg
erythromycin stearate*	Erythrocin / Generic	Tablet: 250 mg
erythromycin ethylsuccinate*	EES, Eryped / EES, Pediazole	Granules, for oral suspension: 200 mg/5 mL, 400 mg/5 mL Tablet: 400 mg, 600 mg[‡]
erythromycin lactobionate*	Erythrocin / Generic	Powder, for injection: 500 mg, 1 g
Ketolides		
telithromycin	Ketek / Not available	Tablet: 300 mg, 400 mg

*Generic available.
[†]Strength available in the United States only.
[‡]Strength available in Canada only.

PHARMACOKINETICS

Macrolides are formulated for oral, parenteral, and ophthalmic use. Several salts of erythromycin are in use, including erythromycin base, erythromycin ethylsuccinate, erythromycin stearate, and erythromycin lactobionate. Erythromycin base is formulated for immediate release and delayed release. Delayed-release tablets have a lower incidence of gastrointestinal side effects than immediate-release tablets.

The expiration date of powder for the oral suspension of erythromycin, clarithromycin, and azithromycin is shortened once the drug is reconstituted. Refrigeration is recommended for oral suspensions of erythromycin; storage at room temperature is recommended for clarithromycin and azithromycin.

ADVERSE REACTIONS

Gastrointestinal (GI) upset is common with the use of macrolides. It occurs in up to 21% of those who take erythromycin. The incidence of GI upset is less with clarithromycin (10%) and azithromycin (5%). Erythromycin and clarithromycin can cause arrhythmias by prolongation of the QT interval. Other adverse reactions include headache and tinnitus. Macrolides may decrease the effectiveness of oral contraceptives.

In 2007, the U.S. Food and Drug Administration (FDA) required the package label for telithromycin to indicate that the drug is contraindicated in individuals with myasthenia gravis because of the risk of fatal respiratory failure. The drug may also cause liver toxicity.

OXAZOLIDINONES

Linezolid is a newer antimicrobial agent indicated for the treatment of gram-positive bacterial pneumonia and skin structure infections. Its use is limited because of adverse side effects and to limit the development of bacterial resistance.

MECHANISM OF ACTION AND PHARMACOKINETICS

Linezolid inhibits bacterial protein synthesis. Its action on the bacterial ribosome blocks a key step in the translation process, which inhibits bacterial replication. The metabolism of linezolid is not well understood. Its $t_{1/2}$ is 4 to 5 hours and approximately 30% of the drug is eliminated unchanged in the urine. Most of the drug is eliminated by nonrenal mechanisms, of which only 9% is in the feces. Linezolid has no effect on cytochrome P-450 (CYP450) isoenzymes.

ADVERSE REACTIONS

Linezolid inhibits monoamine oxidase, the enzyme responsible for the breakdown of monoamine neurotransmitters (e.g., norepinephrine). Drug or drug-food interactions may cause an increase in blood pressure. More common side effects are skin rash, itching, change in taste, headache, mild diarrhea, dizziness, mild stomach upset, nausea, vomiting, and temporary tongue discoloration.

PENICILLINS AND CARBAPENEMS

Penicillin is one of the first antibiotics discovered. It is a naturally occurring substance originally produced by the mold *Penicillium chrysogenum* (also known as *Penicillium notatum*) and can grow on stale bread and fruit. Oral penicillins are used to treat many infections, including URIs, otitis media, skin infections, and strep throat. It is also prescribed to prevent recurrent rheumatic fever. Penicillins may be administered before dental and other medical procedures to prevent bacterial endocarditis in individuals with prosthetic heart valves. Ampicillin may be prescribed for pelvic

TECH ALERT!
A common ending of the penicillin family of drugs is *-cillin*.

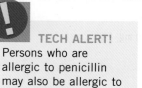

TECH ALERT!
Persons who are allergic to penicillin may also be allergic to cephalosporins.

Oxazolidinones		
	U.S. Brand Name(s)	
Generic Name	**Canadian Brand Name(s)**	**Dosage Forms and Strengths**
linezolid	Zyvox	Powder, for suspension: 100 mg/5 mL
	Zyvoxam	Solution, for injection: 2 mg/mL
		Tablet: 600 mg

Penicillins

Generic Name	U.S. Brand Name(s) Canadian Brand Name(s)	Dosage Forms and Strengths
Standard Penicillins		
penicillin G potassium*	Pfizerpen	Powder, for injection: 20 million units, 5 million units
	Not available for human use	Solution, for injection: 20,000 units/mL, 40,000 units/mL, 60,000 units/mL
phenoxymethyl penicillin potassium* (penicillin VK)	Generics	Powder for oral suspension: 125 mg/5 mL, 250 mg/5 mL[†], 300 mg/5 mL[‡]
	Generics	Tablets: 250 mg, 300 mg[‡], 500 mg
procaine penicillin G*	Generics	Suspension, for IM injection: 300,000 units/mL, 600,000 units/mL
	Not available for human use	
benzathine penicillin G*	Bicillin L-A	Suspension, for IM injection: 300,000 units/mL[†], 600,000 units/mL
	Bicillin L-A	
benzylpenicillin (penicillin G sodium)	Generics	Powder, for injection: 1,000,000 units/vial[‡], 5,000,000 units/vial, 10,000,000 units/vial[‡]
	Crystapen	
Aminopenicillins: Extended-Spectrum		
amoxicillin*	Amoxil, Larotid, Moxatag	Capsule: 250 mg, 500 mg
	Generics	Powder for oral suspension: 50 mg/mL, 125 mg/5 mL, 200 mg/5 mL[†], 250 mg/5 mL, 400 mg/5 mL[†]
		Tablet: 500 mg, 875 mg[†]
		Tablet, chewable: 125 mg, 200 mg[†], 250 mg, 400 mg[†]
		Tablet, extended-release (Moxatag): 775 mg[†]
ampicillin*	Generics	Capsule: 250 mg, 500 mg
	Generics	Powder, for injection: 125 mg[†], 250 mg, 500 mg, 1 g, 2 g, 10 g[†]
		Powder, for oral suspension: 125 mg/5 mL, 250 mg/5 mL, 500 mg/5 mL[‡]
Antistaphyloccocal Penicillins: Penicillinase-Resistant		
cloxacillin*	Not available	Capsule: 250 mg, 500 mg
	Generics	Powder, for oral suspension: 125 mg/5 mL
		Powder, for injection: 0.5 g, 1 g, 2 g
dicloxacillin*	Generics	Capsule: 125 mg, 250 mg, 500 mg
	Not available	
nafcillin*	Nallpen	Powder, for injection: 1 g, 2 g, 10 g
	Not available	Solution, for injection (Nallpen): 20 mg/mL
oxacillin*	Bactocill	Powder, for injection: 1 g, 2 g, 10 g
	Not available	Solution, for injection (Bactocill): 20 mg/mL, 40 mg/mL
Antipseudomonal Penicillins		
piperacillin*	Generic	Powder for injection: 2 g, 3 g, 4 g, 40 g[†]
	Generic	

Continued

Penicillins—cont'd

Generic Name	U.S. Brand Name(s) / Canadian Brand Name(s)	Dosage Forms and Strengths
Penicillin Combinations		
amoxicillin + clavulanic acid*	Augmentin, Augmentin ES, Augmentin XR / Clavulin	**Powder for oral suspension:** amoxicillin 125 mg + clavulanic acid 31.25 mg amoxicillin 200 mg + clavulanic acid 28.5 mg amoxicillin 250 mg + clavulanic acid 62.5 mg amoxicillin 400 mg + clavulanic acid 57 mg amoxicillin 600 mg + clavulanic acid 42.9 mg (Augmentin ES) **Tablet:** amoxicillin 250 mg + clavulanic acid 125 mg amoxicillin 500 mg + clavulanic acid 125 mg amoxicillin 875 mg + clavulanic acid 125 mg **Tablet, chewable (Augmentin):** amoxicillin 125 mg + clavulanic acid 31.25 mg amoxicillin 200 mg + clavulanic acid 28.5 mg amoxicillin 250 mg + clavulanic acid 62.5 mg amoxicillin 400 mg + clavulanic acid 57 mg amoxicillin 500 mg + clavulanic acid 125 mg **Tablet, extended-release (Augmentin XR):** amoxicillin 1000 mg + clavulanic acid 62.5 mg
ampicillin + sulbactam	Unasyn / Not available	**Powder, for injection:** ampicillin 1 g + sulbactam 0.5 g ampicillin 2 g + sulbactam 1 g ampicillin 10 g + sulbactam 5 g
piperacillin + tazobactam	Zosyn / Tazocin	**Powder, for injection:** piperacillin 2 g + tazobactam 0.25 g piperacillin 3 g + tazobactam 0.375 g piperacillin 4 g + tazobactam 0.5 g piperacillin 12 g + tazobactam 1.5 g[‡] piperacillin 36 g + tazobactam 4.5 g **Solution, for injection:** piperacillin 2 g + tazobactam 0.25 g/50 mL[†] piperacillin 3 g + tazobactam 0.375 g/50 mL[†] piperacillin 4 g + tazobactam 0.5 g/100 mL[†]
ticarcillin + clavulanic acid	Timentin / Timentin	**Powder, for injection:** ticarcillin 3 g + clavulanic acid 100 mg ticarcillin 30 g + clavulanic acid 1 g **Solution, for injection:** ticarcillin 3 g + clavulanic acid 100 mg/100 mL[†]

*Generic available.
[†]Strength available in the United States only.
[‡]Strength available in Canada only.

Carbapenems

Generic Name	U.S. Brand Name(s) / Canadian Brand Name(s)	Dosage Forms and Strengths
imipenem + cilastatin*	Primaxin / Primaxin	**Powder, for injection:** imipenem 500 mg + cilastatin 500 mg imipenem 250 mg + cilastatin 250 mg
meropenem*	Merrem / Merrem	**Powder, for injection:** 500 mg, 1 g

*Generic available.

inflammatory disease (see Chapter 34). Parenteral penicillins are also used for the treatment of numerous infections, including bone and joint infections, diabetic foot ulcers, infectious arthritis, sexually transmitted infections, meningitis, and septicemia.

MECHANISM OF ACTION

Penicillins are β-lactam antibiotics; they inhibit the synthesis of the cell wall of sensitive microbes by inhibiting the cross-linkage of peptide side chains of the bacterial cell wall. All penicillins have a sulfur-containing ringlike structure. Side chains on this structure alter the antibacterial and pharmacological properties of the basic penicillin molecule. The side chains can extend the antimicrobial spectrum. For example, amoxicillin and ticarcillin are effective against more types of bacteria than penicillin. Staphylococci are bacteria that have developed resistance to penicillin-type anti-infectives. Antistaphylococcal penicillins are penicillinase-resistant and are not inactivated by penicillinase (staphylococcal β-lactamase), a substance produced by the bacteria that destroys the antibiotic's β-lactam ring.

Carbapenems have a β-lactam ring fused with a penem ring. Carbapenems inhibit the third step in bacterial cell wall synthesis. Their spectrum of activity is broad and they resist inactivation by microbial enzymes (e.g., β-lactamase). Carbapenems are more effective against gram-negative bacteria than other β-lactam antibiotic agents because they have a greater ability to penetrate the outer membrane of the bacteria.

PHARMACOKINETICS

Standard penicillins lack stability in gastric acids, which is why most are administered intramuscularly or must be taken on an empty stomach. The exception is penicillin VK, which is relatively acid-stable.

Procaine penicillin G and benzathine penicillin G are formulated to delay absorption and achieve prolonged blood levels. Levels of benzathine penicillin G can be detected in the blood up to 1 month after an intramuscular injection of the drug is given.

Penicillins that are formulated as powders for reconstitution have shortened expiration dates once mixed with water. Expiration dates range from 10 to 14 days, depending on the drug. Most suspensions should be refrigerated once they are reconstituted.

ADVERSE REACTIONS

GI side effects such as diarrhea, loss of appetite, nausea, vomiting, sore mouth, stomach gas, and heartburn are the most common adverse reactions to penicillins. Other adverse effects include superinfection and hypersensitivity and hematological and neurological reactions. Penicillins may decrease the effectiveness of oral contraceptives.

SULFONAMIDES

Sulfonamides are the oldest antimicrobial agents. They were developed in the 1930s, but their use did not spread until the 1940s in World War II. Sulfonamides are commonly called sulfa drugs because the generic name of all agents begins with sulf-. Sulfonamides and trimethoprim are used in the treatment of various upper respiratory, urinary tract, and skin infections. They are also indicated for the treatment of AIDS-related pneumonia (caused by *Pneumocystis jiroveci* [formerly known as *Pneumocystis carinii*]).

MECHANISM OF ACTION AND PHARMACOKINETICS

Sulfonamides and trimethoprim are antifolate drugs. They interfere with the microbial synthesis of folic acid at separate steps in the biosynthetic pathway that ultimately leads to bacterial DNA synthesis (see Figure 35-4). Food may slightly decrease the absorption of sulfonamides; however, the drug may be taken with small amounts of food to reduce GI upset.

ADVERSE REACTIONS

Adverse reactions common with the use of sulfonamides are nausea, vomiting, abdominal pain, headache, drowsiness, dizziness, diarrhea, and photosensitivity. Sulfonamides may promote the formation of crystals in the urine (crystalluria), especially if taken with acidic foods or beverages.

TECH ALERT!
The following drugs have look-alike and sound-alike issues:
    ampicillin and amoxicillin;
    penicillin G and penicillin VK;
    Ticar and Tigan;
    Augmentin and Augmentin XR

TECH ALERT!
The quantity of clavulanic acid varies widely between products. It is important to read the stock bottle label carefully before making product substitutions.

TECH ALERT!
Primaxin and Premarin have look-alike and sound-alike issues.

TECH ALERT!
A common beginning for sulfonamides *sulf-*.

TECH ALERT!
The warning label "Take with Lots of Water" is put on prescription vials for sulfonamides. This reduces the risk of kidney damage caused by crystalluria.

Sulfonamides

Generic Name	U.S. Brand Name(s) / Canadian Brand Name(s)	Dosage Forms and Strengths
Sulfonamides		
sulfadiazine*	Generics	Tablet: 500 mg
	Not available	
sulfamethoxazole*	Not available	Tablet: 500 mg
	Generics	
sulfisoxazole*	Not available	Tablet: 500 mg
	Generics	
Combination Sulfonamides		
sulfisoxazole + erythromycin ethylsuccinate*	Generics	Granules for suspension: sulfisoxazole 600 mg/5 mL + erythromycin ethylsuccinate 200 mg/5 mL
	Pediazole	
sulfamethoxazole + trimethoprim* (SMX-TMP; Cotrimox)	Bactrim, Bactrim DS, Septra, Septra DS	Solution for injection: sulfamethoxazole 80 mg/mL + trimethoprim 16 mg/mL
	Septra, Sulfatrim	Tablet: sulfamethoxazole 100 mg + trimethoprim 20 mg‡ sulfamethoxazole 400 mg + trimethoprim 80 mg sulfamethoxazole 800 mg + trimethoprim 160 mg
		Suspension: sulfamethoxazole 200 mg/5 mL + trimethoprim 40 mg/5 mL

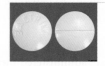

*Generic available.
‡Strength available in Canada only.

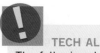

TETRACYCLINES

Tetracylines are ***broad-spectrum antibiotic*** (antibacterial) agents. They may be bactericidal or bacteriostatic. They are used for the treatment of acne, sexually transmitted infections such as chlamydia, Lyme disease, and Rocky Mountain spotted fever.

MECHANISM OF ACTION AND PHARMACOKINETICS

Tetracyclines inhibit protein synthesis. Their site of action is the 30S ribosomal unit (see Figure 35-3). They block the binding of tRNA to the mRNA-ribosome complex. Tetracycline interacts with dairy products, calcium, aluminum, and ferrous supplements to form a chelated complex. The complex significantly reduces the absorption of tetracycline and should be avoided.

Doxycycline and minocycline are more stable in the acidic stomach contents than tetracycline. They also have a longer duration of action. They are given once or twice daily compared with tetracycline, which is given four times daily.

ADVERSE REACTIONS

The tetracyclines can cause nausea, vomiting, diarrhea, and photosensitivity. Serious but less common side effects include hepatotoxicity, pseudomembranous colitis, and kidney disease. Outdated tetracycline becomes toxic. Patients should be advised to discard old medicines. Tetracyclines may decrease the effectiveness of oral contraceptives.

MISCELLANEOUS ANTIBACTERIALS

Isoniazid is used for the treatment of tuberculosis. It inhibits the synthesis of mycolic acid, an important constituent of the highly lipid cell wall of mycobacteria. Isoniazid may cause liver disease and nerve damage. Concurrent administration of vitamin B6 is recommended to prevent neurotoxicity. Isoniazid is abbreviated as INH, but the use of acronyms may cause medication errors.

Tetracyclines

Dosage Forms and Strengths	U.S. Brand Name(s)	Dosage Forms and Strengths
	Canadian Brand Name(s)	
demeclocycline*	Declomycin	Tablet: 150 mg, 300 mg
	Not available	
doxycycline anhydrous	Orecea	Capsule, immediate + delayed release (Orecea): 40 mg
doxycycline calcium	Vibramycin	Capsule: 50 mg, 100 mg
	Not available	Powder, for oral suspension: 25 mg/5 mL, 50 mg/5 mL
doxycycline hyclate*	Atridox, Doryx, Periostat, Vibramycin	Capsule: 50 mg†, 100 mg (Vibramycin) Gingival gel (Atridox): 44 mg/unit Powder, for injection: 100 mg/vial Tablet: 20 mg (Periostat), 100 mg (Vibra-tabs) Tablet, delayed release (Doryx): 75 mg, 100 mg, 150 mg
	Atridox, Periostat, Vibra-Tabs Vibramycin	
doxycycline monohydrate*	Monodox	Tablet: 50 mg, 75 mg, 100 mg (Monodox)
	Not available	
minocycline*	Arestin, Dynacin, Minocin, Soladyn	Capsule (Minocin): 50 mg, 75 mg†, 100 mg Powder, for injection (Minocin): 100 mg/vial† Powder, periodontal-sustained release (Arestin): 1 mg/4 mg Tablet (Dynacin): 75 mg, 100 mg Tablet, extended-release (Soladyn): 45 mg, 55 mg, 65 mg, 80 mg, 90 mg, 105 mg, 115 mg, 135 mg
	Arestin, Minocin	
tetracycline*	Generics	Capsule: 100 mg†, 250 mg, 500 mg† Ophthalmic ointment: 1%‡
	Generics	
tigecycline	Tygacil	Powder, for injection: 50 mg, vial
	Tygacil	

*Generic available.
†Strength available in the United States only.
‡Strength available in Canada only.

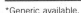

TECH ALERT!
Apply the following warning label to prescription vials for tetracycline: "Avoid Antacids and Dairy Products within 2 Hr of Dose."

TECH ALERT!
Apply the following warning label to prescription vials for tetracycline: "Avoid Tanning and Prolonged Exposure to Sunlight."

TECH ALERT!
Tetracyclines are contraindicated in pregnancy and small children because they can weaken fetal bone, retard bone growth, weaken tooth enamel, and stain teeth.

TECH ALERT!
The following drugs have look-alike and sound-alike issues:
Bactroban, baclofen, and bacitracin;
Cleocin and Clinoril

Metronidazole is an amebacide. It destroys the protozoa that cause giardiasis (traveler's diarrhea) and trichomoniasis (a sexually transmitted infection). It is the drug of choice for the treatment of *Clostridium difficile* enteritis, a condition that may cause pseudomembranous colitis. Topical preparations are used for the treatment of acne rosacea. It is formulated for oral, parenteral, vaginal, and topical use. Alcoholic beverages or medicines containing high levels of alcohol may produce nausea, vomiting, stomach pains, headache, and dizziness. The drug may also produce a metallic taste.

Mupirocin is a topically applied antimicrobial used to treat staphylococcal infections of the skin, such as impetigo.

Chloramphenicol is a broad-spectrum antimicrobial agent that inhibits protein synthesis. Its use is limited and is indicated when other less toxic drugs cannot be used (e.g., for drug allergy). It may be used for the treatment of bacterial meningitis, brain abscess, and Rocky Mountain spotted fever. Neonates are unable to metabolize the drug fully and toxic levels may accumulate. Its use in children may produce gray baby syndrome or cyanosis.

Clindamycin is an antimicrobial agent used topically for the treatment of acne and vaginosis. Systemic use of clindamycin is associated with the development of *C. difficile*, a bacteria that causes diarrhea and pseudomembranous colitis. Drinking lots of fluids can lower the risk of the development of this condition.

Miscellaneous Antibacterial Agents

Generic Name	U.S. Brand Name(s) / Canadian Brand Name(s)	Dosage Forms and Strengths
isoniazid*	Generics / Generics	Powder, oral: 500 g/bottle Solution, for injection: 100 mg/mL† Syrup, oral: 50 mg/5 mL Tablet: 100 mg, 300 mg
metronidazole*	Flagyl, Metrocreme, Metrogel, Metrolotion, Noritate, Vandazole / Flagyl, Flagyl Cream, Flurazole ER, Metrocreme, Metrogel, Metrolotion, Noritate, Rosasol	Capsule (Flagyl): 375 mg† Cream: 0.75% (Metrocreme, Vitazol), 1% (Noritate, Rosasol), 10% (Flagyl Cream) Gel, topical: 0.75% (Metrogel, Nydamax), 1% (Metrogel)† Lotion: 0.75% (Metrolotion) Gel, vaginal (Metrogel, Nidagel, Vandazole): 0.75% Powder, for injection: 500 mg/vial† Solution, for injection: 5 mg/mL Tablet (Flagyl): 250 mg, 500 mg Tablet, extended-release (Flagyl ER, Flurozole ER): 750 mg
mupirocin*	Bactroban, Centany / Bactroban, Bactroban Cream	Cream: 2% Ointment, topical: 2%
chloramphenicol*	Generics / Chloroptic, Chloromycetin, Pentamycetin	Powder, for injection (Chloromycetin): 1 g Ophthalmic solution: 0.5%‡ (Chloroptic), 0.25%‡ (Pentamycetin) Ophthalmic ointment (Chloroptic): 1%‡
clindamycin* 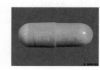	Cleocin, Cleocin T, Cleocin Ovules, Clindagel, Clindesse, Clindamax, Evoclin / Clindets, Dalacin C, Dalacin T 1%	Capsule (Cleocin, Dalacin C): 75 mg†, 150 mg, 300 mg Foam (Evoclin): 1%† Pledgets (Cleocin T, Clindets): 1% Powder, solution for injection (Cleocin): 900 mg/6 mL Solution, for injection (Cleocin, Dalacin C): 150 mg/mL, Solution, for injection in 5% dextrose: 6 mg/mL, 12 mg/mL, 18 mg/mL Powder, for oral solution (Cleocin, Dalacin C): 75 mg/5 mL Topical gel, lotion (Cleocin T, Clindagel, Clindamax): 1% Topical solution (Cleocin T, Dalacin T): 1% Vaginal cream (Clindesse, Cleocin, Dalacin): 2% Vaginal suppositories (Cleocin Ovules): 100 mg
telavancin	Vibativ / Not available	Powder, for injection: 250 mg, 750 mg
vancomycin	Vancocin / Vancocin	Capsule: 125 mg, 250 mg Powder, for injection: 500 mg, 750 mg†, 1 g, 5 g, 10 g

*Generic available.
†Strength available in the United States only.
‡Strength available in Canada only.

Summary of Drugs Used for the Treatment of Bacterial Infections

Generic Name	Brand Name	Usual Dose and Dosing Schedule	Warning Labels
Cephalosporins			
cefadroxil	Duricef	1-2 g orally/day given in one or two daily doses until course of therapy is finished (max, 2 g/day)	COMPLETE FULL COURSE OF THERAPY (ALL). TAKE WITH FOOD (CEFADROXIL). REFRIGERATE, SHAKE WELL, AND DISCARD AFTER 14 DAYS (CEFADROXIL, CEPHALEXIN, CEFACLOR ORAL SUSPENSIONS). REFRIGERATE, SHAKE WELL, AND DISCARD AFTER 10 DAYS (CEFUROXIME SUSPENSION). REFRIGERATE OR STORE AT ROOM TEMPERATURE, SHAKE WELL, AND DISCARD AFTER 14 DAYS (CEFIXIME ORAL SUSPENSION). SWALLOW WHOLE; DON'T CRUSH OR CHEW (EXTENDED-RELEASE). TAKE WITH FOOD (EXTENDED-RELEASE).
cephalexin	Keflex	Varies (max, 4 g/day)	
cefaclor	Ceclor	**Immediate-release:** 250-500 mg orally every 8 hr until course of therapy is finished **Extended release:** 375-500 mg every 12 hr until course of therapy is finished (max, 1.5 g/day)	
cefuroxime	Ceftin	250-500 mg orally every 12 hr until course of therapy is finished. (max, 1 g/day)	
cefixime	Suprax	400 mg orally divided every 12-24 hr until course of therapy is finished (max, 800 mg/day)	
Fluoroquinolones			
ciprofloxacin	Cipro Cipro XR	**Immediate-release:** 500-750 mg orally every 12 hr until course of therapy is finished **Extended-release:** 500-1000 mg once daily until course of therapy is finished (max, 1.5 g/day)	COMPLETE FULL COURSE OF THERAPY. TAKE WITH LOTS OF WATER. AVOID PROLONGED EXPOSURE TO SUNLIGHT. MAY CAUSE DIZZINESS OR DROWSINESS; DO NOT DRIVE OR USE MACHINERY. AVOID ANTACIDS AND VITAMINS CONTAINING IRON AND ZINC. REFRIGERATE, SHAKE WELL, AND DISCARD AFTER 14 DAYS (SUSPENSION). SWALLOW WHOLE; DON'T CRUSH OR CHEW (EXTENDED-RELEASE). TAKE ON AN EMPTY STOMACH.
levofloxacin	Levaquin	250-500 mg every 24 hr (max, 750 mg/day) until course of therapy is finished	
moxifloxacin	Avelox	400 mg orally or IV once daily until course of therapy is finished	
norfloxacin	Noroxin	400 mg orally twice daily until course of therapy is finished	
Macrolides			
azithromycin	Zithromax	500 mg the first 1 to 3 days of therapy, followed by 250 mg once daily for 4 days	COMPLETE FULL COURSE OF THERAPY. STORE AT ROOM TEMPERATURE AND DISCARD IN 14 DAYS (CLARITHROMYCIN AND AZITHROMYCIN EXTENDED-RELEASE SUSPENSION). SHAKE WELL (SUSPENSION). REFRIGERATE; DISCARD IN 10 DAYS (AZITHROMYCIN SUSPENSION, IMMEDIATE-RELEASE). TAKE ON AN EMPTY STOMACH (AZITHROMYCIN SUSPENSION). MAY DECREASE THE EFFECTIVENESS OF ORAL CONTRACEPTIVES. TAKE WITH FOOD (DELAYED-RELEASE).
clarithromycin	Biaxin, Biaxin XL	**Immediate-release:** 250-500 mg every 12 hr up to 1000 mg once daily until course of therapy is finished **Extended-release:** 1000 mg once daily until course of therapy is finished	
erythromycin base, delayed-release	Ery-Tab, ERYC, PCE	250-500 mg every 6-8 hr until course of therapy is finished (max, 4 g/day)	
erythromycin ethylsuccinate	EES	400-800 mg every 6-8 hr until course of therapy is finished (max, 4 g/day)	

Continued

Summary of Drugs Used for the Treatment of Bacterial Infections—cont'd

Generic Name	Brand Name	Usual Dose and Dosing Schedule	Warning Labels
Ketolides			
telithromycin	Ketek	800 mg once daily until course of therapy is finished	COMPLETE FULL COURSE OF THERAPY.
Sulfonamides and Sulfonamide Combinations			
sulfisoxazole	Gantrisin	Varies; 2-4 g initially, then 4-8 g/day in four to six equally divided doses until course of therapy is finished (max, 12 g/day)	COMPLETE FULL COURSE OF THERAPY. TAKE WITH LOTS OF WATER. AVOID PROLONGED SUNLIGHT.
sulfisoxazole + erythromycin ethylsuccinate	Pediazole	400 mg erythromycin + 1200 mg sulfisoxazole every 6 hr until course of therapy is finished (max, 4 g/day erythromycin base or 12 g/day sulfisoxazole)	SHAKE WELL (SUSPENSION). REFRIGERATE; DO NOT FREEZE (SULFISOXAZOLE + ERYTHROMYCIN ETHYLSUCCINATE SUSPENSION). STORE AT ROOM TEMPERATURE (SULFAMETHOXAZOLE + TRIMETHOPRIM SUSPENSION).
sulfamethoxazole + trimethoprim	Septra, Bactrim	40-160 mg trimethoprim + 800 mg sulfamethoxazole every 12 hr until course of therapy is finished	
Penicillins			
ampicillin	Generics	250-1000 mg orally every 6 hr until course of therapy is finished (max, 3.5 g/day)	COMPLETE FULL COURSE OF THERAPY. TAKE ON AN EMPTY STOMACH (AMPICILLIN, CLOXACILLIN, DICLOXACILLIN). REFRIGERATE, SHAKE WELL, AND DISCARD AFTER 14 DAYS (SUSPENSION AMPICILLIN, DICLOXACILLIN, PENICILLIN VK). MAY DECREASE EFFECTIVENESS OF ORAL CONTRACEPTIVES. REFRIGERATE, SHAKE WELL, AND DISCARD AFTER 10 DAYS (SUSPENSION, AMOXICILLIN + CLAVULANIC ACID).
amoxicillin	Amoxil	Varies; 500-875 mg every 12 hr or 250-500 mg PO every 8 hr until course of therapy is finished (max, 1750 mg/day)	
dicloxacillin	Generics	125-500 mg orally every 6 hr until course of therapy is finished (max, 4 g/day)	
penicillin VK	Generics	125-500 mg orally every 6 hr until course of therapy is finished (max, 2 g/day)	
amoxicillin + clavulanic acid	Augmentin	Varies; 250-500 mg every 8 hr or 500-875 mg every 12 hr until course of therapy is finished (max, Augmentin tablets, chewable tablets, or suspension, 1750 mg/day [amoxicillin component[, Augmentin XR tablets 4 g/day [amoxicillin component])	
penicillin G benzathine	Bicillin L-A	Varies	REFRIGERATE; DO NOT FREEZE.
Tetracyclines			
doxycycline	Vibramycin, Monodox	Varies; commonly 100 mg bid on day 1 followed by 100 mg daily or 100 mg bid until course of therapy is completed	COMPLETE FULL COURSE OF THERAPY. TAKE WITH LOTS OF WATER. AVOID PROLONGED SUNLIGHT. AVOID ANTACIDS AND VITAMINS CONTAINING IRON AND ZINC. MAY DECREASE EFFECTIVENESS OF ORAL CONTRACEPTIVES. SHAKE WELL (TETRACYCLINE SUSPENSION). TAKE ON AN EMPTY STOMACH (TETRACYCLINE).
minocycline	Minocin	Varies (max, 350 mg on day 1, then 200 mg/day)	
tetracycline	Generics	Varies (max, 4 g/day)	

Summary of Drugs Used in the Treatment of Anxiety Disorders—cont'd

Generic Name	Brand Name	Usual Dose and Dosing Schedule	Warning Labels
Miscellaneous			
metronidazole	Metrogel, Metrocreme, Noritate	**Acne rosacea:** Apply a thin film once or twice daily.	COMPLETE FULL COURSE OF THERAPY.
	Metrogel	**Bacterial vaginosis:** One applicatorful once daily at bedtime	COMPLETE FULL COURSE OF THERAPY.
	Flagyl	**Other infections:** 500-750 mg PO bid or 250 mg PO tid until course of therapy is completed (max, 4 g/day)	COMPLETE FULL COURSE OF THERAPY. TAKE WITH A FULL GLASS OF WATER. AVOID ALCOHOL. MAY CAUSE DIZZINESS OR DROWSINESS; DO NOT DRIVE OR USE MACHINERY.
isoniazid	Generics	**Tuberculosis prophylaxis:** 300 mg orally once daily or 900 mg/day twice weekly with pyridoxine (50 mg once daily or 100 mg twice weekly) for 9 mo	COMPLETE FULL COURSE OF THERAPY. AVOID ANTACIDS. AVOID ALCOHOL.
clindamycin	Cleocin	150-450 mg orally every 6 hr until course of therapy is completed (max, 2700 mg/day)	COMPLETE FULL COURSE OF THERAPY. TAKE WITH A FULL GLASS OF WATER.
mupirocin	Bactroban	Apply tid or bid for intranasal infections.	COMPLETE FULL COURSE OF THERAPY.

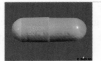

Chapter Summary

- Chronic noninfectious disease is a leading cause of disability and death in developed, industrialized countries; however, infectious disease is still one the leading causes of morbidity and mortality globally.
- Poverty, malnutrition, the lack of clean water, poor sanitation, and inadequate housing increase the risk for infectious disease and decrease the likelihood for adequate treatment.
- Antibiotics have played a key role in improving the survival of those with bacterial infections.
- Microbes can learn how to resist the effects of antibiotics; superbugs are resistant to some currently available antimicrobial agents. Multidrug resistance is a serious problem.
- Microbial resistance is the ability of bacteria to overcome the bactericidal effects of an antibiotic. Resistance traits are encoded on bacterial genes on chromosomal or plasmid DNA and can be transferred to other bacteria.
- Causes of microbial resistance are the following: (1) inappropriate prescribing; (2) failure to complete the full course of therapy; (3) administration of antibacterial agents for viral infections (e.g., the common cold); (4) antibiotics in the food chain (agriculture, animal husbandry, fish farms); and (5) lack of guidelines for preventing the spread of infections in institutional care settings.
- Examples of mechanisms of antimicrobial resistance are the following: (1) secretion of enzymes that inactivate the antibiotic; (2) modification of the target site for antibiotic binding; (3) production of antibiotic-modifying enzymes; and (4) mutations that affect antibiotic transport into the cell.
- Bactericidal agents are able to destroy rapidly proliferating, pathogenic bacteria.

- Bacteriostatic agents slow the growth of bacteria enough for the host's (our body's) defense mechanism to destroy the invading bacteria.
- β-Lactam antibiotics target the bacterial cell wall. Penicillins, cephalosporins, carbapenems, and monobactams are β-lactam antibiotics that inhibit cell wall synthesis.
- Vancomycin is a glycopeptide antibiotic that inhibits cell wall synthesis.
- Antibiotics that inhibit the function of the bacterial cell wall increase cell membrane permeability causing cell contents to leak out.
- There are five classes of anti-infective agents that act to inhibit bacterial protein synthesis—the aminoglycosides, macrolides, tetracyclines, amphenicols, and oxazolidinones.
- Fluoroquinolones and nitroimidazoles are classes of anti-infectives capable of inhibiting DNA synthesis.
- Rifampin inhibits bacterial RNA synthesis.
- Bacteria must synthesize folic acid.
- Sulfonamides are antifolate drugs; trimethoprim is a dihydrofolate reductase inhibitor that interferes with bacterial folic acid synthesis.
- Aminoglycosides are not absorbed systemically when administered by mouth but may be given orally to reduce the number of bacteria in the bowel prior to colorectal surgery.
- The most serious adverse reactions linked to aminoglycoside use are hearing loss (ototoxicity) and kidney damage (nephrotoxicity).
- A common beginning for cephalosporin drugs is *ceph-* or *cef-*.
- Cephalosporins are classified as first-, second-, third-, and fourth-generation agents.
- First-generation cephalosporins are most effective against gram-positive aerobic bacteria. Second-generation cephalosporins have effectiveness against gram-positive and gram-negative bacteria, but third-generation cephalosporins are the most effective against gram-negative anaerobic bacteria. Fourth-generation cephalosporins are used for the treatment of community-acquired and nosocomial pneumonia.
- A common ending of fluoroquinolones is *-floxacin*.
- Oral and parenteral fluoroquinolones are contraindicated in pregnant women and children younger than 16 to 18 years because of the risk for cartilage malformations.
- A common ending for macrolides is *-thromycin*.
- Clarithromycin is a key component of treatment regimens for peptic ulcer disease caused by the bacterium *H. pylori*.
- Gastrointestinal upset is common with the use of macrolides. It occurs in up to 21% of those who take erythromycin.
- Macrolides, penicillins and tetracyclines may decrease the effectiveness of oral contraceptives.
- Penicillins may also be administered before dental and other medical procedures to prevent bacterial endocarditis in individuals with prosthetic heart valves.
- Antistaphylococcal penicillins are penicillinase-resistant.
- Standard penicillins lack stability in gastric acids, which is why most are administered intramuscularly or must be taken on an empty stomach.
- A common beginning for sulfonamides *sulf-*.
- Sulfonamides are indicated for the treatment of AIDS-related pneumonia (caused by *P. jiroveci*), urinary tract infections, and upper respiratory infections.
- Sulfonamides may promote the formation of crystals in the urine (crystalluria), especially if taken with acidic foods or beverages.
- Tetracyclines are used for the treatment of acne, sexually transmitted infections such as chlamydia, Lyme disease, and Rocky Mountain spotted fever.
- Tetracyclines are contraindicated in pregnancy and small children because they can weaken fetal bone, retard bone growth, weaken tooth enamel, and stain teeth.
- Isoniazid is used for the treatment of tuberculosis. Vitamin B6 should be taken with isoniazid to reduce neurotoxicity.
- Metronidazole is the drug of choice for the treatment of *C. difficile* enteritis, a condition that may cause pseudomembranous colitis.
- Individuals taking metronidazole should avoid drinking alcoholic beverages or taking medicines containing alcohol.

- Mupirocin is a topically applied antimicrobial used to treat staphylococcal infections of the skin such as impetigo.
- The systemic use of clindamycin is associated with the development of *C. difficile* bacteria that cause diarrhea and pseudomembranous colitis. Drinking plenty of fluids can lower the risk for the development of this condition.

REVIEW QUESTIONS

1. Antibiotics are used to treat_____.
   a. Strep throat
   b. Cold sores
   c. The common cold
   d. Viral pneumonia

2. Misuse of antimicrobial agents is a major cause for the development and spread of microbial resistance.
   a. True
   b. False

3. Antibacterial agents may be classified as _____.
   a. Bactericidal
   b. Bacteriolytic
   c. Bacteriostatic
   d. a and c

4. Fluoroquinolones and nitroimidazoles are classes of antibiotics capable of inhibiting _____ synthesis.
   a. RNA
   b. DNA
   c. tPA
   d. GABA

5. Second-generation cephalosporins have effectiveness only against gram-positive bacteria.
   a. True
   b. False

6. Fluoroquinolones are formulated for oral, ophthalmic, and parenteral use.
   a. True
   b. False

7. Macrolide antibiotics are primarily used for the treatment of upper respiratory infections (URIs) and lower respiratory infections (LRIs).
   a. True
   b. False

8. Oral penicillins are used to treat many infections, including _____.
   a. Upper respiratory infections
   b. Otitis media, skin infections
   c. Strep throat
   d. All of the above

9. Outdated tetracycline becomes toxic and should be discarded.
   a. True
   b. False

10. Isoniazid is used for the treatment of _____.
    a. Upper respiratory infections
    b. AIDS
    c. Tuberculosis
    d. Peptic ulcers

TECHNICIAN'S CORNER

1. With microbial resistance developing against antibiotics, what steps should be taken by the pharmaceutical and food industries, patients, and health care providers to combat this problem?
2. Can the practice of universal precautions (e.g., handwashing) reduce the incidence of nosocomial infections?

Bibliography

Elsevier: Gold Standard Clinical Pharmacology. Retrieved June 19, 2011, from https://www.clinical pharmacology.com/. 2010.

FDA: FDA Approved Drug Products. Retrieved June 23, 2012, from http://www.accessdata.fda.gov/scripts/cder/drugsatfda/index.cfm?fuseaction=Search.Search_Drug_Name. 2012.

Health Canada: Drug Product Database. Retrieved June 23, 2012, from http://www.hc-sc.gc.ca/dhp-mps/prodpharma/databasdon/index-eng.php. 2010.

Kalant H, Grant D, Mitchell J: *Principles of medical pharmacology*, ed 7, Toronto, 2007, Elsevier Canada, pp 671-686, 702-707, 713.

Lance L, Lacy C, Armstrong L, et al: *Drug information handbook for the allied health professional*, ed 12, Hudson, OH, 2005, APhA Lexi-Comp.

Page C, Curtis M, Sutter M, et al: *Integrated pharmacology*, Philadelphia, 2005, Elsevier Mosby, pp 111-134.

USP Center for the Advancement of Patient Safety: USP Quality Review No. 79: Use caution: Avoid confusion, Rockville, MD, 2004, USP Center for the Advancement of Patient Safety.

36

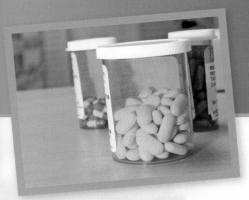

Treatment of Viral Infections

KEY TERMS

Adherence: Closely following or adhering to the treatment regimen.

AIDS (acquired immunodeficiency syndrome): The most severe form of human immunodeficiency virus (HIV) infection. HIV-infected patients are diagnosed with AIDS when their CD4 cell count falls below 200 cells/mm^3 or if they develop an AIDS-defining illness (an unusual illness in someone who is not HIV- positive).

Antiretroviral: Medication that interferes with the replication of retroviruses. HIV is a retrovirus.

Antiviral: Medication that is able to inhibit viral replication.

Antiviral resistance: Ability of a virus to overcome the suppressive action of antiviral agents.

CD4 count: Number of CD4 cells in a sample of blood.

CD4 T lymphocyte: White blood cells that fight infection.

Cross-resistance: Development of resistance to one drug in a particular class that results in resistance to other drugs in that class.

Drug resistance testing: Laboratory test to determine whether an individual's HIV strain is resistant to any anti-HIV medications.

Highly active antiretroviral therapy: Combination of three or more antiretroviral medications taken in a regimen.

Host: Individual infected with a virus.

Human immunodeficiency virus: Virus that causes acquired immunodeficiency syndrome

Mother-to-child transmission: Transmission of the HIV from an HIV-infected mother to her baby during pregnancy, delivery, or through breast milk (also called perinatal transmission).

Oncovirus: A virus that is a causative agent in a cancer.

Viral load: Amount of materials from the virus that get released into the blood when the HIV reproduces.

Virion: Infectious particles of a virus.

Virustatic: Able to suppress viral proliferation.

Virus: Intracellular parasite that consists of a DNA and RNA core surrounded by a protein coat and sometimes an outer covering of lipoprotein.

Overview

A *virus* is an intracellular parasite that consists of a DNA or RNA core surrounded by a protein coat and sometimes an outer covering of lipoprotein. The infectious particle (*virion*) does not have the cellular components necessary for reproduction, so they use the host's cellular machinery to replicate (Figure 36-1). The virus attaches itself to the host's cell and then releases viral genetic material (RNA and DNA) into the host cell. The viral material takes control of the host cell machinery for replication. The host cell eventually dies because the virus keeps it from performing its normal functions. When it dies, the cell releases replicated viruses that proliferate and attack more and more host cells.

Viruses may cause minor illnesses such as the common cold and warts, as well as serious infections such as *human immunodeficiency virus* (HIV), smallpox, and hepatitis C infections. Some viral infections are linked to cancers. For example, human papillomavirus (HPV) is linked to cervical cancer. Epstein-Barr virus (EBV) is associated with nose and throat cancers, and hepatitis B and C viruses are associated with liver cancer. Viruses that can cause cancer are called *oncoviruses*.

An *antiviral* is a medication that is able to inhibit viral replication. All antiviral agents work best when the *host* (the individual with the infection) has a healthy immune system. This is because antivirals do not destroy viruses; they are *virustatic*. When the rate of virus proliferation is slowed, the macrophages, immunoglobulins, T cells, interleukins, interferons, and other cells released by the host in response to the virus's attack ultimately are responsible for recovery from the infection (see Unit X). Like bacterial infections, effective treatment of viral infections is dependent on host factors, viral factors, and drug factors. Figure 35-1 shows factors that influence successful therapy.

The following factors influence the outcome of antiviral therapy: (1) stage of illness at the time of initiation of therapy; (2) dose of antiviral agent used; (3) ability of the virus to penetrate the central nervous system; (4) ability of the virus to remain latent within its host; and (5) development of antiviral resistance. Herpes simplex virus types 1 and 2 (HSV-1, HSV-2) is an example of a virus that demonstrates the importance of timing as related to the initiation of drug therapy. The severity of the infection and symptoms are reduced only when antiviral therapy is initiated within the first 24 to 48 hours of exposure to the virus or onset of symptoms. Other viral infections that are improved by early initiation of antiviral therapy are influenza (Box 36-1) and varicella zoster virus (VZV). HSV-1, HSV-2, and VZV are also examples of viruses that lay dormant in host cells and periodically awaken to cause recurrent disease.

Antiviral agents are typically effective against specific viral strains. For example, amantadine acts against influenza A but not influenza B. Oseltamivir (Tamiflu) is indicated for the treatment of influenza but is not effective for the treatment of HIV, HPV, or HSV. Antibiotics are not effective against viral infections.

Antiviral Resistance

The growth of viral colonies involves viral replication. In the process of replication, the virus may mutate. Although mutations may result in a virus that is not able to reproduce, mutations often result in adaptations that make it easier for the virus to exist in new environments and hosts. *Antiviral resistance* is the ability of a virus to overcome the suppressive action of antiviral agents. It may occur when an individual taking an antiviral drug skips doses or takes them irregularly. Vomiting is an additional cause for subtherapeutic levels. Rather than having drug levels in the body high enough to suppress viral replication, levels of residual drug are low enough to allow the virus to reproduce. The virus may accidentally mutate into a form that is resistant to the antiviral drug(s) taken.

Because viruses continually mutate, it is difficult to develop a vaccine to prevent virus infection. For example, each year, a new flu vaccine must be developed to the latest virulent strain of influenza. A triple cocktail of drugs is administered for highly active antiretroviral therapy (HAART) to decrease mutations and improve antiretroviral therapy for the treatment of HIV and AIDS. Vaccines have

BOX 36-1   **CDC Recommendations for Antiviral Treatment of Influenza**

- Early treatment is recommended for patients who are hospitalized or who have severe, complicated, or progressive illness, or are at high risk for influenza complications.
- Treatment is recommended for the following:
  - Children < 2 yr
  - Adults ≥ 65 yr
  - Immunocompromised persons (HIV or drug-induced)
  - Persons with chronic pulmonary (e.g., asthma), cardiovascular (e.g., hypertension), renal hepatic, hematological (e.g., sickle cell anemia), metabolic (e.g., diabetes), and neurological disorders (e.g., seizures), and stroke
  - Pregnant women or 2 wk post-partum
- Early treatment prevents complications and results in greatest benefit. Treatment within 48 hr of onset of influenza illness.
- Treatment may be considered for non–high-risk, symptomatic outpatients with confirmed or suspected influenza following the guideline for initiating treatment within 48 hr of illness onset.

Adapted from Centers for Disease Control and Prevention. (2011) Morbidity and Mortality Weekly Report. In R. Moolenaar (Series Ed.): Vol. 60. *Antiviral Agents for the Treatment and Chemoprophylaxis of Influenza.*

been developed to prevent HPV. Cervarix and Gardasil are effective against HPV types 16 and 18 oncovirus, which cause most cervical cancers. Gardasil is also effective against HPV types 6 and 11.

Mechanisms of Antiviral Action

Antivirals inhibit virus-specific steps in the replication cycle; they aim to do the following:
- Interfere with the virus attachment to the host cell receptors, cell penetration, and viral uncoating
- Inhibit reverse transcriptase, transamidase, and other virion-associated enzymes
- Inhibit viral transcription
- Inhibit viral messenger RNA (mRNA)
- Interfere with virus regulatory proteins
- Interfere with virus cleavage
- Interfere with viral assembly
- Interfere with the release of virus

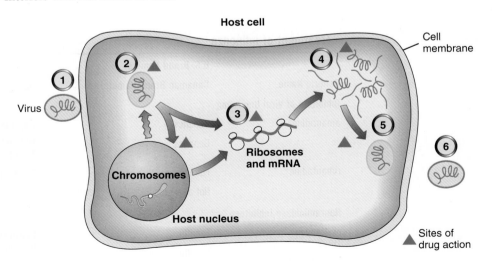

1. Attachment to host cell
2. Uncoating of virus, and entry of viral nucleic acid into host cell nucleus
3. Control of DNA, RNA, and/or protein production
4. Production of viral subunits
5. Assembly of virions
6. Release of virions

FIGURE 36-1 Virus invasion of a host cell, viral replication, and release of virions. (Adapted from Brody TM, Larner J, Minneman KP: *Human pharmacology: Molecular to clinical*, ed 3, St. Louis, 1998, Mosby.)

Treatment of Influenza

Adamantanes and neuraminidase inhibitors are antivirals that prevent and treat influenza. Adamantanes inhibit viral uncoating and neuraminidase inhibitors inhibit viral release and proliferation.

INHIBITORS OF VIRAL UNCOATING

Amantadine and rimantadine are classified as adamantanes and are used for the prevention and treatment of influenza A. They are not effective against influenza B. Because of antiviral resistance to H1N1 and H3N3 influenza A flu strains, amantadine and rimantadine were not recommended by the Centers for Disease Control (CDC) for use during the 2010 flu season.

MECHANISM OF ACTION AND PHARMACOKINETICS

Amantadine and rimantadine interfere with the uncoating of the influenza A virus, a necessary step in the viral replication process. More specifically, they inhibit the activity of the influenza virus M2 protein, which forms a channel in the virus membrane and enables replication after the virus enters the host cell. Amantadine is rapidly absorbed and peak plasma levels are achieved within 2 to 4 hours of an oral dose. Peak plasma levels for rimantadine occur in approximately 6 hours. Rimantadine is approximately 40% protein-bound. It is also highly metabolized in the liver and has active metabolites that account for the drug's long half-life of 13 to 65 hours.

ADVERSE REACTIONS

Amantadine and rimantadine may produce anxiety, irritability, nervousness, drowsiness, confusion, and headache. They can also cause diarrhea or constipation, difficulty sleeping or nightmares, dry mouth, loss of appetite, nausea or vomiting, unusual tiredness, and, rarely, kidney damage.

NEURAMINIDASE INHIBITORS

Oseltamivir and zanamivir are indicated for the treatment of influenza A and influenza B. The H1N1 and H3N3 strains of influenza A are susceptible to the effects of oseltamivir and zanamivir; however, a strain of H1N1 influenza resistant to oseltamivir and zanamivir has been identified.

MECHANISM OF ACTION AND PHARMACOKINETICS

The surfaces of influenza viruses are dotted with neuraminidase proteins. Neuraminidase inhibitors inhibit viral release by inhibiting the enzyme that breaks the bonds that hold the virus particle to

Treatment of influenza

Generic Name	U.S. Brand Name(s) Canadian Brand Name(s)	Dosage Forms and Strengths
Inhibitors of Viral Uncoating		
amantidine*	Generics	Capsule: 100 mg
	Generics	Oral solution: 50 mg/5 mL Tablet: 100 mg[†]
rimantadine*	Flumadine	Tablet (generics): 100 mg
	Not available	
Neuraminidase Inhibitors		
oseltamivir	Tamiflu	Capsule: 30 mg, 45 mg, 75 mg
	Tamiflu	Powder, for suspension: 6 mg/mL[†], 12 mg/mL[‡]
zanamivir	Relenza	Powder, for inhalation: 5 mg
	Relenza	

*Generic available.
[†]Strength available in the United States only.
[‡]Strength available in Canada only.

the outside of the infected cell. They inhibit virus proliferation by blocking virus release from the host cell. This limits the spread of the virus. Oseltamivir (Tamiflu) is formulated for oral use and zanamivir (Relenza) is formulated as a powder for oral inhalation.

ADVERSE REACTIONS
Side effects common to the use of oseltamivir and zanamivir are nausea and vomiting, coughing, dizziness, and headache. Psychosis and other emotional changes have been reported with the use of neuraminidase inhibitors. Zanamivir is not recommended for patients with pulmonary disease because it has been reported to produce bronchospasm and deterioration in pulmonary function. Allergic reactions include oropharyngeal or facial edema.

Treatment of Hepatitis B and Hepatitis C Viruses

Interferons, nucleoside analogues, nucleotide analogues, and protease inhibitors are used for the treatment of viral hepatitis. Interferons are used for the treatment of hepatitis B virus (HBV) and hepatitis C virus (HCV), nucleoside and nucleotide analogues are used to treat HBV, and protease inhibitors interfere with HCV viral replication.

INHIBITORS OF TRANSCRIPTION
Interferons
There are approximately 2000 interferon receptors on each normal and malignant cell. These receptors recognize and bind interferons that are released as part of the body's normal immune response. Interferons may also be produced by recombinant DNA technology. They are not technically antiviral agents. Instead, they protect uninfected cells by promoting resistance to virus infection.

Interferon alfa-2b, interferon alfacon-1, peginterferon alfa-2a, and peginterferon alfa-2b are administered to treat viral infections. Interferon alfacon-1 and peginterferon alfa-2b are indicated for the treatment of HCV. Interferon alfa-2b and peginterferon alfa-2a may be used for the treatment of HBV and HCV.

MECHANISM OF ACTION AND PHARMACOKINETICS
Interferons inhibit viral transcription by activating enzymes that cleave single-stranded viral RNA. Depending on the virus and cell type, they may also inhibit viral uncoating, inhibit the synthesis of mRNA, and interfere with the translation, assembly, and release of viral proteins.

ADVERSE REACTIONS
The most common adverse reactions associated with interferons are flulike symptoms—fever, chills, headache, fatigue, muscle aches, and joint pain. They may also cause nausea, vomiting, diarrhea, dizziness, and depression. More serious adverse affects are a drop in white blood cell count (neutropenia) and in platelet count (thrombocytopenia).

Nucleoside Analogues
Entecavir, lamivudine, ribavirin, and telbivudine are nucleoside analogues used for the treatment of HBV. Ribavirin is indicated for the treatment of hepatitis C when combined with peginterferon alfa. Ribavirin is also indicated for the treatment of respiratory syncytial virus (RSV).

MECHANISM OF ACTION
Entecavir and lamivudine inhibit HBV reverse transcriptase. Entecavir is effective against lamivudine-resistant HBV. Telbivudine inhibits HBV DNA polymerase, resulting in DNA chain termination and inhibition of viral replication.

Ribavirin is effective against RNA and DNA viruses. The mechanism of action is not completely understood, but it is believed that the drug increases the mutation rate of the virus, leading to a growing number of viruses unable to replicate.

TECH ALERT!
The following drugs have look-alike and sound-alike issues:
   peginterferon alfa-2a and peginterferon alfa-2b;
   interferon alfa and interferon alfacon

Treatment of Hepatitis B and Hepatitis C

Generic Name	U.S. Brand Name(s) Canadian Brand Name(s)	Dosage Forms and Strengths
Interferons		
interferon alfa-2b	Intron-A Intron-A	Powder, for injection: 10 million international units (mIU)/vial, 18 mIU/vial, 25 mIU/vial[†] Solution for injection, vial: 6 mIU/mL[‡], 10 mIU/mL[‡], 15 mIU/mL[‡], 18 mIU/mL[‡], 25 mIU/mL[‡] Solution for injection, prefilled syringe (Pen): 18 mIU/Pen, 30 mIU/Pen, 60 mIU/Pen
interferon alfacon-1	Infergen Infergen	Solution for injection: 30 mcg/mL vial
peginterferon alfa-2a	Pegasys Pegasys	Solution for injection, vial: 180 mcg/0.5 mL[‡], 180 mcg/mL Solution for injection, prefilled syringe: 180 mcg/0.5 mL
peginterferon alfa-2b	PegIntron, Sylatron Not available	Powder for injection: 50 mcg, 80 mcg, 120 mcg, 150 mcg, 296 mcg, 444 mcg, 888 mcg Powder for injection, Redipen: 50 mcg, 80 mcg, 120 mcg, 150 mcg
Nucleoside Analogues		
entecavir	Baraclude Baraclude	Solution, oral: 0.05 mg/mL[†] Tablet: 0.5 mg, 1 mg[†]
lamivudine	Epivir HBV Heptovir	Solution, oral: 5 mg/mL Tablet: 100 mg
ribavirin*	Copegus, Rebetol, Ribapak, Ribasphere, RibaTab Not available	Capsule (Rebetol, Ribasphere): 200 mg Oral solution (Rebetol): 40 mg/mL Tablet (Copegus): 200 mg, 400 mg, 500 mg, 600 mg
telbivudine	Tyzeka Sebivo	Tablet: 600 mg
Nucleotide Analogues		
adefovir	Hepsera Hepsera	Tablet: 10 mg
Protease Inhibitor		
boceprevir	Victrelis Victrelis	Capsule: 200 mg
telaprevir	Incivek Incivek	Tablet: 375 mg

*Generic available.
[†]Strength available in the United States only.
[‡]Strength available in Canada only.

Treatment of Respiratory Syncytial Virus: Inhibition of DNA and RNA Replication

Generic Name	U.S. Brand Name(s) Canadian Brand Name(s)	Dosage Forms and Strengths
ribavirin*	Virazole Virazole	Powder, for inhalation: 6 g/vial

*Generic available.

ADVERSE EFFECTS

The most common adverse effects of entecavir and lamivudine are headache, fatigue, dizziness, and nausea. Entecavir and telbivudine have a boxed warning regarding the risks for lactic acidosis, hepatomegaly, and exacerbation of hepatitis when the drug is discontinued. Hepatic function should continue to be monitored for several months after entecavir and telbivudine are discontinued.

Nucleotide Analogues

Adefovir is a prodrug. It inhibits HBV DNA polymerase, resulting in DNA chain termination and inhibition of viral replication.

ADVERSE EFFECTS

Headache, abdominal pain, diarrhea, nausea, dyspepsia, flatulence, and asthenia are the most common side effects associated with adefovir. Adefovir may also cause nephrotoxicity, and hepatitis may worsen on discontinuation.

Protease Inhibitors

Boceprevir and telaprevir are selective protease inhibitors. Both drugs were U.S. Food and Drug Administration (FDA)–approved in 2011 for the treatment of HCV.

MECHANISM OF ACTION

Boceprevir and telaprevir selectively interfere with the virus cleavage of HCV protein, inhibiting viral replication.

ADVERSE EFFECTS

Fatigue, anemia, nausea, and headache are the most common effects of boceprevir. Drug reaction with eosinophilia and systemic symptoms (DRESS) are associated with the use of telaprevir. DRESS symptoms include rash, fever, facial edema, hepatitis and nephritis.

INHIBITION OF DNA AND RNA REPLICATION

Antivirals that inhibit DNA and RNA replication are used for the treatment of herpes simplex type 1 and type 2, herpes zoster, and cytomegalovirus (CMV).

MECHANISM OF ACTION AND PHARMACOKINETICS

The genetic code is stored in DNA. RNA regulates specific cell functions, such as editing strands of code, carrying the code (mRNA), and transferring the code accurately. These are essential steps in the process of viral replication.

Acyclovir inhibits viral DNA synthesis. It is used for the treatment of herpes simplex virus (HSV-1), the virus that causes cold sores; herpes genitalis (HSV-2), one of the viruses that cause genital warts; and varicella zoster virus (VZV), the virus that causes chickenpox and shingles. Acyclovir is approximately 10 times more potent against HSV-1 and -2 than against VZV. Higher doses are required for the treatment of chickenpox and shingles. Acyclovir may be administered topically, orally, or parenterally. GI absorption is poor and bioavailability of orally administered acyclovir is much lower than parenterally administered acyclovir. Systemic effects from topical administration are limited.

Valacyclovir is an ester of acyclovir. It has greater oral absorption. It treats the same conditions as acyclovir but requires less frequent dosing.

Cidofovir is an acyclic phosphonate nucleotide analogue. Nucleotides are the individual units that make up RNA and DNA. Cidofovir inhibits viral DNA polymerase, the enzyme responsible for the replication of new viral RNA and DNA. It is indicated for the treatment of cytomegalovirus retinitis in patients with AIDS.

Foscarnet inhibits the viral-specific DNA polymerases and reverse transcriptases. It inhibits HIV reverse transcriptase and hepatitis B DNA polymerase. It also inhibits replication of the herpes simplex virus, varicella-zoster virus, EBV, human herpesvirus 6, and CMV. It is indicated for the

Treatment of Herpes and Cytomegalovirus: Inhibition of DNA and RNA Replication

Generic Name	U.S. Brand Name(s)	Dosage Forms and Strengths
	Canadian Brand Name(s)	
acyclovir*	Zovirax	Capsule: 200 mg
	Zovirax	Cream: 5%
		Ointment: 5%
		Powder, for injection: 500 mg, 1000 mg/vial†
		Solution, for injection: 25 mg/mL‡, 50 mg/mL
		Suspension: 200 mg/5 mL
		Tablet: 200 mg‡, 400 mg, 800 mg
cidofovir	Vistide	Solution, for injection: 75 mg/mL
	Not available	
famciclovir*	Famvir	Tablet: 125 mg, 250 mg, 500 mg
	Famvir	
foscarnet*	Generics	Solution, for injection: 24 mg/mL
	Not available	
ganciclovir*†	Cytovene, Vitrasert, Zirgan	Gel, ophthalmic (Zirgan): 0.15%†
		Powder, for injection: 500 mg/vial
	Cytovene	Invitreal implant (Vitrasert): 4.5 mg/implant†
penciclovir	Denavir	Cream: 1%
	Denavir	
trifluridine* (trifluorothymidine)	Viroptic	Ophthalmic solution: 1%
	Viroptic	
valacyclovir*	Valtrex	Tablet: 500 mg, 1 g
	Valtrex	
valganciclovir	Valcyte	Powder, for oral solution: 50 mg/mL
	Valcyte	Tablet: 450 mg

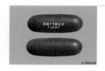

*Generic available.
*†Generic available in the United States only.
†Strength available in the United States only.
‡Strength available in Canada only.

treatment of CMV retinitis in those with AIDS. It is also indicated for the treatment of acyclovir-resistant HSV-1, HSV-2, and herpes labialis.

Ganciclovir is also used for the treatment of CMV. It is similar in structure to acyclovir. Ganciclovir is a competitive inhibitor of viral DNA polymerases that results in the inhibition of viral DNA synthesis.

Famciclovir is metabolized to penciclovir. It has a similar spectrum of activity to acyclovir and is also indicated for the treatment of HSV-1, HSV-2, and acute herpes zoster infections. It has a longer duration of action than acyclovir.

Penciclovir is an active metabolite of famciclovir. It is indicated for the treatment of herpes labialis, commonly known as a cold sore. It is administered topically.

Trifluridine is indicated for the treatment of keratoconjunctivitis of the eye caused by HSV-1 and HSV-2 (see Chapter 20).

TECH ALERT!
The following drugs have look-alike and sound-alike issues:
    Zovirax and Zostrix;
    Denavir and indinavir;
    Virotic and Timoptic

TECH ALERT!

The FDA requires a boxed warning for cidofovir regarding the risk for renal failure resulting in death. Renal function must be monitored 48 hours prior to administration of cidofovir infusion and dosage adjusted as appropriate.

ADVERSE REACTIONS

Adverse reactions that are common to acyclovir, famciclovir, ganciclovir, penciclovir, valacyclovir, and cidofovir are diarrhea, nausea, vomiting, headache, fatigue, dizziness, and confusion. Penciclovir may also cause irritation and discoloration of the skin. Cidofovir may produce neutropenia, hair loss, tinnitus, and hearing loss. Foscarnet has a side effect profile similar to that of cidofovir but can also cause arrhythmias, heart failure, and peripheral neuropathy.

Summary of Drugs Used for the Treatment of Influenza, Herpes, Hepatitis, Respiratory Syncytial Virus, and Cytomegalovirus Viral Infections

Generic Name	Brand Name	Usual Dose and Dosing Schedule	Warning Labels
Influenza A or B Treatment			
amantidine	Generics	Influenza A treatment and prophylaxis: 200 mg/day as one or two divided doses; begin 24-48 hr of onset of signs or symptoms and continue for 24-48 hr after symptoms resolve or for prophylaxis at least 10 days	MAY CAUSE DIZZINESS OR DROWSINESS. COMPLETE FULL COURSE OF THERAPY.
rimantadine	Flumadine	Influenza A treatment and prophylaxis: 100 mg bid; begin 24-48 hr of onset of signs or symptoms, continue for 5-7 days	
oseltamivir	Tamiflu	Influenza A or B treatment and prophylaxis: 75 mg bid for 5 days for acute infection, once daily for 10 days—prophylaxis	REFRIGERATE; SHAKE WELL; DISCARD AFTER 10 DAYS (OSELTAMIVIR SUSPENSION). COMPLETE FULL COURSE OF THERAPY.
zanamivir	Relenza	Influenza A treatment: Two doses to start; then two oral inhalations bid for 5 days; begin within 48 hr of onset of signs or symptoms Influenza A prophylaxis: Two oral inhalations daily for 10 or 28 days, as directed	INHALE USING DISKHALER DELIVERY DEVICE (ZANAMIVIR).
Herpes Infections			
acyclovir	Zovirax	Varies according to type of infection (HSV-1, HSV-2, VZV) and acute versus recurrent infection Dosage range: IV: 5-10 mg/kg every 8 hr for 5-10 days Oral: 200 mg five times/day or 400 mg tid for 5-10 days Topical: Apply every 3 hr for 7 days	SHAKE WELL (ACYCLOVIR SUSPENSION). COMPLETE FULL COURSE OF THERAPY; BEGIN THERAPY WITHIN 72 HR OF ONSET OF SYMPTOMS. SWALLOW WHOLE; DON'T CRUSH OR CHEW (GANCICLOVIR). AVOID PREGNANCY (GANCICLOVIR). TAKE WITH FOOD (GANCICLOVIR). WASH YOUR HANDS WITH SOAP AND WATER AFTER USING (PENCICLOVIR).
famciclovir	Famvir	Varies according to type of infection (HSV-1, HSV-2, VZV) and acute versus recurrent infection Dosage range: 125-500 mg bid or tid for 5-10 days or 1000-1500 mg bid for 1 day	
ganciclovir	Cytovene	Varies according to acute or recurrent CMV infection Dosage range: IV: 5 mg/kg IV every 12-24 hr for 7-21 days Oral: 1000 mg tid or 500 mg six times daily	
penciclovir	Denavir	Cold sores: Apply every 2 hr while awake for 4 days; start within 1 hr of symptom onset	
valacyclovir	Valtrex	Varies according to type of infection (HSV-1, HSV-2, VZV) and acute versus recurrent infection Dosage range: 500 mg-2 g bid or tid for 5-10 days	

Continued

Summary of Drugs Used for the Treatment of Influenza, Herpes, Hepatitis, Respiratory Syncytial Virus, and Cytomegalovirus Viral Infections—cont'd

Generic Name	Brand Name	Usual Dose and Dosing Schedule	Warning Labels
foscarnet	Foscavir	Varies according to type of infection (HSV-1, HSV-2, VZV, CMV) and acute versus recurrent infection Dosage range: 40-90 mg/kg IV every 8-12 hr for 2-3 wk	STORE AT ROOM TEMPERATURE; DISCARD DISCOLORED SOLUTION.
trifluridine	Viroptic	1 drop in affected eye(s) every 2 hr while awake (max, 9 drops/day)	REMOVE CONTACT LENSES BEFORE USE.
Hepatitis B or C Virus			
interferon alfa-2b	Intron A	**Hepatitis B:** 30-35 mIU weekly SC or IM for 16 wk **Hepatitis C:** 3 mIU SC or IM three times weekly for up to 18-24 mo	REFRIGERATE; DO NOT FREEZE.
interferon alfacon-1	Infergen	**Hepatitis C:** 9-15 mcg SC three times/wk for 24 wk; at least 48 hr should elapse between doses	
peginterferon alfa-2a	Pegasys	**Hepatitis B and hepatitis C:** 180 mcg SC once weekly for 48 weeks	
peginterferon alfa-2b	PEG-Intron	**Hepatitis C:** 1 mcg/kg once weekly for 1 yr	
Nucleoside Analogues			
entecavir	Baraclude	**Hepatitis B:** 0.5-1 mg once daily	TAKE ON AN EMPTY STOMACH.
lamivudine	Epivir HBV, Heptovir	**Hepatitis B:** HIV negative patients—100 mg once daily for up to 1 yr	TAKE WITH OR WITHOUT FOOD.
ribavirin	Copegus	**Hepatitis C monoinfection:** 600 mg bid with 3 mIU interferon alfa-2b SC or IM three times weekly for 24-48 wk or 600 mg morning and 800 mg evening with 1.5 mcg/kg SC peginterferon alfa-2b weekly for 48 weeks **Hepatitis C coinfections with HIV:** 800 mg PO daily plus 180 mcg SC weekly peginterferon alfa-2b for 48 wk	TAKE WITH FOOD—SOLID DOSAGE FORMS ONLY. DO NOT CRUSH OR CHEW CAPSULES.
telbivudine	Tyzeka, Sebivo	**Hepatitis B:** 600 mg once daily	TAKE WITH OR WITHOUT FOOD.
Nucleotide Analogues			
adefovir	Hepsera	**Hepatitis B:** 10 mg once daily	TAKE WITH OR WITHOUT FOOD.
Protease Inhibitor			
boceprevir	Victrelis	**Hepatitis C:** Following 4 wk of peginterferon alfa and ribavirin, add 800 mg boceprevir tid for 32 wk; then stop boceprevir, continue peginterferon alfa and ribavirin for an additional 12 wk	TAKE WITH FOOD.
telaprevir	Incivek	**Hepatitis C:** 750 mg tid along with peginterferon alfa and ribavirin for 12 wk, followed by therapy with peginterferon alfa and ribavirin only for an additional 12 wk	TAKE WITH FOOD (NOT LOW FAT).
Cytomegalovirus			
cidofovir	Vistide	**CMV retinitis:** 5 mg/kg IV once weekly for 2 wk with probenecid; prophylaxis 5 mg/kg IV once every other week	USE WITHIN 24 HR OF PREPARATION. REFRIGERATE OR STORE AT ROOM TEMPERATURE.
Respiratory Syncytial Virus			
ribavirin	Virazole	**RSV:** 20 mg/mL administered as continuous aerosol administration for 12-18 hr/day for 3 to 7 days	RECONSTITUTE WITH STERILE WATER FOR INJECTION. USE WITHIN 24 HR OF PREPARATION. STORE AT ROOM TEMPERATURE.

Human Immunodeficiency Virus and Acquired Immunodeficiency Syndrome

HIV-AIDS (*acquired immunodeficiency syndrome*) is a global public health issue. According to the Joint United Nations Programme on HIV/AIDS (UNAIDS) 2010 estimates, almost 34 million people were infected with HIV and 2.5 million were children. Millions more are affected by the disease. Women accounted for 52% of all adults living with HIV worldwide. HIV-AIDS is worsened by poverty. Poverty creates the following conditions: individuals knowingly engage in risky sexual behaviors such as the sex trade; it increases malnutrition, which can weaken the immune system; it decreases access to health care and HIV medicines, which can increase drug resistance; and many HIV medicines should be taken with food, and access to regular meals may be limited.

HIV is the virus that causes AIDS. The virus attacks **CD4 T lymphocytes** and weakens the immune system. As the **CD4 count** declines below 200 cells/mm^3 and the **viral load** increases, HIV-infected individuals are at increasing risk for developing opportunistic infections such as tuberculosis (TB), candidiasis, and CMV and other AIDS-defining conditions. The viral load is commonly believed to be the amount of HIV in the blood, but actually it is the amount of materials from the virus that are released into the bloodstream when the HIV reproduces.

HIV LIFE CYCLE

HIV, like other viruses, lacks the cellular machinery to reproduce itself. It incorporates its DNA into the DNA of the host cell; then, when the host cell tries to make new proteins, it accidentally makes new HIV as well. The steps in the HIV life cycle are briefly described here:

Step 1: Binding. The HIV binds to CD4 surface receptors.

Step 2: Fusion. The HIV is activated by proteins on the cell's surface, allowing the HIV envelope to fuse to the outside of the cell.

Step 3: Uncoating. The virus is uncoated, permitting the contents of the viral capsid (viral RNA and enzymes) to be released into the infected host cell.

Step 4: Reverse transcription. A viral enzyme called reverse transcriptase makes a DNA copy of the viral RNA.

Step 5: Integration. Viral DNA is incorporated into the host cellular DNA.

Step 6: Genome replication. The strands of viral DNA in the nucleus separate and mRNA provides instructions for making new virus (genome). This process is called transcription.

Step 7: Protein synthesis. The HIV mRNA genome acts as a template for synthesizing viral proteins needed to make a new virus in a process called translation.

Step 8: Protein cleavage and viral assembly. Protease is an enzyme that cuts the long chain of viral protein into smaller individual proteins. Some of the cleaved proteins become structural elements of new HIV and others become enzymes, such as reverse transcriptase. The new particles are assembled into new HIV.

Step 9: Virus release. New virus buds off from the host cell.

PHARMACOLOGICAL TREATMENT

Antiretrovirals are medicines that interfere with the replication of retroviruses. HIV is a retrovirus. Antiretrovirals are administered to reduce viral load, increase CD4 counts, delay the development of AIDS-related conditions and opportunistic infections, and improve survival. Antiretrovirals fall into six classes:

- Nucleoside/nucleotide reverse transcriptase inhibitors (NRTIs)
- Non-nucleoside reverse transcriptase inhibitors (NNRTIs)
- Protease inhibitors (PIs)
- Fusion inhibitors
- Chemokine receptor antagonist, type 5
- HIV integrase strand inhibitor

The initiation of drug therapy with antiretrovirals is in accordance with international guidelines. Therapy is initiated in adults when CD4 counts fall below 200 cells/mm^3 and symptoms are present. Antiretroviral therapy should be offered or considered for asymptomatic or mildly symptomatic HIV-infected adults when the CD4 count range is between 200 and 350 cells/mm^3. Antiretroviral therapy is generally not necessary if the individual is asymptomatic and the CD4 count exceeds 350 cells/mm^3. Different guidelines exist for children. Antiretroviral therapy is a lifelong commitment and requires strict adherence to treatment regimens.

To reduce antiviral resistance, ***highly active antiretroviral therapy*** (HAART)—a combination of three or more medications in a regimen also known as an AIDS cocktail—is prescribed. The medications administered for HAART therapy fall into two or more antiretroviral classes. Combination therapy increases adverse reactions, but ***adherence*** to antiviral therapy is essential to decrease the risk of developing resistance. Antiretroviral ***drug resistance testing*** is recommended prior to the initiation of therapy with antiretrovirals and prior to changing therapy.

Nucleoside and Nucleotide Reverse Transcriptase Inhibitors (NRTIs)

Many nucleoside and nucleotide reverse transcriptase inhibitors are prodrugs. They are activated by intracellular phosphorylation by host cell enzymes. They competitively inhibit reverse transcriptase, the enzyme that makes a DNA copy of the viral RNA.

ABACAVIR

Abacavir is an NRTI. It is an ingredient in the triple antiretroviral therapy that combines abacavir with zidovudine and lamivudine. It is also formulated with lamivudine as a dual combination therapy. It is linked to a fatal hypersensitivity reaction that necessitates discontinuation of the drug. Symptoms include fever and chills, muscle and joint pain, fatigue and feeling rundown, nausea and vomiting, skin rash, and shortness of breath.

DIDANOSINE

Didanosine (DDI) is an NRTI. It is metabolized to an active metabolite that has an intracellular half-life ($t_{1/2}$) of 25 to 40 hours; therefore, the drug can be dosed once daily. It is acid-labile, so it must be buffered to prevent inactivation by gastric acids. Didanosine is formulated for pediatric use as a powder for solution and as delayed-release capsules. Side effects such as pancreatitis and peripheral neuropathy limit the use of didanosine.

EMTRICITABINE

Emtricitabine (FTC) is an NRTI similar to lamivudine. ***Cross-resistance*** occurs between lamivudine and emtricitabine. Cross-resistance refers to the development of resistance to one drug in a particular class that results in resistance to the other drugs in that class. Emtricitabine is formulated as an oral capsule and oral solution. Refrigeration is recommended for the oral solution; however, the solution is stable at room temperature for 3 months if refrigeration is not available.

LAMIVUDINE

Lamivudine (3TC) is an NRTI that is effective against HIV, including zidovudine-resistant strains of HIV. Lamivudine also inhibits replication of HBV. It is a good choice of therapy for those who have HIV and HBV coinfections. Lamivudine is an ingredient in HIV combination therapies. (All antiretrovirals should be used in combination.) The drug has good oral absorption, and the relatively long intracellular $t_{1/2}$ (12 hours) permits once-daily dosing.

STAVUDINE

Stavudine (d4T) is an NRTI. It is similar to zidovudine; however, a drug interaction occurs between stavudine and zidovudine that reduces the effectiveness of stavudine because zidovudine inhibits the activation of stavudine. Stavudine has a short $t_{1/2}$ and must be administered more frequently than some of the other NRTIs. It is formulated for oral administration and food does not interfere with absorption.

TENOFOVIR

Tenofovir (TDF) is an NRTI. It is administered orally. Food increases bioavailability of the drug. It has a long intracellular $t_{1/2}$, up to 50 hours.

TABLE 36-1 **World Health Organization Perinatal Mother-to-Child Transmission Guidelines (2012)**

Option	Treatment for CD4 count ≤350 cells/mm³	Prophylaxis for CD4 count >350 cells/mm³
A	**Mother:** Triple antiviral therapy beginning at diagnosis and continued for life	**Mother (during pregnancy):** zidovudine (AZT) starting as early as 14 weeks' gestation **Mother (during delivery):** single dose nevirapine (sdNVP) and 1st dose AZT + 3TC **Mother (postpartum):** Daily AZT + 3TC until 7 days postpartum
	Infant: Daily nevirapine (NVP) continuous from birth through 4-6 weeks (if infant is not breast-feeding) *or* **Infant:** Daily NVP continuous until 1 week after end of breast-feeding period (if infant is breast-feeding)	
B	**Mother:** Triple antiviral therapy beginning at diagnosis and continued for life	**Mother:** Three-drug regimen of ARVs beginning as early as 14 weeks' gestation, and continued during pregnancy, delivery, and 1 week after ending breast-feeding.
	Infant: Daily AZT or NVP antiretroviral drug regimen for 4-6 weeks after birth, whether or not infant is breast-feeding	
B+	**Mother:** Triple antiviral therapy (regardless CD4 count) beginning at diagnosis and continued for life	
	Infant: Daily AZT or NVP antiretroviral drug regimen for 4-6 weeks after birth, whether or not infant is breast-feeding	

First-line triple-antiretroviral regimen for pregnant women:
AZT + 3TC + NVP
or
AZT + 3TC + EFV
or
TDF + 3TC (or FTC) + NVP *or* TDF + 3TC (or FTC) + EFV

3TC, Lamivudine; FTC, emtricitabine; NVP, nevirapine; TDF, tenofovir; EFV, efavirenz.
Adapted from World Health Organization: WHO HIV & AIDS guidelines for PMTCT & breastfeeding 2010 (http://www.avert.org/pmtct-guidelines.htm) and WHO PMTCT update 2012 (www.who.int/hiv/PMTCT_update.pdf).

ZIDOVUDINE

Zidovudine (AZT) was the first available antiretroviral. It was introduced in 1987. It is an NRTI. It is formulated for oral and parenteral administration. The drug may be administered orally to pregnant women and intravenously during delivery and as a suspension to neonates. It has been shown to decrease perinatal *mother-to-child transmission* (PMTCT) of HIV from 25% to 8%. PMTCT regimens should begin at 14 weeks of pregnancy or as soon as possible thereafter. PMTCT 2012 guidelines are shown in Table 36-1.

ADVERSE REACTIONS

Possible side effects from NRTI therapy are liver problems, muscle inflammation and weakness, diabetes, abnormal fat distribution (lipodystrophy syndrome), high cholesterol, decreased bone density caused by osteonecrosis and osteopenia, skin rash, pancreatitis (inflammation of the pancreas), peripheral neuropathy (especially with DDI and d4T), leukopenia (a drop in white blood cell count), and increased bleeding in patients with hemophilia. Side effects associated with almost all NRTIs are headache, stomach upset, fatigue or insomnia, muscle ache, and diarrhea. Additionally, zidovudine may cause nail discoloration.

Non-Nucleoside Reverse Transcriptase Inhibitors (NNRTIs)

NNRTIs bind to viral transcriptase. They differ from NRTIs in three important ways:
1. NNRTIs are noncompetitive inhibitors of reverse transcriptase.
2. They do not need to be activated by host enzymes.
3. They are not effective against HIV-2.

With the exception of nevirapine, NNRTIs are only used in combination therapy with NRTIs and PIs because resistance develops rapidly. All NNRTIs are metabolized by cytochrome P-450 (CYP450) hepatic enzymes and reduce their own $t_{1/2}$ as well as the $t_{1/2}$ of other drugs coadministered with them that are metabolized by the same enzymes. Numerous drug interactions are seen when NNRTIs are administered concurrently with benzodiazepines, HMG-CoA inhibitors (-*statins*), and proton pump inhibitors (-*prazoles*).

DELAVIRDINE

Delavirdine has a short half-life and must be given in multiple daily doses. It is administered three times daily compared with nevirapine and efavirenz, which are dosed once daily. Cross-resistance, frequency of dosing, and the number of tablets per dose (four tablets) have limited the use of delavirdine.

EFAVIRENZ

Efavirenz is an ingredient in the fixed-dose combination medicine Atripla used for the treatment of HIV-1 infection. It is also available as a single-ingredient product; however, monotherapy is not recommended because of the rapid development of resistance. The drug is administered by mouth and, because of its long $t_{1/2}$ (40 to 55 hours), may be given once daily.

Efavirenz is teratogenic and classified in pregnancy category D. The drug should not be administered in the first trimester of pregnancy and women taking the drug should be advised to avoid pregnancy.

NEVIRAPINE

Nevirapine is the one NNRTI that may be administered as monotherapy for the PMTCT of HIV. It is administered as a single dose. Controversy exists about the use of single-dose nevirapine therapy because of the risk of development of drug resistance. Treatment of mothers with triple antiretroviral therapy reduces the risk of antiretroviral resistance.

Nevirapine is associated with fatal liver toxicity and the FDA has required changes in the package labeling to warn of this adverse effect. Risk for the development of liver toxicity with the use of single doses of nevirapine to the mother and child for the prevention of perinatal HIV infection is minimal.

ADVERSE REACTIONS

Rash is a common side effect of all NNRTIs. Nevirapine is associated with fatal hepatotoxicity. The risk is greatest in the first 6 to 18 weeks of therapy and is more common in women than in men. Efavirenz may cause dizziness, drowsiness or insomnia, abnormal dreams, confusion, abnormal thinking, impaired concentration, amnesia, agitation, hallucinations, depersonalization, and euphoria.

Protease Inhibitors

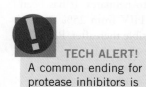

TECH ALERT!
A common ending for protease inhibitors is *-navir*.

PIs interfere with step 8 of the HIV life cycle (see earlier). They block cleavage of long-chain viral proteins into individual proteins that are assembled to make new virus. PIs are administered as combination therapy; most are recommended to be given along with ritonavir.

FOSAMPRENAVIR

Fosamprenavir is indicated for the treatment of HIV-1 infection. Fosamprenavir is a prodrug that is metabolized to the active drug amprenavir. The effect of fosamprenavir is boosted with the coadministration of ritonavir.

ATAZANAVIR

Atazanavir is another PI that is effective against HIV-1. Its effectiveness is increased when the drug is coadministered with ritonavir. Concurrent administration with the NNRTI efavirenz can decrease its bioavailability. Atazanavir may be given orally once daily. Administration with a light meal increases bioavailability compared with a heavy meal or fasting. Atazanavir does not produce hyperlipidemia like other proteases, although it can increase cholesterol levels and blood glucose levels. The drug may produce jaundice but does not cause liver toxicity.

DARUNAVIR

Darunavir was approved by the FDA in 2006. It has advantages over other PIs in that cross-resistance is low and it produces a greater reduction in viral load after 24 weeks of treatment. Like other PIs, it must be administered along with ritonavir.

INDINAVIR

Indinavir must be administered in three daily doses. Absorption is affected by food so the drug is taken on an empty stomach. To avoid the formation of kidney stones, indinavir should be taken with at least 1.5 liters of water daily. The effects of indinavir are boosted by the coadministration of ritonavir.

NELFINAVIR

Nelfinavir is a competitive inhibitor of HIV protease. Current CDC recommendations advise that nelfinavir be administered as part of a three-drug regimen that usually also includes indinavir, efavirenz, and/or abacavir. Unlike indinavir and atazanavir, absorption of nelfinavir is enhanced by a fatty meal. Nelfinavir should be taken with food. Nelfinavir oral powder is stable for 6 hours, once mixed with food or liquid, if refrigerated.

RITONAVIR

Ritonavir is a competitive inhibitor of HIV protease. It differs from other PIs in that it is effective against HIV-1 and HIV-2 proteases. Ritonavir boost the effects of other PIs by inhibiting their metabolism. Ritonavir inhibits the metabolic enzyme CYP3A4. Most PIs must be coadministered with ritonavir. Ritonavir is also formulated as a fixed-dose combination with lopinavir (Kaletra). Resistance to ritonavir appears to occur more slowly than with other PIs. The drug has excellent oral bioavailability and is given twice daily. A disadvantage is that adverse effects are common and occur in more than 85% of those taking the drug.

SAQUINAVIR

Saquinavir is formulated as a hard gelatin capsule and a film-coated tablet. Bioavailability following oral administration is low for both formulations. Extensive first-pass metabolism further reduces the actions of the drug. Similar to other PIs, saquinavir's effects are boosted by coadministration with ritonavir. Saquinavir should be taken with food.

TIPRANAVIR

Tipranavir is a sulfonamide that selectively binds to HIV-1 protease. It was approved in 2005 and currently has a lower rate for the development of resistance than some other PIs. The drug should be taken with food to increase absorption.

The FDA has required the manufacturer of tipranavir to provide a boxed warning in the package labeling regarding reports of fatal and nonfatal intracranial hemorrhage. Like other PIs, tipranavir is not used for monotherapy but is administered with other antiretrovirals.

ADVERSE REACTIONS

PIs can elevate triglyceride, cholesterol (see Chapter 24), and blood glucose levels and produce insulin resistance (see Chapter 33). They also cause the redistribution of fat, causing its accumulation in the abdomen and loss in the face and limbs. All PIs produce nausea, vomiting, and diarrhea.

Fusion Inhibitors

Fusion inhibitors are some of the latest medicines in the arsenal of antiretrovirals to treat HIV infection. Enfuvirtide is currently the only drug in this class. It interferes with step 2 in the HIV life cycle, attachment of the HIV to the host cell membrane. Fusion is required for the virus capsid to release its contents (genetic material) into the host cell. As with other HIV medicines, enfuvirtide is intended to be administered in combination with other antiretrovirals.

Enfuvirtide must be administered by SC injection in the thigh, arm, or abdomen. It is formulated as a powder that is reconstituted prior to administration. Once reconstituted, the solution is stable for only 24 hours if refrigerated.

ADVERSE REACTIONS

Irritation, pain, redness, itchiness, and the formation of nodules and cysts at the site of injection are common adverse reactions. Allergic reactions also occur and produce rash, chills, fever, stiffness, hypotension, nausea, and vomiting.

Chemokine Receptor Type 5 Antagonist

Maraviroc is a human chemokine receptor antagonist, type 5 (CCR5). It is the only agent in this class and is a novel drug for the treatment of HIV. It inhibits HIV entry into host cells.

MECHANISM OF ACTION

Maraviroc is a selective CCR5 antagonist of the G protein–coupled receptor found on the cell surface. It is associated with entry of the HIV virus into human host cells. Maraviroc binding to the CCR5 receptor prevents CCR5-tropic HIV-1 entry into cells. It does not prevent cell entry mediated by CXCR4 receptor binding of dual or mixed receptor binding.

ADVERSE EFFECTS

The most common side effects of maraviroc are colds, cough, fever, rash, and dizziness. Myocardial infarction, hepatotoxicity, and increased infections or cancers have also been reported.

HIV Integrase Strand Inhibitors

Raltegravir is an HIV integrase strand inhibitor and is another novel approach to combating HIV infection. In January 2011, phase III clinical trials for a second HIV integrase inhibitor, elvitegravir, were extended. HIV resistance to raltegravir can develop quickly so it is indicated only in combination with other antiretroviral agents.

MECHANISM OF ACTION

HIV integrase strand inhibitors block the final step in the process of human host cell infection by HIV. The HIV-1 integrase viral enzyme binds to the double-stranded viral DNA and mediates its integration into the infected host cell's DNA to produce a functional provirus.

ADVERSE EFFECTS

Raltegravir side effects include headache, dizziness, diarrhea, and gastrointestinal (GI) upset. Rhabdomyolysis, depression, suicide ideation, thrombocytopenia, and increased cancers have also been reported.

Drugs Used for the Treatment of HIV and AIDS

Generic Name	U.S. Brand Name(s) Canadian Brand Name(s)	Dosage Forms and Strengths
Nucleoside Reverse Transcriptase Inhibitors		
abacavir (ABC)	Ziagen	Tablet: 300 mg
	Ziagen	Solution: 20 mg/mL
didanosine* (DDI)	Videx, Videx EC	Powder, for pediatric solution: 10 mg/mL[†]
	Videx EC	Tablet, delayed-release (Videx EC): 125 mg, 200 mg, 250 mg, 400 mg
emtricitabine (FTC)	Emtriva	Capsule: 200 mg
	Emtriva	Solution: 10 mg/mL[†]
lamivudine* (3TC)	Epivir	Solution: 10 mg/mL
	Epivir	Tablet: 150 mg, 300 mg
stavudine* (d4T)	Zerit	Capsule, immediate-release: 15 mg, 20 mg, 30 mg, 40 mg
	Zerit	Powder, for oral solution: 1 mg/mL[†]

Drugs Used for the Treatment of HIV and AIDS—cont'd

Generic Name	U.S. Brand Name(s) / Canadian Brand Name(s)	Dosage Forms and Strengths
tenofovir DF (TDF)	Viread / Viread	Powder, for oral suspension: 40 mg/scoopful Tablet: 150 mg[†], 200 mg[†], 250 mg[†], 300 mg
zidovudine* (AZT)	Retrovir / Retrovir	Capsule: 100 mg Solution, injection: 10 mg/mL Syrup: 50 mg/5 mL Tablet: 300 mg[†]
Fixed-Dose Combinations		
abacavir + lamivudine	Epzicom / Kivexa	Tablet: 600 mg abacavir + 300 mg lamivudine
emtricitabine + tenofovir	Truvada / Truvada	Tablet: 200 mg emtricitabine + 300 mg tenofovir
lamivudine + zidovudine*	Combivir / Combivir	Tablet: 150 mg lamivudine + 300 mg zidovudine
efavirenz + emtricitabine + tenofovir	Atripla / Atripla	Tablet: 600 mg efavirenz + 200 mg emtricitabine + 300 mg tenofovir
abacavir + lamivudine + zidovudine	Trizivir / Trizivir	Tablet: 300 mg abacavir + 150 mg lamivudine + 300 mg zidovudine
emtricitabine + rilpivirine + tenofovir	Complera / Complera	Tablet: 200 mg emtricitabine + 25 mg rilpivirine + 300 mg tenofovir
Non-Nucleoside Reverse Transcriptase Inhibitors		
delavirdine (DLV)	Rescriptor / Rescriptor	Tablet: 100 mg, 200 mg[†]
efavirenz (EFV)	Sustiva / Sustiva	Capsule: 50 mg, 200 mg Tablet: 600 mg
etravirine	Intelence / Intelence	Tablet: 25 mg[†], 100 mg, 200 mg
nevirapine*	Viramune, Viramune XR / Viramune	Suspension: 50 mg/5 mL[†] Tablet: 200 mg Tablet, extended-release (Viramune XR): 400 mg
rilpivirine	Edurant / Edurant	Tablet: 25 mg
Protease Inhibitors		
atazanavir (ATV)	Reyataz / Reyataz	Capsule: 100 mg[†], 150 mg, 200 mg, 300 mg
darunavir (TMC114)	Prezista / Prezista	Suspension: 100 mg/mL[†] Tablet: 75 mg, 150 mg, 400 mg, 600 mg
fosamprenavir (FPV)	Lexiva / Telzir	Suspension: 50 mg/5 mL Tablet: 700 mg
indinavir (IDV)	Crixivan / Crixivan	Capsule: 100 mg[†], 200 mg, 400 mg
nelfinavir (NFV)	Viracept / Viracept	Powder for oral suspension: 50 mg/scoopful Tablet: 250 mg, 625 mg

Continued

Drugs Used for the Treatment of HIV and AIDS—cont'd

Generic Name	U.S. Brand Name(s) / Canadian Brand Name(s)	Dosage Forms and Strengths
ritonavir (RTV)	Norvir / Norvir, Norvir Sec	Capsule: 100 mg Solution, Oral: 80 mg/mL Tablet: 100 mg
saquinavir mesylate (SQV)	Invirase / Invirase	Capsule: 200 mg Tablet: 500 mg
tipranavir	Aptivus / Aptivus	Capsule: 250 mg Solution, oral: 100 mg/mL†
Combination		
lopinavir + ritonavir	Keletra / Keletra	Solution, oral: 80 mg/mL lopinavir + 20 mg/mL ritonavir Tablet: 100 mg lopinavir + 25 mg ritonavir; 200 mg lopinavir + 50 mg ritonavir
Fusion Inhibitors		
enfuvirtide (T-20)	Fuzeon / Fuzeon	Powder, for solution: 90 mg/vial†, 108 mg/vial‡
CCR5 Antagonist		
maraviroc	Selzentry / Celsentri	Tablet: 150 mg, 300 mg
HIV Integrase Strand Inhibitors		
raltegravir	Isentress / Isentress	Tablet, chewable: 25 mg†, 100 mg† Tablet: 400 mg

*Generic available.
†Strength available in the United States only.
‡Strength available in Canada only.

Summary of Drugs Used for the Treatment of HIV-AIDS

Generic Name	Brand Name	Usual Dose and Dosing Schedule	Warning Labels
Nucleoside Reverse Transcriptase Inhibitors			
abacavir	Ziagen	300 mg bid or 600 mg once daily	TAKE EXACTLY AS DIRECTED; DON'T SKIP DOSES. AVOID ALCOHOL. PROTECT FROM MOISTURE.
didanosine	Videx	Varies according to body weight and dosage form **Extended-release capsule:** 400 mg once daily (>60 kg) **Oral solution:** 250 mg bid (>60 kg)	SWALLOW WHOLE; DON'T CRUSH OR CHEW (EXTENDED-RELEASE). TAKE ON AN EMPTY STOMACH. REFRIGERATE; DISCARD 30 DAYS AFTER RECONSTITUTION (ORAL SOLUTION). TAKE EXACTLY AS DIRECTED; DON'T SKIP DOSES.
emtricitabine	Emtriva	Varies according to body weight and dosage form **Capsule:** 200 mg once daily (>33 kg) **Oral solution:** 6 mg/kg up to 240 mg once daily	TAKE EXACTLY AS DIRECTED; DON'T SKIP DOSES. REFRIGERATE; DO NOT FREEZE (SOLUTION).

Summary of Drugs Used for the Treatment of HIV-AIDS—cont'd

Generic Name	Brand Name	Usual Dose and Dosing Schedule	Warning Labels
lamivudine	Epivir	300 mg once daily or 150 mg bid	TAKE EXACTLY AS DIRECTED; DON'T SKIP DOSES. AVOID EXCESSIVE ALCOHOL.
stavudine	Zerit	Varies according to body weight and dosage form **Capsule, extended-release:** 100 mg once daily (>60 kg) or 75 mg once daily (<60 kg) **Oral solution or capsule:** 40 mg every 12 hr (>60 kg) or 30 mg every 12 hr (<60 kg)	TAKE EXACTLY AS DIRECTED; DON'T SKIP DOSES. PROTECT FROM MOISTURE (CAPSULES). REFRIGERATE; DISCARD 30 DAYS AFTER RECONSTITUTION.
tenofovir DF	Viread	300 mg once daily	TAKE EXACTLY AS DIRECTED; DON'T SKIP DOSES. TAKE WITH FOOD.
zidovudine	Retrovir	**Oral:** 300 mg PO bid or 200 mg PO tid **IV:** 1 mg/kg IV given five or six times daily, around the clock	TAKE EXACTLY AS DIRECTED; DON'T SKIP DOSES. TAKE WITH LOTS OF WATER. REFRIGERATE DILUTED IV SOLUTION; DISCARD AFTER 48 HR (STABLE FOR 24 HR AT ROOM TEMPERATURE).
lamivudine + zidovudine	Combivir	1 tablet bid	TAKE EXACTLY AS DIRECTED; DON'T SKIP DOSES. AVOID EXCESSIVE ALCOHOL.
abacavir + lamivudine	Epzicom	1 tablet once daily	TAKE EXACTLY AS DIRECTED; DON'T SKIP DOSES.
emtricitabine + tenofovir	Truvada	1 tablet once daily	
efavirenz + emtricitabine + tenofovir	Atripla	1 tablet daily at bedtime	TAKE EXACTLY AS DIRECTED; DON'T SKIP DOSES. TAKE ON AN EMPTY STOMACH.
abacavir + lamivudine + zidovudine	Trizivir	1 tablet bid	TAKE EXACTLY AS DIRECTED; DON'T SKIP DOSES.
Non-Nucleoside Reverse Transcriptase Inhibitors			
delavirdine	Rescriptor	400 mg tid	TAKE EXACTLY AS DIRECTED; DON'T SKIP DOSES. AVOID ANTACIDS WITHIN 1 HR OF DOSE.
efavirenz	Sustiva	600 mg once daily at bedtime	TAKE EXACTLY AS DIRECTED; DON'T SKIP DOSES. TAKE ON AN EMPTY STOMACH. MAY CAUSE DIZZINESS OR DROWSINESS; ALCOHOL INTENSIFIES THIS EFFECT. AVOID PREGNANCY.
nevirapine	Viramune	200 mg once daily for the first 14 days, then 200 mg bid	TAKE EXACTLY AS DIRECTED; DON'T SKIP DOSES. SHAKE GENTLY (SUSPENSION).

Continued

Summary of Drugs Used for the Treatment of HIV-AIDS—cont'd

Generic Name	Brand Name	Usual Dose and Dosing Schedule	Warning Labels
Protease Inhibitors			
atazanavir	Reyataz	300 mg once daily (taken with ritonavir)	TAKE EXACTLY AS DIRECTED; DON'T SKIP DOSES. TAKE WITH LIGHT MEAL. AVOID ANTACIDS WITHIN 1 HR OF DOSE. SWALLOW WHOLE; DON'T CRUSH OR CHEW.
darunavir	Prezista	600 mg bid (taken with ritonavir)	TAKE EXACTLY AS DIRECTED; DON'T SKIP DOSES. TAKE WITH FOOD.
fosamprenavir	Lexiva, Telzir	700 mg bid (taken with ritonavir)	TAKE EXACTLY AS DIRECTED; DON'T SKIP DOSES. TAKE WITH FOOD (ORAL SUSPENSION, CHILDREN). TAKE WITHOUT FOOD (ORAL SUSPENSION, ADULTS).
indinavir	Crixivan	800 mg every 8 hr or 400 mg bid with ritonavir	TAKE EXACTLY AS DIRECTED; DON'T SKIP DOSES. TAKE ON AN EMPTY STOMACH. MAINTAIN ADEQUATE HYDRATION. PROTECT FROM MOISTURE.
nelfinavir	Viracept	1250 mg bid or 750 mg tid	TAKE EXACTLY AS DIRECTED; DON'T SKIP DOSES. TAKE WITH FOOD. MIX ORAL POWDER WITH SMALL AMOUNT OF FOOD OR NONACIDIC LIQUID. CONSUME ENTIRE DOSE; MIXTURE STABLE FOR 6 HR IF REFRIGERATED.
ritonavir	Norvir	600 mg bid	TAKE EXACTLY AS DIRECTED; DON'T SKIP DOSES. TAKE WITH FOOD. REFRIGERATE, DON'T FREEZE; CAPSULE STABLE FOR 30 DAYS AT ROOM TEMPERATURE. SHAKE WELL (SUSPENSION). STORE AT ROOM TEMPERATURE (SUSPENSION). DISPENSE IN MANUFACTURER'S ORIGINAL CONTAINER.
saquinavir	Invirase	1000 mg bid (taken with ritonavir)	TAKE EXACTLY AS DIRECTED; DON'T SKIP DOSES. TAKE WITH FOOD.
tipranavir	Aptivus	500 mg bid (taken with ritonavir)	TAKE EXACTLY AS DIRECTED; DON'T SKIP DOSES. TAKE WITH FOOD. REFRIGERATE, DON'T FREEZE; CAPSULE STABLE FOR 60 DAYS AT ROOM TEMPERATURE.
lopinavir + ritonavir	Keletra	3 capsules, 5 mL, or 2 tablets bid (400 mg lopinavir + 100 mg ritonavir) *or* 6 capsules, 10 mL, or 4 tablets once daily (800 mg lopinavir + 200 mg ritonavir)	TAKE EXACTLY AS DIRECTED; DON'T SKIP DOSES. SWALLOW WHOLE; DON'T CRUSH OR CHEW (TABLETS). TAKE WITH FOOD. REFRIGERATE, DON'T FREEZE; SOLUTION STABLE FOR 60 DAYS AT ROOM TEMPERATURE. DISPENSE TABLETS IN MANUFACTURER'S ORIGINAL CONTAINER.

Summary of Drugs Used for the Treatment of HIV-AIDS—cont'd

Generic Name	Brand Name	Usual Dose and Dosing Schedule	Warning Labels
Fusion Inhibitor			
enfuvirtide	Fuzeon	90 mg subcut bid	TAKE EXACTLY AS DIRECTED; DON'T SKIP DOSES. REFRIGERATE DILUTED SOLUTION, DON'T FREEZE; DISCARD AFTER 24 HR.
CCR5 Antagonist			
maraviroc	Selzentry, Celsentri	150 mg bid	MAY CAUSE DIZZINESS OR DROWSINESS. TAKE WITH OR WITHOUT FOOD.
HIV Integrase Strand Inhibitor			
raltegravir	Isentress	400 mg bid	TAKE WITH OR WITHOUT FOOD. SWALLOW WHOLE; DON'T CRUSH OR CHEW.

Chapter Summary

- A virus is an intracellular parasite that consists of a DNA or RNA core surrounded by a protein coat and sometimes an outer covering of lipoprotein.
- The infectious particles (virions) do not have the cellular components necessary for reproduction, so they use their host's cellular machinery to replicate.
- Viruses may cause minor illness such as the common cold and warts or serious infections such as human immunodeficiency virus (HIV) infection, smallpox, and hepatitis C.
- Some viruses are linked to cancer; for example, human papillomavirus (HPV) is associated with cervical cancer.
- An antiviral is a medication that is able to inhibit viral replication.
- All antiviral agents work best when the host (the individual with the infection) has a healthy immune system.
- Effective treatment of viral infections is dependent on host, viral, and drug factors.
- The severity of influenza, herpes, and varicella viral infection and severity of symptoms are reduced when antiviral therapy is initiated within the first 24 to 72 hours of exposure to the virus or onset of symptoms.
- Some viruses can lay dormant in host cells and periodically awaken to cause recurrent disease.
- Antivirals are only effective against a specific virus.
- Antibiotics are not effective against viral infections.
- Antiviral resistance is the ability of a virus to overcome the suppressive action of antiviral agents.
- Because viruses continually mutate, it is difficult to develop a vaccine to prevent virus infection.
- Antivirals inhibit virus-specific steps in the replication cycle.
- A common ending for antivirals that inhibit viral uncoating and are administered to prevent influenza A infection is -*mantidine*. Amantidine and rimantadine inhibit viral uncoating.
- Uncoating of the influenza A virus is a necessary step in the virus replication process.
- Oseltamivir and zanamivir are indicated for the treatment of influenza A and influenza B. They are neuraminidase inhibitors.
- Neuraminidase inhibitors inhibit viral release.
- Zanamivir (Relenza) is formulated as a powder for oral inhalation.
- Interferons protect uninfected cells by promoting a resistance to virus infection.
- Interferon alfacon-1 and peginterferon alfa-2b are indicated for the treatment of hepatitis C virus.
- Interferon alfa-2b and peginterferon alfa-2a may be used for the treatment of hepatitis B and hepatitis C.
- A common ending for antivirals used for the treatment of herpes virus infections is -*cyclovir* and -*ciclovir*.

- Acyclovir, famciclovir, and valacyclovir are used for the treatment of herpes simplex virus (HSV-1), the virus that causes cold sores, herpes genitalis (HSV-2), one of the viruses that cause genital warts, and varicella zoster virus (VZV), the virus that causes chickenpox and shingles.
- Cidofovir is indicated for the treatment of cytomegalovirus (CMV) retinitis in individuals with AIDS.
- Foscarnet is indicated for the treatment of CMV retinitis in individuals with AIDS. It is also indicated for the treatment of acyclovir-resistant HSV-1, HSV-2, and herpes labialis infections.
- Ganciclovir is indicated for the treatment of CMV.
- Penciclovir is a metabolite of famciclovir used for the treatment of cold sores.
- Trifluridine is indicated for the treatment of keratoconjunctivitis of the eye caused by herpes virus.
- Ribavirin is indicated for the treatment of respiratory syncytial virus and hepatitis C when combined with interferon alfa.
- HIV-AIDS is a global public health issue. According to 2010 estimates, almost 34 million people are infected with the HIV.
- HIV is the virus that causes AIDS. The virus attacks CD4 T lymphocytes and weakens the immune system.
- The steps in the HIV life cycle are (1) binding, (2) fusion, (3) uncoating, (4) reverse transcription, (5) integration, (6) genome replication, (7) protein synthesis, (8) protein cleavage and assembly, and (9) virus release.
- Antiretrovirals are medicines that interfere with the replication of retroviruses. HIV is a retrovirus.
- Antiretrovirals fall into six classes: (1) nucleoside and nucleotide reverse transcriptase inhibitors (NRTIs); (2) non-nucleoside reverse transcriptase inhibitors (NNRTIs); (3) protease inhibitors (PIs); (4) fusion inhibitors; (5) chemokine receptor antagonists, type 5 (CCR5); and (6) HIV integrase strand inhibitors.
- To reduce antiviral resistance, highly active antiretroviral therapy (HAART), a combination of three or more medications in a regimen known as an AIDS cocktail, is prescribed.
- Many nucleoside and nucleotide reverse transcriptase inhibitors (NRTIs) are prodrugs.
- NRTIs competitively inhibit reverse transcriptase, the enzyme that makes a DNA copy of the viral RNA.
- Abacavir, didanosine, emtricitabine, lamivudine, stavudine, tenofovir, and zidovudine are NRTIs.
- Zidovudine may be administered to pregnant women and neonates and is used to prevent mother-to-child transmission (PMTCT) of HIV.
- NNRTIs differ from NRTIs in three important ways: (1) NNRTIs are noncompetitive inhibitors of reverse transcriptase; (2) they do not need to be activated by host enzymes; and (3) they are not effective against HIV-2.
- With the exception of nevirapine, NNRTIs are only used in combination therapy with NRTIs and protease inhibitors because resistance develops rapidly.
- Delavirdine, efavirenz, and nevirapine are NNRTIs.
- Nevirapine is administered as a single dose for the PMTCT of HIV. Controversy exists about the use of single-dose nevirapine therapy because of the risk of development of drug resistance.
- Nevirapine is associated with fatal liver toxicity; the FDA has required changes in the package labeling to warn of this adverse effect.
- A common ending for protease inhibitors is *-navir*.
- PIs interfere with step 8 of the HIV life cycle. They block the cleavage of long-chain viral proteins into individual proteins that are assembled to make new virus.
- PIs are administered as combination therapy.
- Fosamprenavir, atazanavir, darunavir, indinavir, nelfinavir, ritonavir, saquinavir, and tipranavir are PIs.
- Ritonavir is effective against HIV-1 and HIV-2 proteases.
- Tipranavir is a sulfonamide that selectively binds to HIV-1 protease.
- The FDA has required the manufacturer of tipranavir to provide a boxed warning in the package labeling regarding reports of fatal and nonfatal intracranial hemorrhage.

- Efuvirtide is a fusion inhibitor and interferes with step 2 in the HIV life cycle, attachment of HIV to the host cell membrane.
- CCR5 antagonists inhibits HIV entry into host cells. Maraviroc is the only drug in this class.
- HIV integrase strand inhibitors block the final step in the process of human host cell infection by HIV.

REVIEW QUESTIONS

1. _____ is the most severe form of HIV infection.
   a. CMV
   b. AIDS
   c. HPV
   d. HSV

2. The individual who infects another with a virus is a host.
   a. True
   b. False

3. An antiviral is a medication that is able to _____ viral replication.
   a. Stimulate
   b. Inhibit
   c. Proliferate
   d. Induce

4. Interferons are not technically antiviral agents.
   a. True
   b. False

5. Which of the following is (are) indicated for the treatment of cytomegalovirus?
   a. Acyclovir
   b. Ganciclovir
   c. Cidofovir
   d. b and c

6. Human immunodeficiency virus (HIV) is the virus that causes acquired immunodeficiency syndrome (AIDS). The virus attacks _____ and weakens the immune system.
   a. CD4 monocytes
   b. CD4 T lymphocytes
   c. CD2 T lymphocytes
   d. None of the above

7. Antiretroviral therapy for HIV-AIDS is a short-term commitment and requires strict adherence to treatment regimens.
   a. True
   b. False

8. Lamivudine is an NRTI that is effective against _____.
   a. HIV
   b. HBV
   c. CMV
   d. a and b

9. Which of the following drugs does the FDA require the manufacturer to provide a black box warning in the package labeling regarding reports of fatal and nonfatal intracranial hemorrhage?
   a. Acyclovir
   b. Famciclovir
   c. Tipranavir
   d. Foscarnet

10. Enfuvirtide is currently the only drug in class of fusion inhibitors to treat HIV infection.
   a. True
   b. False

TECHNICIAN'S
CORNER

1. We have yet to find a cure for the common cold. Why is it to difficult to find that cure?
2. We have publicized and provided education worldwide about preventing the spread of AIDS, yet more cases are seen every year. What else can be done to stop the spread of this deadly disease?

Bibliography

Canadian AIDS Treatment Information Exchange: HIV viral load testing, 2007 http://www.catie.ca/sites/default/files/Viral%20Load.pdf.

Centers for Disease Control and Prevention. (2011) Morbidity and Mortality Weekly Report. In R. Moolenaar (Series Ed.): Vol. 60. *Antiviral Agents for the Treatment and Chemoprophylaxis of Influenza.*

Dorr P, Westby M, Dobbs S, et al: Maraviroc (UK-427,857), a potent, orally bioavailable, and selective small-molecule inhibitor of chemokine receptor CCR5 with broad-spectrum anti-human immunodeficiency virus type 1 activity, *Antimicrob Agents Chemother* 49:4721-4732, 2005.

Elsevier: *Gold Standard Clinical Pharmacology. Overview: Anti-retroviral non-nucleoside reverse transcriptase inhibitors (NNRTIs)*, Retrieved December 6, 2011, from https://www.clinicalpharmacology.com/, 2010.

FDA: FDA Approved Drug Products. Retrieved June 25, 2012, from http://www.accessdata.fda.gov/scripts/cder/drugsatfda/index.cfm?fuseaction=Search.Search_Drug_Name, 2012.

Fiore AE, Fry A, Shay D, et al: Centers for Disease Control and Prevention (CDC): Antiviral agents for the treatment and chemoprophylaxis of influenza—recommendations of the Advisory Committee on Immunization Practices (ACIP), *MMWR Recomm Rep* 60:1-24, 2011.

Health Canada: Drug product database. Retrieved June 25, 2012, from http://www.hc-sc.gc.ca/dhp-mps/prodpharma/databasdon/index-eng.php, 2010.

Joint United Nations Programme on HIV-AIDS: (2010). Global report: UNAIDS report on the global AIDS epidemic 2010, Geneva 2010, Joint United Nations Programme on HIV-AIDS.

Kalant H, Grant D, Mitchell J: *Principles of medical pharmacology*, ed 7, Toronto, 2007, Elsevier Canada, pp 739-759.

Lance L, Lacy C, Armstrong L, et al: *Drug information handbook for the allied health professional*, ed 12, Hudson, OH, 2005, APhA Lexi-Comp.

McColl DJ, Chen X: Strand transfer inhibitors of HIV-1 integrase: Bringing in a new era of antiretroviral therapy, *Antiviral Res* 85:101-118, 2010.

National Institute of Allergy and Infectious Disease: Flu (influenza): Advances in treatment, 2011 (http://www.niaid.nih.gov/topics/Flu/Research/AdvancesTreatment/Pages/default.aspx).

Page C, Curtis M, Sutter M, et al: *Integrated pharmacology*, Philadelphia, 2005, Elsevier Mosby, pp 91-109.

U.S. Department of Health and Human Services: AIDS info: HIV and its treatment, 2011 (http://aidsinfo.nih.gov/contentfiles/HIVandItsTreatment_cbrochure_en.pdf).

U.S. Food and Drug Administration, Center for Drug Evaluation and Research: FDA public health advisory for nevirapine (Viramune), 2005 (http://www.fda.gov/Drugs/DrugSafety/PostmarketDrugSafetyInformationforPatientsandProviders/DrugSafetyInformationforHeathcareProfessionals/PublicHealthAdvisories/ucm051674.htm).

USP Center for the Advancement of Patient Safety: *USP Quality Review No. 79: Use caution: Avoid confusion*, Rockville, MD, 2004, USP Center for the Advancement of Patient Safety.

World Health Organization (WHO): Antiretroviral drugs for treating pregnant women and preventing HIV infection in infants: Towards universal access. Recommendations for a public health approach, 2006 (http://www.who.int/hiv/pub/mtct/antiretroviral/en/index.html).

World Health Organization: (2012). Programmatic Update: Use of Antiretroviral Drugs for Treating Pregnant Women and Preventing HIV Infections in Infants, from www.who.int/hiv/PMTCT_update.pdf.

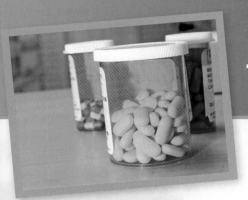

37

Treatment of Cancers

KEY TERMS

Benign: Refers to a tumor that is not cancerous and does not spread to surrounding tissues or other parts of the body.

Biopsy: Removal of cells or tissues for examination by a pathologist. The three types of biopsies are (1) incisional, (2) excisional, and (3) fine-needle aspiration.

Cancer: Term for diseases in which abnormal cells divide without control. Specific cancers are named according to the site at which the cancerous growth begins.

Chemotherapy: Treatment with drugs that kill cancerous cells.

Complementary and alternative medicine: Treatments that may include dietary supplements, herbal preparations, acupuncture, massage, magnet therapy, spiritual healing, and meditation.

Computed tomography scan: Diagnostic examination by a computer linked to an x-ray machine in which a series of detailed pictures are taken of areas inside the body.

Double-contrast barium enema: Diagnostic test to examine the colon and rectum in which an individual is given a barium-containing enema and radiographs are then taken.

Excisional biopsy: Surgical procedure in which an entire lump or suspicious looking tissue is removed for diagnosis.

External radiation: Radiation therapy that uses a machine to aim high-energy rays at the cancer site.

Fecal occult blood test: Test to check for blood in stool.

Implant radiation: Procedure, also known as brachytherapy, in which radioactive material sealed in needles, seeds, wires, or catheters is placed directly into or near a tumor.

Ionizing radiation: Type of high-frequency radiation produced by x-ray procedures, radioactive substances, and ultraviolet light that can lead to health risks at certain doses, including cancer.

Leukemia: Cancer that starts in blood-forming tissue such as the bone marrow.

Lymphoma: Cancer that begins in cells of the immune system.

Magnetic resonance imaging: A procedure that uses a large circular magnet and radio waves to generate signals from atoms in the body to produce an image.

Malignant: Cancerous tumors that can invade and destroy nearby tissue and spread to other parts of the body.

Mammography: Screening examination to detect breast cancer in which a radiograph of the breast is taken.

Melanoma: Form of skin cancer that arises in melanocytes, the cells that produce pigment.

Metastasis: Spread of cancer from one part of the body to another.

Neoplasm: Tumor.

Oncovirus: Virus that is a causative agent of a cancer.

Pap test (Pap smear): Screening test in which cells from the cervix are examined to detect cancer and changes that might lead to cancer.

Polyp: Growth that protrudes from a mucous membrane.

Positron emission tomography scan: Diagnostic examination to detect cancer cells in the body in which a small amount of radioactive glucose (sugar) is injected into a vein and a scanner is then used to make detailed computerized pictures of areas inside the body in which the glucose is distributed.

Primary tumor: Original tumor or initial tumor.

Prostate-specific antigen test: Test that measures the level of free prostate-specific antigen, a protein produced by the prostate gland. Levels are elevated in men who have prostate cancer, infection, or inflammation of the prostate gland and benign prostatic hyperplasia.

Radiation therapy: Use of high-energy radiation from x-rays, gamma rays, neutrons, and other sources to kill cancer cells and shrink tumors.

Radionuclide scan: Diagnostic test in which an individual is given a small amount of radioactive material. A scanner is used to take pictures of the internal parts of the body to detect where the radiation concentrates.

Radon: Radioactive gas that if inhaled in sufficient quantity can lead to lung cancer.

Sonography: Screening examination using ultrasound that results in a computer image of internal organs and tissues.

Stage: Extent of a cancer within the body. Staging is based on the size of the tumor, whether lymph nodes contain cancer, and whether the disease has spread from the original site to other parts of the body.

Stem cell: Type of cell from which other types of cells develop; for example, blood cells develop from blood-forming stem cells.

Stem cell transplantation: Procedure used to replace cells that were destroyed by cancer treatment.

Tumor: Mass of excess tissue that results from abnormal cell division. Tumors may be benign or malignant.

Tumor marker: Substance sometimes found in the blood, other body fluids, or tissues that may signal the presence of a certain type of cancer; for example, a high level of prostate-specific antigen is a signal for possible prostate cancer.

What Is Cancer?

Cancer is a disease that occurs when the normal cell renewal process fails. When old cells fail to die and new cells form more rapidly than needed, the cells may accumulate and form a mass called a *neoplasm* or *tumor*. Tumors are caused by abnormal cell division. They may be benign or

BOX 37-1   **Risk Factors for Cancer**

- Increasing age
- Tobacco
- Environmental pollutants
- Ionizing radiation
- Sunlight and tanning salons (UV light)
- Carcinogenic chemicals (e.g., benzene)
- Viruses (e.g., HPV, EBV)
- Bacteria (e.g., *Helicobacter pylori*)
- Hormone therapy (e.g., DES)
- Family history
- Alcohol

malignant. A ***malignant*** tumor is cancerous and can invade and destroy nearby tissue and spread via ***metastasis*** to other parts of the body, whereas a ***benign*** tumor is not cancerous and does not spread. Specific cancers are named according to the site at which the cancerous growth began. This is the site of the ***primary tumor***. For example, carcinoma begins in skin or tissues covering internal organs, ***leukemia*** begins in blood-forming tissues, and ***lymphoma*** begins in cells of the immune system.

RISK FACTORS FOR CANCER

There are many risk factors for cancer, including age, tobacco use, and exposure to ionizing radiation (Box 37-1).

Age

The risk for developing cancer increases with age. Cancers are more prevalent in persons over the age of 65 years.

Tobacco

Inhalation of cigarette, cigar, and pipe tobacco smoke may increase the risk for developing cancer of the lungs, larynx, mouth, esophagus, bladder, kidney, throat, stomach, pancreas, and cervix and acute myeloid leukemia. Smokers as well as nonsmokers exposed to second-hand tobacco smoke are at increased risk. Chewing tobacco may increase the risk for oral cancer.

Ionizing Radiation and Sunlight

X-rays, nuclear fallout (from atomic weapons testing or leaks from nuclear power plants), and radon gas are examples of ***ionizing radiation***. ***Radon*** is a radioactive gas that is odorless, colorless, and tasteless. High levels may be found in mine shafts and in some homes. Exposure to radioactive fallout increases the risk for the development of leukemia, thyroid cancer, and breast cancer. Exposure to radon gas may increase the risk for developing lung cancer.

Ultraviolet (UV) radiation comes from the sun. The ozone layer of the atmosphere provides protection from excessive exposure to UV radiation, prompting concerns over depletion of the earth's ozone layer. Exposure to UVA and UVB radiation can increase the risk for skin cancer (***melanoma***). UVA levels are highest during midday, whereas UVB levels are found throughout the day. Exposure to UV light from sunlamps and tanning booths also increases cancer risk. Excess exposure to UV radiation is a cancer risk; however, some exposure to sunlight is necessary for the skin to make the hormone vitamin D.

Hazardous Chemicals and Environmental Pollutants

Cancer-causing chemicals (carcinogens) are found in the workplace, home, and environment through pollution. Industrial solvents, cleaning fluids, pesticides, and used engine oil are examples of hazardous chemicals. Known workplace carcinogens include benzene, vinyl chloride, polychlorinated biphenyls (PCBs), asbestos, cadmium, and nickel. These carcinogens may get into the environment through improper disposal or chemical spills or are released into the air in the process of incineration.

Bacterial and Viral Infection

Helicobacter pylori is a bacteria known to cause peptic ulcer disease (PUD). It is also associated with stomach cancer. Exposure to some viruses may increase the risk of developing certain cancers. Viruses that cause cancer are called ***oncoviruses***. Epstein-Barr virus (EBV) is a common virus that remains dormant in most people; however, it has been associated with lymphomas such as Burkitt's lymphoma and immunoblastic lymphoma. The virus is also linked to nasopharyngeal carcinoma. Hepatitis B virus (HBV) and hepatitis C virus (HCV) are linked to liver cancer. Human papillomavirus (HPV) is a virus that causes genital warts and cancer of the cervix. Human immunodeficiency virus (HIV) and human herpesvirus 8 (HHV8) can cause Kaposi's sarcoma. Human T cell leukemia virus, type 1, is another retrovirus; it can cause leukemia and lymphoma.

Hormone Therapy

Hormone replacement therapy (HRT) and diethylstilbestrol (DES) have been linked to specific cancers. HRT, once the principal treatment for menopausal symptoms and also prescribed to reduce osteoporosis and heart disease, is now limited because of the risk for the development of breast cancer, heart attack, stroke, and blood clots. Diethylstilbestrol is an estrogen-type drug that was taken by pregnant women between 1940 and 1971. Girls born to women who took DES have a higher risk for cancer of the cervix than girls born to women who did not take the drug. Women who took DES have a higher incidence of breast cancer.

Family History

In the absence of contact with tobacco, carcinogenic chemicals and drugs, aging, and exposure to certain viruses and bacteria, it is not known why one individual will develop cancer whereas another does not. With the exception of cancers of the breast, ovary, prostate, skin, and colon, most cancers do not run in families. For example, if a father develops stomach cancer, his children have no greater risk for stomach cancer than would a non–family member.

Alcohol

Chronic alcohol consumption (up to two drinks daily over a period of years) may increase the risk for cancer of the liver, mouth, throat, esophagus, larynx, and breast.

Diet, Physical Inactivity, and Obesity

A diet is that is high in fat may increase the risk of cancers of the colon, uterus, and prostate. Cancers of the breast, colon, esophagus, kidney, and uterus are higher in individuals who have little physical activity and are overweight.

TYPES OF CANCERS

Breast Cancer

In 2010, almost 2,632,005 women were diagnosed with breast cancer. Approximately 124 of every 100,000 women will be diagnosed with the disease. The median age at the time of diagnosis is 61 years. One or both breasts may be involved. The mortality rate is approximately 24/100,000 women, accounting for 39,840 deaths in 2010. The following are risk factors for breast cancer: (1) family history; (2) nulliparity (no pregnancies); (3) early onset of menses (periods); (4) advanced age; (5) a personal history of breast cancer; and (6) history of HRT. Signs and symptoms of breast cancer are listed in Box 37-2.

Cancer of the Cervix, Endometrium, and Ovaries

Cancer of the cervix is linked to HPV and exposure to the drug DES while the fetus is still in the uterus. Approximately 8.1/100,000 women are diagnosed annually with cancer of the cervix, and it was estimated that in 2010, almost 12,200 women were diagnosed and 4210 women died from the disease. Ovarian cancer is more common than cervical cancer, with an incidence of 13.5/100,000

BOX 37-2   **Signs and Symptoms of Breast Cancer**

- Nipple tenderness
- Lump or mass in the breast near the underarm area
- Fluid coming out of nipples
- Nipple that has turned inward
- Changes in size of shape of the breast

BOX 37-3   **ABCDE Signs of Skin Cancer**

BOX 37-3   **ABCDE Signs of Skin Cancer**

- **A**symmetry: A mole that looks different on one half than the other half.
- **B**order: The edges of the mole are blurry or jagged.
- **C**olor: The color of a mole changes (e.g., darkens, spreads, loses color, or appears as multiple colors, such as blue, red, white, pink, purple, or gray).
- **D**iameter: The mole is larger than $\frac{1}{4}$ inch in diameter.
- **E**levation: The mole is raised above the skin and has an uneven surface.

women annually. It was estimated that in 2010, almost 21,880 women were diagnosed and 13,850 women died from the disease. The endometrium is the lining of the uterus. Endometrial cancer most commonly affects postmenopausal women.

Skin Cancer

Skin cancer is one of the most common types of cancer. It was estimated that 68,130 men and women (38,870 men and 29,260 women) were diagnosed with the disease in 2010 and 8700 men and women died of cancer of the skin. Skin cancer is divided into two categories, melanoma and nonmelanoma. The most treatable form is nonmelanoma.

Skin cancer is associated with excessive exposure to ultraviolet light from the sun or UV lights used in tanning salons. UV light and ionizing radiation are described earlier ("Risk Factors for Cancer"). Protection from harmful UV light is the best way to prevent skin cancer. This can be achieved by wearing protective clothing when outdoors or by using sunscreen. Warning signs for skin cancer are shown in Box 37-3.

Lung Cancer

Lung cancer is the most common form of cancer. It was estimated that 75/100,000 men and 52/100,000 women were diagnosed with cancer of the lung and bronchus in 2010, almost 222,520 men and women. Almost 157,300 men and women were anticipated to die of cancer of the lung and bronchus in 2010.

There are two types of lung cancer, small cell lung cancer (SCLC) and non–small cell lung cancer (NSCLC). Antineoplastic agents used in the treatment of lung cancer are typically effective against one but not both forms of the disease. A history of smoking tobacco is almost always the cause of small cell lung cancer.

Colorectal Cancer

Cancer of the colon and rectum affects an estimated 47.2/100,000 men and women annually, a total of 142,570 new cases each year. The first signs of colon cancer may be the appearance of a small polyp and blood in the stool. Early detection through the administration of screening examinations helps reduce the numbers of deaths from the disease. Colonoscopy and a *fecal occult blood test* (FOBT) are screening tests for colorectal cancer.

Prostate Cancer

The incidence of prostrate cancer increases as men grow older. Approximately 0.5% of men will be diagnosed with prostate cancer between the age of 35 to 44 years; this increases to 36.7% between 65 and 74 years of age. Levels begin to slowly decline again after the age of 75. It was estimated that approximately 217,730 men were diagnosed with prostate cancer in 2010. Prostate disease, diagnosis, and treatment are described in Chapter 30.

Cancer Screening Tests and Staging

SCREENING TESTS

Early diagnosis is critical to successful treatment. Screening tests are recommended for the early diagnosis of breast cancer, colorectal cancer, cancer of the cervix, and prostate cancer. A *mammography* is a screening examination used to detect breast cancer. A radiograph is taken of the breast and inspected for evidence of tumors. *Sonography* is an alternative method for screening for breast cancers. If a lump is found, a biopsy is performed. A ***biopsy*** is a procedure whereby the cells or tissue is (are) removed for examination by a pathologist. The three types of biopsies are incisional, excisional, and fine-needle aspiration. Regular self-examination of the breast is another important method for screening for breast cancer.

Several tests exist to screen for colorectal cancer. They are the FOBT, colonoscopy, sigmoidoscopy, double-contrast barium enema, and digital rectal examination (DRE). The FOBT is a test that screens for blood in stool. Bleeding may indicate the presence of polyps or cancer. A ***polyp*** is a growth that protrudes from a mucous membrane. A colonoscopy and sigmoidoscopy involve insertion of a lighted tube into the colon to inspect for abnormal growths. Radiographs may be taken of the colon. With this screening procedure, the individual is given a ***double-contrast barium enema*** to permit greater visualization of the bowel. A DRE is a screening test for colon and prostate cancers (see Chapter 30). Some cancers may have a ***tumor marker*** which is a substance sometimes found in the blood, other body fluids, or tissues that may signal the presence of a certain type of cancer; for example, a high level of prostate-specific antigen is a signal for possible prostate cancer. A ***prostate-specific antigen*** (PSA) test is performed to screen for prostate cancer. PSA is a protein produced by the prostate gland. Levels are elevated in men who have prostate cancer, infection, or inflammation of the prostate gland and benign prostatic hyperplasia (BPH; see Chapter 30). A ***Pap test (Pap smear)*** is a screening test for cancer of the cervix. The Pap test is a simple procedure in which cells from the cervix are removed and examined to detect cancer and changes that may lead to cancer.

The results of the screening test may indicate that more diagnostic examinations are warranted. Before a diagnosis of cancer is made, the individual may undergo additional radiographs, ***computed tomography*** (CT) ***scans***, biopsy, ***sonogram***, ***radionuclide scan***, ***magnetic resonance imaging*** (MRI), or ***positron emission tomography scan*** (PET) scan.

STAGING

Staging is a method used to describe how far the cancer has progressed within the body. Staging is based on the size of the tumor, whether lymph nodes contain cancer, and whether the cancer has spread from the original site to other parts of the body.

Treatment of Cancer

Cancer may be treated with chemotherapy, biologic therapy, radiation therapy, and surgery. ***Chemotherapy*** is the use of drugs to kill or slow the growth of cancerous cells. Biologic therapy is the administration of immune system modulators to boost the body's natural defense against abnormal, invasive, and cancerous cells. ***Radiation therapy***, the use of high-energy radiation from x-rays, gamma rays, neutrons, and other sources can be used to kill cancer cells and shrink tumors. Other types of treatments using radiation are ***external radiation*** that uses a machine to aim high-energy rays at the cancer and ***implant radiation*** a procedure, also known as brachytherapy, in which radioactive material sealed in needles, seeds, wires, or catheters is placed directly into or near a tumor.

Some patients may try ***complementary and alternative medicine*** which may include dietary supplements, herbal preparations, acupuncture, massage, magnet therapy, spiritual healing, and meditation and ***stem cell transplantation*** which is a procedure used to replace cells that were destroyed by cancer treatment. The ***stem cell*** is a type of cell from which other types of cells develop; for example, blood cells develop from blood-forming stem cells.

The following factors influence the selection of treatment options: (1) type of cancer; (2) ***stage*** of cancer; (3) individual tolerance for adverse effects of treatment; (4) patient's age; (5) histological and nuclear grade of the primary tumor; and (6) capacity of the cancer to metastasize. This chapter focuses on chemotherapy and biological therapy.

Chemotherapeutic or antineoplastic agents may be administered parenterally or by mouth. They work by various mechanisms to interrupt the cell replication cycle. Some agents are cell cycle–specific; they interrupt a specific stage of the cell cycle (Table 37-1). Examples include mitotic inhibitors, microtubule inhibitors, and DNA synthesis inhibitors. Other antineoplastic agents are nonspecific. The site of action of chemotherapeutic agents is shown in Figure 37-1.

TABLE 37-1   Summary of the Cell Life Cycle

Phase of Cell Life Cycle	Description
Cell Growth	Interphase
Protein synthesis	Proteins are manufactured according to the cell's genetic code; functional proteins, the enzymes, direct the synthesis of other molecules in the cells and thus the production of more and larger organelles and plasma membrane; sometimes called the first growth phase or G1, phase of interphase.
DNA replication	Nucleotides, influenced by newly synthesized enzymes, arrange themselves along the open sides of an unzipped DNA molecule, thereby creating two identical daughter DNA molecules; produces two identical sets of the cell's genetic code, which enables the cell later to split into two different cells, each with its own complete set of DNA; sometimes called the (DNA) synthesis stage or S phase of interphase.
Protein synthesis	After DNA is replicated, the cell continues to grow by means of protein synthesis and the resulting synthesis of other molecules and various organelles; this second growth phase is also called the G2 phase.
Cell Reproduction	M phase
Mitosis or meiosis	The parent cell's replicated set of DNA is divided into two sets separated by an orderly process into distinct cell nuclei; mitosis is subdivided into at least four phases—prophase, metaphase, anaphase, and telophase.
Cytokinesis	The plasma membrane of the parent cell pinches in and eventually separates the cytoplasm and two daughter nuclei into two genetically identical daughter cells.

From Thibodeau G, Patton K: *Anatomy and physiology,* ed 6, St. Louis, 2007, Mosby.

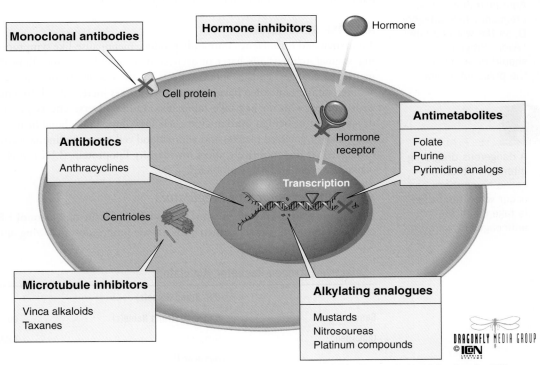

FIGURE 37-1 Site of action of chemotherapeutic agents. (From Raffa RB, Rawls SM, Beyzarov EP: *Netter's illustrated pharmacology*, Philadelphia, 2005, WB Saunders.)

Antineoplastic Agents

HORMONE THERAPY

Hormone therapy is a treatment of choice for breast cancer. The treatment choice is influenced by the woman's menopausal status, affinity of the tumor for estrogen receptors and progesterone receptors, and human epidermal growth factor receptor 2 (HER2/neu) status (overexpression), in addition to the other factors listed earlier.

The hormones estrogen and progesterone can promote the growth of estrogen receptor positive–(ER-positive) and/or progesterone receptor–positive (PR-positive) breast cancer. The administration of an estrogen receptor antagonist (antiestrogen) can reduce the risk of breast cancer recurrence for up to 5 years after treatment of the primary tumor.

Selective Estrogen Receptor Modulators (Antiestrogens)

Tamoxifen is indicated for the treatment of ER-positive breast cancer that is noninvasive or invasive (metastatic). It is approved for the treatment of metastatic breast cancer in premenopausal and postmenopausal women. It is also approved for the treatment of metastatic breast cancer in men. Toremifene is a derivative of tamoxifen that is indicated for the treatment of metastatic breast cancer in postmenopausal women.

MECHANISM OF ACTION AND PHARMACOKINETICS

Tamoxifen and torimefene are antiestrogens. Tamoxifen is a selective ER modulator (SERM) that has antiestrogenic and estrogenic activities. Tamoxifen is an estrogen antagonist in breast tissue. It induces maspin, a tumor suppression gene that is abundant in normal breast cells and lacking in cancerous breast tissue. This may prevent the tumor from becoming invasive. Tamoxifen acts as a partial agonist in the endometrium (lining of the uterus). Its agonist effects on bone cells increase bone turnover (remodeling) and can decrease postmenopausal bone loss. Tamoxifen also has agonist effects on cholesterol metabolism and genitourinary epithelium. Tamoxifen has an active metabolite and long half-life and accumulates with continued administration. It may be given once or twice daily. The action of torimefene is primarily antiestrogenic.

ADVERSE REACTIONS

Tamoxifen and torimefene commonly produce menopause-like symptoms such as hot flashes, sweating, vaginal itchiness, discharge or dryness, nausea, and vomiting. Tamoxifen may additionally cause menstrual changes, and its agonist effects on the endometrium may result in endometrial cancer. Women taking tamoxifen have a two to seven times increased risk for endometrial cancer compared with women who do not take tamoxifen. Other adverse effects produced by tamoxifen include development of benign ovarian cysts, hair loss, impotence, bone or muscle pain, deep vein thrombosis (DVT), lowered platelet and white blood cell count, pulmonary embolism, and visual changes (cataracts). It may positively affect low-density lipoprotein (LDL) levels. Torimefene may produce ocular, vascular, and heart problems.

Estrogen Receptor Downregulators

Fulvestrant is an ER downregulator. It is indicated for the treatment of ER-positive metastatic breast cancer in postmenopausal women with disease progression following antiestrogen therapy.

Selective Estrogen Receptor Modulators

Generic Name	U.S. Brand Name(s)	Dosage Forms and Strengths
	Canadian Brand Name(s)	
tamoxifen*	Generics	Tablet: 10 mg, 20 mg (Nolvadex-D)
	Nolvadex-D	
toremifene	Fareston	Tablet: 60 mg
	Not available	

*Generic available.

Estrogen Receptor Downregulators

Generic Name	U.S. Brand Name(s)	Dosage Forms and Strengths
	Canadian Brand Name(s)	
fulvestrant	Faslodex	Solution, for injection: 50 mg/mL
	Faslodex	

Aromatase Inhibitors

Generic Name	U.S. Brand Name(s)	Dosage Forms and Strengths
	Canadian Brand Name(s)	
anastrozole*	Arimidex	Tablet: 1 mg
	Arimidex	
exemestane*	Aromasin	Tablet: 25 mg
	Aromasin	
letrozole*	Femara	Tablet: 2.5 mg
	Femara	

*Generic available.

MECHANISM OF ACTION AND PHARMACOKINETICS

Fulvestrant is an analogue of estradiol. It acts as a competitive antagonist. When fulvestrant binds to ERs, it inhibits estrogen activity, causes changes in ER function, and triggers ER degradation. Fulvestrant is administered intramuscularly. Plasma concentrations are maintained at therapeutic levels for up to 1 month.

ADVERSE REACTIONS

Adverse effects caused by fulvestrant include pain at the injection site, generalized bone and back pain, hot flashes, headache, nausea and vomiting, diarrhea or constipation, and weakness.

Aromatase Inhibitors

Anastrozole, exemestane, and letrozole are aromatase inhibitors. They may be prescribed alone or in combination with tamoxifen. They are FDA-approved for the first-line treatment of advanced or metastatic ER-positive breast cancer in postmenopausal women. They are also approved as an adjuvant for the treatment of early-stage breast cancer.

MECHANISM OF ACTION AND PHARMACOKINETICS

The adrenal gland is the primary source of estrogen after menopause. Aromatase is an enzyme responsible for converting androgens produced by the adrenal gland into the estrogens estrone and estradiol in the peripheral tissues. Aromatase inhibitors block this process. Anastrozole and letrozole are nonsteroidal aromatase inhibitors and are potent inhibitors of serum estradiol levels. Exemestane is a steroidal aromatase inhibitor. It is a more potent inhibitor of estrogen than the other aromatase inhibitors.

ADVERSE REACTIONS

Like tamoxifen, aromatase inhibitors produce menopause-like symptoms, nausea, and vomiting. Additional adverse effects include dizziness, cough, headache, hair loss, constipation, mood changes, and bone pain. Administration of steroid aromatase inhibitors requires adrenal hormone replacement therapy to replenish depleted glucocorticoids (cortisol) and mineralocorticoids (aldosterone). Symptoms may be fatigue, weight gain, and swelling.

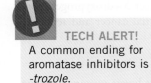

TECH ALERT!
A common ending for aromatase inhibitors is -trozole.

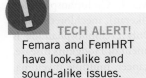

TECH ALERT!
Femara and FemHRT have look-alike and sound-alike issues.

Luteinizing Hormone–Releasing Hormone and Gonadotropin-Releasing Hormone Agonists

Generic Name	U.S. Brand Name(s)	Dosage Forms and Strengths
	Canadian Brand Name(s)	
goserelin	Zoladex	Implant (1 mo): 3.6 mg
	Zoladex, Zoladex LA	Implant (3 mo): 10.8 mg

Progestins Used in the Treatment of Cancer

Generic Name	U.S. Brand Name(s)	Dosage Forms and Strengths
	Canadian Brand Name(s)	
megestrol acetate*	Megace, Megace ES	Suspension, oral: 40 mg/mL (Megace, Megace OS); 125 mg/mL (Megace ES)
	Megace, Megace OS	Tablet: 20 mg†, 40 mg, 160 mg‡

*Generic available.
†Strength available in the United States only.
‡Strength available in Canada only.

Gonadotropin-Releasing Hormone Agonists and Luteinizing Hormone–Releasing Hormone Agonists

Gonadotropin-releasing hormone (GnRH) is also known as luteinizing hormone–releasing hormone (LHRH). Goserelin is a GnRH agonist indicated for the treatment of advanced breast cancer in premenopausal and perimenopausal women with ER-positive disease. The drug initially increases hormone levels and is followed by desensitization to the hormone's effects. GnRH and its analogues are described in depth in Chapter 34. GnRH agonists may be prescribed to treat premenopausal women, whereas SERMs and aromatase inhibitors are only indicated for use in postmenopausal women.

Progestins

Megestrol acetate is a progestin approved for the treatment of breast cancer. It is indicated for the treatment of inoperable, advanced metastatic breast cancer following treatment with tamoxifen or aromatase inhibitors. It is also indicated for the treatment of endometrial cancer. Medroxyprogesterone acetate is approved for the treatment of inoperable, metastatic endometrial cancer and renal cell cancer.

TECH ALERT!
Megesterol suspension is prescribed to increase appetite and combat wasting syndrome in patients with AIDS.

MECHANISM OF ACTION

It is not fully known how megestrol works to suppress estrogen-dependent breast tumors; however, suppression of LH release from the pituitary and increased metabolism of estrogen are believed to be involved.

ADVERSE REACTIONS

The most common adverse effects associated with megestrol use are hot flashes, breakthrough menstrual bleeding, and weight gain. Breast tenderness, hair loss, and hyperglycemia may also occur.

ALKYLATING AGENTS

Alkylating agents are one of the oldest classes of antineoplastic agents. They are related to nitrogen mustard, a lethal gas that was used for chemical warfare in World War I. Cyclophosphamide (Cytoxan), busulfan (Busulfex, Myleran), ifosfamide (Ifex), melphalan (Alkeran), mechlorethamine (Mustargen), and chlorambucil (Leukeran) are all alkylating agents. Only cyclophosphamide is approved for the treatment of breast cancer. It is also indicated for the treatment of Hodgkin's disease, non-Hodgkin's lymphoma, acute lymphocytic leukemia (ALL), ovarian cancer, multiple myeloma, chronic lymphocytic leukemia (CLL), mycosis fungoides, and retinoblastoma.

Alkylating Agents

Generic Name	U.S. Brand Name(s)	Dosage Forms and Strengths
	Canadian Brand Name(s)	
cyclophosphamide*	Cytoxan	Powder, for solution (Cytoxan, Procytox): 200 mg/vial‡, 500 mg/vial, 1000 mg/vial, 2000 mg/vial
	Procytox	Tablet: 25 mg, 50 mg

*Generic available.
‡Strength available in Canada only.

Taxanes

Generic Name	U.S. Brand Name(s)	Dosage Forms and Strengths
	Canadian Brand Name(s)	
docetaxel*	Docefrez, Taxotere	Powder, for injection (Docefrez): 20 mg/vial, 80 mg/vial
	Taxotere	Solution, for injection: 10 mg/mL, 20 mg/mL (Taxotere); 80 mg/4 mL†; 160 mg/8 mL†
		Solution, for injection (concentrate): 20 mg/0.5 mL; 80 mg/2 mL
paclitaxel*	Generics	Solution, for injection: 6 mg/mL
	Taxol	
albumin-bound nanoparticle paclitaxel	Abraxane	Powder, for suspension: 100 mg/vial
	Abraxane	

*Generic available.
†Strength available in the United States only.

MECHANISM OF ACTION AND PHARMACOKINETICS

The alkylating agents vary in their antitumor effects and in toxicity, but their mechanism of action is the same. All alkylating agents damage DNA when they substitute for an alkyl group (saturated carbon atoms) on the amino acid guanine or, in some cases, cytosine. This changes the guanine-cytosine base pair and impairs DNA replication and the growth phase of the cell life cycle (see Table 37-1). Alkylating agents can cause cell mutations and are themselves carcinogenic. They are toxic to cancer cells and noncancerous cells.

Cyclophosphamide is a prodrug. It is available for oral and parenteral use. Resistance can develop to the effects of cyclophosphamide and other alkylating agents.

ADVERSE REACTIONS

Cyclophosphamide commonly causes hair loss, appetite and weight loss, skin discoloration, mouth sores, and fatigue.

MICROTUBULE-TARGETING DRUGS

Epothilones, estramustine, taxanes, and vinca alkaloids target microtubules. They act to inhibit microtubule formation (vinca alkaloids), inhibit microtubule degradation (taxanes), stabilize microtubules (ixabepilone), or suppress microtubule growth and sequester tubulin (eribulin).

Taxanes

Taxanes are cytotoxic drugs that are naturally derived from the Western yew tree (paclitaxel) and European yew tree (docetaxel). They are approved for the treatment of breast cancer.

MECHANISM OF ACTION AND PHARMACOKINETICS

Taxanes interfere with the process of mitosis. Mitosis is a key step in the process of cell division and is the stage at which DNA is organized and distributed. Taxanes are microtubular inhibitors. They

TABLE 37-2 Major Events of Mitosis

Prophase	Metaphase	Anaphase	Telophase
1. Chromosomes shorten and thicken (from coiling of the DNA molecules that compose them); each chromosome consists of two chromatids attached at the centromere. 2. Centrioles move to opposite poles of the cell; spindle fibers appear and begin to orient between opposing poles. 3. Nucleoli and the nuclear membrane disappear.	1. Chromosomes align across the equator of the spindle fiber at its centromere.	1. Each centromere splits, thereby detaching two chromatids that compose each chromosome from each other elongating (DNA molecules start uncoiling). 2. Sister chromatids (now called chromosomes) move to opposite poles; there are now twice as many chromosomes as there were before mitosis started.	1. Changes occurring during telophase essentially reverse those taking place during prophase; new chromosomes start elongating (DNA molecules start uncoiling). 2. A nuclear envelope forms again to enclose each new set of chromosomes. 3. Spindle fibers disappear.

From Thibodeau G, Patton K: *Anatomy and physiology*, ed 6, St. Louis, 2007, Mosby.

> **TECH ALERT!**
> Paclitaxel is insoluble in water, so it is prepared as an emulsion using hydrogenated castor oil (Cremophor). Allergic reactions to this emulsion are common and can be fatal.

> **TECH ALERT!**
> A common beginning for vinca alkaloids is *vin-*.

bind to tubulin subunits, resulting in overly stable, nonfunctional microtubules that do not dissociate and disappear in the final phase of mitosis. Microtubules or spindles are normally formed during the prophase of mitosis and are supposed to disappear by the end of the telophase. The four phases of mitosis are shown in Table 37-2.

ADVERSE REACTIONS

Common adverse reactions produced by taxanes are diarrhea, total body hair loss, nausea, muscle pain, joint and low back pain, flushing, and sweating. They also decrease white blood cell, red blood cell, and platelet counts. When white blood cell levels drop, individuals may get infections more easily. Docetaxel may also cause discoloration of fingernails and loosening from the nail bed. Paclitaxel may cause mouth sores.

Vinca Alkaloids

Vinorelbine, vincristine, and vinblastine are vinca alkaloids. They are naturally derived from the periwinkle plant. Vinca alkaloids are used for the treatment of NSCLC, breast cancer, Kaposi's sarcoma, Hodgkin's disease, non-Hodgkin's lymphoma, and testicular cancer.

Vinca Alkaloids

Generic Name	U.S. Brand Name(s) / Canadian Brand Name(s)	Dosage Forms and Strengths
vinorelbine*	Navelbine	Solution, for injection: 10 mg/mL
	Navelbine	
vinblastine*	Generics	Powder, for injection†: 10 mg/vial
	Generics	Solution, for injection: 1 mg/mL
vincristine*, vincristine PFS*	Generics	Solution, for injection: 1 mg/mL
	Generics	

*Generic available.
†Strength available in the United States only.

TECH ALERT!
Vinblastine and vincristine have look-alike and sound-alike issues.

TECH ALERT!
Vincristine is usually stored in the refrigerator.

MECHANISM OF ACTION AND PHARMACOKINETICS

The mechanism of action of vinca alkaloids is similar to that of taxanes. Both drugs act on microtubules to inhibit mitosis. Vinca alkaloids inhibit microtubule formation (taxanes inhibit microtubule degradation).

ADVERSE REACTIONS

Side effects linked to vinca alkaloids are similar to those for taxanes and include hair loss, nausea and vomiting, constipation, joint and muscle pain, mouth sores, increased risk for infections, and pain at the injection site.

Epothilones

Ixabepilone is a unique class of microtubule inhibitors called epothilones. It is indicated, in combination with capecitabine or as monotherapy for the treatment of metastatic or locally advanced breast cancer that is resistant or refractory to anthracyclines, taxanes, and capecitabine.

Eribulin

Eribulin is isolated from the marine sponge. It suppresses microtubule growth and sequesters tubulin. It disrupts mitotic spindles, leading to apoptotic cell death. It is used for the treatment of metastatic breast cancer.

ADVERSE REACTIONS

Nausea, vomiting, constipation, neutropenia, weight loss, anorexia, and diarrhea are the most common side effects of eribulin. Muscle, joint, and bone pain may also occur.

Estramustine

Estramustine is an antimicrotubule agent. It is also listed as alkylating agent and believed to have a dual mechanism of action—antimitotic effect (microtubule-stabilization) and antigonadotropic effect. Estramustine may also inhibit DNA synthesis and cause dose-related DNA strand breaks. It is approved for the treatment of hormone-refractory prostate cancer in Canada and the United States.

ADVERSE REACTIONS

The most common side effects of estramustine are breast tenderness, gynecomastia, elevated liver function tests, nausea, myalgia, and edema.

ANTHRACYCLINES

TECH ALERT!
A common ending for anthracyclines is *-rubicin*.

Doxorubicin, epirubicin, and idarubicin are anthracyclines. Mitoxantrone is a related compound and is classified as an anthracenedione. Only doxorubicin and epirubicin are indicated for the treatment of breast cancer, typically in combination with other antineoplastic agents. Doxorubicin is

Miscellaneous Microtubule Inhibitors

Generic Name	U.S. Brand Name(s)	Dosage Forms and Strengths
	Canadian Brand Name(s)	
eribulin	Halaven	Solution, for injection: 1 mg/2 mL
	Not available	
estramustine	Emcyt	Capsule: 140 mg
	Emcyt	
ixabepilone	Ixempra	Powder, for injection: 15 mg/vial, 45 mg/vial
	Not available	

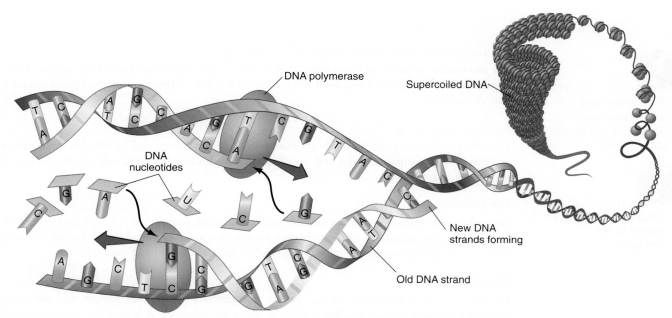

FIGURE 37-2 DNA replication. (From Thibodeau G, Patton K: *Anatomy and physiology*, ed 6, St. Louis, 2007, Mosby.)

also approved for the treatment of numerous other cancers such as bladder cancer, lung cancer, Hodgkin's disease, leukemia, gastric cancer, ovarian cancer, soft tissue sarcoma, and thyroid cancer. Doxorubicin liposomal is approved for the treatment of ovarian cancer, Kaposi's sarcoma, and multiple myeloma. Idarubicin and mitoxantrone are approved for the treatment of acute myelogenous leukemia (AML).

MECHANISM OF ACTION AND PHARMACOKINETICS

Anthracyclines damage cellular DNA. They form a complex with DNA that changes the shape of the helix-shaped strand and results in inhibition of the DNA and RNA enzymes that promote protein synthesis (Figure 37-2). This impairs DNA replication and the growth phase of the cell life cycle (see Table 37-1).

Anthracyclines also inhibit the activity of the enzyme topoisomerase (see later, "Topoisomerase Inhibitors"). Secondary mechanisms for cellular destruction involve the formation of free radicals and complexes with iron. Doxorubicin is a prodrug. It is metabolized to the active metabolite idarubicin (Idamycin PFS). It has a long half-life and may be administered as a weekly or monthly infusion. Mitoxantrone is a related compound that damages DNA by producing breaks in the strand.

TECH ALERT!
Doxorubicin and doxorubicin lisosomal are not substitutable.

Anthracyclines

Generic Name	U.S. Brand Name(s) / Canadian Brand Name(s)	Dosage Forms and Strengths
doxorubicin*	Generics	Powder for injection: 10 mg/vial, 20 mg/vial[†], 50 mg/vial, 150 mg/vial[‡]
	Adriamycin PFS	Solution for injection: 2 mg/mL
doxorubicin liposomal	Doxil	Solution, for injection: 2 mg/mL
	Caelyx, Myocet	
epirubicin*	Ellence	Powder, for injection: 50 mg/vial
	Pharmorubicin PFS	Solution, for injection (Ellence, Pharmorubicin PFS): 2 mg/mL
mitoxantrone*	Generics	Solution for injection: 2 mg/mL
	Generics	

*Generic available.
[†]Strength available in the United States only.
[‡]Strength available in Canada only.

Topoisomerase Inhibitors

Generic name	U.S. brand name(s) / Canadian brand(s)	Dosage forms and strengths
etoposide*	Etopophos	Capsule (VePesid): 50 mg[‡]
	VePesid	Powder, injection (Etopophos): 100 mg/vial[†]
		Solution, injection: 20 mg/mL
teniposide	Vumon	Solution, injection: 10 mg/mL
	Vumon	
irinotecan*	Camptosar	Solution, injection: 20 mg/mL, 40 mg/2 mL[†], 100 mg/5 mL[†], 300 mg/15 mL[†]
	Camptosar	
topotecan*	Hycamtin	Capsule: 0.25 mg[†], 1 mg[†]
	Hycamtin	Powder, injection: 4 mg/vial
		Solution, for injection: 1 mg/mL

*Generic available.
[†]Strength available in the United States only.
[‡]Strength available in Canada only.

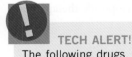

TECH ALERT!
The following drugs have look-alike and sound-alike issues: doxorubicin and doxorubicin liposomal; Ellence and Elase

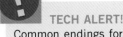

TECH ALERT!
Common endings for topoisomerase inhibitors are -poside and -tecan.

ADVERSE REACTIONS

Doxorubicin is cardiotoxic and may cause heart failure. Mitoxantrone produces less cardiotoxicity. Other side effects produced by the anthracyclines and anthracenediones include heartburn, mouth sores, hair loss, diarrhea, flushing, red or watery eyes, flulike symptoms, and decreased red and white blood cells and platelets. The anthracyclines may turn urine and nails red, whereas mitoxantrone causes them to turn blue-green.

TOPOISOMERASE INHIBITORS

Etoposide, teniposide, irinotecan, and topotecan are topoisomerase inhibitors. Topoisomerase inhibitors are derived from natural and semisynthetic sources. Etoposide and teniposide are semisynthetic derivatives of an extract from the mandrake plant. Irinotecan and topotecan are camptothecin derivatives and are extracted from Camptotheca accuminata (a Chinese tree). Irinotecan is a prodrug. Etoposide is approved for the treatment of testicular cancer and SCLC. Teniposide is approved for the treatment of ALL. Topotecan is indicated for the treatment of ovarian and cervical cancers and SCLC. Irinotecan is only indicated for the treatment of colorectal cancer.

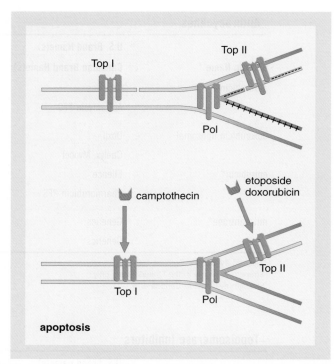

FIGURE 37-3 Site of action of topoisomerase inhibitors. *Top I,* Topoisomerase I; *Top II,* topoisomerase II; *Pol,* DNA polymerase. (From Page C, Curtis M, Sutter M, et al: *Integrated pharmacology,* ed 3, Philadelphia, 2006, Mosby.)

TECH ALERT!
Hycamtin and hycomine have look-alike and sound-alike issues.

TECH ALERT!
Platinum compounds have the common ending *-platin.*

TECH ALERT!
The following drugs have look-alike and sound-alike issues:
carboplatin and cisplatin;
Eloxatin and Aloxi;
Platinol AQ, Plaquenil, Paraplatin AQ, and Patanol

MECHANISM OF ACTION AND PHARMACOKINETICS

Topoisomerases are enzymes that cleave DNA strands, a step needed for DNA replication and RNA transcription (Figure 37-3). Topoisomerase I cleaves one strand of DNA and topoisomerase II cleaves two strands. Topoisomerase II also plays a role in successful mitosis. Oral absorption of the drugs is good but penetration in the central nervous system (CNS) is poor.

ADVERSE REACTIONS

Etoposide and teniposide may cause diarrhea, hair loss, nausea, skin rash, fatigue, irritation at injection site, flulike symptoms, bleeding, or bruising. Irinotecan and topotecan produce similar side effects plus headache, gas, and weight loss. Rarely, individuals on high-dose etoposide therapy may develop acute nonlymphocytic leukemia.

Platinum Compounds

Carboplatin, cisplatin, and oxaliplatin are platinum compounds. Cisplatin is FDA- approved for the treatment of testicular and ovarian cancers. Carboplatin is approved for the treatment of ovarian cancer and oxaliplatin is approved for the treatment of colorectal cancer.

MECHANISM OF ACTION AND PHARMACOKINETICS

The action of platinum compounds on purine bases (adenine and guanine) results in the formation of faulty cross-linkages and defective DNA.

ADVERSE REACTIONS

Side effects of platinum compounds are fatigue, loss of appetite, loss of hair, metallic taste, pain at the site of injection, increased infections, bleeding, bruising, and nausea. Cisplatin may also cause irreversible hearing loss and neurotoxicity. Sensory neurotoxicity produced by oxaliplatin is reversible.

Platinum Compounds

Generic Name	U.S. Brand Name(s) Canadian Brand Name(s)	Dosage Forms and Strengths
carboplatin*	Generics	Powder, for injection: 50 mg/vial†, 150 mg/vial†, 450 mg/vial†
	Generics	Solution for injection: 10 mg/mL
cisplatin*	Generics	Solution for injection: 1 mg/mL
	Generics	
oxaliplatin*†	Eloxatin	Powder, for injection: 50 mg/vial, 100 mg/vial
	Eloxatin	Solution for injection: 5 mg/mL, 50 mg/10 mL†, 100 mg/20 mL†; 200 mg/40 mL†

*Generic available.
*†Generic available in the United States only.
†Strength available in the United States only.

Fluoropyrimidines Used in the Treatment of Colorectal Cancer

Generic Name	U.S. Brand Name(s) Canadian Brand Name(s)	Dosage Forms and Strengths
capecitabine	Xeloda	Tablet: 150 mg, 500 mg
	Xeloda	
fluorouracil (5-FU)*	Carac, Efudex, Fluroplex	Cream: 0.5% (Carac)†, 1% (Fluroplex)†, 5% (Efudex)
	Generics	Solution, for injection: 50 mg/mL Solution, topical (Efudex): 2%†, 5%†
cytarabine*	Cytosar-U	Powder, for injection: 100 mg/vial, 500 mg/vial, 1 g/vial, 2 g/vial
	Cytosar	Solution, for injection: 20 mg/mL, 100 mg/mL
cytarabine liposomal	Depocyt	Suspension, for intrathecal injection: 10 mg/mL
	Depocyt	
fludarabine*	Generics	Powder, for injection: 50 mg/vial
	Fludara	Solution, for injection: 25 mg/mL Tablet: 10 mg‡
gemcitabine*	Gemzar	Powder for injection: 200 mg, 1 g/vial
	Gemzar	

*Generic available.
†Strength available in the United States only.
‡Strength available in Canada only.

TECH ALERT!
The following drugs have look-alike and sound-alike issues:
  cytarabine and cytarabine liposomal;
  cytarabine, Cytoxan, Cytosar, vidarabine, and Cytovene;
  Fludarabine and Flumadine

FLUOROPYRIMIDINES

Capecitabine, cytarabine, gemcitabine, and 5-fluorouracil (5-FU) are fluoropyrimidines, also known as fluorinated pyrimidines. These drugs are indicated for the treatment of several cancers such as colorectal cancer (capecitabine, 5-FU), leukemia (cytarabine), gastric cancer (5-FU), basal cell carcinoma (5-FU), metastatic breast cancer (capecitabine, gemcitabine, 5-FU), lung cancer (gemcitabine), ovarian cancer (gemcitabine), and pancreatic cancer (gemcitabine, 5-FU).

MECHANISM OF ACTION AND PHARMACOKINETICS

Capecitabine and 5-FU are prodrugs. Capecitabine is converted to 5-FU by an enzyme that is present in high levels in tumors. 5-FU must also be activated. Once activated, 5-FU inhibits the enzyme responsible for making thymidine (a DNA nucleoside), inhibits RNA formation, and causes mismatched DNA base pairs (see Figure 37-2).

ADVERSE REACTIONS

Adverse effects linked to capecitabine and 5-FU are stomach upset, loss of appetite, diarrhea or constipation, fatigue, muscle and bone pain, insomnia, headache, and dry, itchy skin. Additional adverse reactions include paresthesia (prickling or tingling sensation) in the hands and feet, jaundice, bone marrow suppression, fatal autoimmune anemias, increased opportunistic infections and cardiotoxicity (capecitabine, 5-FU, and fludarabine).

ANTIMETABOLITES

Methotrexate (MTX) is the principal drug in this class. Pemetrexed is a related compound. Methotrexate is indicated for the treatment of lung cancer, breast cancer, bladder cancer, ALL, cutaneous T-cell lymphoma, lung cancer, non-Hodgkin's lymphoma, and osteogenic sarcoma. It is also indicated for the treatment of rheumatoid arthritis (see Chapter 15). The purine antimetabolites 6-mercaptopurine and 6-thioguanine are primarily indicated for the treatment of acute lymphocytic leukemia. Pentostatin is a structural analogue of the purine adenosine and is indicated for the treatment of hairy cell leukemia.

MECHANISM OF ACTION AND PHARMACOKINETICS

Antimetabolites are chemotherapeutic agents that work most effectively against rapidly dividing cancerous cells. They inhibit normal DNA synthesis by forming abnormal nucleic acid base pairs, resulting in abnormal DNA. Methotrexate is structurally similar to the vitamin folic acid and inhibits folate metabolism, which is essential to the formation of the purines. Pentostatin, 6-mercaptopurine, and 6-thioguanine are purine analogues. Purine bases, along with pyrimidine bases, make up the DNA strand. Methotrexate also causes the depletion of thymidine, a DNA nucleoside, so DNA synthesis ceases and cells die.

ADVERSE REACTIONS

Methotrexate and pemetrexed commonly cause hair loss, photosensitivity, loss of appetite, and nausea. They also decrease the numbers of white and red blood cells and platelets. When white blood cell levels drop, individuals may get infections more easily. Similar adverse reactions are produced by 6-mercaptopurine and 6-thioguanine, with the exception of photosensitivity. Folic acid is commonly prescribed to patients being treated for rheumatoid arthritis with methotrexate. It has been shown to reduce gastrointestinal (GI) side effects and risks for megaloblastic anemia. Supplementation with folic acid is controversial in patients treated for cancer with

TECH ALERT!
The warning label "Avoid aspirin, APAP, and NSAIDs" should be applied to prescription vials for methotrexate because these drugs may decrease methotrexate clearance and cause toxicity. (APAP is acetaminophen; NSAIDs are nonsteroidal anti-inflammatory drugs.)

Antimetabolites

Generic Name	U.S. Brand Name(s) / Canadian Brand Name(s)	Dosage Forms and Strengths
methotrexate* (MTX)	Trexall / Metoject	Powder for injection (generics): 1 g/vial## Solution, for injection: 10 mg/mL (Metoject), 25 mg/mL Tablet (Trexall): 2.5 mg, 5 mg##, 7.5 mg##, 10 mg, 15 mg##
pemetrexed	Alimta / Alimta	Powder for injection: 100 mg/vial, 500 mg/vial
mercaptopurine*	Purinethol / Purinethol	Tablet: 50 mg
thioguanine	Thioguanine / Lanvis	Tablet: 40 mg
pentostatin*	Nipent / Not available	Powder for injection: 10 mg/vial

*Generic available.
##Available in the United States only.

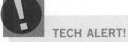
methotrexate. Folic acid may reduce the effectiveness of methotrexate by interfering with its antifolate action.

Miscellaneous Agents

Bleomycin, dactinomycin, and mitomycin are antineoplastic agents approved for the treatment of various cancers. Bleomycin is indicated for the treatment of cervical, penile, testicular, and vulvar cancers in addition to Hodgkin's disease and head and neck cancers. Dactinomycin is indicated for the treatment of testicular cancer, choriocarcinoma, and rhabdomyosarcoma. Mitomycin is approved for gastric and pancreatic cancer treatment. Mytomycin (as Mitosol) is also indicated as an adjunct to glaucoma surgery where it is used to reduce scarring that might result in increased intraocular pressure. Hydroxyurea is indicated for the treatment of head and neck cancers, ovarian cancer, leukemia, and sickle cell anemia. Porifimer is used for the treatment of NSCLC.

MECHANISM OF ACTION AND PHARMACOKINETICS

The primary mechanism of action for bleomycin is to produce breaks in single and double DNA strands. The breaks result in chromosomal gaps and deletions that impair DNA replication. This group of drugs binds reduced iron (Fe^{2+}), which is a secondary mechanism of action. For example, a complex is formed between $Fe2^+$, bleomycin, and oxygen (O_2) in the DNA strand, reducing the O2 necessary for cleavage of the DNA strand. The action of dactinomycin on DNA causes the DNA helix to uncoil and inhibits DNA, RNA, and protein synthesis. Mitomycin therapy results in DNA breaks. Mitomycin also binds to DNA to form abnormal cross-links. Porfimer produces its cytotoxic and antitumor effects only after exposure to light. Photodynamic therapy (PDT) is administered 40 to 50 hours after administration to activate the drug.

ADVERSE REACTIONS

Bleomycin, dactinomycin, and mitomycin may produce pain at the injection site, fatigue, nausea, vomiting, decreased appetite, hair loss, and darkened skin color. Mitomycin may discolor the urine and nails. Mitomycin and bleomycin therapy may result in pulmonary fibrosis and death. Bleomycin and mitomycin may also cause myocardial infarction (MI) and stroke. Dactinomycin and hydroxyurea may cause bone marrow suppression and severe anemias, increasing the risk for infection. Bone marrow suppression and severe anemias are also linked to hydroxyurea.

Miscellaneous Antineoplastic Agents

Generic Name	U.S. Brand Name(s) / Canadian Brand Name(s)	Dosage Forms and Strengths
bleomycin*	Generics	Powder, for injection: 15 units/vial, 30 units/vial[†]
	Generics	
dactinomycin*[†] (actinomycin D)	Cosmegen	Powder, for injection: 500 mcg/vial
	Cosmegen	
mitomycin*	Mitosol	Powder, for injection: 5 mg/vial, 20 mg/vial, 40 mg/vial[†]
	Generics	Solution, topical (Mitosol): 0.2 mg/vial[†]
hydroxyurea*	Droxia, Hydrea	Capsule (Droxia): 200 mg[†], 300 mg[†], 400 mg[†], 500 mg (Hydrea)
	Hydrea	
porfimer	Photofrin	Powder, for injection: 15 mg/vial[‡], 75 mg/vial
	Photofrin	

*Generic available.
*[†]Generic available in the United States only.
[†]Strength available in the United States only.
[‡]Strength available in Canada only.

BIOLOGICAL RESPONSE MODIFIERS

Bevacizumab and trastuzumab are monoclonal antibodies used for the treatment of cancer. Trastuzumab (Herceptin) is used in the treatment of metastatic breast cancer (when tumors overexpress the HER2 protein). Bevacizumab (Avastin) is used for the treatment of several cancers, including colorectal cancer with 5-FU, NSCLC in combination with carboplatin and paclitaxel, renal cancer, and glioblastoma. The mechanism of action of monoclonal antibodies is described in Chapter 15.

Lapatinib (Tykerb) is a biological response modifier that inhibits the kinase components of the epidermal growth factor receptor and HER2 receptors. It is classified as a kinase inhibitor. It is approved for the treatment of breast cancer when taken with capecitabine.

Biological Response Modifiers

Generic Name	U.S. Brand Name(s) Canadian Brand Name(s)	Dosage Forms and Strengths
bevacizumab	Avastin Avastin	Powder, for injection: 100 mg/vial†, 400 mg/vial† Solution, for injection: 25 mg/mL‡
lapatinib	Tykerb Tykerb	Tablet: 250 mg
trastuzumab	Herceptin Herceptin	Powder, for injection: 440 mg/vial

†Strength available in the United States only.
‡Strength available in Canada only.

Summary of Drugs Used for the Treatment of Select Cancers

Generic Name	U.S. Brand Name	Usual Dose And Dosing Schedule	Warning Labels
Hormones			
Selective Estrogen Receptor Modulators			
tamoxifen	Soltamox	Breast cancer: 20-40 mg po twice a day in divided doses	SWALLOW WHOLE (TAMOXIFEN). AVOID PREGNANCY. AVOID GRAPEFRUIT JUICE (TOREMIFENE).
toremifene	Fareston	Breast cancer: 60 mg po once a day	
Estrogen-Receptor Downregulators			
fulvestrant	Faslodex	Breast cancer: 500 mg IM as two 5 mL injection, on day 1, 15, 29 and once monthly thereafter.	AVOID PREGNANCY. REFRIGERATE; DO NOT FREEZE. STORE IN ORIGINAL CONTAINER. PROTECT FROM LIGHT.
Aromatase Inhibitors			
anastrozole	Arimidex	Breast cancer: 1 mg po once daily	AVOID PREGNANCY. TAKE AT THE SAME TIME EACH DAY WITH A DRINK OF WATER. TAKE WITH MEALS (EXEMESTANE). MAY CAUSE DIZZINESS OR DROWSINESS (LETROZOLE).
exemestane	Aromasin	Breast cancer: 25 mg po once daily. Increase to 50 mg daily if taken with CYP3A4 inhibitor	
letrozole	Femara	Breast cancer: 2.5 mg po once daily	

Summary of Drugs Used for the Treatment of Select Cancers—cont'd

Generic Name	U.S. Brand Name	Usual Dose And Dosing Schedule	Warning Labels
Gonadotropin-Releasing Hormone Agonist			
goserelin	Zoladex	**Breast cancer:** 3.6 mg subcut into upper abdominal wall every 28 days **Prostate cancer (advanced):** 3.6 mg subcut implanted into upper abdominal wall every 28 days or 10.8 mg every 12 weeks. **Locally confined Stage T2b-T4 (Stage B2-C):** 8 wks prior to radiation therapy- 3.6 mg SC implant into upper abdominal wall; in 28 days give 10.8 mg implant subcut	AVOID PREGNANCY. STORE AT ROOM TEMPERATURE. INJECT ACCORDING TO PRESCRIBED SCHEDULE.
Progestins			
megestrol acetate*	Megace	**Breast cancer:** 40 mg po four times daily **Endometrial cancer:** 40-320 mg po daily in divided doses	SHAKE WELL (SUSPENSION).
Anthracyclines			
doxorubicin	Adriamycin	**Breast cancer:** 50-60 mg/m^2 IV bolus on day 1 of every 21 days with other agents, this is one of several dosage regimens used in combination with other agents (e.g., cyclophosphamide and fluorouracil, paclitaxel, docetaxel) **Ovarian and SCLC lung cancer:** 40-50 mg/m^2 per dose IV once monthly in combination with various other antineoplastics **Thyroid cancer:** 60-75 mg/m^2 as a single IV dose every 3 weeks, or 25-30 mg/m^2 as a single dose on days 1-3 of a 4-week cycle. May also give 20 mg/m^2 IV once weekly Regimens also for bladder cancer, gastric cancer, and leukemia.	AVOID PREGNANCY. SHAKE WELL (POWDER, FOR INJECTION). REFRIGERATE (DOXORUBICIN, EPIRUBICIN). PROTECT FROM LIGHT (DOXORUBICIN, EPIRUBICIN). MAY CAUSE DISCOLORATION OF URINE (DOXORUBICIN). EXERCISE PRECAUTIONS FOR HANDLING, PREPARING, AND ADMINISTERING CYTOTOXIC DRUGS. STORE AT ROOM TEMPERATURE (MITOXANTRONE). SHAKE VIGOROUSLY TO DISSOLVE (EPIRUBICIN POWDER, FOR INJECTION).
epirubicin	Ellence	**Breast cancer:** 100 mg/m2 IV on day 1 in combination with fluorouracil and cyclophosphamide (FEC regimen) every 21 days for 6 cycles or 60 mg/m^2 IV on days 1 and 8 in combination with oral cyclophosphamide and fluorouracil every 28 days for 6 cycles	
mitoxantrone	generics	**Prostate cancer:** 12-14 mg/m^2 IV every 21 days in combination with prednisone or hydrocortisone.	

Continued

Summary of Drugs Used for the Treatment of Select Cancers—cont'd

Generic Name	U.S. Brand Name	Usual Dose And Dosing Schedule	Warning Labels
Taxanes			
docetaxel	Taxotere	**Breast Cancer (advanaced, metastatic):** 60-100 mg/m^2 IV over 1 hour once every 3 weeks	AVOID PREGNANCY. DO NOT SHAKE (DOCETAXEL). REFRIGERATE; DON'T FREEZE (DOCETAXEL). RECONSTITUTED SOLUTION IS STABLE FOR A CERTAIN LENGTH OF TIME: DOCETAXEL (4 HR); PACLITAXEL (27 HR), NANOPARTICLE ALBUMIN-BOUND PACLITAXEL (8 HR). STORE AT ROOM TEMPERATURE (PACLITAXEL). PROTECT FROM LIGHT (DOCETAXEL, PACLITAXEL). DO NOT MIX IN PVC BAGS OR USE PVC SETS (DOCETAXEL, PACLITAXEL). EXERCISE PRECAUTIONS FOR HANDLING, PREPARING, AND ADMINISTERING CYTOTOXIC DRUGS (DOCETAXEL, PACLITAXEL). AVOID ASPIRIN, APAP, AND NSAIDS.
paclitaxel	Taxol	**Breast Cancer (metastatic):** 175 mg/m^2 IV over 3 hours every 3 weeks	
nanoparticle albumin bound paclitaxel	Abraxane	**Breast Cancer:** 100 mg-260 mg/m^2 IV over 30 minutes once per week for 3 weeks, then one week off, every 28 days (dose depends on previously untreated or taxane-refractory)	
Fluoropyrimidines			
5-fluorouracil	Adrucil	**Breast cancer (metastatic):** 400-600 mg/m^2 IV bolus on days 1 and 8 of every cycle in combination with cyclophosphamide and methotrexate or 600 mg/m^2 IV bolus on day 1 in combination with cyclophosphamide and methotrexate (CMF) every 21-28 days. Regimens also for colorectal, gastric, and pancreatic cancer.	EXERCISE PRECAUTIONS FOR HANDLING, PREPARING, AND ADMINISTERING CYTOTOXIC DRUGS. ONCE THE PHARMACY BULK VIAL IS OPENED, ANY UNUSED PORTION SHOULD BE DISCARDED AFTER 1 HR. AVOID PREGNANCY. AVOID PROLONGED EXPOSURE TO SUNLIGHT. AVOID ASPIRIN, APAP, AND NSAIDS. STORE AT ROOM TEMPERATURE. PROTECT FROM LIGHT.

Summary of Drugs Used for the Treatment of Select Cancers—cont'd

Generic Name	U.S. Brand Name	Usual Dose And Dosing Schedule	Warning Labels
capecitabine	Xeloda	**Breast cancer:** 2500 mg/m²/day PO in 2 divided doses for 2 weeks, repeated every 3 weeks **Colorectal cancer:** 1250 mg/m² PO twice daily within 30 minutes for 2 weeks, repeated every 3 weeks for a total of 8 cycles.	TAKE WITH FOOD (CAPECITABINE). AVOID PREGNANCY. AVOID ASPIRIN, APAP, AND NSAIDS. EXERCISE PRECAUTIONS FOR HANDLING, PREPARING, AND ADMINISTERING CYTOTOXIC DRUGS. REFRIGERATE; DO NOT FREEZE (CYTARABINE, FLUDARABINE POWDER, FOR INJECTION). STORE AT ROOM TEMPERATURE (GEMCITABINE). RECONSTITUTED SOLUTIONS ARE STABLE FOR 8 HR (FLUDARABINE). SWALLOW WHOLE (FLUDARABINE TABLETS).
cytarabine, liposomal (ARA-C)	Depocyt	**Leukemia:** 50 mg intrathecally over 1-5 minutes every 14 days during induction and consolidation weeks 1,3,5,7, and 9, give and additional 50 mg intrathecally at week 13.	
fludarabine	Fludara	**Chronic Lymphocytic Leukemia:** **IV:** 25 mg/m² IV once daily for 5 days every 28 days (Continue 3 cycles after maximum response achieved) **PO:** 40 mg/m²/day PO on days 1-5 given every 4 weeks (Continue 3 cycles after maximum response achieved)	
gemcitabine	Gemzar	**Breast cancer (metastatic):** 1250 mg/m² IV over 30 minutes on days 1 and 8 of a 21-day cycle in combination with paclitaxel **Lung cancer (NSCLC):** 1000 mg/m² IV on days 1, 8, 15 of a 28-day cycle or 1250 mg/m² on days 1 and 8 of a 21-day cycle. Cisplatin (100 mg/m² IV) is given following the gemcitabine infusion on day 1 of either regimen. **Ovarian cancer:** 1000 mg/m² IV over 30 minutes on days 1 and 8 of a 21-day cycle in comination with carboplatin on day 1 after gemcitabine infusion **Pancreatic cancer:** 1000 mg/m² IV over 30 minutes once weekly for up to 7 consecutive weeks, followed by one week of rest	

Continued

Summary of Drugs Used for the Treatment of Select Cancers—cont'd

Generic Name	U.S. Brand Name	Usual Dose And Dosing Schedule	Warning Labels
Antimetabolites			
methotrexate	Generics	**Lung cancer (SCLC): PO:** 10 mg/m2 PO twice weekly x4 doses every 3 weeks in combination with lomustine and cyclophosphamide **IV:** 20 mg/m2 IV as a single dose with cisplatin, doxorubicin, and cyclophosphamide, every 28 days or numerous other regimens. **Breast cancer:** 40-60 mg/m² IV given on day 1 of every 21-28 days along with cyclophosphamide and fluorouracil. Also regimens for bladder cancer, Non-Hodgkin's lymphoma, and acute lymphocytic leukemia.	PROTECT FROM LIGHT (METHOTREXATE). STORE AT ROOM TEMPERATURE. RECONSTITUTE POWDER IMMEDIATELY BEFORE USE AND DISCARD ANY UNUSED PORTION (METHOTREXATE). TAKE WITH A FULL GLASS OF WATER. MAY MAKE SKIN MORE SENSITIVE TO SUNLIGHT. AVOID PREGNANCY. DO NOT DRINK ALCOHOLIC BEVERAGES (METHOTREXATE). EXERCISE PRECAUTIONS FOR HANDLING, PREPARING, AND ADMINISTERING CYTOTOXIC DRUGS. REFRIGERATE AND USE WITHIN 24 HR OF RECONSTITUTION; DISCARD ANY UNUSED PORTION (PEMETREXED).
pemetrexed	Alimta	**Lung cancer (NSCLC):** 500 mg/m² over 10 minutes on day 1 of each 21-day cycle.	
6-mercaptopurine	Purinethol	**Acute lymphocytic leukemia:** 2.5 mg- 5 mg /kg/day PO once daily. Maintenance dose: 1.5-2.5 mg/kg/day once daily.	TAKE WITH A FULL GLASS OF WATER. AVOID ASPIRIN, APAP, AND NSAIDS. AVOID PREGNANCY. PROTECT FROM MOISTURE (MERCAPTOPURINE). TAKE AS DIRECTED; DON'T SKIP DOSES.
6-thioguanine	Tabloid	**Acute lymphocytic leukemia:** 2-3 mg/kg/day PO or 100 mg/m²/day PO every 12 hours for 5-10 days, usually in combination with cytarabine.	
Vinca Alkaloids			
vinorelbine	Navelbine	**Breast Cancer:** 30 mg/m2 IV over 6 to 10 minutes weekly or on days 1 and 8 repeated every 21 days **Lung cancer (NSCLC):** 30 mg/m² IV over 6-10 minutes once weekly or 25-30 mg/m² once weekly with cisplatin	REFRIGERATE; DO NOT FREEZE (VINORELBINE). PROTECT FROM LIGHT (VINORELBINE). AVOID ASPIRIN, APAP, AND NSAIDS. EXERCISE PRECAUTIONS FOR HANDLING, PREPARING, AND ADMINISTERING CYTOTOXIC DRUGS. SYRINGES MUST BE LABELED "FATAL IF GIVEN INTRATHECALLY. FOR IV USE ONLY."
vinblastine	Generics	**Breast Cancer:** 4.5 mg/m² IV on day 1 of every 21 days in combination with doxorubicin and thiotepa Regimens also for NSCLC, Hodgkin's disease, non-Hodgkin's lymphoma, and testicular cancer	
vincristine	Vincasar PFS	**Acute Lymphocytic Leukemia:** 1.4 - 2 mg/m² IV weekly for 4 weeks during the induction phase.	

Summary of Drugs Used for the Treatment of Select Cancers—cont'd

Generic Name	U.S. Brand Name	Usual Dose And Dosing Schedule	Warning Labels
Platinum Compounds			
carboplatin	Generics	**Ovarian cancer:** 300 mg/m² IV on day 1 in combination with cyclophosphamide, repeated every 4 weeks for 6 cycles or 360 mg/m² IV on day 1, repeated every 4 weeks. Other regimens also recommended.	AVOID PREGNANCY. AVOID ASPIRIN, APAP, AND NSAIDS. EXERCISE PRECAUTIONS FOR HANDLING, PREPARING, AND ADMINISTERING CYTOTOXIC DRUGS. STABLE FOR 28 DAYS ONCE VIAL IS PENETRATED (CISPLATIN). PROTECT FROM LIGHT. STORE AT ROOM TEMPERATURE. RECONSTITUTED SOLUTION IS STABLE FOR 8 HR (CARBOPLATIN). RECONSTITUTED SOLUTION AND IVS ARE STABLE FOR 24 HR IF REFRIGERATED.
cisplatin	Generics	**Lung cancer (NSCLC):** 75 mg/m² IV as a single dose following administration of paclitaxel or docetaxel every 3 weeks. Other regimens also recommended. **Testicular cancer:** 20 mg/m² IV as a single dose once daily for 5 days with bleomycin and etoposide, repeated every 3 weeks for 2 cycles or more. **Ovarian cancer:** 50-60 mg/m² IV as a single dose once every 21 days in combination with cyclophosphamide or 75 mg/m² IV as a single dose once every 21 days in combination with paclitaxel	
oxaliplatin	Eloxatin	**Colorectal cancer:** Day 1, oxaliplatin 85 mg/m² IV infusion with leucovorin IV infusion given over 2 hours, followed by 5-FU IV bolus over 2-4 minutes; then 5-FU IV infusion over 22 hours. Day 2, leucovorin 200 mg/m² IV over 2 hours followed by 5-FU IV bolus over 2-4 minutes, then 5-FU IV continuous infusion over 22 hours. The 2-day regimen is repeated every 2 weeks.	
Topoisomerase Inhibitors			
etoposide	VePesid	**Testicular cancer:** 100 mg/m²/day on days 1-5 in combination with bleomycin and cisplatin or 100 mg/m²/day IV on days 1, 3, and 5. Repeated every 3 or 4 weeks. **Lung cancer (SCLC):** 35 mg/m²/day IV for 4 days to 50 mg/m²/day IV for 5 days in combination with other antineoplastics.	TAKE WITH A FULL GLASS OF WATER (ETOPOSIDE CAPSULE). SWALLOW WHOLE; DON'T CRUSH OR CHEW (ETOPOSIDE CAPSULE). AVOID PREGNANCY. RECONSTITUTED SOLUTION IS STABLE FOR 24 HR AT ROOM TEMPERATURE. EXERCISE PRECAUTIONS FOR HANDLING, PREPARING, AND ADMINISTERING CYTOTOXIC DRUGS MAY CAUSE DIZZINESS OR DROWSINESS. AVOID ASPIRIN, APAP, AND NSAIDS.
teniposide	Vumon	**Acute lymphocytic leukemia in children:** 165 mg/m² IV twice weekly for 8-9 doses or 250 mg/m² IV once weekly for 4-8 weeks.	

Continued

Summary of Drugs Used for the Treatment of Select Cancers—cont'd

Generic Name	U.S. Brand Name	Usual Dose And Dosing Schedule	Warning Labels
irinotecan	Camptosar	**Colorectal cancer:** 125 mg/m² IV over 90 minutes, once weekly for 4 weeks, every 6 weeks or 350 mg/m² by IV infusion over 90 minutes, once every 3 weeks. Other regimens with irinotecan followed by leucovorin and 5-FU.	SWALLOW WHOLE; DON'T CRUSH OR CHEW (TOPOTECAN CAPSULES). TAKE WITH A FULL GLASS OF WATER (TOPOTECAN CAPSULES). PROTECT FROM LIGHT. AVOID ASPIRIN, APAP, AND NSAIDS. EXERCISE PRECAUTIONS FOR HANDLING, PREPARING, AND ADMINISTERING CYTOTOXIC DRUGS. RECONSTITUTED SOLUTION IS STABLE FOR 24 HR AT ROOM TEMPERATURE (TOPOTECAN).
topotecan	Hycamtin	**Ovarian cancer:** 1.5 mg/m²/day IV on days 1-5 of a 21-day course. **Cervical cancers:** 0.75 mg/m² IV on days 1-3 in combination with cisplatin IV day 1 only, every 3 weeks **Lung cancer (SCLC):** 1.5-2.3 mg/m²/day PO on days 1-5 of a 21-day course.	

Epothilones

ixabepilone	Ixempra	**Breast cancer:** 40 mg/m² IV over 3 hours, given every 3 weeks in regimens with and without capcitabine.	AVOID PREGNANCY. MAY CAUSE DIZZINESS OR DROWSINESS. AVOID ASPIRIN, APAP, AND NSAIDS. RECONSTITUTED SOLUTION IS STABLE FOR 6 HR AT ROOM TEMPERATURE.

Biologic Response Modifiers

bevacizumab	Avastin	**Colorectal cancer:** 5 or 10 mg/kg IV every 14 days in combination with 5-FU. **Lung cancer (NSCLC):** 15 mg/kg IV every 3 weeks in combination with carboplatin and paclitaxel.	REFRIGERATE; DO NOT FREEZE. AVOID PREGNANCY.
lapatinib	Tykerb	**Breast cancer:** 1250 mg (5 tablets) PO once daily on days 1-21 plus capecitabine 2000 mg/m²/day PO in 2 divided doses on days 1-14 in a repeating 21 day cycle.	TAKE WITH A FULL GLASS OF WATER. TAKE ON AN EMPTY STOMACH. AVOID GRAPEFRUIT JUICE. AVOID PREGNANCY. PROTECT FROM MOISTURE.
trastuzumab	Herceptin	**Metastatic breast cancer:** 4 mg/kg IV infused over 90 minutes on week 1; if tolerated, at week 2, decrease to 2 mg/kg over at least 30 minutes once weekly. Several other recommended regimens.	AVOID PREGNANCY. REFRIGERATE; DON'T FREEZE.

Summary of Drugs Used for the Treatment of Select Cancers—cont'd

Generic Name	U.S. Brand Name	Usual Dose And Dosing Schedule	Warning Labels
Miscellaneous Agents			
actinomycin D (dactinomycin)	Cosmegen	Testicular cancer: 1000 mcg/m^2 IV as a single dose on day 1 as part of a combination regimen with cyclophosphamide, bleomycin, vinblastine, and cisplastin.	AVOID PREGNANCY. AVOID ASPIRIN, APAP, AND NSAIDS. PROTECT FROM LIGHT (DACTINOMYCIN). EXERCISE PRECAUTIONS FOR HANDLING, PREPARING, AND ADMINISTERING CYTOTOXIC DRUGS. RECONSTITUTED SOLUTION IS STABLE FOR 24 HR (BLEOMYCIN). REFRIGERATE; DO NOT FREEZE (BLEOMYCIN POWDER). MAY DISCOLOR URINE (MITOMYCIN).
bleomycin	Blenoxane	Cervical, head & neck, and vulvar cancers: 5-20 units/m^2 (0.25-0.5 units/kg) IV, IM, SC 1 or 2 times per week. Testicular cancer: 10-20 units/m^2 (0.25-0.5 units/kg) IV, IM or subcut given 1 or 2 times per week.	
mitomycin	Generics	Gastric and pancreatic cancer: 20 mg/m^2 IV every 6-8 weeks in combination with other chemotherapeutic agents	
hydroxyurea	Droxia	Ovarian & head and neck cancer: 80 mg/kg PO every third in combination with radiation therapy. Leukemia (CML): 50-100 mg/kg PO daily initially, then 10-30 mg/kg PO once daily maintenance.	TAKE WITH LOTS OF WATER. AVOID ASPIRIN, APAP, AND NSAIDS.
eribulin	Halaven	Breast cancer: 1.4 mg/m^2 IV over 2 to 5 minutes on days 1 and 8, repeated every 21 days.	AVOID PREGNANCY. AVOID ASPIRIN, APAP, AND NSAIDS. STORE AT ROOM TEMPERATURE.
estramustine	Emcyt	Prostate cancer: 14 mg/kg/day or 600 mg/m^2/day PO in 3-4 divided doses.	AVOID PREGNANCY. AVOID ASPIRIN, APAP, AND NSAIDS. TAKE ON AN EMPTY STOMACH. AVOID DAIRY PRODUCTS WITHIN 2-3 HR OF DOSE.
porfimer	Photofrin	Lung cancer (NSCLC): 2 mg/kg IV administered over 3-5 minutes followed 40-50 hours later by laser illumination at the site(s) of tumor involvement.	AVOID PREGNANCY. PROTECT EYES FROM SUNLIGHT.

Chapter Summary

- Cancer is a disease that occurs when new cells form more rapidly than needed; the cells accumulate and form a mass called a tumor.
- A malignant tumor is cancerous and can invade and destroy nearby tissue and spread to other parts of the body; a benign tumor is not cancerous and does not spread.
- Cancers are named according to the site at which the cancerous growth began. This is the site of the primary tumor.
- Age, tobacco smoking or chewing, ionizing radiation and sunlight, hazardous chemicals, environmental pollutants, bacterial and viral infection, hormone therapy, family history, alcohol consumption, and diet, obesity, and lack of physical activity are all risk factors for cancer.

- Advancing age (>61 years) and a history of hormone replacement therapy increase the risk for breast cancer.
- Mammography and breast self-examination are important screening examinations used to detect breast cancer.
- Cancer of the cervix is linked to human papillomavirus and exposure to the drug diethylstilbestrol.
- A Pap test (Pap smear) is a screening test for cancer of the cervix.
- Endometrial cancer most commonly affects postmenopausal women.
- Skin cancer is one of the most common types of cancer.
- Skin cancer is divided into two categories, melanoma and nonmelanoma. The most treatable form is nonmelanoma.
- Skin cancer is associated with excessive exposure to ultraviolet light from the sun or UV lights used in tanning salons. Wearing protective clothing or using a sunscreen when outdoors is recommended.
- There are two types of lung cancer, small cell lung cancer and non–small cell lung cancer.
- A history of smoking tobacco is almost always the cause of small cell lung cancer.
- Colonoscopy and the fecal occult blood test are screening tests for colorectal cancer.
- The incidence of prostrate cancer increases as men grow older.
- Screening tests are recommended for the early diagnosis of breast cancer, colorectal cancer, cancer of the cervix, and prostate cancer.
- A digital rectal examination and a PSA test are screening tests for prostate cancer.
- Staging is a method used to describe how far the cancer has progressed within the body.
- Cancer may be treated with chemotherapy, biological therapy, radiation therapy, and surgery.
- Chemotherapy is the use of drugs to kill or slow the growth of cancerous cells.
- Biological therapy is the administration of immune system modulators to boost the body's natural defense against abnormal, invasive, and cancerous cells.
- The following factors influence the choice for treatment: (1) type of cancer; (2) stage of cancer; (3) individual tolerance for adverse effects of treatment; (4) patient's age; (5) histological and nuclear grade of the primary tumor; and (6) capacity of the cancer to metastasize.
- The hormones estrogen and progesterone can promote the growth of estrogen receptor–positive (ER-positive) and/or progesterone receptor–positive (PR-positive) breast cancer.
- Antiestrogens are used for the treatment of ER–positive breast cancer.
- Tamoxifen and toremifene are selective ER modulators indicated for the treatment of ER–positive breast cancer.
- Most antineoplastic agents are classified in FDA pregnancy risk category D. The warning label "Avoid Pregnancy" should be applied to the prescription vial.
- Fulvestrant is an ER downregulator approved for the treatment of breast cancer.
- A common ending for aromatase inhibitors is -trozole.
- Anastrozole, exemestane, and letrozole are aromatase inhibitors approved for the treatment of breast cancer.
- Goserelin is a gonadotropin-releasing hormone agonist indicated for the treatment of advanced breast cancer in premenopausal and perimenopausal women with ER-positive disease and for prostate cancer in men.
- Megestrol acetate is a progestin approved for the treatment of breast cancer.
- Medroxyprogesterone acetate is approved for the treatment of inoperable metastatic endometrial cancer and renal cell cancer.
- Cyclophosphamide (Cytoxan), busulfan (Busulfex, Myleran), ifosfamide (Ifex), melphalan (Alkeran), mechlorethamine (Mustargen), and chlorambucil (Leukeran) are all alkylating agents.
- A common ending for taxanes is -taxel.
- Taxanes are cytotoxic drugs that are naturally derived from the Western yew (paclitaxel) and the European yew (docetaxel) trees.
- Vinorelbine, vincristine, and vinblastine are vinca alkaloids. They are naturally derived from the periwinkle plant. A common beginning for vinca alkaloids is vin-.
- A common ending for anthracyclines is -rubicin.
- Doxorubicin, epirubicin, and idarubicin are anthracyclines. Mitoxantrone is a related compound and is classified as an anthracenedione.

- Doxorubicin and epirubicin are indicated for the treatment of breast cancer.
- Doxorubicin liposomal is approved for the treatment of ovarian cancer, Kaposi's sarcoma, and multiple myeloma.
- The anthracyclines may turn urine and nails red, whereas mitoxantrone causes them to turn blue-green.
- Common endings for topoisomerase inhibitors are *-poside* and *-tecan*.
- Etoposide, teniposide, irinotecan, and topotecan are topoisomerase inhibitors.
- Teniposide is approved for the treatment of acute lymphocytic leukemia. Topotecan is indicated for the treatment of ovarian, cervical, and small cell lung cancers. Irinotecan is only indicated for the treatment of colorectal cancer.
- Platinum compounds have the common ending *-platin*.
- Cisplatin is approved for the treatment of testicular and ovarian cancer, carboplatin is approved for the treatment of ovarian cancer, and oxaliplatin is approved for the treatment of colorectal cancer.
- Capecitabine, cytarabine, gemcitabine, and 5-fluorouracil are fluoropyrimidines, also known as fluorinated pyrimidines.
- Antimetabolites are chemotherapeutic agents that work by inhibiting normal DNA synthesis by forming abnormal nucleic acid base pairs, resulting in abnormal DNA.
- Pentostatin, 6-mercaptopurine, and 6-thioguanine are purine analogues. Purine bases, along with pyrimidine bases, make up the DNA strand.
- Bleomycin, dactinomycin, and mitomycin are antineoplastic agents approved for the treatment of various cancers. They interfere with DNA, RNA, and protein synthesis.
- A common ending for monoclonal antibodies is *-mab*.
- Bevacizumab (Avastin) and trastuzumab (Herceptin) are monoclonal antibodies used for the treatment of metastatic breast cancer.
- Porfimer produces its cytotoxic and antitumor effects only after exposure to light.

REVIEW QUESTIONS

1. Leukemia is cancer that starts in the _____.
   a. Immune systems
   b. Bones
   c. Blood-forming tissues
   d. Skin

2. Cancerous tumors that can invade and destroy nearby tissue and spread to other parts of the body are termed _____.
   a. Benign
   b. Malignant
   c. Invasive
   d. Tumors

3. Cancers are more prevalent in persons older than 65 years.
   a. True
   b. False

4. Cancer of the cervix is linked to the _____.
   a. Herpes simples virus
   b. Human immunodeficiency virus
   c. Varicella zoster virus
   d. Human papillomavirus

5. Early diagnosis is really not associated with successful treatment of cancer.
   a. True
   b. False

6. Cancer may be treated with _____.
   a. Chemotherapy
   b. Biological therapy
   c. Radiation therapy
   d. All of the above

7. Hormone therapy is a treatment of choice for _____ cancer.
   a. Breast
   b. Lung
   c. Cervical
   d. Skin

8. _____ are one of the oldest classes of antineoplastic agents. They are related to nitrogen mustard, a lethal gas that was used for chemical warfare in World War I.
   a. Antimetabolites
   b. Antitumor antibiotics
   c. Alkylating agents
   d. Hormones

9. Which one of the following is not a vinca alkaloid?
   a. Vinorelbine
   b. Vincristine
   c. Vinblastine
   d. Venlafaxine

10. These drugs commonly cause hair loss, photosensitivity, loss of appetite, and nausea. They also decrease the numbers of white and red blood cells and platelets.
    a. Methotrexate
    b. Pemetrexed
    c. Paclitaxel
    d. a and b

TECHNICIAN'S CORNER

1. There have been many reports of the destruction of the rain forests and the possibility of losing potential cures for cancer. What can we do to prevent this from happening?
2. What are some new innovations being used to deliver chemotherapeutic agents in doses that will not harm good cells?

Bibliography

Elsevier: Gold Standard Clinical Pharmacology. Retrieved December 9, 2011, from https://www.clinicalpharmacology.com/, 2010.

FDA: FDA Approved Drug Products. Retrieved June 29, 2012, from http://www.accessdata.fda.gov/scripts/cder/drugsatfda/index.cfm?fuseaction=Search.Search_Drug_Name, 2012.

Health Canada: Drug Product Database. Retrieved June 29, 2012, from http://www.hc-sc.gc.ca/dhp-mps/prodpharma/databasdon/index-eng.php, 2010.

Kalant H, Grant D, Mitchell J: *Principles of medical pharmacology*, ed 7, Toronto, 2007, Elsevier Canada, pp 777-790.

Lance L, Lacy C, Armstrong L, et al: *Drug information handbook for the allied health professional*, ed 12, Hudson, OH, 2005, APhA Lexi-Comp.

National Cancer Institute: What you need to know about cancer (NIH Publ.No. 06-1566), htttp://www.cancer.gov/cancertopics/wyntk/cancer/WYNTK_Cancer.pdf, 2005.

National Cancer Institute, Surveillance Epidemiology and End Results (SEER): Cancer stat fact sheets, http://seer.cancer.gov/statfacts, 2011.

Page C, Curtis M, Sutter M, et al: *Integrated pharmacology*, Philadelphia, 2005, Elsevier Mosby, pp 163-185.

Thibodeau G, Patton K: *Anatomy and physiology*, ed 6, St. Louis, 2007, Mosby, pp 121-133.

USP Center for the Advancement of Patient Safety: USP Quality Review No. 79: Use caution: Avoid confusion, Rockville, MD, 2004, USP Center for the Advancement of Patient Safety.

38

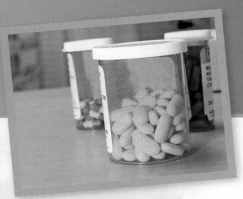

Vaccines, Immunomodulators, and Immunosuppressants

KEY TERMS

Antigen: Substance, usually a protein fragment, that causes an immune response.

Cold chain: Set of safe handling practices ensuring that vaccines and immunologicals requiring refrigeration are maintained at the required temperature from the time of manufacture until the time of administration to patients.

Conjugate vaccine: Vaccine that links antigens or toxoids to the polysaccharide or sugar molecules that certain bacteria use as a protective device to disguise themselves.

Immunomodulator: Chemical agent that modifies the immune response or the functioning of the immune system.

Immunosuppressant: Drug that inhibits proliferation of the cells of the immune system; also known as immunopharmacological.

Immunization: Deliberate artificial exposure to disease to produce acquired immunity.

Inactivated killed vaccine: Killed vaccine. It provides less immunity than a live vaccine but has fewer risks for vaccine-induced disease.

Live attenuated vaccine: Living, but weakened, version of the invader that does not cause disease in nonimmunocompromised individuals (nonvirulent).

Toxoid vaccine: Vaccine that stimulates the immune system to produce antibodies to a specific toxin that causes illness.

Vaccine: Substance that prevents disease by taking advantage of your body's ability to make antibodies and prime killer cells to fight disease.

Overview

An *immunization* is defined as a deliberate artificial exposure to disease to produce acquired immunity. Immunization is achieved by administering vaccines. Vaccines prevent disease by taking advantage of your body's ability to make antibodies and prime killer cells to disease-causing microbes and viruses. Under normal circumstances, cells of your immune system can distinguish between the cells that are part of your body, harmless bacteria normally found in your body, and harmful invaders that need to be destroyed. The first time that your body is exposed to a harmful virus or bacterium, the immune system releases macrophages, cytotoxic T cells, and B cells. The macrophages digest most parts of the virus or bacterium, but not the *antigens*. B cells secrete antibodies to the antigens and, if the person is exposed to the virus or bacteria again, the antibodies will inactivate the antigen. Cytotoxic T cells designed to destroy the virus or bacteria are also released on exposure to antigens. A *vaccine* is an altered antigen injected into your body that does not cause disease but stimulates your immune system's production of antibodies and cytotoxic T cells, and therefore provides protection against the disease if you are exposed to it again.

Types of Vaccines

Live attenuated vaccines are a living, but weakened, version of the invader, so they do not cause disease (are nonvirulent) in healthy individuals. They can, however, mutate to a virulent strain of the virus. Polio, measles, mumps, and rubella vaccines are live vaccines. *Inactivated killed vaccines* are advantageous because they cannot mutate, but they produce less immunity compared with live vaccines. Booster shots are usually required to ensure continued immunity. Flu, hepatitis A, and polio vaccines are inactivated killed vaccines. *Toxoid vaccines* stimulate the immune system to produce antibodies to the toxins that cause illness (e.g., tetanus and diphtheria). *Conjugate vaccines* link antigens or toxoids to the polysaccharide or sugar molecules that certain bacteria use as a protective device to disguise themselves. Conjugate vaccines allow the immune system to recognize and attack these disguised bacteria. *Haemophilus influenzae* type B (Hib) is a conjugate vaccine.

Special Handling Conditions for Vaccines

THE COLD CHAIN

Vaccines and immunologicals requiring refrigeration (Box 38-1) must be protected from extremes in temperature. Exposure to freezing temperatures or heat can destroy their integrity and make them unusable.

TECH ALERT!
Pharmacies, pharmacists, and pharmacy technicians play a key role in ensuring that breaches in the cold chain are avoided.

BOX 38-1   **Vaccines Requiring Refrigeration***

- Diphtheria and tetanus toxoids (DT)
- Diphtheria and tetanus toxoids, and pertussis (adsorbed) (DPT)
- Diphtheria toxoid + hepatitis B surface antigen + pertussis vaccine (adsorbed) + poliovirus vaccine (inactivated) + tetanus toxoid
- Diphtheria and tetanus toxoids, adsorbed pertussis vaccine (adsorbed), inactivated polio vaccine, and *Haemophilus influenzae* type b (Hib) conjugate vaccine
- Hepatitis A vaccine
- Hepatitis B vaccine
- Hib conjugate vaccine
- Inactivated polio vaccine
- Influenza vaccine
- Measles, mumps, and rubella (MMR) vaccine
- Meningococcal A/C/Y/W vaccine
- Pneumococcal polysaccharide 7-polyvalent vaccine
- Pneumococcal polysaccharide 23-polvalent vaccine
- Rabies vaccine
- Tuberculosis testing solution

*At 2°-8° C (36°-46° F).

The *cold chain* refers to a set of safe handling practices that ensure vaccines and immunologicals requiring refrigeration are maintained at the required temperature from the time of manufacture until the time of administration to patients. This means that they must be maintained at a constant temperature from 2° to 8° C (36° to 46° F) throughout the transport process and placed in appropriate storage units once they are delivered to their final destination.

WHY COLD STORAGE IS IMPORTANT

Disruption of the cold chain is a public health threat. When the cold chain is disrupted, the effectiveness and shelf life of vaccines are reduced. The stability of the vaccine decreases exponentially with each increase in temperature. Once the integrity of the vaccine is compromised, it cannot be restored by returning the vaccine to the refrigerator. Loss of potency and effectiveness is cumulative. Each time the cold chain is breached, the vaccine's effectiveness is further reduced. Ultimately, patients are placed at risk when suboptimal vaccines are administered. In addition to vaccine failure, patients may experience increased reactions at the injection site. The severity of problems linked to disruption of the cold chain is dependent on whether the vaccine is chemical or biological and whether the dosage form is an aqueous solution, suspension, or dry powder. Dry powders and chemicals are least affected by breaches in the cold chain. Vaccines and other biological solutions and suspensions are most sensitive to breaches in the cold chain. They are more sensitive to degradation. Disruption of the cold chain is also costly. Vaccines that expire or that have been stored improperly must be destroyed.

COLD CHAIN MAINTENANCE

Maintenance of the cold chain involves appropriate selection and maintenance of refrigeration units and transport containers capable of storing drug products at required temperatures.

Refrigeration Units

When feasible, the pharmacy should place vaccines in a refrigerator designated solely for vaccines. If a separate refrigerator is not feasible, vaccines should be kept separate from other refrigerated pharmaceuticals. Pharmacies that handle a large volume of vaccines should purchase a walk-in refrigeration unit. If the refrigerator is overstocked, air circulation is insufficient to maintain constant temperatures. The refrigeration unit should be equipped with a minimum-maximum thermometer to monitor temperature fluctuations and a continuous temperature-recording device. An alarm that signals when the refrigeration unit is out of range should be installed in the refrigerator. Monitors and thermometers should be calibrated routinely.

It is important to place the refrigerator in a location away from a heat source because this can affect the performance of the unit. The refrigerator cord should also be strategically placed to avoid accidental unplugging from the electrical outlet.

Protocols for Receiving, Stocking, and Storing Drugs

An important component of the cold chain is establishment and adherence to protocols for receiving, stocking, storing, and transporting drugs requiring refrigeration. The pharmacy team should develop these protocols in accordance with national guidelines. Protocols for receiving vaccines should include accurate assessment of the condition of vaccines received by the pharmacy. Pharmacy personnel should be alert for warning signs that the cold chain has been broken during shipment. This might be as simple as noticing that freezer packs have thawed or that the dry ice placed in the transport container with a vaccine has evaporated. Unfortunately, exposure to heat or freezing that results in damage to the vaccine is not easy to detect because no changes in color or appearance occur. There are no visual indicators. Shaking the vaccine may reveal clumps in the vaccine that indicate freezing; often, however, no clumps are visible, making this method unreliable.

A procedure should be established to ensure that vaccines stocked are rotated to avoid wastage caused by outdated supplies. Expiration dates should be checked and vaccines stocked so that those that expire soon are placed in front of vaccines that expire later. Vaccines should not be removed from the refrigerator until the time of dispensing, unless the vaccine must be transported. This is especially important for pneumococcal or influenza vaccines that are purchased in multidose vials.

Transport

Pharmacy personnel in charge of transporting vaccines are responsible for making sure that vaccines arrive at their destination at the proper temperature. How long the vaccine will be out of the refrigerator must be considered when determining the type of transport container. In most cases, vaccines should be transported in an insulated container. Protocols should be followed regarding the number of ice packs needed. Vaccines should always be positioned to avoid direct contact with the ice packs. Heat and cold monitors should also be included in the transport container, if necessary.

Vaccines should be dispensed to patients with accurate advice for transport and storage. Extremes in heat and cold must be avoided; vaccines should never be placed in the hot glove compartment of a car. If the travel time between the pharmacy and the patient's destination, where a refrigerator is located, is less than 20 minutes, the vaccine should be dispensed in an insulated bag. If transport time is longer than 20 minutes, the vaccine should be transported with ice packs in an insulated container. See Figure 38-1 for a diagram explaining the importance of the pharmacy technician in cold chain management.

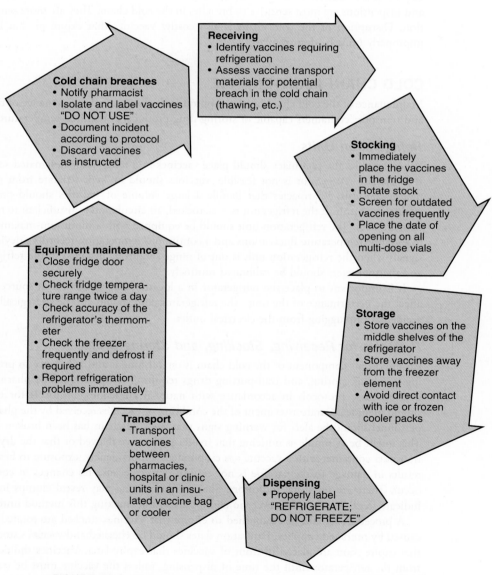

FIGURE 38-1 Pharmacy technician's role in maintaining the cold chain.

Immunizations

Vaccines are administered to provide immunity to a wide variety of childhood diseases, as well as influenza, hepatitis, pneumonia, viral meningitis, rabies, and other conditions. Sufficient immunity may be achieved after a single immunization; however, many vaccines must be administered as a series or require a booster shot. Epidemiologists track flu infections from sentinel sites around the globe to determine which strains of the flu virus are most virulent. Vaccines are developed for the most infectious strains of the virus. Flu vaccines must be reformulated each year. See Figure 38-2 for age-specific immunization schedules recommended by the Centers for Disease Control and Prevention (CDC).

Selected Vaccines, Dosage Forms, and Strength

Generic Name	U.S. Brand Name(s) / Canadian Brand Name(s)	Dosage Forms and Strengths
diphtheria and tetanus toxoids (Td)	DECAVAC (Adult) / TD Adsorbed	**Suspension for injection (all)** **DECAVAC prefilled syringe:** 2 Lf diphtheria toxoid (adsorbed) + 5 Lf tetanus toxoid (adsorbed)/0.5 mL **Pediatric suspension:** 6.7 Lf diphtheria toxoid (adsorbed) + 5 Lf tetanus toxoid (adsorbed)/0.5 mL
diphtheria and tetanus toxoids, and pertussis (acellular) (DTaP)	Infanrix, Adacel, Boostrix, Daptacel, Tripedia / Adacel, Boostrix	**Suspension for injection (all)** **Infanrix:** 25 Lf diphtheria toxoid (adsorbed) + 25 mcg of inactivated pertussis toxin + 10 Lf tetanus toxoid (adsorbed)/0.5 mL dose **Adacel:** 2 Lf diphtheria toxoid (adsorbed) + 2.5 mcg inactivated pertussis toxin + 5 Lf tetanus toxoid (adsorbed)/0.5 mL dose **Boostrix:** 2.5 Lf diphtheria toxoid (adsorbed) + 8 mcg pertussis (adsorbed) + 5 Lf tetanus toxoid (adsorbed)/0.5 mL dose **Daptacel:** 15 Lf diphtheria toxoid (adsorbed) + 10 mcg pertussis (adsorbed) + 5 Lf tetanus toxoid (adsorbed)/0.5 mL **Tripedia:** 6.7 Lf diphtheria toxoid (adsorbed) + 23.4 mcg pertussis (adsorbed) + 5 Lf tetanus toxoid (adsorbed)/0.5 mL
diphtheria toxoid + hepatitis B surface antigen + pertussis vaccine (adsorbed) + poliovirus vaccine (inactivated) + tetanus toxoid	Pediarix / Not available	**Suspension, for injection (Pediarix):** 25 Lf diphtheria toxoid (adsorbed); 10 mcg hepatitis B surface antigen; + 25 mcg pertussis (adsorbed) + 80 D antigen units (DAgU) poliovirus vaccine (inactivated) + 10 Lf tetanus toxoid (adsorbed)/0.5 mL dose
diphtheria + tetanus toxoids (adsorbed) + pertussis vaccine (acellular) + tetanus toxoid conjugate vaccine	TriHIBit (ActHIB reconstituted with Tripedia) / Not available	Tripedia (see above) + ActHIB (see below)
Tetanus toxoid polysaccharide conjugate vaccine	ActHIB, Hiberix / ActHIB	**ActHIB:** 10 mcg of Hib purified capsular polysaccharide conjugated to 24 mcg inactivated tetanus toxoid **Hiberix (booster dose only):** 10 mcg of Hib purified capsular polysaccharide conjugated to 25 mcg inactivated tetanus toxoid

Continued

Selected Vaccines, Dosage Forms, and Strength—cont'd

Generic Name	U.S. Brand Name(s) / Canadian Brand Name(s)	Dosage Forms and Strengths
haemophilus influenzae b (HiB) conjugate vaccine	PedvaxHIB / PedvaxHIB	**Suspension, for injection:** 7.5 mcg HiB PRP + 125 mcg meningococcal protein conjugate/0.5 mL dose
inactivated polio vaccine	IPOL / Imovax Polio	**Suspension, for injection, trivalent, inactivated:** 40 DAgU (Mahoney, Type 1); 8 DAgU (MEF-1, Type 2); 32 DAgU (Saukett, Type 3)/0.5 mL dose
measles, mumps, and rubella (MMR) vaccine	M-M-R II / M-M-R II	**Powder for injection solution:** 1000 tissue culture infective dose (TCID50) measles virus vaccine (live attenuated); 12,500 TCID50 mumps virus vaccine (live); 1000 TCID50 rubella virus vaccine (live)[†], 1000 cell culture infectious dose (CCID) measles virus vaccine (live attenuated); 5000 CCID50 mumps virus vaccine (live); 1000 CCID50 rubella virus vaccine (live)[‡]
hepatitis A vaccine (inactivated)	Havrix, VAQTA / Avaxim, Epaxal, Havrix, Havrix Jr., VAQTA	**Suspension for injection:** 720 Elisa units ELU/0.5 mL (Havrix Jr.); 1440 ELU/mL **Suspension for injection (VAQTA):** 25 units adsorbed/0.5 mL (pediatric); 50 units adsorbed/mL (adult) **Suspension for injection:** 160 units/0.5 mL (Avaxim), 500 units/mL (Epaxal)
hepatitis B vaccine surface antigen, recombinant	Energix-B, Recombivax HB / Energix-B, Recombivax HB	**Suspension for injection, recombinant (Energix-B):** 10 mcg/0.5 mL (pediatric); 20 mcg/mL **Suspension for injection, recombinant (Recombivax HB):** 5 mcg/0.5 mL (pediatric)[†], 10 mcg/mL (adult)[†], 40 mcg/mL (dialysis)
hepatitis A vaccine + hepatitis B vaccine	Twinrix / Twinrix, Twinrix Jr.	**Suspension for injection, recombinant:** 360 ELU (hepatitis A) + 10 mcg (hepatitis B)/0.5 mL (Twinrix Jr.), 720 ELU (hepatitis A) + 20 mcg (hepatitis B)/mL
influenza vaccine (formulated for selected strains each flu season)	Afluria, Agriflu, Fluarix, FluMist, FluLaval, Fluvirin / Agriflu, Flumist	**Solution, nasal (Flumist), quadravalent types A and B (2011-2012 season):** H1N1, H3N3, B/Yamagata/16/88, and B/Victoria/2/87/0.2 mL dose[†]; Trivalent: H1N1, H3N3, B/Brisbane/60/2008/0.2 mL dose[‡] **Suspension for IM injection:** Influenza virus vaccine, trivalent, types A and B (2011-2012 season): A/California1 (H1N1), A/Victoria (H3N2) (an A/Perth-like strain), and B/Brisbane/0.5 mL dose (Afluria, Agriflu, Fluarix, FluLaval, Fluvirin) Influenza virus vaccine, trivalent, types A and B (2011-12 season): A/California1 (H1N1), A/Victoria (H3N2) (an A/Perth-like strain), and B/Texas/6/2011 (a B/Wisconsin/1/2010-like virus)/0.5 mL dose (Fluzone) **Suspension, for intradermal injection:** Influenza virus vaccine, trivalent (types A and B), avian, preservative-free, 2011-2012: A/California1 (H1N1), A/Victoria (H3N2) (an A/Perth-like strain), and B/Texas/6/2011 (a B/Wisconsin/1/2010-like virus)/0.1 mL (Fluzone-intradermal)
meningococcal vaccine	Menomune A/C/Y/W-135 / Meningitec, Menomune A/C/Y/W-135	**Powder, for SC injection:** meningococcal polysaccharide vaccine A, C, Y, W-135, 50 mcg each/0.5 mL dose

Selected Vaccines, Dosage Forms, and Strength—cont'd

Generic Name	U.S. Brand Name(s) Canadian Brand Name(s)	Dosage Forms and Strengths
meningococcal vaccine conjugated with diphtheria toxoid	Menactra Menactra, Meningitec,	**Solution, for IM injection:** 4 mcg meningococcal polysaccharide vaccine A, C, Y, W-135 + 48 mcg diphtheria toxoid conjugate each/0.5 mL dose (Menactra), 10 mcg meningococcal group C + 15 mcg diphtheria toxoid
pneumococcal polysaccharide polyvalent vaccine	Prevnar 13 Prevnar, Prevnar 13	**Suspension for IM injection:** **Prevnar:** 2 mcg/0.5 mL each of polysaccharide serotypes of *Streptococcus pneumoniae* (types 14, 18C, 19F, 23F, 4, 9V) and 4 mcg of serotype 6B **Prevnar 13:** 2.2 mcg/0.5 mL each of 13 saccharide serotypes of *S. pneumoniae* (types 1, 3, 4, 5, 6A, 7F, 9V, 14, 18C, 19A, 19F, 23F) and 4.4 mcg of serotype 6B
pneumococcal polysaccharide 23-polyvalent vaccine	Pneumovax 23 Pneumovax 23	**Solution, for IM or SC injection:** 25 mcg/0.5 mL each of 23 serotypes of *S. pneumoniae* purified capsular polysaccharides
rabies vaccine	HyperRAB S/D, Imovax rabies, RabAvert Imovax rabies, RabAvert	**Powder, for injection:** ≥2.5 units rabies antigen/dose (Imovax rabies, RabAvert) **Solution, for injection, antirabies immune globulin:** 150 units/mL (HyperRAB S/D)
varicella vaccine (live)	Varivax Varivax III, Varilrix, Zostavax	**Powder, for injection:** 1350 PFU (plaque-forming units)/0.5 mL (Varivax, Varivax III, Varilrix), 19400 PFU/0.65mL (Zostavax)
varicella-zoster virus vaccine (live) + rubella virus vaccine (live) + mumps virus vaccine (live) + measles virus vaccine (live attenuated)	ProQuad Priorix-Tetra	**Powder, for injection:** 1000 $TCID_{50}$ measles virus vaccine (live attenuated); 20,000 $TCID_{50}$ mumps virus vaccine (live); 1000 $TCID_{50}$ rubella virus vaccine (live); 9772 units varicella-zoster virus vaccine (ProQuad), 1000 $CCID_{50}$ measles virus vaccine (live attenuated); ≥14,000 $CCID_{50}$ mumps virus vaccine (live); 1000 $CCID_{50}$ rubella virus vaccine (live); 1350 PFU varicella-zoster virus vaccine (Priorix-Tetra)

PRP, polyribosylribitol phosphate capsular polysaccharide; TCID, tissue culture infective dose.; ELU, Elisa Unit.; CCID, cell culture infectious dose.; PFU, plaque forming unit.
†Strength available in the United States only.
‡Strength available in Canada only.

TECH ALERT!
Pharmacists and pharmacy technicians play an important role in increasing community awareness of the importance of vaccination against vaccine-preventable illnesses. Pharmacists are authorized to administer select immunizations in community pharmacies.

Immunosuppressants

Immunosuppressants inhibit the proliferation of cells of the immune system. Corticosteroids, antineoplastics, cyclosporine, macrolides, mycophenolate mofetil, antithymocyte globulin (ATG), monoclonal antibodies, intravenous immunoglobulin (IVIG), Rho(D) immunoglobulin, belatacept, and cytokine inhibitors are all categorized as immunopharmacologicals. Their actions may be cell-specific or nonspecific. Antineoplastic and cytotoxic drugs, also called chemotherapeutic agents, generally act against any type of proliferating cell and are used for the treatment of a variety of cancers. Drugs that have their primary action on cells of the immune system are used for the treatment of autoimmune diseases, such as multiple sclerosis, rheumatoid arthritis, systemic lupus erythematosus (see Chapter 15), and Crohn's disease (see Chapter 27). They are also used to prevent tissue or organ rejection after transplantation surgery. When drugs that are immune cell–specific are used for the treatment of cancers, they are typically administered in high doses at 3- to 6-week intervals.

Drugs that specifically target cells of the immune system are discussed in this chapter. Antineoplastic agents are described in Chapter 37.

A

Vaccine ▼ / Age ►	Birth	1 month	2 months	4 months	6 months	12 months	15 months	18 months	19–23 months	2–3 years	4–6 years
Hepatitis B	HepB	HepB			HepB				HepB Series		
Rotavirus			Rota	Rota	Rota						
Diphtheria, Tetanus, Pertussis			DTaP	DTaP	DTaP		DTaP				DTaP
Haemophilus influenzae type b			Hib	Hib	Hib*	Hib		Hib			
Pneumococcal			PCV	PCV	PCV	PCV				PCV / PPV	
Inactivated Poliovirus			IPV	IPV	IPV						IPV
Influenza					Influenza (Yearly)						
Measles, Mumps, Rubella						MMR					MMR
Varicella						Varicella					Varicella
Hepatitis A						HepA (2 doses)				HepA Series	
Meningococcal										MPSV4	

Range of recommended ages

Catch-up immunization

Certain high-risk groups

B

Vaccine ▼ / Age ►	7–10 years	11–12 YEARS	13–14 years	15 years	16–18 years
Tetanus, Diphtheria, Pertussis		Tdap	Tdap		
Human Papillomavirus		HPV (3 doses)	HPV Series		
Meningococcal	MPSV4	MCV4	MCV4[3] / MCV4		
Pneumococcal		PPV			
Influenza		Influenza (Yearly)			
Hepatitis A		HepA Series			
Hepatitis B		HepB Series			
Inactivated Poliovirus		IPV Series			
Measles, Mumps, Rubella		MMR Series			
Varicella		Varicella Series			

Range of recommended ages

Catch-up immunization

Certain high-risk groups

C

VACCINE ▼ / AGE GROUP ►	19–49 years	50–64 years	≥65 years
Tetanus, diphtheria, pertussis (Td/Tdap)	1-dose Td booster every 10 yrs		
	Substitute 1 dose of Tdap for Td		
Human papillomavirus (HPV)	3 doses (females) (0, 2, 6 mos)		
Measles, mumps, rubella (MMR)	1 or 2 doses	1 dose	
Varicella	2 doses (0, 4–8 wks)		
Influenza	1 dose annually	1 dose annually	
Pneumococcal (polysaccharide)	1–2 doses		1 dose
Hepatitis A	2 doses (0, 6–12 mos or 0, 6–18 mos)		
Hepatitis B	3 doses (0, 1–2, 4–6 mos)		
Meningococcal	1 or more doses		
Zoster		1 dose	

*Covered by the Vaccine Injury Compensation Program.

For all persons in this category who meet the age requirements and who lack evidence of immunity (e.g., lack documentation of vaccination or have no evidence of prior infection)

Recommended if some other risk factor is present (e.g., on the basis of medical, occupational, lifestyle, or other indications)

FIGURE 38-2 A-C, CDC-recommended immunization schedules. (**A, B** from Centers for Disease Control and Prevention: Childhood schedule [birth to 6 years old] and adolescent schedule [7 to 18 years old], 2011 [http://www.cdc.gov/vaccines/schedules/hcp/child-adolescent.html]; and **C** from Centers for Disease Control and Prevention: Recommended adult immunization schedule—United States, 2012 [www.cdc.gov/mmwr/preview/mmwrhtml/mm6104a9.htm?s_cid=mm6104a9_w].)

Cyclosporine

Generic Name	U.S. Brand Name(s) Canadian Brand Name(s)	Dosage Forms and Strengths
cyclosporine* (cyclosporin)	Gengraf, Neoral, Restasis, Sandimmune Sandoz cyclosporine	Capsule (Sandimmune): 25 mg, 50 mg, 100 mg Capsule, modified (Gengraf, Neoral, Sandoz cyclosporine): 10 mg‡, 25 mg, 50 mg, 100 mg Solution, for injection (Sandimmune): 50 mg/mL Solution, oral (Sandimmune): 100 mg/mL Solution, modified, oral (Gengraf, Neoral): 100 mg/mL Emulsion, ophthalmic (Restasis): 0.05%

*Generic available.
‡Strength available in Canada only.

CYCLOSPORINE

Cyclosporine is produced by a fungus (*Tolypocladium inflatum*) and is used to improve survival rates for individuals with organ transplants. It suppresses cell destruction in graft-versus-host reactions.

MECHANISM OF ACTION AND PHARMACOKINETICS

Cyclosporine acts on T lymphocyte cells. It blocks the cellular activation of mature, immunocompetent T cells and suppresses interferon-gamma (IFN-γ). IFN-γ suppression reduces cellular responsiveness to inflammatory stimuli by suppressing macrophage activation. Cyclosporine is formulated as capsules, modified and nonmodified oral solutions, and solution for injection. Cyclosporine-modified solution has greater absorption than capsules. Cyclosporine inhibits cytochrome P-450 (CYP450) microsomal pathways, which are responsible for several drug-drug interactions.

TECH ALERT!
Cyclosporine, oral liquid nonmodified (Sandimmune), is not substitutable for cyclosporine, oral liquid modified (Neoral, Gengraf).

ADVERSE REACTIONS

Adverse reactions of cyclosporine include acne, bleeding or tender gums, overgrowth of gum tissue, diarrhea, hirsutism, headache, leg cramps, anorexia, nausea and vomiting, and tremors. More serious adverse reactions are nephrotoxicity, neurotoxicity, and seizures. Because cyclosporine is an immunosuppressant, it can increase risk for infections.

MACROLIDE IMMUNOSUPRESSANTS

Tacrolimus is another immunosuppressant derived from a fungus (*Streptomyces tsukubaensis*). Everolimus, pimecrolimus, sirolimus, temsirolimus, and tacrolimus and are classified as immunosuppressant macrolides. Everolimus and sirolimus are used to prevent transplant rejections. Pimecrolimus and tacrolimus ointments are used for the treatment of eczema (see Chapter 42). Temsirolimus is indicated for the treatment of advanced renal cancer.

TECH ALERT!
A common ending for macrolides used for immunosuppression is *-limus*.

MECHANISM OF ACTION AND PHARMACOKINETICS

Tacrolimus inhibits the enzyme that is involved in the gene transcription of interleukins (e.g., IL-2), interferons (e.g., IFN-γ), and cytokines. It interferes with the first phase of T cell activation. Tacrolimus is more potent than cyclosporine. Everolimus also inhibits IL-2– and IL-15–stimulated activation and proliferation of T and B lymphocytes. Sirolimus interferes with a key enzyme that regulates the second phase of T cell activation and proliferation. It decreases the levels of immunoglobulins IgM, IgG, and IgA. Temsirolimus is a mammalian target of rapamycin (mTor) antagonist. Sirolimus is its active metabolite. Pimecrolimus inhibits T cell activation by blocking transcription of early cytokines and inhibits IL-2, IL-4, IL-10, and IFN-γ synthesis. It is similar to tacrolimus.

Sirolimus tablets and oral solution are not bioequivalent and thus are not substitutable. A meal high in fats can reduce the absorption of tacrolimus and sirolimus.

TECH ALERT!
Sirolimus should not be administered within 4 hours of cyclosporine.

ADVERSE REACTIONS

Everolimus, tacrolimus, and sirolimus may increase the risk for bacterial, fungal, protozoal, and viral infections (e.g., thrush, urinary tract infection [UTI], upper respiratory infection [URI],

Macrolide Immunosuppressants

Generic Name	U.S. Brand Name(s) Canadian Brand Name(s)	Dosage Forms and Strengths
everolimus	Afinitor, Zortress	Tablet: 0.25 mg, 0.5 mg, 0.75 mg (Zortress); 2.5 mg, 5 mg, 7.5 mg†, 10 mg (Afinitor)
	Afinitor	
pimecrolimus	Elidel	Cream: 1%
	Elidel	
sirolimus	Rapamune	Solution, oral: 1 mg/mL
	Rapamune	Tablet: 0.5 mg†, 1 mg, 2 mg†
tacrolimus	Prograf, Protopic	Capsule: 0.5 mg, 1 mg, 5 mg
	Advagraf, Prograf, Protopic	Capsule, extended release (Advagraf): 0.5 mg, 1 mg, 3 mg, 5 mg Solution, for injection: 5 mg/mL Ointment (Protopic): 0.03%, 0.1%
temsirolimus	Torisel	Solution, for injection: 25 mg/mL
	Torisel	

†Strength available in the United States only.

Mycophenolate Mofetil

Generic Name	U.S. Brand Name(s) Canadian Brand Name(s)	Dosage Forms and Strengths
mycophenolate mofetil	CellCept, Myfortic	Capsule: 250 mg Powder, for injection: 500 mg Powder, for oral suspension: 200 mg/mL Tablet: 500 mg Tablet, delayed-release (Myfortic): 180 mg, 360 mg
	CellCept, Myfortic	

pneumonia) and produce gastrointestinal adverse reactions such as diarrhea or constipation, loss of appetite, nausea, and vomiting. Other side effects are mouth ulcers and stomatitis, insomnia, dizziness or drowsiness, hair loss or unusual hair growth, headache, mood changes, depression, confusion, and tremor. More serious adverse reactions include seizures, hepatitis, and hemolytic anemias.

MYCOPHENOLATE MOFETIL

Mycophenolate is used in conjunction with corticosteroids and cyclosporine to decrease the rejection of transplanted organs.

MECHANISM OF ACTION AND PHARMACOKINETICS

Mycophenolate mofetil is a prodrug. It is metabolized to mycophenolic acid. Mycophenolic acid is an immunosuppressive agent that inhibits the enzyme required for the synthesis of purines needed for T cell and B cell proliferation.

ADVERSE REACTIONS

Gastrointestinal side effects are common and include constipation, diarrhea or soft stools, gas, loss of appetite, nausea, vomiting, stomach pain, or indigestion. Mycophenolate mofetil, like other immunosuppressives, can increase the risk of bacterial and viral infections. Other serious adverse effects are leukopenia, infections, lymphomas, and other malignancies.

Immunomodulators

An *immunomodulator* is a chemical agent that modifies the immune response or the functioning of the immune system. Vaccines, monoclonal antibodies, and T cell costimulation

TECH ALERT!
A common ending for monoclonal antibody immunomodulators is -mab.

Monoclonal Antibody Immunomodulators

Generic Name	U.S. Brand Name(s) Canadian Brand Name(s)	Dosage Forms and Strengths
basiliximab	Simulect	Powder, for injection: 10 mg†, 20 mg
	Simulect	
muromonab-CD3	Orthoclone OKT3	Solution, injection: 1 mg/1 mL
	Not available	

†Strength available in the United States only.

Antithymocyte Globulin

Generic Name	U.S. Brand Name(s) Canadian Brand Name(s)	Dosage Forms and Strengths
antithymocyte globulin	Atgam, Thymoglobulin	Powder, for injection (Thymoglobulin): 25 mg/vial Solution, for injection (Atgam): 50 mg/mL
	Atgam, Thymoglobulin	

blockers are immunomodulators. Immune globulins are classified as immunomodulators and immunosuppressants.

MONOCLONAL ANTIBODIES
Basiliximab, daclizumab, and muromonab are monoclonal antibody immunomodulators used to reduce transplant rejections and prolong the life of transplanted organs. They are active against a variety of leukocyte surface antigens, including CD3, CD4 (T helper cells), and T cell activation markers (IL-2, CD20, and CD25). Muromonab CD3 is administered with cyclosporine to reduce transplant rejection. Basiliximab is used to prolong the life of transplanted organs. Additional monoclonal antibody immunomodulators are described in Chapters 15 and 37.

MECHANISM OF ACTION
Basiliximab binds to and blocks the IL-2 receptor–alpha chain receptor (IL-2Rα), also known as CD25 antigen. Daclizumab blocks T cell activation by binding to the alpha subunit of IL-2Rα and inhibiting the binding of IL-2 to IL-2Rα. Muromonab-CD3 blocks T cell function by binding to T lymphocytes that lead to cytokine release and T cell activation.

ADVERSE REACTIONS
Administration of basiliximab, daclizumab, muromonab, and other monoclonal antibody immunomodulators may produce nausea, stomach pain, headache, redness, itching at the site of infusion, chest pain, hypertension, dyspnea, increased susceptibility to opportunistic infections, reactivation of dormant infections (e.g., tuberculosis [TB]), or worsening of existing infection.

ANTITHYMOCYTE GLOBULIN
ATG is prepared by immunizing horses or rabbits with human thymocytes. The resulting horse immunoglobulin (Atgam) or rabbit immunoglobulin (Thymoglobulin) that fights against human T cells is then collected and purified. ATG is primarily administered to reduce the rejection associated with organ and bone marrow transplantation.

MECHANISM OF ACTION AND PHARMACOKINETICS
ATG reduces the number of T cell lymphocytes. T cell depletion persists for several days following a single dose of ATG and takes approximately 2 months before T cell levels return to normal.

ADVERSE REACTIONS

Side effects associated with ATG administration are fever, chills, leukopenia, and skin rash. Additional adverse reactions are headache, dizziness, tiredness, and diarrhea.

INTRAVENOUS IMMUNOGLOBULIN

IVIG is collected from human plasma. It is classified as a biological response modifier. IVIG is used for the treatment of a variety of infections and chronic lymphatic leukemia. Immunoglobulins are described in the Unit X introduction.

$RH_o(D)$ IMMUNE GLOBULIN

$Rh_o(D)$ immune globulin is administered to pregnant women who are Rh-negative and have been exposed to blood that is Rh-negative. This may occur through exposure to fetal blood, amniocentesis, ectopic pregnancy, abdominal trauma during pregnancy, or whole blood transfusions. When an Rh incompatibility exists between the pregnant woman and fetus, maternal antibodies are produced that act against the fetal red blood cells. This condition is called erythroblastosis fetalis. It is a severe hemolytic disease of the fetus (see Unit V introduction). Anti-D, administered within 72 hours of delivery, can prevent erythroblastosis fetalis in a subsequent pregnancy. $Rh_o(D)$ is also used in the treatment of idiopathic thrombocytopenic purpura (ITP), a condition that causes excessive bruising or bleeding.

MECHANISM OF ACTION AND PHARMACOKINETICS

The mechanism of action for how $Rh_o(D)$ immune globulin (Anti-D), administered to an $Rh_o(D)$ mother suppresses the immune response to exposure to $Rh_o(D)$-positive RBCs is unclear. Antibodies contained in $Rh_o(D)$ immune globulin interact directly with the $Rh_o(D)$ antigens, thereby preventing the interaction between the antigens and maternal immune system. In the treatment of ITP, anti-D blocks platelet destruction and increases platelet count in patients with a spleen. Anti-D binding to $Rh_o(D)$ is thought to result in a anti-D coated RBC complex. It may cause immunosuppression by stimulating cytokines. It is formulated for IM and IV administration.

Intravenous Immunoglobulin

Generic Name	U.S. Brand Name(s) Canadian Brand Name(s)	Dosage Forms and Strengths
IV immunoglobulin (IVIG)	Carimune NF, Flebogamma, Gammagard S/D, Gammagard, Gamastan S/D, Hizentra, Privigen, Vivaglobulin	Powder, for injection: 3 g, 6 g, 12 g (Carimune NF), 0.5 g‡, 2.5 g‡, 5 g, 10 g (Gammagard S/D) Solution, for IM injection: 5% (Flebogamma), 15% (Baygam), 18% Gamastan S/D
	Gammagard S/D, Gammagard, Gamastan S/D, Gammunex, IGIVnex, Privigen, Vivaglobulin	Solution, for subcut injection: 160 mg/mL (Vivaglobulin), 200 mg/mL (Hizentra) Solution, for IV use: 10% (Gammagard, Gammunex, IGIVnex, Privigen)

‡Strength available in Canada only.

Rh_o Immune Globulin

Generic Name	U.S. Brand Name(s) Canadian Brand Name(s)	Dosage Forms and Strengths
Rh_o immune globulin	HyperRHO S/D, MICRhoGAM, RhoGAM, Rhophylac, WinRho SDF	Powder, for injection (WinRho SDF), IM or IV: 600 units, 1500 units, 5000 units/vial Solution, for IM injection only: 250 units (HyperRHO S/D, MICRhoGAM); 1500 units (HyperRHO S/D, RhoGAM, Rhophylac)
	WinRho SDF	Solution, for injection: 600 units/0.5 mL, 1500 units/1.3 mL, 2500units/2.2 mL, 5000 units/4.4 mL, 5000 units/13 mL (WinRho SDF)

ADVERSE REACTIONS

Side effects are headache, muscle aches and pains, pain and tenderness at the injection site, chills, fever, and allergic reactions. Dizziness, weight gain, and difficulty breathing are additional side effects.

T CELL COSTIMULATION BLOCKER

Belatacept is a new, selective, T cell costimulation blocker, U.S. Food and Drug Administration (FDA)–approved in June 2011. It is indicated to prevent post-transplantation rejection in adults receiving a kidney transplant. Adverse effects include anemia, diarrhea, urinary tract infection, peripheral edema, constipation, hypertension, pyrexia, graft dysfunction, cough, nausea, vomiting, headache, hypokalemia, hyperkalemia, and leukopenia. Persons who are Epstein-Barr virus seronegative should not receive belatacept. Persons taking belatacept should not receive immunizations with live viruses.

T-cell Costimulation Blocker

Generic Name	U.S. Brand Name(s) / Canadian Brand Name(s)	Dosage Forms and Strengths
belatacept	Nulojix	Powder, for injection: 250 mg/vial
	Not available	

Summary of Immunosuppressants and Immunomodulators

Generic Name	Brand Name	Usual Dose and Dosing Schedule	Warning Labels
Cyclosporine			
cyclosporine	Neoral, Sandimmune	**Heart and kidney transplantation prophylaxis, oral:** 15 mg/kg as a single dose 4-12 hr before transplantation. For maintenance therapy, continue initial daily in two divided doses or adjust dose downward. **IV:** 5-6 mg/kg IV as a single dose 4-12 hr before transplantation as a slow infusion	AVOID PREGNANCY. DILUTE ORAL SOLUTION IN LIQUID. SWALLOW CAPSULES WHOLE, DON'T CRUSH OR CHEW. AVOID GRAPEFRUIT JUICE. DO NOT REFRIGERATE. ORAL SOLUTION MUST BE USED WITHIN 2 MO OF OPENING. DISCARD DISCOLORED OR CLOUDY SOLUTION FOR INJECTION.
Macrolide Immunosuppressants			
everolimus	Zostress	**Kidney transplantation prophylaxis:** 0.75 mg PO every 12 hr with basiliximab induction and reduced doses of cyclosporine, modified, and corticosteroids	AVOID PREGNANCY. AVOID PROLONGED EXPOSURE TO SUNLIGHT; USE SUNSCREEN. AVOID ASPIRIN, ACETAMINOPHEN, AND NSAIDS. AVOID GRAPEFRUIT JUICE.
pimecrolimus	Elidel	For eczema and atopic dermatitis, see Chapter 42.	SEE CHAPTER 42.
sirolimus	Rapamune	**Kidney transplantation prophylaxis, oral:** 6 mg as soon as possible following transplantation, then 2 mg PO once daily	AVOID PREGNANCY. AVOID GRAPEFRUIT JUICE. AVOID PROLONGED EXPOSURE TO SUNLIGHT; USE SUNSCREEN. DILUTE ORAL SOLUTION WITH WATER OR ORANGE JUICE. REFRIGERATE; DISCARD WITHIN 30 DAYS OF OPENING (ORAL SOLUTION).

Continued

Summary of Immunosuppressants and Immunomodulators—cont'd

Generic Name	Brand Name	Usual Dose and Dosing Schedule	Warning Labels
tacrolimus	Prograf	Kidney transplantation prophylaxis, oral: 0.2 mg/kg/day in 2 divided doses, every 12 hr, within 24 hr of transplantation, with azathioprine or mycophenolate mofetil Heart transplantation prophylaxis, oral: 0.075 mg/kg/day in two divided doses, every 12 hr. May initiate with 0.01 mg/kg/day continuous IV infusion until oral dose is tolerated. For eczema and atopic dermatitis, see Chapter 42.	AVOID GRAPEFRUIT JUICE. TAKE ON AN EMPTY STOMACH.
temsirolimus	Torisel	For renal cell cancer, see Chapter 37.	SEE CHAPTER 37.
Antithymocyte Globulin			
antithymocyte globulin	Atgam	Kidney transplantation prophylaxis: 15 mg/kg/day IV given within 24 hr of transplantation, then once daily for the next 14 days Bone marrow transplantation prophylaxis: 10-20 mg/kg/day IV infusion for 8-14 days, continuing with every other day dosing up to a total of 21 doses	GENTLY ROTATE SOLUTION; DO NOT SHAKE. REFRIGERATE DILUTED SOLUTION.
Mycophenolate Mofetil			
mycophenolate mofetil	CellCept	Kidney transplantation prophylaxis, oral: 1 g bid IV: 1 g IV over at least 2 hr bid given within 24 hr of transplantation Heart or liver transplantation prophylaxis, oral: 1-1.5 g bid with cyclosporine and corticosteroids IV: 1.5 g IV over at least 2 hr bid with cyclosporine and corticosteroids	SHAKE WELL (SUSPENSION). SWALLOW WHOLE; DON'T CRUSH OR CHEW. TAKE ON AN EMPTY STOMACH. STORE RECONSTITUTED SUSPENSION AT ROOM TEMPERATURE AND DISCARD IN 60 DAYS.
Monoclonal Antibody Immunomodulators			
basiliximab	Simulect	Kidney transplantation prophylaxis: 20 mg IV 2 hr prior to transplantation, then 20 mg IV 4 days after transplantation; includes concurrent cyclosporine and corticosteroids	REFRIGERATE; DO NOT FREEZE. MIX GENTLY; DO NOT SHAKE. SOLUTION SHOULD BE USED WITHIN 4 HR OF PREPARATION OR MAY BE REFRIGERATED FOR UP TO 24 HR (DACLIZUMAB, BASILIXIMAB).
muromonab CD3	Orthoclone OKT3	Heart, kidney, and liver transplantation prophylaxis: 5 mg IV once daily for 10-14 day	

Summary of Immunosuppressants and Immunomodulators—cont'd

Generic Name	Brand Name	Usual Dose and Dosing Schedule	Warning Labels
Rh$_0$ Immune Globulin			
Rh$_0$ immune globulin	RhoGAM	**Rh isoimmunization prophylaxis, IM:** [BayRh$_0$(D)] (HyperRHO S/D; full dose, RhoGAM): 300 mcg IM at 28 wk gestation. Repeat within 72 hr of delivery of a confirmed Rh$_0$(D)-positive infant. **IV, IM:** (WinRho SDF, Rhophylac): 300 mcg IM or IV at 28-30 wk of gestation. Repeat dose within 72 hr of delivery of a confirmed Rh$_0$(D)-positive infant (repeat dose for WinRho SDF is 120 mcg).	REFRIGERATE; DO NOT FREEZE. PROTECT FROM LIGHT.
T Cell Costimulation Blocker			
belatacept	Nujolix	**Kidney transplantation prophylaxis:** 10 mg/kg/day IV infusion on day of transplantation (prior to transplantation), day 5, and the end of weeks 2, 4, 8, and 12 after transplantation. Maintenance dose is 5 mg/kg/day (prescribed dose must be evenly divisible by 12.5 mg).	AVOID PROLONGED EXPOSURE TO SUNLIGHT. REFRIGERATE; DON'T FREEZE. PROTECT DRUG FROM LIGHT.

Chapter Summary

- An immunization is defined as a deliberate artificial exposure to disease to produce acquired immunity.
- Vaccines prevent disease by taking advantage of your body's ability to make antibodies and prime killer cells to combat disease-causing microbes and viruses.
- Live attenuated vaccines are a living, but weakened, nonvirulent version of the invader microbe or virus.
- Inactivated killed vaccines are advantageous because they cannot mutate but they produce less immunity than live vaccines.
- Toxoid vaccines stimulate the immune system to produce antibodies to the toxins that cause illness.
- Conjugate vaccines link antigens or toxoids to the polysaccharide or sugar molecules that certain bacteria use as a protective device to disguise themselves.
- The cold chain refers to a set of safe handling practices that ensure that vaccines and immunologicals requiring refrigeration are maintained at the required temperature from the time of manufacture until the time of administration to patients.
- When the cold chain is disrupted, the effectiveness and shelf life of vaccines are reduced.
- Loss of potency and effectiveness is cumulative. Each time the cold chain is breached, the vaccine's effectiveness is further reduced.
- Patients are placed at risk when suboptimal vaccines are administered.
- Vaccines and other biological solutions and suspensions are most sensitive to breaches in the cold chain.
- Vaccines should be placed in a refrigerator designated solely to vaccines or, if a separate refrigerator is not feasible, vaccines should be separated from other refrigerated pharmaceuticals.
- An important component of the cold chain is establishment and adherence to protocols for receiving, stocking, storing, and transporting drugs requiring refrigeration.
- Pharmacy personnel should be alert for warning signs that the cold chain has been broken during shipment. This might be as simple as noticing that freezer packs have thawed or that dry ice placed in the transport container with a vaccine has evaporated.

- Vaccine stock should be rotated to avoid wastage because of outdated supplies. Expiration dates should be checked frequently.
- Vaccines should not be removed from the refrigerator until the time of dispensing or until the vaccine must be transported.
- In most cases, vaccines should be transported in an insulated container.
- Extremes in heat and cold must be avoided; vaccines should never be placed in the hot glove compartment of a car.
- Vaccines are administered to provide immunity to a wide variety of childhood diseases, influenza, hepatitis, pneumonia, viral meningitis, rabies, and other conditions.
- Immunosuppressants inhibit proliferation of cells of the immune system.
- Drugs that have their primary action on cells of the immune system are used to treat autoimmune diseases such as multiple sclerosis, rheumatoid arthritis, systemic lupus erythematosus, and Crohn's disease, prevent tissue or organ rejection after transplantation surgery, and treat cancer.
- Corticosteroids, antineoplastics, cyclosporine, macrolides, mycophenolate mofetil, antithymocyte globulin, monoclonal antibodies, intravenous immunoglobulin, $Rh_o(D)$ immunoglobulin, and cytokine inhibitors are all categorized as immunopharmacologicals.
- Cyclosporine is produced by a fungus (*Tolypocladium inflatum*); it is used to improve survival rates for individuals with organ transplants.
- Cyclosporine acts on T lymphocyte cells.
- Everolimus, tacrolimus, and sirolimus are classified as macrolides. Like cyclosporine, they are used to prevent transplant rejection.
- Tacrolimus interferes with the first phase of T cell activation and sirolimus interferes with a key enzyme that regulates the second phase of T cell activation and proliferation.
- Antithymocyte globulin is prepared by immunizing horses or rabbits with human thymocytes and then collecting the immunoglobulins.
- T cell depletion persists for several days following a single dose of ATG and takes approximately 2 months before T cell levels return to normal.
- Mycophenolate mofetil is a prodrug. It inhibits T cell and B cell proliferation.
- Basiliximab, daclizumab, and muromonab are monoclonal antibody immunomodulators that are used to reduce transplant rejections and prolong the life of transplanted organs.
- They are active against a variety of leukocyte surface antigens.
- Intravenous immunoglobulin is collected from human plasma. It is used for the treatment of a variety of infections and chronic lymphatic leukemia.
- $Rh_o(D)$ immune globulin is administered to pregnant women who are Rh-negative and have been exposed to blood that is Rh-positive.
- When an Rh incompatibility exists between the pregnant woman and fetus, maternal antibodies are produced that act against fetal red blood cells.
- Etanercept is a genetically engineered inhibitor of tumor necrosis factor-α that blocks the inflammatory process triggered by high concentrations of tissue necrosis factor-α.

REVIEW QUESTIONS

1. A living but weakened version of an invader that does not cause disease (nonvirulent) is called a _____.
   a. Live attenuated vaccine
   b. Dead attenuated vaccine
   c. Live encapsulated vaccine
   d. Live strengthened vaccine

2. Drugs that inhibit proliferation of cells of the immune system, also known as immunopharmacologicals, are termed _____.
   a. Immunostimulants
   b. Immunosuppressants
   c. Immunologicals
   d. Immunostabilizers

3. Immunization is not always achieved by administering vaccines.
   a. True
   b. False

4. Examples of inactivated killed vaccine(s) are _____ vaccines.
   a. Flu
   b. Hepatitis A
   c. Polio
   d. All of the above

5. These vaccines stimulate the immune system to produce antibodies to the toxins that cause illnesses such as tetanus and diphtheria.
   a. Conjugated vaccine
   b. Live attenuated vaccines
   c. Toxoid vaccines
   d. Inactivated killed vaccines

6. Disruption of the cold chain is not a public health threat.
   a. True
   b. False

7. Which of the following drugs are not categorized as immunopharmacologicals?
   a. Corticosteroids
   b. Antineoplastics
   c. antivirals
   d. Intravenous immunoglobulin

8. Cyclosporine is produced by a bacteria (*Tolypocladium inflatum*) and is used to improve the survival rates for individuals with organ transplants.
   a. True
   b. False

9. A common ending for monoclonal antibody immunomodulators is _____.
   a. *-tan*
   b. *-mab*
   c. *-ine*
   d. *-olol*

10. Rh$_o$(D) immune globulin is administered to pregnant women who are Rh _____ who have been exposed to blood that is Rh _____.
    a. Negative; positive
    b. Positive; negative
    c. Both a and b
    d. Rh$_o$(D), negative

TECHNICIAN'S CORNER

1. If a patient receives a vaccine, can that patient still become ill with the disease related to the vaccine?
2. Why does the body reject transplanted organs and not manufactured parts?

Bibliography

Childhood Immunization Division, Bureau of Communicable Disease Epidemiology, Laboratory Centre for Disease Control, Canada: National guidelines for vaccine storage and transportation, *Can Commun Dis Rep* 21:93-97, 1995.

Dimayuga R, Scheifele D, Bell A: Effects of freezing on DPT and DPT-IPV vaccines, adsorbed, *Can Commun Dis Rep* 21:101-103, 1995.

Elsevier: Gold Standard Clinical Pharmacology. Rh$_o$(D) immune globulin, 2007. Retrieved April 2, 2011, from https://www.clinicalpharmacology.com/, 2010.

FDA: FDA Approved Drug Products. Retrieved July 7, 2012, from http://www.accessdata.fda.gov/scripts/cder/drugsatfda/index.cfm?fuseaction=Search.Search_Drug_Name, 2012.

Health Canada: Drug product database. Retrieved July 7, 2012, http://www.hc-sc.gc.ca/dhp-mps/prodpharma/databasdon/index-eng.php, 2010.

Kalant H, Grant D, Mitchell J: *Principles of medical pharmacology*, ed 7, Toronto, 2007, Elsevier Canada, pp 546-552.

Lance L, Lacy C, Armstrong L, et al: *Drug information handbook for the allied health professional*, ed 12, Hudson, OH, 2005, APhA Lexi-Comp.

Moscou K: The vaccine cold-chain, 2007 (http://www.canadianhealthcarenetwork.ca/files/2009/10/tt_ce_e_jan_feb07.pdf).

Murdoch J: Chill out: What pharmacists need to know about the room temperature stability of refrigerated pharmaceutical products, *Pharm Pract* 22:32-42, 2006.

National Institute of Allergy and Infectious Disease: Understanding vaccines: What they are, how they work (NIH Publ. No. 08-4219), 2008 (http://www.niaid.nih.gov/topics/vaccines/Documents/undvacc.pdf).

National Library of Medicine: Daily med, 2011(http://dailymed.nlm.nih.gov/dailymed/about.cfm).

Seto J, Marra F: *Keeping it cool: A pharmacist's guide. Executive summary*, University of British Columbia, Continuing Pharmacy Professional Development, Home Study Program, 2005, Rogers, pp 1-7.

Weir E, Hatch K: Preventing cold-chain failure: Vaccine storage and handling, *JAMC* 171, 2004.

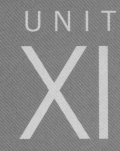

UNIT
XI

Drugs Affecting the Integumentary System

LEARNING OBJECTIVES

1 Identify the layers of the skin and its accessory structures.
2 Understand the function of each part of the integumentary system.
3 Identify the different types of cells of the integumentary system and their function.

KEY TERMS

Ceruminous glands: Produce cerumen, a brown waxy substance.

Dermis: Provides a reservoir or storage area for water and important electrolytes.

Eccrine sweat glands: Produce perspiration or sweat.

Epidermis: Outermost layer of skin.

Hypodermis: Subcutaneous layer that forms a connection between the skin and underlying structures of the body.

Integument: Another name for skin.

Keratinocytes: Cells that contain a fibrous protein called keratin.

Melanocytes: Cells containing melanin.
Sebaceous glands: Secrete oil for the hair and skin.

Overview

The terms *vital, diverse, complex,* and *extensive* describe the largest, thinnest, and one of the most important organs of the body, the skin. It forms a self-repairing and protective boundary between the internal environment of the body and an often external hostile world. *Integument* is another name for skin, and **integumentary system** is a term used to denote the skin and its appendages (hair, nails, and skin glands).

Structure of the Skin

The skin is classified as a cutaneous membrane with two primary layers, the ***epidermis*** (superficial, thinner layer) and ***dermis*** (deep, thicker layer). The specialized area at which the cells of the epidermis meet the connective cells of the dermis is called the ***dermal-epidermal junction***. Beneath the dermis lies a loose ***hypodermis*** (subcutaneous tissue), rich in fat and areolar tissue.

EPIDERMIS

The ***epidermis*** is the outermost layer of the skin that is composed of squamous epithelium. Epithelium is the covering for the internal and external surfaces of the body. The outer layer of the skin is arranged in several layers (strata) and is therefore called stratified squamous epithelium. The epidermis lacks blood vessels, lymphatic vessels, and connective tissue (elastic fibers, cartilage, and fat) and is therefore dependent on the deeper dermis layer and its rich network of capillaries for nourishment.

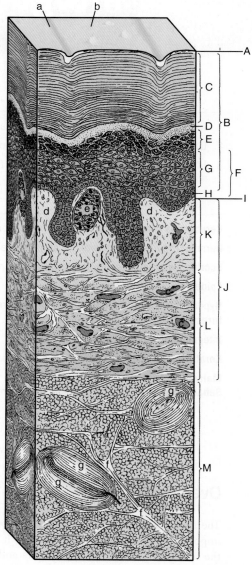

Structure of the skin. (From Thibodeau GA, Patton KT: *Anatomy and physiology*, ed 6, St. Louis, 2007, Mosby.)

Structure of the Skin

Structure	Name	Description
A	Surface film	Thin film coating the skin; made up of a mixture of sweat, sebum, desquamated cells and fragments, various chemicals; protects the skin
B	Epidermis	Superficial primary layer of the skin; made up entirely of keratinized stratified squamous epithelium; includes also hairs, sweat glands, sebaceous glands
C	Stratum corneum (horny layer)	Several layers of flakelike dead cells mostly made up of dense networks of keratin fibers cemented by glycophospholipids and forming a tough waterproof barrier
D	Stratum lucidum (clear layer)	A few layers of squamous cells filled with eleidin, a keratin precursor that gives this layer a translucent quality
E	Stratum granulosum (granular layer)	Two to five layers of dying, somewhat flattened cells filled with darkly staining keratohyalin granules and multilayered bodies of glycophospholipids
F	Stratum germinativum (growth layer)	General name for the stratum spinosum and stratum basale together
G	Stratum spinosum (spiny layer)	Eight to ten layers of cells pulled by desmosomes into a structure with a spiny appearance
H	Stratum basale (base layer)	Single layer of mostly columnar cells capable of mitotic cell division; includes keratinocytes and some melanocytes
I	Dermal-epidermal junction	Basement membrane, a complex arrangement of adhesive components that glue the epidermis and dermis together
J	Dermis	Deep primary layer of the skin; made up of fibrous tissue; also includes some blood vessels (C), muscles, and nerves
K	Papillary region	Loose fibrous tissue with collagenous and elastic fibers; forms nipple-like bumps (papillae, D); includes tactile corpuscles (touch receptors, E) and other sensory receptors
L	Reticular region	Tough network (reticulum) of collagenous dense irregular fibrous tissue (with some elastic fibers); forms most of the dermis
M	Hypodermis (subcutaneous layer; superficial fascia)	Loose, ordinary (areolar) connective tissue and adipose tissue; under the skin (not part of the skin); includes fibrous bands (F) that connect the skin strongly to underlying structures; includes lamellar corpuscles (pressure receptors, G) and other sensory receptors

(From Thibodeau GA, Patton KT: *Anatomy and physiology*, ed 6, St. Louis, 2007, Mosby.)

Epidermal Cells

The epidermis is composed of several types of epithelial cells. *Keratinocytes* are filled with a tough fibrous protein called *keratin*. *Melanocytes* contribute to the color of the skin and serve to decrease the amount of ultraviolet (UV) light that can penetrate into the deeper layers of the skin. *Langerhans cells* are branched cells that play a role in immunity. The cells of the epidermis are found in up to five distinct layers or strata.

Epidermal Growth and Repair

The epidermis has the ability to create new cells and repair itself after injury or disease. New cells must be formed at the same rate that old keratinized cells flake off from the stratus corneum to maintain a constant thickness of the epidermis. The regeneration time required for completion of mitosis, differentiation, and movement of new keratinocytes from stratum basale to the surface of the epidermis is approximately 35 days.

DERMAL-EPIDERMAL JUNCTION

This basement membrane is a complex arrangement of adhesive components that glue together the epidermis and dermis. It serves as a partial barrier to the passage of some cells and large molecules,

Layers of the Epidermis

Layer	Description
Stratum basale (base layer)	Single layer of mostly columnar cells capable of mitotic cell division; keratinocytes and melanocytes are derived from this layer
Stratum spinosum (spiny layer)	Eight to ten layers of irregularly shaped cells that are rich in ribonucleic acid (RNA) and well equipped to initiate the protein synthesis required for production of keratin
Stratum granulosum (granular layer)	Two to five layers of dying, somewhat flattened cells filled with intensely staining granules called keratohyalin, which is required for keratin formation
Stratum lucidum (clear layer)	A few layers of squamous cells filled with eleidin, a keratin precursor that gives this layer a translucent quality
Stratum corneum	Several layers of flakelike dead cells mostly made of keratin fibers cemented by glycophospholipids and forming a tough, waterproof barrier

Layers of the Dermis

Layer	Description
Papillary region	Loose fibrous tissue with collagenous and elastic fibers; form nipple-like bumps (papillae); papillae include tactile corpuscles (e.g., touch receptors) and other sensory receptors
Reticular region	Tough network (reticulum) of collagenous dense irregular fibrous tissue (with some elastic fibers); forms most of the dermis

preventing the passage of chemicals or disease-causing organisms through the skin from the external environment.

DERMIS

The *dermis*, or corium, is sometimes called the true skin. In addition to serving a protective function against mechanical injury and compression, this layer of skin provides a reservoir or storage area for water and important electrolytes. A specialized network of nerves and nerve endings in the dermis called somatic sensory receptors also process the sensory information, such as pain, pressure, touch, and temperature. A variety of muscle fibers, hair follicles, sweat and sebaceous glands, and many blood vessels are embedded in the dermis.

HYPODERMIS

The hypodermis is sometimes called the *subcutaneous layer*, or *superficial fascia*. It lies deep in the dermis and forms a connection between the skin and underlying structures of the body. The hypodermis is mainly composed of loose fibrous and adipose (fat) tissue. Bands of fibers running through the hypodermis help hold the skin to underlying structures, such as deep fascia and muscles.

SKIN COLOR

The main determinant of skin color is the quantity of melanin deposited in the cells of the epidermis. Prolonged exposure to the UV radiation in sunlight in light-skinned individuals causes melanocytes to increase melanin production and darken skin color. UV radiation can also reach into the DNA of the melanocyte and cause severe damage, which could lead to skin cancer. Unless protected by melanin, UV radiation can also break down the vitamin folic acid. Other pigments such as beta-carotene (found in vegetables and roots) also contribute to skin color. Beta-carotene can be converted by the body to vitamin A, a critically important nutrient for skin growth that is stored in skin tissue.

Functions of the Skin

The major functions of the skin are protection, sensation, growth, synthesis of important chemicals and hormones (e.g., vitamin D), excretion, temperature regulation, and immunity.

Functions of the Skin

Function	Example	Mechanism
Protection	From microorganisms From dehydration From UV radiation From mechanical trauma	Surface film, mechanical barrier Keratin Melanin Tissue strength
Sensation	Pain Heat and cold Pressure Touch	Somatic sensory receptors
Body growth and movement	Body growth and change in body contours during movement	Elastic and recoil properties of skin and subcutaneous tissue
Endocrine	Vitamin D production	Activation of precursor compound in skin cells by UV light
Excretion	Water Urea Ammonia Uric acid	Regulation of sweat volume and content
Immunity	Destruction of microorganisms and interaction with immune cells (helper T cells)	Phagocytic cells and Langerhans cells
Temperature regulation	Heat loss or retention	Regulation of blood flow to the skin and evaporation of sweat

Appendages of the Skin

Appendages of the skin consist of the hair, nails, and skin glands.

HAIR

Only a few areas of the skin are hairless. These are the palms of the hands, soles of the feet, lips, nipples, and some areas of the genitalia. Hair growth begins when cells of the epidermis spread down into the dermis to form a small tube, the follicle part of the hair. The root lies hidden in the follicle and the visible part is called the shaft. Deposited in the cells of the hair are varying amounts of melanin, which is responsible for hair color. Two or more *sebaceous glands* secrete *sebum*, an oily substance, into each hair follicle. The sebaceous gland secretions lubricate and condition the hair and surrounding skin to keep it from becoming dry, brittle, and easily damaged.

NAILS

Heavily keratinized epidermal cells comprise the fingernails and toenails. The visible part of each nail is called the *nail body*. The root of the nail lies in the flat sinus hidden by a fold of skin bordered by the *cuticle*. The nail body near the root has a crescent-shaped white area known as the *lunula*, or little moon. Under the nail lies a layer of epithelium called the nail bed.

SKIN GLANDS

The skin glands include three kinds of microscopic glands—sweat, sebaceous, and ceruminous.

SWEAT GLANDS

Sweat or *sudoriferous glands* are the most numerous of the skin glands. They are classified as eccrine and apocrine. *Eccrine sweat glands* are distributed over the entire body surface, except the lips, ear canal, glans penis, and nail beds. They function throughout life to produce a transparent watery liquid (perspiration [sweat]) rich in salts, ammonia, uric acid, urea, and other wastes. Sweat plays a critical role in maintaining a constant core temperature. Eccrine sweat glands are also numerous on the soles of the feet, forehead, and upper part of the torso. *Apocrine sweat glands* are located deep

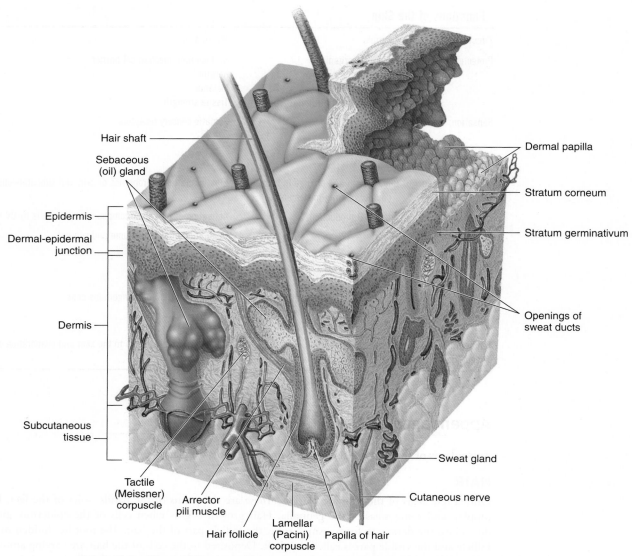

Labels:
Hair shaft
Sebaceous (oil) gland
Epidermis
Dermal-epidermal junction
Dermis
Subcutaneous tissue
Tactile (Meissner) corpuscle
Arrector pili muscle
Hair follicle
Lamellar (Pacini) corpuscle
Papilla of hair
Dermal papilla
Stratum corneum
Stratum germinativum
Openings of sweat ducts
Sweat gland
Cutaneous nerve

Hair follicle. (From Thibodeau GA, Patton KT: *Structure and function of the body*, ed 13, St. Louis, 2008, Mosby Elsevier.)

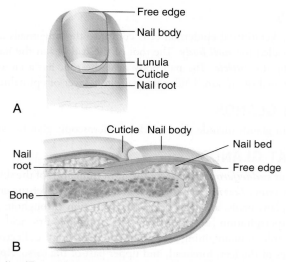

Labels:
Free edge
Nail body
Lunula
Cuticle
Nail root
A
Cuticle
Nail body
Nail root
Nail bed
Free edge
Bone
B

Structure of the nails. (From Thibodeau GA, Patton KT: *Structure and function of the body*, ed 13, St. Louis, 2008, Mosby Elsevier.)

in the subcutaneous layer of the skin in the armpit (axilla), areola of the breast, and pigmented skin areas around the anus. Apocrine glands enlarge and begin to function at puberty.

SEBACEOUS GLANDS

Sebaceous glands secrete oil for the hair and skin. The oil, or sebum, keeps the hair supple and the skin soft and pliant. Sebaceous glands are found in the dermis, except in the skin of the palms and soles. Some sebaceous glands open directly to the skin surface in areas such as the glans penis, lips, and eyelids. Sebum secretion during adolescence is stimulated by the increased production of sex hormones. Overactive secretion with blocked ducts and inflammation produce common acne, or acne vulgaris.

CERUMINOUS GLANDS

Ceruminous glands are a special variety of apocrine sweat glands. They appear as excretory ducts that open onto the free surface of the skin in the external ear canal or with sebaceous glands into the necks of hair follicles in this area. The mixed secretions of sebaceous and ceruminous glands form a brown waxy substance called **cerumen**. It serves a useful purpose in protecting the skin of the ear canal from dehydration.

Summary

Everyone is aware of dramatic changes in the skin from birth to adulthood. The aging process reduces the elasticity and flexibility of the skin that is characteristic in infancy and childhood, often causing the development of wrinkles on the skin, especially in areas of frequent movement such as on the hands, around the mouth, and around the eyelids. However, it is important to remember that changes in the skin are more than cosmetic. The integumentary system protects the internal environment of the body from the external environment. For example, dryness and cracking of the skin can increase the risk for infection and loss of function in the sweat glands as adulthood advances adversely affects the body's ability to cool itself during exercise and when the external temperature is high. The various organ systems of the body operate with the structural and functional assistance of the integumentary system.

39

Treatment of Fungal Infection

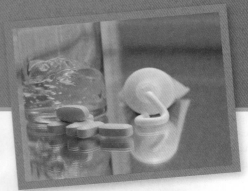

LEARNING OBJECTIVES

1 Learn the terminology associated with fungal infections.
2 Identify risk factors for fungal infections.
3 List and categorize medications used for the treatment of fungal infections.
4 Describe the mechanism of action for drugs used for the treatment of fungal infections.
5 List common endings for drug classes used for the treatment of specific fungal infections.
6 Identify significant drug look-alike and sound-alike issues.
7 Identify warning labels and precautionary messages associated with medications used for the treatment of fungal infections.

KEY TERMS

Antifungal: Drug used to treat a fungal infection.

Candida: Genus of a type of fungus. It is also called yeast.

Dermatophytes: Group of fungi responsible for most fungal infections of the skin, hair, and nails.

Fungus (*pl.*, fungi): Organism similar to plants but lacking chlorophyll and capable of producing mycotic (fungal) infections,

Mycosis: General term for a fungal infection.

Onychomycosis: Fungal infection involving the fingernails or toenails, also known as tinea unguium.

Ringworm: Group of tinea infections involving the body or scalp that have a characteristic ring-like shape. Ringworm is spread person-person and animal-person.

Vulvovaginal candidiasis: Yeast vaginitis.

What Are Fungi and Yeast?

Fungi are organisms similar to plants but lacking chlorophyll and capable of producing mycotic (fungal) infections, Thousands of different fungi exist. Mold, mildew, yeast, and mushrooms are all types of fungi. Many fungi are beneficial and do not cause disease. For example, some mushrooms and fungi are edible. The antibiotic penicillin is derived from a mold, and yeast causes bread to rise. Other fungi can cause severe illness. *Pneumocystis jiroveci* (formerly known as *Pneumocystis carinii*) is a fungus that can cause pneumonia in individuals who have a decreased immune system response (are immunocompromised); *Aspergillus fumigatus* is a mold that also causes serious respiratory infection.

Fungal Infections of the Skin and Nails

The general term used to describe a fungal infection is **mycosis**. Most fungal infections of the skin are caused by a group of fungi called dermatophytes. **Dermatophytes** thrive on dead keratin, a tough protein substance found in the top layer of skin, nails, and hair. They are not typically found in the mouth or vaginal mucosa. **Candida**, also called yeast, is a type of fungus that thrives in warm moist areas and is responsible for fungal infections in the vagina, groin, and mouth. To identify *Candida*, a potassium hydroxide (KOH) stain is applied to a sample of cells from the infected area. A *Candida* stain is shown in Figure 39-1.

Mycoses caused by the dermatophyte tinea are named for the site of the infection. For example, tinea manus is a fungal infection on the hands, tinea corporis is an infection on the body, and tinea capitis is located on the head (hence, cap). Tinea infections are also commonly called **ringworm**.

Dermatophyte infections are common and affect up to 20% of the population. This is because fungi are ubiquitous (found everywhere). They are found in the air, soil, plants, and water. They are also found on surfaces in the home, office, schools, and gyms and even occur normally on our bodies. Fungi that are part of the normal body flora may become pathogenic (cause infection) only when the normal balance of flora is upset. For example, women who take broad-spectrum antibiotics may get a yeast infection because the bacteria and fungi that keep the yeast normally present in the vagina from overgrowing are killed by the antibiotic.

ATHLETE'S FOOT

Athlete's foot (tinea pedis; Figure 39-2) is a common fungal infection that affects athletes and non-athletes. Symptoms are peeling, flaking skin between the toes, redness, itchiness, burning or stinging, and blisters and thickening of skin on the soles of the feet and heels. It may be accompanied by a foul odor. If severe, it may cause cracking of the skin, oozing, and secondary bacterial infection.

Individuals who have abrasions on the feet, as caused by improperly fitted shoes that rub against the skin, are more susceptible to athlete's foot should they walk barefoot across an infected surface. Tips for prevention of athlete's foot are listed in Box 39-1.

Ringworm infections are caused by tinea fungi (*Tinea mentagrophytes*, *Tinea rubrum*, and *Microsporum canis*) and may occur on the scalp, body, feet, fingernails, or toenails. Ringworm is contagious and is spread person-to-person by physical contact with infected surfaces or lesions. Ringworm can also spread between humans and animals. Cats and dogs may be carriers of the fungus.

Ringworm of the body is also known as tinea corporis. Patches and plaques appear pink to red, with raised scaly borders. They form in a distinctive circular pattern that gives the name of "ring" worm (Figure 39-3).

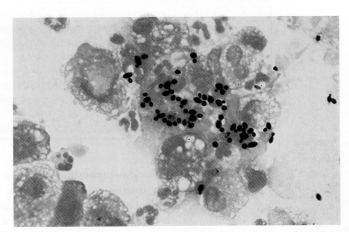

FIGURE 39-1 *Candida* stain (potassium hydroxide stain), http://www.nlm.nih.gov/medlineplus/ency/imagepages/1053.htm (From Mahon CR, Lehman DC, Manuselis G: *Textbook of diagnostic microbiology*, ed 3, St. Louis, 2007, Saunders.)

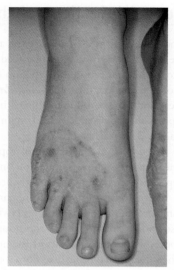

FIGURE 39-2 Athlete's foot. (From Callen JP, Greer KE, Hood A, et al: *Color atlas of dermatology*, Philadelphia, 1993, WB Saunders.)

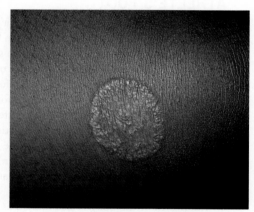

FIGURE 39-3 Tinea corporis. (From Zitelli BJ, Davis HW: *Atlas of pediatric physical diagnosis*, ed 5, Philadelphia, 2008, Mosby.)

BOX 39-1 **Prevention of Athlete's Foot**

- Keep your feet clean and dry.
  - Dry between your toes after swimming or bathing.
  - Wear leather shoes or sandals that allow your feet to breathe.
  - When indoors, wear socks without shoes.
  - Wear cotton socks to absorb sweat. Change your socks twice a day. (White socks do not prevent athlete's foot, as some people believe.)
  - Use talcum or antifungal powder on your feet.
- Allow your shoes to air for at least 24 hours before you wear them again.
- Wear shower sandals in public pools and showers.

TECH NOTE!
Frequent removal and replacement of artificial nails can cause thinning of the nail bed, increasing susceptibility to onychomycosis.

Tinea capitis is also called ringworm of the scalp. It occurs more frequently in children than in adults and is spread by sharing contaminated hats, combs, clothing, bedding, and linens. It may also be spread from animal to person. The fungus can cause bald patches on the scalp (Figure 39-4).

Tinea manus affects the hands and tinea unguium affects the nails. A fungal infection of the nails is also called **onychomycosis**. Infected nails become discolored and thick and may crumble or fall off. Onychomycosis is hard to treat with topically applied **antifungals** because it is difficult for drugs to penetrate the nails and nail bed.

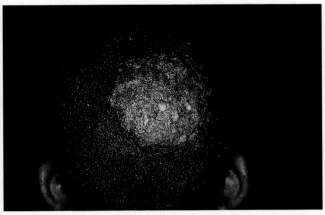

FIGURE 39-4 Ringworm of the scalp. (From Callen JP, Greer KE, Paller LJ, et al: *Color atlas of dermatology*, ed 2, Philadelphia, 2000, Saunders.)

BOX 39-2   **Risk Factors for Vulvovaginal Candidiasis**

- Age
- Decreased immune status
- Diabetes
- Drug therapy (e.g., hormone replacement therapy, oral contraceptives, antibiotics, immunosuppressives, corticosteroids)
- Douching
- Diet
- Menses
- Pregnancy
- Sexual activity
- Stress
- Tight-fitting clothing and synthetic underwear

BOX 39-3   **Signs of Vulvovaginal Candidiasis**

- Itching
- Cottage cheese–like vaginal discharge
- Burning
- Pain during intercourse

CANDIDIASIS

Candida is yeast that can cause infections of the skin and mucus membranes. Sites of infection are the groin, mouth, vagina, penis, skin folds, corners of the mouth, and nail beds. *Candida* is normally present in the gastrointestinal tract and vagina but only causes infection when conditions are favorable for the overgrowth of yeast.

Vulvovaginal candidiasis is also known as yeast vaginitis. The risk for getting yeast vaginitis increases with age. Changes in hormone levels, such as occurs during pregnancy or when taking oral contraceptives or hormone replacement therapy, can also increase the risk of infection. When the body's ability to fight infection is suppressed because of infections like HIV or if taking immunosuppressive drugs (e.g., corticosteroids, antineoplastic agents), fungal infections may flourish. Risk factors of vulvovaginal candidiasis are listed in Box 39-2. Signs and symptoms of vulvovaginal candidiasis are shown in Box 39-3.

Candida can also cause infections in the oral cavity and in the area surrounding the mouth. A *Candida* infection in the oral cavity is termed *thrush* (Figure 39-5). Thrush is most common in infants. A thrush infection in adults is a sign that the immune system is compromised. Thrush is an opportunistic infection that occurs in individuals with diseases that affect the immune system

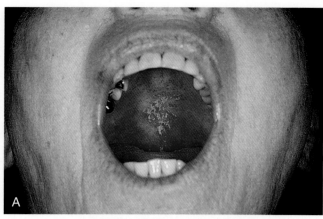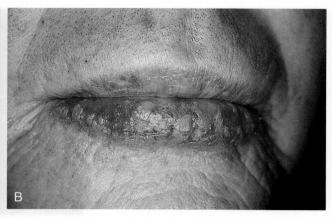

FIGURE 39-5 **A,** Thrush. **B,** Oral candidiasis. (From Callen JP, Greer KE, Paller LJ, et al: *Color atlas of dermatology*, ed 2, Philadelphia, 2000, Saunders.)

TECH ALERT!
A common ending for some antifungal agents is -*azole*.

TECH ALERT!
The following drugs have look-alike and sound-alike issues:
   Mycelex, Myoflex, and Mycolog;
   Lotrimin and Lotrisone;
   Diflucan, Diprivan, and Dilantin;
   Nizoral, Nasarel, and Neoral;
   Miconazole and metronidazole;
   Terconazole and tioconazole

TECH ALERT!
Fluconazole, itraconazole, ketoconazole, and posaconazole are strong to moderate inhibitors of CYP3A4, 5, and 7 and 2C19, resulting in numerous potential drug interactions. Watch for interactions with macrolide antibiotics, quinidine, protease inhibitors, statins, cimetidine, and calcium channel blockers.

such as HIV, persons who take immunosuppressive medicines for cancer treatment or after stem cell and organ transplantation, and individuals taking broad-spectrum anti-infective agents.

Treatment of Fungal and Yeast Infections

Many fungal infections can be treated with nonprescription antifungal agents. Fungal infections that are cured using over-the-counter (OTC) drugs are ringworm, vulvovaginal candidiasis, jock itch, and athlete's foot.

There are three primary mechanisms of action for antifungal agents. Most antifungal agents act by destroying the fungus's cell membrane. The cell membrane of fungi differs from the cell membrane of human cells, so destruction of fungi does not destroy human cells. A second mechanism is interference with the synthesis of nucleic acids needed for replication. A third mechanism is inhibiting the synthesis of the fungal cell wall.

IMIDAZOLES AND TRIAZOLES

Imidazoles and triazoles are formulated for the treatment of cutaneous (skin) fungal infections and systemic infections. Several imidazoles are available for topical use, without prescription. Clotrimazole and miconazole are OTC in the United States and Canada. Butoconazole, ketoconazole and tioconazole are OTC in the United States and prescription only in Canada. These azoles are used to treat athlete's foot, vulvovaginal candidiasis, jock itch, ringworm, and oral candidiasis. The remaining imidazoles (econazole, oxiconazole, sulconazole, sertaconazole) are restricted to prescription use in both countries. Fluconazole, itraconazole, posaconazole, terconazole, and voriconazole are triazoles. All require a prescription in the United States. Fluconazole is available without prescription in Canada.

MECHANISM OF ACTION AND PHARMACOKINETICS

The imidazoles and triazoles interfere with ergosterol, an essential component needed for the synthesis of the fungal cell membrane. This causes cellular contents to leak out and the cell dies. Topical azoles are formulated for application to the skin (creams, gel, lotion), mucous membranes (vaginal creams, suppositories), and scalp (shampoo).

ADVERSE EFFECTS

Adverse effects linked to the topical use of imidazoles and triazoles are stinging or burning at the application site, redness, itchiness, or blistering. Nausea and vomiting, skin rash, liver toxicity, and photophobia are adverse reactions linked to oral use of ketoconazole.

Imidazoles and Triazoles

Generic Name	U.S. Brand Name(s) Canadian Brand Name(s)	Dosage Forms and Strengths
butoconazole	Gynezole-1, Femstat 3♦	Cream, vaginal: 2%
	Gynezole-1	
clotrimazole*	Cruex, Desenex AF, Fungicure Intensive, Gyne-Lotrimin, Gyne-Lotrimin Combo Pak and 3 Day Combo Pak, Gyne-Lotrimin 3 Day Cream, Lotrimin, Lotrimin AF Jock Itch, Lotrimin AF, Mycelex	Cream, topical: (Canesten, Clotrimaderm, Cruex, Lotrimin AF)♦: 1% Lozenge (Mycelex): 10 mg Solution, Topical (Fungicure Intensive, Lotrimin AF, Mycelex)▲: 1% Cream, vaginal: 1% (Gyne-Lotrimin, Mycelex 7)▲, 2% (Gyne-Lotrimin 3, Canesten Cream 3)‖, 10% (Canesten cream 1)‡
	Canasten, Canesten cream 1, Canesten cream 3, Canasten Combi-Pak-1, Canasten Combi-Pak-3, Canesten Comfortab 1, Canesten Comfortab 3, Canesten Combi-pak Comfortab 1, Canesten Combi-pak Comfortab 3, Clotrimaderm	Tablet, vaginal tab: 100 mg (Gyne Lotrimin)▲, 200 mg (Canesten Comfortab 3, Gyne-Lorimin 3)‖, 500 mg (Canesten Comfortab 1)‖ Vaginal tab + cream: Canesten Combi-pak Comfortab, Gyne Lotrimin Combo Pak: 100 mg vaginal tab + 1% cream▲ 200-mg vaginal tab + 1% cream‖ 500-mg vaginal tab + 1% cream‖
econazole*	Generics	Cream: 1%
	Not available	
fluconazole*	Diflucan	Capsule (Canesoral, Diflucan One): 150 mg‖ Powder, for oral suspension: 10 mg/mL; 40 mg/mL† Solution, for injection: 2 mg/mL in dextrose 5% or normal saline Tablet: 50 mg, 100 mg, 150 mg, 200 mg†
	Canesoral, Diflucan, Diflucan One	
itraconazole*	Sporonox, Onmel	Capsule: 100 mg Tablet (Onmel): 200 mg Solution, oral: 10 mg/mL Solution, for injection: 250 mg/25 mL†
	Sporonox	
ketoconazole*	Extina, Nizoral, Nizoral A-D, Xolegel	Cream (Ketoderm, Nizoral Cream♦): 2% Gel (Xolegel): 2% Shampoo (Nizoral A-D, Nizoral): 1%♦, 2% Tablet: 200 mg Topical foam (Extina): 2%
	Ketoderm, Nizoral Cream	
miconazole*	Desenex, Desenex Jock Itch, Lotrimin AF Deodorant Spray, Micatin, Monistat 1 Combination Pack, Monistat 1 Triple Action System Combination Pack, Monistat 1 Day or Night Combination Pack, Monistat 3 Vaginal cream, Monistat 3 combination pack, Monistat 3 Triple Action System Combination Pack, Monistat 7, Oravig, Ting, Zeasorb	Cream (Micatin Derm, Monistat Derm): 2%♦ Lotion (Zeasorb)♦: 2% Ointment♦: 2% Buccal tablet (Oravig): 50 mg Powder, topical (Lotrimin AF, Micatin, Desenex, Zeasorb AF)♦: 2% Spray, solution (Lotrimin AF)♦: 2% Spray, powder (Cruex, Desenex Jock Itch, Lotrimin AF Deodorant, Ting)♦: 2% Vaginal cream♦: 2% (Monistat-7), 4% (Monistat-3) Vaginal suppository: 100 mg† (Monistat 7), 200 mg† (Monistat 3), 400 mg‖ (Monistat 3), 1200 mg (Monistat 1)
	Micatin Derm, Monistat 1 Combination Pack, Monistat 1 Vaginal Ovule, Monistat 3 Vaginal Ovules, Monistat 3 Dual-Pak, Monistat 3 Vaginal cream, Monistat 7, Monistat 7 Dual-Pak, Monistat Derm	Vaginal suppository + cream: 100-mg suppository + 2% cream (Monistat 7 Dual-Pak); 200-mg suppository + 2% cream (Monistat 3 Triple Action System Combination Pack, Monistat 3 combination pack); 400-mg suppository + 2% cream (Monistat 3 Dual-Pak); 1200-mg suppository + 2% cream (Monistat Day or Night Combination Pack, Monistat 1 combination pack) Vaginal cream 2% + topical cream (Monistat 7 Triple Action Pack, Monistat 7 Dual-Pak)♦: 100 mg suppository + 2% cream

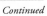

Continued

Imidazoles and Triazoles—cont'd

Generic Name	U.S. Brand Name(s) / Canadian Brand Name(s)	Dosage Forms and Strengths
oxiconazole	Oxistat	Cream: 1%
	Not available	Lotion: 1%
posaconazole	Noxafil	Oral suspension: 40 mg/mL
	Posanol	
sertaconazole	Ertaczo	Cream: 2%
	Not available	
sulconazole	Exelderm	Cream: 1%
	Not available	Topical solution: 1%
terconazole*	Terazol 3, Terazol 7	Vaginal cream: 0.8% (Terazol 3), 0.4% (Terazol 7)
	Terazol 3, Terazol 7	Vaginal suppository: 80 mg
tioconazole*	Vagistat-1	Vaginal ointment: 6.5%◆
	Not available	
voriconazole*†	Vfend	Powder, for injection: 200 mg
	Vfend	Powder, for oral suspension: 40 mg/mL Tablet: 50 mg, 200 mg
clotrimazole + fluconazole	Not available	Vaginal cream + capsule◆: 1% clotrimazole cream +
	Canesoral Combipak	150 mg fluconazole

*Generic available.
*†Generic available in the United States only.
†Strength available in the United States only.
‡Strength available in Canada only.
◆Available OTC in the United States and Canada.
▲Available OTC in the United States only.
ǁAvailable OTC in Canada only.

TECH ALERT!
Terbinafine and terbutaline have look-alike and sound-alike issues.

ALLYLAMINE ANTIFUNGALS

Butenafine, naftifine, and terbinafine are classified as allylamine antifungals. Lamisil (terbinafine) is effective for treating fungal infections involving the nails.

MECHANISM OF ACTION AND PHARMACOKINETICS

Allylamines distort hyphae and stunt the growth of susceptible fungi by blocking an enzyme needed for the synthesis of ergosterol. Butenafine and naftifine are only available for topical application. Terbinafine is formulated for topical and oral use. When administered orally, therapeutic levels are reached within 3 to 18 weeks. Therapeutic levels persist in the skin for 2 to 3 weeks after terbinafine has been discontinued.

ADVERSE EFFECTS

Orally administered terbinafine may produce nausea, vomiting, altered taste, headache, and tiredness. Topical application of terbinafine, butenafine, or naftifine may produce burning, stinging, redness, itchiness, and drying of the skin.

POLYENE CLASS OF ANTIFUNGALS

Nystatin, natamycin, and amphotericin B are all derived from the fungi-like bacteria *Streptomyces*. They belong to the class of antifungals called polyenes. Nystatin is used for the treatment of *Candida* infections on the skin and mucous membranes. Nystatin suspension is commonly prescribed for the treatment of thrush. Amphotericin B is prescribed for systemic infections caused by various fungi, including candidiasis, histoplasmosis, and aspergillosis. Natamycin is used to treat fungal infections in the eye (e.g., blepharitis, conjunctivitis, keratitis). These infections are described in Chapter 20.

Allylamines

Generic Name	U.S. Brand Name(s) / Canadian Brand Name(s)	Dosage Forms and Strengths	Rx (Prescription) or OTC Status
butenafine	Mentax, Lotrimin Ultra Jock Itch, Lotrimin Ultra Athlete's Foot	Cream: 1%	Rx (Mentax)
	Not available		OTC (all Lotrimin Ultra formulations)
naftifine	Naftin	Cream: 1%, 2%	Rx
	Not available	Gel: 1%	
terbinafine*	Lamisil, Lamisil AT Gel, Lamisil AT Athlete's Foot Cream, Lamisil AT for Women, Lamisil AT Jock Itch	Cream: 1% Gel: 1% Granules: 125 mg, 187.5 mg Tablet: 250 mg Spray: 1%	Rx
	Lamisil	Topical solution: 1%	OTC (all Lamisil AT formulations)[†]

*Generic available.
[†]Strength available in the United States only.

Polyenes

Generic Name	U.S. Brand Name(s) / Canadian Brand Name(s)	Dosage Forms and Strengths	Rx or OTC Status
amphotericin B*	Abelcet, Ambisome, Amphotec	Cream (Fungizone): 3%[†] Lotion (Fungizone): 3%[†]	Rx
	Abelcet, Ambisome, Amphotec, Fungizone	Powder, for injection (Ambisome, Amphotec, Fungizone): 50 mg/vial, 100 mg/vial Suspension, oral (Fungizone): 100 mg/mL[†] Suspension, for IV (Abelcet): 5 mg/mL	
natamycin	Natacyn	Ophthalmic suspension: 5%	Rx
	Not available		
nystatin*	Nilstat, Nystop Nyaderm	Cream (Nyaderm): 100,000 units Tablet, oral: 500,000 units Ointment (Nyaderm): 100,000 units Powder, topical (Nystop): 100,000 units Suspension, oral (Nilstat, Nyaderm): 100,000 units Vaginal cream (Nyaderm): 25,000 units/g Vaginal tablet: 100,000 units/tablet	Rx

*Generic available.
[†]Strength available in the United States only.

MECHANISM OF ACTION AND PHARMACOKINETICS

Nystatin, natamycin, and amphotericin B inhibit the synthesis of the fungal cell membrane by binding irreversibly to ergosterol. Nystatin is only available for oral and topical use. Oral absorption of amphotericin B is low so the drug is administered parenterally. Natamycin is formulated for ophthalmic use.

ADVERSE EFFECTS

Systemic absorption of nystatin is low when administered topically and orally, so adverse effects are minimal. Oral administration may produce nausea or diarrhea. Amphotericin B may produce nausea, vomiting, kidney damage, fever, chills, headache, and thrombophlebitis when administered intravenously. Amphotericin B may also cause potassium loss (hypokalemia).

Thiocarbamates

Generic Name	U.S. Brand Name(s) Canadian Brand Name(s)	Dosage Forms and Strengths
tolnaftate*	Lamisil Defense AF, Tinactin, Tinactin Jock Itch	Cream (Pitrex, Tinactin, Tinactin Jock Itch): 1% Gel (Absorbine Jr Antifungal, Fungicure): 1%
	Absorbine Jr Antifungal, Dr Scholl's Athlete's Foot, Fungicure Gel, Pitrex, Tinactin, Tinactin Liquid Chill, Zeasorb AF	Spray (Lamisil Defense AF, Tinactin, Tinactin Liquid Chill): 1% Topical powder (Dr Scholl's Athlete's Foot, Lamisil AF, Tinactin, Zeasorb AF): 1% Topical solution: 1%

*Generic available.

THIOCARBAMATES

Tolnaftate is the only antifungal belonging to the thiocarbamate class. It is approved for the treatment and prevention of athlete's foot. It is also indicated for the treatment of ringworm and jock itch. Tolnaftate is available without prescription.

MECHANISM OF ACTION AND PHARMACOKINETICS

The mechanism of action for tolnaftate is similar to that of terbinafine and naftifine. It stunts the growth of susceptible dermatophytes.

ADVERSE EFFECTS

Adverse reactions are mild; they include irritation at the site of application, itching, or burning.

ECHINOCANDINS

TECH ALERT!
A common ending for echinocandin antifungals is *-fungin*.

Anidulafungin, caspofungin, and micafungin belong to a class of antifungal agents called echinocandins. They are effective for treating infections caused by *Candida* and *Aspergillus*.

MECHANISM OF ACTION AND PHARMACOKINETICS

Echinocandins interfere with the synthesis of the fungal cell wall. They are not toxic to human cells because their target is a cell wall component that does not exist in human cells. Oral absorption is poor, so echinocandins are formulated for parenteral use.

ADVERSE EFFECTS

Echinocandins have fewer adverse effects and drug interactions than other oral or parenterally administered antifungals. They can cause elevated liver enzyme levels, diarrhea, and hypokalemia.

Echinocandins

Generic Name	U.S. Brand Name(s) Canadian Brand Name(s)	Dosage Forms and Strengths
anidulafungin	Eraxis	Powder for injection: 50 mg/vial†, 100 mg/vial
	Eraxis	
caspofungin	Cancidas	Powder for injection: 50 mg/vial, 70 mg/vial
	Cancidas	
micafungin	Mycamine	Powder for injection: 50 mg/vial, 100 mg/vial
	Mycamine	

†Strength available in the United States only.

Miscellaneous Agents

The remaining antifungal agents work by various mechanisms of action. Ciclopirox and undecylenic acid are effective for treating athlete's foot and jock itch. Ciclopirox is a broad-spectrum antifungal agent and is also approved for the treatment of ringworm and mild onychomycosis. Griseofulvin is an orally administered drug used to treat onychomycosis.

MECHANISM OF ACTION AND PHARMACOKINETICS

Ciclopirox, povidone-iodine, and undecylenic acid are topical antifungal agents. Griseofulvin is administered orally. Ciclopirox interferes with DNA and RNA synthesis. Undecylenic acid and zinc undecylate are combined to produce a drug the decreases the spread of susceptible fungi. Formulations must contain at least 10% undecylenate to be effective (between 10% and 27% undecylenate). Also, zinc undecylenate is an astringent and reduces irritation.

Griseofulvin is an orally administered antifungal agent. It interferes with fungal mitosis (see Table 37-2). This disrupts the ability of the fungus to replicate. Griseofulvin formulations made with ultramicronized crystals (Gris-PEG) offer the best absorption. Absorption is also increased when the drug is taken with a fatty meal.

Povidone-iodine is used to treat thrush and is also used as an antiseptic wash (orally and topically).

ADVERSE EFFECTS

Topically applied antifungals may produce mild burning, stinging, itching, swelling, or other signs of skin irritation. Common adverse effects caused by the administration of griseofulvin are nausea, vomiting, headache, dizziness, gas, and heartburn.

TECH ALERT!
Griseofulvin microsize and griseofulvin ultramicrosize have look-alike and sound-alike issues.

Miscellaneous Antifungal Agents

Generic Name	U.S. Brand Name(s) Canadian Brand Name(s)	Dosage Forms and Strengths	Rx or OTC Status
ciclopirox*	Loprox, Penlac Loprox, Penlac, Steiprox	Cream: 0.77%, 1%‡ Gel: 0.77% Lotion: 1%‡ Nail lacquer (Penlac): 8% Shampoo: 1% (Loprox), 1.5% (Steiprox) Suspension, topical: 0.77%	Rx
griseofulvin*	Grifulvin V, Gris-PEG Not available	Suspension: 125 mg/5 mL Tablet, microcrystalline (Grifulvin V): 500 mg Tablet, ultramicrocrystalline (Gris-PEG): 125 mg, 250 mg	Rx
povidone-iodine*	Betadine Betadine	Ointment: 10% Ophthalmic solution: 5% Scrub, cleanser: 7.5% Solution: 10% Spray: 5% Swab stick: 10%†	Rx—ophthalmic and swab stick OTC—all other formulations
undecylenic acid*	Fungicure Liquid, Gordochrom Desenex Ointment, Desenex Antifungal Powder, Fungicure Liquid, Fungicure Professional	Solution, topical: 10%, 12.5% (Fungicure), 25% (Gordochrome) Ointment: undecylenic acid 5.4% + undecylenate 20% (Desenex)‡ Powder: undecylenic acid 2% + undecylenate 27.1%‡	OTC

*Generic available.
†Strength available in the United States only.
‡Strength available in Canada only.

Summary of Drugs Used for the Treatment of Fungal and Yeast Infections

Generic Name	U.S. Brand Name(s)	Usual Dose and Dosing Schedule[a]	Warning Labels
Imidazoles and Triazoles			
butoconazole	Gynezole-1	**Vaginal:** One applicatorful vaginally at bedtime for 3-7 days depending on product formulation	COMPLETE THE FULL COURSE OF THERAPY.
clotrimazole	Lotrimin	**Vaginal:** One applicatorful at bedtime for 3-14 days depending on product formulation **Topical:** Apply bid.	
econazole	Spectazole	**Topical:** Apply bid.	
fluconazole	Diflucan	**Oral or IV:** 200 mg on day 1, then 100 mg daily for 2 wk (esophageal or oropharyngeal candidiasis) *or* 150-200 mg as a single dose or three doses for 3 days each (vulvovaginal candidiasis)	COMPLETE THE FULL COURSE OF THERAPY. SHAKE WELL (SUSPENSION).
itraconazole	Sporonox	**Oral:** 100-400 mg once daily	COMPLETE THE FULL COURSE OF THERAPY. TAKE WITH FOOD. AVOID GRAPEFRUIT JUICE.
ketoconazole	Nizoral	**Oral:** 200-400 mg once daily **Topical:** Apply daily for up to 6 wk. **For dandruff:** Use shampoo every 3-4 days for up to 8 wk.	TAKE WITH FOOD (TABLETS). AVOID ALCOHOL. COMPLETE THE FULL COURSE OF THERAPY.
miconazole	Monistat	**Vaginal:** One applicatorful or one suppository at bedtime for 1-14 days depending on product formulation **Topical:** Apply bid.	COMPLETE THE FULL COURSE OF THERAPY.
oxiconazole	Oxistat	**Topical:** Apply once or twice daily.	COMPLETE THE FULL COURSE OF THERAPY.
posaconazole	Noxafil	**Oral:** 200 mg tid	COMPLETE THE FULL COURSE OF THERAPY. SHAKE WELL. TAKE WITH FOOD.
sulconazole	Exelderm	**Topical:** Apply once or twice daily.	COMPLETE THE FULL COURSE OF THERAPY.
terconazole	Terazol 3, Terazol 7	**Vaginal:** One applicatorful or one suppository at bedtime for 3-7 days depending on product formulation	
tioconazole	Vagistat	**Vaginal:** One applicatorful as a single dose	
sertaconazole	Ertaczo	Apply a thin layer of 2% cream to cleansed, dry, infected area bid for 4 wk.	
voriconazole	Vfend	**Parenteral:** 6 mg/kg IV every 12 hr	AVOID GRAPEFRUIT JUICE. TAKE ON AN EMPTY STOMACH. AVOID ALCOHOL.
		Oral: 400 mg every 12 hr loading dose on day 1, followed by 200 mg every 12 hr	

Summary of Drugs Used for the Treatment of Fungal and Yeast Infections—cont'd

Generic Name	U.S. Brand Name(s)	Usual Dose and Dosing Schedule[a]	Warning Labels
Allylamines			
butenafine	Mentax	**Topical:** Apply once daily for 2-4 wk.	COMPLETE THE FULL COURSE OF THERAPY.
naftifine	Naftin	**Topical:** Apply cream once daily and apply gel bid.	
terbinafine	Lamisil	**Topical:** Apply cream bid and apply gel once daily for 1 to 4 wk. **Oral:** 250 mg once daily for 6-12 wk	COMPLETE THE FULL COURSE OF THERAPY. TAKE WITH FOOD (TABLETS).
Polyenes			
amphotericin B	Fungizone	**IV:** 0.25-1.5/kg/day (max, 1.5 mg/day)	PROTECT FROM LIGHT (IV SOLUTION). REFRIGERATE.
natamycin	Natacyn	**Ophthalmic:** See Chapter 20.	SHAKE WELL.
nystatin	Generics	**Capsule:** One cap tid **Suspension:** 4-6 mL swished in mouth qid **Topical:** Apply bid. **Vaginal:** One insert nightly for 14 days	COMPLETE THE FULL COURSE OF THERAPY. SHAKE WELL (SUSPENSION).
Thiocarbamates			
tolnaftate	Tinactin	**Topical:** Apply bid for 2-4 wk.	COMPLETE THE FULL COURSE OF THERAPY.
Echinocandins			
anidulafungin	Eraxis	100-mg IV loading dose on day 1, followed by 50 mg IV daily for 7 days after symptoms resolve	REFRIGERATE; DON'T FREEZE (CASPOFUNGIN, ANIDULAFUNGIN).
caspofungin	Cancidas	70-mg IV infusion as a loading dose on day 1, followed by 50 mg IV infusion once daily for at least 14 days	
micafungin	Mycamine	150 mg IV daily for 10-30 days	TO MIX, GENTLY SWIRL; DO NOT SHAKE. MAY BE STORED AT ROOM TEMPERATURE FOR 24 HR.
Miscellaneous Agents			
griseofulvin	Gris-PEG	**For tinea unguium** **Oral:** 660-750 mg (ultramicrosize) or 750 mg-1 g (microsize) once daily or in 2-4 divided doses	COMPLETE THE FULL COURSE OF THERAPY. TAKE WITH FOOD. SHAKE WELL.
ciclopirox	Loprox	**Topical:** Apply twice daily.	COMPLETE THE FULL COURSE OF THERAPY.

[a]Usual dose for candidiasis or tinea.

Chapter Summary

- Fungal organisms are similar to plants but lack chlorophyll and can cause mycotic (fungal) infections.
- Some fungi are beneficial to humans, whereas others cause serious infections.
- The general term used to describe a fungal infection is *mycosis*.
- Most fungal infections of the skin are caused by a group of fungi called dermatophytes.
- Mycoses caused by the dermatophyte tinea are named for the site of the infection. For example, tinea manus is a fungal infection on the hands, tinea corporis is an infection on the body, and tinea capitis is located on the head (cap).
- Women who take broad-spectrum anti-infectives may get a yeast infection because the bacteria and fungi that keep the yeast normally present in the vagina from overgrowing are killed by the antibiotic.
- Athlete's foot (tinea pedis) is a common fungal infection that affects athletes and nonathletes.
- Athlete's foot can be prevented by the following: (1) keeping feet clean and dry; (2) wearing open sandals to permit feet to breathe; (3) not walking barefoot across the floor of public facilities; (4) wearing cotton socks and changing socks daily; and (5) using antifungal powders to prevent recurrent infections.
- Tinea infections are also called ringworm. Ringworm has a characteristic ringlike shape and may affect the body, scalp, nails, or feet.
- Ringworm is contagious and is spread via person-to-person and animal-to-person contact.
- *Candida*, also called yeast, is a type of fungus that thrives in warm moist areas and is responsible for fungal infections in the vagina, groin, and mouth.
- Vulvovaginal candidiasis is also known as yeast vaginitis.
- A *Candida* infection in the oral cavity is called thrush.
- Many fungal infections can be treated with nonprescription antifungal agents.
- Fungal infections such as vulvovaginal candidiasis, jock itch, and athlete's foot can be cured using OTC drugs. Some of these drugs can also be used as prophylaxis.
- There are three primary mechanisms of action for antifungal agents: (1) destroy the cell membrane of the fungus; (2) interfere with the synthesis of nucleic acids needed for replication; and (3) inhibit the synthesis of the fungal cell wall.
- A common ending for many antifungal agents is *-azole*.
- The imidazoles and triazoles interfere with ergosterol, an essential component needed for the synthesis of the fungal cell membrane.
- Topical azoles are formulated for application to the skin (creams, gel, lotion), mucous membranes (vaginal creams, suppositories), and scalp (shampoo).
- Butenafine, naftifine, and terbinafine are classified as allylamine antifungals.
- Nystatin, natamycin, and amphotericin B are all derived from the fungi-like bacteria *Streptomyces* and belong to the class of antifungals called polyenes.
- Nystatin, natamycin, and amphotericin B inhibit the synthesis of the fungal cell membrane.
- Tolnaftate is the only antifungal belonging to the thiocarbamate class. It is approved for the treatment and prevention of athlete's foot.
- Anidulafungin, caspofungin, and micafungin belong to a class of antifungal agents called echinocandins.
- Echinocandins interfere with the synthesis of the fungal cell wall.
- The bioavailability of griseofulvin formulations varies. Formulations made with ultramicronized crystals (Gris-PEG) have better absorption than formulations made from micronized crystals. Absorption is also increased when the drug is taken with a fatty meal.

1. *Candida* is a type of _____. It is also called yeast.
   a. Virus
   b. Bacteria
   c. Fungus
   d. Protozoan

2. The antibiotic _____ is derived from a mold.
   a. Tetracycline
   b. Penicillin
   c. Doxycycline
   d. Cephalosporin

3. Ringworm is caused by a _____.
   a. Worm
   b. Fungus
   c. Bacteria
   d. Insect

4. Fungal infections of the _____ are called onychomycosis.
   a. Hair
   b. Skin
   c. Scalp
   d. Nails

5. Which of the following is the primary mechanism of action for antifungal agents?
   a. Destroying the cell membrane of the fungus
   b. Interfering with the synthesis of nucleic acids needed for replication
   c. Inhibiting the synthesis of the fungal cell wall
   d. All of the above

6. _____ is effective for treating fungal infections involving the nails.
   a. Lamisil
   b. Tioconazole
   c. Nystatin
   d. Clotrimazole

7. Nystatin suspension is commonly prescribed for the treatment of thrush.
   a. True
   b. False

8. Natamycin is formulated for _____ use.
   a. Topical
   b. Ophthalmic
   c. Otic
   d. Oral

9. Echinocandins are formulated for oral use.
   a. True
   b. False

10. Griseofulvin is a(n) _____ administered antifungal agent.
    a. Topically
    b. Orally
    c. Parenterally
    d. All of the above

1. There are many reports of onychomycosis caused by artificial nails. What is causing these infections, and how can they be prevented?
2. How did the term *athlete's foot* come about?

Bibliography

Aetna InteliHealth: Candidiasis, 2012 (http://www.intelihealth.com/IH/ihtIH/WSIHW000/9339/31092.html).

Cappelletty D, Eiselstein-McKitrick K: The echinocandins, *Pharmacotherapy* 27:369-388, 2007.

Elsevier: Gold Standard Clinical Pharmacology. Retrieved April 2, 2011, from https://www.clinicalpharmacology.com/, 2010.

FDA: FDA Approved Drug Products. Retrieved July 5, 2012, from http://www.accessdata.fda.gov/scripts/cder/drugsatfda/index.cfm?fuseaction=Search.Search_Drug_Name, 2012.

Health Canada: Drug product database, 2010. Retrieved July 5, 2012 (http://www.hc-sc.gc.ca/dhp-mps/prodpharma/databasdon/index-eng.php).

Kalant H, Grant D, Mitchell J: *Principles of medical pharmacology*, ed 7, Toronto, 2007, Elsevier Canada, pp 688, 691-695.

Lance L, Lacy C, Armstrong L, et al: *Drug information handbook for the allied health professional*, ed 12, Hudson, OH, 2005, APhA Lexi-Comp.

MedlinePlus: Cutaneous candidiasis, 2012 (http://www.nlm.nih.gov/medlineplus/ency/article/000880.htm).

MedlinePlus: Tinea infections (ringworm), 2011 (http://www.nlm.nih.gov/medlineplus/tineainfections.html).

Merck Manual Online Professional Library: Dermatophytoses, 2011 (http://www.merck.com/mmpe/sec10/ch120/ch120c.html?qt=ringwormandalt=sh).

National Institute of Allergy and Infectious Diseases: Vaginal yeast infection, 2008 (http://www.niaid.nih.gov/topics/vaginalYeast/Pages/default.aspx).

National Institute of Allergy and Infectious Diseases: Vaginitis, 2011 (http://www.niaid.nih.gov/topics/vaginitis/Pages/default.aspx).

National Institute of Allergy and Infectious Diseases: Sexually transmitted diseases (STDs), 2012 (http://www.niaid.nih.gov/topics/std/Pages/default.aspx).

National Institute of Allergy and Infectious Diseases: Understanding microbes in sickness and in health, 2006 (https://scholarworks.iupui.edu/bitstream/handle/1805/747/Understanding%20microbes%2c%20in%20sickness%20and%20in%20health.pdf?sequence=1).

Pray W: *Nonprescription product therapeutics*, Baltimore, 1999, Lippincott Williams and Wilkins, pp 542-551.

USP Center for Advancement of Patient Safety: Use caution—avoid confusion, USP Quality Review No. 79, Rockville, MD, 2004, USP Center for Advancement of Patient Safety.

40

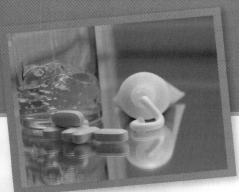

Treatment of Decubitus Ulcers and Burns

1 Learn the terminology associated with decubitus ulcers and burns.

2 Describe the stages of decubitus ulcers and degrees of burns.

3 List and categorize medications used to treat decubitus ulcers and burns.

4 Describe the mechanism of action for each class of drugs used to treat decubitus ulcers and burns.

5 Identify significant drug look-alike and sound-alike issues.

6 Identify warning labels and precautionary messages associated with medications used to treat decubitus ulcers and burns.

KEY TERMS

Blister: Collection of fluid below or within the epidermis.

Débridement: Surgical removal of foreign material and dead tissue from a wound in order to prevent infection and promote healing.

Decubitus ulcer: Pressure sore or "bedsore."

Dehiscent wound: A wound that has reopened after it has been closed surgically.

Eschar: Blackened necrotic tissue of a decubitus ulcer.

Escharotomy: Removal of necrotic skin and underlying tissue.

First-degree burn: Minor discomfort and reddening of the skin.

Fourth-degree burn: Burn that involves underlying muscles, fasciae, or bone.

Full-thickness burn: Third-degree burn where the epidermis and dermis are destroyed.

Partial-thickness burns: First- and second-degree burns.

Rule of palms: Rule for determining the extent of a burn surface area. A palm size of a burn victim is about 1% of total body surface area.

Rule of nines: Formula for estimating the percentage of adult body surface covered by burns dividing the body into 11 areas, each representing 9% of the body surface area.

Second-degree burn: Burn that involves deep epidermal layers and causes damage to the upper layers of dermis.

Third-degree burn: Burn that is characterized by destruction of the epidermis and dermis.

Decubitus Ulcers

A *decubitus ulcer* is a pressure sore, commonly called a "bedsore" (Figure 40-1). Decubitus means "lying down," a name that hints at a common cause of pressure sores, lying in a prone position for long periods. Pressure sores typically occur in patients who are confined to a bed or chair. Patients with sensory or mobility deficits such as spinal cord injury, stroke, coma, multiple sclerosis, peripheral vascular disease, or diabetes, hospitalized older patients, nursing home residents, and malnourished patients are all at risk. Decubitus ulcers can range from a mild pink coloration of the skin, which disappears in a few hours after pressure is relieved on the area, to a deep wound extending to and sometimes through a bone into internal organs. These ulcers, as well as other wound types, are classified in stages according to the severity of the wound.

All decubitus ulcers have a course of injury similar to a burn wound. This can be a mild redness of the skin and/or blistering, such as a first-degree burn, to a deep open wound with blackened tissue, such as a third-degree burn. This blackened tissue is called an *eschar*.

MECHANISM OF FORMATION

A decubitus ulcer typically forms from continuous pressure to an area, however, it can also occur from friction caused by rubbing against something such as a bed sheet, cast, or brace or prolonged exposure to cold. The most common places for pressure ulcers to form are over bones close to the skin, such as the elbows, heels, hips, sacrum, ankles, shoulders, back, and back of the head. The weight of a body presses on the bone and the bone presses on the tissue and skin that it covers. This tissue begins to decay from lack of blood circulation, resulting in the formation of a decubitus ulcer.

WOUND STAGES

Wounds are often categorized according to severity by the use of stages. This is similar to the staging system used to classify burns.

Stage I

This stage is characterized by a surface reddening of the skin. The skin is unbroken and the wound is superficial. Examples of stage I wounds are a light sunburn, a first-degree burn, or a decubitus ulcer. The burn heals spontaneously or the decubitus ulcer quickly fades when pressure is relieved

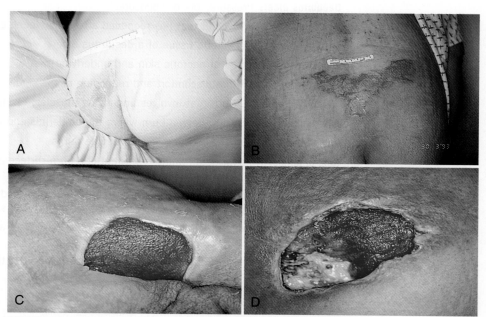

FIGURE 40-1 Decubitus ulcers. **A,** Stage I. **B,** Stage II. **C,** Stage III. **D,** Stage IV. (From Potter PA, Perry AG: *Fundamentals of nursing*, ed 4, St. Louis, 1997, Mosby.)

on that area. The key factors to consider in a stage I wound are the causes of the wound and how to alleviate the pressure on the area to prevent it from worsening. Improving the nutritional status of the individual should also be considered early to prevent wound worsening. The presence of a stage I wound is an indication or early warning of a problem and a signal to take preventive action.

Stage II

This stage is characterized by a **blister**, either broken or unbroken. A partial layer of the skin is injured. Involvement is no longer superficial. The goal of care is to cover, protect, and clean the area. Coverings designed to insulate, absorb, and protect are used. Close attention to prevention, protection, nutrition, and hydration is important also. With quick attention, a stage II wound can heal rapidly. Generally, decubitus ulcers or pressure wounds developing beyond stage II are the result of lack of aggressive intervention when first noted at stage I.

Stage III

In stage III, the wound has extended through all layers of the skin. It is the primary site for a serious infection to occur. The goal of treatment is to alleviate pressure and cover and protect the wound, as with stage II, and an increased emphasis on nutrition and hydration is applied. Medical care is necessary to promote healing and treat and prevent infection. This type of wound will progress rapidly if left unattended. Infection is of grave concern.

Stage IV

Stage IV wounds extend through the skin and involve underlying muscle, tendons, and bone. The diameter of the wound is not as important as the depth. This is very serious and can produce a life-threatening infection, especially if not treated aggressively. All the goals of protecting, cleaning, and alleviating pressure on the area still apply. Nutrition and hydration are now critical. Without adequate nutrition, this wound will not heal.

Anyone with a stage IV wound requires medical care by someone skilled in wound care. Surgical removal of the necrotic or decayed tissue is often necessary for wounds of larger diameter. A skilled wound care physician, physical therapist, or nurse can sometimes successfully treat a smaller diameter wound without surgery. Surgery is the usual course of treatment for larger stage IV wounds. Amputation may be necessary in some cases.

CARE, PREVENTION, AND TREATMENT OF DECUBITUS ULCERS

The Norton or Braden scale (Table 40-1) is a simple assessment tool used to determine a patient's risk for developing a decubitus ulcer.

The most important principle is to prevent initial skin damage, which promotes ulceration. In at-risk patients, aggressive nursing practices, such as frequent turning of immobile patients, changing position every 2 hours or more frequently if needed, and the application of skin protection to bony body parts, is frequently effective. This 2-hour time frame is generally accepted as the maximum interval that the tissue can tolerate pressure without damage. Maintaining hydration, nutrition high in protein, and hygiene are also important parts of prevention and treatment. Range-of-motion exercises and early ambulation are encouraged; low-pressure mattresses and special beds are also used.

TABLE 40-1 **The Norton Scale***

Physical Condition	Mental State	Activity	Mobility	Incontinence	Total Score
Good, 4	Alert, 4	Ambulatory, 4	Full, 4	Not, 4	
Fair, 3	Apathetic, 3	Walks with help, 3	Slightly limited, 3	Occasional, 3	
Poor, 2	Confused, 2	Chair-bound, 2	Very limited, 2	Usual urinary output, 2	
Very bad, 1	Stuporous, 1	Confined to bed, 1	Immobile, 1	Double urinary output, 1	

*The patient is rated from 1 to 4 on the five risk factors listed. A score ≤ 14 indicates a risk for decubitus ulcers or pressure sores.

BOX 40-1   **Topical Treatment of Decubitus Ulcers**

- Occlusive hydrocolloid dressings
- Polyurethane films
- Absorbable gelatin sponges
- Karaya gum patches
- Antiseptic irrigations
- Antibiotic ointments
- Air-permeable occlusive clear dressings (allow aspiration of collected fluids)
- Supportive adhesive-backed foam padding
- Absorptive dextranomer beads

The treatment for a decubitus ulcer involves keeping the area clean and removing necrotic (dead) tissue, which can form a breeding ground for infection. There are many procedures and products available for this purpose. Topical treatments aid the healing of partial-thickness sores (Box 40-1). Some deep wounds even require surgical removal or **débridement** of necrotic tissue. In some cases, amputation may be necessary.

Collagenase

Collagenase is used to promote débridement of necrotic tissue in dermal ulcers and severe burns. Collagenase is a water-soluble proteinase that specifically breaks down collagen into gelatin, allowing less specific enzymes to act. Collagenase is most effective within a narrow pH range of 6 to 8. The two commercially available preparations of collagenase (Santyl, Xiaflex) are derived from the bacterium *Clostridium histolyticum*. In addition, there is evidence that elastin and fibrin are also degraded by collagenase, but to a lesser degree.

Papain and Urea

Papain and urea are used as an enzymatic débridement ointment for the treatment of chronic and acute wounds. Papain is derived from the carica papaya fruit. Papain and urea–based products are most commonly used. The mechanism of action is for papain to attach to and break down any proteins containing cysteine residues. This process is nonselective because most proteins, including growth factors, contain cysteine residues. Collagen contains no cysteine residues and is therefore unaffected by papain. The primary use of a papain-urea product is for nonspecific bulk débridement with a broad pH range (3 to 12).

Trypsin, Balsam Peru, and Castor Oil

Trypsin, balsam Peru, and castor oil are used in the treatment of decubitus ulcers, varicose ulcers, sunburns, **dehiscent wounds** that have come apart, and for débridement of eschar. Trypsin is used to débride necrotic tissue, balsam Peru stimulates circulation at the wound site and may be mildly bactericidal, and castor oil improves epithelialization, acts as a protectant covering, and helps reduce pain. Local application may produce temporary stinging at the application site.

Antibacterials

Antibacterial drugs may be used if the decubitus ulcer is not healing or it continues to ooze after 2 weeks of proper cleansing and bandage changes. Some antibacterial preparations can be applied directly to the skin. Anti-infectives given by mouth or injection are needed for those who have sepsis or infections in the skin or underlying bone. Anti-infectives are also given to prevent diseased heart valves from getting infected, or when the ulcer needs surgical repair.

Burns

Typically, we think of a burn as a thermal injury or lesion caused by contact of the skin with some hot object or fire. In addition, overexposure to ultraviolet light (sunburn) or contact with an electric current, corrosive chemical, or radioactive agents causes injury or death to skin cells. The injuries that result can be classified as burns; the effects may be local or systemic, involving primary shock (which occurs immediately after injury and rarely is fatal) or secondary shock (which develops insidiously following severe burns and is often fatal). In the United States and Canada, approximately

TECH ALERT
The following drugs have look-alike and sound-alike issues:
 Granulex and Regranex;
 Gentamycin, Garamycin, Terramycin, and Kanamycin;
 Betadine, Betagan, and betaine;
 Bactroban, bacitracin, and Baclofen;
 metronidazole and metformin

Treatment of Decubitus Ulcers

Generic Name	U.S. Brand Name(s) / Canadian Brand Name(s)	Dosage Forms and Strengths
collagenase	Santyl, Xiaflex / Santyl	Ointment (Santyl): 250 units/g Powder, for injection (Xiaflex): 0.9 mg/vial
papain and urea	Accuzyme, Ethezyme-830, Gladase, Kovia, Ziox / Not available	Ointment: 830,000 units papain + 10% urea (Accuzyme, Ethezyme-830, Gladase, Kovia); 521,700 units papain + 10% urea + chlorophyllin copper complex (Ziox)
trypsin, balsam Peru, and castor oil	Optase, Granul-Derm, Allan Derm-T, Xenaderm, Granulex / Not available	Aerosol: trypsin 0.1 mg, balsam Peru 72.5 mg, castor oil 650 mg (Granulex, Granul-Derm); trypsin 0.12 mg, balsam Peru 87 mg, castor oil 788 mg Granulex) Gel (Optase): trypsin 0.12 mg, balsam Peru 87 mg, castor oil 788 mg Ointment: balsam Peru 87 mg/g, castor oil 788 mg/g, trypsin 90 USP units/g (Allan Derm-T, Xenaderm)
Topical Antibacterials		
bacitracin zinc*	Generics / Bacitin	Ointment: 500 units/g
gentamicin*	Generics / Generics	Cream: 0.1% Ointment: 0.1%
metronidazole*	Metrocreme, Metrogel, Metrolotion, Noritate / Flagyl Cream, Metrocreme, Metrogel, Metrolotion, Noritate, Rosasol	Cream: 0.75% (Metrocreme), 1% (Noritate, Rosasol) Gel, topical: 0.75% (Metrogel), 1% (Metrogel, Rosasol) Lotion: 0.75% (Metrolotion)
mupirocin*	Bactroban, Centany / Bactroban, Bactroban Cream	Cream: 2% Ointment: 2%
Antiseptics		
povidone-iodine*	Betadine / Betadine	Ointment: 10% Suspension, topical: 7.5% Pad: 10% Solution: 7.5%, 10% Spray: 5% Sponge: 10%, 20%[†] Swab sticks: 10%[†]

*Generic available.
[†]Strength available in the United States only.

1.25 million persons receive medical treatment for burns annually. More than 50,000 of these burn victims are hospitalized as a result of a severe burn injury.

ESTIMATING BODY SURFACE AREA

When burns involve large areas of skin, treatment and the prognosis for recovery depend in large part on the total area involved and severity of the burn. The severity of a burn is determined by the depth and extent (percentage of body surface area [BSA]) of the lesion. There are several ways to estimate the extent of BSA burned. One method is called the rule of palms and is based on the assumption that the palm size of a burn victim is about 1% of the total BSA. Therefore, estimating the number of palms that are burned approximates the percentage of BSA involved.

The rule of 9s (Figure 40-2) is another, more accurate method of determining the extent of a burn injury. In this technique, the body is divided into 11 areas of 9%, with the area around the

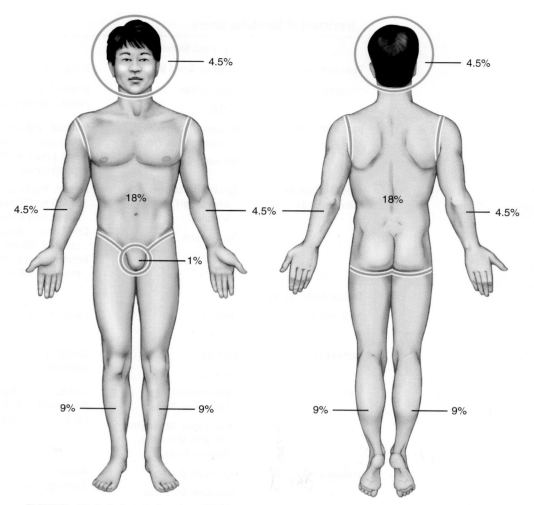

FIGURE 40-2 Rule of 9s. (From Thibodeau GA, Patton KT: *Anatomy and physiology*, ed 6, St. Louis, 2007, Mosby.)

genitals, called the perineum, representing the additional 1% of BSA. As Figure 40-2 shows, 9% of the skin covers the head and upper extremities, including the front and back surfaces. Twice as much, or 18%, of the total skin area covers the front and back of the trunk and each lower extremity, including the front and back surfaces. The rule of 9s works well with adults but does not reflect the differences of BSA in small children. Special tables called Lund-Browder charts, which take the large surface area of certain body areas (e.g., the head) in a growing child into account, are used by physicians to estimate burn percentages in children.

The depth of a burn injury depends on the tissue layers of the skin that are involved (Figure 40-3). A first-degree burn (typical sunburn) causes minor discomfort and some reddening of the skin. Although the surface layers of the burned area may peel in 1 or 2 days, no blistering occurs, and the actual tissue destruction is minimal. First- and second-degree burns are called partial-thickness burns.

Second-degree burns involve the deep epidermal layers and always cause injury to the upper layers of the dermis. In deep second-degree burns, damage to sweat glands, hair follicles, and sebaceous glands may occur, but tissue death is not complete. Blisters, severe pain, generalized swelling, and edema characterize this type of burn. Scarring is common.

Third-degree, or full-thickness, burns are characterized by destruction of both the epidermis and dermis. Tissue death extends below the follicles and sweat glands. If the burn involves underlying muscles, fasciae, or bone, it may be called a fourth-degree burn. A distinction between a second- and third- or fourth-degree burn is that a third- or fourth-degree lesion is insensitive to pain immediately after injury because of destruction of the nerve endings. Scarring is a serious problem. Third- and fourth-degree burns are best managed in specialized burn centers.

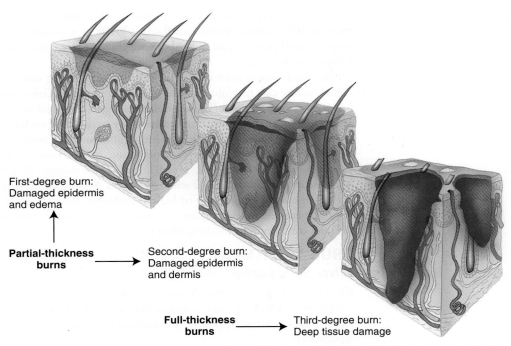

First-degree burn:
Damaged epidermis
and edema

Partial-thickness burns

Second-degree burn:
Damaged epidermis
and dermis

Full-thickness burns

Third-degree burn:
Deep tissue damage

FIGURE 40-3 Classification of burns. (From Thibodeau GA, Patton KT: *Anatomy and physiology*, ed 6, St. Louis, 2007, Mosby.)

COMPLICATIONS

Sloughing of skin, gangrene, scarring, erysipelas (skin infection caused by group A staphylococci), nephritis (kidney infection), pneumonia, immune system impairment, and intestinal disturbances are possible complications. The risk of complication is greatest when more than 25% of the body surface is burned. Two common complications of burns are infection and dehydration.

Signs of infection are as follows:
- Change in color of the burned area or surrounding skin
- Purplish discoloration, particularly if swelling is also present
- Change in thickness of the burn
- Greenish discharge or pus
- Fever

Signs of dehydration are as follows:
- Thirst
- Lightheadedness or dizziness (when moving from lying or sitting to standing)
- Weakness
- Dry skin
- Urinating less often than usual

PRECAUTIONS

Sunburn can be prevented by using sunscreen or sunblock and avoiding excess exposure to ultraviolet (UV) radiation. Chemical-related skin burns can be prevented by avoiding strong chemicals. "Stop, drop, and roll" should be the first actions if a person is on fire. A rug, blanket, or anything within reach can be used to smother flames. Care must be taken so that the individual does not inhale the smoke. Clothing must be carefully cut away so that skin is not pulled away. Blisters should not be opened, because this will increase the chance for infection. All burned patients must receive appropriate tetanus prophylaxis.

TREATMENT

The first step in the care of the burn patient is to check for airway injury or impaired breathing. Airway injury is most likely to occur after facial burns or smoke inhalation in closed spaces.

The second step in burn care is to ensure cardiac output and tissue perfusion. Volume replenishment with crystalloid intravenous fluids is given by standard protocol; at the same time, urinary output, blood pressure and pulse, body weight, and renal function are closely monitored to ensure adequate hydration.

The third step in burn care is the removal of overlying clothing and the irrigation of affected tissues, taking care to avoid excessive cooling of the body. Gentle tissue débridement should be followed by the application of nonadherent dressings, skin substitutes, topical antiseptics, or autografts, as dictated by circumstances. An **escharotomy** (removal of necrotic skin and underlying tissue) for circumferential burns (burns that extend right around the body), antibiotic therapy for infections, IV analgesics, pressor support for hypotension, and/or nutritional support may be needed. Fluid balance is carefully monitored, as well as nutritional therapy. Beta blockers are given to reduce the hypermetabolic state associated with large burns. Emotional support is offered to help patients cope with their altered body image or lifestyle concerns. Burned tissues are positioned per protocol to minimize edema and contractures. Treatment is instituted to prevent venous thrombosis, pneumonia, and complications resulting from immobility.

DRUG TREATMENT

Silver Sulfadiazine

Silver sulfadiazine is the most frequently used topical agent for burns. It is thought to act via the inhibition of DNA replication and modification of the cell membrane and cell wall. The drug is bactericidal against gram-positive and gram-negative organisms, but resistance has occasionally been reported.

ADVERSE EFFECTS

Local skin reactions such as pain, burning, itching, and hypersensitivity are occasionally reported. Transient leukopenia occurs in 5% to 15% of patients, but there is no increased incidence of infectious complications.

Mafenide

Mafenide appears to act on bacterial cellular mechanisms. It interferes with bacterial folic acid synthesis through competitive inhibition of para-aminobenzoic acid. With topical application, mafenide is bacteriostatic against gram-positive and gram-negative bacteria.

ADVERSE EFFECTS

Pain or a burning sensation following mafenide application is the most frequently reported adverse effect. Mafenide is a strong carbonic anhydrase inhibitor. Carbonic anhydrase inhibitors block carbonic anhydrase, an enzyme that affects acid-base balance by its ability to form carbonic acid from water and carbon dioxide. Mafenide may cause alkaline diuresis, leading to acid-base abnormalities. It also inhibits epithelial regeneration (growth of new tissue).

Silver Nitrate

Silver nitrate is a broad-spectrum agent. It is bacteriostatic at a concentration of 5%. The effects of silver nitrate may result from silver ions readily combining with several biologically important chemical groups.

ADVERSE EFFECTS

Silver nitrate is prepared with distilled water. The hypotonic solution may lead to electrolyte imbalance.

Povidone-Iodine

Povidone-iodine acts by destroying microbial protein and DNA. This drug has excellent in vitro antimicrobial activity but is inactivated by wound exudates. In vitro refers to a test that is done in glass or plastic vessels in the laboratory.

ADVERSE EFFECTS

Systemic absorption of iodine results in renal and thyroid dysfunction.

Topical Treatment of Burns

Generic Name	U.S. Brand Name(s) Canadian Brand Name(s)	Dosage Forms and Strengths
mafenide	Sulfamylon Not available	Cream: 85 mg/g Powder, for topical solution: 5%
silver sulfadiazine	Silvadene, Thermazene, SSD, SSD AF Dermazin, Flamazine	Cream: 1%

Summary of Drugs Used in the Treatment of Decubitus Ulcers and Burns

Generic Name	Brand Name	Usual Dose and Dosing Schedule	Warning Labels
Débriding Agents			
collagenase	Santyl	Apply once daily (more if dressing becomes soiled).	DO NOT TOUCH THE TIP OF THE TUBE TO ANY SURFACE, INCLUDING A FINGER, THE WOUND, OR STERILE GAUZE PAD. FLAMMABLE; AVOID OPEN FLAME (GRANUL-DERM SPRAY).
papain and urea	Allanenzyme, Ethezyme, Gladase	Apply directly to wound once or twice daily; secure into place.	
trypsin, balsam peru, and castor oil	Granul-derm	Apply a minimum of bid or as often as necessary.	
Topical Antibacterials			
bacitracin	Baciguent	Apply one to five times daily for up to 7 days.	NOT TO BE USED FOR LONGER THAN 1 WK UNLESS PRESCRIBED.
gentamicin*		**Topical:** apply three or four times daily to affected area.	REPORT ANY DIZZINESS OR SENSATIONS OF RINGING OR FULLNESS IN EARS.
mupirocin	Bactoban	Apply small amount to affected area tid for 7 to 14 days.	FOR TOPICAL USE ONLY DISCONTINUE IF RASH, ITCHING, OR IRRITATION OCCURS.
silver sulfadiazine	Silvadene	Apply bid with a sterile-gloved hand; apply to thickness of $\frac{1}{16}$ inch.	FOR EXTERNAL USE ONLY
mafenide	Sulfamylon	Apply once or twice daily with a sterile-gloved hand; apply to thickness of $\frac{1}{16}$ inch. The burned area should be covered with cream at all times.	DISCONTINUE AND REPORT IMMEDIATELY IF RASH, BLISTERS, OR SWELLING APPEAR WHILE USING CREAM. FOR EXTERNAL USE ONLY
silver nitrate	Generics	Apply a cotton applicator dipped in solution on the affected area two or three times/wk for 2-3 wk.	DISCONTINUE IF REDNESS OR IRRITATION DEVELOPS.
Antiseptics			
povidone-iodine	Betadine	Apply as needed for treatment and prevention of susceptible microbial infections.	DO NOT SWALLOW. FOR EXTERNAL USE AVOID CONTACT WITH THE EYES.

*Generic available.

Rehabilitation

During rehabilitation, individually fitted elastic garments are used to prevent hypertrophic scar formation, and joints are exercised to promote a full range of motion. Referrals for occupational therapy, psychological counseling, support groups, or social services are often necessary to assist the patient with life adjustments.

Chapter Summary

- Decubitus ulcers can range from a very mild pink coloration of the skin, which disappears in a few hours after pressure is relieved on the area, to a very deep wound extending to and sometimes through a bone into internal organs.
- Decubitus ulcers form on area of the body that is exposed to continuous pressure. However it can also occur from friction by rubbing against something such as a bed sheet, cast, or brace or prolonged exposure to cold.
- Stage I of a decubitus ulcer is characterized by a surface reddening of the skin.
- Stage II is characterized by a blister, broken or unbroken.
- In stage III, the wound has extended through all layers of the skin.
- Stage IV wounds extend through the skin and involve underlying muscle, tendons, and bone.
- The treatment for a decubitus ulcer involves keeping the area clean and removing necrotic (dead) tissue, which can form a breeding ground for infection.
- Collagenase is used to promote débridement of necrotic tissue in dermal ulcers and severe burns.
- Papain and urea ointment are used for enzymatic débridement of chronic and acute wounds.
- Trypsin, balsam Peru, and castor oil are used for the treatment of decubitus ulcers, varicose ulcers, débridement of eschar, dehiscent wounds, and sunburns.
- Antibacterial drugs may be used if the decubitus ulcer is not healing or it continues to ooze after 2 weeks of proper cleansing and bandage changes.
- The injuries that result from electrical, chemical, or radioactive agents can be classified as burns. The effects may be local or systemic involving primary shock (which occurs immediately after injury and rarely fatal) or secondary shock (which develops insidiously following severe burns and is often fatal).
- The severity of a burn is determined by the depth and extent (percentage of body surface area) of the lesion.
- There are several ways to estimate the extent of body surface area burned. One method is called the rule of palms and is based on the assumption that the palm size of a burn victim is approximately 1% of the total body surface area.
- The rule of 9s is another and more accurate method of determining the extent of a burn injury. With this method, the body is divided into 11 areas of 9%, with the area around the genitals, called the perineum, representing the additional 1% of body surface area.
- A first-degree burn (typical sunburn) causes minor discomfort and some reddening of the skin.
- Second-degree burns involve the deep epidermal layers and always cause injury to the upper layers of the dermis.
- Third-degree, or full-thickness, burns are characterized by destruction of both the epidermis and dermis.
- If burning involves underlying muscles, fasciae, or bone, it may be called a fourth-degree burn.
- Two common complications of burns are infection and dehydration.
- The procedure for the care of the burn patient includes assessing the airway to ensure that breathing is unimpaired, ensuring cardiac output and tissue perfusion; removing overlying clothing, and irrigating affected tissues. Gentle tissue débridement should be followed by application of nonadherent dressings, skin substitutes, topical antiseptics, or autografts, as dictated by circumstances.
- Silver sulfadiazine is the most frequently used topical agent for burns. It is thought to act via the inhibition of DNA replication and modification of the cell membrane and cell wall.
- Mafenide appears to act on bacterial cellular mechanism. It interferes with bacterial folic acid synthesis through competitive inhibition of para-aminobenzoic acid.
- Silver nitrate is a broad-spectrum agent. It is bacteriostatic at a concentration of 5%.

1. Pressure sores typically occur in patients who are _____.
   a. Confined to the bed
   b. Chair-bound
   c. Ambulatory
   d. a and b

2. The usual mechanism of forming a decubitus ulcer is from _____.
   a. Pressure
   b. Infection
   c. Inflammation
   d. Laceration

3. In stage _____ of a decubitus ulcer, the wound has extended through all layers of the skin.
   a. I
   b. II
   c. III
   d. IV

4. Frequent turning is optional to alleviate pressure on the wound and to promote healing.
   a. True
   b. False

5. The severity of a burn is determined by the _____ (percentage of body surface area) of the lesion.
   a. Depth
   b. Width
   c. Extent
   d. a and c

6. The rule of 9s is a more accurate method of determining the extent of a burn injury than the rule of palms.
   a. true
   b. false

7. Third-degree, or _____, burns are characterized by destruction of both the epidermis and dermis.
   a. Partial-thickness
   b. Full-thickness
   c. Total thickness
   d. All of the above

8. Common complications of burns are _____ and _____.
   a. infection, dehydration
   b. infection, stroke
   c. dehydration, stroke
   d. stroke, shock

9. _____ is the most frequently used topical agent for burns.
   a. Gentamycin
   b. Silver sulfadiazine
   c. Silver nitrate
   d. Mupirocin

10. The removal of necrotic skin and underlying tissue from a burn or decubitus ulcer is termed _____.
    a. Escharectomy
    b. Escharotomy
    c. Necrotomy
    d. Ulcerectomy

TECHNICIAN'S
CORNER

1. Aloe vera is widely used to treat minor burns. Which active ingredient in the aloe vera promotes healing of burns?
2. Can decubitus ulcers be prevented from developing? If so, how?

Bibliography

Elsevier: Gold Standard Clinical Pharmacology. 2010. Retrieved April 2, 2011, from https://www .clinicalpharmacology.com/ Health Canada: Drug product database, 2010 (http://www.hc-sc.gc.ca/dhp-mps/prodpharma/databasdon/index-eng.php).

DA: FDA Approved Drug Products. Retrieved April 21, 2012, from http://www.accessdata.fda.gov/scripts/cder/drugsatfda/index.cfm?fuseaction=Search.Search_Drug_Name, 2012.

Lance L, Lacy C, Armstrong L, et al: *Drug information handbook for the allied health professional*, ed 12, Hudson, OH, 2005, APhA Lexi-Comp.

LDHP Medical Review Services Corporation: Decubitus ulcer information and wound stages, 1999 (http://www.expertlaw.com/library/malpractice/decubitus_ulcers.html).

MedLinePlus: Pressure ulcer, 2012 (http://www.nlm.nih.gov/medlineplus/ency/article/007071.htm).

Moore J, Jensen P: Assessing the role and impact of enzymatic debridement, 2004 (http://www.podiatrytoday.com/article/2785).

Noronha C, Almeida A: Local burn treatments, 1999 (http://www.medbc.com/annals/review/vol_13/num_4/text/vol13n4p216.htm).

Sussman C, Bates-Jensen B: *Wound care*, Gaithersburg, MD, 1998, Aspen Publishers.

Thibodeau G, Patton K: *Anatomy and physiology*, ed 6, St. Louis, 2007, Mosby.

Wolf SE: Burns, 2009 (http://www.merckmanuals.com/home/injuries_and_poisoning/burns/burns.html?qt=burns&alt=sh). https://ufandshands.org/burns

Review Date: 1/13/2010 Reviewed By: Jacob L. Heller, MD, MHA, Emergency Medicine, Virginia Mason Medical Center, Seattle, Washington. Also reviewed by David Zieve, MD, MHA, Medical Director, A.D.A.M., Inc.

41

Treatment of Acne

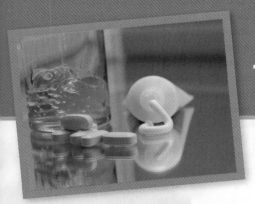

LEARNING OBJECTIVES

1 Learn the terminology associated with acne.

2 Describe the types and causes of acne.

3 List and categorize medications used to treat acne.

4 Describe mechanism of action for each class of drugs used to treat acne.

5 Identify significant drug look-alike and sound-alike issues.

6 Identify warning labels and precautionary messages associated with medications used to treat acne.

KEY TERMS

Acne: Disorder resulting from the action of hormones and other substances on the skin's oil glands (sebaceous glands) and hair follicles.

Acne vulgaris: Most common form of acne.

Blackhead: Trapped sebum and bacteria partially open to the surface that turn black because of changes in sebum as it is exposed to air; also called an open comedone.

Comedone: Enlarged and plugged hair follicles; the most characteristic sign of acne.

Cysts: Deep, painful, pus-filled lesions that can cause scarring.

Desquamation: The shedding of the outer layers of the skin.

Keratolytic: A peeling agent that causes the softening and shedding of the horny outer layer of the skin.

Milia: Tiny little bumps that occur when normally sloughed skin cells become trapped in small pockets on the surface of the skin.

Nodule: Large, painful, solid lesions that are lodged deep within the skin.

Papule: Obstructed follicle that becomes inflamed.

Pilosebaceous units: These consist of sebaceous glands connected to a canal, called a follicle, and that contain fine hairs.

Pustule: Larger lesions that are more inflamed than papules and can be superficial or deep.

Whitehead: Trapped sebum and bacteria that stay below the skin surface; may show up as tiny white spots, or they may be so small that they are invisible to the naked eye; also called a closed comedone.

Acne

Acne is a disorder resulting from the action of hormones and other substances on the skin's oil glands (sebaceous glands) and hair follicles (Figure 41-1). These factors lead to plugged pores and outbreaks of lesions, commonly called pimples or "zits." Acne lesions usually occur on the face, neck, back, chest, and shoulders. Although acne is usually not a serious health threat, it can be a source of significant emotional distress. Severe acne can lead to permanent scarring.

Acne is a disease of the *pilosebaceous units* (PSUs). Found over most of the body, PSUs consist of sebaceous glands connected to canals, called follicles, that contain fine hairs (Figure 41-2). These units are most numerous on the face, upper back, and chest. The sebaceous glands make an oily substance called sebum that normally empties onto the skin surface through the opening of the follicle, commonly called a pore. Cells called keratinocytes line the follicle.

The hair, sebum, and keratinocytes that fill the narrow follicle may produce a plug, which is an early sign of acne. The plug prevents sebum from reaching the surface of the skin through a pore. The mixture of oil and cells allows bacteria called *Propionibacterium acnes* that normally live on the skin to grow in the plugged follicles. These bacteria produce chemicals and enzymes and attract white blood cells that cause inflammation. Inflammation is a characteristic reaction of tissues to disease or injury and is marked by four signs—swelling, redness, heat, and pain. When the wall of

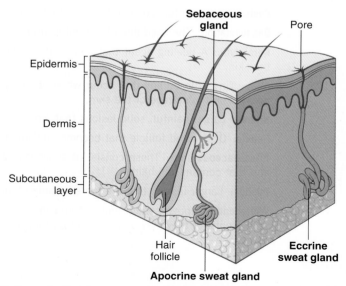

FIGURE 41-1 Adult acne. (From Callen JP, Paller AS, Greer KE, Swinyer LF: *Color atlas of dermatology*, ed 2, Philadelphia, 2000, WB Saunders.)

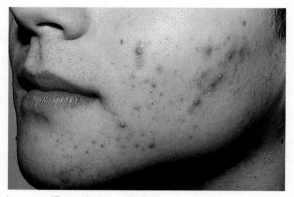

FIGURE 41-2 Normal pilosebaceous unit. (From Chabner DE: *The language of medicine*, ed 8, St. Louis, 2007, WB Saunders.)

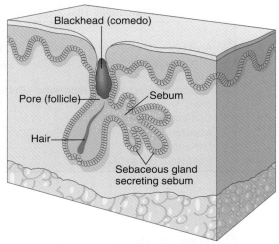

FIGURE 41-3 Open comedone. (From Chabner DE: *The language of medicine*, ed 8, St. Louis, 2007, WB Saunders.)

the plugged follicle breaks down, it spills sebum, shedding skin cells and bacteria into the nearby skin, leading to lesions or pimples.

Common acne, or ***acne vulgaris***, occurs most frequently during adolescence as a result of overactive secretion by the sebaceous glands, accompanied by blockages and inflammation of their ducts. People of all races, ages, and ethnic backgrounds get acne. An estimated 80% of all people between the ages of 11 and 30 years have acne outbreaks at some point. The rate of sebum secretion increases more than fivefold between 10 and 19 years of age. For most people, acne tends to go away by the time they reach their 30s; however, some people in their 40s and 50s continue to have this skin problem.

People with acne frequently have a variety of lesions. The basic acne lesion, called the ***comedone***, is simply an enlarged and plugged hair follicle and is the most characteristic sign of acne. If the plugged follicle, or comedone, stays beneath the skin, it is called a closed comedone and produces a white bump called a ***whitehead***. A comedone that reaches the surface of the skin and opens up is called an open comedone or ***blackhead*** because it looks black on the skin's surface (Figure 41-3). This black discoloration is caused by changes in sebum as it is exposed to air. It is not caused by dirt. Whiteheads and blackheads may stay in the skin for a long time and are considered to be noninflammatory acne.

Pus-filled pimples, or pustules, result from secondary infections within or beneath the epidermis, often in a hair follicle or sweat pore. Troublesome acne lesions can develop, including the following:

- ***Papules***—inflamed lesions that usually appear as small pink bumps on the skin; can be tender to the touch
- ***Pustules*** (pimples)—papules topped by white or yellow pus-filled lesions that may be red at the base
- ***Nodules***—large, painful, solid lesions that are lodged deep within the skin
- ***Cysts***—deep, painful, pus-filled lesions that can cause scarring

Blackheads and whiteheads normally release their contents at the surface of the skin and then heal. If the follicle wall ruptures, inflammatory acne can ensue. This rupture can be caused by random occurrence or by picking or touching the skin. This is why it is important to leave acne-prone skin relatively untouched.

Milia are tiny little bumps that occur when normally sloughed skin cells get trapped in small pockets on the surface of the skin. They are common in newborns across the nose and upper cheeks and can also be seen on adult skin. The bumps disappear as the surface is worn away and the dead skin is sloughed. In newborns, the bumps usually disappear within the first few weeks of life. However, for adults, milia may persist indefinitely. Treatment is not indicated for children. Adults can have them removed by a physician for cosmetic reasons.

BOX 41-1   **Medications That Trigger or Exacerbate Acne**

MORE COMMON	LESS COMMON
• Anabolic steroids (e.g., danazol [Danocrine], testosterone)	• Azathioprine (Imuran)
• Bromides	• Cyclosporine (Sandimmune, Neoral)
• Corticosteroids (e.g., prednisone [Deltasone])	• Disulfiram (Antabuse)
• Corticotropin (H.P. Acthar)	• Phenobarbital
• Isoniazid	• Quinidine
• Lithium	• Tetracycline
• Phenytoin (Dilantin)	• Vitamins B_1, B_6, B_{12}, and D

Causes of Acne

The exact cause of acne is unknown; however, it is believe to result from several related factors. One important factor is an increase in hormones called androgens (sex hormones). These increase in boys and girls during puberty and cause the sebaceous glands to enlarge and make more sebum. Hormonal changes related to pregnancy or starting or stopping birth control pills can also cause acne.

Another factor is heredity or genetics. Researchers believe that the tendency to develop acne can be inherited from parents. For example, studies have shown that many school-age boys with acne have a family history of the disorder. Other risk factors for acne are the use of certain drugs, including androgens and lithium (Box 41-1) and the use of comedogenic greasy cosmetics. They may alter the cells of the follicles and make them stick together, producing a plug.

FACTORS THAT CAN WORSEN ACNE

Factors that can cause an acne flare include the following:
• Changing hormone levels in adolescent girls and adult women 2 to 7 days before their menstrual period starts
• Oil from skin products (moisturizers or cosmetics) or grease encountered in the work environment (e.g., a kitchen with fry vats)
• Pressure from sports helmets or equipment, backpacks, tight collars, or tight sports uniforms
• Environmental irritants (e.g., pollution, high humidity)
• Squeezing or picking at blemishes
• Hard scrubbing of the skin
• Stress

MYTHS ABOUT THE CAUSES OF ACNE

There have been many theories concerning the causes of acne. Because adolescents commonly suffer from acne and indulge in fast food, junk food, and sweets, these food items are often blamed as the causes of acne. Not keeping one's skin clean is also blamed for causing blackheads but that also is a myth. Another supposed cause of acne is stress. Stress in itself does not cause acne but can compound existing acne, making it worse.

Treatment of Acne

The goals of treatment are to heal existing lesions, stop new lesions from forming, prevent scarring, and minimize the psychological stress and embarrassment caused by this disease. Drug treatment is aimed at reducing several problems that play a part in causing acne:
• Abnormal clumping of cells in the follicles
• Increased oil production
• Bacteria
• Inflammation

All medicines can have side effects; some may be more severe than others. Pharmacy technicians should remind customers to review the package insert that comes with the medicine and ask the pharmacist if they have any questions about possible side effects. Depending on the severity of the acne, the physician may recommend one of several over-the-counter (OTC) and/or prescription medicines. Some of these may be topical (applied to the skin) and others may be oral (taken by mouth). One or more topical medicines may be used, or combined therapy with oral and topical medicines may be recommended.

Mild acne consists of small lesions, such as blackheads, whiteheads, or pustules, which appear at or near the surface of the skin. As such, mild cases of acne can sometimes be controlled at home by gently washing the affected area(s) with warm water and a mild soap twice daily to remove dead skin cells and excess oil and use of the products described below.

TREATMENT OF MILD ACNE WITH OVER-THE-COUNTER MEDICATIONS

Topical OTC medicines are available in many forms, such as gels, lotions, creams, soaps, or pads. At home treatment with OTC topical medicines may take up to 8 weeks before noticeable improvement can be seen. Once acne clears, treatment must be continued to prevent new lesions from forming. If the acne does not respond to at-home treatment, a dermatologist can assess the situation and determine an appropriate alternative therapy. In these cases, combination therapy of two or more treatments may be used. Combination therapy may include the use of a prescription topical antimicrobial or topical retinoid. These prescription topicals can be effective for clearing mild acne.

Comedolytics (Keratolytics)

SALICYLIC ACID

Salicylic acid is a mild comedolytic agent that provides a milder, less effective alternative to the prescription agent tretinoin. In cleansing preparations, salicylic acid is considered an adjunctive treatment.

Mechanism of Action and Pharmacokinetics. Salicylic acid is a surface **keratolytic** (peeling agent). It helps break down blackheads and whiteheads. It also helps cut down the shedding of cells lining the hair follicles. Absorption of topically applied salicylates is variable and depends on the dosage formulation (range, 9% to 25%). The absorbed drug is 95% eliminated in urine. Treatment for 8–12 weeks is needed before improvement.

Adverse Effects. The adverse effects are burning, redness, and peeling of skin.

SULFUR-RESORCINOL COMBINATION

Combinations of sulfur 3% to 8% with resorcinol 2%, which enhances the effects of the sulfur, are available without prescription for the treatment of acne.

Mechanism of Action and Pharmacokinetics. Sulfur and resorcinol function as keratolytics, fostering cell turnover and **desquamation** and helping break down blackheads and whiteheads. Sulfur is a weak keratolytic and antibacterial agent. Resorcinal primarily acts as an adjuvant boosting the effectiveness of sulfur.

Pharmacokinetic data for the sulfur-resorcinol combination (Acnomel) are unavailable.

Adverse Effects. The adverse effects are redness and peeling of skin. The odor of sulfur limits its use. Resorcinol may produce brown, scaly areas which is reversible.

Antimicrobials

SULFUR-SULFACETAMIDE COMBINATION

Sodium sulfacetamide is an antibacterial agent used for the treatment of acne, rosacea, and seborrheic dermatitis, a red flaking skin rash.

Mechanism of Action and Pharmacokinetics. Sodium sulfacetamide interferes with the growth of bacteria on the skin. Sulfur may also inhibit the growth of bacteria on the skin and may cause drying of the skin. Pharmacokinetic data for sodium sulfacetamide are limited. Approximately 4% is absorbed through the skin. The absorbed drug is excreted unchanged in the urine.

Adverse Effects. The adverse effects are redness, warmth, swelling, itching, stinging, burning, and/or irritation of the treated area.

Over-the-Counter Acne Products

Generic Name	U.S. Brand Name(s) Canadian Brand Name(s)	Dosage Forms and Strengths
benzoyl peroxide*	Clearplex, PanOxyl Bar, BenzEFoam, Oscion, BPO, Clearasil Ultra Vanishing Rapid Action, NeoBenz Micro, Oxy Daily Wash Maximum, Oxy Spot Treatment, Lavoclen, BenzacAC, Triaz, Neutrogena on the Spot, Pacnex, DesQuam, ZapZyt Maximum Strength, AcneFree, Proactiv	**Cream:** 3.5%, 5.5%, 8.5% (NeoBenz Micro), 10% (Clearasil Ultra Vanishing Rapid Action) **Gel (Adasept B.P.5, Benzac AC, Desquam E, Neutrogena on the Spot, Solugel):** 2.5%, 3%, 4%, 5%, 6%, 7%, 8%, 9%, 10% **Suspension, wash:** 2.5%, 4%, 4.25%, 4.5%, 5%, 5.25%, 7%, 8%, 10% **Lotion:** 4%, 5%, 10%, 20%
	Adasept B.P.5 gel, Benoxyl, Benzac AC, Benzac W 5 Gel, Benzac W Wash, Benzagel, Clean & Clear Continuous Control, Clean & Clear Persagel, Clearasil BP, Desquam X, Oxy Cover Up, Oxy Vanishing Formula Acne, PanOxyl 5 Bar, PanOxyl 5 Wash, PanOxyl Aquagel, Proactiv, Solugel 4, Spectro Acne Care Deep Pore Vanishing Lotion	**Soap (PanOxyl):** 5%‡, 10%† **Emulsion:** 4%, 8% (LavoClen), 10% (Panoxyl Creamy Wash) **Pad:** 3%, 6%, 9% (Oscion, Triaz), 4.25%, 7% (Pacnex LP, Pacnex HP), 4%, 8% **Foam (BenzEFoam):** 5.3%, 9.8%
resorcinol and sulfur	Acnomel Acne Cream, Clearasil Daily Clear	**Cream:** resorcinol 2%, sulfur 8%
	Acnomel Cream	
salicylic acid*	Clearasil Acne Fighting Foaming Cleanser, Clearasil Total Deep Pore Cleanser, Clearasil Overnight Acne Defense Gel, Clearasil 3 in 1 Acne Defense Cleanser, Clearasil Blackhead Clearing Scrub, Neutrogena Acne Wash Oil-Free, ZapZyt Wash	**Cream (Clearasil Total Deep Pore Cleanser), Neutrogena Acne Wash Oil-Free Cream):** 2% **Cloths (Neutrogena Acne Oil-Free Cloths):** 2% **Foam (Clearasil Acne Fighting Foaming Cleanser):** 2% **Gel (Clearasil Overnight Acne Defense Gel):** 2%
	AcneFree 24/7 Severe Acne Wash, Clearasil Cleanser, Clearasil ClearStick, Neutrogena Acne Wash Foam Cleanser, Clean and Clear Blackhead Clearing Scrub, Oxy Daily Cleaning Pads, Panoxyl Clear Acne Cleansing Gel	**Suspension (Clearasil 3 in 1 Acne Defense Cleanser, Clearasil Blackhead Clearing Scrub, Neutrogena Acne Wash Oil-Free Cleanser):** 2%
sulfur and sulfacetamide*	AVAR e LS, AVAR Green, Clenia, Rosanil, Prascion, Prascion TS, Prascion FC, SE 10-5, Suphera, BP 10-1, SulZee, Clarifoam, Sumaxin, Sumaxin TS, SulfaCleanse 8/4	**Cream (Clenia):** sulfur 5%, sulfacetamide sodium 10% **Foam (Clarifoam):** sulfur 5%, sulfacetamide sodium 10% **Gel:** sulfur 5%, sulfacetanide sodium 10% **Topical emulsion (BP, SulZee):** sulfacetamide sodium 10%, sulfur 1%
	Sulfacet-R	**Lotion (Prascion FC, Sulfacet R):** sulfur 5%, sulfacetamide 10% **Pad:** sulfur 5%, sulfacetamide 10%, sulfur 4%, sulfacetamide 10% **Solution (Sumaxin):** sulfur 4%, sulfacetamide 9% **Suspension:** sulfur 4%, sulfacetamide 8% (SulfaCleanse 8/4, Sumaxin TS), sulfur 5%, sulfacetamide 10% (Prascion TS, Rosanil)

*Generic available.
†Strength available in the United States only.
‡Strength available in Canada only.

BENZOYL PEROXIDE

Benzoyl peroxide is the most effective and widely used nonprescription medication currently available for the treatment of noninflammatory acne.

Mechanism of Action and Pharmacokinetics. Benzoyl peroxide causes irritation and desquamation that prevents closure of the pilosebaceous duct. Its irritant effects cause an increased turnover rate of epithelial cells lining the follicular duct, which then increases sloughing and promotes resolution of the comedones. When benzoyl peroxide combines with proteins in the comedones, oxygen is released. *P. acne* is anaerobic and is destroyed in the presence of oxygen. Pharmacokinetic data for benzoyl peroxide are limited. Approximately 5% of a topical dose is absorbed systemically.

Adverse Effects. The adverse effects are dryness and irritation of the skin. Benzoyl peroxide may also bleach clothing or hair that it comes in contact with.

TREATMENT OF MODERATE TO MODERATELY SEVERE ACNE

In moderate to moderately severe acne, numerous whiteheads, blackheads, papules, and pustules appear to cover from 25% to 75% of the face and/or other affected area(s). Up to 100 comedones may be visible with 15-50 inflammatory lesions. Moderate to moderately severe acne usually requires the help of a dermatologist and combination therapy. Treatments used for moderate to moderately severe acne are as follows:

- Physical methods, such as comedone extraction or ultraviolet (UV) light therapy
- Oral antibiotics—help stop or slow the growth of bacteria and reduce inflammation

Drug Treatment for Moderate to Moderately Severe Acne

Generic Name	U.S. Brand Name(s) / Canadian Brand Name(s)	Dosage Forms and Strengths
adapalene	Differin / Differin, Differin XP	Cream: 0.1% / Gel: 0.1%, 0.3% / Lotion: 0.1%
adapalene + benzoyl	Epiduo / Tactuo	Gel: 0.1% adapalene + 2.5% benzoyl peroxide
azelaic acid	Azelex, Finacea / Finacea	Cream (Azelex): 20% / Gel (Finacea): 15%
benzoyl peroxide*	See earlier table for OTC acne products. / See earlier table for OTC acne products.	See earlier table for OTC acne products.
erythromycin base*, topical	Akne-mycin, C-Solve-2, Erythra-derm / Erysol	Gel: 2% / Ointment (Akne-mycin): 2% / Pad: 2% / Solution (C-Solve-2, ErySol, Erythra-derm): 2%
benzoyl peroxide and erythromycin*	Benzamycin, Benzamycin Pak / Benzamycin	Gel: benzoyl peroxide 5%, erythromycin 3%
doxycycline hyclate*	Doryx, Oracea, Vibramycin / Vibra-Tab, Vibramycin	Capsule: 20 mg, 40 mg (Oracea), 100 mg (Vibramycin) / Tablet: 20 mg, 100 mg (Vibra-tabs) / Tablet, delayed-release (Doryx): 75 mg, 100 mg, 150 mg
doxycycline monohydrate	Monodox / Not available	Capsule, (Monodox): 50 mg, 75 mg, 100 mg

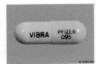

Continued

Drug Treatment for Moderate to Moderately Severe Acne—cont'd

Generic Name	U.S. Brand Name(s)	Dosage Forms and Strengths
	Canadian Brand Name(s)	
benzoyl peroxide and clindamycin*	Acanya, Benzaclin, Duac	**Gel:** benzoyl peroxide 2.5% + clindamycin phosphate 1.2% (Acanya); benzoyl peroxide 5% + clindamycin phosphate 1% (Benzaclin, Clindoxyl), benzoyl peroxide 5% + clindamycin phosphate 1.2% (Duac)
	Benzaclin, Clindoxyl	
minocycline*	Cleervue-M Kit, Dynacin, Minocin, Soladyn	**Capsule (Dynacin, Minocin):** 50 mg, 75 mg[†], 100 mg
	Minocin	**Tablet:** 50 mg[†], 75 mg[†], 100 mg[†] **Tablet ER (Solodyn):** 45 mg, 55 mg, 65 mg, 80 mg, 90 mg, 105 mg, 115 mg, 135 mg **Kit (Cleervue-M):** 30 each Calming Wipes, Medicated Topical pledget, 60 each minocycline HCl 50 mg or 100 mg, oral capsule
tetracycline*	Generics	**Capsule:** 250 mg, 500 mg
	Generics	
tazarotene	Avage, Fabior, Tazorac	**Cream:** 0.05%, 0.1% **Foam (Fabior):** 0.1% **Gel:** 0.05%, 0.1%
	Tazorac	
tretinoin*	Atralin, Avita, Renova, Retin-A, Retin-A Micro	**Cream:** 0.01% (Stieva-A), 0.02%, 0.05% (Renova), 0.025% (Rejuva-A, Retin-A, Stieva-A), 0.05%, 0.1% (Avita, Retin-A, Stieva-A) **Gel:** 0.01%, 0.025% (Avita, Retin-A), 0.04% (Retin-A Micro), 0.05% (Atralin), 0.1% (Retin-A, Retin-A Micro) **Solution:** 0.05% (Retin A)
	Rejuva-A, Retin-A, Retin-A Micro, Renova, Retisol A, Stieva-A	
clindamycin + tretinoin	Veltin, Ziana	**Gel:** clindamycin phosphate 1.2%, tretinoin 0.025%
	Biacna	
tretinoin + erythromycin	Not available	**Gel:** tretinoin 0.01% + erythromycin 4%, tretinoin 0.025% + erythromycin 4%, tretinoin 0.05% + erythromycin 4%
	Stievamycin, Stievamycin Mild, Stievamycin Forte	

*Generic available.
[†]Strength available in the United States only.

- Vitamin A derivatives (retinoids)—unplug existing comedones (plural of comedo), allowing other topical medicines, such as antibiotics, to enter the follicles. Some may also help decrease the formation of comedones. These drugs contain an altered form of vitamin A.
- Prescription-strength topical keratolytics
- Oral contraceptives

Antibiotics

Oral and topical antibiotics may be prescribed for the treatment of acne. Oral antibiotics commonly are initial therapy for patients with moderate to severe inflammatory acne. Systemic antibiotics decrease *P. acnes* colonization and have intrinsic anti-inflammatory effects. First-line oral antibiotics have included tetracycline, doxycycline, and minocycline. Clindamycin, sulfonamides, and erythromycin are less commonly used for the treatment of acne. Because the resistance of *P. acne* to erythromycin has increased, it has become a second-line agent used when treatment with tetracycline antibiotics fails or is not tolerated. The mechanism of action and adverse effects produced by these antibiotics are described in Chapter 35.

Oral antibiotics must be taken for 6 to 8 weeks before results are evident and treatment should be given for 6 months to prevent the development of microbial resistance. Oral antibiotics may be discontinued after inflammation has resolved. Topical antibiotics may be continued for prophylaxis. Some patients may require long-term oral antibiotic therapy to control their acne and prevent scarring.

Dermatologists recommend early treatment for moderate to moderately severe acne because, if not treated early, scars can develop. Acne scars can take two forms, as raised thickened tissue or as a depression, such as pits or pock marks. The only reliable method of preventing or limiting the extent of these scars is to treat acne early in its course and for as long as necessary.

Topical anti-infective agents are used for the treatment of acne to reduce inflammation caused by bacteria rather than having a direct bactericidal effect. Topical anti-infectives used for the treatment of acne are clindamycin, erythromycin, metronidazole, and sulfacetamide.

Retinoids

Retinoids include vitamin A and its derivatives. Adapalene, tretinoin, and tazarotene are retinoids.

ADAPALENE

Adapalene is a retinoid-type drug. It affects the growth of skin cells and thereby reduces the formation of pimples. It is available for topical use only.

Mechanism of Action and Pharmacokinetics. Adapalene modulates cell differentiation and keratinization, which is responsible for the drug's ability to break down comedones. It is also a potent anti-inflammatory. The absorption, distribution, and metabolism of topically applied adapalene are unknown. Excretion appears to be primarily by the biliary route.

Adverse Effects. The adverse effects are irritation, redness, dryness, itching, peeling, and burning. It is also a photo irritant.

TRETINOIN

Tretinoin is a retinoid. It is used for the treatment of mild to moderate acne.

Mechanism of Action and Pharmacokinetics. Tretinoin increases cell turnover in the follicular wall and decreases the cohesiveness of cells, leading to the extrusion of comedones and inhibition of the formation of new comedones. In patients with acne, new cells replace the cells of existing pimples, and the rapid turnover of cells prevents new pimples from forming. Tretinoin is administered topically and orally. The effects of topical administration appear approximately 2 to 3 weeks after initiation of therapy. When applied for cosmetic uses such as wrinkles, beneficial effects may take up to 6 month to be achieved. Tretinoin is well absorbed orally but protein binding is greater than 95%. Tretinoin is metabolized by the cytochrome P450 hepatic enzyme system and the drug appears to induce its own metabolism. An approximately 10-fold increase in the urinary excretion of 4-oxo trans retinoic acid glucuronide is observed after 2 to 6 weeks of continuous dosing.

Adverse Effects. The adverse effects of topical administraton are dry skin, peeling, itching, burning, stinging, redness and photosensitivity.

CLINDAMYCIN-TRETINOIN

Clindamycin and tretinoin are combined as a topical formulation for the treatment of acne.

Mechanism of Action and Pharmacokinetics. Clindamycin binds to the 50S ribosomal subunits of susceptible bacteria and prevents elongation of the peptide chains by interfering with the peptidyl transfer, thereby suppressing bacterial protein synthesis. Tretinoin increases cell turnover in the follicular wall and decreases the cohesiveness of cells, leading to the extrusion of comedones and inhibition of the formation of new comedones. Topical clindamycin has been shown to be systemically absorbed, but minimally. The absorption of clindamycin hydrochloride is greater than clindamycin phosphate; however, commercial topical preparations are in the phosphate form. Tretinoin is minimally absorbed following topical application.

Adverse Effects. The adverse effects are redness, scaling, dryness, itching, burning, and stinging, and sunburn.

TAZAROTENE

Tazarotene is a retinoid prodrug.

Mechanism of Action and Pharmacokinetics. Tazarotene modulates the differentiation and proliferation of epithelial tissue and has some anti-inflammatory and immunological activity. When

TECH ALERT!

The following drugs have look-alike and sound-alike issues:

Akne-Mycin and AK-Mycin;

doxycycline, dicyclomine, doxepin, and doxylamine;

Doxy-100 and Doxil;

Monodox and Maalox;

Dynacin, Dyazide, Dynabac, DynaCirc, and Dynapen;

Minocin, Indocin, Minizide, Mithracin, and niacin;

tretinoin and trientine

administered topically, tazarotene absorption is minimal. It is metabolized rapidly via esterase hydrolysis in the skin to tazarotenic acid, an active metabolite. Tazarotenic acid is hydrophilic. The topical half-life ($t_{1/2}$) of tazarotenic acid is approximately 18 hours.

Adverse Effects. The adverse effects are itching burning, stinging, redness, irritation, swelling, dryness of the skin, and pain.

AZELAIC ACID

Azelaic acid occurs naturally and is found in whole-grain and animal products. It reduces redness and inflammatory papules and pustules associated with rosacea and acne.

Mechanism of Action and Pharmacokinetics. Azelaic acid works by killing the bacteria that infect pores and by decreasing the production of keratin, a natural substance that could lead to the development of acne. Approximately 4% of topically applied azelaic acid is absorbed systemically. Azelaic acid is mainly excreted unchanged in the urine; the $t_{1/2}$ is approximately 12 hours after topical application.

Adverse Effects. Adverse effects are slight stinging or burning, tingling, and redness, and drying of the skin may occur.

Treatment of Severe Acne

Severe acne is characterized by deep cysts, inflammation, extensive damage to the skin, and scarring. Severe acne is characterized by more than 100 comedones, imflammatory lesions and cysts. It requires an aggressive treatment regimen and should be treated by a dermatologist. Severe disfiguring forms of acne can require years of treatment and individuals may experience one or more treatment failures. Almost every case of acne can be successfully treated. People with nodules or cysts should be treated by a dermatologist. Physical methods and medications that dermatologists use to treat severe acne include the following:

* Drainage and surgical excision
* Interlesional corticoid injection
* Isotretinoin
* Oral antibiotics
* Oral contraceptives

Isotretinoin

For patients with severe inflammatory acne that does not improve with the medications discussed earlier, the physician may prescribe isotretinoin, a retinoid (vitamin A derivative). Isotretinoin is an oral drug that is usually taken once or twice daily with food for 15 to 20 weeks. It markedly reduces the size of the oil glands so that much less oil is produced. Thus, the growth of bacteria is decreased. Treatment with isotretinoin can help prevent scarring.

Mechanism of Action and Pharmacokinetics. Isotretinoin reduces the production of sebum and shrinks the sebaceous glands. It stabilizes keratinization and prevents comedones from forming. Isotretinoin works by altering DNA transcription. This decreases the size and output of sebaceous glands and makes the cells that are sloughed off into the sebaceous glands less sticky and therefore less able to form comedones. Isotretinoin is up to 99% protein-bound. Cytochrome P-450 (CYP450) metabolic enzymes (CYP2C8, CYP2C9, CYP3A4, and CYP2B6) metabolize isotretinoin in the

Treatment for Severe Acne

Generic Name	U.S. Brand Name(s) Canadian Brand Name(s)	Dosage Forms and Strengths
isotretinoin	Absorica, Amnesteem, Claravis, Myorisan, Sotret Accutane, Clarus	Capsule: 10 mg, 20 mg[†], 30 mg[†], 40 mg
oral antibiotics	See "Topical Corticosteroids" drug monographs in Chapters 35 and 42.	See "Topical Corticosteroids" drug monograph in Chapter 42.
oral contraceptives	See Chapter 34.	See Chapter 34.

[†]Strength available in the United States only.

liver. Metabolites are eliminated via the kidney and in feces. The $t_{1/2}$ of isotretinoin is approximately 10 to 20 hours. Food increases absorption by 1.5- to 2-fold.

Adverse Reactions. Isotretionin must be used cautiously in women of childbearing age because it can produce fetal abnormalities. Isotretinoin is classified in U.S. Food and Drug Administration (FDA) pregnancy category X. Women must use two separate, effective forms of birth control at the same time for 1 month before treatment begins, during the entire course of treatment, and for 1 full month after stopping the drug.

Other possible side effects of isotretinoin include dry eyes, mouth, lips, nose, or skin (very common), itching, nosebleeds, muscle aches, sensitivity to the sun, poor night vision, changes in mood, depression, suicidal thoughts, changes in the blood lipids (e.g., an increase in fat levels in the blood [triglycerides, cholesterol]), and changes in liver function. Blood tests to determine baseline liver function are taken before isotretinoin is started and periodically during treatment. Side effects usually cease after the medicine is stopped. Oral administration of isotretinoin may produce hyperglycemia.

FDA iPLEDGE PROGRAM FOR ISOTRETINOIN

The FDA announced the approval of a strengthened risk management program, called iPLEDGE, for generic isotretinoin. Wholesalers, prescribers, pharmacies, and patients must agree to accept specific responsibilities designed to minimize pregnancy exposure to distribute, prescribe, dispense, and use isotretinoin. The FDA approved a strengthened risk management plan for isotretinoin on August 12, 2005, to make sure that women do not become pregnant while taking this medicine because isotretinoin causes birth defects. Since March 1, 2006, only prescribers registered and activated in iPLEDGE can prescribe isotretinoin and only patients registered and qualified in iPLEDGE can be given isotretinoin.

The iPLEDGE program is a technology-based, closed system of registered wholesalers, prescribers, pharmacies, and patients. See the following website for more details on the iPLEDGE program: https://www.ipledgeprogram.com/.

TREATMENT OF HORMONALLY INFLUENCED ACNE IN WOMEN

In some women, acne is caused by an excess of androgen hormones. They may exhibit hirsutism (excessive growth of hair on the face or body), premenstrual acne flares, irregular menstrual cycles, and elevated blood levels of certain androgens. The physician may prescribe one of several drugs to treat women with this type of acne.

Oral Contraceptives

Oral contraceptives (OCs) help suppress androgens produced by the ovaries. Side effects are nausea, weight gain, menstrual spotting, and breast tenderness. When an OC is used to treat acne, the physician should prescribe a formulation that contains progestins with a low androgen level. Appropriate progestins include norethindrone, norethindrone acetate, ethynodiol diacetate, and norgestimate. Ultimately, the choice of OC should be based on tolerability and compliance.

Other Treatment Modalities for Acne

Physicians may use other types of procedures in addition to drug therapy to treat patients with acne. For example, the physician may remove the patient's comedones during an office visit. Sometimes, the physician will inject corticosteroids directly into lesions to help reduce the size and pain of inflamed cysts and nodules.

TECH ALERT!
Isotretinoin must be dispensed in the manufacturer's original packaging with the warning label "Avoid Pregnancy."

Treatment of Hormonally Induced Acne in Women

Generic Name	U.S. Brand Name(s) / Canadian Brand Name(s)	Dosage Forms and Strengths
oral contraceptives[a]	See Chapter 34.	See Chapter 34.

[a]A complete listing of oral contraceptives is given in Chapter 34.

If scarring has occurred, dermabrasion (or microdermabrasion), which is a form of sanding down scars, is sometimes used. Another treatment option for deep scars caused by cystic acne is the transfer of fat from another part of the body to the scar. Alternatively, a synthetic filling material may be injected under the scar to improve its appearance.

Summary of Drugs Used for the Treatment of Acne

Generic Name	Brand Name	Usual Dose and Dosing Schedule	Warning Labels
benzoyl peroxide	Various brands and generics see "Over the Counter Acne" products mini-drug monograph	**Cleansers:** Wash once or twice daily. **Topical:** Apply sparingly once daily; increase to two or three times daily if needed.	BLEACHING AGENT; AVOID CONTACT WITH FABRIC AND HAIR.
resorcinol and sulfur	Acnomel	Apply a small amount to affected area as directed by physician.	FOR EXTERNAL USE ONLY.
salicylic acid	Various brands and generics see "Over the Counter Acne" products mini-drug monograph	**Cream, cloth, foam, liquid, gel:** Apply to skin once or twice daily and rinse thoroughly. **Pads:** Apply to affected area one to three times daily. **Patch:** Apply over affected area at night; remove in the morning. **Bath gels or soap:** Wash once daily,	AVOID THE EYES, MOUTH, LIPS, INSIDE THE NOSE.
sulfur and sulfacetamide	Sulfacet-R	Apply a thin film one to three times daily. Cleansing products should be used once or twice daily.	FOR EXTERNAL USE ONLY. AVOID CONTACT WITH EYES, EYELIDS, LIPS, MOUTH.
adapalene	Differin	Apply once daily at bedtime.	FOR EXTERNAL USE ONLY.
azelaic acid	Azelex	Apply and massage a thin film into affected area twice daily.	FOR EXTERNAL USE ONLY. KEEP AWAY FROM EYES, EARS, AND MUCOUS MEMBRANES.
erythromycin	Various brands and generics	**Oral:** 250-500 mg bid **Topical:** Apply over affected area bid.	FOR EXTERNAL USE ONLY.
benzoyl peroxide and erythromycin	Benzamycin, Benzamycin Pak	Apply bid, morning and evening.	FOR EXTERNAL USE ONLY.
doxycycline	Vibramycin	50-100 mg bid or 40 mg (Oracea) once daily	AVOID SUNLIGHT. AVOID TAKING ANTACIDS, IRON, AND DAIRY PRODUCTS.
benzoyl peroxide and clindamycin	BenzaClin, Duac	**BenzaClin:** Apply bid **Duac:** Apply once daily in the evening.	MAY BLEACH HAIR AND FABRIC. FOR EXTERNAL USE ONLY. AVOID CONTACT WITH EYES, NOSE, MOUTH, AND ALL MUCOUS MEMBRANES.
minocycline	Minocin	50-100 mg once or twice daily	AVOID SUNLIGHT. AVOID TAKING ANTACIDS, IRON, AND DAIRY PRODUCTS.
tetracycline	Generics	250-500 mg/dose every 6 hr	AVOID SUNLIGHT AVOID TAKING ANTACIDS, IRON, AND DAIRY PRODUCTS.
tazarotene	Avage, Tazorac / Tazarac	Apply thin film once daily in the evening to the affected area.	DO NOT USE IF PREGNANT. FOR EXTERNAL USE ONLY.

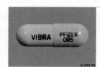

Summary of Drugs Used for the Treatment of Acne—cont'd

Generic Name	Brand Name	Usual Dose and Dosing Schedule	Warning Labels
tretinoin	Renova, Retin-A	Apply to acne lesions once daily before bedtime or on alternate days.	MAY CAUSE SENSITIVITY TO SUNLIGHT.
clindamycin + tretinoin	Ziana, Veltin	Apply to entire face every night at bedtime.	AVOID EXCESSIVE EXPOSURE TO THE SUN, COLD, AND WIND. FOR EXTERNAL USE ONLY.
isotretinoin	Accutane, Amnesteem, Clarus, Clavaris, Sotret	0.5-1 mg/kg/day PO given in two divided doses for 15-20 wk	TAKE WITH FOOD. AVOID PREGNANCY. AVOID USE OF VITAMIN A PRODUCTS.

Chapter Summary

- Acne is a disorder resulting from the action of hormones and other substances on the skin's oil glands (sebaceous glands) and hair follicles.
- Doctors describe acne as a disease of the pilosebaceous units. Found over most of the body, PSUs consist of sebaceous glands connected to canals, called follicles, that contain fine hairs.
- Common acne, or acne vulgaris, occurs most frequently during adolescence as a result of overactive secretion by the sebaceous glands, accompanied by blockages and inflammation of their ducts.
- Pus-filled pimples, or pustules, result from secondary infections within or beneath the epidermis, often in a hair follicle or sweat pore.
- Milia are tiny bumps that occur when normally sloughed skin cells get trapped in small pockets on the surface of the skin.
- The goals of treatment for acne are to heal existing lesions, stop new lesions from forming, prevent scarring, and minimize the psychological stress and embarrassment caused by this disease.
- Benzoyl peroxide is the most effective and widely used nonprescription medication currently available for the treatment of noninflammatory acne.
- Salicylic acid is a mild comedolytic agent (keratolytic) that provides a milder, less effective alternative to the prescription agent tretinoin.
- Topical OTC medicines are available in many forms, such as gels, lotions, creams, soaps, and pads. In some people, OTC acne medicines may cause side effects such as skin irritation, burning, or redness, which often get better or go away with continued use of the medicine.
- Adapalene is believed to affect the growth of skin cells and thereby reduce the formation of pimples.
- Azelaic acid works by killing the bacteria that infect pores and by decreasing the production of keratin, a natural substance that could lead to the development of acne.
- Tazarotene modulates the differentiation and proliferation of epithelial tissue and has some antiinflammatory and immunological activity.
- Tretinoin increases cell turnover in the follicular wall and decreases the cohesiveness of cells, leading to the extrusion of comedones and inhibition of the formation of new comedones.
- Severe acne is characterized by deep cysts, inflammation, extensive damage to the skin, and scarring. It requires an aggressive treatment regimen and should be treated by a dermatologist.
- For patients with severe inflammatory acne a physician may prescribe isotretinoin, a retinoid (vitamin A derivative).
- Early treatment is the best way to prevent acne scars. Once scarring has occurred, dermabrasion may be used to treat irregular scars.
- Medical researchers are working on new drugs to treat acne, like Nicomide-T Gel a vitamin B supplement, to replace some of those in current use, particularly topical antibiotics,. Exactly how Nicomide-T Gel works is unknown.

1. An enlarged and plugged hair follicle, the most characteristic sign of acne, is called a _____.
    a. Milia
    b. Pustule
    c. Comedone
    d. Papule

2. Physicians know the exact cause of acne.
    a. True
    b. False

3. _____ is the most effective and widely used nonprescription medication currently available for the treatment of noninflammatory acne.
    a. Salicylic acid
    b. Benzoyl peroxide
    c. Sulfur
    d. Doxycycline

4. At-home treatment for acne requires _____ to see improvement.
    a. 2 to 4 weeks
    b. 4 to 8 weeks
    c. 6 to 10 weeks
    d. 8 to 10 weeks

5. When acne is resistant to topical therapies, intravenous antibiotics may be used.
    a. True
    b. False

6. Which of the following oral antibiotics is less commonly used for the treatment of moderate to severe acne?
    a. Doxycycline
    b. Tetracycline
    c. Clindamycin
    d. Minocycline

7. _____ works by killing the bacteria that infect pores and by decreasing the production of keratin, a natural substance that could lead to the development of acne.
    a. Azelaic acid
    b. Adapalene
    c. Benzoyl peroxide
    d. a and c

8. _____ is an effective medicine that can help prevent scarring.
    a. Tretinoin
    b. Isotretinoin
    c. Retinoin
    d. All of the above

9. Oral contraceptives are used to treat which type of acne?
    a. Mild
    b. Moderate
    c. Severe
    d. Hormonally induced

10. Which of the following drugs are used for treating hormonally influenced acne?
    a. Corticosteroids
    b. Antiandrogens
    c. Progestins
    d. All of the above

TECHNICIAN'S CORNER

1. There are many OTC and prescription medications available for the treatment of acne. Are there any natural/herbal remedies available?
2. What advice can one give to a teenager with acne?

Bibliography

American Academy of Dermatology: Acne. 2012 (http://www.aad.org/skin-conditions/dermatology-a-to-z/acne).

American Academy of Dermatology: Treating severe acne. 2011(http://www.skincare physicians.com/acnenet/treatsevereacne.html).

American Pharmacists Association: *Handbook of nonprescription drugs*, ed 16, Washington DC, 2009, American Pharmacists Association.

Dlugosz CK, OTC Advisor: *Self care for dermatologic disorder, monograph 6.* 2010, American Pharmacists Association.

Elsevier: Gold Standard Clinical Pharmacology. Retrieved June 24, 2011, from https://www.clinicalpharmacology.com/, 2010.

FDA: FDA Approved Drug Products. Retrieved July 8, 2012, from http://www.accessdata.fda.gov/scripts/cder/drugsatfda/index.cfm?fuseaction=Search.Search_Drug_Name, 2012.

Feldman S, Careccia RE, Barham KL, et al: Diagnosis and treatment of acne, *Am Fam Physician* 69:2123-2130, 2004.

Health Canada: Drug Product Database. Retrieved July 8, 2012, from http://www.hc-sc.gc.ca/dhp-mps/prodpharma/databasdon/index-eng.php, 2010.

Lance L, Lacy C, Armstrong L, et al: *Drug information handbook for the allied health professional*, ed 12, Hudson, OH, 2005, APhA Lexi-Comp.

National Institute of Arthritis and Musculoskeletal and Skin Diseases: Acne (NIH Publ. No. 06-4998), 2010 (http://www.niams.nih.gov/Health_Info/Acne/default.asp). http://www.drugs.com/cdi/nicomide-t-gel.html#aIGDKmBoYLPJ9Zcw.99.

Repchinsky C: *Patient self-care: helping your patinets make therapeutic choices*, ed 2, 2010, Canadian Pharmacists Association, pp 577-596.

Repchinsky C: *Compendium of self care products*, ed 2, 2010, Canadian Pharmacists Association, pp 173-174.

Thibodeau G, Patton K: *Anatomy and physiology*, ed 6, St. Louis, 2007, Mosby.

Wikipedia: Acne vulgaris. 2012 (http://en.wikipedia.org/wiki/Acne_vulgaris).

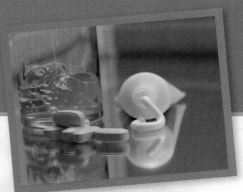

42

Treatment of Eczema and Psoriasis

1 Learn the terminology associated with eczema and psoriasis.

2 Describe the causes of eczema and psoriasis.

3 List the symptoms of eczema and psoriasis.

4 List and categorize medications used to treat eczema and psoriasis.

5 Describe the mechanism of action for drugs used to treat eczema and psoriasis.

6 Identify significant drug look-alike and sound-alike issues.

7 Identify warning labels and precautionary messages associated with medications used to treat eczema and psoriasis.

KEY TERMS

Atopic: Group of diseases in which there is an inherited tendency to develop other allergic conditions.

Atopic dermatitis: Chronic inflammatory disease of the skin.

Cutaneous: Pertaining to the skin.

Dermatitis: Inflammation of the skin.

Eczema: General term used to describe several types of inflammation of the skin.

Exacerbation: Aggravation of symptoms or increase in the severity of the disease.

Phototherapy: Treatment for atopic dermatitis that involves exposing the skin to ultraviolet A or B light waves.

Plaque psoriasis: Most common form of psoriasis. It is characterized by raised, inflamed (red) lesions covered with a silvery white scale.

Psoriasis: Chronic disease of the skin characterized by itchy red patches covered with silvery scales.

Remission: Lessening in severity or an abatement of symptoms.

Overview

Eczema is a general term used to describe several types of inflammation of the skin. It is a common condition affecting millions of Americans and Canadians. There are several types of eczema—atopic dermatitis, allergic contact eczema, contact eczema, dyshidrotic eczema, neurodermatitis, nummular eczema, seborrheic eczema, and stasis dermatitis. These are described in Box 42-1.

Atopic dermatitis is the most common form of eczema, affecting more than 15 million Americans. It is a chronic disease of the skin that often develops in infancy and may continue throughout

BOX 42-1   **Types of Eczema**

- Allergic contact eczema (dermatitis): Red, itchy, weepy reaction in which the skin has come into contact with a substance that the immune system recognizes as foreign (e.g., poison ivy or certain preservatives in creams and lotions)
- Atopic dermatitis: Chronic skin disease characterized by itchy inflamed skin
- Contact eczema: Localized reaction that includes redness, itching, and burning where the skin has come into contact with an allergen (an allergy-causing substance) or with an irritant (e.g., acid, cleaning agent, or other chemical)
- Dyshidrotic eczema: Irritation of the skin on the palms of hands and soles of the feet characterized by clear deep blisters that itch and burn
- Neurodermatitis: Scaly patches of the skin on the head, lower legs, wrists, or forearms caused by localized itch (e.g., insect bite) that become intensely irritated when scratched
- Nummular eczema: Coin-shaped patches of irritated skin—most common on the arms, back, buttocks, and lower legs—that may be crusted, scaling, and extremely itchy
- Seborrheic eczema: Yellowish, oily, scaly patches of skin on the scalp, face, and occasionally other parts of the body
- Statis dermatitis: Skin irritation on the lower legs, generally related to circulatory problems

Adapted from National Institute of Arthritis and Musculoskeletal and Skin Diseases: Types of eczema (dermatitis), 2011 (http://www.niams.nih.gov/Health_Info/Atopic_Dermatitis/default.asp#aa).

BOX 42-2   **Common Irritants**

- Wool or synthetic fibers
- Soaps and detergents
- Perfumes and cosmetics
- Cleaning solvents, mineral oil, and chlorine
- Dust
- Sand

adulthood. Atopic refers a group of diseases in which there is an inherited tendency to develop other allergic conditions. Up to 75% of children with eczema (atopic dermatitis) are prone to developing asthma and hay fever.

Unlike contact dermatitis, in which symptoms appear after exposure to an allergen, the cause of eczema (atopic dermatitis) is unknown. People who live in dry climates and in large cities seem to have a higher incidence of the condition, perhaps because atopic dermatitis appears to be linked to environmental factors. Heredity and a malfunction of the body's immune system are other important factors that are associated with the condition. Atopic diseases are autoimmune disorders; persons with atopic dermatitis have a hyperactive dermal response to irritants. Common irritants are listed in Box 42-2.

Langerhans cells in the skin are potent activators of T cells (see Unit X), and levels are increased in the skin of those with atopic diseases. Psoriasis is also caused by T cell hyperactivity. *Psoriasis* is a condition associated with the rapid turnover of skin cells. Whereas the normal rate of cell turnover is approximately 30 days, the cell turnover rate may be as short as a few days with psoriasis. Individuals with psoriasis have thick silvery scaly patches; this is the most common type, known as *plaque psoriasis*. They may also have some redness and swelling. Itchy psoriatic patches may be found on the neck, elbows, genitals, scalp, hands, and feet. The following factors aggravate psoriasis:

- Stress
- Dry skin
- Environmental factors that produce dry skin (e.g., hot air heating systems, weather)
- Infections
- Some medicines

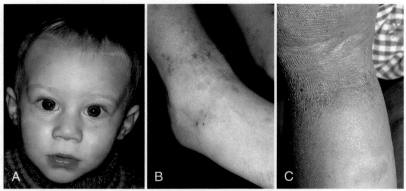

FIGURE 42-1 Eczema. **A,** Infantile phase. **B,** Childhood phase. **C,** Adolescent phase. (**A, B** from Fitzpatrick JE, Morelli JG: *Dermatology secrets in color*, ed 3, Philadelphia, 2007, Mosby; **C,** courtesy of Dr. James E. Fitzpatrick.)

BOX 42-3   **Signs and Symptoms of Eczema**

- Dry, rectangular scales on the skin
- Small rough bumps and papules on arms, legs, face
- Thickened, leathery patches of skin
- Inflammation around the corners of the mouth and face rash
- Darkened eyelids and skin around the eyes
- Extra skin fold under the eye
- Excess creases in the palms of the hands
- Hives (urticaria)
- Intense itching
- Redness

Symptoms of Atopic Dermatitis (Eczema)

Atopic dermatitis commonly produces symptoms of intense itching, redness (from scratching), skin irritation, and inflammation. Eczematous patches may form that are flaky and crusting and may even ooze a clear fluid (Figure 42-1).

Individuals with eczema (atopic dermatitis; Box 42-3) and psoriasis may experience periods when their symptoms worsen (*exacerbation*) and periods when they get better or go away completely (*remission*). It is not uncommon for eczema that has gone into remission in childhood to return with the onset of puberty. Factors that exacerbate symptoms of eczema are as follows:

- Stress
- Contact with environmental pollutants and household cleaning products
- Food allergy (e.g., to eggs, peanuts, milk, fish, soy products, wheat)
- Wearing wool or clothing that rubs and irritates skin
- Factors that cause dry skin (e.g., low-humidity environments, not applying moisturizer, hot baths)
- Scratching

Scratching can break down the protective layer of the skin and increase the risk of developing secondary bacterial or viral infections.

Nonpharmaceutical Treatment of Eczema and Psoriasis

Nonpharmaceutical treatment for eczema involves using skin care regimens (Box 42-4) that reduce irritation and avoiding allergens and irritants. It may also include the use of phototherapy. *Phototherapy* involves exposing the skin to ultraviolet (UV) A or B light waves. It may be used alone or in combination with drug therapy. Phototherapy is only recommended for those older than 12 years. Adverse reactions to the use of UV light therapy are premature aging of the skin and increased risk for skin cancer.

Pharmaceutical Treatment of Eczema and Psoriasis

CORTICOSTEROIDS

The use of topical corticosteroids continues to be a mainstay of therapy for the treatment of eczema. Corticosteroids are also used for the treatment of psoriasis, seborrhea, and other skin conditions if inflammation is present. The use of oral corticosteroids is reserved for severe symptoms.

Topical corticosteroids are categorized into seven groups based on potency (Box 42-5). Class I agents (e.g., diflorasone diacetate [Psorcon]) are superhigh potency. Class VII agents include hydrocortisone, which is mild enough for over-the-counter (OTC) use. The vehicle (base) in which the corticosteroid is suspended may influence the potency. For example, betamethasone dipropionate in an optimized vehicle is superpotent (class II), whereas the same drug in a regular vehicle is classified as potent (class IV). Higher potency corticosteroids have more adverse reactions. Only the mildest potency agents, such as hydrocortisone, should be used on the face.

MECHANISM OF ACTION AND PHARMACOKINETICS

Topical corticosteroids possess anti-inflammatory and immunosuppressive properties and produce vasoconstriction. They reduce the permeability of the cells to T lymphocytes and eosinophils, thereby decreasing the release of mediators of the inflammatory response (e.g., cytokines). They also reduce the number of inflammatory cells, which decreases redness, swelling, and inflammation.

TECH ALERT!
The following drugs have look-alike and sound-alike issues:
fluocinolone and fluocinonide;
hydrocortisone acetate, hydrocortisone butyrate, and hydrocortisone valerate;
betamethasone dipropionate and betamethasone valerate;
betamethasone dipropionate augmented formula and betamethasone dipropionate regular

---

BOX 42-4   **Recommended Skin Care for Persons with Eczema**

- Avoid hot baths or showers.
- Air-dry or gently pat skin dry after bathing (avoid vigorous rubbing).

BOX 42-5   **Potency Classification of Selected Topical Corticosteroids (Generic Names)**

CLASS I: SUPER–HIGH POTENCY
- Clobetasol propionate
- Diflorasone diacetate

CLASS II: SUPER POTENT
- Betamethasone dipropionate (optimized vehicle)
- Halobetasol propionate

CLASS III: VERY POTENT
- Amcinonide
- Desoximetasone
- Halcinonide
- Fluocinonide
- Mometasone furoate
- Diflorasone diacetate (cream)
- Triamcinolone (>0.5%)

CLASS IV: POTENT
- Betamethasone dipropionate (regular vehicle)
- Flurandrenolide (ointment)
- Mometasone furoate

CLASS V: MEDIUM POTENCY
- Beclomethasone
- Betamethasone valerate
- Diflucortolone valerate
- Fluocinolone acetonide
- Flurandrenolide (cream)
- Fluticasone propionate (cream)
- Hydrocortisone butyrate (cream)
- Hydrocortisone valerate (cream)
- Triamcinolone acetonide (>0.5%)

CLASS VI: MILD POTENCY
- Alclometasone dipropionate (cream, ointment)
- Desonide (cream)
- Prednicarbate

CLASS VII: MILDEST POTENCY
- Dexamethasone
- Hydrocortisone base

Adapted from Raymond G, Houle M.-C: A review of corticosteroids for the treatment of psoriasis, Skin Therapy Letter, Vol. 2., 2007 (http://www.skinpharmacies.ca/2_1_2.html).

Topical Corticosteroids

Generic Name	U.S. Brand Name(s) Canadian Brand Name(s)	Dosage Forms and Strengths
alclometasone dipropionate*	Aclovate	Cream: 0.05%
	Not available	Ointment: 0.05%
amcinonide*	Generics	Cream: 0.1%
	Cyclort	Lotion: 0.1% Ointment: 0.1%
betamethasone dipropionate*	Diprolene, Diprolene AF	Cream, augmented: 0.05% Cream (Diprosone): 0.05%
	Diprolene, Diprosone	Gel, augmented: 0.05%† Lotion, augmented: 0.05% Lotion (Diprosone): 0.05% Ointment (Diprosone): 0.05% Ointment, augmented: 0.05%
betamethasone valerate*	Beta-Val, Dermabet, Luxiq, Valnac	Cream: 0.05%‡, 0.1% Lotion: 0.1%
	Betaderm, Luxiq, Prevex B, Ratio-Ectosone-Mild, Ratio-Ectosone Regular, Valisone G	Ointment: 0.05%‡, 0.1% Topical foam (Luxiq): 0.12%
clobetasol propionate*	Clobex, Cormax, Embeline, Embeline E, Olux, Olux-E, Temovate, Temovate-E	Cream: 0.05% Gel (Temovate): 0.05%†
	Clobex, Dermovate	Lotion: 0.05% Ointment: 0.05% Shampoo: 0.05% Spray: 0.05% Solution: 0.05% Topical foam (Olux): 0.05%†
clocortolone	Cloderm	Cream: 0.1%
	Not available	
desonide*	Desowen, Verdeso, Desonate	Cream (Desowen, Desocort): 0.05%
	Desocort, Tridesilon, Verdeso	Gel (Desonate): 0.05% Lotion (Desowen): 0.05% Ointment (Desocort, Desowen): 0.05% Topical foam (Verdeso): 0.05%
desoximetasone*	Topicort	Cream: 0.25%, 0.05% (Topicort Mild)
	Topicort, Topicort Mild	Gel: 0.05% Ointment: 0.25%, 0.05%†
diflucortolone valerate	Not available	Cream: 0.1%
	Nerisone, Nerisone Oily	Oily cream: 0.1% Ointment: 0.1%
diflorasone diacetate*	Generics	Cream: 0.05%
	Not available	Ointment: 0.05%
fluocinolone acetonide*	Capex, DermaSmoothe FS, Synalar	Cream: 0.01%, 0.025% Ointment: 0.025%
	Capex, DermaSmoothe FS, Synalar	Shampoo (Capex): 0.01% Solution: 0.01% Topical oil (DermaSmoothe FS): 0.01%

Topical Corticosteroids—cont'd

Generic Name	U.S. Brand Name(s) / Canadian Brand Name(s)	Dosage Forms and Strengths
fluocinonide*	Lidex, Lidex-E, Vanos	Cream: 0.05% (Lidex), 0.1% (Vanos)
	Lidemol, Lidex, Lyderm, Tiamol, Topactin	Cream, emulsified (Lidex-E, Lidemol, Topactin): 0.05%
		Gel (Lidex, Lyderm): 0.05%
		Ointment (Lidex): 0.05%
		Solution: 0.05%[†]
flurandrenolide	Cordran, Cordran SP, Cordran Tape	Cream (Cordran SP): 0.025%, 0.05%
	Not available	Lotion (Cordran): 0.05%
		Tape: 4 mcg
fluticasone propionate	Cutivate	Cream: 0.05%
	Cutivate	Lotion: 0.05%[†]
		Ointment: 0.005%[†]
halcinonide	Halog	Cream: 0.1%
	Not available	Ointment: 0.1%
halobetasol propionate*	Ultravate	Cream: 0.05%
	Ultravate	Ointment: 0.05%
hydrocortisone base* (only Rx trade names listed)	Nutracort, Stie-cort, Synacort, Texacort	Cream (Cortate, Emo Cort): 1%, 2.5%
	Cortate, Cortoderm, Emo Cort, Prevex HC, Sarna HC	Lotion (Emo Cort, Sarna HC): 1%, 2.5%
		Ointment: 1% (Cortate, Cortoderm)
		Solution: 2.5% (Emo Cort)
hydrocortisone acetate* (only Rx trade names listed)	Micort HC,	Cream: 1% (Hyderm), 2% (Micort HC, Topiderm HC), 2.5% (Micort HC)
	Hyderm, Topiderm HC	
hydrocortisone butyrate*	Locoid	Cream: 0.1%
	Not available	Cream, lipocream: 0.1%
		Lotion: 0.1%
		Ointment: 0.1%
		Solution: 0.1%
Hydrocortisone probutate	Pandel	Cream: 0.1%
	Pandel	
hydrocortisone valerate*[†]	Westcort	Cream (Hydroval): 0.2%
	Hydroval	Ointment: 0.2%
mometasone furoate*	Elocon	Cream: 0.1%
	Elocom	Lotion: 0.1%
		Ointment: 0.1%
prednicarbate*[†]	Dermatop, Dermatop E	Cream, emollient: 0.1%
	Dermatop	Ointment: 0.1%
triamcinolone acetonide*	Kenalog, Triacet, Triderm, Trianex	Cream: 0.025%, 0.05 (Kenalog), 0.1% (Triderm), 0.5% (Aristocort C, Triacet)
	Aristocort C, Aristocort R, Triaderm	Lotion: 0.025%, 0.1%
		Ointment: 0.025%, 0.1% (Aristocort R, Kenaolg, Triderm), 0.5%
		Ointment, augmented: 0.05%
		Topical spray: 0.147 mg/g (Kenalog)

*Generic available.
*[†]Generic available in the United States only.
[†]Strength available in the United States only.
[‡]Strength available in Canada only.

ADVERSE EFFECTS

Long-term use of topical corticosteroids can result in thinning of the skin, stretch marks (striae), spider veins, acne, milia, rosacea (enlarged blood vessels, especially on the nose), bruising, atrophy, lacerations, poor wound healing, and growth suppression (in children). Adverse reactions are more extensive when high-potency corticosteroids are used and they are applied to a large body surface area.

IMMUNOMODULATORS: CALCINEURIN INHIBITORS

Calcineurin inhibitors are immunomodulators. They control inflammation and reduce the immune system response to allergens. Pimecrolimus is indicated for the treatment of mild to moderate eczema. It is approved for short-term and intermittent long-term therapy. Tacrolimus is approved for the treatment of moderate to severe atopic dermatitis that has failed to respond to corticosteroid treatment.

MECHANISM OF ACTION AND PHARMACOKINETICS

Pimecrolimus and tacrolimus inhibit T cell activation and the production of cytokines, interleukins, and interferons, mediators of the inflammatory response. Pharmacokinetic data on pimecrolimus are limited. Absorption through the skin is minimal and *cutaneous* metabolism is negligible. Peak concentration of tacrolimus is achieved within 4 to 9 hours after application. The elimination half-life of tacrolimus is long (71 to 112 hours).

ADVERSE EFFECTS

Common adverse reactions associated with topical application are local burning and stinging of the skin. The U.S. Food and Drug Administration (FDA) and Health Canada require manufacturers to include a boxed warning in the package insert, advising health care providers that pimecrolimus and tacrolimus may increase the risk for the development of lymphoma. The risk for lymphoma is minimal with topical application compared with parenteral use, according to the Canadian Dermatology Association.

Vitamin D Analogues

Calcipotriene is a synthetic analogue of vitamin D. The generic name is calcipotriol in Canada. Calcitriol is an active form of vitamin D_3. Calcitriol, calcipotriene, and calcipotriol are approved for the treatment of psoriasis. Signs of improvement can be seen in approximately 2 weeks after calcipotriene administration; however, maximum effects may take 4 to 8 weeks.

MECHANISM OF ACTION AND PHARMACOKINETICS

Calcipotriene (calcipotriol) inhibits the rapid and repeated production of new skin cells (proliferation). It inhibits the proliferation of T cells and inhibits the release of mediators of inflammation (e.g., cytokines, interleukins, interferons). The mechanism of action for topical calcitriol is unknown.

Calcineurin Inhibitors

Generic Name	U.S. Brand Name(s) / Canadian Brand Name(s)	Dosage Forms and Strengths
pimecrolimus	Elidel	Cream: 1%
	Elidel	
tacrolimus*†	Avagraf, Prograf, Protopic	Capsule, immediate-release (Prograf): 0.5 mg, 1 mg, 5 mg
	Advagraf, Prograf, Protopic	Capsule, extended-release (Advagraf): 0.5 mg, 1 mg, 3 mg, 5 mg
		Ointment (Protoptic): 0.03%, 0.1%
		Solution, for injection (Prograf): 5 mg/mL

*†Generic available in the United States only.

When applied to skin with psoriasis, approximately 6% of the drug is absorbed. Absorption is slightly less through intact skin (5%). Metabolism in the liver is rapid. Calcipotriene is metabolized to vitamin D_3, which is recycled, and inactive metabolites.

ADVERSE EFFECTS

Most adverse reactions are localized to the site of application. Irritation and redness are common. When large areas of the body are covered with the drug, some systemic absorption may occur. Vitamin D plays an important role in calcium absorption. Systemic effects produced by calcipotriene (calcipotriol) are increased calcium levels in the blood and urine.

Furanocoumarins

The psoralens are a class of drugs that increase photosensitivity and are classified as furanocoumarins. Methoxsalen is the only drug in this class. It is approved for the treatment of atopic dermatitis and psoriasis, along with UV light therapy. Methoxsalen and UV light work synergistically. Methoxsalen increases the skin's sensitivity to UV light and UV light activates methoxsalen. A psoralen plus UVA light therapy is also known as PUVA.

MECHANISM OF ACTION AND PHARMACOKINETICS

The action of methoxsalen on pyrimidine bases of the DNA molecule results in the suppression of DNA synthesis, which decreases cell replication and proliferation. DNA photo damage produces cutaneous immunosuppression by affecting leukocyte regulatory mechanisms. Psoralens may be administered orally, topically, or parenterally. Food increases bioavailability. The bioavailability of

Vitamin D Analogues

Generic Name	U.S. Brand Name(s) Canadian Brand Name(s)	Dosage Forms and Strengths
calcipotriene*† (calcipotriol in Canada)	Dovonex, Sorilux Dovonex	Cream: 0.005% Foam (Sorilux): 0.005% Solution, scalp: 0.005% Ointment: 0.005%
calcipotriene + betamethasone dipropionate	Taclonex, Taclonex Scalp Dovobet	Gel (Dovobet): 0.05% betamethasone + 0.005% calcipotriol Ointment: 0.05% betamethasone + 0.005% calcipotriol (Dovobet), 0.064% betamethasone + 0.005% calcipotriene (Taclonex) Suspension (Taclonex): 0.064% betamethasone + 0.005% calcipotriene
calcitriol	Vectical Silkis	Ointment: 3 mcg/g

*†Generic available in the United States only.

Furanocoumarins

Generic Name	U.S. Brand Name(s) Canadian Brand Name(s)	Dosage Forms and Strengths
methoxsalen	8-MOP, Oxsoralen, Oxsoralen Ultra, UVADEX Oxsoralen, Oxsoralen Ultra	Capsule (Oxsoralen^, Oxsoralen Ultra, 8-MOP): 10 mg Lotion (Oxsoralen)^: 1% Solution, for injection (UVADEX): 20 mcg/mL

^The trade name Oxsoralen marketed as a capsule in Canada and a lotion in the United States.

hard gelatin capsules of methoxsalen (8-MOP) and soft gelatin capsules (Oxsoralen-Ultra) is not equivalent, so product substitution is not permitted. 8-MOP should be taken with food or milk, whereas Oxsorelan-Ultra should be taken with low-fat food or milk. Methoxsalen is extensively metabolized in the liver and 90% to 95% is eliminated in urine. The elimination half-life is approximately 2 hours.

ADVERSE EFFECTS

Adverse reactions produced by oral methoxsalen therapy are photosensitivity, insomnia, headache, dizziness, leg cramps, itching, dry skin, nausea, and vomiting. Topical application can cause burning, blistering, and swelling at the site of application.

IMMUNOSUPPRESSIVES AND ANTIMETABOLITES

Atopic dermatitis is believed to be an autoimmune disease; therefore, immune system modulation and immunosuppression can downregulate the body's response to allergens and other irritants. Alefacept, cyclosporine, and azathioprine are immunosuppressants (see Chapter 15). Cyclosporine is FDA-approved for the short-term treatment of severe atopic dermatitis and psoriasis. Alefacept is indicated for the treatment of moderate to severe plaque psoriasis. Azathioprine is also used for the treatment of severe psoriasis, although it is not FDA-approved. Methotrexate is an antimetabolite (see Chapters 15 and 37) that is indicated for the treatment of moderate to severe chronic psoriasis and psoriatic arthritis.

MECHANISM OF ACTION AND PHARMACOKINETICS

Alefacept is a CD2-directed LFA-3/Fc fusion protein. It is created by DNA recombinant technology. Alefacept is administered IM in once weekly injections over a 3-month period. The elimination $t_{1/2}$ is approximately 270 hours and the drug has 63% bioavailability. Alefacept is contraindicated in patients with HIV infection and should not be given if CD4+ T lymphocyte levels are below normal. Cyclosporine selectively interferes with T cell proliferation and interleukin production. The result is a decreased immune system response. Azathioprine and methotrexate slow the rapid rate of skin cell turnover that occurs with eczema and psoriasis. Azathioprine suppresses a T cell–mediated immune system response and blocks the synthesis of RNA and DNA needed for cell replication.

Immunosuppressants

Generic Name	U.S. Brand Name(s) Canadian Brand Name(s)	Dosage Forms and Strengths
alefacept	Amevive	Powder, for IM injection: 15 mg/vial
	Amevive	
azathioprine*	Azasan, Imuran	Injection, powder for reconstitution: 50 mg‡, 100 mg†
	Imuran	Tablet: 25 mg, 50 mg (Imuran), 75 mg†, 100 mg† (Azasan)
cyclosporine* (ciclosporin)	Gengraf, Neoral	Capsule, modified (Gengraf, Neoral): 10 mg‡, 25 mg, 50 mg, 100 mg
	Neoral	Solution, oral, modified (Gengraf, Neoral): 100 mg/mL (See Chapter 15 for additional dosage forms and brand names.)
methotrexate* (MTX)	Metoject, Rheumatrex, Trexall	Powder for injection (generics): 1 g/vial†
	Generics	Solution, for injection (generics): 10 mg/mL (Metoject)†, 25 mg/mL
		Tablet: 2.5-mg dosepak (Rheumatrex); 5 mg†, 7.5 mg†, 10 mg†, 15 mg† (Trexall)

*Generic available.
†Strength available in the United States only.
‡Strength available in Canada only.

Methotrexate also interferes with normal DNA synthesis. The bioavailability of cyclosporine varies between the modified (Neoral) and nonmodified (Sandimmune) formulations. The absorption of the nonmodified formula may be increased by high-fat meals or grapefruit juice. The absorption of modified cyclosporine is decreased by food. Azathioprine is a prodrug. It is well absorbed and extensively metabolized in the liver. The elimination half-life is 5 hours. The absorption of methotrexate is dose-dependent. Absorption from the GI tract occurs by active transport. Absorption decreases at higher doses. Food also delays absorption. Metabolism occurs in the liver, gut, and cells, and methotrexate is subject to first pass metabolism. Because methotrexate is primarily eliminated in the kidney, high dose therapy can cause high urine concentrations and crystalluria; leading to kidney damage. See Chapter 15 for additional pharmacokinetic information.

ADVERSE EFFECTS

Alefacept, cyclosporine, azathioprine, and methotrexate may produce nausea and vomiting. All of the drugs may also may increase the risk for infection. Alefacept additionally produces chills, hoarse throat and cough, dizziness, and myalgia. Pain, pruritus, and inflammation at the injection site also may occur. Azathioprine and methotrexate use may cause a dangerous drop in red and white blood cells. Cyclosporine and methotrexate can cause kidney toxicity, whereas alefacept and azathioprine can cause liver toxicity. Other serious sides effects produced by alefacept are cancers (e.g., skin, leukemia, solid organ) and angioedema. Weight gain and hypertension are other side effects of cyclosporine therapy. See Chapter 15 for a complete listing of adverse reactions.

> **TECH NOTE!**
> Folic acid is commonly prescribed to patients being treated with methotrexate.

Tumor Necrosis Factor-α Inhibitors

Etanercept, infliximab, and adalimumab are tumor necrosis factor (TNF)-α inhibitors indicated for the treatment of psoriasis. TNF-α inhibitors are genetically engineered drugs that block the inflammatory process triggered by high concentrations of TNF. Psoriasis is a condition that is linked to high levels of TNF-α. TNF-α inhibitors prevent cell lysis (destruction) and release of the substances that cause inflammation. Infiltration of inflammatory cells within the plaques is reduced by TNF-α inhibitor administration. Epidermal thickness may also be reduced by infliximab. Adverse reactions of etanercept are nausea, stomach pain, headache, opportunistic infections, redness, and itching at the injection site. Adalimumab, etanercept, and infliximab are also associated with unspecified rashes and possible new-onset psoriasis. See Chapter 15 for additional information.

RETINOIDS

Retinoid analogues are used to treat psoriasis. Acitretin is a synthetic retinoid and tazarotene is a retinoid prodrug (see Chapter 41).

MECHANISM OF ACTION AND PHARMACOKINETICS

When acitretin binds to retinoic acid receptors it modifies epithelial cell growth and differentiation. Tazarotene inhibits epidermal hyperproliferation in treated plaques. The absorption of tazarotene is minimal when applied topically. Metabolism occurs in the skin and results in the active metabolite

Tumor Necrosis Factor-α inhibitors

Generic Name	U.S. Brand Name(s) Canadian Brand Name(s)	Dosage Forms and Strengths
adalimumab	Humira	Prefilled pen kit: 40 mg/0.8 mL
	Humira	
etanercept	Enbrel	Injection, powder for reconstitution: 25 mg/vial
	Enbrel	Injection, solution: 50 mg/mL (0.98-mL prefilled syringe)
infliximab	Remicade	Injection, powder for reconstitution: 100-mg/mL vial
	Remicade	

tazarotenic acid. Tazarotenic acid is systemically absorbed and metabolized further. The half-life ($t_{1/2}$) of tazarotenic acid is approximately 18 hours.

ADVERSE REACTIONS

Itching, burning, stinging or redness, and worsening of psoriasis occur in up to 30% of people using tazarotene. Up to 10% may experience eczema, contact dermatitis, fissures, and/or bleeding. Tazarotene is contraindicated in pregnancy (FDA category X), and a negative pregnancy test should be obtained prior to use. Acitretin use may produce hypervitaminosis A. In addition, up to 75% of people using acitretin develop cheilitis, alopecia, and peeling skin. Redness, itching and dry skin, and a nail disorder may also occur.

Miscellaneous Agents

Anthralin is one of the oldest drugs approved for the treatment of psoriasis. It was approved in 1939 but is no longer marketed for treatment in the United States or Canada.

MECHANISM OF ACTION

Anthralin reduces cell turnover by inhibiting mitosis in skin cells. Mitosis is the part of the cell replication process in which DNA is replicated, divided, and split between the old cell and the new cell.

ADVERSE EFFECTS

Anthralin causes skin discoloration and may cause discoloration of hair and nails.

Retinoids

Generic Name	U.S. Brand Name(s) Canadian Brand Name(s)	Dosage Forms and Strengths
acitretin	Soriatane	Capsule: 10 mg, 17.5 mg[†], 25 mg, 22.5mg[†]
	Soriatane	
tazarotene	Avage, Fabior, Tazorac	Cream: 0.05%, 0.1%
	Tazorac	Foam (Fabior): 0.1% Gel: 0.05%[‡], 0.1%[‡]

[†]Strength available in the United States only.
[‡]Strength Available in Canada only.

Summary of Drugs Used for the Treatment of Eczema and Psoriasis

Generic Name	Brand Name	Usual Dose and Dosing Schedule	Warning Labels
Topical Corticosteroids			
alclometasone dipropionate*	Aclovate	Cream or ointment: Apply a thin film two or three times daily.	FOR EXTERNAL USE.
amcinonide*	Generics	All dosage forms: Apply a thin film two or three times daily.	FOR EXTERNAL USE.
betamethasone dipropionate*	Diprolene AF Diprosone	Cream, lotion, ointment: Apply a thin film two to four times daily.	FOR EXTERNAL USE.
betamethasone valerate*	Betaderm, Luxiq, Valisone	Foam: Apply twice a day. Cream, lotion, ointment: Apply a thin film two to four times daily.	FOR EXTERNAL USE. SHAKE WELL (FOAM, LOTION).
clobetasol propionate*	Clobex	All dosage forms: Apply twice a day.	FOR EXTERNAL USE.

Summary of Drugs Used for the Treatment of Eczema and Psoriasis—cont'd

Generic Name	Brand Name	Usual Dose and Dosing Schedule	Warning Labels
desonide*	Desowen	**Foam:** Apply twice a day.	FOR EXTERNAL USE.
	Desocort	**Cream, lotion, ointment:** Apply a thin film two to four times daily.	
desoximetasone*	Topicort	**Cream, gel, ointment:** Apply a thin film twice a day.	FOR EXTERNAL USE.
diflucortolone valerate	Nerisone	**Cream:** Apply three times a day.	FOR EXTERNAL USE.
diflorasone diacetate*	Psorcon-E	**Nonemollient dosage forms:** Apply a thin film one to four times daily. **Emollient dosage forms:** Apply a thin film one to three times daily.	FOR EXTERNAL USE.
fluocinolone acetonide*	Synalar	**Cream, ointment, solution:** Apply a thin film two to four times daily.	FOR EXTERNAL USE.
	Derma-Smoothe FS	**Oil:** Apply a thin film three times a day.	
halcinonide	Halog	**Cream, ointment, solution:** Apply a thin film two to four times daily.	FOR EXTERNAL USE.
halobetasol propionate*	Ultravate	**Cream or ointment:** Apply a thin film once or twice daily.	FOR EXTERNAL USE.
hydrocortisone, acetate*	Keratol HC	**All dosage forms:** Apply three or four times daily.	FOR EXTERNAL USE.
hydrocortisone butyrate*	Locoid	**All dosage forms:** Apply once or twice daily.	FOR EXTERNAL USE.
hydrocortisone valerate*	Westcort	**All dosage forms:** Apply two to four times daily.	FOR EXTERNAL USE.
mometasone furoate*	Elocon	**Topical dosage forms:** Apply once daily.	FOR EXTERNAL USE.
prednicarbate*	Dermatop	**Cream or ointment:** Apply a thin film twice daily.	FOR EXTERNAL USE.
triamcinolone acetonide*	Generics	**Cream, lotion, ointment:** Apply a thin film two to four times daily.	FOR EXTERNAL USE.
Calcineurin Inhibitors			
pimecrolimus	Elidel	**Eczema:** Apply a thin layer twice a day.	AVOID EXCESS EXPOSURE TO SUNLIGHT.
tacrilimus	Protopic	**Eczema:** Apply a thin layer twice a day.	AVOID GRAPEFRUIT JUICE (CAPSULE).
Immunosuppressives			
alefacept	Amevive	**Psoriasis:** 15 mg IM once weekly for 12 weeks	AVOID PREGNANCY. REPORT SIGNS OF INFECTION, ANGIOEDEMA (FACIAL SWELLING, URTICARIA), JAUNDICE, AND EASY BRUISING.

Continued

Summary of Drugs Used for the Treatment of Eczema and Psoriasis—cont'd

Generic Name	Brand Name	Usual Dose and Dosing Schedule	Warning Labels
cyclosporine	Neoral	Psoriasis: 1.25 mg/kg orally bid up to 4 mg/kg daily	TAKE WITH FOOD. AVOID PREGNANCY. AVOID ALCOHOL. SWALLOW WHOLE; DON'T CRUSH OR CHEW.
methotrexate	Generics	Psoriasis: 10-25 mg PO, IV, or IM given as a single weekly dose or 2.5-5 mg PO every 12 hr for 3 doses every week	AVOID ALCOHOL. AVOID PROLONGED EXPOSURE TO SUNLIGHT. AVOID PREGNANCY. EXERCISE PRECAUTIONS FOR HANDLING, PREPARING, AND ADMINISTERING CYTOTOXIC DRUGS.
Vitamin D Analogues			
calcipotriene	Dovonex	Psoriasis: Apply a thin layer twice a day.	FOR EXTERNAL USE. AVOID EXCESS EXPOSURE TO SUNLIGHT. AVOID FACE.
calcipotriene + betamethasone	Taclonex	Psoriasis: Apply a thin layer once daily.	
calcitriol	Vectical	Mild to moderate psoriasis: Apply twice a day.	
Furanocoumarins			
methoxsalen	Oxsoralen Ultra	Psoriasis: 1 cap 1.5-2 hr before UVA therapy	TAKE WITH FOOD OR MILK. AVOID SUN EXPOSURE FOR 24 HR BEFORE AND 48 HR AFTER TREATMENT.
Tumor Necrosis Factor-α Inhibitors			
adalimumab	Humira	Chronic plaque psoriasis: 80 mg subcut in two injections on day 1, then 40 mg subcut every other week	REFRIGERATE; DO NOT FREEZE.
etanercept	Enbrel	Psoriasis: 50 mg subcut weekly given as one 50-mg subcut injection or as two 25-mg subcut injections 3-4 days apart	PROTECT FROM LIGHT. REFRIGERATE; DON'T FREEZE.
infliximab	Remicade	Psoriasis: 5 mg/kg IV given at week 0, 2, and 6 and repeated every 8 wk thereafter	REFRIGERATE; DON'T FREEZE. GENTLY SWIRL RECONSTITUTED PRODUCT; DO NOT SHAKE. AFTER MIXING, DISCARD ANY UNUSED PORTION.
Retinoids			
acitretin	Soriatane	Recalcitrant psoriasis: 25-50 mg PO once daily	TAKE WITH MAIN MEAL. AVOID ALCOHOL.
tazarotene	Tazorac	Psoriasis: Apply once daily, in the evening, to psoriatic lesions (max, 12 wk)	PROTECT SKIN FROM THE SUN. AVOID PREGNANCY.

*Generic available.

Chapter Summary

- Eczema is a general term used to describe several types of inflammation of the skin.
- Atopic diseases are an autoimmune disorder.
- Atopic dermatitis, allergic contact eczema, contact eczema, dyshidrotic eczema, neurodermatitis, nummular eczema, seborrheic eczema, and stasis dermatitis are all types of eczema.
- Atopic dermatitis is the most common form of eczema.
- Atopic dermatitis is a chronic disease of the skin that often develops in infancy and may continue throughout adulthood.
- Atopic dermatitis commonly produces symptoms of intense itching, redness (from scratching), skin irritation, and inflammation. Eczematous patches may form that are flaky and crusting, and may even ooze a clear fluid.
- People who live in dry climates and in large cities seem to have a higher incidence of atopic dermatitis.
- Psoriasis is a condition associated with the rapid turnover of skin cells and is caused by hyperactivity of the T cells.
- Individuals with psoriasis have thick, silvery, scaly patches. They may also have some redness and swelling.
- Individuals with eczema (atopic dermatitis) and psoriasis may experience periods when their symptoms worsen (exacerbation) and periods when they get better or go away completely (remission).
- Nonpharmaceutical treatment for eczema involves using skin care regimens that reduce irritation and avoid allergens and irritants and may include the use of phototherapy.
- Phototherapy involves exposing the skin to ultraviolet A or B light waves.
- Adverse reactions to the use of UV light therapy are premature aging of the skin and increased risk for skin cancer.
- The use of topical corticosteroids continues to be a mainstay of therapy for the treatment of eczema.
- Corticosteroids are also used for the treatment of psoriasis, seborrhea, and other skin conditions in which inflammation is present.
- Topical corticosteroids are categorized into seven groups based on potency.
- The vehicle (base) in which the corticosteroid is suspended may influence the potency.
- Higher potency corticosteroids cause more adverse reactions.
- Only the mildest potency agents, such as hydrocortisone, should be used on the face.
- Long-term use of topical corticosteroids can result in thinning of the skin, stretch marks (striae), spider veins, acne, milia, rosacea (enlarged blood vessels, especially on the nose), bruising, atrophy, lacerations, poor wound healing, and growth suppression (in children).
- Pimecrolimus and tacrolimus are calcineurin inhibitor immunomodulators that control inflammation and reduce the immune system response to allergens.
- Pimecrolimus is indicated for the treatment of mild to moderate eczema.
- Tacrolimus is approved for the treatment of moderate to severe atopic dermatitis that has failed to respond to corticosteroid treatment.
- The FDA and Health Canada require manufacturers to include a boxed warning in the package insert, advising health care providers that tacrolimus and pimecrolimus may increase the risk for development of lymphoma.
- Calcipotriene is a synthetic analogue of vitamin D. It is known as calcipotriol in Canada.
- Calcipotriene (calcipotriol) inhibits the rapid and repeated production of new skin cells and is used for the treatment of psoriasis.
- Calcitriol is an active form of vitamin D that is used topically for the treatment of psoriasis.
- Psoralens are a class of drugs that increase photosensitivity and are classified as furanocoumarins. Methoxsalen is the only drug in this class.
- Psoralens plus ultraviolet light A therapy is also known as PUVA.
- The bioavailability of methoxsalen hard gelatin capsules (8-MOP) and soft gelatin capsules (Oxsoralen-Ultra) is not equivalent, so product substitution is not permitted.
- Alefacept is a CD2-directed LFA-3/FC fusion protein and is indicated for the treatment of moderate to severe plaque psoriasis.

- Cyclosporine is FDA-approved for the short-term treatment of severe atopic dermatitis and psoriasis. It decreases immune system hyperactivity.
- Methotrexate is an antimetabolite indicated for the treatment of moderate to severe chronic psoriasis and psoriatic arthritis.
- Azathioprine and methotrexate slow the rapid rate of skin cell turnover that occurs with eczema and psoriasis.
- Anthralin is one of the oldest drugs approved for treatment of psoriasis.
- Anthralin causes skin discoloration and may cause discoloration of the hair and nails.
- The retinoids acitretin and tazarotene are used for the treatment of psoriasis.
- Adalimumab, etanercept, and infliximab are TNF-α inhibitors indicated for the treatment of plaque psoriasis.

REVIEW QUESTIONS

1. A chronic disease of the skin characterized by itchy red patches covered with silvery scales is known as _____.
   a. Eczema
   b. Psoriasis
   c. Dermatitis
   d. Rosacea

2. _____ is defined as a group of diseases in which there is an inherited tendency to develop other allergic conditions.
   a. Atopic
   b. Ectopic
   c. Dermatopic
   d. Allergic

3. When symptoms worsen, it is called _____, and periods when they get better or go away completely are called _____.
   a. Exacerbation; metastasis
   b. Exacerbation; remission
   c. Metastasis; inflammation
   d. Allergic; nonallergic

4. Phototherapy reduces the risk for skin cancer.
   a. True
   b. False

5. A mainstay of therapy for the treatment of eczema is the use of _____.
   a. Antibiotics
   b. Corticosteroids
   c. Antihistamines
   d. None of the above

6. Pimecrolimus is indicated for the treatment of moderate to severe eczema.
   a. True
   b. False

7. For which two drugs does FDA require a boxed warning in the package insert, advising health care providers that the drugs may increase the risk for the development of lymphoma?
   a. Desonide
   b. Pimecrolimus
   c. Tacrolimus
   d. b and c

8. Methoxsalen is the only drug in this class.
   a. Immunomodulators
   b. Furanocoumarins
   c. Calcineurin inhibitors
   d. Immunosuppressants

9. _____ is an antimetabolite indicated for the treatment of moderate to severe chronic psoriasis and psoriatic arthritis.
   a. Anthralin
   b. Cyclosporine
   c. Methotrexate
   d. Calcipotriene

10. Anthralin is one of the oldest drugs approved for the treatment of psoriasis.
    a. True
    b. False

TECHNICIAN'S CORNER

1. Because eczema is allergy-related, how can one prevent flare-ups from occurring?
2. How well do calamine lotion and oatmeal soap (both OTC products) work in decreasing the symptoms of atopic dermatitis?

Bibliography

Elsevier: Gold Standard Clinical Pharmacology. Retrieved Dec 12, 2011, from https://www.clinicalpharmacology.com/, 2010.

FDA: FDA Approved Drug Products. Retrieved July 11, 2012, from http://www.accessdata.fda.gov/scripts/cder/drugsatfda/index.cfm?fuseaction=Search.Search_Drug_Name, 2012.

FDA: Amevive product labeling. Available at http://www.accessdata.fda.gov/drugsatfda_docs/label/2012/125036s0144lbl.pdf, 2012.

Health Canada: Drug product database. 2010 (http://www.hc-sc.gc.ca/dhp-mps/prodpharma/databasdon/index-eng.php).

Kalant H, Grant D, Mitchell J: *Principles of medical pharmacology*, ed 7, Toronto, 2007, Elsevier Canada, pp 891-898.

Khandpur S, Sharma VK, Sumanth K: Topical immunomodulators in dermatology, *J Postgrad Med* 50:131-139, 2004.

Lance L, Lacy C, Armstrong L, et al: *Drug information handbook for the allied health professional*, ed 12, Hudson, OH, 2005, APhA Lexi-Comp.

National Institute of Arthritis and Musculoskeletal and Skin Diseases: Atopic dermatitis (NIH Publ. No. 09-4272). 2009 (http://www.niams.nih.gov/hi/topics/dermatitis/index.html).

National Institute of Arthritis and Musculoskeletal and Skin Diseases: Psoriasis (NIH Publ. No. 09-5040). 2009 (http://www.niams.nih.gov/Health_Info/Psoriasis/default.asp).

Page C, Curtis M, Sutter M, et al: *Integrated pharmacology*. Philadelphia, 2005, Elsevier Mosby, pp 506-508, 512-514.

Raymond G, Houle M-C: A review of corticosteroids for the treatment of psoriasis. 2007 (http://www.skinpharmacies.ca/2_1_2.html).

USP Center for Advancement of Patient Safety: *Use caution—avoid confusion, USP Quality Review No. 79.* Rockville, MD, 2004, USP Center for Advancement of Patient Safety.

Vender R: Management of eczema. 2006 (http://www.skinpharmacies.ca/2_1_2.html).

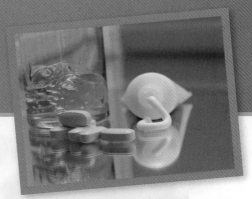

43

Treatment of Lice and Scabies

1 Learn the terminology associated with lice and scabies.

2 Describe the epidemiology of lice and scabies infestation.

3 List the symptoms of lice and scabies infestation.

4 List prevention strategies.

5 List and categorize medications used to treat lice and scabies.

6 Describe mechanism of action for drugs used to lice and scabies.

7 Identify warning labels and precautionary messages associated with medications used to treat lice and scabies.

KEY TERMS

Lice: Group of parasites (*Pediculus humanus capitis, Pediculus humanus corporis, Phthirus pubis*) that can live on the body, scalp, or genital area of humans.

Nits: Head lice eggs.

Nymph: Baby louse.

Ovicidal: Kills eggs.

Parasite: Organism that benefits by living in, with, or on another organism.

Pediculicide: Drug that kills lice.

Scabicide: Drug that kills the scabies mite.

Scabies: Parasitic infection caused by the mite *Sarcoptes scabiei*.

Epidemiology of Lice and Scabies Infestation

Lice and *scabies* infestations affect people worldwide without regard for social status or race. They are caused by parasites and are readily spread person to person. A *parasite* is an organism that benefits by living in, with, or on another organism (host), usually to the detriment of the host.

LICE

Head Lice

Head lice most commonly infests children aged 3 to 11 years and their families, but anyone can become infested (Figure 43-1*A, B*). Infestation is caused by the parasite *Pediculus humanus capitis*. Head lice is spread between individuals through head-to-head contact, as occurs during children's play and sports. Less commonly, transmission occurs by sharing personal items such as combs, brushes, hats, towels, scarves, pillows, and coats with someone who has head lice.

TECH ALERT!
It is a myth that head lice infestation is caused by poor hygiene (lack of cleanliness).

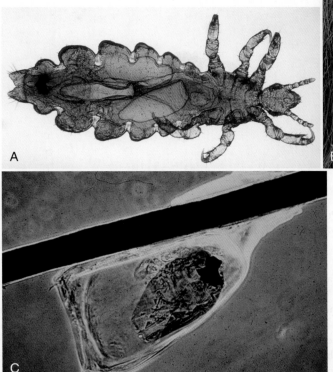

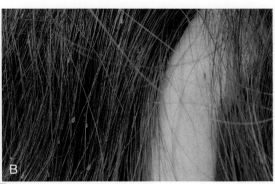

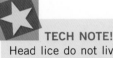

FIGURE 43-1 A, Adult head louse. **B,** Head lice infestation. **C,** Nit attached to hair shaft. (**A,** Courtesy of Dr. Dennis D. Juranek, Centers for Disease Control and Prevention; **B** from Callen J, Greer K, Hood A, et al: *Color atlas of dermatology*, Philadelphia, 1993, WB Saunders; **C** from Kumar V, Abbas AK, Fausto M: *Robbins and Cotran pathologic basis of disease*, ed 7, Philadelphia, 2005, WB Saunders.)

> **TECH NOTE!**
> Head lice do not live on pets, there is no human to pet transmission, and pets need not be treated with pediculicides.

> **TECH NOTE!**
> Pharmacy technicians may have customers coming into the pharmacy asking about head lice treatments. Because these products are available over the counter (OTC), they will be able to direct customers to the pharmacy shelves for available products.

The life cycle of a head louse is approximately 4 to 6 weeks. The adult females lay eggs, also called **nits**, at the base of the hair shaft (see Figure 43-1*C*) within 24 hours of mating. In approximately 7 days, the nits hatch and a nymph emerges. A **nymph** is a baby louse. The nymph becomes an adult in approximately 7 days; and the adult lives for approximately 30 days.

Lice are parasites that feed on blood. This is why eggs are laid close to the base of the hair shaft and nits that are found within $\frac{1}{4}$ inch of the scalp are typically viable eggs. Newly hatched nymphs must be close to a blood source. Nit shells found farther than a fingertip away from the base of the scalp (2 to 5 cm) are likely remains of an earlier infestation; treatment is not necessary. An adult louse can live for up to 3 days away from a human host. Head lice are a nuisance but are not a health risk.

Body Lice

Body lice infestations are caused by the parasite *Pediculus humanus corporis*. Infestations are a serious public health concern because body lice may cause epidemics of typhus and louse-borne relapsing fever. Body lice thrive in crowded environments with chronic poverty and unsanitary conditions, such as refugee camps, temporary housing from natural disasters, and prisons. In the United States and Canada, body lice infestations rarely occur except in homeless populations without access to bathing facilities.

Like head lice, body lice infestation is spread person to person through direct contact with a person who has body lice. Another mode of transmission is through shared bedding or clothes. Body lice can live in the seams of the clothing of infested individuals.

The life cycle of body lice is similar to that of head lice and begins with laying eggs. The nits hatch and nymphs mature to adults in 7 days. Adults can only survive away from a human host for 10 days.

Pubic Lice

Pubic lice, or "crabs," is sometimes classified as a sexually transmitted infection (STI) because it is usually spread through sexual contact (Figure 43-2). It is rare for lice to be spread through contact with bedding, linens, or clothes. Although the life cycle of pubic lice is the same as that of head lice, pubic lice and head lice are different species. Head lice do not inhabit the genitalia and pubic lice do not live in the hair. Lice infestation in the pubic region is caused by the parasite *Phthirus pubis*.

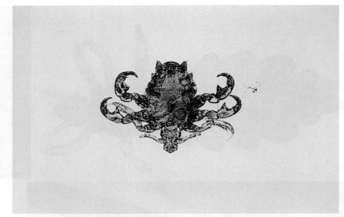

FIGURE 43-2 Pubic lice. (From Mahon CR, Lehman DC, Manuselis G: *Textbook of diagnostic microbiology*, ed 3, St. Louis, 2007, WB Saunders.)

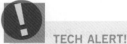

TECH ALERT!

It is a myth that individuals can get pubic lice from sitting on a public toilet seat.

SCABIES

Scabies infestations are common and affect those of all social classes and race. Infestations are caused by a parasitic mite called *Sarcoptes scabiei*. The mite flourishes and spreads by person-to-person contact in environments in which the population density is high, such as hospitals, nursing homes, child care facilities, and schools. Transmission occurs through close contact and sharing bedding, linen, clothing, or sexual relations.

The scabies mite burrows beneath the skin. Sites of infestation can be seen in the webbing between fingers and toes, skin folds of the breast, penis, and shoulder blades, and in the bends of the elbows, knees, and wrists. Like lice, *S. scabiei* feeds on blood and dies if away from a human host for longer than 48 to 72 hours. The adult mite can live for approximately 30 days.

TECH ALERT!

Shaving the head is not necessary to treat head lice!

Symptoms of Lice and Scabies Infestation and Prevention of Lice Reinfestation

Symptoms of lice and scabies infestation are listed in Box 43-1. Methods for the prevention of lice reinfestation are listed in Box 43-2.

BOX 43-1   **Symptoms of Lice and Scabies Infestation**

HEAD AND PUBIC LICE	SCABIES
• Itching	• Intense itching
• Feeling of something moving in hair or genital area	• Pimple-like rash
• Sores (from scratching)	

BODY LOUSE
• Itching
• Rash
• Thickening and discoloration of skin

BOX 43-2   **Strategies to Prevent Reinfestation**

• Treat all infested and probably infested household members simultaneously.
• Use a nit comb to remove eggs. Use daily lice combing between pediculicidal treatments.
• Don't wash the hair for 1-2 days after the treatment is rinsed from the hair.
• Vacuum the floor and furniture in infested household.
• Wash clothing, linens, and bedding in hot water (130° F [54°C]).
• Dry-clean clothing that is not washable.
• Place stuffed toys, clothing, and bedding that cannot be washed or dry-cleaned in a large plastic bag and seal the bag for 2 weeks.

Treatment of Head Lice, Pubic Lice, and Scabies

Head lice may be treated with nonprescription and prescription *pediculicides*. The Centers for Disease Control and Prevention (CDC) and Nova Scotia Public Health Services recommend that all family members with active infestations, as well as those with probable infestations (nits but no live lice), be treated. Treatment is more effective if a fine-toothed nit comb is used to remove eggs from the hair shaft. OTC and prescription agents are effective treatments for head lice and pubic lice. OTC products are more effective and have a lower risk of toxicity than lindane. Drug resistance is a growing problem for OTC and prescription pediculicides, especially permethrin, because of the residue left after treatment.

OVER-THE-COUNTER DRUGS

OTC pediculicides available for the treatment of lice are pyrethrins, permethrin, and isopropyl myristate. They are formulated in various dosage forms, such as shampoo, cream rinse, lotion, and household spray.

Pyrethrins and Permethrin

Pyrethrins are naturally derived from the chrysanthemum flower. Their effectiveness is boosted by the addition of piperonyl butoxide, a petroleum distillate. Pyrethrins are indicated for the treatment of head lice, pubic lice, and body lice. Permethrin is a mixture of synthetic isomers of pyrethrins. It is more effective for the treatment of head lice but less effective against pubic lice (as low as 57% efficacy). It is also effective against the scabies mite.

Pyrethrins are not *ovicidal* (do not kill the eggs), so retreatment is necessary in 7 to 10 days to kill newly hatched nymphs. Permethrin is ovicidal.

MECHANISM OF ACTION AND PHARMACOKINETICS

Pyrethrins and permethrin paralyze and kill lice by blocking the repolarization of sodium channels. Their action is discontinued once the drug is washed off. Permethrin leaves a residue on the hair that can destroy eggs and newly hatched nymphs. Detailed human pharmacokinetic data are limited. Absorption of pyrethrins and permethrin through the skin is minimal. Both drugs are rapidly metabolized by ester hydrolysis in the liver.

ADVERSE EFFECTS

Adverse effects caused by topical application of pyrethrins are redness, itching and stinging, tingling, and minor swelling.

Isopropyl Myristate

Isopropyl myristate 50% is available in Canada for the OTC treatment of head lice. It is not available in the United States.

Pyrethins and Permethrin

Generic Name	U.S. Brand Name(s) Canadian Brand Name(s)	Dosage Forms and Strengths
pyrethrins + piperonyl butoxide*	A-200 Lice treatment, RID Step 1 Lice-Killing shampoo, RID Mousse	**Mousse:** piperonyl butoxide 4%, pyrethrins 0.33% **Shampoo:** pyrethrins 0.33% + piperonyl butoxide 4% **Spray:** pyrethrins 0.3% + piperonyl butoxide 3%
	R&C Shampoo with Conditioner, Licetrol, Pronto	
permethrin*	Nix, Elimite	**Cream rinse:** 1%
	Nix, Kwellada-P	**Lotion:** 1%, 5%‡ **Cream:** 5%

*Generic available.
‡Strength available in Canada only

MECHANISM OF ACTION AND PHARMACOKINETICS

Isopropyl myristate purportedly dissolves the louse exoskeleton, resulting in dehydration and death. It is not ovicidal, so nit removal and retreatment in 10 days are required. Evidence of the effectiveness of isopropyl myristate is lacking. Pharmacokinetic information is unavailable.

ADVERSE EFFECTS

Adverse effects caused by topical application of isopropyl myristate are redness, itching and mild skin irritation.

PRESCRIPTION TREATMENTS

Lindane

Lindane is an organochlorine pesticide known by the chemical name gamma-hexachlorocyclohexane. It is used in agriculture to control pests* and medically to kill lice. It is a ***scabicide*** and pediculicide, killing all type of lice, scabies, and their eggs.

MECHANISM OF ACTION AND PHARMACOKINETICS

Lindane is absorbed through into the body of the scabies mite and lice, where it paralyzes and kills the parasite. Lindane is highly lipid-soluble and absorption through the skin is variable. Absorption of lindane through intact human skin increases with repeated applications; the half-life is long ($t_{1/2}$ = 18 hours). Lindane is stored in body fats and is significantly metabolized in the liver. Repeated use causes accumulation and increases the risk for neurotoxicity.

ADVERSE EFFECTS

Lindane is neurotoxic and can cause illness, vomiting, seizures, and death if accidentally swallowed. The U.S. Food and Drug Administration (FDA) has required manufacturers to place a boxed warning in the package insert to alert health care providers of the following:
- Lindane is not a first-line therapy and repeat applications should be avoided.
- Lindane should not be used by infants, young children, elders, adults weighing less than 110 lb [50 kg], and breast-feeding women.
- The drug should be dispensed in 1- to 2-ounce single-application vials, the maximum amount needed for a treatment.

TECH ALERT!
Malathion is flammable, and those using the product should stay away from open flames, hair dryers, curling irons, and lit cigarettes, cigars, and pipes.

Isopropyl Myristate

Generic Name	U.S. Brand Name(s)	Dosage Forms and Strengths
	Canadian Brand Name(s)	
isopropyl myristate	Not available	Cream rinse: 50%
	Resultz	

Lindane

Generic Name	U.S. Brand Name(s)	Dosage Forms and Strengths
	Canadian Brand Name(s)	
lindane*	Generics	Lotion: 1%
	Hexit	Shampoo: 1%

*Generic available.

*On January 1, 2005, Canada withdrew registration of lindane for agricultural pest control.

Malathion

Malathion is an organophosphate pesticide used in agriculture to control pests and medically to kill head lice and their eggs. It was withdrawn from the U.S. market and then reintroduced in 1999 following labeling changes. It remains withdrawn from the market in Canada.

MECHANISM OF ACTION AND PHARMACOKINETICS

Malathion paralyzes the central nervous system of parasites by causing an accumulation of acetylcholine (ACh). The lotion is applied to dry hair until the hair and scalp are saturated. The drug must be allowed to dry naturally on the head and should be left on for 8 to 12 hours before being rinsed off. Retreatment is only recommended if crawling lice are found 7 to 10 days after initial treatment. The pharmacokinetics of malathion are dependent on the dose and route of exposure. Less than 10% of the applied dose is absorbed systemically. Absorption through the scalp of infants is greater and the use of malathion is contraindicated in this age group. Safety in children less than 6 years old has not been established. The onset of action is 3 seconds to 1 hour. Malathion must be metabolized to its active metabolite malaoxon. The elimination half-life ranges between 8-48 hours.

ADVERSE EFFECTS

The most common adverse effects linked to malathion use are stinging, redness, minor swelling, itching, and tingling.

Crotamiton

Crotamiton is a scabicide. Its mechanism of action is unknown. It is classified in FDA pregnancy category C and is an alternative to lindane. The pharmacokinetics and degree of systemic absorption of crotamiton after topical application have not been determined.

ADVERSE EFFECTS

Crotamiton has few adverse reactions. Reactions are linked to drug allergy and include itchiness, minor swelling, and redness.

Spinosad

Spinosad is a pediculicide indicated for the topical treatment of head lice infestations in patients 4 years of age and older. It is derived from *Saccharopolyspora spinosa*, a bacterium found in soil.

Malathion

| Generic Name | U.S. Brand Name(s) | Dosage Form and Strength |
	Canadian Brand Name(s)	
malathion*	Ovide	Lotion: 0.5%
	Not available	

*Generic available.

Crotamiton

| Generic Name | U.S. Brand Name(s) | Dosage Forms and Strengths |
	Canadian Brand Name(s)	
crotamiton*†	Eurax	Cream: 10%
	Eurax	Lotion: 10% (United States only)

*†Generic available in the United States only.

MECHANISM OF ACTION AND PHARMACOKINETICS

Spinosad produces neuronal excitation in lice, resulting in hyperexcitation, paralysis, and death. The pharmacokinetics and degree of systemic absorption of spinosad after topical application have not been determined. Systemic exposure is not expected.

ADVERSE EFFECTS

Most common adverse reactions are application site redness (3%), redness and irritation of the eyes (2%), and application site irritation (1%).

Spinosad

Generic Name	U.S. Brand Name(s) Canadian Brand Name(s)	Dosage Forms and Strengths
spinosad	Natroba	Topical suspension: 0.9%

Summary of Drugs Used for the Treatment of Lice and Scabies

Generic Name	Brand name	Usual Dose and Dosing Schedule	Warning Labels
Over-the-Counter			
pyrethrins + piperonyl butoxide	RID, R&C various	**Lice, shampoo, cream rinse:** Apply to dry hair. Saturate hair with product. Leave on for as long as instructed on product label. Rinse hair. Use nit comb to remove eggs. **Scabies, lotion, cream:** Apply after bathing to the skin over the entire body from the chin to the toes. Leave on overnight (or 8 hr). Wash off. Repeat treatment in 7-10 days if needed.	SHAKE WELL (LOTION, CREAM RINSE). DO NOT REWASH HAIR FOR 1-2 DAYS AFTER TREATMENT. TREAT ALL INFESTED AND PROBABLY INFESTED HOUSEHOLD MEMBERS . DO NOT OVERUSE PRODUCT. SHAKE WELL.
permethrin	Kwellada, NIX	**Lice, cream rinse:** Apply to dry hair. Apply a sufficient amount of product to saturate the hair and scalp thoroughly. Let set for 10 min; then rinse hair with water and towel-dry. Use lice comb to remove dead lice and nits. Retreat in 10 days.	
isopropyl myristate	Resultz	**Cream rinse:** Apply to dry hair. Apply a sufficient amount of product to saturate the hair and scalp thoroughly. Let set for 10 min; then rinse hair with water and towel dry. Use lice comb to remove dead lice and nits. Retreat in 10 days.	SHAKE WELL.
Prescription Only			
crotamiton	Eurax	Apply after bathing to the skin over the entire body from the chin to the toes. Repeat in 24 hr. Bathe 48 hr *after* second dose. Treatment may be repeated in 7-10 days if needed.	SHAKE WELL.
lindane	Generics	**Shampoo:** Saturate hair with product. Leave on for 4 min; rub until a lather is formed, then rinse hair. Use nit comb to remove eggs. **Lotion, cream:** Apply 1 hr after bathing to the skin over the entire body from the chin to the toes. Leave on 8-12 hr. Wash off.	SHAKE WELL. DO NOT REWASH HAIR FOR 1-2 DAYS AFTER TREATMENT. TREAT ALL HOUSEHOLD MEMBERS. RETREAT IN 7-10 DAYS IF CRAWLING BUGS ARE EVIDENT. DO NOT OVERUSE PRODUCT.

Summary of Drugs Used for the Treatment of Lice and Scabies—cont'd

Generic Name	Brand name	Usual Dose and Dosing Schedule	Warning Labels
malathion	Ovide	Saturate hair with product. Leave on 8-12 hr; then wash hair. Use nit comb to remove eggs.	FLAMMABLE; AVOID FLAMES.
spinosad	Natroba	Apply a sufficient amount of spinosad suspension to cover dry scalp and hair, up to one bottle (120 mL). Leave on for 10 min and then rinse thoroughly. If live lice are still seen 7 days after the first treatment, apply a second treatment.	WASH HANDS AFTER APPLYING.

Chapter Summary

- Lice and scabies infestations affect people worldwide, without regard for social status or race.
- Head lice, body lice, pubic lice, and scabies are spread through direct person-to-person contact.
- Lice and scabies infestations are caused by parasites.
- A parasite is an organism that benefits by living in, with, or on another organism (host), usually to the detriment of the host.
- Head lice most commonly affects children aged 3 to 11 years and their families, but anyone can become infested.
- Head lice infestation is caused by the parasite *Pediculus humanus capitis* it is not caused by poor hygiene (lack of cleanliness).
- Adult head lice and pubic lice can live up to 3 days away from a human host.
- Adult body lice can survive away from a human host for 10 days.
- Body lice infestations are caused by the parasite *Pediculus humanus corporis*.
- Body louse infestations are a serious public health concern because body lice may cause epidemics of typhus and louse-borne relapsing fever.
- Pubic lice, or "crabs," is sometimes classified as an STI because it is most commonly spread through sexual contact.
- Individuals cannot get pubic lice from sitting on public toilet seats.
- Lice infestation in the pubic region is caused by the parasite *Phthirus pubis*.
- Scabies infestations are common and are caused by a parasitic mite called *Sarcoptes scabiei*.
- The mite flourishes and spreads via person-to-person contact in environments in which the population density is high, such as hospitals, nursing homes, child care facilities, and schools.
- Like lice, *S. scabiei* feeds on blood and dies if away from a human host for longer than 48 to 72 hours.
- Strategies to prevent lice and scabies reinfestation include the following: (1) treat all household members; (2) use a nit comb to remove eggs (lice); (3) wash clothing, linens, and bedding in hot water (130° F [54° C]); (4) dry-clean clothing that is not washable; and (5) place stuffed toys, clothing, and bedding that cannot be washed or dry-cleaned in a large plastic bag and seal the bag for 2 weeks.
- Head lice and pubic lice may be treated with nonprescription and prescription pediculicides.
- A pediculicide is a drug that kills lice.
- OTC and prescription agents are both effective and, in the case of lindane lotion, OTC products are more effective and have a lower risk of toxicity.
- Drug resistance is a growing problem for OTC and prescription pediculicides, especially permethrin, because of the residue left after treatment.
- Pyrethrins and permethrin are nonprescription treatments for lice infestation.
- Pyrethrins are naturally derived from the chrysanthemum flower.
- Permethrin is a mixture of synthetic isomers of pyrethrins.
- Pyrethrins are indicated for the treatment of head lice, body lice, and pubic lice, whereas permethrin is only approved for the treatment of head lice.

- Permethrin is ovicidal (kills eggs), whereas pyrethrins are not.
- Lindane and malathion are pesticides used in agriculture to control pests and as agents to kill lice.
- Lindane, also known as gamma-hexachlorocyclohexane, is also a scabicide.
- Absorption of lindane through intact human skin increases with repeated applications. Repeated use causes accumulation and increases the risk for neurotoxicity.
- Lindane can cause illness, vomiting, seizures, and death if accidentally swallowed.
- Pharmacy technicians must apply the warning label "For External Use Only" to prescription vials containing lindane lotion and shampoo.
- Malathion paralyzes the central nervous system of parasites by causing an accumulation of acetylcholine.
- Malathion is flammable; those using it should stay away from open flames, hair dryers, curling irons, and lit cigarettes, cigars, and pipes.
- Crotamiton is a scabicide that is classified in FDA pregnancy category C; it is an alternative to lindane.
- Spinosad is a pediculicide indicated for the topical treatment of head lice infestations in patients 4 years of age and older.

REVIEW QUESTIONS

1. A _____ is an organism that benefits by living in, with, or on another organism (host); usually to the detriment of the host.
   a. Parasite
   b. Protozoan
   c. Proteus
   d. Bacteria

2. The life cycle of a head louse is approximately _____.
   a. 1 to 2 weeks
   b. 2 to 3 weeks
   c. 3 to 5 weeks
   d. 4 to 6 weeks

3. Body lice infestations are a serious public health concern because body lice may cause epidemics of typhus and louse-borne relapsing fever.
   a. True
   b. False

4. _____, or crabs, is sometimes classified as a sexually transmitted infection.
   a. Scabies
   b. Head lice
   c. Pubic lice
   d. Body lice

5. The scabies mite lives on the surface of the skin.
   a. True
   b. False

6. _____may be treated with nonprescription and prescription pediculicides.
   a. Scabies
   b. Head lice
   c. Pubic lice
   d. b and c

7. Pyrethrins are naturally derived from the _____flower.
   a. Passion
   b. Chrysanthemum
   c. Periwinkle
   d. Coneflower

8. Lindane _____.
   a. Is neurotoxic
   b. Should not be used by anyone weighing less than 100 lb (50 kg)
   c. In only dispensed in 1- or 2-oz applicator bottles
   d. All of the above

9. Malathion, an organophosphate pesticide used in agriculture to control pests and as an agent to kill head lice and their eggs, is sold in the U.S. market and in Canada.
   a. True
   b. False

10. Crotamiton is a(n) _____. It is classified in FDA pregnancy category C and is an alternative to lindane.
   a. Scabicide
   b. Pediculocide
   c. Insecticide
   d. Pesticide

TECHNICIAN'S CORNER

1. Crotamiton is a scabicide that is classified in FDA pregnancy category C. What types of effects would it have on a developing fetus?
2. Why is a boxed warning put on some drugs, such as lindane?

Bibliography

Center for Drug Evaluation and Research: Lindane shampoo and lindane lotion: Questions and answers, 2000 (http://www.fda.gov/Drugs/DrugSafety/PostmarketDrugSafetyInformationforPatientsandProviders/ucm110848.htm).

Centers for Disease Control and Prevention: Parasites, lice, head lice, 2010 (http://www.cdc.gov/parasites/lice/head/index.html).

Centers for Disease Control and Prevention: *Parasites, lice, head lice,* Malathion, 2010, Frequently asked questions, (http://www.cdc.gov/parasites/lice/head/gen_info/faqs_malathion.html).

Centers for Disease Control and Prevention: Parasites, lice, pubic "crab" lice, 2010 (http://www.cdc.gov/parasites/lice/pubic/index.html).

Centers for Disease Control and Prevention: Parasites, scabies, 2010 (http://www.cdc.gov/parasites/scabies).

Centers for Disease Control and Prevention (CDC): Unintentional topical lindane ingestions—United States, 1998-2003, *MMWR Morb Mortal Wkly Rep* 54:533-535, 2005.

Elsevier. (2010). Gold Standard Clinical Pharmacology. Retrieved April 2, 2011, from https://www.clinicalpharmacology.com/.

FDA. (2012). FDA Approved Drug Products. Retrieved July 3, 2012, from http://www.accessdata.fda.gov/scripts/cder/drugsatfda/index.cfm?fuseaction=Search.Search_Drug_Name.

Health Canada. (2010). Drug Product Database. Retrieved July 3, 2012, from http://www.hc-sc.gc.ca/dhp-mps/prodpharma/databasdon/index-eng.php.

Lance L, Lacy C, Armstrong L, Goldman M: *Drug information handbook for the allied health professional,* ed 12, Hudson, OH, 2005, APhA Lexi-Comp.

Micromedex: Clinical Resource Database (http://www.thomsonhc.com).

Public Health Services, Nova Scotia: Guidelines for treatment of pediculosis capitis (head lice), 2008 (http://www.gov.ns.ca/hpp/publications/head_lice_guidelines_for_treatment.pdf).

USP Center for Advancement of Patient Safety: Use caution—avoid confusion, USP Quality Review No. 79, Rockville, MD, April 2004, USP Center for Advancement of Patient Safety.

Glossary

Absorption: Process involving movement of drug molecules from the site of administration into the circulatory system.

Accommodation: Ability of the lens to contract and relax to adjust for vision to see things from close up.

Acetylcholine (ACh): Neurotransmitter involved in muscle contraction.

Acetylcholinesterase: Enzyme that degrades acetylcholine and reverses acetylcholine-induced depolarization.

Acne vulgaris: Most common form of acne.

Acne: Disorder resulting from the action of hormones and other substances on the skin's oil glands (sebaceous glands) and hair follicles.

Acupuncture: Nonpharmacological treatment for pain that involves the application of needles to precise points on the body.

Acute pain: Sudden pain that results from injury or inflammation; usually self-limiting.

Additive effect: Increased drug effect produced when a second similar drug is added to therapy that is greater than the effects produced by either drug alone.

Adenosine triphosphate: Nucleotide that supplies the energy required for muscle contraction.

Adherence: Closely following or adhering to a treatment regimen.

Adjunct: Drug used to complement the effects of another drug.

Affinity: Attraction that the receptor site has for the drug.

Agonist: Drug that binds to its receptor site and stimulates a cellular response.

AIDS (acquired immunodeficiency syndrome): Most severe form of human immonodeficiency virus (HIV) infection. HIV-infected patients are diagnosed with AIDS when their CD4 cell count falls below 200 cells/mm^3 or develop an AIDS-defining illness (an illness that is very unusual in someone who is not HIV-positive).

Aldosterone: Hormone that promotes sodium and fluid reabsorption.

Allergen: Substance that produces an allergic reaction.

Allergic asthma: Asthma symptoms induced by a hypersensitivity reaction caused by overexpression of immunoglobulin E antibodies on exposure to environmental allergens.

Allergic conjunctivitis: Inflammation of the tissue lining the eyelids caused by the reaction to an allergy-causing substance.

Allergic rhinitis: Seasonal condition characterized by inflammation and swelling of the nasal passageways (rhinitis) accompanied by a runny nose (rhinorrhea).

Allergy: Hypersensitivity reaction by the immune system on exposure to an allergen.

Alzheimer's disease: Neurodegenerative disease that causes memory loss and behavioral changes.

Amenorrhea: Absence of normal menstruation.

Amphiarthroses: Slightly moveable joint (e.g., symphysis pubis in pelvic area).

Amyotrophic lateral sclerosis: Degenerative disease that causes muscle wasting and muscle weakness; also known as Lou Gehrig's disease.

Analgesic: Drug that reduces pain.

Anaphylactic shock: Acute, life-threatening allergic reaction that produces peripheral vasodilation.

Anaphylaxis: Life-threatening allergic reaction.

Aneurysm: Weakened spot of the artery wall that has stretched or burst, filling the area with blood.

Angina pectoris: Symptomatic manifestation of ischemic heart disease characterized by a severe squeezing or pressure-like chest pain; brought on by exertion or stress.

Angioedema: Allergic skin disease characterized by patches of circumscribed swelling involving the skin and its subcutaneous layers, the mucous membranes, and sometimes the viscera.

Angiotensin-converting enzyme: Enzyme that catalyzes the conversion of angiotensin I to angiotensin II.

Angiotension II: Potent vasoconstrictor that is produced when the renin-aldosterone-angiotensin system is activated.

Angle-closure glaucoma: Sudden increase in intraocular pressure caused by obstruction of the drainage portal between the cornea and iris (angle); can rapidly progress to blindness.

Anion: Negatively charged particle.

Anoxia: Absence of oxygen supply to cells that results in cell damage or death.

Antagonism: Drug-drug interaction or drug-food interaction that causes decreased effects (e.g., when a pharmacological antagonist is administered to block the effect of another drug).

Antagonist: Drug that binds to the receptor site and does not produce an action. An antagonist prevents another drug or natural body chemical from binding and activating the receptor site.

Antibiotic: Naturally occurring substance produced by a microorganism or semisynthetic substance derived from a microorganism capable of destroying or inhibiting the growth of another microorganism.

Anticoagulant: Drug that prolongs coagulation time and is used to prevent clot formation.

Antidiarrheal: Drug that prevents or relieves diarrhea.

Antifungal: Drug used to treat a fungal infection.

Antigen: Substance, usually a protein fragment, that causes an immune response.

Antimicrobial: Substance capable of destroying or inhibiting the growth of a microorganism.

Antinuclear antibody: Autoantibody or abnormal antibody that attacks the nucleus of normal cells.

Antiplatelet drug: Drug that prevents accumulation of platelets, thereby blocking an important step in the clot formation process.

Antiretroviral: Medication that interferes with the replication of retroviruses (e.g., HIV is a retrovirus).

Antithrombotic: Drug that inhibits clot formation by reducing the coagulation action of the blood protein thrombin.

Antithyroid drug: Drug administered to treat hyperthyroidism.

Antiviral resistance: Ability of a virus to overcome the suppressive action of antiviral agents.

Antiviral: Medication that is able to inhibit viral replication.

Anxiety: Condition associated with tension, apprehension, fear, or panic.

Anxiolytic: Drug used to treat anxiety.

ApoE4 allele: Defective form of apolipoprotein E associated with Alzheimer's disease.

Appendicular skeleton: Bone of upper extremities (arms, hands) and lower extremities (hip, legs, feet).

Aqueous humor: Portion of anterior cavity that lies in front of the lens and is filled with a clear watery liquid.

Arterial plaque: Hardened lipid streak within an artery formed by deposits of cholesterol, lipid material, and lipophages.

Arteriosclerosis: Loss of elasticity (hardening) of the arteries. Thickening and loss of elasticity of arterial walls; sometimes called hardening of the arteries.

Arthritis: Condition that is associated with joint pain.

Asthma: Chronic disease that affects the airways and causes irritation, inflammation, and difficulty breathing.

Astigmatism: Irregular curvature of the cornea or lens that results in the inability to form a well-focused image in the eye.

Ataxia: Condition in which the muscles fail to function in a coordinated manner.

Atheromas: Hard plaque formed within an artery.

Atherosclerosis: Process in which plaques (atheromas) containing cholesterol, lipid material, and lipophages are formed within arteries, impeding the flow of blood and oxygen.

Atherothrombosis: Formation of a blood clot in an artery.

Atopic dermatitis: Chronic inflammatory disease of the skin.

Atopic: Group of diseases where there is an inherited tendency to develop other allergic conditions.

Adenosine triphosphate (ATP): Nucleotide that supplies the energy required for muscle contraction.

Atrial fibrillation: Rapid and uncoordinated contractions during which the heart may beat from 300 to 400 beats/min.

Atrial flutter: Irregular heart beat in which contractions in the atrium exceed the number of contractions in the ventricle. T he heart rate is from 160 to 350 beats/min.

Atrophic vaginitis: Postmenopausal thinning and dryness of the vaginal epithelium related to decreased estrogen levels.

Aura: Unusual sensation and/or auditory, visual, or olfactory hallucination experienced just before the onset of a seizure.

Autoantibody: Abnormal antibody that attacks healthy cells and tissue.

Autoimmune disease: Disease that occurs when the immune system turns against the parts of the body it is designed to protect.

Automaticity: Spontaneous depolarization (contraction) of heart cells.

Autonomic nervous system (ANS): Division of nervous system that controls involuntary body functions; consists of sympathetic and parasympathetic divisions.

Axial skeleton: Consists of the cranium and bones of the face, ear, vertebral column, ribs, sternum, and hyoid.

Bactericidal: Able to destroy bacteria.

Bacteriostatic: Able to inhibit bacterial proliferation; host defense mechanisms destroy the bacteria.

Basal ganglia: Subcortical nuclei located in the forebrain and brainstem that initiate, control, and modulate movement and posture.

Benign prostatic hyperplasia: Noncancerous growth of cells in the prostate gland.

Benign: Tumor that is not cancerous and does not spread to surrounding tissues or other parts of the body.

Bicarbonate: Substance used as a buffer to maintain the normal levels of acidity (pH) in blood and other fluids in the body.

Bioavailability: Fraction of administered drug dose that enters the systemic circulation and is available to produce a drug effect.

Bioequivalent drug: Drug that shows no statistical differences in the rate and extent of absorption when it is administered in the same strength, dosage form, and route of administration as the brand name product.

Biofeedback: Nonpharmacological treatment for pain that involves relaxation techniques and gaining self-control over muscle tension, heart rate, and skin temperature.

Biopharmaceutical: Pharmaceutical derived from biological sources (e.g., proteins, gene sequences) and manufactured using biotechnology methods such as recombinant DNA technology.

Biopsy: Removal of cells or tissues for examination by a pathologist. The three types of biopsy are incisional, excisional, and fine-needle aspiration biopsies.

Biotransformation: Process of drug metabolism in the body that transforms a drug to a more active, equally active, or inactive metabolite.

Bipolar disorder: Mental illness associated with sudden swings in mood between depression and periods of mania, racing thoughts, distractibility, and increased goal-directed behavior.

Blackhead (open comedone): Trapped sebum and bacteria partially open to the surface that turn black due to changes in sebum as it is exposed to air.

Blepharitis: Chronic disease of the eye that produces distinctive flaky scales that form on the eyelids and eyelashes.

Blepharoptosis: Condition that causes the eyelid muscles to droop.

Blister: Collection of fluid below or within the epidermis.

Bone mineral density test: Test carried out to measure the degree of bone loss.

Bone resorption: Process during which bone is broken down into mineral ions (e.g., calcium).

Botulinum toxin: Toxin produced by the bacterium *Clostridium botulinum* that causes muscle paralysis.

Bradykinesia: Slowness in initiating and carrying out voluntary movements.

Breakthrough pain: Pain that occurs in between scheduled doses of analgesics.

Broad-spectrum antibiotic: Antimicrobial capable of destroying a wide range of bacteria.

Bronchodilator: Drug that relaxes tightened airway muscles and improves air flow through the airways.

Cancer: Term for diseases in which abnormal cells divide without control. Specific cancers are named according to the site where the cancerous growth begins.

Candida: Type of fungus; also called yeast.

Cardiac output: Volume of blood ejected from the left ventricle in 1 minute.

Cardioglycosides: Class of drugs, generally derived from the foxglove plant, that can alter cardiovascular function. Digitalis is representative of this class of drugs.

Cardiomyopathy: Heart disease that causes abnormal enlargement of the heart.

Catatonia: Symptom of schizophrenia associated with unresponsiveness and immobility.

Cation: Positively charged electrolyte.

CD4 count: Number of CD4 cells in a sample of blood.

CD4 T lymphocyte: White blood cell that fights infection.

Central nervous system (CNS): Consists of the brain and spinal cord.

Central vision: What is seen when you look straight ahead or read.

Central-acting muscle relaxant: Drug that produces relaxation of muscles through central nervous system depression blocking nerve transmission between the spinal cord and muscles.

Cephalgia: Head pain.

Cerebral palsy: Neurologic disorder that affects muscle movement and coordination.

Cerumen: Waxlike substance secreted by modified sweat glands in the ear.

Chemotherapy: Treatment with drugs that kill cancer.

Chloride: Major anion (negatively charged ion) found in the fluid outside of cells and in blood.

Cholesterol: Naturally occurring waxy substance produced by the liver and found in foods that maintain cell membranes; needed for vitamin D production. Excess cholesterol can cause atherosclerosis.

Chronic obstructive pulmonary disease: Progressive disease of the airways that produces gradual loss of pulmonary function.

Chronic pain: Pain that persists for a long period that is worsened by psychological factors and is resistant to many medical treatments.

Circadian rhythms: Biological changes that occur according to time cycles.

Clonus: Involuntary rhythmic muscle contraction that causes the feet and wrists to flex and relax involuntarily.

Cluster headache: Intensely painful vascular headache that occurs in groups and produces pain on one side of the head.

Cognitive function: Ability to take in information via the senses, process the details, commit the information to memory, and recall it when necessary.

Cold chain: Set of safe handling practices that ensure that vaccines and immunologicals requiring refrigeration are maintained at the required temperature from the time of manufacture until the time of administration to patients.

Colloids: Proteins or other large molecules that remain suspended in the blood for a long period and are too large to cross membranes.

Colonoscopy: Examination of the colon for signs of inflammation and damage; performed by inserting a thin tube with a small light and camera at the end (i.e., endoscope) into the anus.

Comedone: Enlarged and plugged hair follicle; the most characteristic sign of acne.

Complementary and alternative medicine (CAM): Treatments that may include dietary supplements, herbal preparations, acupuncture, massage, magnet therapy, spiritual healing, and meditation.

Complex focal seizure: Seizure disorder that produces a blank stare, disorientation, repetitive actions, and memory loss.

Computed tomography (CT): Diagnostic examination in which a series of detailed pictures are taken of areas inside the body; created by a computer linked to an x-ray machine.

Condom: Thin, flexible, penile sheath made of synthetic or natural material that is placed over the penis; used to prevent pregnancy and some sexually transmitted infections.

Conduction impairment: Blocking of air waves as they are conducted through the external and middle ears to the sensory receptors of the inner ear.

Conjugate vaccine: Vaccine that links antigens or toxoids to polysaccharide or sugar molecules; used by certain bacteria as a protective device to disguise themselves.

Conjunctivitis (pink eye): Common, self-limiting ailment that causes itching, burning, and teary outflow.

Constipation: Abnormally delayed or infrequent passage of dry hardened feces.

Controlled substance: Drug whose possession and distribution is restricted because of its potential for abuse as determined by federal or state law. Controlled substances are placed in schedules according to their abuse potential and effects if abused.

Convulsions: Sudden contraction of muscles caused by seizures.

Cornea: Clear part of the eye located in front of the iris.

Coronary artery disease: Condition that occurs when the arteries that supply blood to the heart muscle become hardened and narrowed.

Crohn's disease: Irritable bowel disease that produces inflammation and damage anywhere along the gastrointestinal tract.

Cross-resistance: Development of resistance to one drug in a particular class that results in resistance to other drugs in that class.

Crystalloid: Intravenous solution that contains electrolytes in concentrations similar to those of plasma.

Cutaneous: Pertaining to the skin.

Cyclooxygenase-2 inhibitor: Analgesic antiinflammatory drug that preferentially blocks cyclooxygenase-2, an enzyme that produces prostaglandin, which is a substance involved in mediating pain.

Cysts: End products of pustules or nodules.

Cytomegalovirus retinitis: Viral opportunistic infection of the eye that can cause pain and blindness.

Débridement: Surgical removal of foreign material and dead tissue from a wound to prevent infection and promote healing.

Decubitus ulcer: Pressure sore, or bed sore.

Deglutition: Swallowing.

Dehydration: Condition that results from excessive loss of body water.

Delusion: Irrational thoughts or false beliefs that dominate a person's behavior and viewpoint and do not change, even when evidence is provided that these beliefs are not valid.

Dementia: Condition associated with loss of memory and cognition.

Demyelination: Damage caused by recurrent inflammation of myelin that results in nervous system scars that interrupt communication between the nerves and the rest of the body.

Deoxyribonucleic acid (DNA): DNA is the repository of hereditary characteristics; it is a nucleic acid that contains the genetic blueprint.

Depolarization: Process during which the heart muscle conducts an electrical impulse, causing a contraction.

Depolarizing neuromuscular blocker: Drug that acts as an agonist at acetylcholine receptor sites and produces sustained depolarization, causing the receptors to convert to an inactive state.

Depressant: Drug that decreases activity in the brain; used as a sedative or hypnotic to promote drowsiness and relaxation.

Dermatitis: Inflammation of the skin.

Dermatomyositis: Form of myositis that affects muscles and the skin.

Dermatophytes: Group of fungi responsible for most fungal infections of the skin, hair, and nails.

Desquamation: Shedding of the outer layers of the skin.

Diabetes mellitus: Chronic condition in which the body is unable to use glucose (sugar) as energy effectively.

Diabetic neuropathy: Nerve disorder caused by uncontrolled diabetes. It leads to pain or a loss of feeling in the toes, feet, legs, hands, and/or arms.

Diaphoresis (hyperhidrosis): Excessive sweating.

Diaphragm: Rubber or plastic cup that fits over the cervix; used for contraception.

Diarrhea: Abnormally frequent passage of loose and watery stools.

Diarthroses: Freely moveable joints (e.g. knee, hip, elbow, shoulder).

Diastolic blood pressure: Blood pressure measured when the heart is at rest (diastole).

Diffusion: Passive movement of molecules across cell membranes from an area of high drug concentration to an area of lower concentration.

Digestion: Complete process of altering the physical and chemical composition of ingested food materials so they can be absorbed and used by the body's cells.

Digital rectal examination: Screening examination involving palpation of the prostate gland; conducted by insertion of a gloved lubricated finger into the rectum.

Digitalization: Process of rapidly increasing the initial dose of digoxin until the therapeutic dose is achieved.

Disinhibition: Opposite of inhibited.

Distribution: Process of movement of the drug from the circulatory system across barrier membrane(s) to the site of drug action.

Diuretic: Drug that produces diuresis (urination).

Dosage form: Drug formulation (e.g., capsule, tablet, solution).

Dose: Amount of a drug required for one application or administration.

Dosing schedule: How frequently a drug dose is administered (e.g., "four times a day").

Double-contrast barium enema: Diagnostic test to examine the colon and rectum in which an individual is administered a barium-containing enema and then radiographs are taken.

Drug delivery system: Dosage form or device designed to release a specific amount of drug.

Drug dependence: Occurs when a person taking a drug does not continue to take it and suffers from physical or psychological withdrawal symptoms, or both.

Drug resistance testing: Laboratory test to determine whether an individual's HIV strain is resistant to any anti-HIV medications.

Drug: Substance used to diagnose, treat, cure, prevent, or mitigate disease in humans or other animals.

Drug-disease contraindication: No rationale for drug use; drug administration should be avoided because it may worsen the patient's medical condition.

Drug-drug interaction: Reaction that occurs when two or more drugs are administered at the same time.

Drug-food interaction: Altered drug response that occurs when a drug is administered with certain foods.

Drug receptor theory: Theory that states that a drug must interact or bind with targeted cells in the body if drug action is to be produced.

Duodenal ulcer: Ulcer located in the upper portion of the small intestine or duodenum.

Duration of action: Time between the onset of drug action and discontinuation of drug action.

Dysfunctional uterine bleeding: Irregular or excessive uterine bleeding that results from a structural problem or hormonal imbalance.

Dysmenorrhea: Difficult or painful menstruation.

Dysphoria: Feeling of emotional or mental discomfort, restlessness, and depression; the opposite of euphoria.

Eclampsia: Life-threatening condition that can develop in pregnant women that causes high blood pressure and seizures.

Ectopic: Occurring in an abnormal location.

Eczema: General term used to describe several types of inflammation of the skin.

Edema: Presence of abnormally large amounts of fluid in the intercellular tissue spaces of the body.

Efficacy: Measure of a drug's effectiveness.

Ejaculation: Release of semen from the penis during orgasm.

Ejection fraction: Percentage of blood ejected from the left ventricle with each heartbeat.

Electrical cardioversion: Process of applying an electrical shock to the heart with a defibrillator to convert the heart to a normal rhythm.

Electrolytes: Small charged molecules essential for homeostasis that play an important role in body chemistry.

Elimination: Process that results in the removal of drug from the body.

Embolic stroke: Stroke caused by an emboli obstructing the flow of blood through an artery.

Embolus: Moving blood clot.

Endometriosis: Presence of functioning endometrial tissue outside the uterus.

Endorphins, enkephalins, and dynorphin: Substances released by the body in response to painful stimuli that act as natural painkillers.

Endoscope: Thin flexible tube with a small video camera and light attached to one end.

Endoscopy: Test used to look for ulcers inside the stomach and small intestine using an endoscope.

Endotracheal intubation: Process of inserting a tube into the trachea or windpipe to facilitate mechanical ventilation.

Endplate: Projection extending off the end of a motor neuron where the neurotransmitter acetylcholine is released.

Enteral: Refers to a drug dosage form that is administered orally.

Enuresis: Bedwetting or uncontrollable urination during sleep.

Enzyme: Protein capable of causing a chemical reaction. Enzymes are involved in the metabolism of some drugs.

Epilepsy: Recurrent seizure disorder characterized by a sudden, excessive, disorderly discharge of cerebral neurons.

Equilibrium: Steadiness or balance accompanied by a sense of knowing where the body is in relationship to surroundings.

Erectile dysfunction: Persistent inability to achieve and/or maintain an erection sufficient for satisfactory sexual intercourse.

Erythrocytes: Red blood cells.

Erythropoiesis: Formation of red blood cells.

Eschar: Blackened necrotic tissue of a decubitus ulcer.

Escharotomy: Removal of necrotic skin and underlying tissue.

Euphoria: State of intense happiness or well-being; the opposite of dysphoria.

Exacerbation: Aggravation of symptoms or increase in the severity of the disease.

Excisional biopsy: Surgical procedure in which an entire lump or suspicious-looking tissue is removed for diagnosis.

External radiation: Radiation therapy that uses a machine to aim high-energy rays at the cancer.

Extracellular fluid: Type of fluid that surrounds the cells; consists mainly of the plasma found in blood vessels.

Extrapyramidal symptoms: Excessive muscle movement (motor activity) associated with the use of neuroleptics; includes muscular rigidity, tremor, bradykinesia (slow movement), and difficulty in walking.

Fasting blood glucose: Blood glucose level after a person has not eaten for 8 to 12 hours (usually overnight).

Febrile seizure: Seizure associated with a sudden spike in body temperature.

Fecal occult blood test (FOBT): Test to check for blood in stool.

Fertility: Being fertile; able to reproduce.

First-degree burn: Minor discomfort and reddening of the skin.

First-pass effect: Process whereby only a fraction of an orally administered drug reaches the systemic circulation because much of the drug is metabolized in the liver to an inactive metabolite before entering the general circulation.

Fistula: Ulcer that tunnels from the site of origin to surrounding tissues.

Fontanels: Soft spots found in a baby's skull.

Forced expiratory volume (FEV): The maximum volume of air that can be breathed out in 1 second; also called forced vital capacity.

Fourth-degree burn: Burn that involves underlying muscles, fasciae, or bone.

Full-thickness burn: Third-degree burn in which the epidermis and dermis are destroyed.

Fungus (*pl.*, fungi): Organism similar to a plant but lacking chlorophyll; capable of producing mycotic (fungal) infection.

Fusarium keratitis: Rare fungal infection that occurs in soft contact lens wearers; can result in blindness.

Gastric ulcer: Ulcer located in the stomach.

Gastroenteritis: Inflammation of the lining membrane of the stomach and intestines.

Gastroesophageal reflux disease (GERD): Motility disorder associated with impaired peristalsis that results in the backflow of gastric contents into the esophagus.

Generalized anxiety disorder: Condition associated with excessive worrying and tension that is experienced daily for more than 6 months.

Generalized seizures: Seizures that spread across both cerebral hemispheres; include tonic-clonic seizures.

Gestational diabetes: Diabetes that may be caused by the hormones of pregnancy or a shortage of insulin.

Gingival hyperplasia: Excess growth of gum tissue that could grow over the teeth.

Glial cells: Cells that form the blood-brain barrier and support function of the neurons.

Gout: Disease associated with deposits of urate crystals in the joints that produces inflammation; caused by hyperuricemia.

Graves' disease: Autoimmune disorder that causes hyperthyroidism.

Gynecomastia: Painful breast enlargement in men.

Half-life ($t_{1/2}$): Length of time it takes for the plasma concentration of an administered drug to be reduced by 50%.

Hallucination: Visions or voices that exist only in a person's mind and cannot be seen or heard by others.

Hashimoto's disease: Autoimmune disorder that causes hypothyroidism.

Heart failure: Clinical syndrome in which the heart is unable to pump blood at a rate necessary to meet the body's metabolic needs.

Helminthes: Group of parasitic worms that can cause eye infection and blindness.

Hemoglobin A1c test: Blood test that measures a person's average blood glucose level over a period of 2 to 3 months.

Hemoglobin: Red pigment made up of iron atoms; transports oxygen and carbon dioxide in the body.

Hemorrhagic stroke: Sudden bleeding into or around the brain.

Hemostasis: Process of stopping the flow of blood.

Hepatoxicity: Serious adverse reaction that occurs in the liver.

Herpes simplex keratitis: Painful eye infection caused by a herpesvirus that can lead to blindness.

Herpes zoster ophthalmicus: Painful eye infection caused by a herpesvirus that can lead to blindness.

Hiatal hernia: Condition in which the lower esophageal sphincter shifts above the diaphragm.

High-density lipoprotein: Lipoprotein that transports cholesterol, triglycerides, and other lipids from blood to body tissues; known as good cholesterol.

Highly active antiretroviral therapy (HAART): Combination of three or more antiretroviral medications taken in a regimen.

Hirsutism: Excessive hair growth in women.

Histamine: Organic nitrogen compound involved in local immune responses; has a regulating physiological function in the gut and acts as a neurotransmitter.

Homeopathic medicine: Medical field in which drugs are administered in minute quantities to stimulate natural body healing systems.

Homeostasis: Constancy or balance maintained by the body despite constant changes.

Host: Individual infected with a virus.

Huntington's disease: Progressive and degenerative disease of neurons that affects muscle movement, cognitive functions, and emotions.

Hydrophilic: Having a strong affinity for water; water-loving; able to dissolve in and absorb water.

Hydrophobic: Lacking an affinity for water; water-hating; resistant to wetting.

Hyperalgesia: Heightened sensitivity to pain that can result from treatment of chronic pain with high-dose opioids.

Hypercalcemia: Condition in which the serum calcium level is higher than 5.5 mEq/L.

Hyperchloremia: Condition in which the serum chloride level is higher than 107 mEq/L.

Hyperglycemia: Condition of elevated blood glucose levels.

Hyperkalemia: Condition in which the serum potassium level is higher than 5.5 mEq/L.

Hyperlipidemia: Increased concentration of cholesterol and triglycerides in the blood associated with the development of atherosclerosis.

Hypermagnesemia: Condition in which the serum level of magnesium is higher than 2.5 mEq/L.

Hypernatremia: Condition in which the serum sodium concentration is higher than 145 mEq/L.

Hyperopia: Farsightedness.

Hyperplasia: Abnormal increase in the number of cells in an organ or tissue.

Hypertension: High blood pressure; elevated diastolic or systolic blood pressure, or both.

Hyperthyroidism: Condition in which there is an excessive production of thyroid hormones.

Hypertonic: Refers to fluids with a higher osmolarity than serum.

Hyperuricemia: Condition in which urate levels build up in the blood.

Hypnotic: Drug that induces sleep.

Hypocalcemia: Condition in which the serum calcium level is lower than 4.5 mEq/L.

Hypochloremia: Condition in which the serum chloride level is lower than 97 mEq/L.

Hypoglycemia: Low blood glucose levels.

Hypogonadism: Inadequate production of sex hormones.

Hypokalemia: Condition in which potassium is lost from the body, resulting in a serum potassium level lower than 3.5 mEq/L.

Hypomagnesemia: Condition in which the serum level of magnesium is lower than 1.5 mEq/L.

Hyponatremia: Condition of decreased serum sodium concentration below the normal range (<136 mEq/L).

Hypophosphatemia: Condition in which the serum phosphate level is defined as mild (2 to 2.5 mg/dL, or 0.65 to 0.81 mmol/L), moderate (1 to 2 mg/dL, or 0.32 to 0.65 mmol/L), or severe (<1 mg/dL, or 0.32 mmol/L).

Hypothyroidism: Condition in which there is insufficient production of thyroid hormones.

Hypotonic: Refers to fluid with lower osmolarity than serum.

Hysterectomy: Surgical removal of the uterus.

Idiosyncratic reaction: Unexpected drug reaction.

Immunization: Deliberate artificial exposure to disease to produce acquired immunity.

Immunoglobulin E: Antibody associated with allergies.

Immunomodulator: Chemical agent that modifies the immune response or functioning of the immune system.

Immunosuppressant: Drug that inhibits proliferation of the cells of the immune system; also known as an immunopharmacological.

Implant radiation: Procedure, also known as brachytherapy, in which radioactive material sealed in needles, seeds, wires, or catheters is placed directly into or near a tumor in the body.

Inactivated killed vaccine: Killed vaccine; provides less immunity than live vaccines but has fewer risks for vaccine-induced disease.

Incontinence: Loss of bladder or bowel control.

Infarction: Sudden loss of blood supply to an area that results in cell death. A myocardial infarction (MI) is known as a heart attack. A cerebral infarction is also known as a stroke.

Infertility: Inability to achieve pregnancy during 1 year or more of unprotected intercourse.

Inflammation: Response to tissue irritation or injury marked by signs of redness, swelling, heat, and pain.

Inflammatory bowel disease (IBD): Chronic disorder of the gastrointestinal tract characterized by inflammation of the intestines; results in abdominal cramping and persistent diarrhea.

Insomnia: Condition characterized by difficulty falling asleep, staying asleep, or both.

Insulin resistance: Condition in which the body does not respond to insulin; contributes to the development of type 2 diabetes.

Interferon: Antiviral protein that enhances T cell recognition of antigens (interferon-γ) and produce immune system suppression (interferon-α, interferon-β).

Intracellular fluid: Fluid inside cells.

Intraocular pressure: Inner pressure of the eye. Normal intraocular pressure ranges from 12 to 22 mm Hg.

Intrauterine device (IUD): Device inserted in the uterus to prevent pregnancy.

Inverse agonist: Drug that has affinity and activity at the receptor site. The drug can turn off a receptor that is activated or turn on a receptor that is not currently active.

Ionization: Chemical process involving the gain or release of a proton (H^+). Ionized drug molecules may have a positive or negative charge.

Ionizing radiation: Type of high-frequency radiation produced by x-ray procedures, radioactive substances, and ultraviolet (UV) light that can lead to health risks, including cancer, at certain doses.

Ions: Charged particles.

Iris: Colored part of the eye that can expand or contract to allow the correct amount of light to enter the eye.

Iritis: Condition associated with inflammation of the iris.

Irritable bowel syndrome: Condition that causes abdominal distress and erratic movement of the contents of the large bowel resulting in diarrhea and/or constipation.

Ischemia: Reduction of blood supplied to tissues; typically caused by blood vessel obstruction due to atherosclerosis, stenosis, or plaque.

Ischemic heart disease: Any condition in which heart muscle is damaged or works inefficiently because of an absence or relative deficiency of its blood supply.

Ischemic stroke: Ischemia in the brain.

Isolated systolic hypertension: Condition involving only elevated systolic blood pressure. Diastolic blood pressure is within the normal range.

Isotonic: Refers to fluid close to the same osmolarity as serum.

Kallman's syndrome: Congenital disorder that causes hypogonadism and loss of the sense of smell.

Keratitis: Severe infection of the cornea that may be caused by bacteria or fungi.

Keratolytic: Pertains to keratolysis, the softening and shedding of the horny outer layer of the skin. A keratolytic agent is a peeling agent.

Klinefelter's syndrome: A chromosomal disorder in males. People with this condition are born with at least one extra X chromosome.

Labyrinth: Bony structure in the inner ear consisting of three parts (vestibule, cochlea, and semicircular canals) involved in balance.

β-Lactamase: Enzyme secreted by some microbes that has the ability to destroy β-lactam antibiotics.

Laryngopharyngeal reflux: Reflux of gastric contents into the larynx and pharynx.

Laxative: Medicine that induces evacuation of the bowel.

Legend drugs: Drugs required by state or federal law to be dispensed by a prescription only. Prescriptions must be written for a legitimate medical condition and issued by a practitioner authorized to prescribe.

Leukemia: Cancer that starts in blood-forming tissue such as the bone marrow.

Leukocytes: White blood cells (WBCs).

Leukocytosis: Abnormally high WBC count.

Leukopenia: Abnormally low WBC count.

Leukotriene: Proinflammatory mediator released as part of the allergic inflammatory response. Leukotrienes also trigger contractions in the smooth muscles of airways.

Lice: Group of parasites *(Pediculus humanus capitis, Pediculus humanus corporis, Phthirus pubis)* that can live on the body, scalp, or genital area of humans.

Lipid: Fatlike substance.

Lipophilic: Having an affinity for lipids; lipid-loving.

Lipoprotein: Small globules of cholesterol covered by a layer of protein.

Live attenuated vaccine: Living, but weakened, version of an invader that does not cause disease in nonimmunocompromised individuals (nonvirulent).

Low-density lipoprotein: Compound consisting of a lipid and protein that carries most of the total cholesterol in the blood and deposits the excess along the inside of arterial walls; also known as bad cholesterol.

Lower esophageal sphincter: Sphincter separating the esophagus and stomach.

Lower motor neurons: Neurons that branch out from the spinal cord to the muscles and tissues of the body.

Lymphoma: Cancer that begins in cells of the immune system.

Magnesium: Fourth most common cation in the body.

Major depression: Mental illness associated with persistent feelings of sadness, emptiness, or hopelessness that lasts for several weeks.

Malignant: Cancerous tumors that can invade and destroy nearby tissue and spread to other parts of the body.

Mammography: Screening examination to detect breast cancer in which a radiograph is taken of the breast.

Mast cells: Granule-containing cells found in connective tissue. They contain many granules rich in histamine, which are released during allergic reactions.

Mastication: Chewing.

Materia medica: Medicinal materials.

Mechanism of action: Manner in which a drug produces its effect.

Medication error: Error made in the process of prescribing, preparing, dispensing, or administering drug therapy.

Melanoma: Form of skin cancer that arises in melanocytes, the cells that produce pigment.

Melatonin: Hormone released by the pineal gland that makes a person feel drowsy.

Ménière's disease: Chronic inner ear disease associated with intermittent buildup of fluid in the inner ear that causes hearing loss and vertigo.

Menopause: Termination of menstrual cycles; an event usually marked by the passage of at least 1 year without menstruation.

Menorrhagia: Excessive menstrual bleeding.

Metabolic syndrome: Important risk factor of hypertension that promotes the development of atherosclerosis and cardiovascular disease.

Metabolism: Biochemical process involving transformation of active drugs to a compound that can be easily eliminated, or the conversion of prodrugs to active drugs.

Metabolite: Product of drug metabolism. Metabolites may be inactivated drugs or active drugs with equal or greater activity than the parent drug.

Metastasis: Spread of cancer from one part of the body to another.

Metered-dose inhaler: Device used for delivering a dose of inhaled medication. A solution or powder is delivered as a mist and inhaled.

Microbial resistance: Ability of bacteria to overcome the bactericidal or bacteriostatic effects of an anti-infective. Resistance traits are encoded on bacterial genes and can be transferred to other bacteria.

Microvilli: Brushlike border of each villus in the small intestine; increases the surface area for absorption.

Migraine: Vascular headache that is often accompanied by nausea and visual disturbances.

Milia: Tiny little bumps that occur when normally sloughed skin cells get trapped in small pockets on the surface of the skin.

Milliequivalent: Unit used to measure the number of ionic charges or electrovalent bonds (electrolytes) in a solution.

Mitral valve stenosis: Disease of the mitral valve involving the buildup of plaquelike material around the valve.

Monoamine oxidase: Enzyme found in the liver, intestine, and terminal neurons; responsible for degradation of monoamine neurotransmitters and dietary amines.

Mother to child transmission: Transmission of a substance or virus (e.g., HIV from an HIV-infected mother) to her baby during pregnancy or delivery, or through breast milk (also called perinatal transmission).

Motor neuron: Neuron that connects to the sarcolemma to form a neuromuscular junction.

Multiple sclerosis: Autoimmune disease that causes progressive damage to nerves resulting in spasticity, pain, mood changes, and other physical symptoms.

Myasthenia gravis: Autoimmune disease in which the immune system attacks the muscle cells at the neuromuscular junction and is characterized by muscle weakness.

Mycosis: General term for a fungal infection.

Myelin: Fatty covering that insulates nerve cells in the brain and spinal cord.

Myocardial infarction: Condition that results in heart muscle tissue death; caused by the occlusion (blockage) of a coronary artery; also referred to as a heart attack.

Myoclonic seizure: Seizure characterized by jerking muscle movements; caused by contraction of major muscle groups.

Myopia: Nearsightedness.

Myositis: Autoimmune disease that causes chronic inflammation of the muscles.

Natriuretic peptides: Hormones that play a role in cardiac homeostasis.

Nebulizer: Device that creates a mist out of a liquid inhalant solution, making drug delivery easier.

Necrosis: Cell death that may be caused by lack of blood and oxygen to the affected area(s).

Negative symptoms: Spasticity symptoms, which may indicate schizophrenia, that can produce muscle weakness, decreased endurance, and reduction in the ability to make voluntary muscle movements.

Neoplasm: Tumor.

Nephrotoxicity: Serious adverse effect that occurs in the kidneys.

Neurodegeneration: Destruction of nerve cells.

Neurodegenerative disease: Disorder that results in progressive destruction of neurons.

Neuroleptic malignant syndrome: Potentially fatal reaction to administration of neuroleptics. Symptoms include stupor, muscle rigidity, and high temperature.

Neuroleptic: Drug used to treat schizophrenia and psychoses.

Neuromuscular junction: Space between motor neuron endplate and muscle sole plate that neurotransmitters must cross.

Neuron: Functional unit of the nervous system, which includes the cell body, dendrites, axon, and terminals.

Neuropathic pain: Type of pain associated with nerve injury caused by trauma, infection, or chronic diseases such as diabetes.

Neuroprotective: Protects nerve cells from damage.

Neurotransmitter: Protein that transmits nerve signals from one neuron to another.

Nigrostriatal pathway: Pathway located in the substantia nigra that stimulates and inhibits movement.

Nits: Head lice eggs.

Nociceptors: Thin nerve fibers in the skin, muscle, and other body tissues that carry pain signals.

Nocturia: Nighttime urination.

Nodule: Ruptured pustules that form abscesses.

Noncompetitive antagonist: Drug that binds to an alternative receptor site that prevents the agonist from binding to and producing its desired action.

Nondepolarizing competitive blockers: Drugs that compete with acetylcholine for binding sites.

Non–rapid eye movement (REM) sleep: Stages 1 through 4 of the sleep cycle.

NSAID: Nonsteroidal anti-inflammatory drug.

Nymph: Baby louse.

Obsessive-compulsive disorder: Condition associated with the inability to control or stop repeated unwanted thoughts or behaviors.

Oncovirus: Virus that is a causative agent in a cancer.

Onset of action: Time it takes for drug action to begin.

Onychomycosis: Fungal infection involving the fingernails or toenails; also known as tinea unguium.

Open-angle glaucoma: Disorder characterized by elevated pressure in the eye that can lead to permanent blindness.

Opiate-naïve: Refers to a person who has no current exposure to opioids.

Opioid: Naturally occurring or synthetically derived analgesic with properties similar to those of morphine.

Optic nerve: Bundle of nerve fibers located in the back of the eye that connects the retina to the brain.

Osmolarity: Osmotic pressure of a solution expressed as milliosmoles per liter (mOsm/L) or millimoles per liter (mmol/L) of the solution.

Osmosis: Movement of water across a semipermeable membrane from an area of higher concentration to an area of lower concentration.

Osteoblast: Cell responsible for bone formation, deposition, and mineralization of the collagen matrix of bone.

Osteoclast: Cell responsible for bone resorption.

Osteolysis: Dissolution or degradation of bone.

Osteopenia: Decrease in bone mineral density that places people at increased risk of developing osteoporosis.

Osteoporosis: Chronic progressive disease of bone characterized by loss of bone density and bone strength; results in increased risk for fractures.

Otitis: Inflammation of the ear.

Otitis externa: Inflammation of the ear canal or external ear.

Otitis media: Infection of the middle ear; typically caused by viral or bacterial infection.

Otoliths: Calcium carbonate crystals found in the utricle and saccule of the inner ear.

Otorrhea: Discharge coming from the external auditory canal or inside the canal.

Otosclerosis: Hardening of the bones of the middle ear.

Ototoxicity: Damage or toxicity to the ear or eighth cranial nerve (associated with hearing).

Over-the-counter (OTC) drugs: Drugs that can be obtained without a prescription.

Ovicidal: Able to destroy eggs.

Panic disorder: Condition associated with repeated sudden onset of feelings of terror.

Pap test (Pap smear): Screening test in which cells from the cervix are examined to detect cancer and changes that may lead to cancer.

Papule: Obstructed follicle that becomes inflamed.

Parasite: Organism that benefits by living in, with, or on another organism.

Parasympathetic nervous system: Division of the autonomic nervous system (ANS) that functions during restful situations; the "rest and digest" part of the ANS.

Parenteral: Refers to a drug dosage form administered by injection or infusion.

Parkinson's disease: Progressive disorder of the nervous system involving degeneration of dopaminergic neurons and causing impaired muscle movement.

Partial agonist: Drug that behaves like an agonist under some conditions and acts like an antagonist under different conditions.

Partial thromboplastin time: Blood test that determines the effectiveness of heparin in reducing antithrombotic activity; measures how long it takes for blood to clot.

Partial-thickness burns: First- and second-degree burns.

Pathophysiology: Study of structural and functional changes produced by disease.

PCA: Patient-controlled analgesia.

Peak effect: Maximum drug effect produced by a given dose of drug after the drug has reached its maximum concentration in the body.

Peak flow meter: Handheld device used to measure the volume of air exhaled and how rapidly the air is moved out.

Pediculicide: Drug that kills lice.

Pelvic inflammatory disease: Infection of the uterus, fallopian tubes, and adjacent pelvic structures that is not associated with pregnancy or surgery.

Peptic ulcer disease: Term used to describe ulcers located in the duodenum or stomach.

Peripheral nervous system (PNS): Division of the nervous system outside the brain and spinal cord.

Peripheral vision: Sometimes called side vision, this is usually the first area of vision to be lost with glaucoma.

Peripheral-acting muscle relaxants: Drugs that block nerve transmission between the motor endplate and skeletal muscle receptors.

Peristalsis: Forceful wave of contractions in the esophagus that moves food and liquids from the mouth to the stomach.

Petit mal seizure: Absence seizure in which the person experiences a brief period of unconsciousness and stares vacantly into space.

Pharmaceutical alternative: Drug that contains the same active ingredient as the brand name drug; however, the strength and dosage form may be different.

Pharmaceutical equivalent: Drug that contains identical amount of active ingredient as a brand name drug but may have different inactive ingredients, be manufactured in a different dosage form, and exhibit different rates of absorption.

Pharmacodynamics: Study of drugs and their actions on a living organism.

Pharmacognosy: Science dealing with the biologic and biochemical features of natural drugs and their constituents. It is the study of drugs of plant or animal origin.

Pharmacokinetics: Science dealing with what the body does to a drug; includes the study of absorption, distribution, metabolism, and elimination.

Pharmacology: Study of drugs and their interactions with living systems, including chemical and physical properties, toxicology, and therapeutics.

Pharmacotherapeutics: Use of drugs in the treatment of disease. It is the study of factors that influence patient response to drugs.

Pharmacotherapy: Use of drugs in the treatment of disease.

Phenylketonuria: Disease marked by failure to metabolize the amino acid phenylalanine to tyrosine; results in severe neurological deficits in infancy if untreated.

Phobia: Irrational fear of things or situations that produce symptoms of intense anxiety.

Phosphodiesterase type 5 inhibitor: Drug used to relax smooth muscle and blood vessels that supply the corpus cavernosum and control penile engorgement.

Photopsia: Condition similar to floaters; associated with flashes of light.

Phototherapy: Treatment for atopic dermatitis that involves exposing the skin to ultraviolet A or B light waves.

Pilosebaceous units (PSUs): These consist of a sebaceous gland connected to a canal, called a follicle; contain fine hairs.

Plaque psoriasis: Most common form of psoriasis characterized by raised inflamed (red) lesions covered with a silvery white scale.

Plaque: Fatty cholesterol deposits; patchy areas of inflammation and demyelination that disrupt nerve signals between the brain and the rest of the body.

Plasticity: Ability of the brain to restructure itself and adapt to injury.

Platelets: Structures found in the blood involved in the coagulation process.

Polycystic ovary disease: Condition characterized by ovaries twice the normal size that contain fluid-filled cysts.

Polymyositis: Form of myositis that affects multiple muscles, particularly the muscles closest to the trunk.

Polyp: Growth that protrudes from a mucous membrane.

Positive inotropic effect: Increase in the force of myocardial contractions.

Positive symptoms: Hallucinations, delusions, or other unusual thoughts or perceptions that are symptoms of schizophrenia; also, spasticity symptoms that cause muscle spasms and hyperexcitable reflexes.

Positron emission tomography (PET): Diagnostic examination used to detect cancer cells in the body in which a small amount of radioactive glucose (sugar) is injected into a vein and a scanner is used to make detailed, computerized pictures of areas inside the body where the glucose is used.

Postprandial: After eating.

Post-traumatic stress disorder: Stress disorder that develops in persons who have participated in, witnessed, or been a victim of a terrifying event.

Postural hypotension: Drop in blood pressure caused by a change in posture.

Potassium: Main electrolyte in extracellular fluid.

Potency: Measure of the amount of drug required to produce a response. It is the effective dose concentration.

Potentiation: Process whereby one drug, acting at a separate site or via a different mechanism of action, increases the effect of another drug but produces no effect when administered alone. Food can also potentiate the effects of a drug.

Prediabetes: Condition of impaired fasting glucose and impaired glucose tolerance in which the body consistently has elevated glucose levels.

Pregnancy: Condition of having a developing embryo or fetus in the body after successful conception.

Premenstrual dysphoric disorder: Disorder characterized by symptoms such as depression, anxiety, hopelessness, sad feelings, and self-depreciation.

Premenstrual syndrome: Condition involving a groupof symptoms (e.g., headache, irritability, depression, fatigue, sleep changes, weight gain) that occur before the start of the menstrual cycle.

Presbycusis: Common in older adults; causes degeneration of nerve tissue in the ear and vestibular nerve.

Presbyopia: Farsightedness caused by the aging process.

Primary tumor: Original tumor or initial tumor.

Prodrug: Drug administered in an inactive form that is metabolized in the body to an active form.

Prolactinoma: Pituitary tumor that produces an excessive amount of prolactin.

Prostate gland: Gland in the male reproductive system just below the bladder, surrounding the urethra.

Prostate-specific antigen (PSA): Protein produced by the prostate gland. Levels are elevated in men who have prostate cancer, infection, or inflammation and tumors of the prostate gland and benign prostate hyperplasia.

Prostate-specific antigen (PSA) test: Blood test to measure PSA. A free PSA test result reports the percentage of PSA that is not attached to another chemical compared with the total amount in a man's blood. Free PSA is linked to benign prostate hyperplasia but not to cancer.

Prostatitis: Inflammation of the prostate gland.

Prothrombin time: Test given to determine the effectiveness of warfarin in reducing clotting time.

Pseudoparkinsonism: Adverse reaction to the administration of neuroleptics; characterized by symptoms mimicking those of Parkinson's disease.

Psoriasis: Chronic disease of the skin characterized by itchy red patches covered with silvery scales.

Psychosis: Mental state characterized by disorganized behavior and thought, delusions, hallucinations, and loss of touch with reality.

Purine: One of two nitrogen-containing bases found in DNA and RNA. Purine bases are metabolized.

Pustule: Larger lesions that are more inflamed than papules; can be superficial or deep.

Radiation therapy: Use of high-energy radiation from x-rays, gamma rays, neutrons, and other sources to kill cancer cells and shrink tumors.

Radioactive iodine uptake: Test using radioactive iodine to screen for thyroid disease.

Radionuclide scan: Diagnostic test in which an individual is administered a small amount of radioactive material. A scanner is used to take pictures of the internal parts of the body to detect where the radiation concentrates.

Radon: Radioactive gas that if inhaled in sufficient quantity can lead to lung cancer.

Rapid eye movement (REM) sleep: Stage of sleep when dreaming occurs.

Rebound hypersomnia: Condition associated with excessive sleep that follows long-term insomnia or the use of drugs that depress REM and non-REM sleep.

Receptor site: Location of drug-cell binding.

Reflux: Backflow of gastric contents into the esophageal or laryngopharyngeal region.

Refraction: Deflection or bending of light rays through the cornea, aqueous humor, lens, and vitreous humor.

Refractory period: Time between contractions that it takes for repolarization to occur.

Remission: Lessening in severity or abatement of symptoms.

Remodeling: Process of continual turnover of bone.

Repolarization: Period of time when the heart is recharging and preparing for another contraction.

Rh factor: Antigen present in the red blood cells of Rh-positive individuals.

Rhabdomyolysis: Breakdown of muscle fibers and release of muscle fiber contents into the circulation.

Rheumatoid arthritis: Chronic disease characterized by inflammation and remodeling of the joints.

Rheumatoid factor: Immunoglobulin (antibody) present in many people who have rheumatoid arthritis.

Ribonucleic acid (RNA): Nucleic acid involved in protein synthesis that carries and transfers genetic information and assembles proteins.

Ringworm: Group of tinea infections involving the body or scalp that have a characteristic ringlike shape. Ringworm is spread by person to person and animal to person contact.

Rule of nines: Formula for estimating the percentage of adult body surface covered by burns; divides the body into 11 areas, each representing 9% of the total body surface area.

Rule of palms: Rule for determining the extent of a burn surface area. A palm size of a burn victim is about 1% of the total body surface area.

Saccule: Saclike inner ear structure that senses vertical motion of the head.

Salpingitis: Inflammation of the fallopian tube, usually as a result of a sexually transmitted infection.

Sarcolemma: Plasma membrane of a muscle fiber.

Sarcomere: Basic contractile unit of the muscle cell.

Sarcoplasmic reticulum (SR): Networks of tubules and sacs contained in muscle cells.

Scabicide: Drug that kills the scabies mite.

Scabies: Parasitic infection caused by the mite *Sarcoptes scabei*.

Second-degree burn: Burn that involves deep epidermal layers and causes damage to the upper layers of the dermis.

Sedative: Drug that causes relaxation and promotes drowsiness.

Seizure threshold: Measure of a person's susceptibility to seizures.

Semen: Fluid containing sperm and secretions from glands of the male reproductive tract.

Serotonin syndrome: Potentially life-threatening adverse drug reaction that produces symptoms of confusion, agitation, diarrhea, tremors, and increased blood pressure; caused by excessive serotonin.

Shingles: Recurring and painful skin rash caused by the herpes zoster virus.

Simple focal seizures: Seizure that affects only one part of the brain; causes the person to experience unusual sensations or feelings.

Sinus cavity: Mucous-lined, air-filled space found in the frontal bone (frontal sinuses), sphenoid, ethmoid, maxillae (paranasal sinuses), and middle and inner ear (mastoid sinuses).

Sodium: Major electrolyte in the interstitial fluid.

Soleplate: Portion of the membrane of muscle cells that receives messages transmitted by motor neurons.

Somatic nervous system: Division of the nervous system that carries information to the somatic effectors or skeletal muscles.

Sonogram: Computer image of internal organs and tissues produced by ultrasound.

Spacer: Device attached to the end of a metered-dose inhaler that facilitates drug delivery into the lungs (rather than to the back of the throat).

Spasticity: Motor disorder that causes increased muscle tone, exaggerated tendon jerks, and hyperexcitable muscles.

Spirometry: Test that measures the volume of air that is expired (blown out of the lungs) after taking a deep breath and how rapidly the volume of air is expired.

Stage: Refers to the extent of a cancer within the body. Staging is based on the size of the tumor, whether lymph nodes contain cancer, and whether the disease has spread from the original site to other parts of the body (metastasis).

Status epilepticus: Medical emergency brought on by repeated generalized seizures that can deprive the brain of oxygen.

Stem cell: Type of cell from which other types of cells develop; for example, blood cells develop from blood-forming stem cells.

Stem cell transplantation: Procedure used to replace cells that were destroyed by cancer treatment.

Stroke volume: Equal to the volume of blood ejected by the left ventricle during each cardiac contraction minus the volume of blood in the ventricle at the end of systole.

Stye: Painful lump located on the eyelid margin caused by an acute self-limiting infection of the oil glands of the eyelid.

Substance P: Peptide involved in the production of pain sensations; controls pain perception.

Substantia nigra: Part of the basal ganglia containing clusters of dopamine-producing neurons.

Supraovulation: Simultaneous rupture of multiple mature follicles.

Supraventricular tachycardia: Heart rate up to 200 beats/min that originates in an area above the ventricles.

Sympathetic nervous system: Division of the ANS that functions during stressful situations; fight-or-flight part of the ANS.

Synapse: Gap between neurons where nerve information is transmitted from one neuron to another.

Synarthrosis: Immovable joint (skull).

Synergistic effect: Drug-drug or drug-food interaction that produces an effect greater than the effect that would be produced if either drug were administered alone.

Synovium: Thin layer of tissue that lines the joint space.

Systemic lupus erythematosus (SLE): Autoimmune disease that affects almost all body systems.

T tubules: Transverse tubules that extend across the sarcoplasm.

Tangles: Twisted fibers made up of clumps of a protein called tau that interfere with nerve signal transmission.

Tear deficiency: Also known as dry eyes.

Tetanus: Potentially fatal condition characterized by a continuous muscle spasm caused by exposure to the nerve toxin produced by the bacterium *Clostridium tetani*. It is also known as lockjaw.

Tetraiodothyronine (T$_4$): Most abundant thyroid hormone; contains four atoms of iodine; also known as thyroxine.

Tetraiodothyronine test: Test to measure the level of free circulating thyroid hormone.

Therapeutic alternative: Drug that contains different active ingredient(s) than the brand name drug but produces the same desired therapeutic outcome.

Therapeutic duplication: Administration of two drugs that produce similar effects and side effects.

Therapeutic index (TI): Ratio of the effective dose to the lethal dose.

Third-degree burn: Burn characterized by destruction of the epidermis and dermis.

Thrombocytes: Platelets.

Thrombocytopenia: Condition that results from a deficiency in the platelet count.

Thrombolytic: Drug used to dissolve blood clots.

Thrombopoeisis: Formation of platelets.

Thrombosis: Formation of a blood clot.

Thrombotic stroke: Stroke caused by thrombosis.

Thrombus: Stationary blood clot.

Thyroid antibody test: Diagnostic test used to measure levels of thyroid antibodies; diagnostic for autoimmune thyroid disease.

Thyroid-releasing factor: Hormone released by the hypothalamus that stimulates the pituitary gland to release thyroid-stimulating hormone.

Thyroid-stimulating hormone (TSH): Hormone released by the pituitary gland that stimulates the thyroid gland to produce and release thyroid hormones.

Thyroid-stimulating hormone test: Diagnostic test used to measure the level of TSH in the blood; low level signals hyperthyroidism.

Tinnitus: Intermittent or continuous whistling, crackling, squeaking, or ringing noise in the ears.

Tissue plasminogen activator: Naturally occurring thrombolytic substance.

Tolerance: Increasing doses of a drug are required to achieve the same effects as were achieved previously at lower doses.

Tonic-clonic (grand mal) seizure: Generalized seizure that causes stiffening of the limbs, difficulty breathing, and jerking movements; is followed by disorientation and limbs that become limp.

Tonometry: Use of a device to measure the pressure in the eye.

Toxic megacolon: Life-threatening condition characterized by a very inflated colon, abdominal distention, and sometimes fever, abdominal pain, or shock.

Toxic shock syndrome: Rare disorder caused by certain *Staphylococcus aureus* strains that occurs in women using tampons.

Toxicology: Science dealing with the study of poisons.

Toxoid vaccine: Vaccine that stimulates the immune system to produce antibodies to a specific toxin that causes illness.

Trabecular meshwork: Small openings around the outer edge of the iris that form meshlike drainage canals surrounding the iris; sometimes referred to as the canal of Schlemm.

Transient ischemic attack (TIA): Stroke that typically lasts for a few minutes; also known as a ministroke.

Trigeminal neuralgia: Painful condition that produces intense stabbing pain in areas of the face innervated by branches of the trigeminal nerve.

Triglycerides: Storage form of energy found in fat tissue muscle; metabolize to very low-density lipoproteins.

Triiodothyronine (T$_3$): Hormone secreted by the thyroid gland; contains three atoms of iodine.

Tumor marker: Substance sometimes found in the blood, other body fluids, or tissues that may signal the presence of a certain type of cancer; for example, a high level of PSA is a signal for possible prostate cancer.

Tumor necrosis factor (TNF): Inflammatory cytokine released as part of the immune response; found in the synovial fluid of people with rheumatoid arthritis.

Tumor: Abnormal mass of tissue that results from excessive cell division. Tumors may be benign (not cancerous) or malignant (cancerous).

Turner's syndrome: Congenital endocrine disorder caused by failure of the ovaries to respond to pituitary hormone (gonadotropin) stimulation.

Tympanic membrane: Eardrum.

Type 1 diabetes: Autoimmune disease that results in high blood glucose levels. Pancreatic beta cells are destroyed and insufficient amounts of insulin are produced.

Type 2 diabetes: Condition that results in high blood glucose levels. People with type 2 diabetes have insulin resistance.

Ulcer: Open wound or sore.

Ulcerative colitis: Irritable bowel disease that results in inflammation, ulcers, and damage to the colon.

Upper esophageal sphincter: Sphincter separating the pharynx and esophagus. It relaxes to permit passage of food and liquids during swallowing, prevent air from entering the esophagus during breathing, and prevent gastric secretions from entering the pharynx.

Upper motor neurons: Neurons that carry messages from the brain down to the spinal cord.

Urate: Product of purine metabolism. Urate crystals may accumulate in joints and produce inflammation and pain.

Uricosuric: Drug that increases the renal clearance of urates.

Urinalysis: Microscopic and chemical examination of a fresh urine sample.

Urinary frequency: Need to urinate more often than is normal.

Urticaria: Hives.

Utricle: Saclike inner ear structure that senses forward and backward motion and side to side motion of the head.

Uveitis: Serious eye condition that produces inflammation of the uvea; can cause scarring of the eye and blindness if untreated.

Vaccine: Substance that prevents disease by taking advantage of the body's ability to make antibodies and prime killer cells to fight disease.

Vaginitis: Inflammation of the vagina.

Vasospasm: Spasms that constrict blood vessels and reduce the flow of blood and oxygen.

Ventricular fibrillation: Life-threatening arrhythmia during which the heart beats up to 600 beats/min.

Ventricular tachycardia: Condition in which ventricles beat faster than 200 beats/min.

Vertigo: Feeling of spinning in space (dizziness and loss of balance).

Viral load: Amount of materials from the virus that get released into the blood when HIV reproduces.

Virion: Infectious particles of a virus.

Virostatic: Able to suppress viral proliferation.

Virus: Intracellular parasite that consists of a DNA and RNA core surrounded by a protein coat and sometimes an outer covering of lipoprotein.

Vitreous floaters: Particles that float in the vitreous and cast shadows on the retina; these appear as spots, cobwebs, or spiders.

Vulvovaginal candidiasis: Yeast vaginitis.

Wheal: Raised blister-like area on the skin.

Whitehead (closed comedo): Trapped sebum and bacteria that stay below the skin surface; may show up as tiny white spots or may be so small that they are invisible to the naked eye.

Index

Page numbers followed by "f" indicate figures, "t" indicate tables, and "b" indicate boxes.

Sulfur-resorcinol combination, 731, 732t, 738

Sulfur-sulfacetamide combination, 731, 732t, 738

Sulindac, 161
  for gout, 269t

Sumatriptan, 167t–168t, 169

Sunburn, 721

Superficial fascia, **696**

Superovulation, **580**

Suppositories, 13, 13f

Suppressor T cells, **597**

Supraventricular tachycardia (SVT), **405**

Surfactant, **453–454**

Suspensions, 12

Sustained-release tablets, 12

SVT. *See* Supraventricular tachycardia

Sweat glands, **697–699**

Swimmer's ear, 295, 296t

Sympathetic system, **73**

Sympathomimetics, 75t, **190**

Synapse, **70**

Synarthroses, **198**

Synergistic effects, **55**

Synovial fluid, 509t

Synovial joint, **232–233**, 232f

Syrups, 12

Systemic lupus erythematosus (SLE), **233**
  osteoporosis and, 254

Systolic blood pressure (SBP), **342**

Systolic heart failure (SHF), **371**

T

T lymphocytes, **476**, **594**, **597**

T₃. *See* Triiodothyronine

T₄. *See* Tetraiodothyronine

Tablets, 11–12

Tacrolimus, 683–684, 684t, 688, 748t, 753

Tadalafil, 499, 500t, 502

Tamoxifen, 652, 652t, 664t–671t

Tamsulosin, 496t, 497

Tangles, **175**, 176f

TAO. *See* Thyroid-associated ophthalmopathy

Tardive dyskinesia, **109**
  Huntington's disease and, 127

Taste buds, **416**

Taxanes, 655–656, 655t, 664t–671t

Tazarotene, 733t–734t, 735–736, 738, 752t, 754

Tazobactam, 609t–610t

TCAs. *See* Tricyclic antidepressants

T-cell costimulation blocker, 687, 687t, 689

TCMs. *See* Central memory T cells

Tear deficiency, **277**

Telaprevir, 626t, 627, 630

Telavancin, 614t

Telbivudine, 625, 626t, 630

Telithromycin, 4, 607t, 616

Telmisartan, 353t–354t, 361t–366t

Temazepam, 186t, 189t
  half-life of, 80t, 187t

TEMs. *See* Effector memory T cells

Temsirolimus, 684t, 688

Tenecteplase, 391t, 397

Teniposide, 659t, 664t–671t

Tenofovir, 632, 636t–638t, 639

TENS. *See* Transcutaneous electrical stimulation

Teratogenicity, 48

Terazosin, 75t, 356t, 361t–366t, 496t, 497

Terbinafine, 705t–706t, 711

Terbutaline, 460t, 468

Terconazole, 705t–706t, 710

Teriparatide, 261t
  for osteoporosis and Paget's disease, 262t–264t
  PTH and, 260

Tertiary bronchi, **453**

Testosterone, 583, 583t, 587–588
  as controlled substance, 584b
  for hypogonadism, 581t
  through transdermal patches, 18

Tetanus, **208**
  vaccine for, 679t–681t

Tetrabenazine, 127t–128t
  hypotension from, 127

Tetracycline, 59t, 430, 600, 612, 613t, 616, 733t–734t, 738
  calcium and, 55
  for STIs, 578t

Tetraiodothyronine (T₄), **524–525**, **532**
  test of, **532–533**

Theophylline, 464–465, 465t, 470
  serum blood level modifiers for, 465b

Therapeutic alternative, **37**

Therapeutic duplication, **61**

Therapeutic index (TI), **45**

Thiabendazole, 307

Thiamazole, 535t

Thiazide diuretics, 4, 348, 348t, 361t–366t, 376t–377t

Thiazolidinediones, 255b, 554–555, 555t, 559t–560t

Thin film tablets, 12

Thioamides, 535, 535t

Thiocarbamates, 708, 708t, 711

Thioguanine, 662–663, 662t, 664t–671t

Thioridazine, 109t, 110, 113

Thiothixene, 109t–110t, 114

Thiouracil, 535t

Thioxanthenes, 108, 110t, 113t–115t

Third-degree burns, 720

Thoracic cavity, 454–455

Thorax, **454–455**

Thrombocytes, **318**, 318f, 320

Thrombocytopenia, **321**

Thrombolytics, **391–392**, 391t, 397

Thrombophlebitis, **325**

Thrombosis, **385–386**

Thrombotic stroke, **382**

Thromboxane A2 (TXA₂), 386

Thrombus, 329b

Thrush, 704f

Thymus gland, **595**

Thyroid antibody test, **532–533**

Thyroid-associated ophthalmopathy (TAO), 532

Thyroid cartilage, **452**

Thyroid gland, 527
  disorders of, 531–541, 537t–538t
    diagnosis of, 532–533
    types of, 534–537

Thyroid hormones
  control of, 532
  interactions with, 537b
  physiological actions of, 532b
  structural formula of, 533f
  synthesis of, 532

Thyroid-releasing factor (TRF), **532**

Thyroid-stimulating hormone (TSH), **524–525**, **532**
  test of, **532–533**, 533f

Thyroid-stimulating immunoglobulins (TSIs), **534**

TI. *See* Therapeutic index

TIA. *See* Transient ischemic attack

Tiagabine, 138, 138t

Ticarcillin, 609t–610t

Ticlopidine, 387t, 396

Tigecycline, 613t

Tiludronate, 257–258, 259t
  for osteoporosis and Paget's disease, 262t–264t

Time-release tablets, 12

Timolol, 361t–366t

Timolol hemihydrate, 282t–283t, 285t–287t, 355t

Timolol maleate, 286t–287t

Tinctures, 12

Tinea capitis, 702

Tinea corporis, 702f

Tinnitus, **292–293**
  quinidine and, 407

Tinzaparin, 390, 397

Tioconazole, 705t–706t, 710

Tiotropium bromide, 461t, 464t, 467, 469

Tipranavir, 635, 636t–638t, 640

Tirofiban, 386, 387t, 396

Tissue plasminogen activator (t-PA), 326

Tizanidine, 224, 224t, 226t

TNF-α. *See* Tumor necrosis factor

Tobacco. *See* Cigarette smoking

Tobramycin, 303t–305t, 308–309, 603t
  for blepharitis, 301

Tocilizumab, 241, 241t, 247

Tolcapone, 122, 123t, 125–126

Tolerance, 48
  for antidepressants, 83
  for benzodiazepines, **80**

Tolmetin, 162

Tolnaftate, 708, 708t, 711

Valproates, 136
    liver disease and, 136
    for migraine headache, 169t–170t
    for seizure disorders, 136, 137t, 142t–144t
Valsartan, 353t–354t, 360t–366t, 376t–377t
Vancomycin, 599–600, 614t
Vancomycin-resistant enterococci (VRE), **601–602**
Vardenafil, 499, 500t, 502
Variant angina, 330
    calcium channel blockers for, 334
Varicella zoster virus (VZV), 622
    vaccine for, 679t–681t
Varicose veins, **325**
Vascular layer, **276**
Vasoconstriction, from triptans, 166
Vasodilators, 360t–366t, 376t–377t
    direct, 359
    for heart failure, 376
Vasospasm, **330**
Vasospastic angina, **330**
VCF. *See* Vaginal contraceptive film
Vecuronium, 210t, 212t–213t
Veins, **323**
Venlafaxine, 81, 82t–84t, 98t, 100t–101t
Venous thromboembolism (VTE), 258
Ventricles, **321**
Ventricular fibrillation, 404–405
Ventricular tachycardia, **405**
Verapamil, 59t, 335t–337t, 357t–358t, 409t–410t
Vertebral column, 198
Vertigo, 293, 294t–295t
    treatment for, 294
Very low-density lipoprotein (VLDL), 394
Vestibule, **452**
Vigabatrin, 138, 138t, 143
Villus epithelium, 28f
Vinblastine, 656, 657t, 664t–671t

Vinca alkaloids, 656–657, 657t, 664t–671t
Vincristine, 656, 657t, 664t–671t
Vinorelbine, 656, 657t, 664t–671t
Vinyl chloride, 647
Viral infections, 621–644
    antibiotics and, 622
    cancer and, 647–648
    of eye, 306t
Viral load, **631**
Virus, 622
    in host, 623f
Virustatic, **622**
Visceral pleura, **454–455**
Vitamin B_2, 34
Vitamin B_3. *See* Niacin
Vitamin B_{12}, 320
Vitamin D, 253–254
    for eczema and psoriasis, 748–749, 749t, 754
Vitreous floaters, **305**
Vitreous humor, **276–277**, 509t
VLDL. *See* Very low-density lipoprotein
Voriconazole, 705t–706t, 710
VRE. *See* Vancomycin-resistant enterococci
VTE. *See* Venous thromboembolism
Vulvovaginal candidiasis, **703**
    risk factors for, 703b
VZV. *See* Varicella zoster virus

W

Warfarin, 59t, 388, 390, 397
    bleeding from, 55
    overdose of, 390
    pregnancy and, 390
    TI of, 45
Warning labels, 16b, 49, 49b
    for neuroleptics, 110b
Water-clogged ears, 295, 296t
WBCs. *See* White blood cells

Weak acids, 26, 56–57
    cell membranes and, 27f
Weak bases, 26–27, 56–57
    cell membranes and, 27f
Weight, pharmacotherapeutics and, 46
Wheals, **478**
White blood cells (WBCs), 319–320
    disorders of, 321
White coat hypertension, 345
Whiteheads, **729**
World Health Organization, 8
    PMTCT and, 633t

X

Xanthines, 458–459, 464–465, 465t, 470
    GERD and, 420
    half-life of, 464–465
Xanthine oxidase inhibitors, 270

Y

Yeast, **700**
Yohimbe, 502

Z

Zafirlukast, 463, 463t
Zaleplon, 186, 187t, 189
    half-life of, 187t
Zanamivir, 624–625, 624t, 629
Zidovudine, 633, 636t–638t, 639
Zileuton, 463, 463t
Ziprasidone, 112t, 114
Zoledronic acid, 259t
    for osteoporosis and Paget's disease, 262t–264t
Zolmitriptan, 167t–168t, 169
Zolpidem, 186, 187t, 189
    half-life of, 187t
Zonisamide, 140–141, 141t–144t
Zopiclone, 186, 187t, 189
    half-life of, 187t